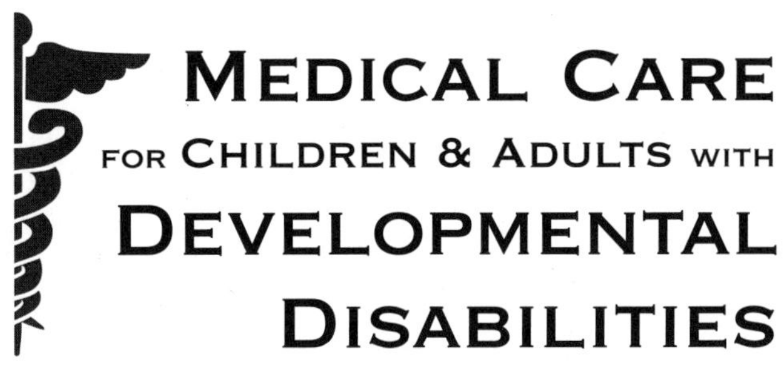
MEDICAL CARE
FOR CHILDREN & ADULTS WITH
DEVELOPMENTAL
DISABILITIES
SECOND EDITION

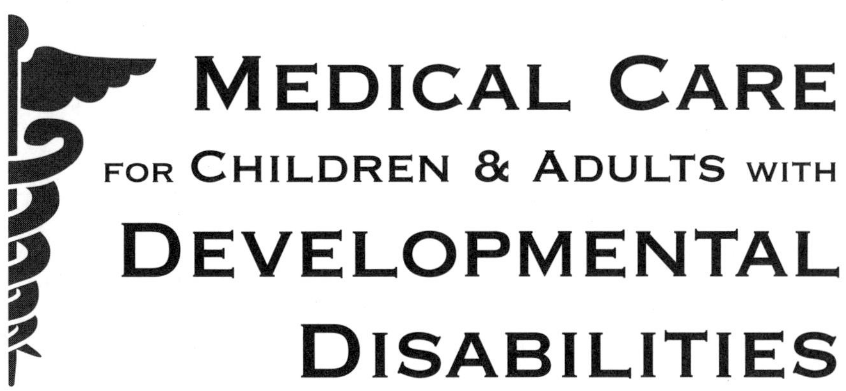

Medical Care for Children & Adults with Developmental Disabilities

Second Edition

edited by

I. Leslie Rubin, M.D.
Visiting Scholar, Department of Pediatrics
Morehouse School of Medicine
President, Institute for the Study of Disadvantage and Disability
Medical Director, The TEAM Centers and Developmental Pediatric Specialists

and

Allen C. Crocker, M.D.
Associate Professor of Pediatrics, Harvard Medical School
Associate Professor of Society, Human Development, and Health
Harvard School of Public Health
Senior Associate in Medicine, Children's Hospital Boston

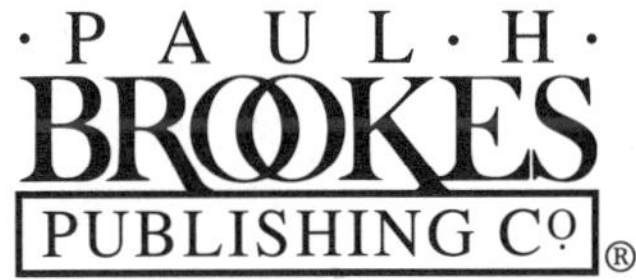

Baltimore • London • Sydney

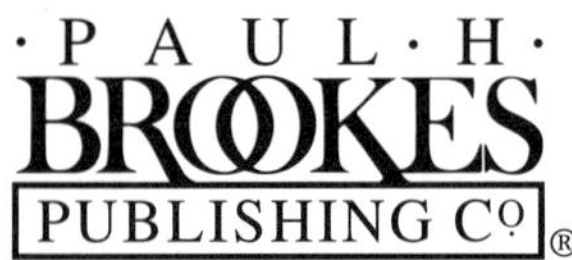

Paul H. Brookes Publishing Co.
Post Office Box 10624
Baltimore, Maryland 21285-0624

www.brookespublishing.com

Typeset by Integrated Publishing Solutions, Grand Rapids, Michigan.
Manufactured in the United States of America by
Sheridan Books, Inc., Chelsea, Michigan.

Clinical vignettes are derived from the authors' actual experiences. In most instances, pseudonyms have been used and identifying details have been changed to protect confidentiality. Real names and identifying details are used by permission.

Library of Congress Cataloging-in-Publication Data

Medical care for children and adults with developmental disabilities / edited by I. Leslie Rubin and Allen C. Crocker.—2nd ed.
p.; cm.
Rev. ed. of: Developmental disabilities. 1989.
Includes bibliographical references and index.
ISBN-13: 978-1-55766-766-3 (hardcover)
ISBN-10: 1-55766-766-7 (hardcover)
1. Developmentally disabled children—Medical care. 2. Developmentally disabled—Medical care. [DNLM: 1. Developmental Disabilities. 2. Adult. 3. Child. 4. Delivery of Health Care. 5. Mentally Disabled Persons. WA 300 M4893 2006]
I. Rubin, Isadore Leslie. II. Crocker, Allen C. III. Developmental disabilities.
RJ506.D47D485 2006
618.92'89—dc22 2005033047

British Library Cataloguing in Publication data are available from the British Library.

Contents

About the Editors

I. Leslie Rubin, M.D., Visiting Scholar, Department of Pediatrics, Morehouse School of Medicine; President, Institute for the Study of Disadvantage and Disability; Medical Director, TEAM Centers and Developmental Pediatric Specialists, 776 Windsor Parkway, Atlanta, Georgia 30342

Dr. Rubin is originally from South Africa, where he was sensitized to inequity and injustice. These elements have shaped and guided his personal and professional life. After graduation from the University of Witwatersrand Medical School, in Johannesburg, South Africa, he trained in pediatrics, taking care of many infants and children with potentially preventable conditions.

He came to the United States in 1976 to specialize in neonatology and in care of children with disabilities at Case Western Reserve University in Cleveland, Ohio. He joined the faculty at Case Western until 1980, when he migrated to Boston to work with Allen C. Crocker at Children's Hospital Boston and Harvard Medical School. There, he actively participated in clinical and academic programs and provided outreach consultation to a number of the regional schools and centers serving children and adults with developmental disabilities.

Dr. Rubin moved to Atlanta, Georgia, in 1994 to help develop clinical and academic programs at the Marcus Institute and Emory University. In 1998, he developed interdisciplinary clinical programs in cerebral palsy and autism and for children with sickle cell disease who have had strokes at the Hughes Spalding Children's Hospital in downtown Atlanta. Since 1998, he has been part of the Southeast Pediatric Environmental Health Specialty Unit at Emory University. In 1999, he began to work at TEAM Centers in Chattanooga, Tennessee.

In May 2004, Dr. Rubin founded the Institute for the Study of Disadvantage and Disability, which is dedicated to improving awareness and understanding of the relationship between social and economic disadvantage and disabilities. In September 2004, he left Emory University and the Marcus Institute and joined the Morehouse School of Medicine to work more closely in academic and clinical programs relating to community and public health to help reduce health disparities for children and adults with developmental disabilities as well as those who live in circumstances of social and economic disadvantage.

Allen C. Crocker, M.D., Associate Professor of Pediatrics, Harvard Medical School; Associate Professor of Society, Human Development, and Health, Harvard School of Public Health; Senior Associate in Medicine, Children's Hospital Boston, 300 Longwood Avenue, Boston, Massachusetts 02115

Dr. Crocker was born and lived thereafter in Boston. He was educated at Massachusetts Institute of Technology and Harvard Medical School (1948). His houseofficership was at Children's Hospital Boston, with postwar military service in Germany.

Dr. Crocker then began a long career at Children's Hospital Boston, which became the principal site of his vocation. There, he learned about development, both child and personal. He spent 15 years with Sidney Farber, involved especially with children who had inborn errors of metabolism.

Since 1967, he has directed a series of Maternal and Child Health Bureau training programs relating to mental retardation and developmental disabilities, including much clinical energy. He has had great joy in community programs for children and parents, and with a wide variety of advocacy groups. He has been unaccountably fortunate in professional opportunities.

CONTRIBUTORS

Randell Alexander, M.D., Ph.D.
Professor and Chief
Division of Child Protection and Forensic Pediatrics
University of Florida
1650 Prudential Drive, Suite 100
Jacksonville, Florida 32207

Deborah Allen, Sc.D.
Associate Professor
Department of Maternal and Child Health
Senior Research Associate
Health and Disability Working Group
Boston University School of Public Health
715 Albany Street
Boston, Massachusetts 02118

Norberto Alvarez, M.D.
Assistant Professor of Neurology
Harvard Medical School
Children's Hospital Boston
Medical Director
Wrentham Developmental Center
Post Office Box 144
Wrentham, Massachusetts 02093

Jack L. Arbiser, M.D.
Assistant Professor of Dermatology
Emory University School of Medicine
5309 Woodruff Memorial Building
Atlanta, Georgia 30322

Linda L. Barnes, Ph.D., M.A., M.T.S.
Associate Professor of Pediatrics and Public Health
Boston University School of Medicine
91 East Concord Street
Boston, Massachusetts 02118

Stuart B. Bauer, M.D.
Professor of Surgery
Harvard Medical School
Senior Associate in Urology
Children's Hospital Boston
300 Longwood Avenue
Boston, Massachusetts 02115

Joan B. Beasley, Ph.D.
Consultation and Training Services
184 Bonad Road
Chestnut Hill, Massachusetts 02467

Lauren C. Berman, M.S.W., L.I.C.S.W.
Director of Social Work
LEND Program
Children's Hospital Boston
300 Longwood Avenue
Boston, Massachusetts 02115

Arnold Birenbaum, Ph.D.
Professor of Pediatrics
Albert Einstein College of Medicine
Rose F. Kennedy Center
1410 Pelham Parkway South
Bronx, New York 10461

Diego Botero, M.D.
Instructor, Harvard Medical School
Staff Physician, Endocrinology Program
Children's Hospital Boston
300 Longwood Avenue
Boston, Massachusetts 02115

Athos Bousvaros, M.D., M.P.H.
Assistant Professor of Pediatrics
Harvard Medical School
Associate Director, Inflammatory Bowel Disease Center
Children's Hospital Boston
300 Longwood Avenue
Boston, Massachusetts 02115

Alfred Brann, Jr., M.D.
Professor of Pediatrics
Emory University School of Medicine
Director, World Health Organization Collaborating Center in Reproductive Health in Atlanta
49 Jesse Hill Jr. Drive
Atlanta, Georgia 30303

Nathan A. Call, Ph.D.
Assistant Professor of Psychology
Louisiana State University
232 Audubon Hall
Baton Rouge, Louisiana 70803

Karen L. Carter, M.D.
Assistant Professor of Pediatrics
Medical College of Georgia
1120 15th Street
Augusta, Georgia 30912

Sharon A. Cermak, Ed.D., OTR/L
Professor of Occupational Therapy
Sargent College
Boston University
635 Commonwealth Avenue
Boston, Massachusetts 02115

Bartley G. Cilento, Jr., M.D.
Assistant Professor of Surgery (Urology)
Harvard Medical School
Children's Hospital Boston
300 Longwood Avenue
Boston, Massachusetts 02115

Herbert J. Cohen, M.D.
Professor of Pediatrics and Rehabilitation Medicine
Albert Einstein College of Medicine
Rose F. Kennedy Center
1410 Pelham Parkway South
Bronx, New York 10461

Stanley A. Cohen, M.D.
Adjunct Clinical Professor of Pediatrics
Emory University School of Medicine
Pediatric Gastroenterology and Nutrition
Children's Center for Digestive Health Care
Children's Healthcare of Atlanta
993D Johnson Ferry Road, Suite 440
Atlanta, Georgia 30342

John M. Costello, M.A., CCC-SLP
Director, Communication Enhancement Center
Children's Hospital Boston
300 Longwood Avenue
Boston, Massachusetts 02115

David L. Coulter, M.D.
Associate Professor of Neurology
Harvard Medical School
LEND Program
Children's Hospital Boston
300 Longwood Avenue
Boston, Massachusetts 02115

Gerald Cox, M.D., Ph.D.
Senior Medical Director
Genzyme Corporation
500 Kendall Street
Cambridge, Massachusetts 02142

Susan R. Cusack, M.Ed.
Project Director, Educational Technology Leadership Institute
Lesley University
29 Everett Street
Cambridge, Massachusetts 02138

Kenneth J. Dooley, M.D.
Associate Professor of Pediatrics
Emory University School of Medicine
Sibley Heart Center
2835 Brandywine Road
Atlanta, Georgia 30341

Mohamed El-Defrawi, M.D.
Southern Illinois University School of Medicine
901 West Jefferson Street
Springfield, Illinois 62702

Marc T. Emmerich, M.D.
Primary Care and Consulting Physician
Liberty Healthcare, Children's Hospital, and Boston's Community Medical Group
Dowling North 5108
Boston, Massachusetts 02118

Theodor Feigelman, M.D.
Director, Center for Human Development
Atlantic Health System
100 Madison Avenue
Morristown, New Jersey 07962

Paul M. Fernhoff, M.D.
Associate Professor of Human Genetics and Pediatrics
Medical Director
Emory Genetics
Emory University School of Medicine
2165 N. Decatur Road NE
Decatur, Georgia 30033

Wayne Fisher, Ph.D.
Director, Center for Autism Spectrum Disorders
H.B. Munroe Professor of Behavioral Research
Munroe-Meyer Institute
University of Nebraska Medical Center
985450 Nebraska Medical Center
Omaha, Nebraska 68198

Laurie N. Fishman, M.D.
Assistant Professor of Pediatrics
Harvard Medical School
Attending in Gastroenterology
Children's Hospital Boston
300 Longwood Avenue
Boston, Massachusetts 02115

Amy Fleischman, M.D., M.M.Sc.
Instructor in Medicine
Division of Endocrinology
Children's Hospital Boston
300 Longwood Avenue
Boston, Massachusetts 02115

Linda Freeman, M.S., M.B.A.
Director of Family Initiatives
New England SERVE
101 Tremont Street, Suite 812
Boston, Massachusetts 02108

Sandra L. Friedman, M.D., M.P.H.
Instructor in Pediatrics
Harvard Medical School
Director of Pediatric Training
LEND Program
Director of Neurodevelopmental Disabilities
Children's Hospital Boston
300 Longwood Avenue
Boston, Massachusetts 02115

Anne B. Fulton, M.D.
Harvard Medical School
Senior Associate in Ophthalmology
Children's Hospital Boston
300 Longwood Avenue
Boston, Massachusetts 02115

J. Carolyn Graff, Ph.D., RN
Chief of Nursing
Boling Center for Developmental Disabilities
University of Tennessee Health Science Center
711 Jefferson Avenue
Memphis, Tennessee 38105

Robert J. Graham, M.D.
Associate in the Division of Critical Care Medicine
Department of Anesthesiology, Perioperative and Pain Medicine
Children's Hospital Boston
300 Longwood Avenue
Boston, Massachusetts 02115

Jason C. Hadley
Emory University School of Medicine
5001 Woodruff Memorial Building
Atlanta, Georgia 30322

Ronald M. Hansen, Ph.D.
Research Associate, Department of Ophthalmology
Harvard Medical School
Children's Hospital Boston
300 Longwood Avenue
Boston, Massachusetts 02115

Nancy Hatch-Warner, M.A.
Parent
161A East Beach Road
Charlestown, Rhode Island 02813

Susan Havercamp, Ph.D.
Assistant Professor, Department of Psychiatry
University of North Carolina at Chapel Hill
Clinical Psychologist
Developmental Disabilities Consulting and Psychological Services
Post Office Box 4202
Chapel Hill, North Carolina 27515

Daniel J. Hedequist, M.D.
Assistant Professor of Orthopedic Surgery
Harvard Medical School
Children's Hospital Boston
300 Longwood Avenue
Boston, Massachusetts 02115

David T. Helm, Ph.D.
Director, Interdisciplinary Training
LEND Program
Institute for Community Inclusion
University of Massachusetts Boston and Children's Hospital Boston
300 Longwood Avenue
Boston, Massachusetts 02115

Adria Hodas, M.S.N., RNC, FNP
Director of Health Services
Toward Independent Living and Learning, Inc.
20 Eastbrook Road
Dedham, Massachusetts 02026

Robert A. Jacobs, M.D.
Professor of Pediatrics
University of Southern California (USC)
Keck School of Medicine
Head, Division of General Pediatrics
USC University Center for Excellence in Developmental Disabilities
Childrens Hospital Los Angeles
4650 Sunset Boulevard
Los Angeles, California 90027

Matthew P. Janicki, Ph.D.
Research Associate Professor of Human Development
College of Associated Health Professions
University of Illinois at Chicago
1640 West Roosevelt Road
Chicago, Illinois 60608

Lawrence C. Kaplan, M.D., Sc.M.
Associate Professor of Pediatrics
Dartmouth Medical School
Director, Division of Genetics and Child Development
Children's Hospital at Dartmouth
1 Medical Center Drive
Lebanon, New Hampshire 03756

Eliot S. Katz, M.D.
Instructor, Harvard Medical School
Massachusetts General Hospital
Division of Pediatric Pulmonology
55 Fruit Street
Boston, Massachusetts 02114

Michael E. Kelley, Ph.D.
Psychologist
Marcus Institute
1920 Briarcliff Road
Atlanta, Georgia 30329

Frances Dougherty Kendall, M.D.
Medical Genetics
Horizon Molecular Medicine
1 Dunwoody Park, Suite 250
Atlanta, Georgia 30338

Margaret A. Kenna, M.D.
Associate Professor of Otology and Laryngology
Harvard Medical School
Children's Hospital Boston
300 Longwood Avenue
Boston, Massachusetts 02115

Harry L. Keyserling, M.D.
Professor of Pediatrics
Emory University School of Medicine
2015 Uppergate Drive
Atlanta, Georgia 30322

Imran Khan, M.D.
Southern Illinois University School of Medicine
901 West Jefferson Street
Springfield, Illinois 62702

Michele Kiely, Dr.P.H.
Chief, Collaborative Studies Unit
National Institute of Child Health and Human Development
National Institutes of Health
6100 Executive Boulevard
Rockville, Maryland 20892

Bruce R. Korf, M.D., Ph.D.
Wayne H. and Sara Crews Finley Professor of Medical Genetics
Chairman, Department of Genetics
University of Alabama at Birmingham
Kaul Human Genetics Building, Room 230
720 20th Street South
Birmingham, Alabama 35294

Donald J. Lollar, Ed.D.
Senior Research Scientist
Centers for Disease Control and Prevention
1600 Cliffon Road E-87
Atlanta, Georgia 30333

Yona Lunsky, Ph.D.
Department of Psychiatry
University of Toronto
Dual Diagnosis Program
Centre for Addiction and Mental Health
1001 Queen Street West, Unit 4-4
Toronto, Ontario M6J 1H4
Canada

William Mahle, M.D.
Associate Professor of Pediatrics
Emory University School of Medicine
Children's Healthcare of Atlanta
1405 Clifton Road NE
Atlanta, GA 30322

Deborah Marsden, M.B.B.S.
Assistant in Medicine (Genetics and Metabolism)
Metabolism Program
Children's Hospital Boston
300 Longwood Avenue
Boston, Massachusetts 02115

D. Luisa Mayer, Ph.D.
Assistant Professor, Harvard Medical School
Clinical Associate, Department of Ophthalmology
Children's Hospital Boston
300 Longwood Avenue
Boston, Massachusetts 02115

Raun Melmed, M.D.
Medical Director
Southwest Autism Research and Resource Center
Director, Melmed Center
5020 East Shea Boulevard, Suite 100
Scottsdale, Arizona 85254

Kathryn B. Miller, O.D.
Optometrist
Children's Hospital Boston
300 Longwood Avenue
Boston, Massachusetts 02115

Michael Millis, M.D.
Associate Professor of Orthopedic Surgery
Harvard Medical School
Children's Hospital Boston
300 Longwood Avenue
Boston, Massachusetts 02115

Kerim Munir, M.D., M.P.H., D.Sc.
Director of Psychiatry
LEND Program
Institute for Community Inclusion
Division of General Pediatrics
Children's Hospital Boston
300 Longwood Avenue
Boston, Massachusetts 02115

Aruna Navathe, M.A., RD, LD, CSP, CDE
Clinical Nutritionist
Nutrition Coordinator
Children's Healthcare of Atlanta
1001 Johnson Ferry Road NE
Atlanta, Georgia 30342

Marilyn W. Neault, Ph.D.
Department of Otolaryngology and Communication Disorders
Children's Hospital Boston
300 Longwood Avenue
Boston, Massachusetts 02115

Priscilla S. Osborne, PT, M.S., PCS
Director of Physical Therapy Training
LEND Program
Institute for Community Inclusion
Children's Hospital Boston
300 Longwood Avenue
Boston, Massachusetts 02155

Matthew Parvin, M.D.
Southern Illinois University School of Medicine
901 West Jefferson Street
Springfield, Illinois 62702

Robert J. Pary, M.D.
Professor of Clinical Psychiatry
Clerkship Director
Southern Illinois University School of Medicine
901 West Jefferson
Springfield, Illinois 62702

Joel Pearlman, D.M.D.
Associate Clinical Professor and Preceptor
Tufts University School of Dental Medicine
Director of Dentistry and Associate Chief Dentist
Tufts Dental Facility Serving Persons with Special Needs
Wrentham Developmental Center
Emerald Street, Box 144
Wrentham, Massachusetts 02093

Alan K. Percy, M.D.
Professor of Pediatrics
University of Alabama at Birmingham
Associate Director
Civitan International Research Center
Director, Sparks Clinics
1530 3rd Avenue S
Birmingham, Alabama 35294

Cathleen C. Piazza, Ph.D.
Director, Pediatric Feeding Disorders Program
Munroe-Meyer Institute
University of Nebraska Medical Center
985450 Nebraska Medical Center
Omaha, Nebraska 68198

Brian P. Pollack, M.D., Ph.D.
Resident Physician
Emory University School of Medicine
5001 Woodruff Memorial Building
Atlanta, Georgia 30322

Lisa Albers Prock, M.D., M.P.H.
Instructor, Harvard Medical School
Associate in Medicine
Director, Adoption Program
Children's Hospital Boston
300 Longwood Avenue
Boston, Massachusetts 02115

Alya Reeve, M.D.
Associate Professor of Psychiatry and Neurology
University of New Mexico
2400 Tucker Road NE
Albuquerque, New Mexico 87131

Henry Roane, Ph.D.
Director, Severe Behavior Disorders Program
Emory University School of Medicine
Marcus Institute
1920 Briarcliff Road
Atlanta, Georgia 30329

Howard S. Schub, M.D.
Section Chief, Neurology
Children's Health Care of Atlanta at Scottish Rite
Child Neurology Associates
5505 Peachtree Dunwoody Road, Suite 500
Atlanta, Georgia 30342

Kathryn Pekala Service, M.S., RNC/NP, CDDN
Nurse Practitioner
Massachusetts Department of Mental Retardation
1 Roundhouse Plaza
Northampton, Massachusetts 01060

John M. Shoffner, M.D.
Horizon Molecular Medicine
Neurology, Biochemical Genetics, Molecular Genetics
1 Dunwoody Park, Suite 250
Atlanta, Georgia 30338

Peter J. Smith, M.D., M.A.
Assistant Professor of Pediatrics
University of Chicago
5841 South Maryland, MC0900
Chicago, Illinois 60637

Deborah Spitalnik, Ph.D.
Professor of Pediatrics and Executive Director
The Elizabeth M. Boggs Center on Developmental Disabilities
University of Medicine and Dentistry of New Jersey
Robert Wood Johnson Medical School
335 George Street
New Brunswick, New Jersey 08903

Edward Sterling, D.D.S.
Director, Nisonger Center Dental Program
The Ohio State University
1581 Dodd Drive
Columbus, Ohio 43210

Peter Tanguay, M.D.
Spafford Ackerly Endowed Professor of Child and Adolescent Psychiatry, Emeritus
School of Medicine
University of Louisville
Louisville, Kentucky 40292

Elizabeth Thiele, M.D., Ph.D.
Associate Professor of Neurology
Harvard Medical School
Director, Pediatric Epilepsy Program
Director, Carol and James Herscot Center for Tuberous Sclerosis Complex
Massachusetts General Hospital
175 Cambridge Street, Suite 340
Boston, Massachusetts 02114

Carl V. Tyler, Jr., M.D., M.S., CAQ-Geriatrics
Coordinator of Geriatric Education and Research
Fairview/Cleveland Clinic Family Medicine Residency
18200 Lorain Avenue
Cleveland, Ohio 44111

Jeannie Visootsak, M.D.
Assistant Professor
Developmental Pediatrician
Department of Human Genetics
Emory University School of Medicine
2165 N. Decatur Road
Decatur, Georgia 30033

Joseph Wagstaff, M.D., Ph.D.
Clinical Genetics Program
Department of Pediatrics
Carolinas Medical Center
Post Office Box 32861
Charlotte, North Carolina 28232

David A. Waltz, M.D.
Assistant Professor of Pediatrics
Harvard Medical School
Assistant in Medicine (Respiratory Diseases)
Children's Hospital Boston
300 Longwood Avenue
Boston, Massachusetts 02115

Sheryl White-Scott, M.D.
Assistant Clinical Professor of Medicine
New York Medical College
Director, Program for the Disabled
Sister Thea Bowman
Kingsbrook Jewish Medical Center
1205 Sutter Avenue
Brooklyn, New York 11208

Sarah Winter, M.D.
Clinical Associate
Professor of Pediatrics
Ohio State University College of Medicine
Neurodevelopmental Pediatrician
Section of Developmental and Behavioral Pediatrics
Columbus Children's Hospital
700 Children's Drive
Columbus, Ohio 43205

Mark L. Wolraich, M.D.
CMRI/Shaun Walters Professor of Pediatrics
OU Child Study Center
University of Oklahoma Health Sciences Center
1100 NE 13th Street
Oklahoma City, Oklahoma 73117

Foreword

It was my privilege to serve as the 16th U.S. Surgeon General from 1998 to 2002. For 3 of those years, I also served as Assistant Secretary for Health (ASH) in the U.S. Department of Health and Human Services. As ASH, I was able to lead the development of Healthy People 2010—the nation's health plan for this decade. One of the two goals of Healthy People 2010 was to improve the quality and years of healthy life. There are some specific objectives related to the need to improve the *quality* of life and experiences of persons with developmental disabilities throughout the life span. The second goal was that of eliminating disparities in health among different racial and ethnic groups as well as other groups who suffer disproportionately.

The Healthy People 2010 Plan was released to the nation in January 2000, but it was not until March 2001 that I fully appreciated the significance of the goal of improving the quality of life of persons with developmental disabilities. It was then that I was invited to testify at a Senate Subcommittee Hearing in Anchorage, Alaska, chaired by Senator Ted Stevens and held in conjunction with the 2001 Special Olympics. At the Special Olympics, I was not only able to observe persons with developmental disabilities at their best but also witness the tremendous unmet needs of this group of persons for health maintenance and health care. At the invitation of Dr. Timothy Shriver, son of Eunice Kennedy Shriver, I had lunch with a group of parents of persons with developmental disabilities and listened to them detail their experiences with the current health care system. Their indictment of the health care system left me without speech or appetite.

In addition, a group of health care providers who served the Special Olympics and took care of patients with developmental disabilities in their own practices took me on rounds. During this session, I observed some of the major health problems of this group ranging from decayed teeth and periodontal disease to severe cardiovascular disease at a young age. By the time I testified before Senator Stevens's committee, I had changed my prepared speech to one in which I expressed concern and embarrassment for the health experience of persons with developmental disabilities, and I announced my intent to prepare and release a Surgeon General's Report on the health care needs of persons with developmental disabilities.

In October 2001, I held a Surgeon General's Listening Session on the topic of developmental disabilities and had the opportunity to listen to persons with developmental disabilities, their families, their caregivers, health professionals, and policy makers. This listening session was followed in December 2001 by a Surgeon General's Conference on the health needs of children and adults with developmental disabilities. It was out of that conference, along with contributions from my colleagues at the National Institute of Child Health and Human Development, that we were able to prepare our report. In February 2002, I had the opportunity to release what would be my last report as Surgeon General. It was entitled *Closing the Gap: A National Blueprint to Improve the Health of Persons with Mental Retardation.*

I am pleased that the findings, goals, and major actions recommended in that report are dealt with so well in this comprehensive textbook of medical care for children and adults with developmental disabilities. Thus, I will not repeat them in this statement. Clearly, the needs, challenges, and opportunities for intervention to enhance the health and well-being of persons with developmental disabilities are present throughout the life span. Optimally, care is provided with an appreciation for the complexity of challenges faced by the person with disabilities but also within the context of a dynamic family structure. Equally dynamic is the health care system upon which persons with disabilities rely for their care. Thus, enhancement in the knowledge, the technologies, and the systems available for care can have a dramatic impact on life expectancy and quality of life for persons with developmental disabilities—a condition the contributors to this volume have illustrated throughout the text.

Yet there is not, and never will be, a substitute for the so-called *medical home*, which provides a large portion of the care needed for persons with developmental disabilities. Moreover, this medical home coordinates access to all other care needed while maintaining meaningful and therapeutic relationships with the individuals and their families. A primary care or medical home still remains critical to quality health care for this population. But the care of persons with developmental disabilities also takes place in the context of community—a community not only of resources, but of knowledge, attitudes, and values, all important to the quality of life of persons with developmental disabilities.

I am pleased that a community of experts have come together to create *Medical Care for Children and Adults with Developmental Disabilities, Second Edition*, dealing with the health care needs of persons with developmental disabilities. It is a very comprehensive, timely, and thorough book, bringing to bear the latest knowledge and technologies related to this field. Perhaps never before has this topic been dealt with so comprehensively and so insightfully.

David Satcher, M.D., Ph.D.
Interim President
Morehouse School of Medicine
16th U.S. Surgeon General

PREFACE

For the editors, this book has sentimental aspects, both from history and from content. Its concerns and its outreach are connected to a larger fellowship. Individuals with disabilities are a crucial part of the human family; in this volume their activities, their impact, and their persona are vigorously recognized. The reader will find sharing as well as caring on behalf of people with special needs. Those of you who practice, study, or plan in this area, come be with us.

The first edition of the book (then called *Developmental Disabilities: Delivery of Medical Care for Children and Adults*, 1989, Lea & Febiger) was, in many ways, a campaign. It had some "gee whiz" intonation and gave primary attention to basic principles. Now, nearly 17 years later, responsibility and expectation are the tone. The mood is one of "yes, indeed." Health care planning is the characteristic mode.

For workers in this field, we welcome you. We express alliance with your hopes. The book has been designed to capture a sequence of interests. First, there is material on foundations of the clinical work, with presentation of the guides and bases. Then follows a review of the settings and systems in which the work is carried out. The clinical chapters are, predictably, the heart of the work and the most extensive. These utilize, as far as feasible, a life-span orientation. And finally is some reflective material on the practice world, supports, sociological issues, and values. Most of the authors are new to this edition, and their collaboration is earnestly appreciated; they are dearly valued colleagues. Thanks further for those who are repeat allies in the authorship and once more have assisted critically in working for a successful volume.

There are many common resolutions encompassed in this conglomeration of contributions. Their presentation together, as formulation of a knowledge base, gives justification for a specialized and separate volume. Further, in this form, it permits a continuing theme of advocacy. Developmental disabilities now have relevant training and clinical centers, public agencies, and dedicated supports. We offer this focused text as part of the infrastructure. We have all been inspired by the personal richness and the positive features of individuals with disabilities. Our own preparation and capabilities should be encouraged thereby. This book is directed at forming a more accurate stewardship, and, as we proceed, there is room for times of wonder.

The medical practitioner is the ultimate target of our treatise; other clinicians will find the language and technology fully manageable. Our gratification would be double if the book is also helpful to educators, public planners, the clergy, legal colleagues, and program designers. A pediatric bias cannot be denied, but we urge other medics (family practitioners, internists, adult specialists) to join the studies and seek outreaching service goals. Ultimately, our ambitions rest strongly for relevant training in family medicine. Teaching for the care of grown-ups with disabilities badly needs reinforcement, as does related public health and community supports.

Being a book created for the assistance of clinical workers (and teachers), the medical theme is dominant, but the reader will recognize our interest in associated supportive areas. Particularly, we wish to assert the humanistic roots and effects. This does not purport to be a "disease" book but rather a chronicle of helpful health information and ideas for people in the world of developmental disabilities. The yearning for wellness is central. It is our belief that health care can serve as a facilitator, and we have great respect for the accessibility of happiness.

Allen C. Crocker, M.D.

Acknowledgments

Both Allen and I would like to recognize and acknowledge all who have gone before us and paved the way and upon whose knowledge and experiences our understanding and appreciation are based. In *The Pirkei Avos Treasury: Ethics of the Fathers* (Lieber & Sherman, 1995, Messorah Publications), there are three specific teachings that are relevant to our mission:

1:6 Provide yourself with a teacher, get yourself a colleague and judge all [people] favorably.

4:1 Who is wise? [One] who learns from all [people].

6:6 One who learns in order to teach will be enabled to learn and teach; but one who learns in order to practice will be enabled to learn and to teach, to preserve and to practice.

Indeed, we have learned as much from our patients as from our mentors, and from the children as much as from the adults, and from our students as much as from our teachers. We are, therefore, grateful to all of the "patients"—children and adults—who gave us the opportunity and privilege of being able to practice our profession and to their families who provided us with valuable insights.

Through all our experiences, we have learned two critical lessons:

1. There is a value system that is fundamental to what we do; it is the essence that keeps us together and the guiding light that keeps us focused and, at all times, striving to do better.
2. The "practice of medicine" is a truth in that we learn from each experience, and with each experience we appreciate what works and what does not work and what we should do the next time; it is the experiential building block of the term *evidence-based medicine.*

A big vote of thanks goes to those who have subjected experience and practice to the scrutiny of the scientific method, thus giving us the confidence that what we are doing has validity and that we constantly need to examine and reexamine what we do both through personal experience and through the scientific method and most importantly through the sharing of experiences, practices, and ideas.

We would like to recognize Dr. David Satcher and the role he has played in bringing to our national consciousness the notion of *disparities* in health care in general and disparities in health care for children and adults with developmental disabilities in particular. His work as Surgeon General and Assistant Secretary of Health to articulate the *blueprint* to improve the health of people with developmental disabilities has inspired and energized us all and in part is the *raison d'être* for this book. May the spirit with which the initiative was launched continue to have a positive impact for many years to come until there are no longer *disparities* in our society, certainly not in health care. We thank him for agreeing to write the foreword and for his endorsement of the efforts of everyone who contributed to this book.

I would personally like to thank all those who helped in one way or another to put this book together—the unsung heroes—wherever I have been and learned; from my original home in South Africa, most significantly in this context thanks to David Saffer; through my learning experiences in Cleveland, Ohio, especially with Bob Bilenker, who introduced me to the systems of delivery of health care for people with developmental disabilities; and on to my rich sojourn at the Children's Hospital in Boston from 1980 to 1994 with my mentor and friend, Allen Crocker, for an appreciation of the interdisciplinary process and the many valuable colleagues and the programs for children and adults with developmental disabilities, especially the Children's Extended Care Center, Berkshire Meadows, the Wrentham Developmental Center, and the many other schools and programs that were part of the wider circle of our clinical and academic interactions.

Since 1994, I have been in Atlanta and the Southeast and would like to thank the many creative and energetic people and programs in those areas, particularly the family support programs and advocacy groups who continue to strive to improve the quality of life for children and adults with developmental disabilities and their families.

We also have a particular appreciation for our colleagues around the country in other parts of the world who are part of our global village. We are all indeed part of a substantially larger community engaged in the process of living together and working together to promote health and create harmony in our societies.

Both Allen and I have a deep sense of gratitude to all of our colleagues and friends whose contributions made this book come to life and to the staff at Paul H. Brookes Publishing Co., who have been supportive of our project and patient with our initial measured pace and then with the organization and editing of the book—particularly to Heather Shrestha and Janet Betten, who were there with us to the final breathless stages of publication.

I. Leslie Rubin, M.D.

I would like to dedicate this book to my family—to my parents, who gave me the foundation to become who I am personally and professionally; to my wife, Barbara, who has been my enduring support and constant when all else at times seemed uncertain and daunting; to my children, Justine, Laila, Xandy, and Mandy; to Mandy's husband, Tiran; and to their daughter (my granddaughter), Mikayla. All of them continue to inspire me and keep me young. Last, but not least, to all the friends, extended families, and communities who provide us all with a sense of purpose and belonging.

—*I.L.R.*

I would like to express indebtedness to my wife, Marga, who gave love and support; gratitude for the cheer and inspiration of our children, Elli, Philip, and Monica; and a hurrah to our grandchildren, Rita, Alex, Sonya, Britt, Irene, Evan, Kelsey, Ethan, and Chloe.

—*A.C.C.*

The World of Care

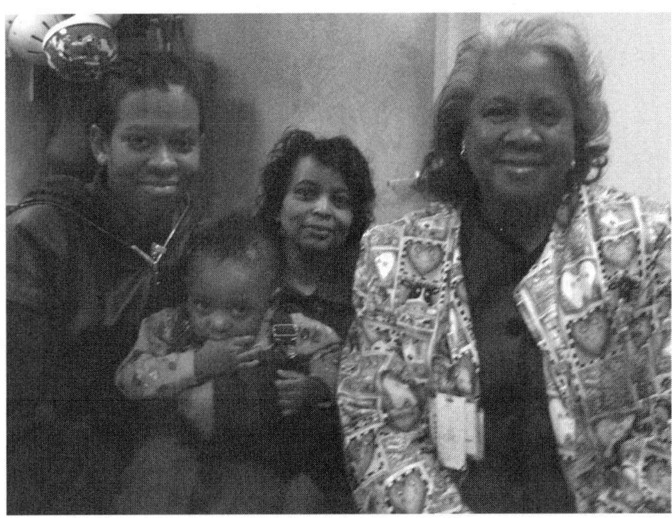

Little Sekhem, who attends the Interdisciplinary Cerebral Palsy Clinic; his mother, who has serious hearing impairment; his grandmother, who works at Hughes Spalding Children's Hospital; and his great-grandmother, who works at Grady Hospital, all in Atlanta, Georgia.

Section I

Programs of Care

Chapter 1

The Foundations of Medical Care

Allen C. Crocker

The particular health care needs of people with developmental disabilities have not been considered extensively in medical teaching. This book, its editors, and its authors are here, with much heart, to improve and reinforce the resources in this field. Mental retardation, or intellectual disability, has cultural, phenomenological, and sometimes biomedical special ground. The provider of medical care in this setting, either in a specialized fashion or, more commonly, as part of a larger practice, has rich opportunities to work for best vitality and to share broadly felt hopes.

Attention to the medical aspects of intellectual disabilities grew in the 1960s as the backgrounds and causation of various developmental disabilities were identified, with implications both for prevention and management. There was excitement about the discovery of chromosomal aberrations, Rh sensitization, lead toxicity, phenylketonuria in newborns, rubella vaccine, the effects of alcohol on fetuses, and the effects of other disadvantageous circumstances on little children. Long-term support services for children with intellectual disabilities developed slowly, pressed by the growth of consumer advocacy (e.g., The Association for Retarded Children), the leadership of the Kennedy administration, founding of the network of University Affiliated Facilities (as they were first called), and the sustaining urgency of the social revolution. In the 1970s, the fields of developmental and behavioral pediatrics arose, and more guidance was offered to primary practice.

For some decades, health care for adults with intellectual disabilities did not receive regular consideration. Indeed, such individuals were almost invisible in the medical world. The largest block of physicians caring for adults with developmental disabilities were those on staff in the state residential facilities (the "institutions"), and they tended to be much removed from mainstream medicine. To some extent, there was an identified focus in membership of the Medicine Division of what is now the American Association on Mental Retardation. Scholarly studies, however, and education of new professionals were sparse.

Actually, even at the height of involvement of state residential facilities (the 1960s), only about 10% of Americans with significant intellectual disabilities were living in institutions. The vast majority were with their families and/or residing in the community, and health care they received was from usual local practitioners. A handful of journal articles (and no books) appeared in the 1960s and early 1970s on medical issues in adults with intellectual disabilities, but by the late 1970s and early 1980s, there were earnest considerations published about best care.

Again, as had been the situation for children, a combination of factors affected the field of medical care for adults with intellectual disabilities. Individuals were leaving the institutions as criticisms built up about the circumstances of congregate care. This persuasion became much enhanced as consumer groups began what was to be a long series of class action suits against state governments and superintendents (about 50 of these in the late 1970s and on into the 1990s). Often, a prominent element in the legal challenge was the quality of medical care received by residents. Byproducts of these actions were the hiring of more health care providers, use of consultation services with academic centers, and development of medical agencies who could be contracted to provide on-site care. Furthermore, many people were identified now to be in their communities, and continuing education about special needs was provided for local physicians and hospitals. Among this atmosphere, the first edition of this book was published (at that time the initial one to consider medical care for adults with developmental disabilities).

In these discussions, it is misleading to imply the presence of a uniform or "usual" set of health care needs relevant to individuals with intellectual disabilities. Some general practice principles derive for the social and personal circumstances of exceptionality, which are discussed later in the chapter. But the heterogeneity of the group in the setting of medical care provisions is appropriate to note, in that it affects need and patterns of use. The terminology of Cole (1987) is helpful here. He recognized a "Level I, low-consuming group" of adults who typically needed 1–3 medical encounters per year; these individuals constituted about 45% of the clients in his state agency. He also spoke of a "Level II, intermediate group" (40% of the clients at his agency), who occasionally required medical specialty consultants, and "Level III, high-consuming group" (about 15% of the clients at his agency), who needed ongoing monitoring and access to tertiary care. Most of the individuals at Level I and some at Level II can be reasonably accommodated by the generic community medical system.

In a regional survey carried out by Minihan and Dean (1990), nearly half of the medical conditions among the 330 individuals they studied could be appropriately cared for by usual primary care physicians. Many of the rest needed more specialized attention. Put another way, the medical care needs of adults with mild intellectual disabilities typically are modest and similar to those of the general population, though some thoughtful support and interpretation is often required. Individuals whose developmental disorders are more pervasive may have important additional organic features and need assistance in best care and guidance. Much of the energy of this book is addressed to particular biomedical issues in this high-consuming group.

In many ways, the unrest in the medical care segments of the state institutions is gratifying because it precipitates an activation of study, planning, and teaching for adults with intellectual disabilities generally. One sees now an area in which there is a lively interest (in fact, it is now a *field*). The combination of good medical care and appropriate social responsibility is at hand. Consumer groups and families generally are articulate; service vendors are including medical issues and health promotion in individualized service plans (ISPs) and other planning; state agencies acknowledge the obligation to support health needs; nursing groups have a wonderful activist view; and medical systems are looking at education and practice. The scene for adults is slowly emulating some of the strength that had developed for guidance and assistance to children with special needs.

ORIGINS OF GOOD MEDICAL CARE

The foundations on which sound and just medical care are built derive from two conceptual issues—rights and values—complemented, of course, by a knowledge base that is robust. The medical field now has a commanding legacy in all three. Much of this has been secured in the universe of children with special needs. The application then to adult services can be direct.

The Right to Treatment

The matter of "the right to treatment," which is structured terminology for assurance of appropriate care, is a complex one. In the United States, health care is an expectation but not strictly an entitlement (except regarding emergencies, prisons, and some public health efforts). A particular social urgency exists for individuals (of any age) who are notably vulnerable. In this regard, the personal circumstance of intellectual disabilities draws a compassionate outreach to good services, though some extensions of this are still in development. A model "right to treatment" premise appears in Article II of the "Declaration of General and Special Rights of the Mentally Retarded," promulgated on October 24, 1968, by the International League of Societies for the Mentally Handicapped (a union of associations for retarded citizens from many countries) and adopted by the United Nations 3 years later. By its simplicity, it can stand as a guidepost for reinforced caring:

> The mentally retarded person has the right to proper medical care and physical restoration and to such education, training, habilitation, and guidance as will enable him to develop his ability and potential to the fullest possible extent, no matter how severe his degree of disability. No mentally handicapped person should be deprived of such services by reason of the cost involved. (International League of Societies for the Mentally Handicapped, 1968)

This International League rights statement captures the essentials:

1. A specific and dedicated effort will be made to bring appropriate care to these individuals.
2. A way must be found to prevent cost from being a barrier.
3. Discrimination shall not exist based on severity of personal involvement or limitations in prognosis.

It stands proudly, along with other critical human rights declarations, as a product of yearning and deep deliberation. Obviously, the actualization of such rights requires a system of ethical resolves, cultural acceptance, assisting financial supports, and some key pieces of legislation. The progress of the medical field has been substantial. The cost issues are discussed in Chapter 35. Ultimately, in the United States Medicaid is the most crucial support available, commonly funding health maintenance organization (HMO) managed care enrollment. Kastner, Walsh, and Criscione (1997) noted that individuals with disabilities constituted 15% of Medicaid's rolls but 37% of the medical care costs therein.

Other managed care systems, state Children's Health Insurance Programs, Medicare, and various indemnity plans have significance, but omissions and hardships persist.

Several thoughtful legislative landmarks have provided a grounding for right-to-treatment assurance. One of unexpected utility was Section 504 of the Rehabilitation Act of 1973 (PL 93-112), which noted that "no otherwise qualified handicapped individual in the United States . . . shall, solely by reason of his handicap, be excluded" from care programs that involve federal assistance (e.g., Medicaid). This intent was carried further in the Americans with Disabilities Act of 1990 (PL 101-336), in which a broadly conceived protection was specified for community resources and programs in the lives of individuals of all ages with disabilities.

Application of Section 504, and also later certain child abuse regulations, engendered a dramatic response to a tragic failure to respond to the care needs of a newborn infant with serious disabilities in Indiana in 1982 (the so-called "Baby Doe" dilemma). A resolution called "Principles of Treatment of Disabled Infants" was jointly signed on November 29, 1983, by both professional and consumer groups (e.g., American Academy of Pediatrics, National Down Syndrome Congress, The Association for Retarded Citizens of the United States, Spina Bifida Association of America, The Association for Persons with Severe Handicaps, American Association on Mental Deficiency, American Coalition of Citizens with Disabilities). This remarkable document asserted,

> When medical care is clearly beneficial, it should always be provided. When appropriate medical care is not available, arrangements should be made to transfer the infant to an appropriate medical facility. Consideration such as anticipated or actual limited potential of an individual and present or future lack of available community resources are irrelevant and must not determine the decisions concerning medical care. The individual's medical condition should be the sole focus of the decision. These are very strict standards. (American Academy of Pediatrics, 1984, pp. 559–560)

Ethical considerations bear on discussions of rights as well. In Chapter 33, the concept of "exceptional bioethics" is explored as a sound infrastructure for services in the setting of important exceptionality.

The Assurance of Values

Beyond the basic rights, there is also a requirement for ensuring those concurrent values that will make medical practice most supportive and effective. In the present reference, this implies securing service behaviors and attributes that will allow the person with disabilities and his or her family or important collaborators to best build for health and wellness.

For children with chronic problems, planning of this sort was focused in the early days of Title V ("Crippled Children") of the Social Security Act of 1935 (PL 74-271) but more energetically expanded in the 1980s by Surgeon General C. Everett Koop and Vince Hutchins and Merle McPherson of the Maternal and Child Health Bureau (MCHB). Ways were considered to bring humanizing and responsible characteristics to child health care, including a developmental orientation, integration, comprehensiveness, and freedom from discrimination. Finally, the simple phrase was agreed on—"family-centered, community-based, coordinated care"—which has now been extensively used as a benchmark for programs for children with special health care needs. MCHB also provided a table of guidance for care, originally prepared so as to be equally applicable for children with or without special needs (Healy & Lewis-Beck, 1987; see Table 1.1). A study project based in Boston with support from MCHB went further in producing an evaluative system called "Enhancing Quality (Standards and Indicators of Quality Care for Children with Special Health Care Needs)" (Epstein et al., 1989). This document has special concern with family centeredness; provides 68 standards; and is designed to be used with individual professionals, health care teams, clinics or hospitals, state health departments, and community programs.

Table 1.1. Principles of health care for children

Optimal health care for children should

1. Consider the child and his or her family as the focus of health care services
2. Be based on child and family needs that are determined by comprehensive and relevant evaluations
3. Encourage normal patterns of living within the home and community
4. Provide guidance in creating an environment that supports and nurtures developmental progress
5. Ensure access to a comprehensive range of health, educational, and social services
6. Encourage the child and the family to become educated consumers by fostering their knowledge and understanding of the health care system
7. Reflect an efficient and effective allocation of resources
8. Contribute to an ongoing process of coordination and communication between the child and family, the school, and all other relevant agencies
9. Improve the functional independence of the child and his or her family
10. Protect the fiscal integrity of the family unit

Adapted from Healy, A., & Lewis-Beck, J.A. (1987). *Guidelines for physicians: Improving health care for children with chronic illness* (Monograph). Washington, DC: U.S. Department of Health and Human Services, Maternal and Child Health Bureau.

Table 1.2. Means by which service programs, including systems of medical care, are devised and guided

	Origins	Effects
Regulations	Legislation Agency interpretation Judicial decisions	Process Management
Standards	Professional groups	Accreditation Approval
Codes, affirmations, values statements, and declarations of rights	Various studies, projects, and conferences	Behavioral guidelines Routes for suasion
Ethical precepts	Academic settings Teaching and inquiry	Quality assurance Accountability
Public opinion	Cultural	Ultimate support

Looking at values statements for health care practice for adults with disabilities is a repeated concern in many specific chapters of this book. The collective philosophical statements would, understandably, much resemble those for children. Although there has been no literal conversion of the MCHB phrase "family-centered, community-based, coordinated care" for adult consideration, equivalents would be apparent, such as "personalized, integrated, and inclusive." Elements that are relevant include individualized evaluation, continuity, family partnership, and alliance with habilitative resources.

Ultimate proposals of values can be generated in many modes and have different lives. Table 1.2 lists the conception of a virtual network of guidance materials, with different beginnings and different degrees of energy and enforcement. Completeness of services could be reflected, for example, in compliance with the accreditation rules of the Council on Quality and Leadership for People with Disabilities (formerly AC/DD). Attention to strategic concerns, however, could be reflected in the guidelines for Title XIX (Medicaid). Many of the other items can seem more arbitrary or philosophical, or even problematic (as in the phenomenon of public opinion). A thoughtful and practical "Principles of Care" schema for adults in Table 1.3 has proven helpful in defining expectations in certain federal class action suits.

Attainment of a Knowledge Base

As movement grew for ethical, accurate, and loving care, there was an obvious need for scholarly foundation as well. This has indeed been coming, but slowly and deliberately. Before 1960, systematic published materials on the medical care of individuals with developmental disabilities were sparse. The field was basically established between 1960 and 1990, and the elements of this period are summarized here.

A landmark review on mental retardation was edited by Gardner, Tarjan, and Richmond (1965) and published as a 40-page handbook in the *Journal of the American Medical Association.* The material included holds well today. In this handbook, one finds a record of the pioneering contributions of Carter (1964); Garrard and Richmond (1964); Masland, Saranson, and Gladwin (1958); Penrose (1963); Stevens and Heber (1964); and Tarjan (1966).

Assistance to medical professionals was provided in those early times by thoughtful elucidation of the genetic foundations of key disorders. Hsia's (1959) *Inborn Errors of Metabolism* was an inspired analysis of biochemical illnesses, with a great deal of further information provided by the astonishing *The Metabolic Basis of Inherited Disease* (Stanbury, Wyngaarden, & Fredrickson, 1960), now with seven further editions. Also valuable was Gardner's (1961) *Molecular Genetics and Human Disease* and Milunsky's (1975) *The Prevention of Genetic Disease and Mental Retardation.* Students and clinicians found in the atlases, and similar books, the most prominent presentation of the biomedical syndromes, an essential though limited venue. Gellis and Feingold began it with their atlas in 1968; much that was systematic was added by Smith in 1970 (*Recognizable Patterns of Human Malformation*); Holmes, Moser, and colleagues (1972) reflected on phenotypes from Fernald State School in their atlas; and Bergsma (1973) launched the National Foundation sequence with his *Birth Defects: Atlas and Compendium.* Present day workers would find these historic works to be engaging.

By the 1980s, the first reports began to appear on the experience of providing medical services for children and adults with intellectual disabilities. Nelson and Crocker (1978) wrote on medical services in a state school. The challenge of community-based care was discussed by Garrard (1982), McDonald (1985), Minihan (1986), and Ziring et al. (1988). An extensive symposium on community health care for adults with intellectual disabilities was reported in 1987 (Crocker & Yankauer). Pueschel launched a new industry by bringing out a scientifically and clinically accurate parent guide for individuals with Down syndrome in 1978 and then a professional's book in 1982 (Pueschel & Rynders).

The number of volumes on medical care in the developmental disabilities gradually increased. An early volume was Johnston and Magrab's (1976) *Developmental*

Table 1.3. Principles of care for an adult with developmental disabilities

1. A thoughtful consideration of etiology for the person's developmental disorder shall have been made or be made, recorded in defensible and available form, shared with the family and the medical providers, and updated if new technology suggests a potential value.
2. A problem-related, continuing care record shall be established and maintained and be viewed as a central and valued component of the person's life accouterments. This record will be handy, portable, legible, and interesting.
3. Provision of primary care shall be based in a location that is proximate, stable and accessible, and graced by love.
4. Referral for specialty care shall be generated by the quest for accuracy and draw on quality, dedicated resources.
5. Signs of worsening cortical disorder experienced in the domains of cognition, language, mobility, sensory function, or structure shall be viewed with alarm, and explanations and intervention will be sought.
6. Common secondary conditions that diminish health, such as aspiration, urinary tract infection, bowel problems, poor nutrition, periodontal diseases, skeletal changes, seizures, and sleep disturbances, shall be foreseen and treated considerately.
7. Preventive care approaches shall be invoked for avoidable or detectable health impairments such as untoward cardiovascular, gynecologic, or infectious ailments.
8. Medications that alter mood or behavior shall be considered double-edged swords, justifying particular caution in prescription and watchfulness.
9. Habilitative, rehabilitative, and assistive therapies and technologies shall be richly provided for the goals of joy, action, and extension.
10. The person, family members, and/or their surrogates shall share in all decision making, with extraordinary attention shown to display options, risks, and benefits.
11. Care will be coordinated across facilities and agencies and financial counseling shall be provided regarding assistance for reimbursing the costs of care.
12. Supportive health care services shall be minimally obtrusive, shall celebrate the presences of wellness, and shall look as well to buttressing the state of personal happiness.

From Crocker, A.C. (1999). Community-based and managed health care. In M.L. Wehmeyer & J.R. Patton (Eds.), *Mental retardation in the 21st century* (pp. 268–269). Austin, TX: PRO-ED; reprinted by permission.

Disorders: Assessment, Treatment, and Education. The most widely used of the books on children became 1) Accardo and Capute's (1979) *The Pediatrician and the Developmentally Delayed Child,* which morphed to a sequence by Capute and Accardo (1991) called *Developmental Disabilities in Infancy and Childhood*; 2) Scheiner and Abroms's (1980) notable *The Practical Management of the Developmentally Disabled Child*; and 3) Batshaw and Perret's (1986) *Children with Handicaps: A Medical Primer,* now *Children with Disabilities, Fifth Edition* (Batshaw, 2002). The mental health area had major early attention, including Menolascino (1970) and Szymanski and Tanguay (1980). Developmental-behavioral pediatrics was launched as a study area by Levine, Carey, and Crocker (1983). The first edition of *Medical Care for Children and Adults with Developmental Disabilities* (then *Developmental Disabilities: Delivery of Medical Care for Children and Adults,* Rubin & Crocker, 1989) brought a life-span consideration. Valuable related texts included Thompson, Rubin, and Bilenker (1983) on cerebral palsy; Birenbaum and Cohen (1985) on community services; and Haynie, Porter, and Palfrey (1989, now Porter, Haynie, Bierle, Caldwell, & Palfrey, 1997) on children assisted by medical technology.

PROVISION OF MEDICAL CARE FOR DEVELOPMENTAL DISABILITIES

Stewardship

Health care workers engaged with individuals with developmental or other disabilities are collaborating in a significant supportive force, acknowledging widespread human specialness and assisting in endeavors of life enrichment. Supportive health care workers enriched the experiences of a girl named Gia (see Figure 1.1). Her story, presented next, is told by her parents, Flora and Joe Bellofatto.

Our daughter came into the world, as do others with Down syndrome, with a preordained destiny that would inevitably include a myriad of developmental challenges. However, as medical complications quickly and dramatically came to the fore, concerns regarding developmental disabilities disappeared, and the quest to preserve her life became the paramount struggle. Her ultimate survival can be attributed to an irrepressible will to live coupled with a series of astute, proactive decisions made without prejudice by the many medical professionals she encountered on her journey.

Shortly after her birth, a precautionary echocardiogram was performed, which revealed the presence of a complete atrioventricular canal (CAVC). The plan was to perform heart surgery later that year, but when Gia suddenly fell into severe respiratory distress at 1 week of age, her battle to live began. She was diagnosed with necrotizing enterocolitis (NEC) and by all accounts had a tenuous hold on life. She overcame that episode but experienced several life-threatening recurrences.

Though she valiantly fought the virulent infection, her heart began to fail. Because she was a full-term 7-pound baby, the doctors were baffled by the origin of the NEC and its relentless recurrences. While the CAVC was not typically associated with poor blood flow, it was thought that her heart was somehow causally related to the NEC. After weeks of exhaustive deliberation with and among her doctors, the decision was made to perform cardiac surgery despite her precarious condition, in an effort to prevent further episodes of NEC.

At 2 months of age, she underwent cardiac surgery, and her heart was successfully repaired. Two weeks later, extensive strictures were found during intestinal surgery, resulting in the loss of half of her colon and a portion of her small bowel. She was left with an ileostomy that was reversed when she was 6 months old.

Throughout the 4-month ordeal, we as parents were tortured by our inability to render direct care to our daughter. Though forced to relinquish our role as primary caregivers, we refused to become bystanders. Our newly assigned position was that of advocate, and our principal obligation was to be ever present. We endeavored to become informed, albeit it at the most rudimentary level, about the numerous health issues she confronted. Prior to consenting to even minor procedures, we gathered multiple opinions and questioned every doctor incessantly, undaunted by the exceptional medical prowess in our midst.

With each devastating setback Gia experienced, we were brought to our knees, disheartened and discouraged about her ability to overcome what was thrust upon her. Though we had unwavering confidence in her doctors, her palpable desire to live enabled us to persevere and imbued us with hope. Her eyes conveyed a steadfast resolve that she would not succumb. She has a unique ability to inspire not only us but also all those who entered her orbit to fight for her. In turn, we believe that the simple act of holding her for countless hours each day, month after month, gave her solace and strength and that our bedside vigils instilled in her a worthwhile reason to fight.

Throughout her struggle, the doctors and nurses who treated her demonstrated a genuine commitment to delivering the highest caliber of care. Her chromosomal make-up was a consideration only in terms of approach and was a never regarded as a disincentive for utilizing aggressive, lifesaving measures. The acumen and compassion of these progressive-minded individuals supported Gia's unrelenting will to live, allowing her body and spirit to triumph.

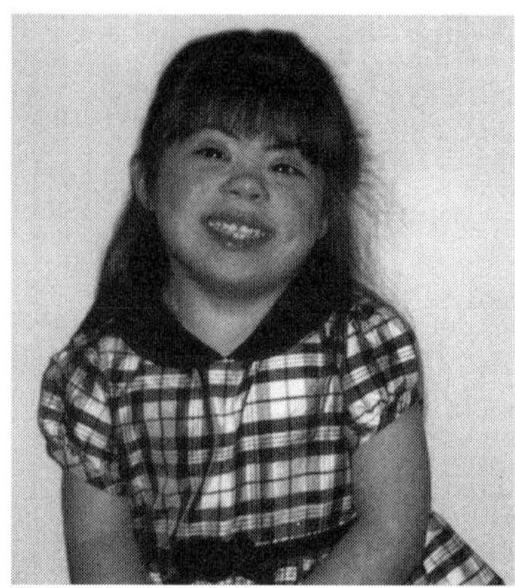

Figure 1.1. Although she had a tumultuous beginning, Gia continues to thrive and relish life.

Although she had a tumultuous beginning, she continues to thrive and relish life. Eager to move and explore her world, Gia learned to crawl at 9 months of age and, by 2½ years, perfected her walking skills. Now, at 3½, she expresses herself primarily through sign language, with a vocabulary of 75 words that grows steadily. Her achievements reflect a steely determination inherent in a personality that continues to captivate like a kaleidoscope with infinite facets and brilliant colors.

The long-term alliance between health care workers and individuals with disabilities is a good one. Advocacy becomes a notable (and creative) activity. In disability work, there is so much to learn, and one finds oneself with a remarkable team. Part of the experience also is the consumer activists, whose promotion is a great value. For medical workers, these are circumstances of discovery.

The opportunity exists to reinforce health and to add to the holistic supports that surround the person with disabilities. Safety, including pharmacologic safety, can be secured, with additional reflection on risks and needs. The biomedical environment can be helpful for study, referral, and search (including causation). Particular trust may be available, and catalytic, especially for introduction of interventions. Different pieces of a medical base may be fashioned and may assist in coordination. One looks to a growth of common feeling and a supportive amity.

Some Thoughts on Words

In both the worlds of service and of friendship there exists a continuing opportunity for nurturing use of language, the right terms used warmly. Because speech reveals enthusiasms or biases, it is appropriate to secure those terminologies that are heartening. Some provider discipline vocabularies are overly concrete (this can include medical terminology) and can portray stigma.

Clinicians should reach out to women, men, boys, and girls, not to males, females, cases, or subjects and seek sisters and brothers, rather than siblings. They can find ways to empathize with exceptionality (see Chapter 27.2) and use descriptive terms that look to pluses and are gentle and respectful. "People-first" phraseology (e.g., *a child with Down syndrome*) is now mainstream and is the preeminent use in this book. The term *handicap* is archaic in its earlier utilization and has a limited employment to describe social or environmental disadvantage. See Table 1.4 for further comments.

On July 25, 2003, a press release signed by President George W. Bush declared that the "President's Committee on Mental Retardation" has been retitled the "President's Committee for People with Intellectual Disabilities." With that significant change, one puts aside a class name that had become onerous and attempts to establish a less-troubling usage—although this new one will doubtless become hurtful eventually. This redoubtable achievement by the nation's self-advocates deserves endorsement. A major national commission had been sorely challenged on the nomenclature assignment; it appears that there will be an inscrutable, though piecemeal, dismissal of *mental retardation*. The American Association on Mental Retardation is in an earnest transition frame of mind. It became the American Association of Mental Deficiency in 1933, changed to the American Association on Mental Retardation in 1987, and will see a new shift soon. This book will understandably bridge the terminology evolution while acknowledging the technical usefulness of the earlier language.

Table 1.4. Style guide for disability issues

Always use person-first nomenclature (e.g., *a child with Down syndrome,* not *a Down syndrome child*).
Descriptive adjectives cannot become class names (nouns) (e.g., do not use *the disabled* or *the retarded*).
Avoid deprecatory descriptors such as *low functioning, affliction,* or *slowness.*
Eponyms do not take the possessive form (e.g., *Klinefelter,* not *Klinefelter's*).
Handicapped refers to social constrictions, not personal status. *Disabled* is preferred but is used thoughtfully.
An individual is never a *case,* which is a legal term or a part of public health statistics.
Male or *female* should not be a primary identifier. Use *woman, man, girl,* and *boy.* Use *brother* and/or *sister* rather than *sibling.*

Story of the Medical Model

While saluting the productive collaboration of medical strengths with the disability world, it is also appropriate to acknowledge that the relationship has sometimes been awkward. Much of disability is not health linked, and the use of medical terms ("medicalization") for the circumstances of a person with disabilities can be disturbing. An emphasis on insinuated disease or disorder in exceptionality can divert from social goals or self-worth. Medical partnership, however, should be respectful and minimally intrusive. The aims for wellness may require a thoughtful design to use medical resources gently.

The medical model has been particularly considered in two settings. The first is the traditional involvement of physicians as superintendents (state schools) or as commissioners in the intellectual disability field. These regulations have now largely been discontinued, assisting in an orientation to developmental and social services. The other relates to the Independent Living Movement (especially physical disability), in which there is a superior self-direction, with reflective medical alliance as needed (Crocker, 1999a, 1999b).

CONTINUING EFFORTS TO ENSURE QUALITY

Privacy and HIPAA

The Health Insurance Portability and Accountability Act (HIPAA) of 1996 (PL 104-191) has added a vigorous new level of explicit regulation of privacy for personal medical records. The general principles are not new, but the current extensions are complex and a considerable source of pressure in private and public transactions (Annas, 2003). The major guidance became effective in April 2003.

Patients have the right to have their personal medical information kept private, and physicians have an obligation to keep medical information secret. Transfer is permitted for health care operations, but nontreatment uses of protected health information require patient authorization. Transfer for payment activities is accepted, of course, with notable regulation for public health uses, law enforcement, abuse issues, and emergencies. Patients or guardians now have enhanced access to inspect their own health information, amend it if needed, request restriction, and seek accounting of disclosure. The widespread notification of private citizens (and/or guardians) about HIPAA regulations has brought privacy into focus.

Medical Home

A modern conception of pediatric practice as it reaches out to children with special health care needs (CSHCN) is that of providing a so-called *medical home*. This was first mentioned in the late 1960s, slowly grew in interest in the next two decades, and became a strong model of planning in 1992 (Sia, Tonniges, Osterhus, & Taba, 2004). This concept embodies many of the pediatric values that were emerging in the early 1980s with the support of MCHB.

In the earliest versions of the medical home, the primary emphasis was on achieving expert and uninterrupted care for a child with multiple health issues, incorporation of family expertise in planning, and coordination for procurement of community services. Sometimes, this involved subsidization for nurse practitioner or social work collaboration in the pediatric office to bring particular help to children with multiple special needs. Gradually, other means were found for such coverage, and the features of the medical home became notable for an office change in attitude and service patterns.

The five most important special provisions have come to be *usual source of care* (familiarity and access for the child with special needs), *personal doctor or nurse* (continuity and a sustained relationship), *coordinated care* (discussion, planning, relation to school), and *family-centered care* (respect, feedback) (Strickland et al., 2004). In the National Survey of Children with Special Health Care Needs, about half of the children were receiving these components of support (Centers for Disease Control and Prevention, 2001). Efforts of this sort are correlated with a reduction in delayed care, unmet needs, school days missed per illness, and family supports unattained. A new listing has now been formulated of the central values for care planning: accessible, family-centered, continuous, comprehensive, coordinated, compassionate, and culturally effective (American Academy of Pediatrics, 2004).

Developmental Pediatrics

Since 2002, there has been a major enhancement of training directives and certification in developmental pediatrics. The American Board of Pediatrics surprisingly established two related sub-boards for specialized qualification after general pediatrics. That for Developmental-Behavioral Pediatrics is a 3-year process resembling programs that had been present, in varying length, in university centers for some time. The one in Neurodevelopment Disabilities (NDD) acknowledges the considerable relationship to child neurology in much of this work and plans jointly with that specialty. NDD can start after 2 years of general pediatrics and runs 4 years, incorporating a year of adult neurology, experience in child neurology, and laboratory studies. Both sub-boards have curriculum content with a contemporary philosophy, involving interdisciplinary relationships, community organizations, and child advocacy. These new training opportunities will unquestionably reinforce the professionalism of developmental pediatrics and influence the placement of personnel in faculty and research positions. It remains to be seen what the effects will be on the numbers of available colleagues.

A Word on Current Planning

Despite the ambient concerns about access and quality of medical services for individuals with intellectual disabilities, appropriate analysis is underway. Two exemplary national conferences took place at the beginning of the millennium. The Surgeon General's Conference on Health Disparities and Mental Retardation produced the report *Closing the Gap* (Office of the Surgeon General, 2002). A remarkable national "Listening Session" of early comments, in network format, occurred on October 10, 2001. The other was the National Goals Conference of The Arc of the United States *Keeping the Promises* (January 6, 2003).

Some excerpts from *Closing the Gap* (Office of the Surgeon General) indicate the level of apprehension:

- Even a quick glimpse at the health status of person with mental retardation, both children and adults, reveals glaring deficiencies that must be addressed. (2002, p. iv)

- Compared with other populations, adults, adolescents, and children with MR experience poorer health and more difficulty in finding, getting to, and paying for appropriate health care. These challenges are even more daunting for people with MR from minority communities with many cultures and languages and whose culture and primary language may not be reflected in available health services. (2002, p. xii)

- A provider's willingness to treat people with intellectual disabilities is influenced by public, private, and advocacy groups; access to technical support and professional allies; and evidence that it is financially viable to treat people with intellectual disabilities. (2002, p. A-3)

- Physicians and other providers often lack training and experience in treating individuals with mental retardation and are reluctant to assume clinical responsibility for them. Cultural sensitivity may be lacking. Financing for health care services is often inadequate, and scientific knowledge about the efficacy of care for this population is far from complete. Services may be poorer in quality because of societal assumptions that people with mental retardation cannot participate appropriately in their own health care. (2002, p. D-1)

The Surgeon General's Conference went on to identify goals and action steps for consideration, at many levels. The goals are listed in Table 1.5, with selections from some of the action items.

Keeping the Promises utilized many work groups. The Health Service work group suggested significant areas with incomplete knowledge and urged work to be done on many, including the following:

- Strategies to enhance participation of individuals with intellectual disabilities in their own health promotion activities
- Inquiry about the utility of guidelines and standards regarding health outcomes
- Examination of the impact of different models of state-based health care financing
- More information about health status and risks across the lifespan
- Identification of effective health care provider training methods
- Determination of the usefulness of alternative medicine approaches
- Consideration of the methods of transferring user-friendly information that can assist in health care decisions (The Arc of the United States, 2003, pp. 22–23)

Table 1.5. Goals and action steps from the Surgeon General's Conference on Health Disparities and Mental Retardation

Goal 1: Integrate health promotion into community environments of people with intellectual disabilities
- Education on self-care and wellness
- Assessment of the effects of health promotion activities

Goal 2: Increase knowledge and understanding of health and intellectual disabilities, ensuring that knowledge is made practical and easy to use
- Enable individuals and families to partner with investigators
- Create a national research agenda that identifies gaps
- Collect data on health status
- Enhance the visibility of health and mental retardation research

Goal 3: Improve the quality of health care for people with intellectual disabilities
- Identify priority areas of health care quality improvement
- Develop standards of care
- Ensure practice and financing that promotes improvement

Goal 4: Train health care providers in the care of adults and children with intellectual disabilities
- Integrate didactic and clinical training
- Provide interdisciplinary training and continuing education

Goal 5: Ensure that health care financing produces good health outcomes for adults and children with intellectual disabilities
- Encourage relationships among diverse financing mechanisms
- Define *effective, cost effective,* and *health outcome*
- Identify models for leveraging

Goal 6: Increase sources of health care services for adults, adolescents, and children with intellectual disabilities, ensuring that health care is easily accessible for them
- Increase number of professionals with appropriate training, especially for socioeconomically and linguistically diverse communities
- Integrate health care into diverse community programs
- Make access to care less complicated
- Support supplementary services for physicians
- Ensure continuity of services throughout life

Adapted from Office of the Surgeon General. (2002). *Closing the gap: A national blueprint to improve the health of persons with mental retardation.* Rockville, MD: U.S. Department of Health and Human Services.

CONCLUSION

This chapter presents a medley of the factors supporting medical care, including historical developments and persistent concerns. It provides the underlying principles for the specifics of care that are presented in the rest of the book.

REFERENCES

Accardo, P.J., & Capute, A.J. (1979). *The pediatrician and the developmentally delayed child.* Baltimore: University Park Press.

American Academy of Pediatrics. (1984). Joint policy statement: Principles of treatment of disabled infants. *Pediatrics, 73*(4), 559–560.

American Academy of Pediatrics. (2004). *What's a medical home?* [Information sheet]. Elk Grove Village, IL: Author.

Americans with Disabilities Act (ADA) of 1990, PL 101-336, 42 U.S.C. §§ 12101 *et seq.*

Annas, G.J. (2003). HIPAA regulations—a new era of medical-record privacy? *New England Journal of Medicine, 348,* 1486–1490.

The Arc of the United States. (2003). *Keeping the promises.* Silver Spring, MD: Author.

Batshaw, M.L. (Ed.). (2002). *Children with disabilities* (5th ed.). Baltimore: Paul H. Brookes Publishing Co.

Batshaw, M.L., & Perret, Y.M. (1986). *Children with handicaps: A medical primer.* Baltimore: Paul H. Brookes Publishing Co.

Bergsma, D. (Ed.). (1973). *Birth defects: Atlas and compendium.* Baltimore: Lippincott, Williams & Wilkins.

Birenbaum, A., & Cohen, H.J. (1985). *Community services for the mentally retarded.* Totowa, NJ: Bowman & Allenheld.

Capute, A.J., & Accardo, P.J. (Eds.). (1991). *Developmental disabilities in infancy and childhood.* Baltimore: Paul H. Brookes Publishing Co.

Carter, C.H. (Ed.). (1964). *Medical aspects of mental retardation.* Springfield, IL: Charles C Thomas.

Centers for Disease Control and Prevention. (2001). *The national survey of children with special health care needs chartbook, 2001.* Hyattsville, MD: Author.

Cole, R.F. (1987). Community-based prepaid medical care for adults with mental retardation: Proposal for a pilot project. *Mental Retardation, 25,* 233–235.

Crocker, A.C. (1999a). Community-based and managed health care. In M.L. Wehmeyer & J.R. Patton (Eds.), *Mental retardation in the 21st century* (pp. 265–279). Austin, TX: PRO-ED.

Crocker, A.C. (1999b). The medical model: A mostly historical discussion. In H. Bersani, Jr. (Ed.), *Responding to the challenge* (pp. 3–9). Cambridge, MA: Brookline Books.

Crocker, A.C., & Yankauer, A. (Eds.). (1987). Community health care services for adults with mental retardation: The Sterling D. Garrard Memorial Symposium. *Mental Retardation, 25,* 189–242.

Epstein, S.G., Taylor, A.B., Halberg A.S., Gardner, J.D., Walker, D.K., & Crocker, A.C. (1989). *Enhancing quality: Standards and indicators of quality care for children with special health care needs.* Boston: New England SERVE.

Gardner, G.E., Tarjan, G., & Richmond, J.B. (Eds.). (1965). Mental retardation: A handbook for the primary physician. *Journal of the American Medical Association, 191,* 117–156.

Gardner, L. (1961). *Molecular genetics and human disease.* Springfield, IL: Charles C Thomas.

Garrard, S.D. (1982). Health services for mentally retarded people in community residences. *American Journal of Public Health, 72,* 1226.

Garrard, S.D., & Richmond, J.B. (1964). Diagnosis in mental retardation. In C.H. Carter (Ed.), *Medical aspects of mental retardation.* Springfield, IL: Charles C Thomas.

Gellis, S.S., & Feingold, M. (1968). *Atlas of mental retardation syndromes.* Washington, DC: U.S. Department of Health, Education, and Welfare.

Haynie M., Porter, S.M., & Palfrey, J.S. (1989). *Children assisted by medical technology in educational settings.* Boston: Children's Hospital.

Health Insurance Portability and Accountability Act (HIPAA) of 1996, PL 104-191, 110 Stat. 1936.

Healy, A., & Lewis-Beck, J.A. (1987). *Guidelines for physicians: Improving health care for children with chronic illness* [Monograph]. Washington, DC: U.S. Department of Health and Human Services, Maternal and Child Health Bureau.

Holmes, L.B., Moser H.W., Halldorsson, S., Mack, C., Pant, S., & Matzilevich, B. (1972). *Mental retardation: An atlas of diseases with associated physical abnormalities.* New York: Macmillan.

Hsia, D.Y.Y. (1959). *Inborn errors of metabolism.* Chicago: Year-Book Publishers.

International League of Societies for the Mentally Handicapped. (1968). *The rights of the mentally retarded: Principles and programs.* Helsinki, Sweden: Author.

Johnston, R.B., & Magrab, P.R. (Eds.). (1976). *Developmental disorders: Assessment, treatment, and education.* Baltimore: University Park Press.

Kastner, T.A., Walsh, K.K., & Criscione, T. (1997). Overview and implications of Medicaid managed care for people with developmental disabilities. *Mental Retardation, 35,* 257–269.

Levine, M.D., Carey, W.B., & Crocker, A.C., (1983). *Developmental behavioral pediatrics.* Philadelphia: W.B. Saunders.

Masland, R.L., Saranson, S.P., & Gladwin, T. (1958). *Mental subnormality.* New York: Basic Books.

McDonald, E.P. (1985). Medical needs of severely developmentally disabled persons residing in the community. *American Journal of Mental Deficiency, 90,* 171–176.

Menolascino, F.S. (1970). *Psychiatric approaches to mental retardation.* New York: Basic Books.

Milunsky, A. (1975). *The prevention of genetic disease and mental retardation.* Philadelphia: W.B. Saunders.

Minihan, P.M. (1986). Planning for community physician services prior to deinstitutionalization of mentally retarded persons. *American Journal of Public Health, 76,* 1202–1206.

Minihan, P.M., & Dean, D.H. (1990). Meeting the needs for health services of persons with mental retardation living in the community. *American Journal of Public Health, 80,* 1043–1048.

Nelson, R.P., & Crocker, A.C. (1978). The medical care of mentally retarded persons in public residential facilities. *New England Journal of Medicine, 299,* 1039.

Office of the Surgeon General. (2002). *Closing the gap: A national blueprint to improve the health of persons with mental retardation.* Rockville, MD: U.S. Department of Health and Human Services.

Penrose, L.S. (1963). *Biology of mental defect* (2nd ed.). New York: Grune & Stratton.

Porter, S. Haynie, M., Bierle, T., Caldwell, T.H., & Palfrey, J.S. (1997). *Children and youth assisted by medical technology in educational settings: Guidelines for care* (2nd ed.). Baltimore: Paul H. Brookes Publishing Co.

Pueschel, S.M. (Ed.). (1978). *Down syndrome: Growing and learning.* Kansas City, MO: Sheed Andrews & McMeel.

Pueschel, S.M., & Rynders, J.E. (Eds.). (1982). *Down syndrome: Advances in biomedicine and the behavioral sciences.* Cambridge, England: The Ware Press.

Rehabilitation Act of 1973, PL 93-112, 29 U.S.C. §§ 701 *et seq.*

Rubin, I.L., & Crocker, A.C. (Eds.). (1989). *Developmental disabilities: Delivery of medical care for children and adults.* Philadelphia: Lea & Febiger.

Scheiner, A.P., & Abroms, I.F. (Eds.). (1980). *The practical management of the developmentally disabled child.* St. Louis: C.V. Mosby.

Sia, C., Tonniges, T.F., Osterhus, E., & Taba, S. (2004). History of the medical home concept. *Pediatrics, 113,* 1473–1478.

Smith, D.W. (1970). *Recognizable patterns of human malformation.* Philadelphia: W.B. Saunders.

Social Security Act of 1935, PL 74-271, 42 U.S.C. §§ 301 *et seq.*

Stanbury, J.B., Wyngaarden, J.B., & Fredrickson, D.S. (Eds.). (1960). *The metabolic basis of inherited disease.* New York: McGraw-Hill.

Stevens, H.A., & Heber, R. (1964). *Mental retardation: Review of research.* Chicago: University of Chicago Press.

Strickland, B., McPherson, M., Weissman, G., van Dyck, P., Huang, Z.J., & Newacheck, P. (2004). Access to the medical home: Results of the national survey of children with special health care needs. *Pediatrics, 113,* 1485–1492.

Szymanksi, L.S., & Tanguay, P.E. (Eds.). (1980). *Emotional disorders of mentally retarded persons: Assessment, treatment, and consultation.* Baltimore: University Park Press.

Tarjan, G. (1966). Cinderella and the prince: Mental retardation and community psychiatry. *American Journal of Psychiatry, 122*, 1057–1059.

Thompson, G.H., Rubin, I.L., & Bilenker, R.M. (Eds.). (1983). *Comprehensive management of cerebral palsy*. New York: Grune & Stratton.

Ziring, P.R., Kastner T., Friedman, D.L, Pond, W.S., Barnett, M.L., Sonnenberg, E.M., et al. (1988). Provision of health care for persons with developmental disabilities living in the community. *Journal of the American Medical Association, 260*, 1439–1444.

CHAPTER 2

THE DEVELOPMENTAL DISABILITIES

Allen C. Crocker

The term *developmental disabilities* has been slowly increasing in use since its introduction by the pioneer advocate Elizabeth Boggs in the late 1960s. It gathers together a group of challenging conditions with early onset, long-term duration, developmental implications, and continuing service needs. Individuals with intellectual disabilities are a prominent component within the group, but a widely varying cluster of other situations are also pertinent, such as musculoskeletal disorders, palsies, seizure syndromes, visual impairments, hearing impairments, autism, and multiple congenital anomalies. When used in legislation, *developmental disabilities* joins the interests of children with intellectual disabilities with those of children with less prevalent disorders but comparable service needs. The Developmental Disabilities Services and Facilities Construction Amendments of 1970 (PL 91-517, also called the Kennedy-Yarborough Act) created a number of new supports. These include Developmental Disabilities Planning Councils (citizen and professional groups) to advise on services in every state, protection and advocacy mechanisms to monitor and intervene in rights issues (i.e., Disability Law Centers), support for training programs (i.e., then called "University Affiliated Facilities") on numerous campuses, and provision of some limited funds for strategic projects.

Families welcomed into the Developmental Disabilities system were those who had a family member with intellectual disabilities, cerebral palsy, epilepsy, or autism. Families who had members with other disabilities, however, were excluded, and revisions were made to add serious neurological disorders and severe learning disabilities to the list. The resulting situation was ambiguous and created a call for a more rational nosology. Lengthy deliberation by a commission from Abt Associates of Cambridge, Massachusetts, settled on a functional grid that has proved to be effective and equitable. The commission's definition of *Developmental Disability* was recorded in the Rehabilitation Act Amendments of 1978 (PL 95-602):

> A severe, chronic disability of a person which (A) is attributable to a mental or physical impairment or combination of mental and physical impairments; (B) is manifested before the person attains the age twenty-two; (C) is likely to continue indefinitely; (D) results in substantial functional limitations in three or more of the following areas of major life activity: (i) self-care, (ii) receptive and expressive language, (iii) learning, (iv) mobility, (v) self-direction, (vi) capacity for independent living, and (vii) economic sufficiency; and (E) reflects the person's need for a combination and sequence of special interdisciplinary, or generic care, treatment, or other services which are life-long or extended duration and are individually planned and coordinated.

This categorization is well considered because it implies a biological or constitutional origin, includes disabilities beginning in the developmental period and continuing throughout a person's life, addresses issues that are important in a person's developmental progress, and values the provision of services. *THESE ARE THE PEOPLE OF THIS BOOK.* The definition of *developmental disabilities* has remained stable since 1978. Note, however, that this conceptualization states that in order to receive continuing services from public and professional agencies, an individual must have a disability that has a specific developmental aspect and is of significant magnitude. It is commonly stated about 3% of the population (at diverse age groups) falls into this category.

Additional developmental disabilities acts and/or amendments removed the capacity for construction, allowed satellites to exist with certain University Affiliated Facilities, strengthened protection and advocacy activities, and began regular reports to the U.S. Congress. Bill of Rights elements were added, and goals of independence, productivity, and integration into the community were enunciated. In addition, diversity was emphasized, and underserved populations were identified. In these fashions, the humanistic intentions of the effort were established.

OTHER CLASSIFICATION SYSTEMS AND FREQUENCIES

Numerous other systems of organization are parallel or analogous to the developmental disabilities system. Various agencies and programs use additional ways to gather and to count. The two largest categories to note are 1) the biomedical, clinical, or functional challenge elements and 2) the public planning or policy groups.

Generic Clinical Groupings

Mental retardation was one of the first labels used to categorize individuals by personal attributes and, therefore, has meaning for individuals, families, and scholars as well as a historic precedence. Many confoundments and responsibilities quickly come forward in this sensitive area of nomenclature. In the 15 years since the publication of the first edition of this book, the term *mental retardation* has gradually evolved into a less comfortable (or even partially unacceptable) designation that has a personally devaluing tone in the views of many individuals. The stigma attached to *mental retardation* is beginning to limit the term's accepted use. The term *intellectual disability* has found much value as an alternative term (see Chapter 1). In this book, both terms appear. The term *mental retardation* is eliminated on a social or personal basis but acknowledged as having strong traditions and utility in a clinical, scientific, or nosologic setting.

The medical field has long looked to the Committee on Terminology and Classification of the American Association on Mental Retardation for thoughtful derivation of a consensus definition for *mental retardation.* This term is typically revised about every 10 years as new perceptions become established. The 2002 version (see Table 2.1) gives strong consideration to the qualifying elements of context, culture, and needs for support. Co-existent strengths and some potential for functional evolution with time are thoughtfully noted. The same basic definition would apply to the term *intellectual disability.*

In this regard, this condition is the largest functional component within the developmental disabilities. Ascertainment of its incidence has long been sought for use in educational planning, advocacy, and epidemiology. Kiernan and Bruininks (1986) have provided a valuable summary of the methods in which prevalence (and, in a related fashion, incidence) of a disability such as mental retardation can be estimated. There are five primary techniques:

1. Key informants (individuals with knowledge of patterns in the community)
2. Community forum (individuals in a public meeting)
3. Rates under treatment (listings of individuals using services)
4. Social indicators (analysis of factors that correlate)
5. Direct survey (standardized contact with the direct population)

Furthermore, conclusions about prevalence for any given population will be influenced by the effects of features such as age, culture, availability of service programs, and enrollment criteria. These authors consider 1.0% to be the most reasonable prevalence figure for intellectual disability for all ages in the general population. They acknowledge that many other studies report 2½%–3%.

Looking further at notable clinical groupings, Kiernan and Bruininks (1986) suggested prevalence rates of 0.75% (7.5/1,000) for epilepsy and 0.35% for cerebral palsy. Gortmarker and Sappenfield (1984) put these levels at 0.35% and 0.25%. Many individuals with mild expression of seizure disorder or cerebral palsy have limited service needs and are not counted within the community total for developmental disabilities. Sensory disabilities have a wide range of occurrence. In developed countries, an estimated 0.1%–0.2% of children have moderate or greater bilateral sensorineural hearing impairment, and 5–10 times that many have lesser degrees of hearing impairment (Kelly, 1999). For North America, 3–6 children per 10,000 are blind or have severe vi-

Table 2.1. A definition for mental retardation

Mental Retardation is a disability characterized by significant limitation both in intellectual functioning and in adaptive behavior as expressed in conceptual, social, and practical adaptive skills. This disability originates before age 18.

The following five assumptions are essential in the application of this definition:

1. Limitation in present functioning must be considered within the context of community environments typical of the individual's age peers and culture.
2. Valid assessment considers cultural and linguistic diversity as well as differences in communication, sensory, motor, and behavioral factors.
3. Within an individual, limitations often coexist with strengths.
4. An important purpose of describing limitations is to develop a profile of needed supports.
5. With appropriate personalized supports over a sustained period, the life functioning of the person with mental retardation generally will improve.

From Luckasson, R., Borthwick-Duffy, S., Buntinx, W.H.E., Coulter, D.L., Craig, E.M., Reeve, A., Schalock, R.L., & Snell, W.E. (2002). *Mental retardation: Definition, classification, and systems of supports* (10th ed., p. 1). Washington, DC: American Association on Mental Retardation; reprinted by permission.

sual impairment, and several times that many have important limitations (Davidson & Burns, 1999).

Tabulation is further complicated by the presence of concurrent disabilities. Accardo and Capute (1979) commented that of all children with developmental disabilities, approximately one third have a single difficulty, another third have two difficulties, and the remaining third have three or more difficulties. Thirty to seventy percent of children with cerebral palsy are anticipated to also have intellectual disabilities (generally the more limbs involved, the more significant the retardation), and 25%–35% are anticipated to have seizures (Shapiro, Palmer, Wachtel, & Capute, 1983). This author's experience in hospital developmental referrals is that about a tenth of children with intellectual disabilities will have seizures, and about a quarter of those referred for epilepsy will have intellectual disabilities. In considerable degree, these phenomena can be viewed as so-called "comorbidities," or an added disability being derived from the same background as the first one (see Chapter 4). Clearly the effects of early stress on the central nervous system are not discrete.

Counting in the clinical area also involves reckoning with the so-called birth defects or congenital anomaly syndromes, as well as some of the genetic conditions. Many of these conditions have a truly low incidence. Down syndrome, congenital heart disease, facial or palate clefts, and neural tube defects are often regarded as epidemiologic markers and are the most frequently occurring conditions, with rates of about 1 per 1,000 live births. Many of the other syndromes are unusual variants, and some of these conditions are well known despite the fact that they affect few individuals. Fetal alcohol syndrome is found to be common when looked for (1–2/1,000 births), and fragile X syndrome has a similar rate (1 per 1,250 males). Many other syndromes are rare:

- Prader-Willi syndrome (1:10,000)
- Rett syndrome (1:20,000)
- Cornelia de Lange syndrome (1:30,000)
- Cri-du-chat (5p–) syndrome (1:50,000)
- Hurler syndrome (1:100,000)

All of these would be part of the developmental disabilities world.

Finally, estimates of developmental disabilities in the medical area acknowledge children with chronic illnesses that in some settings have significant developmental implications. The classic Vanderbilt Study (Hobbs, Perrin, & Ireys, 1985) concluded that 10%–15% of children in the United States are chronically ill and 10% of those children have problems that are pressing and have serious service needs. Newacheck and Halfon (1998) looked at a great variety of health conditions tracked in the National Health Interview Survey and concluded that 6.5% of U.S. children had health-related disabilities.

Children in Programs or Services

Young people with disabilities also come to be counted in specific settings, often where supports will be provided. The most structured of these is education, which features personalized program planning with considerable investment for quality improvement (see Chapter 6.4). The primary guide for intervention at school is the individualized education program (IEP), and the establishment of that document affirms the child's dedicated enrollment. Presence of an IEP certifies the need for special curriculum planning for the child. The percentage of children for whom an IEP has been written is a marker of special needs among pupils in the school district but also reflects educational philosophy, local economic conditions, and the role of consumer convictions. Traditionally, this rate varies between 8% and 15% of all students, or around 10% for most states. Children with learning disabilities and speech-language impairments are the largest group who receive IEPs. Children with intellectual disabilities are the third largest group (i.e., approximately 18%–20% of the total).

A remarkable cohort of children whose developmental disabilities are linked to compelling program needs are those assisted by medical technology. Included here are boys and girls (and some adults) who require special procedures, such as oxygen administration, portable ventilator use, gastrointestinal tube feedings, urostomy or colostomy care, clean intermittent catheterization, intravenous medications or feedings (with pumps), and renal dialysis. Many of these young people are graduates of severe preterm birth, complex surgical repair of congenital anomalies, or early trauma (see Chapter 10). Their enrollment in school and community requires special teams and resources (Crocker & Porter, 2001). A total state census of children who used 1 or more of 12 specific supports was undertaken in Massachusetts in 1987 and 1990, using data from hospitals, schools, nursing homes, visiting nurse associates, and other sources (Palfrey et al., 1994; Palfrey et al., 1991). Table 2.2 lists the diverse supporting technology required for these children, who can be said to epitomize thoughtful interdisciplinary planning. The majority of these children were enrolled in school-

Table 2.2. Census results for Massachusetts children with medical technology assistance, 1990s

Technology	Adjusted estimate
Overall	2237
Tracheostomy	219
Suctioning	434
Respirator	70
Oxygen	405
Nasogastric tube	121
Gastrostomy tube	972
Ileo-colostomy	118
Jejunostomy tube	67
Urostomy	42
Catheterization	526
Intravenous line	299
Dialysis	48

From Palfrey, J.S., Haynie, M., Porter, S., Fenton, T., Cooperman-Vincent, P., Shaw, D., Johnson, B., Bierle, T., & Walker, D.K. (1994). Prevalence of medical technology assistance among children in Massachusetts in 1987 and 1990. *Public Health Reports, 109,* 226–233; reprinted by permission.

based settings. The total prevalence was 0.16%. Their developmental levels are bimodal in distribution; a little more than half had normal intelligence, but development is challenged in many ways.

Another group of infants and toddlers with special needs are children who have disorders often associated with delayed courses. These little ones are regarded as *at risk,* which is an important early descriptor that carries with it an assumption that assistance will be provided to ensure the best learning (i.e., early intervention). Tjossem (1976) suggested that there were three major groups: infants with conditions known to be associated with developmental liability ("infants with established disability"), infants whose early history has troubled elements or whose courses were slowed ("infants at biologic risk"), and infants for whom circumstances of early care were limited ("infants at environmental risk"). Established conditions included many of the so-called birth defects, chromosomal disorders, and genetic syndromes. Many of the children at biological risk had preterm births or unknown types of personal restrictions. Environmental risks included troubled family settings, such as very young mothers and significant social disadvantage.

Estimates of incidence vary widely, in part because of different ratings and interpretations given to events in early childhood by responsible agency personnel. In Massachusetts, for example, about 30,000 very young children are enrolled in more than 60 programs of early intervention (about 7% of children from birth to 3 years of age). Some other states have enrolled fewer children (2%, or even 0.7%). In many states, early intervention is now an entitlement.

Through the inspired leadership of Martha Eliot, children with particular needs were identified in 1935 for so-called *Crippled Children's Services (CCS),* part of the Social Security Act of 1935 (PL 74-271). State-administered care programs were established, particularly for youngsters with physical disabilities and those who lived in rural settings. The CCS programs grew under the guidance of the Children's Bureau and administered to children with a variety of chronic illness diagnoses. The programs assisted a total of 650,000 children by 1979 (Crocker, 1989b). Gradually, a conviction was reached that other designs of public health planning and supports could be more efficacious, and direct care was phased out by most state departments. A more broadly applicable categorization was determined for children who would appropriately benefit from governmental guidance, support, and special services—still with Maternal and Child Health Bureau supervision. This system was codified in the Omnibus Budget Reconciliation Act of 1989 (PL 101-239) as *Children with Special Health Care Needs (CSHCN).*

CSHCN is a mouthful as an acronym, but the concept has proven to be a valuable one. Planning and quality control services were needed for children with special health care needs, children with special needs, and children with chronic or ongoing health conditions. Stein's (Stein, Bauman, Westbrook, Coupey, & Ireys, 1993) definition of these children is provided in Table 2.3. These children have some special needs and limitations on their activities (compared with typically developing peers) and need continuing service supports of various degrees. Among children as a whole, multiple surveys have shown CSHCNs to be at 14%–18% of the total. This lively and important group of children needs to be given thoughtful regard for a number of reasons. A variety of education and social support issues are involved, but health care needs require particular attention.

Obvious personal and cultural elements affect the language used to describe disabilities, many of which are included in other sections of this book. The focus on disability produced by the landmark achievement of the Americans with Disabilities Act of 1990 (PL 101-336) is important. In the education of the public that was carried out in preparation of this astonishing legislation, it was repeatedly affirmed that there were 43,000,000 Americans with disabilities. Such a compilation (of all manner of special needs in all age groups) comes to about 14% of the U.S. population. In many settings where special needs are discussed, it is often ex-

Table 2.3. Characteristics of chronic or ongoing health conditions

1. Have a biological, psychological, or cognitive basis and
2. Have lasted or are virtually certain to last for at least one year and
3. Produce one or more of the following sequelae:
   a. Limitation of function, activities, or social role in comparison with healthy age peers in the general area of physical, cognitive, emotional, and social growth and development
   b. Dependency on one of the following to compensate for or minimize limitation of function, activities, or social role:
      1. Medications
      2. Special diet
      3. Medical technology
      4. Assistive device
      5. Personal assistance
   c. Need for medical care or related services, psychological services or educational services over and above the usual for the child's age, or special ongoing treatments, intervention, or accommodations at home or in school

Reprinted from *Journal of Pediatrics, 122*(3), Stein, R.E.K., Bauman, L.J., Westbrook, L.E., Coupey, S.M., & Ireys, H.T., "Framework for Identifying Children Who Have Chronic Conditions: The Case for a New Definition," p. 345. Copyright 1993, with permission from Elsevier.

pressed that "disability" in the macro sense (all 14%) should be given support as needed in most planning efforts, rather than the subdivisions (e.g., Down syndrome, hearing impairments). The editors of this book agree with much of that philosophy, but there is an earnest service world (developmental disabilities) that has lessons right now.

ETIOLOGY OF DEVELOPMENTAL DISABILITIES

Both care providers and theorists in the field of developmental disabilities benefit from a working conception of the origins of these human conditions. Parents need a hypothesis for their child's exceptionality, educators need references to children with similar learning experiences, physicians need good information on expected special health concerns, and public health workers need to know epidemiologic or preventive implications. A real hypothesis about etiology is often elusive, however. Special needs generally have multiple elements, and, in many instances, the true nature of the cause is unknown. It is possible, though, to make a best conjecture about the timing of the aberration (e.g., prenatal, perinatal) and thus about the relevant circumstances.

Table 2.4 presents a conception arranged principally by the time in child development when the major influence occurred that changed the child's life; these elements have, to some extent, their own natural history. In Table 2.4, figures are given for relative frequency in a study population with intellectual disabilities (at this author's Developmental Evaluation Center). In childhood, ascertaining the pattern of developmental abnormality, and hence its presumed onset, is relatively simple. For adults (e.g., individuals within a state residential facility) determination of the cause of disability is less certain.

Table 2.4. Schematic consideration of the mechanisms of intellectual disabilities (with relative prevalence in a hospital referral experience)

I. Hereditary disorders **(5)**

Preconceptional origin, multiple somatic effects, frequently a progressive course

- Inborn errors of metabolism and other recessive transmission
  - Tay-Sachs disease, Hurler syndrome, phenylketonuria
- Varying dominant expression syndromes
  - Neurofibromatosis, tuberous sclerosis
- Hereditary chromosomal aberrations
  - Translocation, fragile X syndrome
- Mitochondrial inheritance

II. Early alterations affecting chromosomes or embryonic development **(32)**

Sporadic events, phenotypic changes, usually stable developmental modification

- Chromosomal changes, including trisomy, deletions
  - Down syndrome, Williams syndrome
- Prenatal influence syndromes
  - Multiple congenital anomalies, intrauterine infection
- Multifactorial syndromes
  - Neural tube defects, autism

III. Other pregnancy problems and perinatal morbidity **(11)**

Impingement on progress of fetus during last two trimesters or newborn, neurologic abnormalities frequent, disability usually stable

- Fetal malnutrition/placental insufficiency
- Perinatal difficulties
  - Prematurity, hypoxia, central nervous system hemorrhage

IV. Acquired childhood conditions **(4)**

Acute effects on developmental status, variable potential for functional recovery

- Infection
  - Encephalitis, meningitis
- Cranial trauma
- Other
  - Asphyxia, near drowning, intoxication

V. Environmental problems and behavioral syndromes **(18)**

Dynamic influences, operational throughout development

- Psychosocial deprivation
- Parental neurosis, psychosis, personality disorder
- Certain emotional and behavioral disorders

VI. Unknown causes **(30)**

No definite hereditary, gestational, perinatal, acquired, or environmental issues, or multiple elements present

From Crocker, A.C. (1989a). The causes of mental retardation. *Pediatric Annals, 10,* 623–636; adapted by permission.

Hereditary Disorders

Inheritance of disability by a Mendelian pattern of single gene transmission is uncommon but concrete, exemplified by the inborn errors of metabolism (see Chapter 7). A variety of neurologic syndromes can have family passage, including the diversely expressed phakomatosis disorders. On rare occasions, polygenic patterns are seen in affected families. A complicated replication of mutated genes causes cogent abnormality in families with a history of fragile X syndrome (see Chapter 9.3).

Early Alterations Affecting Chromosomes or Embryonic Development

Vastly more common among the origins of disability syndromes is the sporadic occurrences of significant change in the germ cells of young embryos near the time of conception. As could be expected, these events produce a significant alteration of the phenotype and hence are signaled by special physical findings. Postnatally, the resulting disability proceeds in a stable course. Many of the chromosomal shifts are not compatible with survival through pregnancy (trisomy 21 has a significant mortality, but many children do make it). Children with "minor" or "major" birth defects have a form of embryodysgenesis that may include abnormalities in the central nervous system with resultant functional changes. Researchers are learning that many of these conditions are accompanied by small changes in chromosomes, or potentiating genes.

Other Pregnancy Problems and Perinatal Morbidity

Fetal malnutrition refers to diminished support for fetal growth as pregnancy proceeds, especially regarding placental integrity or vascular configuration. Uterine bleeding, early onset of labor, or reduced size of infant may result, sometimes with untoward developmental consequences. Perinatal stresses (premature birth, obstetrical complications in full-term infants) particularly affect vulnerable infants because of potentially compromising events—trauma, central nervous system hemorrhage, pulmonary difficulties, acidosis, hypoglycemia, seizures, and sometimes infection that may operate negatively on the extrauterine adjustment of the immature infant brain. The role of perinatal problems in postnatal outcome can be difficult to determine, except in extremes; some infants with very harrowing courses escape cerebral complications. A period of follow-up in an infant development clinic helps to identify children who need particular supportive services.

Acquired Childhood Conditions

Now that measles encephalitis is controlled, most episodes of encephalitis that come to the developmentalist's attention are from organisms that are not identified. There is an extraordinary boon from the virtual obliteration of pneumococcal and *H. influenzae* meningitis currently. The most publicized causes of cranial injury are those involving motor vehicles, but a greater incidence occurs from household accidents. Child abuse is also a significant cause.

Environmental Problems and Behavioral Syndromes

Interpreting the role of varying environmental circumstances or the effects of certain behavioral disorders on the ultimate developmental outcome of children is particularly challenging. Of equal puzzlement is the potential for repair or reversal of intellectual disabilities when better circumstances for living or learning can be created. Psychosocial deprivation implies an incomplete nurturance of a child's requisites, a frustration of his or her promise or legacy. This situation may involve frank parental dysfunction, including abuse or neglect, or an unkind environment beyond the control of the family (see Chapter 34). Ironically, the prior presence of other developmental disabilities may potentiate the likelihood of troubled nurturance, with additional difficulties resulting. Much less frequently, a specific qualifying circumstance such as parental psychosis or character disorder is present.

Unknown Causes

Thoughtful study of a child with developmental impairments generally allows some workable conclusions about the timing and nature of special issues in the child's life, which can be helpful for the family's understanding. In many instances, however, one cannot be more specific, and it is appropriate to list the etiology as *unknown.* This term is also justified when several issues of relatively minor nature are present and the situation appears to be multifactorial or obscure. Modern genetic studies, including testing for biochemical abnormalities, changes in genes, or alterations in gene products, have

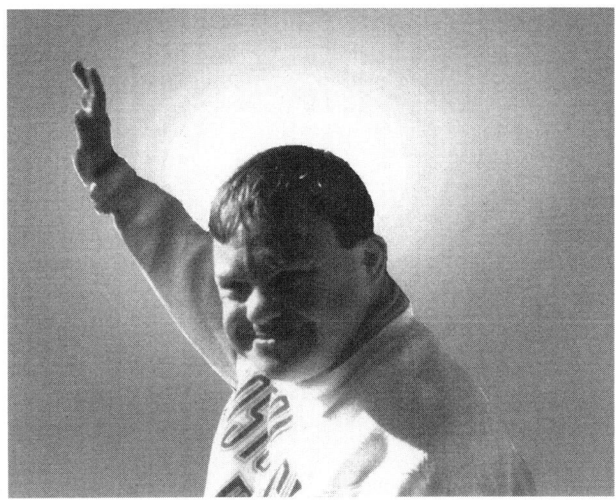

Figure 2.1. Mike's good nature captivated the hearts of everyone.

for some children elucidated a discrete constitutional factor (consultation with clinical genetics experts can be valuable) (Roberts, Palfrey, & Bridgemohan, 2004). In others, particularly with mild expression of disability, interpretation may require postponement.

CONCLUSION

This chapter explores the types of developmental disabilities and their occurrence rates. Considering people with disabilities from a medical perspective, however, should not overshadow the fact that people with disabilities are individuals. They have names and stories. Angela and Dan Becker share the story of their son, Mike (see Figure 2.1).

Our son, Mike, who died at age 38, made the most of his life with Down syndrome; diabetes; and, finally, kidney failure. He did it with the help of loving family, friends, and caregivers—and with an unquenchable zest for life that endeared him to virtually everyone within smiling distance. Mike was born in September 1964—a time of Dark Ages for people with Down syndrome. Distressed as most parents would be, we agonized over Mike's care and future and spent months consulting specialists. Meanwhile, we took him everywhere we went. His smiling good nature captivated the hearts of everyone. At age 3, another major health problem beset Mike—diabetes—which in time would become the dominant issue of his life.

Our search for schooling led us to the Cardinal Cushing School in Hanover, Massachusetts. Starting at age 7, Mike lived in a dorm at Cardinal Cushing School, attended classes, learned to read and write, improved his speech, produced intriguing artwork, joined the Cub Scouts, took dates to proms, and excelled at Special Olympics. He spent weekends, vacations, and holidays with us. He stopped at the Health Center three times a day for his tests and insulin shots and made great friends of the nurses. Two weeks each summer, he attended the Joslin Camp for diabetics to monitor his control. He was the only child with Down syndrome there but got along famously with staff and fellow campers. In 1986, a beaming Mike graduated from high school. We couldn't have been prouder if he had gotten his diploma from Harvard.

Mike was now ready for a group home. He lived on campus until a Cushing residence opened in 1993. He was blessed with wonderful staff and trained by his nurses in diabetic management. He learned to do his own tests and shots (but not calibrations). He refused to let his intrusive routine dampen his spirits and viewed his medical appointments as opportunities to make new friends. He enjoyed a varied, productive, and happy life. He had a fine workshop and several good jobs within his limits. He continued to be a sports and music junkie and was a great traveler (to Disney World, Branson, Opryland, and Cooperstown, among other places). He had a great sense of humor. His favorite phrase was, "Nobody's perfect."

From day one, he loved to do things for people—bestow gifts, host parties, share with others, deliver meals to seniors, participate in "walks"—but as years passed, Mike's blood levels became harder to control, and his reactions more frequent and severe. His creatinine levels soared; his kidneys failed. He had his first dialysis in February 2001. The next 28 months were really tough for Mike, with frequent hospitalizations, amputation of two toes and a finger, major surgery on an arm and an eye, and much more. His pill intake set an all-time record.

During this time, Mike had a zillion medical appointments in addition to dialysis. Mostly what kept him going was the compassion and patience of the medical staff at Harvard Vanguard Medical Associates. Wherever he went, the nurses were his "buddies." His doctors spoke to him, not just his parents, and joked with him and explained treatments in simple, nonfrightening terms. To coordinate efforts and help Mike tolerate dialysis, the medical center provided a case manager who proved to be indispensable.

In the face of his grueling regimen, Mike still did a lot. He attended church, went to sports events and shows, bowled well, took two dialysis sea cruises with us, and visited Gillette Stadium as a special guest of the New England Patriots. And he never stopped smiling. But his health problems were finally too much for him. On May 22, 2003, he died, peacefully, of a stroke. Our hearts broke in half.

Hundreds attended his funeral service and burial. We remain most proud of Mike for facing adversity with such courage and good humor, for the many friendships he made and for his indomitable optimism. Our beloved Mike lived a short life, but it was a life full of love, joys, and more precious moments that we could ever count.

REFERENCES

Accardo, P.J., & Capute, A.J. (1979). *The pediatrician and the developmentally delayed child.* Baltimore: University Park Press.

Americans with Disabilities Act (ADA) of 1990, PL 101-336, 42 U.S.C. §§ 12101 *et seq.*

Crocker, A.C. (1989a). The causes of mental retardation. *Pediatric Annals, 10,* 623–636.

Crocker, A.C. (1989b). Services for children with special health care needs (formerly called Crippled Children's Services). In I.L. Rubin & A.C. Crocker (Eds.), *Developmental disabilities: Delivery of medical care for children and adults* (pp. 61–64). Philadelphia: Lea & Febiger.

Crocker, A.C., & Porter, S.M. (2001). Inclusion of young children with complex health care needs. In M.J. Guralnick (Ed.), *Early childhood inclusion: Focus on change* (pp. 399–412). Baltimore: Paul H. Brookes Publishing Co.

Davidson, P.W., & Burns, C.M. (1999). Visual impairment and blindness. In M.D. Levine, W.B. Carey, & A.C. Crocker (Eds.), *Developmental behavioral pediatrics* (pp. 571–578). Philadelphia: W.B. Saunders.

Developmental Disabilities Services and Facilities Construction Amendments of 1970, PL 91-517, 84 Stat. 1316.

Gortmarker, S.L., & Sappenfield, W.M. (1984). Chronic childhood disorders: Prevalence and impact. *Pediatric Clinics North America, 31,* 3.

Hobbs, N., Perrin, J.M., & Ireys, H.T. (1985) *Chronically ill children and their families.* San Francisco: Jossey-Bass.

Kelly, D.P. (1999). Hearing impairment. In M.D. Levine, W.B. Carey, & A.C. Crocker (Eds.), *Developmental behavioral pediatrics* (pp. 560–570). Philadelphia: W.B. Saunders.

Kiernan, W.E., & Bruininks, R.H. (1986). Demographic characteristics. In W.E. Kiernan & J. A. Stark (Eds.), *Pathways to employment for adults with developmental disabilities* (pp. 21–50). Baltimore: Paul H. Brookes Publishing Co.

Luckasson, R., Borthwick-Duffy, S., Buntinx, W.H.E., Coulter, D.L., Craig, E.M., Reeve, A., Schalock, R.L., & Snell, W.E. (2002). *Mental retardation: Definition, classification, and systems of supports* (10th ed.). Washington, DC: American Association on Mental Retardation.

Newacheck, P.W., & Halfon, N. (1998). Prevalence and impact of disabling chronic conditions in childhood. *American Journal of Public Health, 88,* 610–617.

Omnibus Budget Reconciliation Act (OBRA) of 1989, PL 101-239, 42 U.S.C. §§ 1396 *et seq.*

Palfrey, J.S., Haynie, M., Porter, S., Fenton, T., Cooperman-Vincent, P., et al. (1994). Prevalence of medical technology assistance among children in Massachusetts in 1987 and 1990. *Public Health Reports, 109,* 226–233.

Palfrey, J.S., Walker, D.K., Haynie, M., Singer, J.D., Porter, S., Bushey, B., et al. (1991). Technology's children: Report of a statewide census of children dependent on medical supports. *Pediatrics, 87,* 611–618.

Rehabilitation Act Amendments of 1978; PL 95-602, 29 U.S.C. §§ 701 *et seq.*

Roberts, G., Palfrey, J., & Bridgemohan, C. (2004). A rational approach to the medical evaluation of a child with developmental delay. *Contemporary Pediatrics, 21,* 76–100.

Shapiro, B.K., Palmer, F.B., Wachtel, R.C., & Capute, A.J. (1983). Associated dysfunctions. In G.H. Thompson, I.L. Rubin, & R.M. Bilenker (Eds.), *Comprehensive management of cerebral palsy.* New York: Grune & Stratton.

Social Security Act of 1935, PL 74-271, 42 U.S.C. §§ 301 *et seq.*

Stein, R.E.K., Bauman, L.J., Westbrook, L.E., Coupey, S.M., & Ireys, H.T. (1993). Framework for identifying children who have chronic conditions: The case for a new definition. *Journal of Pediatrics, 122*(3), 342–347.

Tjossem, T. (Ed.). (1976). *Intervention strategies for high risk infants and young children.* Baltimore: University Park Press.

CHAPTER 3

THE SPECTRUM OF MEDICAL CARE

Allen C. Crocker

The conceptualization that special needs have lifetime duration and require a partnership for best accommodation is fundamental to the definition of developmental disabilities. This chapter reflects on the continuing personal exploration and interaction of individuals with developmental disabilities and acknowledges the lifelong nature of collaboration and support.

THE COMMITMENT FOR CARE

Informed primary and specialty medical care is necessary for individuals with developmental disabilities; a balance must be sought between the appropriateness of providing usual, "generic" care and concern for the special vulnerabilities. Much of the health care is usual, but specialized knowledge is needed. The necessary considerations in providing medical care can be illustrated by examining four types of disorders: hereditary disease (Hurler syndrome), chromosomal aberration (Down syndrome), prenatal influence syndrome (myelodysplasia), and possible perinatal difficulties (cerebral palsy).

Hurler Syndrome

The inborn error of mucopolysaccharide (MPS) metabolism represents homozygous expression (autosomal recessive transmission) of L-iduronidase deficiency, and the clinical difficulties center around altered MPS functions in key locations (see Chapter 7.2). In the proband child, diagnosis is typically established during the second half of the first year of life and confirmed by enzyme assay on white blood cells. As is usual for large-molecule inborn errors, there is an early period of reasonable personal progress (1–2 years) and a middle time of slowed development (2–4 years). Functional losses then occur, and death comes typically in middle childhood. Good resolve is required by the family and community to acknowledge the involved limitations and embrace the special existence and charm embodied by these children.

Table 3.1 presents a HEALTHWATCH synopsis of the special needs of children with Hurler syndrome (Crocker, 1974). This field has become enormously active for therapeutic intervention; bone marrow transplantation has literally given new life to dozens of such children, and enzyme infusion therapy has important ameliorative effects. These are very fundamental achievements, accessible to more recently diagnosed children. For further information and resources, contact the National MPS Society (Post Office Box 736, Bangor, ME 04402-0736; telephone 207-947-1445).

Down Syndrome

Down syndrome is the clinical expression of a surfeit of material in chromosome 21 (by trisomy or translocation, enigmatically derived). It occurs widely at an incidence of about 1 per 1,000 births, is diagnosed at birth or prenatally, has high public recognition, and has its own lore (some mythic). Individuals with Down syndrome have been traditional victims of stereotyping and segregation, but in the last several decades vastly improved opportunities have been secured in education, vocation, and independent living.

Significant medical care issues exist, as summarized in Table 3.2; however, early intervention, thoughtful (mostly inclusive) curricula, and enthusiastic advocacy have had critical value. Health care is more accurate; most notably, medical surgical treatment of congenital heart disease now assures good survival (see Chapter 9.2). Parent support, promotion of research, and consideration of rights are energetically watched by two exemplary organizations—the National Down Syndrome Congress (1370 Center Drive, Suite 102, Atlanta, GA 30338; telephone 800-232-6372) and the National Down Syndrome Society (666 Broadway, 8th Floor, New York, NY 10012-2317; telephone 800-221-4602).

Table 3.1. HEALTHWATCH for children with Hurler syndrome

Concern	Clinical expression	When seen	Management
Phenotypic changes	Full forehead; flat nose; joint restriction; synophrys; hirsutism	Gradually apparent in first year	None necessary
Growth pattern	Accelerated at first, then stops (maximum 42 inches)	Appears at 1–2 years of age but stops by 3 years	None necessary
Hernias	Inguinal in most boys; umbilical in both sexes	Early months	Repair optional; will recur if not reinforced
Joint restriction	Flexion contracture of all joints; progressive for some years	Elbows by few months of age; other joints gradually apparent	Range of motion exercises of limited use; encourage general activity
Kyphosis	Beaking of L-1, with angulation of spine	Early months; more when upright	None necessary (no spinal cord pressure)
Corneal clouding	Hazy appearance	1–2 months	None necessary
Hearing problems	Middle ear effusions; ankylosis of ossicles; hearing impairment	1–2 years	Treatment of infection; ventilation tubes; possible amplification
Hepatosplenomegaly	Firm organomegaly; limited progression	During first year	None necessary
Subarachnoid cysts	Increased intracranial pressure; hydrocephalus	Variable; 1–3 years	Shunting may be advisable
Seizures	Primary generalized	2–4 years	Unusual anticonvulsants; will be time limited
Cardiac problems	Thickened valves; coronary narrowing; cardiac myopathy	Murmur in first year; other issues by 3 years	May require treatment for congestive failure
Airway problems	Large adenoids or tonsils; increased secretions; thickening or narrowing of larynx or trachea; obstructive sleep apnea	Slowly progressive	In later years, oxygen therapy; rarely, tracheostomy; great care in anesthesia
Enzyme deficiency	All of the above; consideration of experimental interventions		Bone marrow transplantation; enzyme replacement therapy

Myelodysplasia

The cluster of congenital anomalies identified as neural tube defects (spina bifida, meningocele, myelomeningocele, some hydrocephalus, and anencephaly) are prenatal influence syndromes with apparent multifactorial elements (risk in repeat pregnancies ranges from 1 per 20 to 1 per 40). The term *myelodysplasia* is used to describe spinal defects in which there is cord involvement and loss of nerve function (see Chapter 8.1). This prototypic developmental disability requires a team of devoted professionals to accomplish optimal habilitation. Because the natural history of clinical difficulties in myelodysplasia is variable, no time frame is given in the HEALTHWATCH chart in Table 3.3. Family and individual support materials are available from the Spina Bifida Association of America (4590 MacArthur Boulevard NW, Suite 250, Washington, DC 20007-4226; telephone 800-621-3141).

Cerebral Palsy

The term *cerebral palsy* is applied to a disorder of movement and posture due to a nonprogressive lesion of the immature brain. The diagnosis is a matter of clinical judgment and is useful for the development of services. As with myelodysplasia, significantly involved individuals will make optimal progress when they are provided with guidance from an interdisciplinary specialty team. There is an evolution of motor problems and associated dysfunctions, with difficult times arriving in middle to late childhood. The story becomes more complex in adults because determining the basis for diminishing function in mobility, language, and independence is often perplexing. Important components of care are presented in Table 3.4. Information and resources are available from United Cerebral Palsy (1660 L Street NW, Suite 700, Washington, D.C. 20036-5602; telephone 800-872-5827).

Table 3.2. HEALTHWATCH for individuals with Down syndrome

Concern	Clinical expression	When seen	Prevalence	Management
Congenital heart disease	Atrioventricular canal defects; auricular or ventricular septal defects; tetralogy of Fallot	Newborn	40%–50%	Cardiac consultation; echocardiography; surgical repair; subacute bacterial endocarditis prophylaxis
Hypotonia	Reduced muscle tone; increased range of joints	Throughout life; improvement with maturity	All	Guidance by physical therapy; early intervention; adapted physical education
Delayed growth	Typically at or near third percentile for general population	Throughout life	All	Use Down syndrome growth charts and early nutritional support; check thyroid and heart
Developmental delays	Some global delay of variable degrees; specific language problems	First year; continues	All	Early intervention; educational planning; speech-language therapy
Hearing concerns	Serous otitis media; small ear canals; mostly conductive impairment	Check by 6 months; review regularly in early years	As much as to 50% at some times; 10% sensorineural	Audiology; tympanometry; ear, nose, and throat consultation
Ocular problems	a. Refractive errors b. Strabismus c. Cataracts	Eye exam by 6–12 months, then follow-ups	a. 50% b. 35% c. 5%	Look for cataract; ophthalmologic consultation
Cervical spine abnormality	Atlantoaxial instability; potential neck signs; potential long-tract signs	X-ray by 3 years; repeat in middle childhood	10%, of which 1%–2% are serious	Some neurologic and orthopedic help; possible restriction or fusion
Thyroid disease	Hypothyroidism; decreased growth and development	Some congenital; mostly occurs during 20s; check at 2–3 years and repeat	15%	Endocrine consult; replacement therapy as needed
Overweight	Excessive weight gain	Preschool and adolescent years	Common	Lifestyle adjustment, including diet and activity
Seizure disorders	Primary generalized (also hypsarrhythmia)	Childhood	5%–10%	Electrencephalogram; neurologic consultation
Emotional problems	Inappropriate behavior, depression, and other emotional disturbances	Mid- to late childhood; adult life	Common	Family guidance; mental health assistance
Premature senescence	Behavioral changes; functional losses	40s and 50s	Unknown (increased rate)	Special support

Note: Additional variable occurrences include congenial intestinal obstruction, Hirschsprung disease, alopecia areata, keratoconus, hip dysplasia, diabetes mellitus, missing teeth, obstructive sleep apnea, celiac disease, and mitral valve prolapse.

PASSAGES

Lifelong planning is appropriate for all individuals with developmental disabilities because the special needs manifest themselves before the individual is 21 years old and are likely to persist throughout the person's life. Nevertheless, human services tend to be designed for separate periods in life, with different groups of workers for each period. The potential for discontinuity is troubling.

Table 3.3. HEALTHWATCH for individuals with myelodyplasia

Concern	Clinical expression	Management
Myelomeningocele	Exposed meninges and spinal cord	Repair in first 24–48 hours
Hydrocephalus	Increased intracranial pressure; ventricular enlargement	Scans; ventriculoperitoneal shunting in early weeks
Shunt failure	Vomiting; irritability; headache; drowsiness; strabismus	Consultation; possible revision
Chiari II malformation	Stridor; apnea (central and obstructive); feeding difficulties	Shunt revision; Chiari decompression; airway management; G tube
Spinal cord tethering	Worsening gait; bowel and bladder dysfunction	Magnetic resonance imaging study; urodynamics; surgical detethering
Loss of muscle action	Flaccid paraplegia; degree per motor level; can cause some spasticity	Assisted ambulation (orthoses) or wheelchair
	Muscle imbalance; potential for contractures; dislocations	Training; preventive physical therapy; later, muscle lengthening and transfer; release of contractures
	Scoliosis, plus complications	Bracing; surgery
Loss of sensation	Potential for skin trauma; decubitus; underlying osteomyelitis	Care; inspection; hygiene; bone scans
Neurogenic bladder	Incontinence; poor emptying; reflux; pyelonephritis; renal failure	Renal ultrasound; urodynamic studies; clean intermittent catherization; padding; collecting devices; monitoring of electrolytes and others; anticholinergics; antibiotics; artificial sphincter
Neurogenic bowel	Incontinence; constipation	Training; suppositories; mini-enemas; antegrade colonic enemas
Developmental phenomena	Learning disabilities; attention-deficit disorder; intellectual disabilities; strabismus; seizures; precocious puberty	Early intervention; educational planning; neuropsychology testing; endocrine consultation; anticonvulsants
Chronic deprivation and interruptions of activities	Adjustment problems; obesity	Support by habilitation team; counseling; therapy; nutrition; recreation

Note: Additional difficulties include sexual dysfunction, and other congenital anomalies.

Karen Marie Metzler, a woman with disabilities, shared her insight on the impact of medical care throughout her life. She required medical care from birth and continues to face issues in her adult years. She writes:

My story began on December 12, 1950. Born with multiple birth defects, including spina bifida and facial anomalies, I became a "one-in-a-million live births" occurrence—a premature Christmas present for parents who tried to conceive the "old fashioned" way for 13 years. That first Christmas was spent with our entire family hospitalized. Mother and father eventually went home; I stayed behind for nearly a year undergoing many surgeries. Now, after 53 years and some 110 operations, I am that child who was not to live past the age of 2.

Educated in public schools when not hospitalized, I was generally self-taught due to regulations preventing district-paid tutors without 6 weeks' prior notice. Hospital-based tutors did not exist then. Our family prized education, though our budget forced a trade-off in favor of my medical expenses and the mortgage payments. Only after 13 years of my medical expenses and a then-experimental kidney operation were they forced into near bankruptcy and applied for any state funds. Two years and four jobs between them, they worked their way off it.

My 1969 graduation was marred by bureaucratic resistance to financial aid to college. Even Case Western Reserve's medical dean claimed to my face, "You aren't worth the investment; you'll die on us!" Advocates argued that because more than $300,000 (in old preinflation any dollars) had been spent by my parents alone to keep me alive medically, a college education enabling me to compete for employment at my full intellectual capacity was surely warranted.

I am orphaned now, not by permanent institutionalization so prevalent in 1950, nor the quasi-kind imposed on my childhood, but by countless medical treatments and surgeries. I remain alone because I was born an only child and have lived in the family home since the death of my mother in 1998. My father passed away on Father's Day in 1982. After his death, Mother and I survived on our respective Social Security checks. Hers paid the household expenses; mine paid Medigap premiums and medications. I am among the "cresting generation" of those of us who benefited from earlier medical breakthroughs and beliefs germinating toward our parents' dreams that their child would one day become a full-fledged member of society. Because those of my generation

Table 3.4. HEALTHWATCH for individuals with cerebral palsy

Concern	Clinical expression	Prevalence	Management
Central nervous system abnormality	Infancy—variation in tone, delayed motor milestones, asymmetry, hyperreflexia, primitive reflexes	All	Early intervention programs
	Preschool—development of motor, posture, and movement patterns		Orthopedics and physical therapy (see below)
	Childhood—difficulty with motor tasks, possible deformities		
	May present with spasticity, dyskinesia (athetosis, choreoathetosis, dystonia), ataxia, or mixed syndromes		
Altered muscle function	Slow, weak movements; combination of extremity involvement—diplegia, hemiplegia, and/or quadriplegia	All	Physical therapy—muscle stretching, stimulation, and positioning
	Imbalance leading to contractures, dislocations, leg-length discrepancy, and scoliosis		Orthopedics and physiatry—bracing, corrective surgery, Baclofen/pump, Botox and phenol injections
Associated dysfunctions	Intellectual disability	50%	Assessment; special education
	Visual problems—strabismus, visual field defects, and amblyopia	> 50%	Ophthalmologic collaboration; visual stimulation
	Hearing impairment (sensorineural)	5%–15%	Audiologic collaboration
	Seizures—all forms	30%	Anticonvulsant treatment
	Communication disorders—speech (oromotor function) and language (e.g., central processing)	Common	Speech therapy collaboration; communication enhancement
	Urinary tract infections; urinary retention	Common	Medical surveillance; urology consultation as needed
	Feeding/swallowing disorders—gastroesophageal reflux, aspiration pneumonia, wheezing	Common	Medications; thickened feedings; G-tube; gastrointestinal and pulmonary consults as needed
Emotional and coping issues	Adjustment problems, especially in adolescents and adults	Common	Psychosocial support in many areas
	Loss of function in adults		Rehabilitation; physiatry

are the pioneers, the stages of our growth highlight current neglected needs. However, before the rectifying structures, services, and attitudes are built into place, we continue to age and move on into further barren territory.

My story and the stories of others like me expand the caregiving and aging issues to those of us who are mentally competent adult children who have survived disability and chronic illnesses. Social services are beginning to recognize the aging of our parents and the concern for our caregiving as we remain after their passing; however, there are gaps between the gerontological services our parents need and the availability of independent living services for young adults with disabilities and chronic illnesses. I am positing the reverse position of the adult child with disabilities and chronic illnesses who is capable of assuming responsibility for his or her parents' care at least psychosocially as an advocate, if not physically. We are confronted with some of the same issues as those in mainstream society's sandwiched generation. However, judged incompetent by the powers that be, self-determination and input are denied us—to the very extreme of denial of bedside farewells in the last moments of our parents' lives, as was the case for me.

Often, because of the inability to afford personal care attendants, individuals who have never lived institutionalized outside of the community are forced prematurely into nursing homes during the prime of their adulthood, particularly if they are without family members to subsidize expenses and/or supply caregiving. As parents age, a family choice must be made between their caregiving requirements and those of the adult child with a disability or chronic illness. This necessitates a choice between whose care the family assets are devoted to. My parents, as did others, dreamt of inclusion and community living for me. My cohort was the first generation to experience it. Now, parental dreams and inspiration from the Americans with Disabilities Act of 1990 (PL 101-336) are being lost to a bureaucracy that maintains obsolete funding that puts into bloated administrative costs dollars needed for services that create individually determined independence.

The strength to survive and surmount childhood battles was bolstered by the dream of a normalized future. It is nullified by the present realities faced by my generation. The passage of time seems to steal away opportunities, as the future becomes an unaccomplished past. I write this hoping to engage public awareness and action. In the depths of my private thoughts, it is like the springtime thaw that vacillates between days of clouds and days of sunshine. Our human spirit wants to blossom, rather than wither. To have and to know, the flowering of our potential.

Recently, more attention has been given to the renowned transition from youthful student to young adult worker (leaving the entitlements and the family), but equally jarring are the progressions from early intervention to preschool, from middle school to high school, and from work to retirement and the elder years. Family members share the lifespan journey strategically. Maintaining coordinated medical care coverage is challenging indeed. Understandably, pediatricians tend to continue into some of the adult years because of their personal knowledge of the problems of their patients, but this pattern of care can also be viewed as an abdication of internal medicine; the new group must take over.

A helpful schema that captures the characteristic landmarks was created by Marie Cullinane (1983), a former nurse from the Children's Hospital Boston; it has been used in many discussions and presentations (see Figure 3.1). The six diagrams follow a hypothetical person with early and substantial service requirements (e.g., troubled newborn with Down syndrome in cardiac failure, a severely preterm infant, or a small child with a threatening inborn error of metabolism). The pattern of service needs is indicated by the prominence of the divisions of the diagram, clearly in an arbitrary assignment. Medical, or health care, services are inferred by the black segments and demonstrate the characteristically variable role of the health care component of the team.

The period of *birth to 6 months* is a compelling one, with fundamental and urgent efforts underway. The child may require substantial clinical intervention, with various types of medical assistance (e.g., pediatrics, nursing, physical therapy). Direct support for the parents can be provided by social services, counselors, and other parents. In *infancy and early childhood* important outreach is underway, with consolidation of the health issues and much adventure in developmental intervention. *middle and late childhood,* basically the school years, is a huge period of personal gains. Educational resources bring a wide range of learning experiences, often supported by particular therapies. New emphases on recreational opportunities and social fulfillment acknowledge the individual's broader personal needs. In the years of *youth,* the curriculum may well introduce prevocational or vocational learning. Counseling and guidance are important, and families benefit from assistance as well. Community activities, including possible residential opportunities, can be pertinent. The years of *adult* life will presumably involve moving to a new home and participating in day activities such as employment. Agency guidance is the basis for a quality program. Recreation and leisure activities are important. Health care needs are customarily moderate in youth and early adult life. These may become more significant when the person is *elderly.* Vocational programs decline, but day activities are valuable, and social support can be crucial to a successful life.

INFANCY AND TODDLERHOOD

Except for certain fixed situations, medical professionals working with infants and toddlers with developmental disabilities deal extensively with the concept of "risk" and apply themselves to supporting activities that may be ameliorative. This type of outreach has launched the industry of early intervention, with its love, thoughtfulness, and positive goals. Discussion of eligibility for early intervention services is a form of wake-up call regarding the factors that are operational in the health of young children, such as congenital infections, placental insufficiency, preterm delivery, environmental toxins, and understimulation. Mobilization in early intervention gives regular attention to many infants at risk, team assessment, and dedicated support to families. It also activates the treatment professions and assures enhanced parental resolve and confidence.

The protections and supports for little children with special health care needs are multiple (see Chapter 10). Of pertinence are the therapy programs commenced in the intensive care nurseries; tracking systems; infant follow-up clinics; child-find operations; coordinated care through medical home activities; Early and Periodic Screening, Diagnosis and Treatment (EPSDT); and deployment of American Academy of Pediatrics and "Bright Futures" guidelines. During the infant and toddler years, families feel supported, especially through early intervention. Home visiting is a wonderful comfort; the home-centered program keeps the family integrated and reassured. For many families, the impending transfer to preschool feels like the beginning of adult life for the child!

THE SCHOOL YEARS

Young people with special needs can be expected to proceed into preschool, usually included with typical children, commencing what will be an extended (15+-year) relationship with the school district. This crucially important period of personal development is a generally healthy interval. State and national legislation have brought seminal entitlements for developmental services, with effects on health care also (see Chapter 6.4).

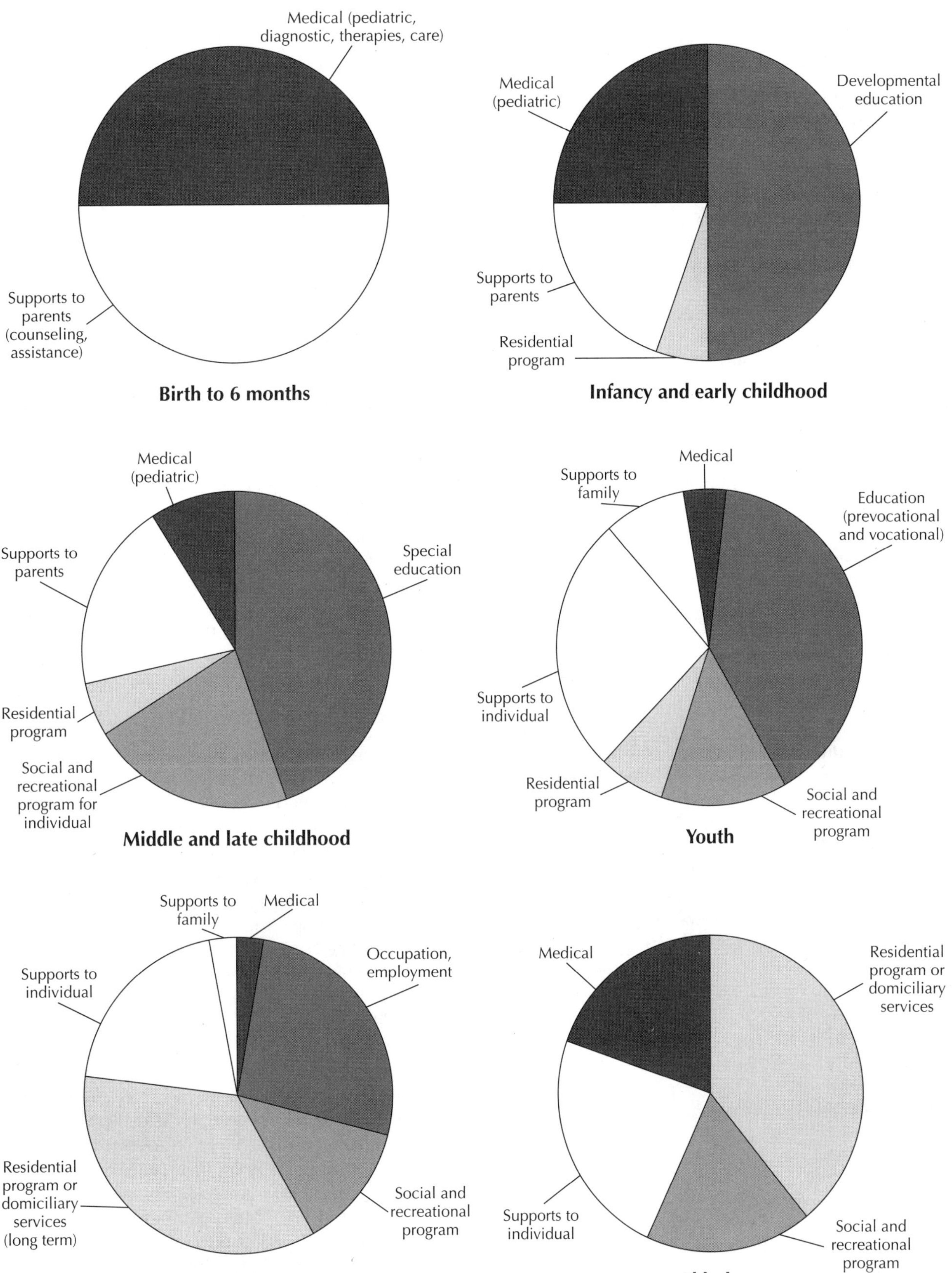

Figure 3.1. Sequential program needs of an individual with intellectual and other developmental disabilities. (Reprinted from *Developmental-Behavioral Pediatrics,* M.D. Levine, W.B. Carey, A.C. Crocker, & R.T. Gross [Eds.], "Coordination of Services," A.C. Crocker & M.M. Cullinane, Copyright 1983, with permission from Elsevier.)

As noted in Figure 3.1, in the segment called Middle and Late Childhood, "special education" support is the predominant influence in the treatment schema. This support includes curricular and special services activities conceived as having value in educational assistance but possibly also affecting health progress (as in behavioral therapy and motor training). Note that the 2000 U.S. Census finding showed that disabilities of all types were reported at increasing rates as age increased (see Table 3.5), a phenomenon shared similarly by each of the major ethnic groups (see Table 3.6) (Waldrop & Stern, 2003).

Of the children considered in the census, about 18% are grouped as children with special health care needs (i.e., chronic or ongoing health conditions). Their characterization (see Table 2.3) includes a need for health and related services of a type or amount beyond that required by children generally. Some more compelling situations are present (Newacheck et al., 1998), including 6.7% of children with limitations in social role activities (e.g., school, play) because of chronic physical or mental conditions, 0.2% (about 149,000) who require assistance or special equipment for activities of daily living, and 0.1% (about 92,000) who have residential care because of a chronic health problem. Children with special health care needs have an average of 6.4 annual physician contacts and about 7.4 school absences each year.

The Family Partners Project of Brandeis University and Family Voices (Krauss, Gulley, Leiter, Minihan, & Sciegaj, 2000) reviewed the health care supports of 2,220 families who had children with special needs. Half of the children were hospitalized at least once, and half were treated in the emergency room during the preceding year. Almost half used durable medical equipment. Nearly half received physical, occupational, or speech-language therapy. A fifth received mental health services, and a quarter required home health services. Particular challenges included getting referrals, finding skilled providers, achieving mental health supports, and filling home health services. The most important physician involved was either the primary care doctor or a specific specialist, and 87% of these physicians were given favorable ratings. Overall, about 83% of families were satisfied with their children's health plans. Clearly, the need for coordinated services remains preeminent.

Table 3.5. Prevalence of disability types by age group based on the 2000 U.S. population census

Disability	Total (%)	Male (%)	Female (%)
Population age 5–15			
Mental disability	4.6	6.0	3.1
Physical disability	1.0	1.1	0.9
Sensory disability	1.0	1.0	0.9
Population age 16–64			
Mental disability	3.8	3.9	3.7
Physical disability	6.2	6.0	6.4
Sensory disability	2.3	2.7	1.9
Population age 65 and older			
Mental disability	10.8	9.9	11.4
Physical disability	28.6	25.8	30.7
Sensory disability	14.2	15.6	13.2

Adapted from Waldrop, J., & Stern, S.M. (2003). *Disability status: 2000.* Washington, DC: U.S. Census Bureau.

Table 3.6. Prevalence of total disability by ethnic group and age group based on the 2000 U.S. population census

Ethnic group	Age 5–15	Age 16–64	Age 65 and older
White	5.7%	16.2%	40.4%
Black or African American	7.0%	26.4%	52.8%
Hispanic or Latino	5.4%	24.0%	48.5%
Asian	2.9%	16.9%	40.8%

Adapted from Waldrop, J., & Stern, S.M. (2003). *Disability status: 2000.* Washington, DC: U.S. Census Bureau.

YOUTH AND YOUNG ADULTHOOD

A child with developmental disabilities achieves so much in childhood services. The onset of adolescence can be disheartening because it involves rapid change as children are transferred out of these childhood services. In some regards, the young person and family are losing a good base, which causes them uncertainty. School and training programs typically emphasize life skill issues and vocational preparation.

Most adolescents experience predictable alterations in sexual feelings, expectations in social behavior, and assumptions of independence. Young adults with special needs experience the same things but also experience a sharply widening gap in opportunities compared with typically developing peers. They often have elements of an identity problem, feel alone, and are depressed. In addition, adolescents with developmental disabilities feel a major obligation to shift their health care support systems. Often, their pediatric care teams are reluctant to let go, and the adult service world is not notably outreaching. "Many families experience this journey into adulthood as uncertain and challenging" (Porter, Freeman, & Griffin, 2000, p. 9).

Numerous guidebooks are now available that assist in the transition to adolescence (e.g., see Porter et al.,

2000). The planning effort commonly focuses strongly on health care, but other areas have parallel considerations, such as education, employment, and recreation. Some common principles can be noted for the modifications:

- The young adult must be a full member of the planning team.
- The medical recommendations should be concrete.
- There should be comfort with the new health care provider.
- Significant elements of health-related self-care are appropriately begun at this time.
- Planning should seek activities that represent normal experiences
- Much emphasis should be placed on establishing a diverse network of service and support connections
- Palpable personal goals need to be configured.

An underlying concept throughout must be avoidance of social isolation. Richard Nelson has captured many of the concerns:

> Youth with chronic illness or disability confront a much more uncertain future. Their childhood has probably created an even greater dependence on parents and other adults than it has for other young people. The arduous adolescent process of exploring limits, reality testing, and self-image development may be seriously delayed or compromised. Future options may be perceived as dependent, not on ability or motivation, but on the status of the health conditions. (1984, personal communication)

ADULT YEARS

As was mentioned in Chapter 1, an early symposium was published on health care services for adults with intellectual disabilities (Crocker & Yankauer, 1987). In a summary section, some basic issues were specified that the symposium hoped would be strengthened in the years to follow to better secure adult services. *Multiple options for service delivery*, with diverse routes of care, are now usual, including generic medical practices. The concept of a *medical home* for coordination has been achieved for many children and has some equivalents for adults through vendors and state agencies. The recommendations for *health care networks* (planning, resource sharing, info base), *resource centers* (some in university or hospital centers), or *health care clearing houses* (e.g., consultants, directories, manuals) are unmet. *Comprehensive and portable medical records* are planned by some states. *Fees* for care depend heavily on Medicare and Medicaid, and personnel *training* on health maintenance is earnestly pursued. Finally, *health services research* is sporadic, but *watchdog components* are interwoven with evaluation.

Carl Tyler looked thoughtfully at care for adults with intellectual disabilities and produced a virtual handbook to serve as a guide (Tyler, 1999). His chapter on "commonly under-recognized health problems" cautions about visual and auditory impairment, chronic and recurrent infections (prostate, bladder, kidney, bronchi, sinuses, ear, and liver), infected teeth and periodontal disease, gastrointestinal problems (dysphagia, esophagitis, constipation), chronic obstructive pulmonary diseases, degenerative joint disease and osteoporosis, and neurological conditions (compressive neuropathies, migraine headaches, seizures). He advised to be wary about "conditions that may cause decline in adaptive functioning," some of which also appear previously:

- Adverse drug effects
- Alzheimer disease
- Auditory impairment
- Bereavement
- Chronic hepatitis
- Chronic sinusitis
- Depression
- Hypothyrodism
- Malnutrition
- Obstructive sleep disorder
- Visual impairment
- Vitamin B_{12} deficiency

THE LATER YEARS

Sentimental names are assigned to the categories of notably senior citizens—they are *aging* at 55–64, *elderly* at 65, and *aged* at 75 years. Another system considers them *young old* at 65–74 and *old old* after 75. This lively nosology is superseded by the Older Americans Act (PL 102-375) that has adopted 60 as "older." Seventeen percent of Americans are older than 60; in earlier considerations this cohort was 1 in 9 citizens but now is close to 1 in 5. A sensitive indicator is the over-75 group, edging up around the world to 4%–7%. Among the almost

10,000 clients enrolled in various residential programs of the Department of Mental Retardation of the Commonwealth of Massachusetts, the statistics are about the same (about 2%–5% are older than 75 years).

Regard for the older person with developmental disabilities is more invested than formerly (see Chapter 26). A particular effort has been to modify the traditional "developmental services" philosophy and allow some personalized retirement. "Aging in place" (growing old where you live) is a hoped-for goal but can be challenging for programs. Health care supports have been given much devotion by community-based nurse practitioners. Attention is needed for aging myopathy (changes in muscle bulk and strength), osteopenia (thinning of bones), and functional changes in joints. Exercise is the central help. Day program assistance for older individuals from the community "aging network" is a modern effort to utilize strong existent activities with a varied degree of success. One looks especially to Senior Centers, Adult Day Health Programs, and Home Care Corporations (Seltzer, Krauss, Litchfield, & Modlish, 1989).

An interesting insight on the effects of aging on individuals with intellectual disability is provided by a survey of 47 verbal men and women with an average age of 62. The individuals were asked, "What does growing old mean to you?" The responses, in order of frequency, included concerns about physical changes, general changes ("I'm getting to be old"), changes in being able to work, reduction in recreational opportunities, a dismissal of the aging concept, or some sadness or concerns about death. For the question "When is a person old?" the answers varied, but most individuals gave an older age than they were at the time (Erickson, Krauss, & Seltzer, 1989).

CONCLUSION

Individuals with developmental disabilities require lifelong medical care. Continual collaboration and support are needed as the person progresses from infancy and toddlerhood, to the school years, to youth and young adulthood, and finally to the adult and later years.

REFERENCES

Americans with Disabilities Act (ADA) of 1990, PL 101-336, 42 U.S.C. §§ 12101 *et seq.*

Crocker, A.C. (1974). Present status of treatment of the mucopolysaccharidoses. In D. Bergsma (Ed.), *Clinical cytogenetics and genetics* (pp. 113–124). Miami, FL: Symposia Specialists.

Crocker, A.C., & Cullinane, M.M. (1983). Coordination of services. In M.D. Levine, W.B. Carey, A.C. Crocker, & R.T. Gross (Eds.), *Developmental-behavioral pediatrics*. Philadelphia: W.B. Saunders.

Crocker, A.C., & Yankauer, A. (1987). Basic issues. *Mental Retardation, 25*, 227–232.

Cullinane, M.M. (1983). Coordination of services. In M.D. Levine, W.B. Carey, A.C. Crocker, & R.T. Gross (Eds.), *Developmental-behavioral pediatrics* (pp. 1117–1118). Philadelphia: W.B. Saunders.

Erickson, M., Krauss, M.W., & Seltzer, M.M. (1989). Perceptions of old age among a sample of aging mentally retarded persons. *Journal of Applied Gerontology, 8*, 251–260.

Krauss, M.W., Gulley, S., Leiter, V., Minihan, P., & Sciegaj, M. (2000). *Report on a National Survey of the Health Care Experiences of Families of Children with Special Health Care Needs.* Waltham, MA: Brandeis University.

Newacheck., P.W., Strickland, B., Shonkoff, J.P., Perrin, J.M., McPherson, M., McManus, M., et al. (1998). An epidemiologic profile of children with special health care needs. *Pediatrics, 102*, 117–123.

Porter, S., Freeman, L., & Griffin, L.R. (2000). *Transition planning for adolescents with special health care needs and disabilities: A guide for health care providers.* Boston: Institute for Community Inclusion.

Seltzer, M.M., Krauss, M.W., Litchfield, L.C., & Modlish, N.J.K. (1989). Utilization of aging network services by elderly persons with mental retardation. *The Gerontologist, 29*, 234–238.

Tyler, C.V. (1999). *Medical issues for adults with mental retardation/developmental disabilities.* Homewood, IL: High Tide Press.

Waldrop, J., & Stern, S.M. (2003). *Disability status: 2000.* Washington, DC: U.S. Census Bureau.

CHAPTER 4

Preventing Secondary Conditions and Promoting Health

Donald J. Lollar

A large portion of this volume addresses purely medical care among people with developmental disabilities. This chapter proposes that the concept of *health* is broader than that of *medicine* alone. The concept of *prevention* is also presented in a broader context so that clinical practice is pivotal to the assessment of and intervention for potentially complicating conditions and the encouragement of behaviors that promote health.

The term *secondary conditions* has evolved since the early 1990s (Lollar, 1999; Pope & Tarlov, 1991). Basically, it can be defined as "any preventable condition to which a person or family is more susceptible by virtue of experiencing a primary diagnosis associated with disability" (Lollar, 1999, p. 43). The term refers to outcomes for which a person is at greater risk due to the presence of a primary disabling condition. That is, the primary diagnosis is a risk factor for the appearance of a secondary condition. *Secondary* refers to timing—when the conditions occur—and does not mean that the conditions are less serious. The term *conditions* is used to suggest that the varied outcomes are not exclusively in the medical or physical domain of function but can also include emotional, social, and environmental dimensions.

Several examples of secondary conditions for individuals with developmental disabilities might help to clarify the concept. For example, urinary tract infections and pressure sores are secondary conditions often connected with spina bifida or spinal cord injury. That is, they are conditions for which the person is at greater risk because of the primary disabling condition. Social isolation and depression, conditions experienced by individuals across varied diagnoses, are also associated with developmental disabilities. Without wishing to stretch the concept too much, reduced access to health care and injuries to family caregivers can also be considered secondary conditions for clinical purposes. In clinical practice, secondary conditions often are more severe and disruptive than the stabilized primary diagnosis and have implicitly negative consequences. The clinician's task is to work with individuals and families to prevent or reduce the impact of such secondary conditions on the person and family.

For congenital conditions such as cerebral palsy and spina bifida, the medical problems and associated secondary conditions often are significant and easily identified; however, to the extent that cognitive impairments are the primary emphasis, medical symptoms are often less easily identified and more difficult to manage. In clinical practice, much, if not most, time is not spent addressing the primary medical condition creating body dysfunction, but rather intervening with the secondary conditions.

In daily appointments at clinics, little distinction might be made between primary symptoms and secondary conditions for the person with disabilities or his or her family. Diagnosis is diagnosis; treatment is treatment; intervention is intervention. The most relevant distinguishable clinical element of secondary conditions is that they are preventable. That is, although there is a greater risk for the occurrence of them, secondary conditions are not part of the primary manifestation(s) of a diagnosis. The evaluation or diagnosis of secondary conditions, therefore, can be as broad or narrow as the clinician chooses. In addition, the less medical the secondary condition, the less attention might be given to assessment and interventions. Crocker (1995) developed a typology of secondary conditions that reflects the complexity often found:

- *Complication*—An untoward occurrence, accidental but resulting from the primary condition (e.g., pressure sore in spina bifida)
- *Contingency*—An event involving another body system but ultimately deriving from the conditions of the primary condition (e.g., conductive hearing impairment associated with Down syndrome)
- *Unexpected progression*—A troubling extension of the potential continuing natural history of the primary condition (e.g., loss of ambulation in cerebral palsy)

- *Comorbidity*—Another parallel condition, deriving from the same background as that producing the first diagnosis (e.g., hydrocephalus and spina bifida).
- *Other health concerns*—Ill health from other origin but perhaps masked or confounded in some fashion by the primary condition (e.g., obesity in Down syndrome)
- *Effects of aging*—Liabilities or dysfunctions due to advancing years, often accelerated by a primary condition (e.g., overuse syndrome related to mobility problems)

In the field of developmental disabilities, the world of secondary conditions is a large and often complicated one. Varied therapeutic, educational, technological, environmental, and social interventions must be considered during encounters with the individual and his or her family. As a matter of course, practitioners working with people with developmental disabilities usually are already aware of the breadth and complexity of secondary conditions and alternative interventions that are part and parcel of these interactions. Nonetheless, the skill and sensitivity of the provider will be challenged beyond the medical issues to the health issues of the person and his or her family. Consider Elizabeth's situation.

Elizabeth is an 18-year-old high school senior who is preparing to go off to college in the fall. She was born at 26 weeks, weighing less than $2\frac{1}{2}$ pounds. She spent 70 days in the neonatal intensive care unit in the early 1980s and developed jaundice in the hospital but required no ventilator. Otherwise, the hospitalization was fairly uneventful, and her parents stayed with her every night and watched apprehensively the progress or setbacks of other babies and families in the unit.

The goal was for Elizabeth to reach 5 pounds in order to go home. When she was discharged, nobody discussed with her family the course or potential complications of her life. The hospital did not follow up, but early events suggested serious problems. Elizabeth had great difficulty eating; she could not coordinate sucking and swallowing, and, therefore, feeding became a daily crisis for her parents. Follow-up care was provided by a community family practice group; even though the physicians were uncertain about Elizabeth's development, they were hesitant to make a referral outside their practice.

At 16 months, Elizabeth was diagnosed with cerebral palsy. For her parents, the diagnosis was something of a relief, and it provided a term to understand their daughter's lack of progress. As Elizabeth got older, she had multiple surgeries, including soft tissue releases, two femoral osteotomies, and a spinal fusion. Her health at about age 16 was complicated by severe, debilitating migraines that necessitated frequent hospitalizations and a strict regimen of medications to control the headaches.

By age 18, Elizabeth used a power chair and was bright and driven to succeed academically. She was expected to graduate in the top 3% of her high school class, and she had already received a full academic scholarship from a nearby liberal arts college. She had traveled internationally and was fluent in French. Her parents took care to make certain that Elizabeth was well groomed and wore fashionable, well-fitting clothing. Her spinal fusion assured that she always sat upright. Elizabeth recognized that many people saw her wheelchair and drew immediate conclusions about her intellect and that others saw her intellect and could not imagine the disabilities she had.

Just as Elizabeth was welcoming the independence that college offered, her hip surgery began to fail, and she experienced unrelenting pain. The medications caused weight gain, which she managed to control, and she developed severe bowel impactions that became increasingly difficult to resolve. The migraine headaches became less severe but not without multiple medications to control them.

In her senior year, Elizabeth found herself making the rounds of physicians, and she and her parents learned the term *secondary conditions*. The distress of addressing the failing hip and the migraines created depression, and she lacked the motivation to exercise. She also found that her 6-year-old seating system no longer provided good support. Although her specialists provided care and attention to her individual concerns, she had no one to address the multiple health problems and the secondary conditions she experienced. No one addressed weight gain, and no one asked about bowel functions. No one encouraged exercise. The medication for depression created greater spasticity, which increased her hip pain.

Elizabeth's story may provide some insight into the care of young adults with disabilities. The great disappointment for Elizabeth and her family was the instability of her health at age 18. Most of what they had read suggested that cerebral palsy did not lead to additional health concerns. This very bright, engaging young's woman academic performance masked her problems so much that many teachers and peers could not imagine that someone so bright could have so many disabilities. Moreover, the increasing health problems that demanded attention drew her physicians away from efforts to integrate health care, that is, to address, depression, weight, conditioning, and bowel function as well as to address her hip problems and her headaches.

SECONDARY CONDITIONS DATA

Horowitz, Kerker, Owens, and Zigler (2001) concluded that there is a lack of research addressing secondary conditions among individuals with cognitive impairments. These investigators emphasized the need for research to highlight the prevalence and impact of secondary conditions among these individuals. Traci, Seekins, Szalda-Petree, and Ravesloot (2002) completed a study in Montana of the prevalence of secondary conditions among a group of 119 adults across a broad spectrum of living arrangements, from independent residences to residential care facilities. Communication difficulties were reported most frequently by the direct care providers who completed the survey, followed (in descending order of importance) by problems with physical fitness and conditioning, persistence or low frustration tolerance for task completion, weight, personal hygiene, dental and oral hygiene, fatigue, depression, mobility, and sleep disturbance. Traci et al. concluded that these limitations all included significant behavioral or lifestyle components; more medically oriented conditions, such as gastrointestinal dysfunction, bowel problems, or respiratory difficulties, were reported substantially less often.

Looking closely at the list, one sees the correlation among several of the conditions—conditioning is related to weight, which is related to appearance, which is related to mobility, which is related to fatigue, which ultimately is related to sleep and depression. This relationship is, of course, just one of a number of cyclical groups that can be generated among the secondary conditions listed in Table 4.1. Although some of these conditions (e.g., depression, sleep disturbance) might have diagnostic codes, several do not (e.g., fitness, low frustration tolerance, personal hygiene). Thus, a clinician's inquiring about some of these conditions would not necessarily be a part of routine patient–clinician encounters.

Table 4.1. Estimated prevalence of secondary conditions in adults with developmental disabilities

Secondary condition	Estimated prevalence/1,000
Physical fitness and conditioning problems	590
Communication difficulties	573
Mobility	509
Persistence or low frustration tolerance	500
Weight problems	479
Personal hygiene or appearance problems	470
Dental and oral hygiene problems	451
Fatigue	422
Depression	369
Sleep problems/disturbance	316
Bowel dysfunction	288
Respiratory	178
Cardiovascular/circulatory	156
Osteoporosis	112

From Traci, M.A., Seekins, T., Szalda-Petree, A., and Ravesloot, C. (2002). Assessing secondary conditions among adults with developmental disabilities: A preliminary study. *Mental Retardation, 40*(2), 125; adapted by permission.

Lollar (1997) amended the Secondary Conditions Surveillance Instrument (Ravesloot, Seekins, & Walsh, 1997) to identify secondary conditions among a sample of adolescents with spina bifida. Table 4.2 provides the rank order of the most problematic secondary conditions for this sample. Incontinence of bladder (ranked first) and bowel (sixth) were the two medically associated secondary conditions, although the definitions for these two conditions included in the instrument clearly related to the preventable negative social aspects of incontinence rather than just the body dysfunction. In addition to limitations in learning (second) and mobility (fourth), secondary problems of everyday living were prominent. Physical fitness (third), motivation (fifth), self-esteem (eighth), and fatigue (ninth) overlapped with the secondary conditions of the adults in the Montana sample (Traci et al., 2002). This exercise showed, as might be expected, that young people with spina bifida contend with the social aspects of bowel and bladder incontinence as well as with the general problems of everyday life. Also, cross-cutting issues related to fitness, motivation, and fatigue emerge.

Havercamp (2001) completed a population-based survey in North Carolina of health needs of adults with developmental disabilities. Information was collected from the adults and their case managers. Physical fitness and obesity were the major problems that emerged. A high rate of mental health problems was found, and more than half of those in the representative state sample were being prescribed medication for mental health problems. Finally, the survey indicated that access to health care services was often difficult, with particular problems in oral health services and in reproductive services for women. The study concluded that lack of physical activity was a risk factor for chronic conditions, such as cardiac disease, and that there was an alarmingly elevated rate of emotional problems associated with inadequate support and high stress. Moreover, the lifestyles of adults with developmental disabilities were found in many ways to closely approximate the lifestyles of the general population, thus creating

Table 4.2. Adolescent spina bifida secondary conditions rank order

1.	Bladder incontinence	7.	Recreational problems
2.	Learning/memory	8.	Self-esteem problems
3.	Physical fitness	9.	Fatigue
4.	Mobility problems	10.	Headaches
5.	Initiation/motivation	11.	Social isolation
6.	Bowel incontinence		

Adapted from Lollar, D.J. (1997, July 6). *Secondary conditions among adolescents with spina bifida.* Paper presented at the meeting of the Society for Research into Hydrocephalus and Spina Bifida, Manchester, United Kingdom.

additional risk factors for stroke, lung cancer, and respiratory disease related to tobacco and alcohol use.

Data clearly indicate that secondary conditions, including problems with access to care, are a part of the life experience of individuals with developmental disabilities. Together, the aforementioned studies indicate that physical fitness, obesity, and emotional issues are major secondary conditions for these groups. Associated with these conditions are motivation, persistence or low frustration tolerance, poor communication, difficulty with personal hygiene, fatigue, mobility limitations, and sleep disturbance. Finally, obtaining oral health services and reproductive services is often difficult; however, services for emotional issues and associated medications seem to be rather well identified and readily available, contrary to anecdotal evidence.

CLOSING THE GAP

The Surgeon General's report *Closing the Gap: A National Blueprint to Improve the Health of Persons with Mental Retardation* concluded that individuals with cognitive impairments experience poorer health and have more problems "finding, getting to, and paying for appropriate health care" (Office of the Surgeon General, 2002). The report set the stage for describing difficulty obtaining services through a vignette of a young woman with cognitive impairments experiencing active seizures. She was triaged as a nonemergency case by emergency department staff because they assumed that her seizures were part of her condition. The Surgeon General's report included the following six goals (and related action steps for each goal) to improve the health of people with cognitive impairments:

1. Integrate health promotion into community environments for people with intellectual disabilities.
2. Increase knowledge and understanding of health and intellectual disabilities, ensuring that knowledge is made practical and easy to use.
3. Improve the quality of health care for people with intellectual disabilities.
4. Train health care providers in the care of adults and children with intellectual disabilities.
5. Ensure that health care financing produces good health outcomes for adults and children with intellectual disabilities.
6. Increase sources of health care services for adults, adolescents, and children with intellectual disabilities, ensuring that health care is easily accessible for them.

Among these goals to improve health, several relate directly to secondary conditions. Specifically, integrating health promotion into community environments, making knowledge practical and easy to use, increasing sources of services to improve accessibility, and training health care providers in the care of people with intellectual disabilities individually and collectively could contribute to reducing the occurrence of secondary conditions and improving health. These goals apply not only to individuals with cognitive impairments but also to the general population of people with developmental disabilities.

The report concluded with a list of under-recognized medical problems—including constipation and impaction, visual and auditory problems, recurrent ear infections, periodontal disease and infected teeth, osteoporosis, and neuropathies—to which individuals with intellectual disabilities are more vulnerable. This list, however, does not include the broader range of secondary conditions (emotional, familial, social, and environmental) encountered in clinical settings.

BARRIERS

Barriers to appropriate evaluation of and intervention for secondary conditions can be both internal and external to the person. Moreover, barriers to assessment and intervention are often a result of the interaction of the person with his or her environment. Environmental barriers can include physical barriers, social or attitudinal barriers, and policy or system barriers. Physical barriers are the most visible ones—particularly if the individual has mobility limitations. The social and attitudinal barriers, however, can be less easy to recognize. For instance, an individual without experience with people with disabilities might be impatient with someone with a disability for being slower at answering questions, completing basic reading tasks, or "looking" different. Health care providers themselves can unwittingly be a barrier to the evaluation of and intervention for secondary conditions. Policy or system barriers most often concern guidelines for reimbursement for services and specific details of treatment coverage. Not only should providers themselves exhibit patience during clinical encounters, but insurers must acknowledge the additional time and attention needed as they adjust economic risks for reimbursement among these individuals.

The greatest of these barriers to evaluation and treatment of secondary conditions, however, might well be the unexamined perceptions of providers and insurers. Individuals with developmental disabilities must be evaluated and subsequently treated with an integrated approach, focusing both on the person and the context in which he or she lives and functions. This process requires attention to factors beyond the individual, including family or other significant individuals in their lives, neighborhood supports or lack thereof, and community resources. Medical conditions are often created and/or exacerbated by factors external to the person.

Although acknowledging that the time limitations for examinations and treatment set by public or private insurers are necessary, the needs of the person with disabilities do not change because such limitations exist. The economy of secondary conditions is sometimes subtle and other times overt. That is, routinely, small intervention strategies can prevent major secondary medical and other conditions from occurring. Looking beyond the medical situation, however, is necessary for the conditions to be identified and interventions to be implemented. Bowel impaction, for example, is a major secondary condition for many but is related to diet, exercise, access to good nutritional and physical activity information, and encouragement to adhere to recommended healthy habits. In such cases, encouragement is what the practitioner provides, and health promotion becomes the cumulative public health outcome.

In dealing with young people with disabilities, health care professionals might be interacting with individuals who have less-developed social and decision-making skills, so the interpersonal skills of the providers become more important and more noted when they are absent. The most basic environmental support for people with disabilities is the respect shown by a health provider. This respect is particularly important for children because they have an inherent drive for competence and the need for autonomy. One of the most basic ways to establish respect is to address or question a person directly; however, health care providers often find it easier to ask questions of a caregiver, family member, or person transporting a younger child or young adult than to ask that person directly. Young people, even children, can usually answer straightforward questions about their lives.

When compared with the amount of time routinely needed to see a person without disabilities, about twice as much time is necessary when seeing a person with disabilities or a member of that person's family (Voelker, 2002). Sometimes, including others for verification or elaboration is important, but the tendency is to overlook the individual in the name of efficiency and credibility. When such behavior occurs, the opportunity to build a relationship and interpersonal competence in a health setting is lost. The effect of an extra investment of time is that the person is more comfortable interacting with a professional in a nonthreatening setting. To this end, patience and attention are needed.

A second and related dynamic is the transition from pediatric to adult care. Often, adult providers do not feel comfortable with individuals with more complex needs. Because developmental disabilities, by definition, begin during childhood or adolescence, pediatric providers begin the process of transition. Baseline functioning across all spheres of living can be accurately obtained, and interventions to reduce or prevent secondary conditions can be established during pediatric visits—whether medical or health related—only to be undermined by lack of follow-up. Pediatricians, both primary care and specialty, usually are torn between continuing care for young people as they mature to adulthood and acknowledging the limits of their own training, experience, and professional comfort.

Crucial in the transition from child to adult practitioners is the reconstruction of resources by the young person and his or her family. This process often requires looking for different medical and health providers, emotional supports, and hospitals because many pediatric medical centers will not admit anyone older than 21 years of age. This change can be particularly difficult for a young adult with disabilities whose pediatric team has not made transition plans and is not on the staff of an adult facility. The dynamics inherent to making a transition, including developmental changes and family relationships, make evaluation of and intervention for secondary conditions particularly significant, especially when the transition is occurring while the young person still lives at home.

Young people with spina bifida, for example, often are interested in and adamant about living independently. Frequently, however, family and other supports needed to maintain bowel and bladder continence and to conduct appropriate skin checks are not handled well during transition by any of the principals—young person, family, or professionals. As a result, continence is lost, pressure sores develop, functioning is lost, and dependence continues. This example shows medical secondary conditions resulting from an interaction, or lack thereof, between the individual, the individual's family, and the health professionals who provide the medical care.

Although these outcomes are not a major responsibility of the medical staff, the resulting conditions are clearly secondary in nature (i.e., bladder dysfunction and loss of sensation are primary conditions associated with spina bifida). As such, treatment—catheterization and weight shifts to prevent social incontinence and pressure sores, respectively—*are* within the scope of responsibility of the medical staff. Therefore, medical staff and family, along with the young person, must establish mutual respect, communication, and a relationship that will allow straightforward analyses of issues related to independence during adolescent development. Involvement beyond the medical is unavoidable if secondary conditions are to be addressed.

IDENTIFICATION AND ASSESSMENT

In 2001, the World Health Organization (WHO) officially adopted a new classification to complement its *International Classification of Diseases–Tenth Revision (ICD)* (1992) that included the general concepts of functioning, disability, and health. Diagnosis alone does not adequately capture the experience of disability. This new classification presents a model that goes beyond the traditional medical model and integrates biological, psychological, and social components. It allows the practitioner to record systematically the functional dimensions of the person's experience. In addition, the model includes environmental factors that affect health and well-being.

Together, this model, classification, and coding system form the *International Classification of Functioning, Disability, and Health (ICF)* (WHO, 2001). The ICF has been formally approved as the second member of the family of classifications, along with ICD, by the World Health Assembly of WHO. Table 4.3 provides a listing of the domains included in each of the dimensions of ICF. The most salient aspects of the coding system for health providers are those under the heading Activities and Participation. Including the functional limitations at the personal level substantially expands information available to the system of care that surrounds the person and family.

Secondary conditions can now be described more clearly using ICF definitions and codes, allowing problems (impairments) in body systems and functions to be coded by body system or structure, such as mental or sensory functions, cardiovascular system, or respiratory system. Personal activity limitations or societal participation restrictions, such as learning, communication, mobility, self-care, work, school, or social relationships, are other dimensions of the coding. In addition, environmental barriers can be described and classified as physical, attitudinal, or systemic in nature.

Table 4.3. Dimensions and one-level classification of the *International Classification of Functioning, Disability and Health*

Body functions
Mental functions
Sensory functions and pain
Voice and speech functions
Functions of the cardiovascular, haematological, immunological, and respiratory systems
Functions of the digestive, metabolic, and endocrine systems
Genitourinary and reproductive functions
Neuromusculoskeletal and movement-related functions
Functions of skin and related structures
Body structure
Structures of the nervous system
The eye, ear, and related structures
Structures involved in voice and speech
Structures of the cardiovascular, immunological, and respiratory systems
Structures related to the digestive, metabolic, and endocrine systems
Structures related to movement
Skin and related structures
Activities and participation
Learning and applying knowledge
General tasks and demands
Communication
Mobility
Self-care
Domestic life
Interpersonal interactions and relationships
Major life areas
Community, social and civic life
Environmental factors
Products and technology
Natural environment and human-made changes to environment
Support and relationships
Attitudes
Services, systems, and policies

From World Health Organization. (2001). *International classification of functioning, disability and health* (pp. 29–30). Geneva: Author; reprinted by permission.

Using this system, assessment of secondary conditions is the implementation of standard clinical evaluation of physiological status, with additional emphasis on prevalent impairments, personal limitations, and restrictions.

Classifying additional health dimensions beyond the etiology reflected in existing ICD codes, therefore, is possible, practical, and useful. The ICF system can be the foundation for organizing and reporting relevant health information beyond diagnosis. Diagnosis is not a proxy for function, and much of medical management requires more functional data. At present, however, these data are not being collected, recorded, or reported. New facts from aggregated health information could inform understanding of appropriate procedures and interventions.

Selected dimensions of the ICF may become part of the patient encounter information needed for health information systems and reimbursement. Functional data, particularly coding for limitations in personal activities, could provide a wealth of new information on secondary conditions when integrated with currently collected demographic, etiologic, and procedural information. Of course, training in the use of this system will be needed. With the advent and utilization of electronic health information, such training can be comfortably integrated into practice settings.

Finally, it is important to remember that assessment of an individual with developmental disabilities and his or her family should also include observable and inherent strengths. Debilitating diagnoses and secondary conditions can create the opportunity for positive outcomes for the individual, family, and even society at large. To make the distinction clear, a term such as *secondary benefits* should also be a part of the clinician's thinking when focusing on the health of individuals with developmental disabilities and their families. For example, greater family cohesion is often a secondary benefit, as well as increased openness by the individual's brothers and sisters to individual differences.

Crocker has suggested the need to be aware of, acknowledge, and encourage "good goals, good relations, good leisure, and appreciation" and outcomes related to happiness (2000, p. 324). Prevention of secondary conditions and health promotion can be greatly enhanced by identifying such positive characteristics and by integrating that information as interventions are being prescribed. Strength identification and integration also add the dimension needed for health promotion—a measure of motivation.

INTERVENTIONS

An intervention is traditionally framed as a treatment for a condition at the time the condition is identified. If evaluation is sufficiently inclusive to identify risk factors for the creation of secondary conditions, interventions need equal breadth. Interventions can be unintentionally limited if evaluations are overly restrictive. Three types of interventions contribute to preventing or reducing secondary conditions among individuals with developmental disabilities and their families: preventive services, health promotion services, and environmental interventions.

Clinical preventive services traditionally include screening tests, immunization, and counseling (U.S. Preventive Services Task Force, 1996). (Because counseling can, and often does, overlap into health promotion services, it is discussed in that context in this section.) A study by Jones and Kerr (1997) indicated, however, that individuals with cognitive impairments did not receive annual health screenings. *The Guide to Clinical Preventive Services* (1996) from the U.S. Preventive Services Task Force should be applied to people with developmental disabilities. The recommendations in that publication cover 80 primary conditions for which all individuals are at risk. It further concludes that, if a segment of the population does not receive the services detailed therein, they are at greater risk for the conditions identified.

Most relevant for individuals with developmental disabilities are coronary disease, cancer, metabolic and nutritional disorders, vision and hearing disorders, emotional problems, and substance abuse. Among children with disabilities, screening for elevated lead levels is cited as important, particularly in lower socioeconomic neighborhoods where lead in paint is frequently found. Children with developmental disabilities often live in those poorer neighborhoods.

Screening for emotional problems in both children and adults with developmental disabilities is a critical assessment given the magnitude of this problem. The *Healthy People 2010* chapter called "Disability and Secondary Conditions" provided two objectives aimed at reducing depression among children and adults with disabilities (U.S. Department of Health and Human Services, 2000). Data for that report from the National Health Interview Survey indicate that 17% of children *without* disabilities are reported to be sad, unhappy, or depressed, whereas 31% of children *with* disabilities report these emotional problems. Likewise, 28% of adults *with* disabilities report that depression prevents them from being active, whereas only 7% of adults *without* disabilities report the same.

Providers may mistakenly conclude from a routine visit that nothing untoward is occurring emotionally for an individual because the problem is not evident. Observational skills notwithstanding, providers need to ask about emotional issues. Although screenings for emotional problems might be routine in most practices for most children or adults, people with developmental disabilities often seem to slip through the clinical cracks, perhaps due to poor communication, reimbursement issues, or the insidious assumption that it does not really matter whether these individuals receive certain services.

Childhood immunizations, however, are relatively well covered for children with developmental disabilities who receive primary care. Often, though, children with relatively complicated diagnoses, such as spina bifida or cerebral palsy, are seen by specialists rather than primary care physicians and, as a result, more routine screenings or immunizations are often overlooked. Even when primary care pediatricians see young people with disabilities, they might have insufficient knowledge to screen for certain problems—latex allergies among children with spina bifida, for example. A common pediatric icebreaker, blowing up a latex glove to form a playful balloon, can result in an anaphylactic reaction.

Health promotion services really begin with helping a person with developmental disabilities to become increasingly responsible for his or her own health. Self-determination is often a long-term goal that may not be reached. Too often, health care professionals do not keep this goal of self-determination utmost in their clinical thinking. Health promotion, when included, is seen as imparting health-related information—from the professional to the individual. Sound bites of accumulated wisdom are presumed to provide the knowledge and incentive for healthy behaviors to begin and continue.

Although people with developmental disabilities are usually quite willing to listen to authority figures, they might have difficulty comprehending the message given. If comprehension is not a problem for the individual, then the person may experience memory problems or difficulty keeping a sequence of instructions in the order necessary for them to be of help. Frustration tolerance can be so low that, if barriers arise, the whole message can be lost. Yet, healthy behaviors provide the greatest opportunity for health care providers to be oriented beyond just medicine and toward health.

Counseling is, by definition, two way in nature—that is, an exchange between or among individuals. Counseling connotes mutuality, rather than more directed terms such as *guidance* or *teaching*. In view of the secondary conditions discussed earlier—poor conditioning, obesity, oral health problems, and so forth—counseling to promote health behaviors and prevent secondary conditions is extremely important, particularly in the areas of physical activity, healthy diet, and tobacco use. Unfortunately, the time required for appropriate counseling interaction on health behaviors is extremely limited during routine clinical visits. It is all but prohibitive if an individual requires more attention, as is often the case with people with developmental disabilities. In addition, such health promotion services are not always covered by insurers, despite the fact that many insurers use prevention as a major thrust of marketing for their plans.

One facet of counseling that is often overlooked involves the discussion of exploitation. From childhood onward, people are vulnerable to being manipulated by others who are more cognitively adept and more emotionally hardened. Whether the outcome of the exploitation involves money, time, work, or even sex, individuals with developmental disabilities are of a more trusting nature, without guile, and therefore more vulnerable to manipulation. Health care providers can offer both the perceived authority and the sense of personal safety to allow someone with a developmental disability to disclose information about being taken unfair advantage of by others.

Environmental facilitation to reduce or prevent secondary conditions can be seen as the outer boundary of clinical practice. Personal assistive technology, however, is routinely provided for vision and hearing impairments in the general population. These devices are so ubiquitous that they are not commonly viewed as disability related but simply a part of functioning. For people with developmental disabilities, assessing what assistance should be provided to keep impairments (body function problems) from becoming personal activity limitations (seeing clearly enough to read) or participation restrictions (seeing well enough to drive in the community) should be a part of clinical encounters. Personal digital assistants (PDAs), for example, are used by a growing segment of the population to organize their lives. Use of PDAs by individuals with developmental disabilities, including cognitive impairments, has the potential to increase community participation substantially. Features such as basic social cues, simple directions (perhaps based on global positioning features), mathematical computation capabilities, or emergency procedures could be included, using symbols, signs, oral instructions, or written material, according to level of functioning of the individual.

Germane to this discussion is the issue of *funding* for technology to assist people with developmental disabilities. *Medical necessity* is the term used by health care professionals to describe the need for various kinds of assistance for restoring function, reducing disease, or restoring physical equilibrium, such as a wheelchair for a person with a mobility limitation or a voice synthesizer for someone with limitations in vocal communication. Determinations are based on the notion that such assistance is needed for improved function—at the level of body functions and structures, using ICF descriptions. The definitions used by third-party payers, however, often differ from those used by health professionals in practice (Ireys, Wehr, & Cooke, 1999). As commonly used, *medical necessity* as a criterion denies needed services to individuals with disabilities.

Many people with cognitive impairments do not need the kinds of assistance routinely covered by the medical necessity criterion. They might, however, need accommodations at home to increase safety or independence or health maintenance programs. These and other needed services are important for what might be called *health necessity*. Health necessity describes the services for maintaining function, preventing secondary conditions, increasing functional independence, and equalizing opportunity for participation. Rehabilitation, even, is at times not deemed a medical necessity except as it serves to restore function. Clinical practice should be vigilant that all possible health necessities are explored for people with developmental disabilities.

Maintaining function and increasing independence to decrease secondary conditions also should be part of the prescription for well-being for these individuals. Care should be taken, however, because the network that maintains assistive technology often is fragmented, the result being technology that is present but nonfunctioning. Under these circumstances, the environmental facilitator becomes a barrier, capable of creating secondary conditions for the individual or family. Fundamental to the success of any environmental facilitator, whether a medical service coordinator, a technological device, or a personal assistance service, is access to it.

The concept of teamwork has focused on one of two notions—the "team" is all of the varied medical specialists involved in an individual's care or the "team" is a group of individuals from varied disciplines (including nursing, social work, the therapies, psychology, and nutrition) who contribute to the individual's well-being and the well-being of the individual's family. In the current environment of managed care, both approaches to teamwork have suffered. Increased secondary conditions for the individual and his or her family have resulted from the approach to management that discourages the inclusion of varied perspectives of the needs of the person and his or her family.

CONCLUSION

The world of secondary conditions is at once familiar and foreign, comfortable and unsettling. Beginning with Pope and Tarlov (1991) through the current volume, promoting health and preventing secondary conditions has grown in importance in public health and medical care. Exploring secondary conditions for people with developmental disabilities and their families requires, first, expanding the notion of medical care to include health. This change requires examining and intervening with dimensions beyond body functions and structures and expanding to include personal activities and community participation. It means paying attention to the environmental context that facilitates or impedes the health and well-being of this population. The task substantially expands traditional boundaries but allows significant improvement in the outcomes important to those people with developmental disabilities and their families.

REFERENCES

Crocker, A.C. (1995). The best kind of health care. In American Association of University Affiliated Programs, *Health promotion and disability prevention for people with disabilities: A companion to Healthy People 2000* (pp. 20–28). Silver Spring, MD: Association of University Centers on Disabilities.

Crocker, A.C. (2000). Introduction: The happiness in all our lives. *American Journal of Mental Retardation, 105*(5), 319–325.

Havercamp, S.M. (2001). *Core indicators project: Health indicators, 2000–2001.* Chapel Hill: University of North Carolina, Center for Development and Learning.

Horowitz, S.M., Kerker, B.D., Owens, P.L., & Zigler, E. (2001). *The health status and needs of individuals with mental retardation.* Washington, DC: Special Olympics.

Ireys, H.T., Wehr, E., & Cooke, R.E. (1999). *Defining medical necessity: Strategies for promoting access to quality care for persons with developmental disabilities, mental retardation, and other special health care needs.* Arlington, VA: National Center for Education in Maternal and Child Health.

Jones, R.G., & Kerr, M.P. (1997). A randomized control trial of an opportunistic health screening tool in primary care for people with intellectual disability. *Journal of Intellectual Disability Research, 41,* 409–415.

Lollar, D.J. (1997, July 6). *Secondary conditions among adolescents with spina bifida.* Paper presented at the meeting of the Society for Research into Hydrocephalus and Spina Bifida, Manchester, United Kingdom.

Lollar, D.J. (1999). Clinical dimensions of secondary conditions. In R.J. Simeonsson & L.N. McDevitt (Eds.), *Issues in disability and health: The role of secondary conditions and quality of life* (pp. 41–50). Chapel Hill: University of North Carolina, FPG Child Development Center.

Office of the Surgeon General. (2002). *Closing the gap: A national blueprint to improve the health of persons with mental retardation.* Washington, DC: U.S. Department of Health and Human Services.

Pope, A.M., & Tarlov, A.R. (1991). *Disability in America.* Washington, DC: National Academies Press.

Ravesloot, C., Seekins, T., & Walsh, J. (1997). A structural analysis of secondary conditions experienced by people with physical disabilities. *Rehabilitation Psychology, 42*(1), 3–16.

Traci, M.A., Seekins, T., Szalda-Petree, A., & Ravesloot, C. (2002). Assessing secondary conditions among adults with developmental disabilities: A preliminary study. *Mental Retardation, 40*(2), 119–131.

U.S. Department of Health and Human Services. (2000). *Healthy People 2010.* Washington, DC: Author.

U.S. Preventive Services Task Force. (1996). *Guide to clinical preventive services* (2nd ed.). Alexandria, VA: International Medical Publishing.

Voelker, R. (2002, July 17). Improved care for neglected population must be "rule rather than exception." *Journal of the American Medical Association, 288*(3), 299–301.

World Health Organization. (1992). *International Classification of Diseases* (10th rev.). Geneva: Author.

World Health Organization. (2001). *International classification of functioning, disability and health.* Geneva: Author.

CHAPTER 5

PEOPLE AND PROGRAMS

Lauren C. Berman, Linda Freeman, and David T. Helm

Families provide the holding environment in which to raise children by offering love, attention, communication, spiritual connection, hope, and interactive relationships. Parenting any child is a challenging endeavor, but for families with children with special health care needs, the demands can be overwhelming. Most families want to take care of their children themselves. No matter how exhausted family members are, they typically devote endless hours to caring and providing for their children. Families bear the ultimate responsibility for raising children with disabilities, but they should not have to do it alone.

This chapter explores how ideas about disabilities have shaped people and programs. It begins by looking at the importance of treating families as partners and understanding families in the context of their lives. Then, it explores emotional issues for families as well as life cycle and developmental issues that may arise. Next, the chapter explains how to set appropriate expectations for an individual with disabilities and how to address the needs of brothers and sisters. The chapter also explores the concept of medical home partnerships and suggests resources for families. Finally, the chapter addresses the transition to adulthood.

FAMILIES AS PARTNERS

Working with families whose children have disabilities is demanding work and takes a special commitment of not only time but also the willingness to open oneself to new ways of thinking and to reach beyond any barriers. The journey professionals take with patients and their families can teach important lessons about life and the strength of the human spirit. Claire McCarthy, a developmental pediatrician whose child was born with a severe developmental disability, described the act of instilling hope as the art of "spinning straw into gold." As a parent, she recognized that hope is a matter of perspective.

> It is possible to have hope, even when there can be no improvement in the disease or condition . . . All of us are faced with some kind of challenge, but what defines us is what we do with what we are given. (McCarthy & Brown, 2003)

Jean Allord, the mother of a child with multiple disabilities described her experience with professionals under the medical model:

> In our early years of dealing with professionals, especially the medical evaluation teams, I often felt as if we were specimens under a glass, to be scrutinized, measured, and judged; to have our every response reported on, and to have tabulations taken to see how we had "accepted" Angela's conditions. It was a subtle tug of war—we withholding, defending; they proclaiming and dispensing from their safe, insulated throne, never at any time did I ever trust them enough to reveal my deepest anguish. In the end, this combative stance was detrimental to all of us. (Allord, 1985, p. 2)

The disability field has evolved from using a biomedical model of providers as "experts" to a more family-centered approach. In this approach, providers work collaboratively with parents and other family members as an integral part of the intervention team. Self-determination and active involvement in making decisions are emphasized. Services are flexible, accessible, and comprehensive. They address the needs of the child in a way that is consistent with the priorities of the family. This approach builds on the strength of families and creates an atmosphere in which cultural traditions, values, and diversity are acknowledged and honored (Beckman, 2002; Seligman & Darling, 1989).

Providers must set the tone for collaboration. Beginning with the initial contact, they should reach out to parents with openness and understanding. For families who are hard to connect with, this may mean making a home visit or having an initial discussion on the telephone or by e-mail. Finding the time to ask families about their concerns and listen to their responses is essential. Exploring their values and circumstances is an investment in a partnership that will benefit the child and family over the long haul.

Building trust in a relationship takes time. Parents may have preconceived notions about the nature of the professional role and expectations of professionals that may interfere with communication (Seligman & Darling, 1989). Beckman (2002) suggested that providers make sure they follow through on their commitments, even ones that seem unimportant. Returning telephone calls, keeping appointments on time, answering questions honestly, offering choices, and giving families enough information so that they can make informed decisions builds trust in the relationship. Even small gestures like a smile or a reassuring word can have an impact on the family's ownership and investment in service goals.

Providers also need to remember that families most often have contact with professionals at points of crisis, when their coping skills are exhausted. The shock and stress of a medical emergency can make families look much less functional than they would normally. For this reason, exploring past coping skills is important (Dillon, 1986). By pointing out areas of strength, providers have a real opportunity to build parent confidence. Shamoon Shanok (2000) talked about an "asymmetrical balance" in the parent–professional relationship. Although the roles are complementary, they are not identical. "Parents often feel that professionals hold all the power, while paradoxically, professionals often feel the converse" (2000, p. 337).

Working as a Team

Teamwork is a critical, yet underestimated, component of working with families with disabilities. A team can offer varied perspectives and can provide the needed flexibility to help families integrate their experience in the medical setting. The interdisciplinary team can achieve more as a group than can be done by the same professionals independently. A functioning team must be nurtured and supported. Formal and informal time spent together, oral and written communication, a clear understanding of each individual's role, and respect for differing opinions all enhance the process of becoming a team. According to Bronstein (2003), the five core components of an interdisciplinary team are 1) interdependence, 2) newly created professional activity, 3) flexibility, 4) collective ownership of goals, and 5) reflection on the process.

Parents should be an integral part of the intervention team. When they are treated with respect, most parents will appreciate being part of the team and will accept that the team will at times meet without them. Having a specific team member act as a bridge, eliciting parents' input and sharing the team's perspectives, can be helpful. There may also be times when team members will work with family members to help them explore new ways of coping and come to a better understanding of the options that are available.

In one situation, a pediatrician was in a battle with two parents who did not want their son, who was in great need of services, to be referred to an early intervention program. The social worker met with the parents and learned that they were mistrustful of doctors and other medical professionals. They lived in a rural community, were isolated, and highly valued their privacy. In a joint meeting with the family, the social worker and the pediatrician had a conversation about the dilemma while the parents observed. The social worker took the family's perspective of wanting to maintain privacy while the pediatrician talked about the importance of early intervention for the child. The discussion started out with each professional taking an opposite stance, but as the conversation evolved, each started to better understand the other's perspective. Gradually, the parents joined in the conversation, offering advice and sharing significant information about their family. By having the opportunity to be observers, the parents were able to be more open in their thinking. At the end of the meeting, they decided they wanted to try the recommended services. They called several months later to thank the team and to report how helpful they found their son's early intervention services.

UNDERSTANDING THE FAMILY IN CONTEXT

A pediatric resident made a home visit to a family of a child with Down syndrome. This visit was a key feature of a hospital program in which residents are linked to families of children with special health care needs to sensitize them to the issues of caring for such a child. Before the visit, the program's coordinator noted that this resident, clearly caring and sensitive, felt deep sadness for families like the one she was about to visit. After the visit, the resident shared what she learned and its impact: "I had always thought my role was to feel sorry for families in this situation. But the family I visited was happy . . . really happy. I now have to rethink everything—the way I work with the family and my perceptions about how they feel about having a child with a special health care need. I don't need to feel sorry for them."

In order to develop a meaningful partnership with families, providers should develop a clear understanding of their own biases and cultural perceptions (ethnic, social, and spiritual), including their understanding of what it means to have a disability or to have a family member with disabilities. Families and their children exist in a broader context whereby perceptions of health and illness, family expectations, dreams, and views of the future vary considerably. The world is socially constructed by people as they forge meaning out of their experience (Berger & Luckman, 1967; Kleinman, 1988). Professionals' views on people who are different or exceptional are conveyed to the families they work with (both overtly and covertly) and often model for the families how to view their children.

Families speak of memories of their first experience seeing their child in the neonatal intensive care unit, tethered to tubes and wrapped in bandages. One family recalls how scared they were and that providers all seemed to be saying how much they pitied the child, whereas another family recalls being soothed when their provider pointed out what beautiful hands their child had and that he would probably grow up to be a piano player. The positive outlook, the focus on "success" and beauty, clearly altered the way the child was perceived. Fortunately, the days of health care workers automatically suggesting a child should be sent to an institution due to his or her having a disability are long gone, but the modern day equivalent may be the provider suggesting only a future of heartache and disappointment rather than one emphasizing success and hope.

Health issues need to fit into the context of the routines of the family's life. The family's encounter with health issues is typically a shock and a disruption from everyday life and dreams of the future. The understanding and perceptions of all of these events are viewed through the lens of culture. For example, one family may perceive their child's disabilities as stigmatizing or a matter of family "shame," whereas another may celebrate the birth of their child with similar disabilities.

A growing number of studies delineate cultural understanding of disability (Jezewski & Sotnik, 2001; Lynch & Hanson, 2004), including accounts of how the clash between Western medicine and Eastern or "third world" perceptions of disability can have disastrous results. Fadiman (1997) told the story of the conflict between doctors in California and a Hmong family from Laos over their daughter with severe epilepsy. Both sides wanted the best for the child, yet their approaches differed so dramatically that a terrible result was inevitable. Without sustained efforts to communicate across cultural barriers, in the midst of frustration and miscommunication, trust was lost, and resentment prevailed. If both parties recognize and understand the cultural gulf, they may be better able to work collaboratively for the child.

An American Indian Parent Group explained cultural conflicts that American Indians may experience with professionals:

> When a serious decision must be made, we talk it through with extended family members or listen to our elders. Then, together we decide what is best for the child. Some doctors get upset with us if we do not make an immediate decision for our child, but others respect our cultural way of making decisions. They invite family members to take part in the discussion and give us time to decide which makes it easier for us. Our traditional ways are important to us, and we respect them. (Porter et al., 1992)

In some African cultures, families hide the fact that a child has a disability, whereas families in a Somali population in Boston traditionally do not. Rather, they talk broadly to many people in their community, seeking advice and counsel from elders and more experienced neighbors (Beigel & Todd, 2003). Different understandings of the meaning of disability or of human differences (exceptionality) result in diverse reactions from family members and individuals with disabilities (Crocker, 1998). How families view health and illness more generally, and how they cope with these issues, vary considerably with their differing social and economic status, along with their gender, religion, age, education, and spiritual orientation. All these factors need to be taken into consideration along with an understanding of how the family makes health-related decisions (e.g., family dynamics or family or cultural myths or taboos), which may affect the parent–professional relationship.

The result of this family's unique constellation of variables can manifest itself in stigmatizing perceptions and responses to individuals with disabilities and their family members, or, conversely, may result in acceptance, understanding, and support. Health care providers must try to understand how the family is responding to the situation so that they can be aware of the role they can play in minimizing difficulties (e.g., stigma) for the family both in their own actions and in the contacts and connections that they can help the family build.

EMOTIONAL ISSUES FOR FAMILIES

Emotional issues are an integral part of the reality of parenting a child with special health care needs. Featherstone (1981) identified loneliness, fear, guilt, and anger as emotions that all families experience at some point. These feelings can take different shapes in different lives but are universal for parents as well as brothers and sisters. Parents can deny the diagnosis, the impact of the diagnosis, or the permanence of the diagnosis. Denial is a coping strategy that wards off excess anxiety. It takes an enormous amount of energy once someone acknowledges a loss to incorporate and adjust to it (Laborde & Seligman, 1991; Moses, 1987; Seligman & Darling, 1989).

Many parents blame themselves for their child's disability even when it is clear that they are not responsible. They wonder what they might have done differently to prevent or improve their child's condition. At each developmental stage, parents rework their feelings of loss and responsibility. Professionals can help parents by not blaming them and stating that point directly. This action is equally and sometimes more important when professionals feel that the parents might have some responsibility for the child's condition, such as a family where the child's care is not optimal. Professionals need to embrace the idea that parents are doing the best they can given their abilities and life circumstances. Blaming parents only serves to immobilize them. Parents need to separate "negative feeling they have about themselves or their child's disability from their other more positive feelings toward their child" (Laborde & Seligman, 1991, p. 261).

Parents have the difficult task of letting go of the child they had hoped for and building a relationship with the child they have. Grieving for that lost hope has a positive function. Denial, for example, buys the time to find inner strength and external supports: the friends, professionals, and information parents have to learn. These strengths and supports accumulate so that the person has enough of a foundation to accept that the loss or change has occurred (Moses, 1987). Providers will encounter family members in different states of grieving. It helps to put the parent's response in context—to realize that these states are a necessary part of moving forward. Regardless of their backgrounds, parents often become stuck if they resist experiencing and sharing the feelings of grief. Providers need to be sensitive to these challenges and help families identify ways to deal with their feelings.

If providers normalize feelings and respond with empathy, families usually feel accepted. It is also important to be sensitive to and respect the family's timing on dealing with painful feelings. Taking the time to consider a family's readiness and receptivity for hearing difficult information as well as paying attention to the specific words that are used is critical. When a child is very young, most parents are focused on the child's achievement of developmental milestones. Using the word *wheelchair*, for example, in a casual conversation can be devastating, whereas when a child is older, a wheelchair may seem a relative inconvenience compared with all the independence it offers.

Shamoon Shanok pointed out that professionals need to be aware that "having a young child with special needs forces parents to cede some of their rightful centrality," which puts them in the "paradoxical position of giving up a large portion of their autonomy and authority while at the same time their child's particular challenges heighten and lengthen his or her dependency on them" (2000, p. 337). Some parents may deeply love their child but may find their child's condition impossible to accept. These feelings can be heightened at times of stress and can come and go over time. A mental health professional can be helpful in providing a place to express and understand unacceptable wishes and feelings. Parent-to-parent support groups also provide an important forum for parents to address negative feelings and feelings of guilt. Connecting with others in a similar situation provides validation, support, encouragement, and affirmation.

Sharing the Diagnosis

The process of diagnosis is a particularly vulnerable time for families. Whether the diagnosis is given at birth or at some other point, the impact on the family is immense. When a child is diagnosed, parents experience a double shock. Laborde and Seligman explained, "Not only must parents cope with their feelings about their child's disability, but they must also confront their previously held negative attitudes toward those persons they may have considered deviant" (1991, p. 250). Encouraging parents to express their feelings frees up emotional energy that can be used for active participation in the diagnostic process (Klein, 1993; Moses, 1987).

Many families report that the exact moment of diagnosis is etched in their memories and reviewed over and over again (Klein, 1993; Penn, 1983). According to Penn (1983), it is at that moment that all the relationships in the family change to adjust to the illness or disability. For professionals, who are trained to fix things rather than listen, leading the discussion about the diagnosis can be a particularly challenging task (Klein, 1993). Professionals may experience the diagnosis of a child with disabilities as a tragedy and may not feel able to help families at a time when they most need it. One mother dealt with such a professional:

> At age 7 months my daughter was diagnosed with cerebral palsy. The news came in a brief phone call from her former pediatrician. There were no words of comfort, no helpful advice, no offer to meet with my family to discuss a condition I knew little about. She would need to see a neurologist. I was advised that the first available appointment was in three weeks. When I asked for more—more information, an explanation, a little reassurance, I was told, "Well, she's not going to be a vegetable." (Chedd, 1994, p. 9)

In giving a diagnosis, the setting is important. A quiet, private place where parents and family members have the opportunity to express emotion and ask questions is best. Parents need to know what is happening with their child, what the disability is, why it occurred, how it can be treated, and the prognosis (Laborde & Seligman, 1991). The clinician should be clear and specific in presenting information. Klein (1993) suggested that clinicians can empower families and teach them to trust their own perceptions by beginning with a review of the parents' observations and concerns, followed by the clinician's observations that confirm or clarify those of the parents. Instead of lecturing families, developing a dialogue in which parents have a chance to ask questions and add their own ideas and reactions works best (Maynard, 1989).

Sometimes professionals try to protect families by being vague and using euphemisms instead of diagnostic terminology. Many families find this confusing. Not having a specific diagnosis can leave a family in a state of limbo, trying to balance hopefulness against their fears of the unknown. One mother, for example, was relieved when she finally learned that her daughter had Tay Sachs disease. Even though the diagnosis meant that her daughter would regress and eventually die, at least she "knew" what it was and could find out information and connect with support services (Mack & Berman, 1988). A specific diagnosis, no matter how serious, can open the door to educational and support services.

In some instances, no specific diagnosis is available. In this situation, being honest with families and including them in the ongoing process is best. When the diagnosis is possibly terminal, a different approach is needed. One strategy described by Back, Arnold, and Quill (2003) is to help families and patients "hope for the best and prepare for the worst." By giving equal time for hope and preparation, the provider allows the family to talk about the topic that is most important to them. In this way, the professional can align with the family's hopes while supporting the evolution of acceptance and preparation over time.

Even in the best of circumstances, parents may not remember information that is communicated by health professionals. Sometimes having another team member present provides a valuable "witness" to the family's experience. Another provider, preferably someone attuned to nonverbal communication, can help with the integration of information and feelings over time. Klein (1993) suggested preparing a written summary for parents using language understandable to lay people to prevent the confusion and misinformation that can happen over time. Families often report that they find this more valuable than technical clinical reports.

Bonding

New parents are in a time of transition, vulnerability, and potential growth. They feel most competent when they can connect with their child and have a good understanding of his or her experience. One of the first tasks new parents face is bonding with their child. Bonding is a critical part of parenting and has a profound impact on the family as a whole. Research shows that primary reciprocal attachments are fundamental to the development of cognitive and emotional intelligence, language, personality, and relational style (Shamoon Shanok, 2000). A medical crisis can interfere with the process of bonding.

When a child looks different and/or has relational and communication challenges, parents may have a difficult time engaging with the child. The unique match between the child's emotional and cognitive style and the family's needs and expectations is essential. Differences in temperament, communication style, and emotional expression have a strong influence on the parent–child relationship. Providers need to find ways to comfort families and facilitate the process of bonding.

Another issue for parents is communication. Parents need feedback from their child as reinforcement for their actions as parents. A lack of feedback can result in a self-defeating cycle of avoidance and miscommunication. Providers can help families in learning to accurately read their child's cues. One family, for instance, had a daughter with disabilities who was cranky, cried quietly, was listless, and refused to be fed. The parents assumed that like their other children, this child needed stimulation. They were frustrated when their repeated efforts to engage their daughter only caused her to be more irritable. During an office visit, the pediatrician noted that the child got easily overstimulated. With the help of the nurse, the mother discovered that when she wrapped her daughter in a blanket and brought her into a quiet room where the lights were low, feeding went much better.

LIFE CYCLE AND DEVELOPMENTAL ISSUES

Families are evolving and ever-changing systems. The ability to adapt to change is the hallmark of healthy family functioning. The tasks of the whole family at each stage of the family life cycle are different and build on each other. Carter and McGoldrick (1980) have identified six stages of the family life cycle: 1) young adults who are between families, 2) families joined through marriage, 3) families with young children, 4) families with adolescents, 5) families who are launching children, and 6) families in later life. For families with children with disabilities, each life cycle change may have a greater than normal impact. Common events such as the birth of a brother or sister, a family vacation, or the launching of children may engender special problems. Adaptation to these ordinary events cannot be taken for granted and may require extraordinary planning and adaptation (Seligman & Darling, 1989; Stein, 1983).

Families may experience increased distress if stages of the life cycle are not fully reached because the child has not achieved independence. Families may re-experience some of the feeling they had when the child was first diagnosed. According to Roland (1987), the interface of the child's individual development, the life cycle stage of the family, and the progression and nature of the child's disability have a significant impact on the family's experience. Relapsing illness, such as dealing with episodic asthma or recurring seizures, forces families to alternate between periods of drawing closely together and periods of release from the immediate demands of the illness. In many situations, there can be a fundamental clash between the life cycle demands of the family and the ongoing demands of the child's disability.

The primary developmental task for couples, for example, is to separate from their family of origin and form a new couple system. The birth of a child with disabilities can interfere with the process of individuation. For some couples, the unexpected demands of their child's illness may force them into dependence on their family of origin before they have learned to work together as a team. Parents may react differently because of their separate roles in the family system. If one spouse feels deserted due to the partner's intense focus on the child, that spouse may return to his or her family of origin and make the preoccupied partner a scapegoat. The extended family, however, may turn away from the couple because they feel overwhelmed or blame one of the parents and fear social stigma related to the child's disabilities (Dillon, 1986). Professionals have the very difficult task of holding the multiple perspectives of each person in the family, each of the subsystems (e.g., brothers and sisters, parents, grandparents), and the family unit as a whole (Shamoon Shanok, 2000).

SETTING EXPECTATIONS

One of the most challenging tasks for families whose children have disabilities is setting appropriate expectations. Parental expectations need to be in line with the child's abilities and interests, not the parents'. As their child moves through each developmental stage, parents are confronted by the way their child's functioning differs from peers. Bernice Neugarten talked about the concept of "social time clocks" in which the family and its members use culturally determined life cycle markers to compare themselves with others. A crisis is generated when families feel "off time" or "out of synch" with their peers (Neugarten, 1979).

For families whose children have disabilities, the inability of their child to achieve developmental tasks "on time" may constantly remind the family of being "out of step" and may add to a feeling of unresolved resentment and despair, masked by feelings of tiredness, disaffection, or indifference (Dillon, 1986). Often families come to professionals for help in setting expectations. If expectations are too high, the child and the family feel they are always failing. If they are too low, important opportunities may be missed. Family members may also be affected by the demands put on them by health care providers for treatment and home management. According to Stein (1983), this can lead to a realignment of family members with one parent (often the mother) bearing the brunt of the day-to-day responsibility. Brothers and sisters may choose to be more independent or align themselves with the other parent or another adult in the family.

BROTHERS AND SISTERS

The literature on brothers and sisters of children with developmental disabilities shows both positive and negative effects that vary with age, gender, birth order, age spacing, and parent adjustment (Hannah & Midlarsky, 1999; Trevino, 1979; Zetlin, 1986). Grossman (1972) discovered that college students who had a brother or sister with developmental disabilities showed an increased acceptance of differences, greater compassion and awareness of prejudice, as well as higher levels of empathy and altruism. They were more focused on their own futures than were comparable young adults without brothers or sisters with disabilities. Lobato,

Barbour, Hall, and Miller (1987) also found that many brothers and sisters of children with disabilities go into the helping professions.

Orsmond and Seltzer (2000) noted that sisters scored higher than brothers in caregiving, companionship, and positive affect aspects of the relationship, while brothers had different responses depending on whether they had a brother or a sister with a disability. Brothers of boys with developmental disabilities had a more favorable emotional response than brothers of girls with developmental disabilities. Stoneman et al. (1991) found that the most reliable difference between brothers and sisters of children with disabilities is that they eventually assume a more directive, caregiving role toward their brothers and sisters, regardless of birth order and gender. Overall, the literature suggests that adjustment of brothers and sisters depends on many intertwined variables. Most often, a brother's or sister's ability to accept and cope with the child with disabilities is strongly affected by his or her parents' attitude and adjustment (Trevino, 1979).

Crocker (1983) identified six areas that may influence the experience of being a brother or sister of a child with developmental disabilities. These are 1) changes in the normal family rhythms, conformity, and images; 2) competition for parental resource and attention; 3) misconceptions about the cause and/or outcome of the brother or sister's disability, as well as possible genetic implications; 4) increased responsibilities for taking care of their brother or sister and constraints of independence due to requests from parents to include the sister or brother in social activities; 5) parental expectations about accomplishments to make up for losses; and finally 6) bewilderment in response to the parents' feelings of grief and conflict.

Although brothers and sisters of individuals with disabilities often become adults with particular sensitivities and compassion for people of all types, it is important to be attentive to growing pains while acknowledging that each family has its own version of normal. Brothers and sisters may experience the impact of their atypical home life in many ways, including parental stress and anxiety, less time spent with parents who must care for their special child, and disruption of normal routines. For example, David, age 7, told his babysitter that it was not fair that his brother with spina bifida got so much extra attention. When his family was shopping the previous day, a woman they did not know came up and gave his brother a balloon, and the week before, when he went to the doctor's office with his mother and brother, a woman at the office gave his brother extra stickers.

Brothers and sisters may have extra family responsibilities including being an intermediary between the child with disabilities and the outside world (Stein, 1983). They may worry that they will catch the disability or conversely feel guilty that they do not have it themselves. They may be feeling their own anxiety, guilt, and anger as all the normal feelings of sibling rivalry are heightened.

Brothers and sisters need to be reassured that the disability in the family did not result from something they might have done. If children are not given answers, they will make up their own to fill a void. Not understanding the cause of the disability, a child might imagine that something they once did (or even thought) caused it. Providers need to provide age-appropriate information, offer opportunities to meet with brothers and sisters of children with special needs, and help parents to reassure brothers and sisters by planning for the future of their child with special needs (Meyer & Vadasy, 1994). Parents also need to be encouraged to set aside special time for their children who do not have disabilities.

MEDICAL HOME PARTNERSHIPS

Andrea, the mother of a daughter with bipolar disorder and a son with autism, spoke tearfully of the pediatrician who saved her, and her children's, lives. "I owe everything to her. I would not have made it without the resources she told me about, her support and drive. She knew that what was going on with my kids affected me; she took a holistic approach. She got me involved in parent groups. She even asked me for copies of my children's IEPs [individualized education programs] so she could look them over. She always made sure that all the different physicians involved in my children's care talked together."

Because children with complex medical needs have an array of specialists dealing with discrete medical issues, a provider is needed to take responsibility for coordinating care and seeing the child as a whole person. To coordinate and improve health care for children with complex needs, the American Academy of Pediatrics and the federal Maternal and Child Health Bureau endorse the concept of *medical home.* A medical home is an identified consistent primary care practice in which the physician and/or nurse practitioner works in partnership with the individual, his or her family, and other specialists. Ideally, the medical home offers connections to a community-based system of services that is family-centered, comprehensive, coordinated, and culturally competent. The medical providers actively share health information and decision making with families. Patients and families are included in treatment decisions about most aspects of their care. In addition, they receive a written health care plan developed jointly by the clinical staff and the family. The plan identifies unmet needs, sets long- and short-term goals, includes information about resources, and assists families in making the transition from childhood to adulthood. (See Table 5.1 for a checklist of how to make a practice family friendly.)

The Developmental Disabilities Quality Coalition (DDQC), a broad-based coalition of professionals from key organizations involved with developmental disabilities, has expanded the medical home concept to address adults with special health care needs. The DDQC's Community Health Supports Model applies the principle of normalization to health care by emphasizing supports needed to enhance the individual's functioning and full participation in community life (Coulter, Edenzon, & Reiss, 2003). Health is seen as a state of physical, mental, emotional, social, and spiritual well-being, not as the absence of illness or disability. This view is based on the premise that quality lives and quality health care are integrally connected. Therefore, the focus is on having the supports needed to design and achieve lives of quality and meaning, characterized by opportunity, inclusion, and participation.

This model focuses on promoting health through environmental adaptations; technological assistance; and the provision of social, emotional, and spiritual supports, as well as through medical, behavioral, and therapeutic interventions. "These supports are provided in a manner that reflects the personal preferences of each individual, conveys that the person receiving services is a valued, respected, community participant, and assists individuals to achieve self-determined lives of mastery, satisfaction, and meaning" (Coulter et al., 2003). In addition, research, training, public policy, and service delivery practices are expanded to address issues across the life span. This model emphasizes that individuals with disabilities and their families be involved in the planning, conduction, and monitoring of all activities.

Table 5.1. How to know if a practice is family centered

Staff are available after hours, on weekends, and on holidays.
The insurance carried by all patients is accepted.
The office is physically accessible to all children.
Staff are welcoming and accommodating.
Receptionists know the families when they call.
Office and clinical staff recognize and accommodate children's special needs.
Office staff respond quickly to requests for letters to support insurance coverage, medical necessity determinations, or access to specialized medications.
Physicians actively share health information and decision-making with families.
Families receive written health care plans developed jointly by clinical staff and the family.
Families are encouraged to share their knowledge, observations, and information about their child's special needs as partners in planning and evaluating care.
Physicians take the time to ask about and listen to a family's questions and concerns at each visit.
Clinical staff focus on the whole family not just the child's health care status.
Staff help identify unmet needs for the child and family.
Staff share information on resources including recreational, educational, and social services that may be helpful to the "whole child."
Planning for the child and family's medical needs in the future is part of an annual assessment.
Families receive assistance in making the transition from child to adult services.

From New England SERVE, The Medical Home Partnership. (2003). *A new way . . . a better way: Building a home base for your child with special health care needs.* [Brochure]. Boston: Author; adapted by permission.

RESOURCES FOR FAMILIES

The evidence is overwhelming that families benefit from connections to other families who face the same or similar circumstance. Information coming from those who have been or are in "their shoes" seems to be the most powerful and sustaining support network that families report as critical to their moving forward and becoming the best advocate for their child. The alliance with other people who have or are experiencing the same feelings of uncertainty is rewarding and therapeutic. Families can connect to individuals or groups who may represent a specific diagnostic category or group, or more generally to others who are grappling with similar or broad questions of service needs, uncertain futures, or access to resources.

A vast network of family support services exists both nationally and internationally. Families should be connected to others via any and all routes with which they are comfortable. They can meet others face to face, or more anonymously through newsletters, web sites, or telephone conversations. Conferences highlighting information about specific services or supports are a good way for families to connect to the network of support services. Families should be encouraged to use the Internet, telephone book, hospital social workers, discharge planners, or family resource centers as well as friends and friends of friends. (See Table 5.2 for a list of helpful Internet resources.)

Table 5.2. Selected web sites for families

The following are excellent web sites with links to other useful sites:

- Family TIES, http://www.massfamilyties.org, is a statewide information and referral network for families of children with special needs. Although it is based in Massachusetts and funded by the Massachusetts Department of Public Health, its resource directory covers national organizations and services in other states.
- Family Village, http://www.familyvillage.wisc.edu, provides Internet resources for individuals with cognitive or other disabilities and their families, with discussion boards and links for "shopping" for specialized products.
- Family Voices, http://www.familyvoices.org, is a national organization of families and others whose lives have been touched by children with special health care needs. Family Voices has chapters in every state. By visiting Family Voice's home page, families and others can link to these chapters by clicking under Quick Links, Family Voices State by State.
- Internet Resources for Special Children (IRSC), http://www.irsc.org, provides parents, educators, medical professionals, and caregivers with information regarding children with disabilities. This web site includes a comprehensive list of Internet links, with an emphasis on specific disabilities.
- Kids Needs—The Place for Kids with Special Needs, http://www.kidneeds.com, is a resource to provide children with special needs and their families and caregivers with access to information that is categorized by type of disability (e.g., physical disabilities, learning disabilities).
- National Information Center for Children and Youth with Disabilities, http://www.nichcy.org, is a national information and referral center that provides information on disabilities and disability-related issues for families and professionals. It includes information on summer camps and state-by-state agencies serving people with disabilities. It also lists local parent-to-parent programs and contact information. Information is in English and Spanish.

As children develop, educational issues, social supports, and planning for adulthood come into the forefront, even as medical issues may continue to be important. Success in maintaining the child's optimal health status is integrally connected with success in these other developmental, educational, and social areas. Health care providers and families frequently find the array of state and community resources bewildering. Many programs exist locally, regionally, and nationally. State Title V programs, which are mandated to monitor and provide coordinated care, vary from state to state. Although many social agencies and public programs provide case management, services can be difficult to obtain. Providers can play a critical role in advising families on the usefulness of information and programs that exist.

Hospital Services

When a child is in the hospital, families are often unaware of the possible services available to them. Although not all hospitals will have all services, any one of a number of programs should be able to assist a family to get needed support and information. Many hospitals have family resource centers that provide a range of information including referrals to community service, parent groups, parent-to-parent networking, resource specialists, and a resource library. Interpreter services are available for families who speak English as a second language. Bicultural interpreters can provide a bridge by helping medical staff become more aware of relevant cultural and social issues. Pastoral counseling and religious service are often available on site, offering comfort and spiritual counseling. Many hospitals also have financial specialists that can assist in negotiating with health insurance companies and help families to obtain public health insurance and private funding for special health care needs.

Social workers can assess the child or family's needs and provide psychosocial/support services as well as family counseling. Discharge planners can arrange for and coordinate community-based medical services. Child-life specialists can work with the child during the hospitalization, often using play to help the child adapt to the medical setting and deal with the demands of his or her illness or disability. Psychologists and psychiatrists are available to help the child with psychological issues as well as assess the need for psychiatric medication. Because parents use services differently at various times, offering several sources of information and support is important. Then, parents can choose what is right for them in their current situation.

Home-Based Services

A variety of in-home services may be appropriate and needed, depending on the child's health care needs as well as the family's ability to care for their child. Some parents want to do most of the care alone or with other family members, whereas other parents want or need more assistance from outside agencies. In some situations, a child may require skilled nursing care either as a brief home visit to provide teaching and support or as shift nursing care in 4- to 12-hour shifts. Home health aides or personal care attendants can assist with daily life activities. Homemakers can help with household tasks such as cleaning, shopping, and food preparation. At times, a family may need someone to temporarily take over the care of their child in order to get a break or "respite." These services can be planned or on an emergency basis. They can be provided in or out of the home. Many families want to be involved in their child's care but they also need to take care of themselves and the rest of the family. Providers can direct families to the resources they need in order to feel competent and supported in their role as caregiver.

Many people with developmental disabilities use special equipment. Families can usually learn to manage this equipment, even though the idea of introducing this equipment into family life can be upsetting and overwhelming at first. The home care agency or a separate equipment vendor usually takes care of equipment needs. Suggestions for needed equipment and technology can come from a variety of sources including physical and occupational therapists, speech-language therapists, and educators.

Early Intervention and School Services

Joanne says that she has the best pediatrician for her two sons with disabilities because "she is there for whatever I need." The pediatrician's caring extended into the school arena, attending an IEP meeting at the school when the school program wasn't going well. When Joanne's third son was feeling left out because of his two brothers' complex needs, the pediatrician made extra time to talk with him and help him understand more about his brothers' conditions. Even now, after Joanne's sons have made the transition to adult providers, Joanne can call the pediatrician anytime for anything, even just a pep talk.

Physicians and other health care providers can play a key role in both identifying children who may be eligible for services and for supporting families whose children may need specific services to thrive in their school setting. Unfortunately, they are not always fully aware of either the services offered or the system requirements of early intervention (Helm & Shishmanian, 1997; Solomon, 1995). They need both knowledge-based and practice-based information. The former is information that makes the providers aware of what services are available and would include the eligibility criteria for early intervention and how reimbursement works in their state. This information can often be obtained via printed materials (including web sites) or short information training sessions. Practice-based information, however, is more sociological or cultural and reflects attitudes and perceptions. Some providers, for example, might think that middle class parents would find early intervention referrals stigmatizing and therefore not give them in a borderline situation, or they may use developmental screening tests that are not culturally sensitive to diverse childrearing practices and could affect results.

The medical profession has also played a central role in special education services for children with disabilities. Craig noted, "Traditionally, physicians, not educators, have diagnosed the disabilities that made children eligible for special education services . . . . Families often ask physicians for advice about the best placement for their child with learning disabilities or sensory integration problems" (1999, p. 781). Educators and health care providers should work together as part of a team to advise the family on educational planning because it is in the best interest of the child. Familiarity with federal and state laws will assist health care providers with understanding their responsibilities and in facilitating the child's participation in the classroom.

Physicians and other providers can help identify accommodations and needed supports to increase the child's access to and participation in the classroom. Educators often provide initial testing, but physicians are sometimes asked to conduct evaluations outside the school system when parents are uncertain of school-based testing or if the child's situation is deemed more complex and in need of medical assessment. The health care provider's role in the educational team should start early and continue throughout the child's educational experience.

As the child reaches adolescence and begins to see the end of his or her public education tenure, plans should begin to investigate postsecondary educational options. Providers should continue to play a role, as needed, in the adolescent's transition from high school to other settings. The adolescent will take the lead in deciding what is next, and the provider should be part of that team as well. Accommodations, assistive technologies, and health-oriented evaluations may be needed in order for the adolescent to be successful in his or her next educational undertaking. Providers should be informed and ready to assist as necessary.

TRANSITION TO ADULTHOOD

Recently Jon has been seizing every opportunity to assert his independence. I don't mean the little stuff like making his breakfast, taking his medications and paying his bills. I mean the big stuff. He resents my meddling and his sister's bossiness: he is embarrassed by his father's silliness. He is a teenager on the brink of leaving home. While he may be living under our roof for a while longer, he has been trying to separate emotionally for quite some time. (Klein & Shive, 2001, p. 211)

For any child or parent, life has its share of major milestones and points of transition. Starting school, getting a driver's license, going to the high school prom, and graduating from high school are just a few of those transitions. In the world of disability, the word *transition* takes on special meaning. Major life events are charged with emotions because they may not be happening at all, are not happening in the anticipated way, or are segues to an uncertain future. Transitions are times when families rework old issues as they face a new reality. From a practical perspective, transitions are a lot of work. Transition from one school program to another or from school to work, for example, requires years of planning and advocacy on the part of family members and school/public agency staff.

Health care providers play a critical role in successfully preparing adolescents and their families for the transition to adulthood. Providers can be helpful by raising particular topics at certain stages in the young adult's life. For example, when the child is between the ages of 11 and 13, providers can meet privately with him or her for at least part of the office visit to reinforce the concept that young adults begin to take responsibility for their own health care management. Attention needs to be paid to encouraging the individual to assume increasing responsibility for understanding his or her health condition and medications. Anticipatory guidance about sexuality and relationships, substance abuse, and other areas such as smoking can be provided. Providers can broaden their questions beyond the medical arena by asking how to be helpful in the education planning process. They can remind families that when the student is 14 years old, federal law mandates that the individualized transition plan (ITP) focus on developing a vision for employment and education. They can discuss community recreation options with a focus on developing strategies to avoid social isolation and foster friendships.

As the adolescent grows older, the provider can expand the areas of discussion and begin to assess the adolescent's and family's readiness for transfer to an adult health care provider. Educational concerns can include reminding the individual that when he or she is 16 years old, transition services must be included in the school IEP. Discussions about further education and visions for both employment and education can begin. Referrals to community-based vocational opportunities should be introduced. As the student approaches age 17, providers can remind families that special education services end with graduation or at age 22, so future planning becomes more concrete. Families should consider whether their young adult is in a position to make independent decisions or whether legal steps for guardianship (at age 18) need to be taken.

Reaching independence is the essence of becoming an adult. "For individuals with severe developmental disabilities, complete independence may not be a realistic goal" (White, Schuyler, Edelman, Hayes, & Batshaw, 2002). Significant aspects of independence, however, may still be possible. Carrying out activities of daily living (ADLs) with minimal assistance, separating from parents, and employment are all possible goals. Parents need to begin early in helping their child develop a sense of competence. Developmentally appropriate chores such as cleaning one's room, helping to prepare meals, washing dishes, and making decisions about how to spend allowance money should be encouraged. Participation in sports, leisure, and community activities can provide an opportunity to develop a sense of independence and autonomy (White et al., 2002).

The transition from school to work can take many forms. Individuals with disabilities can continue their public education through age 21. The Individuals with Disabilities Education Improvement Act of 2004 (PL 108-446) requires that public schools provide services to support the transition from school to work. These include vocational training, guidance on possibilities for postsecondary education, and help in obtaining adult services. PL 108-446 also mandates that students have an ITP, focused on the skills needed to make the transition into the community and the work force. The planning process involves getting information about the student's abilities, skills, and interests, which is then applied to the formation of future goals.

Vocational rehabilitation counselors must participate in the ITP before the student leaves school. Their purpose is to help individuals acquire and maintain gainful employment. A vocational rehabilitation counselor will work with a young adult to develop an individualized plan for employment (IPE) that includes training and postsecondary education and any disability-related employment needs and accommodations (White et al., 2002). Although there is a range of service options available, the expectation of competitive employment should be explored fully.

For students with good cognitive skills, many colleges have inclusive programs that offer specialized support services to assist students with disabilities. These services include various accommodations such as wheelchair-accessible classrooms, amplification systems for students with hearing disabilities, computerized scanning for students with visual problems, interpreters, tutorial help, and untimed tests. Some schools have a special track for students with disabilities and offer internships that often lead to competitive employment. The Bureau of Vocational Rehabilitation, the Internet, and guidebooks for individuals with learning disabilities are helpful in identifying appropriate programs.

Recreation and socialization are critical ingredients to a full life, allowing opportunities for fun, learning new skills, and developing friendships. Because recreational experiences reduce stress levels and minimize social isolation, the impact on health is positive. Recreational opportunities vary in communities, depending on the part of the country, age of the individual, and type of activity sought.

Community Living Programs

State and federal laws, such as the Americans with Disabilities Act (ADA) of 1990 (PL 101-336), have expanded the range of community living options for adults with disabilities. For some individuals, especially those with physical versus cognitive disabilities, living independently may be the best option. These living situations often need to be wheelchair accessible and have adaptive equipment, such as computers and panic buttons. Individuals with more severe physical disabilities may need a personal assistant to help them with washing, dressing, and preparing meals.

Group homes offer the opportunity for community living within a supervised setting with on-site counselors who provide support with personal living skills, recreation, and access to employment opportunities. Other options include staffed apartments, shared living, and adult foster care placements that provide an opportunity to live with a family that is trained to care for individuals with developmental disabilities (White et al., 2002). Waiting lists for living situations can be long, and parents need to begin early in advocating for their child. In Massachusetts, for example, a class action suit *(Boulet v. Cellucci)* resulted in a settlement for 2,225 people on the waiting list (Sarkissian, 2001).

Family members who choose to have their adult child or brother or sister live with them at home have access to services such as counseling, crisis intervention, respite care, advocacy, day programs and supported employment. Although many residential placements have closed, some residential facilities still specialize in meeting the needs of individuals with multiple, severe disabilities and specific conditions such as blindness and autism. Intermediate Care Facilities (ICFs) are smaller institutions (25 or fewer residents) that are most appropriate for people with significant health problems and limited daily living skills. Compared with other living arrangements, they can be more restrictive and medically oriented.

Employment

Employment options for people with disabilities ranges from full competitive employment in the community to more restricted and supported program settings. Individuals with disabilities should be encouraged to learn about job and employment options at an early age, to explore work environments to discover what they like and what they are good at, and to generally plan for a future that includes employment. Health care providers should work with the individuals, their families, and their school personnel in exploring options, experiences, and in general, the world of work. Through these prolonged explorations, individuals learn the value of work and how to plan for a future that includes employment (Kiernan & Stark, 1986; Wehman & Kregel, 1998). Angela's story illustrates how an adult with developmental disabilities can find a living and work situation in the community that fits her individual needs.

Angela is a 29-year-old high school graduate with a number of part-time job experiences who used to live at home. Her supportive and involved family is committed to helping her follow a typical course into adult life, and agency supports have made all the difference for her. Angela's mild cerebral palsy and cognitive disabilities make her eligible for the services of the state's Department of Mental Retardation.

When Angela left high school at age 22, she was referred to her state's Vocational Rehabilitation Agency in their Work Experience Program. She received a situational assessment (an opportunity to assess her work skills and behavior in a real work setting) and benefited from more work experience. She was then hired full time by a hospital as a central processing aide and, after staff reductions, now works part time as a lab control aide.

Angela had always dreamed of working with animals but did not want to give up her lab job and the hospital benefits. Furthermore, the situational assessment she had earlier participated in helped her to recognize that mobility problems and cognitive limitations made dreams of being an animal technician unrealistic. Now, she has a half-time clerical position in an animal hospital. This job capitalized on her strengths while providing the opportunity to work in the animal care field.

Angela's dreams and goals were further supported and explored when her Employment Specialist helped her to realize her vision of obtaining a driver's license. This meant accommodations for her limited reading skills and identifying a driver's education program with experience with people with disabilities. After taking the course, Angela decided she wasn't comfortable with driving, but the decision was hers.

Angela now has her own apartment and is much more independent in her personal life. With funds from the Department of Mental Retardation to help identify a roommate, she found a roommate and now lives in subsidized housing. With friends in her community, and continuing emotional support from her family, she is happily settled and employed. Even when she confronted extreme emotional strain from her mother's illness and subsequent death, she has been able to get the support she needed from her employer's Employee Assistance Program rather than disability-specific sources.

Angela's experience shows how appropriate supports can nurture integration into the community.

As indicated previously, the transition process is key to successful employment. No one should be considered too disabled to work; thus, everyone needs to be exposed to work, careers, and employment considerations. A host of services are available to assist individuals with disabilities to find employment and to receive the supports they need to be successful. Individuals can use One Stop Career Centers, which are increasingly able to serve all those who seek employment. Similarly the vocational rehabilitation services of the state are often used as a vehicle to employment or training for work. This system can provide a multitude of supports to the job seeker with disabilities (Kiernan & Schalock, 1989; Wehman, 2003; Wehman & Kregel, 1998).

CONCLUSION

Providers can make a significant difference in helping strengthen and support families who have children with special health care needs. The healing words of a caring provider can reverberate throughout all aspects of a family's life. Guiding families in setting realistic goals, recognizing their children's strengths, supporting them in grieving their losses, and helping them to brainstorm creative solutions to difficult problems are central themes in this work. Families need to find meaning in their experience and need hope to build positive expectations for the future. By recognizing and including families as integral partners in intervention teams, providers have a unique opportunity to tap into family and community resources while developing an understanding of the family within the context of their cultural and social norms.

Providers who take the time early in the relationship to build trust and to establish a collaborative approach have more satisfying provider–patient relationships, enhanced compliance, and even improved health for the child. Respecting the particular challenges families face and the individualized nature of their journey yields a rich experience and a deeper understanding of their needs. Providers are in an ideal position to help connect families to the vast—and often overwhelming—array of community (and other) resources and supports. By expanding their perspective and practice beyond the limitations of the biomedical model, providers can play an important role in empowering families as they struggle with the challenges ahead.

REFERENCES

Allord, J. (1985) A parent's perspective on a developmentally disabled child. In V.G. Martin & E.A. Griswold (Eds.), *Look to families* (pp. 1–3). Denver: Health and Human Services.

Americans with Disabilities Act (ADA) of 1990, PL 101-336, 42 U.S.C. §§ 12101 *et seq.*

Back, A.L., Arnold, R.M., & Quill, T.E. (2003). Hope for the best, and prepare for the worst. *Annals of Internal Medicine, 138*(5), 439–443.

Beckman, P.J. (2002). Providing family-centered services. In M.L. Batshaw (Ed.), *Children with disabilities* (5th ed., pp. 683–691). Baltimore: Paul H. Brookes Publishing Co.

Beigel, K., & Todd, S. (2003, May). *Somali development center report.* Presentation at LEND Convocation, Boston.

Berger, P., & Luckman, T. (1967). *The social construction of reality.* Garden City, NY: Doubleday and Co.

Boulet v. Cellucci, 107 F. Supp. 2d 61 (D. Mass. 2000)

Bronstein, L.R. (2003). A model for interdisciplinary collaboration. *Social Work, 48*(3), 297–306.

Carter, E., & McGoldrick, M. (1980). The family lifecycle and family therapy: An overview. In E. Carter & M. McGoldrick (Eds.), *The family lifecycle* (pp. 3–20). New York: Gardner Press.

Chedd, N.A. (1994). The way we see it: Families and caregivers speak out. *NDTA Network, Neurodevelopmental Treatment Association Bulletin.*

Coulter, D., Edenzon, M., & Reiss, S. (2003). *Health promotion and prevention of disabilities.* Presentation at a plenary talk of the American Association of Mental Retardation, Chicago.

Craig, S.E. (1999). Special education services for children with disabilities. In M.D. Levine, W.B. Carey, & A.C. Crocker (Eds.), *Developmental-behavioral pediatrics* (pp. 781–792). Philadelphia: W.B. Saunders.

Crocker, A.C. (1983). Sisters and brothers. In J.A. Mulick & S.M. Pueschel (Eds.), *Parent–professional partnerships in developmental disability services.* Cambridge, MA: Ware Press.

Crocker, A.C. (1998). Exceptionality. *Developmental and Behavioral Pediatrics, 19*(4), 300–305.

Developmental Disabilities Quality Coalition. (2003). *Community health supports model of people with developmental disabilities.* Retrieved from http://www.pediatricservices.com

Dillon, C. (1986). Chronic illness in children: Its impact on the lifecycle. In D.H. Rodman & A.A. Murphy, *A new look at patent social work alliance: improved care and treatment for the chronically ill child* (pp. 5–21). Washington, DC: National Center for Education in Maternal and Child Health.

Fadiman, A. (1997). *The spirit catches you and you fall down: A Hmong child, her American doctors, and the collision of two cultures.* New York: Noonday Press.

Featherstone, H. (1981). *A difference in the family: Living with a disabled child.* New York: Penguin Books.

Grossman, F.K. (1972). *Brothers and sisters of retarded children.* Syracuse, NY: Syracuse University Press.

Hannah, M.E., & Midlarsky, E. (1999). Competence and adjustment of siblings of children with mental retardation. *American Journal of Mental Retardation, 104*(1), 22–37.

Helm, D.T., & Shishmanian, E. (1997). Information pediatricians need about early intervention. *Children's Health Care, 26*(4), 255–264.

Individuals with Disabilities Education Improvement Act of 2004, PL 108-446, 20 U.S.C. §§ 1400 *et seq.*

Jezewski, M.A., & Sotnik, P. (2001). *Culture brokering: Providing culturally competent rehabilitation services to foreign-born persons.* Buffalo, NY: Center for International Rehabilitation Research Information and Exchange.

Kiernan, W.E., & Schalock, R.L. (Eds.). (1989). *Economy, industry, and disability: A look ahead.* Baltimore: Paul H. Brookes Publishing Co.

Kiernan, W.E., & Stark, J.A. (Eds.). (1986). *Pathways to employment for adults with developmental disabilities.* Baltimore: Paul H. Brookes Publishing Co.

Klein, S.D. (1993). The challenge of communicating with parents. *Developmental and Behavioral Pediatrics, 14*(3), 184–191.

Klein, S.D., & Schive, K. (Eds.). (2001). *You will dream new dreams: Inspiring personal stories by parents of children with disabilities.* New York: Kensington Books.

Kleinman, A. (1988). *The illness narratives: Suffering and healing and the human condition.* New York: Basic Books.

Laborde, P.R., & Seligman, M. (1991). Counseling parents with children with disabilities. In M. Seligman (Ed.), *The family with a handicapped child* (pp. 247–274). Boston: Allyn & Bacon.

Lobato, D., Barbour, R.A., Hall, L.J., & Miller, C.T. (1987). Psychosocial characteristics of preschool siblings of handicapped children. *Journal of Abnormal Psychology, 15,* 329–338.

Lynch, E.W., & Hanson, M.J. (Eds.). (2004). *Developing cross-cultural competence: A guide for working with children and their families* (3rd ed.). Baltimore: Paul H. Brookes Publishing Co.

Mack, S., & Berman, L.C. (1988). A group for parents of children with fatal genetic illnesses. *American Journal of Orthopsychiatry, 58*(3), 397–404.

Maynard, D.W. (1989). Notes on the delivery and reception of diagnostic news regarding mental disabilities. In D.T. Helm, W.T. Anderson, A.J. Meehan, & A.W. Rawls (Eds.), *The interactional order: New directions in the study of social order.* New York: Irvington Publishers.

McCarthy, C., & Brown, M. (2003, May). *Hope at the time of diagnosis.* Care Points Conference, Brookline, MA.

Meyer, D., & Vadasy, P.F. (1994). *Sibshops: Workshop for siblings of children with special needs.* Baltimore: Paul H. Brookes Publishing Co.

Moses, K. (1987, Spring). The impact of childhood disability: The parent's struggle. *Ways Magazine,* 1–8.

Neugarten, B. (1979). Time, age, and the lifecycle. *American Journal of Psychiatry, 183*(7), 887–893.

New England SERVE, The Medical Home Partnership. (2003). *A new way . . . a better way: Building a home base for your child with special health care needs* [Brochure]. Boston: Author.

Orsmond, G.I., & Seltzer, M.M. (2000). Brothers and sisters of adults with mental retardation: Gendered nature of the sibling relationship. *American Journal on Mental Retardation, 105*(6), 486–508.

Penn, P. (1983). Coalitions and binding interactions in families with chronic illness. *Family Systems Medicine, 1*(2), 16–25.

Porter, S., Burkely, J., Bierle, T., Lowcock, J., Haynie, L.M., & Palfrey, J. (1992). *Working toward a balance in our lives: A booklet for families of children with disabilities and special health care needs.* Boston: Children's Hospital.

Roland, J. (1987). Chronic illness and the lifecycle: A conceptual framework. *Family Process, 26,* 203–221.

Sarkissian, L.V. (2001). *Building a future: A handbook for families. 2001–2002 waiting list settlement edition: Strategies on supported housing for adults with cognitive disabilities.* Boston: The Arc, Massachusetts.

Seligman, M., & Darling, R.B. (1989). *Ordinary families, special children: A systems approach to childhood disability.* New York: The Guilford Press.

Shamoon Shanok, R. (2000). The action is in the interaction: Clinical practice guidelines for work with parents of children with developmental disorders. In Interdisciplinary Council on Developmental and Learning Disabilities (ICDL) (Ed.), *Clinical practice guidelines: Redefining the standards of care of infants, children, and families with special needs* (pp. 333–371). Bethesda, MD: ICDL Press.

Solomon, R. (1995). Pediatricians and early intervention: Everything you need to know, but are too busy to ask. *Infants and Young Children, 7,* 38–51.

Stein, R. (1983). Growing up with a physical difference. *Children's Health Care, 12*(2) 53–61.

Stoneman, Z., Brody, G., Davis, C.H., Crapps, J.M., & Malone, D.M. (1991). Ascribed role relationships between children with mental retardation and their younger siblings. *American Journal on Mental Retardation, 95,* 537–550.

Trevino, F. (1979). Siblings of handicapped children: Identifying those at risk. *Social Casework, 60,* 488–493.

Wehman, P. (2003). Workplace inclusion: Persons with disabilities and coworkers working together. *Journal of Vocational Rehabilitation, 18*(2), 124–131.

Wehman, P., & Kregel, J. (Eds.). (1998). *More than a job: Securing satisfying careers for people with disabilities.* Baltimore: Paul H. Brookes Publishing Co.

White, P.H., Schuyler, V., Edelman, A., Hayes, A., & Batshaw, M.L. (2002). Future expectations: Transition from adolescence to adulthood. In M.L. Batshaw (Ed.), *Children with disabilities* (5th ed., pp. 693–706). Baltimore: Paul H. Brookes Publishing Co.

Zetlin, A.G. (1986). Mentally retarded adults and their siblings. *American Journal of Mental Deficiency, 91*(3), 217–225.

CHAPTER 6

SYSTEMS OF MEDICAL CARE DELIVERY

6.1 CLINICAL CENTERS AND TEAMS

Allen C. Crocker

Complex personal pictures are common in the developmental disabilities field. Individual challenges are often present in numerous functions and systems, and indeed the territory of human development, whether typical or altered, is an amalgam of contributing features and leading causes. On this basis, utilization of clinical centers, which have multiple types of related personnel, is efficacious for assessment and some follow-along activities. The use of centers has been increasing as the knowledge base has grown and funding supports require accountability. Centers with teams are universal in schools, common in treatment programs, and expected in rehabilitation facilities. It is in developmental centers, especially child development centers, that classical team studies are carried out. These are characteristic of metropolitan areas, especially in children's hospitals and training programs. In the early days of Title V supports, child development clinics were widespread and administered by the departments of health. Since the Kennedy administration, they have often been part of the University Affiliated Facilities (now University Centers for Excellence in Developmental Disabilities).

The Developmental Evaluation Center at the Children's Hospital Boston has been a representative facility for child review (Zadig & Crocker, 1975). The major clinical disciplines have been present; more than 2,000 children are welcomed each year. Referrals derive characteristically from pediatricians, schools, agencies, and families. In addition to general developmental study, a Feeding Team, an Autism Center, an Infant Follow-up Program, a Mucopolysaccharidosis Institute, a Psychopharmacology Program, and numerous further areas exist. Projects in allied departments are concerned with cerebral palsy, myelodysplasia, craniofacial anomalies, and many other disabilities.

The heart of a center, then, is its team or teams, and the essence of each team's work is collaboration (in study, planning, and intervention) on behalf of a child and his or her family. Much variation exists in the dynamics and relationships within the teams; a diagrammatic representation of the configurations is shown in Figure 6.1-1.

Teams ordinarily are based in a central facility. Sometimes, they may be part of outreach activities that work directly in community settings. How a team utilizes the strengths and contributions of its various professional members is a test of the level of mutual respect that exists in that agency among different disciplines. This, in turn, is influenced by local biases, the resolution of the workers involved, and the requirements of funding and reimbursement patterns. In Figure 6.1-1, the size of the individual disks makes reference to the level of the activity, and the one with the darker ring indicates the coordinating or communicating member. Some relevant features follow:

1. *Solo action or practice*—In this model, a single worker accepts the responsibility for identifying the cogent issues and designing relevant management (e.g., physician, social worker, community health nurse). Services for individuals with multiple problems are unlikely to be well guided in this practical, but rather assumptive, mode.
2. *Consultation practice*—The resources of an outside expert (e.g., neurologist) are obtained to enlarge the understanding of the basic problem, but limited continuing contact occurs.
3. *Partnership practice*—The primary clinician may establish a partly shared responsibility with another analogous worker; the scope of interaction with the individual with developmental disabilities is inevitably enhanced.
4. *Multidisciplinary team*—This practical system has been predominant since the 1950s, utilizing the considerations of a cluster of professionals. The various workers (e.g., psychology, psychiatry, speech pathology) may or may not be located in the same facility, and they often do not have the opportunity to confer together directly on behalf of the individual with developmental disabilities. The coordinator must utilize and amalgamate the diverse reports

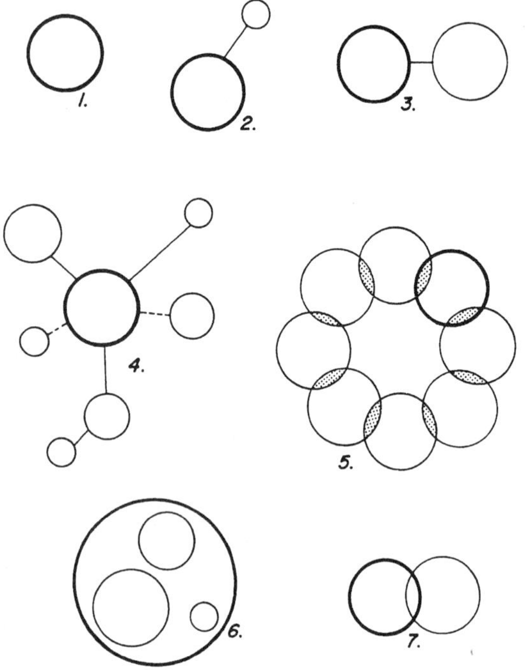

Figure 6.1-1. A representation of the structure of teams involved in the evaluation of children with developmental disabilities: 1) solo practice, 2) consultation, 3) partnership, 4) multidisciplinary team, 5) interdisciplinary team, 6) transdisciplinary team, and 7) collaborative practice. (Reprinted from *Developmental-Behavioral Pediatrics*, M.D. Levine, W.B. Carey, A.C. Crocker, & R.T. Gross [Eds.], "Coordination of Services," A.C. Crocker & M.M. Cullinane, Copyright 1983, with permission from Elsevier.)

and interpret them for the individual and his or her family.

5. *Interdisciplinary team*—The advanced and symmetrical design of the interdisciplinary team was promoted by the training programs of the federal Maternal and Child Health Bureau since the 1970s. In the fully expressed form, the various clinicians work in the same facility, communicate as they proceed, and create an integrated report while working at the same conference table. In this regard, there is a practical and intellectual sharing. An expanded diagram of the possible components is shown in Figure 6.1-2. One worker serves as the coordinator, expedites the report, and chairs the family conference. The views of all professionals are equally valued, and family contact responsibilities are assigned as appropriate. Time requirements are considerable, as are costs, and some degree of subsidization may be required.

6. *Transdisciplinary services*—In the setting of teams that are stable and experienced, one individual will sometimes take on all of the activities of the different disciplines, including coordination and communication, for a given person with developmental disabilities. This person then becomes the interpreter and guide for the person with developmental disabilities and his or her family. A special closeness results as well as good continuity.

7. *Collaborative practice*—There is potential for truly mutual sharing of patients by just two (or possibly three) professionals of different disciplines who maintain a high degree of feedback (and equal position) and divide the tasks of working with patients in a common setting. Examples include physician and nurse practitioner, orthopedist and physical therapist, and physician and psychologist. This break with traditional authoritarian unilateral management requires training and experience but can be extremely rewarding.

Young people with developmental disabilities (and sometimes older ones as well) receive care from a group of professionals, particularly for diagnostic work, assessment, or special therapies. The interdisciplinary design, in some degree, is the prototype. These teams will address clinical management but also educational hopes, special services, social needs, behavioral guidance, and family support (Garner, 1998).

Problem-solving in centers, and specifically by teams, calls for some particular individual contributions and for group synthesis as well. Specific roles for members need to be perceived and agreed on. The team coordinator provides important leadership and deserves respect. Compliance by members is essential regarding completion of clinical or historical studies, report writing, conference attendance, and special communication. For physicians, often accustomed to individual effort, alliance in action plans with inter- or multidisciplinary teams may take some adjustment and experience. The benefits will become quite clear (Crocker, 1998). As the team's service continues, one can expect from all of the members that there will be trust, openness, and mutual reliance.

Team models can have some real limitations, as well. Involvement in the group can be demanding on schedules and is notably time consuming. Some professionals mention experiences in which the team process proved to be wasteful and clumsy. With some anger, they equate teams with committees, and they consider the term *interdisciplinarianism* to be symbolic of unwieldiness. Team activities are very taxing on the time of individuals with developmental disabilities and their families as well, especially if their own resources are reduced. The presence of a team may be intimidating to

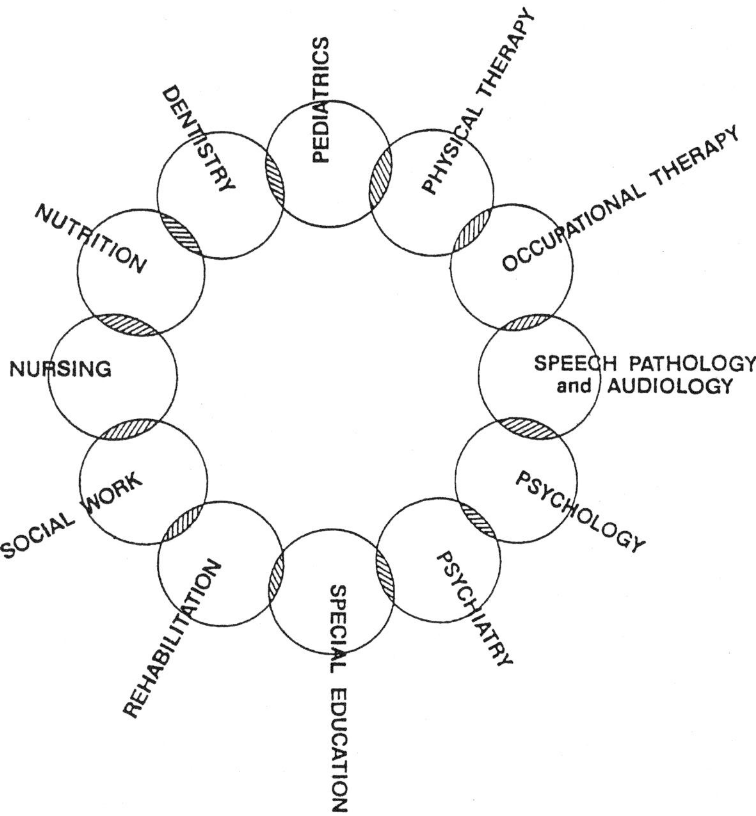

Figure 6.1-2. The array of professional disciplines—the interdisciplinary team—potentially involved in the study of a child with disabilities.

families, including those with language or cultural uncertainty. Some may find the team using "group think," with particular local interpretation.

Mostly, however, a center and its teams are the principal setting for study and support and can be thought of as a haven for involved individuals and families and a source of resources, problem solving, friendship, and advocacy. Teams are fairly abundant for programs with children; regrettably they are sparse for adults with disabilities. For helping professionals, the centers are a guide to special studies, knowledge, and updated therapies. The efforts of centers and teams are the major source of the materials that constitute this volume.

REFERENCES

Crocker, A.C. (1998). Teamwork: Medicine. In F.P. Orlove & H.G. Garner (Eds.), *Teamwork: Parents and professionals speak for themselves* (pp. 55–72). Washington, DC: Child Welfare League of America Press.

Crocker, A.C., & Cullinane, M.M. (1983). The function of teams. In M.D. Levine, W.B. Carey, A.C. Crocker, & R.T. Gross (Eds.), *Developmental-behavioral pediatrics* (pp. 990–993). Philadelphia: W.B. Saunders.

Garner, H.G. (1998). Challenges and opportunities of teamwork. In F.P. Orlove & H.G. Garner (Eds.), *Teamwork: Parents and professionals speak for themselves* (pp. 11–29). Washington, DC: Child Welfare League of America Press.

Zadig, J.M., & Crocker, A.C. (1975). A center for study of the young child with developmental delay. In B.Z. Friedlander, G.M. Sterritt, & G.E. Kirk (Eds.), *Exceptional infant: Vol. 3. Assessment and intervention* (pp. 5–39). New York: Brunner/Mazel.

6.2 THE HEALTH DEPARTMENT

Deborah Allen

Since 1919, federal law has established the framework for state programs to improve maternal and child health. The Sheppard-Towner Act of 1921 (part of the Maternity and Infancy Act) provided federal funding for states to promote maternal and infant health and reduce infant mortality. Funds were to be distributed through "formula grants," based on statistics reflecting level of need in each of the states (U.S. Department of Health and Human Services, 2001). Although conservative lobbying led to its repeal in 1929, the Sheppard-Towner Act provided a model for maternal and child health provisions incorporated into the Social Security Act of 1935 (PL 74-271).

Title V of PL 74-271 included two programs that addressed the well-being of mothers and children. Part 1 established funding for programs to improve prenatal and maternity care. Part 2 established funding for what were called "Crippled Children's Services," responsible for finding children with "crippling" conditions and offering them diagnosis, hospitalization, and aftercare. Part 2 broke new ground in assigning shared responsibility to state and federal governments to serve children with special health care needs (U.S. Department of Health and Human Services, 2001). That model of shared responsibility is still in place; states have considerable discretion to design their own programs for children with special health care needs, but they do so within broad federal guidelines and with a base of federal funding. Parents, clinicians, and others who look to their states' Title V programs for support or leadership can be most effective if they understand the federal framework for the program (see Table 6.2-1 for summary facts about the Title V Children with Special Health Care Needs program at the national level), and the varied approaches to its implementation in different states.

Table 6.2-1. Summary of the National Title V Children with Special Health Care Needs (CSHCN) Program

History
1. Title V of the Social Security Act of 1935 (PL 74-271)—established state-federal Crippled Children's Services Program
2. Omnibus Budget Reconciliation Act (OBRA) of 1981 (PL 97-35)—incorporated Children's Services Program into the Maternal and Child Health Block Grant
3. Omnibus Budget Reconciliation Act (OBRA) of 1989 (PL 101-239)—mandated that states build "systems of services"

National Title V funding levels for 2004
1. $598,938,847 for all Title V programs
2. $208,258,253 for children with special health care needs

National CSHCN Program structure
1. Health Resources and Services Administration Agency
2. Maternal and Child Health Bureau
3. Services for Children with Special Needs Division

CSHCN Division of Services Programs
1. Medical home
2. Family participation
3. Healthy and ready to work
4. Genetics and newborn screening
5. Cultural competence
6. Financing and managed care

Sources: U.S. Department of Health and Human Services (2000, n.d.).

EVOLUTION OF THE TITLE V PROGRAM

The 1935 version of Title V was designed to address issues that were central concerns of families caring for children with special health care needs at that time: limited clinical insight into complex pediatric conditions, lack of a national infrastructure to make the few effective treatments that were available accessible to families, and high cost of therapeutic and custodial care of children with long-term disability. Although gaps in clinical knowledge, access to specialty care, and the cost of caring for a child with special health care needs remain issues for many families today, the environment in which families raise children with special health care needs is dramatically different. The role of Title V has evolved in response to changes in the environment, including

- The emergence of the disability rights movement among adults with disabilities and a parallel movement among parents of children with special health care needs to fight for inclusion of individuals with disabilities in all aspects of community life and for the resources required for accessible housing, personal assistance, and other supports needed to make inclusion feasible (Disability Social History Project, 2003)
- The invention of new medical techniques, new kinds of equipment, and new medications that make survival possible for children with complex conditions and make community living medically feasible for virtually all children with special health care needs (Family Re-Union, 2003)
- The establishment of neonatal and pediatric intensive care units (NICUs and PICUs); children's specialty hospitals; early intervention; and other systems that deliver health, education, and developmental services to children with complex conditions widely throughout the United States (Newacheck & Taylor, 1994)
- The establishment of the Medicaid program in 1965, which provides the capital needed to develop new technologies and support access to these technologies and assures a funding stream for the service systems that make these technologies available to children and families (Smith & Vidyasagar, 1980)

These changes, which have made sophisticated clinical services widely (if imperfectly) available to children with special needs, have made it less necessary for Title V programs to focus on direct medical care. The result has been a gradual shift to a role that focuses more on needs assessment, program and policy planning, and monitoring and improvement of program implementation efforts. This broader role is captured in the mandate defined for Title V in the Omnibus Budget Reconciliation Act (OBRA) of 1989 (PL 101-239), which calls for development of state systems of services for children with special health care needs (N.A.C.H. State Policy Services, 2004).

CURRENT MANDATE OF PROGRAMS

PL 101-239 does not offer any details on what it means to establish "systems of services" for children with special health care needs. It does not tell states what a good system looks like. Nor, for that matter, does it tell states which children comprise "children with special health care needs." Therefore, it does not offer interested constituencies adequate means to hold states accountable. Like PL 101-239, Objectives 16–23 of Healthy People 2010 (n.d.) call for the establishment of state systems of care for children with special health care needs. In the case of Healthy People 2010, however, widespread discussion among parents, providers, and state and federal leaders has fleshed out the system's skeleton, identifying six outcomes that define and may be used to measure implementation of both PL 101-239 and the Health People 2010 mandate.

First, parents participate in decision-making at all levels of the system and are satisfied with services. This outcome operationalizes the concept "family-centered care" by calling for a family role in system design at the clinic, local, state, and federal levels. It acknowledges the challenge inherent in efforts to devise good measures of system quality for children with special health care needs. Children experience such diverse special health needs, and the outcomes of different conditions vary so widely from child to child (and even for the same child over time), that typical quality indicators are inadequate. Parent satisfaction, thoughtfully measured, may be the best way to ascertain quality of care across the full range of diagnoses and service elements.

Second, every child has a medical home. The American Academy of Pediatrics (2002) defines a *medical home* as the hub for the multiple services that may be required by a family caring for a child with special health care needs. A medical home is responsible for primary medical care but also for coordinating all aspects of medical care, linking medical care to school or early intervention, and helping the family get connected to social and support services they may need. These services range from community-based, informal, parent-to-parent networks to Supplemental Security Income or other highly structured federal entitlement programs.

Third, families have insurance coverage that is adequate to meet their child's basic and special health care needs. A child with complex medical needs may require primary and specialty medical care; therapists; and access to acute, long-term, inpatient and outpatient care. Private benefit packages may not cover this wide range of medical needs. In many cases, privately insured families find that a service their child needs is either not covered or is limited by their insurer. Even families of children on Medicaid or other public programs, which are more generous than private benefit packages in most states, experience gaps. This outcome addresses the need to mobilize public and private systems to ensure that no child with special health care needs is uninsured or, as is more frequently the case, underinsured, and thus unable to pay for services that would improve the child's health or ability to function.

Fourth, children receive ongoing screening to identify those with special health care needs. This outcome defines the proactive identification of children with special health care needs as a fundamental measure of system effectiveness. Discussions of this outcome have generally focused on medical screening to identify conditions for which there are clear biochemical or physiological markers (e.g., newborn screening for inborn errors of metabolism or for hearing loss); however, this outcome may be interpreted to include responsibility for screening throughout childhood for developmental as well as physical conditions. It may also be understood to refer to responsibility to "screen" data to identify children with special health care needs within program caseloads.

Fifth, families have access to user-friendly community-based services. Typically, the family of a child with special health care needs faces an ongoing struggle 1) to figure out the nature of their child's condition; 2) to identify and obtain the services he or she needs; 3) to get the child's insurer to cover services that are medical; 4) to find resources to cover the many services that lie outside the realm of health insurance; 5) to design and ensure the implementation of the school-based services the child needs; and 6) to identify national, state, and local public and private programs of potential benefit to themselves and their child. In the process, they find that programs have discordant or even contradictory eligibility requirements, application procedures, and service constraints. The distress involved in confronting these barriers is exacerbated by the interpersonal interactions involved in many system encounters.

Finally, all children and youth have access to services needed to ensure effective transition to adulthood: from school to higher education or work, from parents' home to a desired form of independent living, and from pediatric to adult health care. This outcome calls for interventions that target service providers (e.g., in school and medical settings, in vocational rehabilitation programs), parents, and youth themselves to establish attitudes, expectations, and skills that support transition. It implies effective intervention in the adult, as well as the pediatric service world, because the inadequacies of adult service systems place real limits on the extent to which stakeholders are willing and able to help youth shift away from the relative safety of pediatric services. In the school setting, the Individuals with Disabilities Education Act (IDEA) of 1990 (PL 101-476) mandates transition services. Although no equivalent mandate exists in the medical setting, proactive attention to transition is part of what defines a child's medical home.

In 2002, a parallel set of outcomes was incorporated into the President's "New Freedom Initiative," making their achievement a matter of clear administration policy (U.S. Department of Health and Human Services, 2003). The question, "Who is a child with special health care needs?" has also now been addressed at both national and state levels. Since the passage of PL 74-271, states have been free to identify the population to be served with Title V funds more or less broadly. Some states have identified children of interest for Title V very narrowly—as those with a limited set of diagnoses who receive direct care from a more clinically oriented state program. Other states have used broader definitions, regardless of whether they serve all of the children those definitions include. McPherson et al. (1998) defined *children with special health care needs* as children who have or are at risk for chronic physical, developmental, behavioral, or emotional conditions and who also require health and related services of a type or amount beyond that required by children generally. Table 6.2-2 presents selected findings from a national survey conducted from 2000–2002 to ascertain prevalence of special health care needs based on the American Academy of Pediatrics definition.

For those working within Title V programs, the six outcomes provide benchmarks against which to measure progress. For those outside the system, they provide a way of holding Title V programs accountable and of ensuring that in each state public funds for children with special health care needs are put to best use to address the major obstacles to achieving what, by national consensus, are now the critical challenges.

Table 6.2-2. The epidemiology of special health care needs

Children with special health care needs are those "who have or are at risk for chronic physical, developmental, behavioral or emotional conditions and who also require health and related services of a type or amount beyond that required by children generally" (McPherson et al., 1998).

The national prevalence of special health needs is 9,360,356, or 12.8% (Data and Resource Center for Child and Adolescent Health, n.d.).

West Virginia has the highest prevalence, with 16.7%, and California has the lowest at 10.3%.

Compared with children with no special health care needs, children with special health care needs experience (Newacheck et al., n.d.)

- More "annual bed days"
- More days of school lost
- Slightly greater likelihood of being insured
- Slightly greater likelihood of having a usual source of care
- Almost three times the number of annual physician contacts
- More than three times the number of annual hospitalizations

STATE IMPLEMENTATION OF PROGRAMS

The six Healthy People 2010/New Freedom Initiative outcomes capture the aims of state Title V Children with Special Health Care Needs Programs, but they do not define what the programs do. Great variability exists in the ways states go about "assuring" systems of care for children with special health care needs depending on such variables as demographics; geography and size of the state; the extent and structure of private sector pediatric health services, including specialty care services in the state; and broad social attitudes toward government in the state. Outsiders seeking to work with and ensure maximum effectiveness of a state's program have the right to ask if the state is doing what is needed to build an effective system of care.

The answer varies from state to state. It varies first because needs differ. Some states, generally the more populated and urban states, have tertiary hospitals, including hospitals just for children's care and well-developed networks of primary and specialty care physicians and therapists; however, even the most medically developed states report sharp constraints on their ability to ensure mental health and dental care to children with special health care needs (Association of Maternal and Child Health Programs, 2004). Title V programs in states that lack medical infrastructure may determine that to ensure an adequate "system of services," they must facilitate access to specialists for children with special needs. Title V programs in more medically developed states may be able to rely on private systems to meet children's clinical needs and use their own resources to focus on "enabling" services—such as care coordination, family support, and respite, which are less likely to be reimbursed or provided by health care payers.

Table 6.2-3 presents examples of strategies in different states to improve systems of care and advance the national children with special health care needs agenda. The list may suggest ways a state could improve its system of care for children with special health care needs, but it is just meant to be suggestive. A state may have developed its own innovative strategies to advance the agenda. This information can be determined by contacting the state Title V Children with Special Health Care Needs Director (see https://performance.hrsa.gov/mchb/mchreports/link/state_links.asp). At the national level, Title V supports a set of "centers" that assist states, providers, and parent groups in their efforts to enhance services. Web sites for these centers may suggest other strategies to address needs in a particular state.

CONCLUSION

Beyond the current borders of Title V and other existing state public health programs lies the question of capacity in relation to adults. Although there are government programs that address health and that address employment and personal care assistance for some adults with disabilities, there is no equivalent of Title V. Certainly, many health department programs that promote health of the whole population are relevant to or may be modified to include individuals with disabilities. One state has, for example, made services for women with disabilities a special focus of its breast cancer screening program. Generally, however, adults with disabilities rely on family and friends for help or confront fragmented, uneven health and social service systems alone. The increasing survival of individuals with disabilities through adolescence and into adulthood and old age, the continued inadequacy of service systems, and the complexity of negotiating those systems all suggest that needs in this area will only expand in the years to come. If children and families who leave the pediatric system familiar with Title V join forces with the adult disability movement, they may increasingly demand for government to meet that need—applying the mandate of Title V to address life-span service needs.

Table 6.2-3. Illustrative state Healthy People 2010/New Freedom Initiative strategies

1. *Family participation*—contribution of state support for practice-based family advisory committees (Colorado)
2. *Medical home*—reassignment of state care coordinators to medical home practices (Massachusetts)
3. *Adequate coverage*—use of state funding for tertiary consultation to medical home practices (Illinois)
4. *Screening*—incorporation of screening for special health care needs into emergency room visits (Utah)
5. *User-friendly services*—development of a single application form for multiple child health and family support programs (Wisconsin)
6. *Transition*—creation of a youth advisory group to the Department of Public Health (Maine)

REFERENCES

American Academy of Pediatrics, Medical Home Initiatives for Children with Special Needs Project Advisory Committee. (2002). The medical home. *Pediatrics, 110,*184–186.

Association of Maternal and Child Health Programs. (AMCHP). (2004, March). *AMCHP fact sheet: Mental health.* Retrieved from http://www.amchp.org/aboutamchp/pubs-amchp.htm

Data Resource Center for Child and Adolescent Health. (n.d.). *National Survey of Children with Special Health Care Needs.* Retrieved from http://www.cshcndata.org

Disability Social History Project. (2003, Sept. 23). *Disability history timeline.* Retrieved from http://disabilityhistory.org/timeline_new.html

Family Re-Union. (2003, Nov. 4). *Family-centered health care: A revolution that improves pediatric health systems.* Retrieved from http://www.familyreunion.org/health/arango/fccare.html

Healthy People 2010. (n.d.). *Healthy People 2010 home page.* Retrieved from http://www.healthypeople.gov

Individuals with Disabilities Education Act (IDEA) of 1990, PL 101-476, 20 U.S.C. §§ 1400 *et seq.*

Maternity and Infancy Act, Nov. 23, 1921, ch. 135, 42 Stat. 224.

McPherson, M., Arango, P., Fox, H., Lauver, C., McManus, M., Newacheck, P., et al. (1998). A new definition of children with special health care needs. *Pediatrics, 102,* 137–140.

N.A.C.H. State Policy Services. (2004, March). *Medicaid: Nation's health care safety net for children.* Retrieved from http://www.childrenshospitals.net/Content/ContentGroups/Public_Policy/Fact_Sheets1/20049/Medicaid_Nations_Health_Care_Safety_Net_for_Children.htm

Newacheck, P.W., & Taylor, W.R. (1994). Childhood chronic illness: Prevalence, severity, and impact. [Abstract]. *American Journal of Public Health, 82,* 364–371.

Omnibus Budget Reconciliation Act (OBRA) of 1981, PL 97-35, 35 Stat. 357.

Omnibus Budget Reconciliation Act (OBRA) of 1989, PL 101-239, 42 U.S.C. §§ 1396 *et seq.*

Smith, G.F., & Vadyasagar, D. (1980). *Historical review and recent advances in neonatal and perinatal medicine.* Evansville, IN: Mead Johnson Nutritional Division.

Social Security Act of 1935, PL 74-271, 42 U.S.C. §§ 301 *et seq.*
U.S. Department of Health and Human Services. (2003, Nov. 4). *New Freedom Initiative.* Retrieved from http://www.hhs.gov/newfreedom/
U.S. Department of Health and Human Services, Health Resources and Services Administration, Maternal and Child Health Bureau. (2001). *Celebrating 65 years of Title V: The Maternal and Child Health Program 1935–2000. A review of federal appropriations and allocations to states for Maternal and Child Health Programs under Title V of the Social Security Act.* Washington, DC: Author.
U.S. Department of Health and Human Services, Health Resources and Services Administration, Maternal and Child Health Bureau. (n.d.). *Child health USA 2002: Health services and utilization.* Retrieved from http://mchb.hrsa.gov/chusa02/main_pages/page_52.htm

6.3 COMMUNITY NURSING

J. Carolyn Graff

Nurses in the community provide comprehensive, lifelong care to individuals with developmental disabilities and their families. These services extend beyond those traditionally provided by community health or public health nurses and include settings where children and adults with developmental disabilities live, learn, work, play, and participate in their health care. Individuals with developmental disabilities live in their family homes, supported living arrangements, and residential programs. Supported living arrangements may include an individual's own home or apartment or a group home. Residential programs may include intermediate care and nursing facilities. Given the numerous practice settings for nurses, this chapter addresses nursing education and certification, standards of practice and roles, practice settings and responsibilities, and future roles and responsibilities for nurses working in the community with individuals with developmental disabilities.

NURSING EDUCATION AND CERTIFICATION

Professional registered nurses are prepared to practice following graduation from a school of nursing and after passing a national examination for registered nurse licensure. Registered nurses are prepared in associate, bachelor's, generic master's, or doctoral schools of nursing (see Table 6.3-1). The American Nurses Association has maintained that the bachelor's degree in nursing is the preferred educational preparation for entry into nursing practice. Licensed practical nurses, licensed vocational nurses, and unlicensed assistive personnel (nurse aides) may assist nurses with providing care to individuals with developmental disabilities or provide care with supervision of the professional registered nurse.

Various graduate programs in nursing prepare nurses with a bachelor's degree in nursing to become advanced practice registered nurses and function as clinical nurse specialists or nurse practitioners. Advanced

Table 6.3-1. Nursing education required for various job titles

Title	Licensure	Education program	Usual length of study
Professional registered nurse (R.N.)	R.N. by NCLEX-RN plus state boards of nursing	Associate's degree (A.D.N.)	2 years
	R.N. by NCLEX-RN plus state boards of nursing	Bachelor's degree (B.S.N.)	4–5 years
Advanced practice registered nurse: clinical nurse specialist	R.N. plus certification	Master of Science degree in Nursing (M.S.N.) in clinical specialty	B.S.N. plus 1.5–2 years
Advanced practice registered nurse: nurse practitioner	R.N. plus certification	Master of Science degree in Nursing (M.S.N.) with nurse practitioner specialty track	B.S.N. plus 1.5–2 years
Doctorate in nursing	R.N.	Doctor of Philosophy (Ph.D.)	M.S.N. plus 4–5 years
	R.N.	Doctor of Nursing Practice (D.N.P.)	M.S.N. plus 3 years
	R.N.	Doctor of Nursing Science (D.N.Sc.)	M.S.N. plus 3 years
	R.N.	Doctor of Nursing (N.D.)	B.A. or B.S. plus 3–5 years
Licensed practical (vocational) nurse	Licensed practical nurse or licensed vocational nurse by NCLEX-PN	Vocational training	1–1.5 years

Source: National Council of State Boards of Nursing (2004).
NCLEX-RN = National Council of State Boards of Nursing (NCSBN) NCLEX licensing examination for professional registered nurses.
NCLEX-PN = National Council of State Boards of Nursing (NCSBN) NCLEX licensing examination for licensed practical/vocational nurses.

practice nurses have specialized clinical knowledge and skills and hold a master's or doctoral degree. Clinical nurse specialists are clinical experts in evidence-based nursing practice in specialty areas such as adult health, maternal–child, pediatrics, psychiatric, and oncology nursing. They practice autonomously and integrate their expertise and knowledge of disease and treatments into their care of individuals. As direct care providers, clinical nurse specialists may perform comprehensive health assessments, develop differential diagnoses, prescribe treatments, and order diagnostic tests (American Nurses Association, 2004).

Nurse practitioners perform comprehensive assessments; diagnose; develop differential diagnoses; order, conduct, supervise, and interpret diagnostic tests; and prescribe treatments to manage acute and chronic illnesses (American Nurses Association, 2004). They practice independently and may specialize in areas such as acute, family, geriatric, neonatal, pediatric, and primary care. They collaborate with other health care professionals to promote health, prevent illness and injury, and treat and manage health problems.

All nurses have the responsibility to obtain ongoing education to assure they are knowledgeable and competent to practice nursing. This education may include 1) seeking out experiences and learning activities that will maintain and develop their clinical and professional skills and knowledge, 2) obtaining certification in a specialty area, and 3) pursuing graduate or postgraduate education. Continuing education is required for nursing relicensure in many states (National Council of State Boards of Nursing, 2004). Agencies such as the American Nurses Credentialing Center offer certification examinations in areas such as adult health, child and adolescent health, community health, family health, gerontology, home health, informatics, nursing administration, and pediatrics. Nursing certification in developmental disabilities is available through the Developmental Disabilities Nurses Association.

NURSING STANDARDS

In addition to the laws, rules, and regulations of each state's Nurse Practice Act, nurses' roles and responsibilities are guided by standards of practice outlined by the American Nurses Association (2004). The document "Nursing: Scope and Standards of Practice" guides all nurses in applying their professional knowledge and skills. Specialty standards have been developed for nurses working with individuals with developmental disabilities (Nehring, Roth, Natvig, Betz, Savage, & Krajicek, 2004). These specialty standards emphasize the common and unique needs of individuals with developmental disabilities and the expectations of nurses to address those needs.

The standards of practice specific to nurses working with individuals with developmental disabilities are listed in Table 6.3-2. Given the variability of environments and settings in which nurses work, the link between nurses' work environments and ability to practice and make decisions should be recognized. Nurses

Table 6.3-2. Standards of Intellectual and Developmental Disabilities Nursing Practice

1.	Assessment	The registered nurse who specializes in intellectual and developmental disabilities collects comprehensive data pertinent to the individual's health or situation.
2.	Diagnosis	The registered nurse who specializes in intellectual and developmental disabilities analyzes the assessment data to determine the diagnosis or issues.
3.	Outcome identification	The registered nurse who specializes in intellectual and developmental disabilities identifies expected outcomes for a plan to the patient or the situation.
4.	Planning	The registered nurse who specializes in intellectual and developmental disabilities develops a plan that prescribes strategies and alternatives to attain expected outcomes.
5.	Implementation	The registered nurse who specializes in intellectual and developmental disabilities implements the identified plan.
5a.	Coordination of care	The registered nurse who specializes in intellectual and developmental disabilities coordinates care delivery.
5b.	Health teaching and health promotion	The registered nurse who specializes in intellectual and developmental disabilities employs strategies to promote health and a safe environment.
5c.	Consultation	The registered nurse and the advanced practice registered nurse who specialize in intellectual and developmental disabilities provide consultation to influence the identified plan, enhance the abilities of others, and effect change.
5d.	Prescriptive authority and treatment	The advanced practice registered nurse who specializes in intellectual and developmental disabilities uses prescriptive authority, procedures, referrals, treatments, and therapies in accordance with state and federal laws and regulations.
6.	Evaluation	The registered nurse who specializes in intellectual and developmental disabilities evaluates progress toward attainment of outcomes.

Source: Nehring, Roth, Natvig, Betz, Savage, and Krajicek (2004).

must individualize practice and develop a plan of care with each individual and family that respects and integrates that individual's and family's values and beliefs. They establish a partnership with the individual, family, family support system, and other health care providers to collaborate and coordinate care.

Themes that span all areas of nursing practice and that are fundamental to many of the standards of practice include 1) providing age-appropriate and culturally and ethnically sensitive care, 2) maintaining a safe environment, 3) educating individuals and their families about healthy practices and treatment modalities, 4) assuring continuity of care, and 5) coordinating care across settings and among caregivers. In addition, nurses must be able to effectively manage information, communicate, and use technology (American Nurses Association, 2004). Standards of professional performance are presented in Table 6.3-3. Nurses are responsible for 1) the quality and effectiveness of their practice, 2) evaluating their practice, and 3) their competence to practice.

NURSING ROLES

In their effort to ensure that quality care is provided to all individuals and their families, nurses "blend evidence-based practice with intuition, caring, and compassion" (American Nurses Association, 2004, p. 17). Nursing is the "protection, promotion, and optimization of health and abilities, prevention of illness and injury, alleviation of suffering through the diagnosis and treatment of human response, and advocacy in the care of individuals, families, communities, and populations" (American Nurses Association, 2003, p. 6). In addition to providing direct care, nurses may assist individuals with developmental disabilities and their families in their role as nursing administrator, consultant, educator, or researcher.

Direct Care Provider

Nurses provide direct care to individuals with developmental disabilities following the previously mentioned standards of practice, standards of professional performance, and state Nurse Practice Acts. Nurses who are direct care providers may include care coordinators, case managers, clinic nurses, clinical nurse specialists, community health nurses, home health nurses, hospice nurses, nurse practitioners, occupational health nurses, and school nurses.

As a critical-thinking model, the nursing process serves as a basis for nursing practice and includes assessment, diagnosis, outcomes identification, planning, implementation, and evaluation (American Nurses Association, 2004). Goals of the nursing process are to restore, support, and promote health. Health restoration includes those nursing activities that modify the impact of an illness or disability. This concept is similar to rehabilitation or the process in which an individual relearns a lost skill or behavior. Nursing practice that is supportive includes modifying relationships or the environment to support the individual's health. Health promotion practice includes 1) mobilizing healthy patterns of living, 2) fostering personal and family devel-

Table 6.3-3. Standards of Professional Performance of Intellectual and Developmental Disabilities Nursing

Standard	Description
1. Quality of practice	The registered nurse who specializes in intellectual and developmental disabilities systematically enhances the quality and effectiveness of nursing practice.
2. Education	The registered nurse who specializes in intellectual and developmental disabilities attains knowledge and competency that reflects current nursing practice.
3. Professional practice evaluation	The registered nurse who specializes in intellectual and developmental disabilities evaluates his or her own nursing practice in relation to professional practice standards and guidelines, relevant statutes, rules, and regulations.
4. Collegiality	The registered nurse who specializes in intellectual and developmental disabilities interacts with and contributes to the professional development of peers and colleagues.
5. Collaboration	The registered nurse who specializes in intellectual and developmental disabilities collaborates with the individual with intellectual and developmental disabilities, family, and others in the conduct of nursing practice.
6. Ethics	The registered nurse who specializes in intellectual and developmental disabilities integrates ethical provisions in all areas of practice.
7. Research	The registered nurse who specializes in intellectual and developmental disabilities integrates research findings into practice.
8. Resource utilization	The registered nurse who specializes in intellectual and developmental disabilities considers factors related to safety, effectiveness, cost, and impact on practice in the planning and delivery of nursing services to individuals with intellectual and developmental disabilities.
9. Leadership	The registered nurse who specializes in intellectual and developmental disabilities provides leadership in the professional practice setting and the profession.

Source: Nehring, Roth, Natvig, Betz, Savage, and Krajicek (2004).

opment, and 3) supporting self-defined goals of individuals and their families. This definition of health promotion is similar to habilitation or the process by which individuals develop new skills and abilities (Russell & Free, 1994).

Nursing Administrator

The nursing administrator provides direct and indirect services to individuals with developmental disabilities. Direct services tend to emphasize managing crises, and indirect services emphasize prevention. Indirect services may include developing and implementing 1) performance indicators to evaluate competencies of staff providing nursing care, 2) policies and procedures to ensure consistency in practice and outcomes of care, and 3) quality-assurance activities to determine if staff are performing activities effectively (Graff, Whitaker, Murphy, & McFadden, 2005).

Consultant

As consultants, nurses share their expertise in evaluation, treatment, and planning of health care with individuals with developmental disabilities. Nurses provide consultations in the nurse practice settings described in the next section and other community settings such as government facilities and agencies. Nursing consultation may include 1) coordinating specialty health care, 2) facilitating access to services, 3) involving stakeholders in the decision-making process, 4) monitoring health care financing, 5) planning hospitalizations and emergency services, 6) planning treatment, and 7) sharing pertinent health information (American Academy of Pediatrics, 1999). Nurses may be consultants to screen children with or at risk for developmental disabilities; diagnose the type, scope, and etiology of developmental disabilities; treat primary and secondary medical conditions; and provide treatment on a short-term basis. Nurses providing consultation services to individuals with developmental disabilities should have at least a bachelor's degree in nursing; however, most consultants have master's or doctoral degrees.

Educator

Nurses may serve as educators in the following positions: administrator, direct care provider, faculty member in a nursing program, researcher, and school nurse. School nurses spend significant amounts of time educating students, teachers, parents, and others about the health needs of children with developmental disabilities and the implications for success in school. Nurses may educate parents, individuals with developmental disabilities, and caregivers about the importance of preventive health care and visits for health surveillance. They educate student nurses, other nurses, and service providers about developmental disabilities and the health-related accommodations needed to ensure inclusion and optimal health of individuals with developmental disabilities.

Researcher

Nurses conduct research at a level appropriate to their education (Developmental Disabilities Nurses Association, 1995). Professional registered nurses may be involved in data collection, data analysis, and manuscript preparation. Nurses with doctoral degrees design and conduct research and ensure that findings are disseminated to other professionals. Nurses should possess current knowledge of research conducted in the area of developmental disabilities so that their practice can be based on scientific evidence whenever possible.

Nurses should also possess up-to-date knowledge of research that is being conducted so that they can refer interested individuals and their families to the most appropriate research study. Information on current clinical studies can be located at the National Institutes of Health web site (http://clinicalstudies.info.nih.gov/). Nurses are responsible for assuring that the rights of research participants are protected and that research integrity is sound. The Office for Human Research Protections establishes policy and provides guidelines for protecting the welfare of individuals with developmental disabilities participating in research studies (U.S. Department of Health and Human Services, n.d.). Information about protecting the rights of research participants with developmental disabilities can be found at http://www.hhs.gov/ohrp/irb/irb_chapter6.htm.

NURSE PRACTICE SETTINGS, ROLES, AND RESPONSIBILITIES

Nurses providing care to individuals with developmental disabilities and their families practice in homes, schools, ambulatory care clinics, occupational health clinics, independent nursing practices, and University Centers for Excellence in Developmental Disabilities, Education, Research, and Service (UCEDDs). Nurses' education and practice settings greatly influence their practice. Professional registered nurses specializing in developmental disabilities have an understanding of the concepts and strategies of nursing practice in developmental disabilities and can assess, plan, implement, and evaluate the health and health services of individuals with developmental disabilities. These nurses may serve as care coordinators for individuals with developmental disabilities who have less complex needs. In the absence of an advanced practice registered nurse, professional registered nurses may provide care to individuals with more complex needs in consultation with an advanced practice registered nurse. Advanced practice registered nurses perform many of the same activities as professional registered nurses; however, their practice involves greater depth and breadth of knowledge, greater ability to synthesize data, and increased complexity of skills and interventions.

Homes

According to the Administration on Developmental Disabilities (2000), 88% of the more than 4 million individuals with developmental disabilities in the United States live with their families or in their own households. Children with developmental disabilities grow up with their family members and may continue to live with their parents, brothers, and sisters into adulthood. Many individuals with developmental disabilities, however, live in their own homes with support and assistance from family members, friends, neighbors, and professionals.

Early Intervention and Preschool Programs Early intervention programs offer services to meet the needs of infants and toddlers age 3 or younger who have disabilities in physical, cognitive, communication, social, emotional, and/or adaptive development (Individuals with Disabilities Education Act Amendments of 1997, PL 105-17). Preschool programs offer services to meet the developmental needs of children ages 3–5. Nurses provide services to children enrolled in early intervention and preschool programs as members of or consultants to teams of professionals. They often provide services in the homes of infants and toddlers to ensure that these services occur in "natural environments" or "settings that are natural or normal for the child's age peers who have no disabilities" (U.S. Department of Education, 1999). In addition, they help with the transition from an early intervention program to a preschool program through thoughtful planning and collaboration with the child's parents to ensure that the child's health needs are met in the new setting.

Home Health Home health care includes skilled nursing care and other skilled care services, such as physical and occupational therapy, speech-language therapy, and social services (Centers for Medicare & Medicaid Services, 2004). Skilled nursing care can be short term or long term and refers to services that can only be performed safely and correctly by a professional registered nurse, a licensed practical nurse, or a licensed vocational nurse. Short-term home health care includes treatment for an illness or injury to assist an individual to regain independence or to become as independent as possible. Services may be needed for an acute illness that may or may not be related to developmental disabilities. For example, a child with Down syndrome may have home visits following open-heart surgery for a cardiac defect identified at birth. Short-term home health care is required to monitor the child's postoperative recovery and may extend over several weeks or months.

The goal of long-term home health care is to assist an individual to maintain the highest level of health or ability and to learn to live with the illness or disability. The level and complexity of care an individual requires determines the type of nurse providing the care. For example, a 10-year-old child with cerebral palsy, spastic quadriplegia, and seizure disorder uses gastrostomy tube feedings, has a tracheostomy, and uses a ventilator. This child requires daily ongoing or long-term home health care. This child will require care by a professional registered nurse or licensed practical nurse. Any care provided by a licensed practical nurse, licensed vocational nurse, or unlicensed assistive personnel must be supervised by a professional registered nurse with the proper knowledge and skills.

Hospice Hospice and palliative care occur at the end of life and include care focused on relief of symptoms and on providing psychological and social support to individuals with life-threatening or terminal illness and their family members. This approach addresses these individuals' physical, emotional, social, and spiritual needs and aims to improve their quality of life. Hospice and palliative care can occur in an individual's home, apartment, group home, hospice facility, or hospital.

Interdisciplinary teams of professionals such as chaplains, nurses, physicians, social workers, and other health care professionals offer this care. Major responsibilities of the team include (National Hospice, 2003)

- Managing the individual's pain and symptoms
- Assisting the individual and family with the emotional, psychosocial, and spiritual aspects of dying
- Providing needed drugs, medical supplies, and equipment

- Coaching the family on how to care for the individual
- Delivering special services like speech and physical therapy
- Making short-term inpatient care available when pain or symptoms become too difficult to manage at home or the caregiver needs respite
- Providing bereavement care and counseling to surviving family and friends

Extensive efforts may be needed to prevent and alleviate pain. Pain is an unpleasant subjective sensory and emotional experience that is associated with actual and potential tissue damage or is described in terms of tissue damage (American Pain Society, 1999). Or, as described by McCaffery (1968), pain is what an individual says it is and exists when the individual says it exists.

Nurses may face challenges as they try to identify pain experiences of individuals with developmental disabilities. Because pain is considered multidimensional and affects the emotional and spiritual dimensions of one's life, nurses may be unable to recognize an individual's cues and behaviors indicating pain. Undertreatment of pain occurs more often in individuals who cannot speak for themselves (American Pain Society, 1999). Therefore, nurses must rely on their own observational skills, knowledge of an individual's behavior, and others' knowledge of the individual's behaviors that indicate pain.

Communication between the individual with developmental disabilities and nurses should focus on the individual's preferences for care that will provide the best quality of life during the illness. Whenever possible, individuals with developmental disabilities should discuss their desires for end-of-life care in advance of a crisis. When treatment options are available, the individual should participate fully in making a decision about the type and extent of treatment.

When the individual with developmental disabilities cannot make a decision about care and no advance directive exists, another individual (or individuals) must give direction about the decision. This decision maker, or surrogate, is a close family member or friend or an individual designated by law. Surrogate decisions about care are based on one of these standards and followed in this order:

1. The instructions expressed by the person such as in a living will or orally when the person was capable of making decisions
2. Inferences about what the person would likely want in a particular situation based on what is known about his prior behavior and patterns of decision making
3. What the surrogate and health care team believe is in the person's best interest (which is resorted to when the person's wishes and values are not known.) (*Merck Manual,* 2004)

This last standard may often be the one used with individuals with developmental disabilities. Whenever possible, advance directives (i.e., a living will or durable power of attorney for health care) should be prepared.

Tuffrey-Wijne (2003) reported a lack of empirical data around the palliative care needs of individuals with developmental disabilities. Potential problems in providing palliative care to individuals with developmental disabilities included 1) late presentation of the illness, 2) difficulty assessing symptoms, 3) difficulty in understanding the illness and its implications, and 4) ethical issues around decision making and consent to treatment. They recommended future research on the views and experiences of individuals with intellectual disabilities focusing on symptom assessment, evaluation of current practice and access to services, and development of information and training materials.

Schools

Although schools offer services to meet children's educational needs and ensure children's success in an inclusive environment, school nurses should ensure that needed school and community resources are available to promote children's health and prepare children for full participation in school and society. School nurses 1) provide direct health care to students with developmental disabilities; 2) educate students, teachers, parents, and others about the health needs of the child; 3) develop students' individualized health plans (IHPs); 4) collaborate with educators, parents, and other professionals to ensure that each child's IHP and individualized education program (IEP) meet the child's health needs and are congruent; 5) serve as consultants to educators on health care needs and strategies to integrate the delivery of health services to the child over the school day; and 6) promote activities to prevent serious side effects or complications of the developmental disabilities. For example, the school nurse recognizes the importance of exercise in reducing obesity and suggests exercise for students with Down syndrome or Prader-Willi syndrome to prevent obesity that is associated with these genetic disorders.

Delegation of health-related procedures may be necessary when the school nurse is unavailable to the child during part of the school day. The school nurse has responsibility for training staff to carry out the procedures, supervising these procedures, and assuring that the procedures are modified when necessary. The role of the school nurse in promoting inclusion of students with special health care needs is outlined in Table 6.3-4 and demonstrated in Bruce's story.

Bruce is an 11-year-old boy with spina bifida, Arnold Chiari malformation, and tonic-clonic seizure disorder who attends sixth grade in his neighborhood school. He receives medication for his seizure disorder during the school day and requires monitoring for seizures. He also uses urinary catheterization twice during the school day. The school nurse is a professional registered nurse who is responsible for three schools. Because she cannot be present for Bruce's medication and urinary catheterization procedures, she delegates these responsibilities to a licensed practical nurse who works at Bruce's school. The school nurse has trained the licensed practical nurse, classroom teachers, and a paraprofessional working with Bruce on the procedure to follow if Bruce has a seizure. She supervises these procedures and is responsible for training all school staff working with Bruce in these procedures. The health-related procedures have been integrated into Bruce's activities throughout the school day. Using the nursing process, the school nurse has included information about these procedures in Bruce's IHP and serves as the health expert on his IEP team.

Table 6.3-4. Role of the school nurse in inclusion

Identifies students with health care needs and provides support in developing individualized education programs
Maintains a vital role by serving as case manager and participating in interdisciplinary conferences to promote student success in the classroom
Involves students and families in health care planning and management
Advocates for students' health rights to ensure the school's responsiveness to students' educational and health needs
Individualizes performance expectations based on students' physical, emotional, social, and cognitive abilities
Provides input on modifications to the physical space, program, time, supplies, training, personnel, and curriculum
Develops individual health care plans for students with health needs to provide educational awareness for school staff and give direction in safely managing these concerns in the classroom
Obtains orders from health care providers after assessing students' needs for technological assistance with skilled procedures during the school day
Develops a skilled procedure record, delegating nursing services when appropriate, providing training for school staff, and monitoring periodically the delivery of all skilled procedures in the school setting performed by nonprofessional care providers
Provides peers and their families information to help them understand the diverse health care needs of students in the classroom
Fosters peer acceptance and provides classroom teachers with information and support
Participates in interdisciplinary instruction or team teaching in the classroom to educate students on health issues and promote healthy lifestyle behaviors

Source: National Association of School Nurses (2001).

Ambulatory Care Clinics

Children and adults with developmental disabilities visit ambulatory care clinics located in community health centers, health departments, hospitals, and physician's offices in which primary care or specialty services are provided by nurses and other health care providers. Mobile health services may be available as traveling teams of health care providers who visit remote areas by motor vehicle, plane, helicopter, or boat. Clinics that are convenient and located closer to individuals with developmental disabilities can help with providing high-quality health care and ensure that services are based on the individual's need, preference, and choice (American Association on Mental Retardation & The Arc of the United States, 2002).

Occupational Health

Occupational health nurses provide health services for individuals with developmental disabilities working in business or industry. They provide on-the-job treatment, follow-up, referrals, and emergency care for job-related injuries and illnesses. They also serve as gatekeepers for health services, rehabilitation, and return-to-work issues. These nurses may provide counseling about work-related injuries, substance abuse, and emotional problems and make referrals to employee assistance programs and other community resources. Occupational health nurses teach and encourage workers to take responsibility for their own health, using strategies such as smoking cessation, exercise, nutrition and weight control, and stress management. They monitor the health status of workers to identify workplace exposures, gather health and hazard data, and use data to prevent injury and illness (American Association of Occupational Health Nurses, 2004). Occupational health nurses may ensure appropriate job placements for individuals with developmental disabilities and identify strategies for success in the workplace.

Independent Nursing Practices

Advanced practice registered nurses in independent practice may provide outpatient care as family, geriatric, pediatric, primary care, or women's health nurse practitioners. They may provide services in their own office or during a visit to the home of individuals with developmental disabilities. Providing health care in the home can serve to minimize the trauma experienced by some individuals when their routines are altered and they are forced to visit an unfamiliar environment. Nurses in independent practice collaborate with physicians, therapists, and other health care professionals in the community.

University Centers for Excellence in Developmental Disabilities

UCEDDs, a network of centers affiliated with major research universities, are located in every state and territory in the United States. The goal of UCEDDs is to ensure that all individuals, including individuals with disabilities, participate fully in their communities. UCEDDs offer interdisciplinary training of students and fellows and opportunities for research related to developmental disabilities (Administration on Developmental Disabilities, 2000). Children and adults with developmental disabilities and their families can participate in interdisciplinary, family-centered, culturally competent, and state-of-the-art treatment and evaluations (Association of University Centers on Disabilities, 2001).

Nurses working in UCEDDs participate in all aspects of the center to include providing treatment and evaluations as a single discipline or as a member of a team. Nurses have master's or doctoral degrees and extensive knowledge and skills in the care of individuals with developmental disabilities. They serve as experts to individuals with developmental disabilities, families, and other nurses and professionals. They share their knowledge and skills with students in all disciplines and conduct research related to developmental disabilities. Consider the experiences of Jisele at a UCEDD.

Jisele is a 3-year-old with trisomy 9 who lives with her parents and a 6-year-old sister. Jisele and her parents participated in an interdisciplinary team evaluation at a UCEDD. Recommendations from the team's evaluations included making the transition from home-based early intervention services to a center-based preschool program. The preschool program would offer Jisele opportunities to spend time with other children and allow her mother respite.

Jisele's parents are ready to proceed with developmental services; however, they are unsure how the staff will handle Jisele's tracheostomy, frequent suctioning, gastrostomy tube, and breathing treatments every 4 hours. To work toward a smooth transition into the preschool program, the nurse consultant for the preschool met with Jisele's parents to begin developing an IHP. Jisele's parents took the lead in developing the procedures to be followed at preschool for Jisele's tracheostomy care, gastrostomy tube feedings, and breathing treatments. Her mother visited the preschool to assist the nurse in teaching the procedures to staff.

CONCLUSION

Nurses have a long history of advocating and caring for individuals with developmental disabilities and their families. Factors such as the availability of nurses and other health professionals (Cooper, 2004; Erickson, Holm, & Chelminiak, 2004; Rinne, 2004), genetic and genomic advances (Collins, Green, Guttmacher, & Guyer, 2003), health care costs (Grosse, 2004), the need for ongoing nursing education and certification (Nehring, 2004), the aging nursing workforce (Mitchell, 2003), and the increasing longevity of individuals with developmental disabilities (Braddock, Hemp, & Rizzolo, 2004) create new challenges for individuals with developmental disabilities; their families; nurses; other health care professionals; and the numerous local, state, and national agencies responsible for providing services. Building on their legacy, nurses must move to the forefront as advocates who promote self-determination, independence, and a fulfilling quality of life for individuals with developmental disabilities.

REFERENCES

Administration on Developmental Disabilities. (2000). *Public Law 106–402.* Retrieved November 7, 2004, from http://www.acf.hhs.gov/programs/add/DDA.htm

American Academy of Pediatrics, Committee on Children with Disabilities. (1999). Care coordination: Integrating health and related systems of care for children with special health care needs. *Pediatrics, 104*(4), 978–981.

American Association of Occupational Health Nurses. (2004). *The occupational and environmental health nursing profession.* Retrieved November 7, 2004, from http://www.aaohn.org

American Association on Mental Retardation & The Arc of the United States. (2002). *The Arc and AAMR position statements: Health care.* Retrieved November 7, 2004, from http://www.thearc.org/position-statements.htm

American Nurses Association. (2003). *Nursing's social policy statement* (2nd ed.). Washington, DC: Author.

American Nurses Association. (2004). *Nursing: Scope and standards of practice.* Washington, DC: Author.

American Pain Society. (1999). *Principles of analgesic use in the treatment of acute pain and cancer pain* (4th ed.). Glenview, IL: Author.

Association of University Centers on Disabilities. (2001). *Association of University Centers on Disabilities: Mission and vision.* Retrieved November 7, 2004, from http://www.aucd.org/about/mission.htm

Braddock, D., Hemp, R., & Rizzolo, M.C. (2004). State of the states in developmental disabilities: 2004. *Mental Retardation, 42*(5), 356–370.

Centers for Medicare & Medicaid Services. (2004). *Medicare and home health care* (Publication No. CMS-10969). Washington, DC: U.S. Department of Health and Human Services.

Collins, F.S., Green, E.D., Guttmacher, A.E., & Guyer, M.S. (2003). A vision for the future of genomics research. *Nature, 422*(6934), 835–847.

Cooper, R.A. (2004). Weighing the evidence for expanding physician supply. *Annals of Internal Medicine, 141*(9), 705–714.

Developmental Disabilities Nurses Association. (1995). *Standards of developmental disabilities nursing practice.* Blaine, WA: Author.

Erickson, J.I., Holm, L.J., & Chelminiak, L. (2004). Keeping the nursing shortage from becoming a nursing crisis. *Journal of Nursing Administration, 34*(2), 83–87.

Graff, C., Whitaker, T., Murphy, L., & McFarland, S. (2005). Roles and responsibilities of nurses and other health professionals. In W.M. Nehring (Eds.), *Core curriculum for specializing in intellectual and developmental disabilities* (pp. 83–93). Boston: Jones and Bartlett.

Grosse, S. (2004). Economic costs associated with mental retardation, cerebral palsy, hearing loss, and vision impairment—United States, 2003. *Morbidity and Mortality Weekly Report, 53*(3), 57–59.

Individuals with Disabilities Education Act (IDEA) Amendments of 1997, PL 105–17, 20 U.S.C. §§ 1400 *et seq.*

McCaffery, M. (1968). *Nurse practice theories related to cognition, bodily pain, and man–environment interactions.* Los Angeles: University of California–Los Angeles.

Merck Manual of Medical Information—Second Home Edition. (2004). Decision making (surrogate). Retrieved November 9, 2004, from http://www.merck.com/mmhe/sec01/ch009/ch009f.html?alt=pf

Mitchell, G.J. (2003). Nursing shortage or nursing famine: Looking beyond numbers? *Nursing Science Quarterly, 16*(3), 219–224.

National Association of School Nurses (NASN). (2001). *School health nursing services role in health care: Inclusion.* Retrieved November 8, 2004, from http://www.nasn.org/briefs/briefs.htm

National Council of State Boards of Nursing. (2004). *Nursing regulation: Nursing licensure and certification.* Retrieved November 9, 2004, from http://www.ncsbn.org/regulation/nlc.asp

National Hospice and Palliative Care Organization. (2003). *What is hospice and palliative care?* Retrieved November 9, 2004, from http://www.nhpco.org/i4a/pages/index.cfm?pageid=3281

Nehring, W. (2004). Directions for the future of intellectual and developmental disabilities as a nursing specialty. *International Journal of Nursing in Intellectual and Developmental Disabilities, 1*(1). Retrieved from http://journal.hsmc.org/ijnidd

Nehring, W., Roth, S.P., Natvig, D., Betz, C.L., Savage, T., & Krajicek, M. (2004). *Intellectual and developmental disabilities nursing: Scope and standards of practice.* Silver Spring, MD: Publishing Program of the American Nurses Association.

Rinne, C.A. (2004). Nursing shortage or nursing famine: Looking beyond numbers? *Nursing Science Quarterly, 17*(3), 281.

Russell, F.F., & Free, T.A. (1994). The nurse's role in habilitation. In S.P. Roth & J.S. Morse (Eds.), *A life-span approach to nursing care for individuals with developmental disabilities* (pp. 59–88). Baltimore: Paul H. Brookes Publishing Co.

Tuffrey-Wijne, I. (2003). The palliative care needs of people with intellectual disabilities: A literature review. *Journal of Palliative Medicine, 17*(1), 55–62.

U.S. Department of Education. (1999). *IDEA '97 final regulations.* Retrieved November 8, 2004, from http://www.ed.gov/offices/OSERS/Policy/IDEA/regs.html

U.S. Department of Health and Human Services, Office of Human Research Protections. (n.d.). *Institutional review board guidebook: Chapter VI, Special classes of subjects.* Retrieved November 8, 2004, from http://www.hhs.gov/ohrp/irb/irb_chapter6.htm

6.4 HEALTH ISSUES IN SCHOOL

Peter J. Smith

Clinicians frequently interact with local school system(s) and have a number of critical roles to play for families in their practice whose children require special education services. This chapter 1) briefly reviews the history of the special education laws, 2) outlines provisions of the Individuals with Disabilities Education Act (IDEA) of 1990 (PL 101-476) and its amendments, and 3) discusses implications of the special education process for child health providers.

HISTORY OF SPECIAL EDUCATION LAW

The 20th century experienced a slow, steady progression of legislation and program development acknowledging the citizenship and fundamental rights of individuals with disabilities. The timelines in Tables 6.4-1 and 6.4-2 delineate events that have had a profound effect on the current configuration of services for children with disabilities. In 1935, the passage of Title V of the Social Security Act of 1935 (PL 74-271) created the Crippled Children's Programs in each state to provide services for children identified as having disabilities such as *infantile paralysis* (a term that is now no longer in use). In the 1960s, the first President's Panel on Mental Retardation proposed a new conceptualization of intellectual and developmental disabilities. Rather than making the primary focus a view of what people cannot do, the panel urged celebration of and responsiveness to

6.4 Health Issues in School is reprinted with permission from *Contemporary Pediatrics*, Vol. 9, 2002, pp. 102–127. *Contemporary Pediatrics* is a copyrighted publication of Advanstar Communications Inc.

Table 6.4-1. Selected special education legislation

1935	*Social Security Act of 1935 (PL 74-271)*—This act established federal responsibility for the well-being of children and their mothers; a specific component addressed "Services for Crippled Children."
1963	*Maternal and Child Health and Mental Retardation Planning Amendments (PL 88-156)*—These amendments were the result of John F. Kennedy's presidential commission and provided new federal funding for special projects for children with intellectual disabilities (i.e., early screening).
1966	*Elementary and Secondary Education Act (ESEA) Amendments of 1966 (PL 89-750)*—These amendments added to the ESEA of 1965 (PL 89-10) to establish the first federal grant program for the education of children with disabilities at the local school level. They also established the Bureau of Education for the Handicapped.
1970	*Education of the Handicapped Act of 1970 (PL 91-230)*—This legislation replaced Title VI of PL 89-750.
1973	*Rehabilitation Act of 1973 (PL 93-112)*—This act prohibited federal agencies and any program/activity receiving federal funding from discriminating against someone with a disability.
1975	*Education for All Handicapped Children Act of 1975 (PL 94-142)*—This act passed in perpetuity by an overwhelming majority. It mandated free appropriate public education (FAPE) and was implemented in 1978.
1986	*Education of the Handicapped Act Amendments of 1986 (PL 99-457)*—These amendments established early intervention, which is appropriate services to infants and toddlers with disabilities and their families.
1990	*Americans with Disabilities Act (ADA) of 1990 (PL 101-336)*—National mandate against discrimination based on disability.
	Individuals with Disabilities Education Act (IDEA) of 1990 (PL 101-476)—This act reauthorized PL 91-230 and combined PL 99-457 and PL 94-142.
1997	*IDEA Amendments of 1997 (PL 105-17)*—These amendments reauthorized and expanded IDEA.
2004	*Individuals with Disabilities Education Improvement Act of 2004 (PL 108-446)*—This act reauthorized and further expanded IDEA.

Table 6.4-2. Court cases related to special education

1954	*Brown v. Board of Education of Topeka*—The U.S. Supreme Court ruled that education is a right that must be made available to all on equal terms; in addition, separate facilities were found to be inherently unequal.
1971	*Pennsylvania Association of Retarded Citizens v. Commonwealth of Pennsylvania*—The court ruled that all individuals with intellectual disabilities are capable of benefiting from education.
1972	*Mills v. Board of Education of the District of Columbia*—The court ruled that school systems must educate students with disabilities even if their funds are insufficient. In addition, this ruling noted significant racial disparities within special education.
1982	*Board of Education of the Hendrick Hudson Central School District v. Rowley*—The court ruled that school districts must provide appropriate services that allow a student with disabilities to benefit from instruction. School districts are not required to provide optimal services.
1984	*Irving Independent School District v. Tatro*—The court ruled that school districts must provide school health–related medical services if the qualifications of the three-prong "bright-line" test are met: 1) the child qualifies under the Education for All Handicapped Act of 1975 (PL 94-142) for special education, 2) the service is necessary for the child to benefit from special education, and 3) the service needs to be provided by a qualified person other than a physician.
1985	*Burlington School Committee v. Department of Education*—The court ruled that tuition reimbursement can be given for private school placement when the public school cannot or has not provided an appropriate individualized education program or free appropriate public education.
1994	*Felix v. Cayetano (Felix Consent Decree)*—The court ruled that the Hawaii Departments of Education and Health must establish a new system of care by June 30, 2000, for children with disabilities who are eligible for and in need of education and/or mental health services.
1999	*Cedar Rapids Community School District, Petitioner v. Garret F.*—This ruling affirmed the *Irving Independent School District v. Tatro ruling:* Services provided by nonphysicians, when these services are needed for a child to attend school, are required as related services under PL 94-142.

what children with disabilities can do. Furthermore, the panel responded to the demand from parents and professional advocates that a more systematic response to the educational and functional needs of children with disabilities should be implemented (National Academy of Sciences, 1982; Tjossem, 1976).

The watershed event occurred in 1975 when the U.S. Congress passed the Education for All Handicapped Children Act of 1975 (PL 94-142) by an overwhelming majority. Subsequent amendments and refinements have maintained the law's core tenets and extended its reach to infants, toddlers, and preschoolers with disabilities. States must provide a free appropriate public education (FAPE) to all children with disabilities, and the education should take place in the *least restrictive environment.* This process involves 1) identification and referral of all children with special needs; 2) evaluation and preparation of a detailed plan; 3) implementation of educational and related services; and 4) maintenance of a child's rights through due process.

Identification and Referral of All Children with Special Needs

Children with functionally relevant health concerns (e.g., congenital anomalies, cerebral palsy, hearing loss) or developmental delays are eligible for early intervention under the IDEA Amendments of 1997 (PL 105-17) and can be identified and referred for early intervention services as early as birth. Parents, physicians, or child care providers can refer children for a team evaluation and subsequent service provision (National Early Childhood Technical Assistance System, n.d.). Those who refer children younger than 3 years old, however, need to be aware of the administrative details in their state (Shonkoff & Meisels, 2000). Federal law does not mandate the lead agency for birth to 3 programs, and *disability* is defined state by state. Therefore, referrals should be directed to the state-appointed agency. In some states, the lead agency is the Department of Public Health. In others, it is the Department of Education or another program. States can also change their agency structure at any time (Hebbeler, Spiker, Wagner, Cameto, McKenn, & SRI International, 1999). All identification of children older than 3 years is handled by the state Department of Education. In addition, all school systems are required to have established formal preschool identification procedures to detect developmental concerns as they emerge.

Evaluation and Preparation of a Detailed Plan

Every child involved in special education must have an individualized education program (IEP) that includes information on the child's current performance, annual goals, and planned services with objective criteria for measuring the child's progress on at least an annual basis. A parent must be invited to contribute to the formation of the IEP. In addition, the information in the IEP must be based on the assessment of a multidisciplinary team. Evaluation by child health professionals as part of the IEP is particularly relevant for children with complex medical conditions; children who are receiving nursing care at school; children who are taking medications; and children who have substantial mental health concerns. The actual composition of the team should be tailored to the questions that have arisen for the student.

In carrying out the evaluation, school systems must use a variety of assessments, including appropriate standardized materials that are technically sound and address educational, behavioral, physical, and developmental concerns. The assessments must be free of racial and cultural bias and be administered in the child's own language or mode of communication (e.g., American Sign Language) by personnel who are appropriately trained and experienced in the use of the particular assessments.

Implementation of Educational and Related Services

Early intervention services for young children are delivered by a variety of personnel in a variety of venues as designated through the individualized family service plan (IFSP). The services include home- and center-based interventions by physical and occupational therapists as well as speech-language therapy, deaf and blind education, parent training, and social work services. Increasingly, early intervention programs are providing intervention for children with problematic behavior either as a primary concern or secondary to another disability (e.g., developmental delay, deafness). Special education for preschoolers, school-age children, and adolescents encompasses activities that enhance the forward development of every child. For individuals with severe disabilities, the focus may be on improvement in activities of daily living (ADLs) such as eating, ambulation, transfers, hygiene, toileting, and communicating basic needs. For children with complex learning styles, providers may focus on noticing the subtleties of the children's nonverbal learning disabilities and providing the children with appropriate strategies to deal with their inability to understand simple spatial relationships.

Services for children with disabilities should take place in the least restrictive environment. School systems are required to look carefully at the placement of children with disabilities to ensure that the children have full access to the general education curriculum. PL 105-17 states that

> Each public agency shall ensure (1) that to the maximum extent appropriate, children with disabilities, including children in public or private institutions or other care facilities, are educated with children who are nondisabled; and (2) that special classes, separate schooling or other removal of children with disabilities from the regular educational environment occurs only if the nature or severity of the disability is such that education in regular classes with the use of supplementary aids and services cannot be achieved satisfactorily.

PL 105-17 addresses barriers to education through the provision of special education and related services. The law defines special education as "specially designed instruction, at no cost to parents, to meet the unique needs of a child with a disability." Related services are defined as "transportation, and such developmental, corrective, and other support services as may be required to assist a child with a disability to benefit from special education." Such services may include speech and audiology services, psychological services, physical and occupational therapy, recreation, social work, school health services, counseling, and medical services for diagnostic and evaluation purposes. These services can be provided only if they are related to the child's educational needs.

Maintenance of a Child's Rights Through Due Process

PL 101-476 and its amendments ensure that parents are involved in all decisions regarding education plans, placement, and services for the child with disabilities. Under PL 105-17, parents of children with special needs have the right to dispute the plan that is developed for their child and to request further evaluation and/or the implementation of a different set of services. Due process provisions are carefully delineated. Parents have the right to timeliness in the proceedings, open disclosure of all assessments that may influence the program recommendations, and proper education on the issues at hand. These due process rights have provided a level of educational assurance to children with disabilities that is actually above what is accorded to children without disabilities. Many families have used these mechanisms to protect the rights of their children. A few have even fought their cases as far as the U.S. Supreme Court.

IMPLICATIONS FOR CLINICIANS

Prior to the implementation of PL 94-142 in 1978, health care providers had a limited role with regard to special education. They might have been asked to write a note to keep a child with disabilities out of school or to help find an institutional placement for an infant with intellectual disabilities. This role has changed dramatically, due in large part to the expanding amount of children served by special education (see Figure 6.4-1). Health care providers have clear roles and expectations to serve as active members in the special education process through actions on behalf of individual children or families; through actions in a local region (i.e., on the school board or town council); or through actions at the state and national level (e.g., by writing letters or giving testimony).

When children enter early intervention, the full extent of their health and developmental profile may still not be thoroughly delineated or understood (American Academy of Pedicatrics, 2000, 2001; Green & Pal-

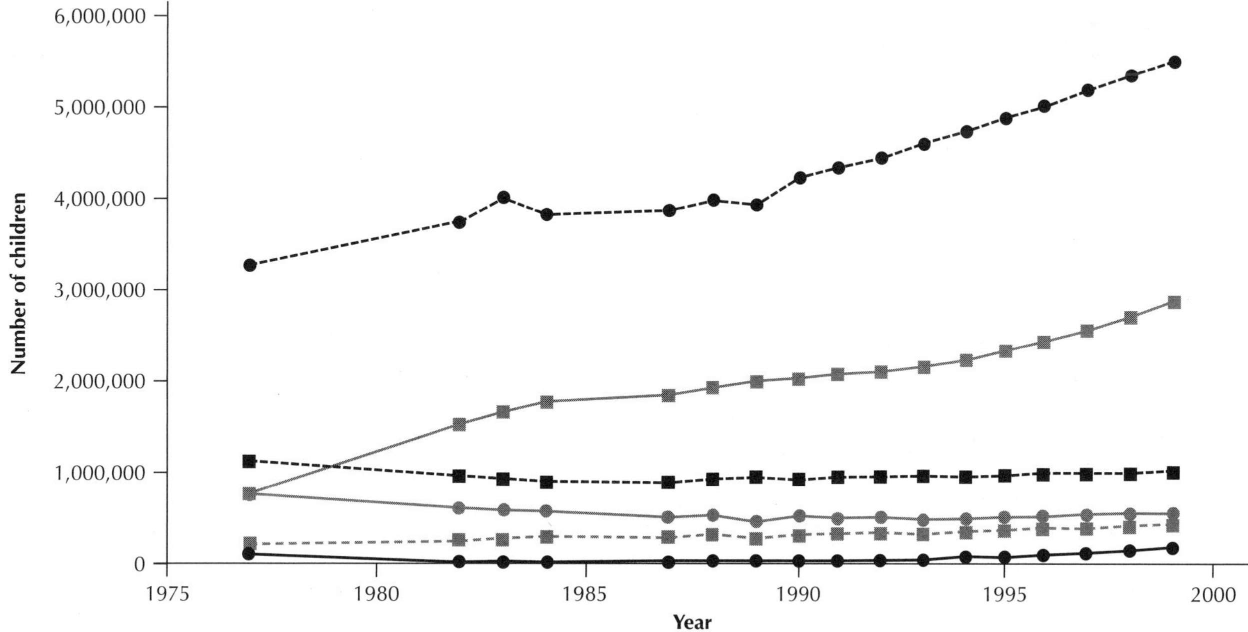

Figure 6.4-1: Number of children (age 6–21) served by the Education for All Handicapped Children Act of 1975 (PL 94-142) and its amendments listed by disability (from the United States and territories/outlying areas).
Source: U.S. Department of Education (2000).
Key: ●---● All disabilities; ■—■ Learning disabilities; ■---■ Speech-language disabilities; ●—● Intellectual disabilities; ■---■ Emotional disturbances; ●—● Other health impairments.

fry, 2000; Levine, 1994; Shonkoff & Phillips, 2000). During the period of early intervention, additional components of disability are often discovered or elucidated. Health care providers can often make or break a school-age child's chances of getting appropriate special education services. Failure to use the appropriate terminology may result in poor communication with the school and lack of services for a given child.

Health care providers who take the care to learn the specific language of the special education eligibility determinations can be extremely helpful to families. If they keep abreast of the special education system developments, then they are in an excellent position to alert parents to their entitlements and to help them to navigate through the complex and lengthy eligibility process (Porter, Haynie, Bierle, Caldwell, & Palfrey, 1997). Specific assistance can be offered by 1) ensuring that the family contacts the local special education office in writing as soon as a difficulty is suspected; 2) requesting a copy of the reports generated by each separate assessment (both to maintain a complete copy in the medical record of the child and to encourage timeliness in reporting); and 3) reviewing the final IEP with the family when it has been produced (but before it has been signed by the family).

Too often, parents feel intimidated during large meetings with school personnel. Occasionally, the physician may need to send a letter to the assessment team or even to attend the meeting with the parents. Most school districts are very interested in the involvement of a child's health care provider, and this type of advocacy for the child can have a large impact on the ultimate substance of the IEP.

Since the first implementation of federal special education legislation, localities and states have struggled with funding special education services. As a result, there have been periods in almost every state of retrenchment as the expense of providing services has increased. One significant challenge comes from the unfulfilled promise of federal sharing in the funding formula. As a result, the funding issue emerges periodically as a congressional debate. Whenever there is a reauthorization of legislation as far reaching as IDEA, professionals must join with parents in advocating to maintain the successful portions of the laws and to improve those areas that remain weak.

CONCLUSION

When budgets are tight, too often education is not seen as a high priority for state governments. In such cases, remembering the nation's history is helpful. One of the original framers of democracy in America, John Adams, realized that in order for democracy to work, citizens must be well educated. To preserve their "rights and liberties" the citizens needed "wisdom, and knowledge, as well as virtue." In addition, he foresaw the need to spread "the opportunities and advantages of education . . . among the different orders of the people" (National Humanities Institute, 1780/1999). In other words, one of the bedrock foundations to the American experience was the universality of a quality education.

The movement for quality special education must be seen in this light. Education for all is not a recently discovered right that sprang from the idealism of the 1960s, but rather a basic right that had not yet been fully realized (like so many of the principles of the founding patriots). Special education is part of the enlightened understanding of American culture—everyone benefits if ALL individuals are empowered by a full education. This insight stems from the simple fact that if all are educated, then there is no wasted talent.

Americans must continue the movement toward appropriate community inclusion of all children, regardless of their condition or disabilities. All of those

Table 6.4-3. On-line resources relating to special education

IDEA Practices Home (http://www.ideapractices.org/) answers questions about the Individuals with Disabilities Education Act (IDEA) of 1990 (PL 101-476) and its amendments, keeps readers informed about "IDEAs That Work," and supports efforts to help all children learn, progress, and realize their dreams.

The Office of Special Education Programs (http://www.ed.gov/offices/OSERS/OSEP/) is dedicated to improving results for infants, toddlers, children, and youth with disabilities age birth through 21 by providing leadership and financial support to assist states and local districts.

Rethinking Special Education for a New Century (http://www.edexcellence.net/library/special_ed/index.html) is a volume of papers examining the past, present, and future of special education. It is intended to help lay the groundwork for the reauthorization of IDEA. The entire volume is available as a single PDF document.

The official web site of the American Academy of Pediatrics (http://www.aap.org/advocacy/medhome/linksorgsgov.htm) contains an advocacy section regarding children with special health care needs.

Information on the Bright Futures Project web site (http://www.brightfutures.org/) is based on published guidelines for health supervision of infants, children, and adolescents. One goal of the project is to establish a partnership between health professionals and families. This site is designed to be used by both health professionals and families and to help users to better understand the diagnostic process and what to expect during health supervision visits. Issues, concerns, and questions are also addressed.

Formed in 1982, the Society for Developmental and Behavioral Pediatrics (http://www.sdbp.org/) is a national, interdisciplinary organization with about 640 members. The web site's goal is to improve the health care of infants, children, and adolescents by promoting research and teaching in developmental and behavioral pediatrics.

who interact with children have the duty to learn about special education, disability legislature, and other issues that are important to individuals they serve (see Table 6.4-3). Of course, this task will not be easy and will require creativity, hard work, and patient persistence.

REFERENCES

American Academy of Pediatrics, Committee on Children with Disabilities. (2001). American Academy of Pediatrics policy statement: Development surveillance and screening of infants and young children (RE0062). *Pediatrics, 108,* 192–196.

American Academy of Pedicatrics, Newborn Screening Task Force. (2000). Serving the family from birth to the medical home—Newborn screening: A blueprint for the future; A call for a national agenda on state newborn screening programs. *Pediatrics, 106*(Suppl.), 389–427.

Americans with Disabilities Act of 1990, PL 101-336, 42 U.S.C. §§ 12101 *et seq.*

Board of Education of the Hendrick Hudson Central School District v. Rowley, 458 U.S. 176 (1982).

Brown v. Board of Education, 347 U.S. 483 (1954).

Burlington School Committee v. Department of Education, 471 U.S. 359 (1985).

Cedar Rapids Community School District, Petitioner v. Garret F., 06 F. 3d 822 (1999).

Education of the Handicapped Act Amendments of 1986, PL 99-457, 20 U.S.C. §§ 1400 *et seq.*

Education for All Handicapped Children Act of 1975, PL 94-142, 20 U.S.C. §§ 1400 *et seq.*

Education of the Handicapped Act of 1970, PL 91-230, 84 Stat. 121–154, 20 U.S.C. §§ 1400 *et seq.*

Elementary and Secondary Education Act Amendments of 1966, PL 89-750, 80 Stat. 1190, 20 U.S.C. §§ 873 *et seq.*

Felix v. Cayetano, No. 93-00367 (D. Haw. Oct. 25, 1994).

Green, M., & Palfrey, J.S. (Eds.). (2000). *Bright futures: Guidelines for health supervision of infants, children, and adolescents* (2nd ed.) Arlington, VA: National Center for Education in Maternal and Child Health.

Hebbeler, K., Spiker, D., Wagner, M., Cameto, R., McKenna, P., & SRI International. (1999). *National Early Intervention Longitudinal Study (NEILS): State-to-state variations in early intervention systems.* Menlo Park, CA: SRI International.

Individuals with Disabilities Education Act (IDEA) Amendments of 1997, PL 105-17, 20 U.S.C. §§ 1400 *et seq.*

Individuals with Disabilities Education Act of 1990, PL 101-476, 20 U.S.C. §§ 1400 *et seq.*

Individuals with Disabilities Education Improvement Act of 2004, PL 108-446, 20 U.S.C. §§ 1400 *et seq.*

Irving Independent School District v. Tatro, 468 U.S. 883 (1984).

Levine, M.D. (1994). *Educational care: A system for understanding and helping children with learning problems at home and in school.* Cambridge, MA: Educators Publishing Service.

Maternal and Child Health and Mental Retardation Planning Amendments of 1963, PL 88-156, 77 Stat. 273.

Mills v. Board of Education of the District of Columbia, 348 F. Supp. 866 (D.D.C. 1972).

National Academy of Sciences. (1982). *Placing children in special education: Strategy for equity.* Washington, DC: Author.

National Early Childhood Technical Assistance System. (n.d.). *Early intervention program for infants and toddlers with disabilities (Part C of IDEA).* Retrieved February 18, 2005, from http://www.nectas.unc.edu/partc/partc.asp

National Humanities Institute. (1999). *Constitution of Massachusetts.* Originally written in 1780. Retrieved August 3, 2005, from http://www.nhinet.org/ccs/docs/ma=1780.htm

Palfrey, J.S. (1994). *Community child health.* Westport, CT: Praeger Publishing.

Pennsylvania Association for Retarded Citizens (PARC) v. Commonwealth of Pennsylvania, 343 F. Supp. 279 (1972).

Porter, S., Haynie, M., Bierle, R., Caldwell, T.H., & Palfrey, J.S. (1997). *Children and youth assisted by medical technology in educational settings: Guidelines for care.* Baltimore: Paul H. Brookes Publishing Co.

Rehabilitation Act of 1973, PL 93-112, 29 U.S.C. §§ 701 *et seq.*

Shonkoff, J.P., & Meisels, S.J. (2000). Early childhood intervention: The evolution of a concept. In J.P. Shonkoff & S.J. Meisels (Eds.), *Handbook of early childhood intervention.* New York: Cambridge University Press.

Shonkoff, J.P., & Phillips, D.A. (Eds.). (2000) *From neurons to neighborhoods: The science of early childhood development.* Washington, DC: National Academies Press.

Smith, P.J., Mathews, K.S., Hehir, T., & Palfrey, J.S. (2002). Educating children with disabilities: How pediatricians can help. *Contemporary Pediatrics, 9,* 102–127.

Social Security Act of 1935, PL 74-271, 42 U.S.C. §§ 301 *et seq.*

Tjossem, T. (Ed.). (1976). *Intervention strategies for high risk infants and young children.* Baltimore: University Park Press.

U.S. Department of Education. (2000). *The twenty-second annual report to Congress on the implementation of the Individuals with Disabilities Education Act.* Washington, DC: Author.

6.5 TRANSITION FROM ADOLESCENCE TO ADULTHOOD

Karen L. Carter

Adolescence is fraught with changes and increasing demands. These changes may be even more dramatic and challenging for teenagers with disabilities. Adolescents with disabilities often are thwarted in their efforts to step into adulthood. When they try to practice new skills and adopt new responsibilities, others may ignore them. In addition, proactive planning is necessary to enable adolescents to achieve independence. Successful transition teams help build the individual's self-advocacy skills, remove the obstacles that could hinder independence, and seek involvement from medical practitioners.

I experienced this transition process firsthand with my son, Judson. I adopted Judson when he was 16 years old and living in an institution. I believed that he would benefit from living full time in the community, so for 2 years I begged for appropriate funding. Although everyone agreed that Judson could live successfully in the community with 24-hour support, no one would provide the funds. Without these funds, Judson would be forced to stay in the institution indefinitely.

A formal hearing was held to determine whether Judson needed to remain in the institution. The judge asked if I wanted to say anything, and I poured out my heart. I doubted that I could say anything that would change the mountain of information stating that Judson should stay in the institution. At the same time, I feared that he would be released into the community with no funding at all. Two weeks later, papers arrived from the judge ordering Judson out of the institution by his eighteenth birthday.

Judson's transition to adolescence would have been smoother if he had had a proactive transition team. Parents or other members of transition teams may not understand the need for proactive transition planning, but crisis management is difficult at best and may cause haphazard intervention. Effective transition planning begins at birth and nurtures the child's self-sufficiency as he or she matures. Communication, decision making, and financial responsibility originate in early childhood. During late childhood, these skills are refined, and children are given increasing responsibility at home, school, and therapy.

PROMOTING SELF-ADVOCACY

Communication skills are essential tools for all people with disabilities. Many adolescents with disabilities continue to look to their parents for all decisions, personal or medical, even though they have opinions and can express them. For this reason, teachers, physicians, and parents should ask children to make and express choices and to indicate disapproval. That way, when individuals with disabilities reach adolescence, they will be able to make their own decisions concerning large issues, such as which physician to see and where to live, as well as small issues, such as choosing what clothes to wear and what to eat (Rubin, Carter, & Twardowski, 1999).

Caregivers must recognize the importance of the burgeoning interests that adolescents with disabilities develop and allow them to explore these interests. They should give adolescents opportunities to develop new interests by joining clubs or taking classes. In addition, adolescents with disabilities should be allowed to make minor mistakes that are not harmful. Young people learn from making small errors in judgment as natural consequences occur. With time, they will learn to make wise decisions and will discover joy when they make successful decisions.

As an individual with disabilities matures, he or she should assume more of a leadership role in the transition team. Team members must recognize the individual's increased sophistication and accept his or her decisions. The individual with disabilities will notice that he or she is succeeding when others respect him or her. When the adolescent makes a decision, other team members must listen and acknowledge the decision. If there is disagreement, team members should negotiate so that the adolescent is still part of the decision-making process.

REMOVING OBSTACLES

Despite the advantages of a proactive transition plan, many obstacles can prevent smooth transition. In an effort to exert their independence and begin to control their behaviors, adolescents may decide to independently care for themselves without reminders. They may begin to neglect any health issue that makes them different from other teenagers. In addition, they may begin to explore negative behaviors such as smoking, taking drugs, and having unprotected sexual experiences. Transition team members should use health education to provide the necessary information to enable a person to make wise health decisions.

Adolescents should also be taught that successful, independent adults need support groups. The team should help an individual to develop a network of friends and family who listen and respond to him or her. Sometimes, after developing a plan and implementing supports, the needs of the individual change. Therefore, obtaining and maintaining adequate supports is a continuous process. Adolescents must decide what services they need and ask for funding for the programs. Often, the funds are available with a well-informed request.

Transition teams should also plan for the fact that insurance regulations may change when an adolescent becomes an adult. Many resources for insurance and other sources of medical support only provide coverage until 21 years of age. Other carriers have strict restrictions on the number of therapy visits. The transition team should research alternative forms of support and seek assistance from people knowledgeable in this area.

PARTICIPATION BY MEDICAL PROFESSIONALS

The American Academy of Pediatrics recommends a strong transition plan (Burush & Rose, 1988; Committee on Children with Disabilities, 1996, 1999, 2000).

Physicians should participate in developing this comprehensive plan. They can educate adolescents about their diagnoses and can assess them to determine their unique abilities. Physicians can encourage self-advocacy skills (e.g., expressing opinions) during medical interviews and physicals.

Multiple systems of care with different criteria for entry and vastly different services are available to adolescents with disabilities. Physicians can help choose which systems are appropriate and can help adolescents get on waiting lists when they turn 14 years old. Physicians can also help adolescents develop a personal system of coordinating their health care needs.

The American Academy of Pediatrics (2004) recommends a medical home for each person with disabilities. This medical home includes people who provide for continuous medical care. Pediatricians often provide care coordination for people with disabilities, which can enhance the transition from adolescence to adulthood (Committee on Children with Disabilities, 2000).

CONCLUSION

The goal for all children with disabilities is to develop into mature, competent adults. This goal can be accomplished through teamwork and planning. Doctors must provide the highest quality of health care. They must recognize that individuals with disabilities need developmentally appropriate anticipatory guidance when making this transition. In addition, pediatricians should participate in transition planning for work, home, and community.

Adults with disabilities can attain rites of passage and embrace their new responsibilities. They can begin social interactions as adults, start work, and initiate citizenship. Physicians must nurture self-determination and self-advocacy. They are in a unique position to help bridge the gap between childhood experiences and mature roles in work, home, and leisure. Health practitioners must support individuals with disabilities' efforts and help them advance to their full potential.

REFERENCES

American Academy of Pediatrics, Medical Home Initiative for Children with Special Needs Project Advisory Committee. (2004). The medical home. *Pediatrics, 113*(Suppl. 5), 154–157.

Bursuch, W., & Rose, E. (1988). *Development, assessment, and education of adolescents with developmental disabilities. Developmental disabilities: A life-span perspective.* Philadelphia: Grune and Stratton.

Committee on Children with Disabilities. (1999). Care coordination: Integrating health and related systems of care for children with special health care needs. *Pediatrics, 104*(4), 978–981.

Committee on Children with Disabilities. (2000). The role of the pediatrician in transitioning children and adolescents with developmental disabilities and chronic illnesses from school to work or college. *Pediatrics, 106*(4), 854–856.

Committee on Children with Disabilities & Committee on Adolescence. (1996). Transition of care provided for adolescents with special health care needs. *Pediatrics, 98*(6), 1203–1206.

Rubin, L., Carter, K., & Twardowski, S. (1999). Self-determination for individuals with disabilities. Unpublished manuscript.

6.6 COMMUNITY PRACTICE FOR ADULTS

Marc T. Emmerich

Provision of medical care for adults with developmental disabilities living in the community presents a number of unique challenges to practitioners. Even those clinicians experienced in the community care of *children* with developmental disabilities and those experienced in the care of adults with developmental disabilities in *institutional* settings will find that *community* care of *adults* with developmental disabilities requires different techniques and strategies, as well as extra time commitments, to help ensure adequate delivery of health care. The following discussion refers almost exclusively to the care of those individuals with more significant intellectual disabilities who have significantly limited means of reliable communication, and, therefore, significantly limited ability to advocate for themselves.

COMMUNICATION ISSUES

A survey by Minihan, Dean, and Lyons (1993) found that Maine physicians caring for people with developmental disabilities considered written and verbal communication issues to pose the greatest obstacles to patient care. In medical practice, the history of an illness is usually critical in determining a diagnosis. When communication about that history is impaired, so is the clinician's ability to establish an appropriate diagnosis and initiate treatment. If individuals cannot communicate their own history, clinicians turn to gathering objective observations from family members who may know the most subtle nuances of their loved one's behavior.

Many adults with developmental disabilities, however, do not live with their families. The only information available may be that given by accompanying direct support staff who 1) may not be very familiar with an individual; 2) may observe the individual only a few hours per day and may not have first-hand accounts (or any information) about the other times of day or night; and 3) may not know the history of the individual's previous episodes of the illness. In fact, sometimes an individual will be accompanied to the clinician's office by a staff member who knows little to nothing about any of the individual's medical history and may not even know why the appointment was made for the individual he or she is accompanying.

Rather than *obtaining* a history from the accompanying staff person, the clinician may find him- or herself *enlightening* the staff person about the individual's medical history. Even with the best possible information provided by familiar supporters, clinicians will find that they may need to rely more heavily than usual on other sources of information, such as lab tests or X-rays, to help establish a diagnosis and/or monitor an illness. In addition to verbal communication with staff, state and/or vendor agencies often request written communication at the time of the office visit to help ensure that the treatment plan is carried out, which requires additional time from the clinician.

Forms brought to the office by familiar and day-to-day supporters, on which *they* have documented an individual's behavior or apparent symptoms over time, can greatly facilitate the information-gathering process at the office visit. For example, a menstrual record (see Figure 6.6-1) can represent an entire year on a single sheet, with each row representing 1 month. A letter is placed in each box representing the date on which menstrual bleeding (B) or spotting (S) occurred.

Sleep data are generally only able to be collected when an individual has overnight awake supporters and can be shown as 1 month of information on a sheet (see Figure 6.6-2). Each column represents one night. Going down the column, for each half-hour interval starting with the top box at 8 P.M., overnight awake supporters fill in an *X* if the individual is awake or an *O* if the individual is asleep (or other symbol for another specific observation, if pertinent for that individual). When the schedules are completed, the clinician can receive information that may not have been available from anyone other than multiple overnight awake supporters, who usually are not readily contacted by clinicians.

The value of collecting the information *all* of the time for *all* individuals who cannot report their own medical history is illustrated by Figure 6.6-1, in which menstrual irregularities increased significantly during the latter part of the time period represented on the sheet. If information collection does not begin until irregularities are noticed and reported, then the clinician must assess the irregularities without the benefit of previous baseline information.

Menstrual cycle record

Name: Teresa Year: 2001

Month/day	1	2	3	4	5	6	7	8	9	10	11	12	13	14	15	16	17	18	19	20	21	22	23	24	25	26	27	28	29	30	31
January															B	B	B														
February																B	B														
March						B	B	B																							
April				B	B	B	B																				B				
May																						B	B	B							
June																															
July																															
August						B																							B	B	B
September	B	B																													
October		B																													
November																					B	B									
December																		B	B												

Figure 6.6-1. Menstrual cycle record for Teresa. *Key:* B = bleeding.

Sleep data sheet

Name: James X = awake O = asleep

Month: March 2005 Other symbols: ______

Day/time	1	2	3	4	5	6	7	8	9	10	11	12	13	14	15	16	17	18	19	20	21	22	23	24	25	26	27	28	29	30	31
8:00 P.M.	X	X	X	X	X	X	X	X	X	X	X	X	X	X	X	X	X	X	X	X	X	X	X	X	O	X	X	X	X	X	X
8:30	X	X	X	X	X	X	X	X	X	X	X	X	X	X	X	X	X	X	X	X	X	X	X	X	X	X	X	X	X	X	X
9:00	X	O	X	X	X	X	X	X	O	X	X	O	X	X	X	X	X	X	X	X	X	O	O	X	X	X	X	X	X	O	X
9:30	X	O	X	O	O	X	O	X	O	O	X	O	O	X	X	X	O	X	X	O	O	O	O	O	X	X	O	X	X	O	O
10:00	X	X	X	O	O	O	O	X	O	X	O	X	O	X	X	X	O	X	X	O	O	X	X	O	X	O	O	X	O	O	O
10:30	X	X	X	O	O	O	O	X	O	X	O	O	O	X	X	X	O	X	O	O	O	X	X	O	X	O	O	X	O	O	O
11:00	X	X	X	O	O	O	O	X	O	X	O	O	O	X	X	X	O	O	O	O	O	X	X	O	X	O	O	X	X	O	O
11:30	X	X	X	O	O	O	O	X	O	X	O	O	O	X	X	O	O	X	O	O	O	X	O	O	X	O	O	X	X	O	O
12:00 A.M.	X	X	X	O	O	O	O	O	O	O	O	O	O	X	X	X	O	X	X	O	O	X	O	O	O	O	O	X	X	O	O
12:30	X	X	O	O	O	O	O	O	O	O	O	O	O	O	O	X	O	X	X	O	O	O	O	O	O	O	O	X	X	O	O
1:00	O	X	O	O	O	O	O	O	O	O	O	O	O	O	O	X	O	X	X	O	O	O	O	O	O	O	O	X	X	O	O
1:30	O	X	O	O	O	O	O	O	O	O	O	O	O	O	O	X	O	O	O	X	O	O	X	O	O	O	O	X	X	O	O
2:00	O	O	O	O	O	O	O	O	O	O	O	O	O	O	O	X	O	O	O	X	O	O	X	O	O	O	O	X	X	O	O
2:30	O	O	O	O	O	O	O	O	O	O	O	O	O	O	O	X	X	O	O	X	O	O	X	O	O	O	O	X	X	O	O
3:00	O	O	O	O	O	O	O	O	O	O	O	O	O	O	O	X	X	O	O	O	O	O	X	O	O	O	O	O	X	O	X
3:30	O	O	O	O	O	O	X	O	O	O	O	O	O	O	O	X	X	O	O	X	O	O	X	O	O	O	O	O	X	X	X
4:00	O	O	O	O	O	O	X	O	O	O	O	X	O	O	O	O	X	O	O	X	O	O	X	O	O	O	O	O	O	X	X
4:30	O	O	X	X	X	O	O	O	X	O	O	X	O	O	O	O	X	O	O	O	O	O	X	O	O	O	O	O	O	O	X
5:00	O	O	X	X	X	O	O	X	X	O	X	O	O	O	O	O	X	X	O	O	O	X	O	X	X	O	O	O	O	O	X
5:30	X	X	X	X	X	X	O	X	X	O	X	O	O	O	X	X	X	X	X	O	X	X	X	X	X	X	O	O	O	O	X
6:00	X	X	X	X	X	X	X	X	X	X	X	X	O	X	X	X	X	X	X	X	X	X	X	O	X	X	X	O	O	O	X
6:30	X	X	X	X	X	X	X	X	X	X	X	X	O	X	X	X	X	X	X	X	X	X	X	O	X	X	X	O	O	X	X
7:00 A.M.	X	X	X	X	X	X	X	X	X	X	X	X	O	X	X	X	X	X	X	X	X	X	X	X	X	X	X	X	O	X	X
Total	4.5	4.5	4	7	7	7.5	7.5	5	7.5	6.5	7	7.5	10	5.5	5	2	5	4	5.5	5.5	7.5	5.5	3.5	8.5	5.5	7.5	8.5	3.5	4.5	8.5	5.5
Staff Initials	FL	FL	FL	FL	FL	EC	EC	EC	FL	FL	FL	EC	FL	FL	EC	FL	FL	FL	FL	FL	EC	FL	FL	EC	FL	EC	EC	EC	FL	FL	FL

Figure 6.6-2. Sleep data sheet for James. *Key:* X = awake; O = asleep.

As part of any evaluation, clinicians should attempt to communicate directly with individuals with disabilities as much as possible. Some individuals who are verbal, however, may not be reliable historians, thereby leading an unsuspecting clinician astray. It may be important to obtain corroborating information from supporters familiar with the individual.

Interactions Between Clinicians and Direct Supporters

Interactions between a clinician and an individual's supporters may be as varied as the number of supporters the clinician encounters for a particular individual, which may be quite a few. In my experience, the majority of individuals attend outpatient appointments with one or two residential staff who may not know much about the individual. Whether present in the office or not, however, other parties may be acutely interested in the outcome of the clinical visit: the individual's mother, father, brothers, sisters, service coordinator, social worker, and/or a behavioral consultant. Despite the fact that day program staff rarely accompany the individual to the physician's office, it is their concerns that often precipitate a visit to the physician. Depending on their varied interactions with the individual, these concerned supporters may have different perspectives and information to offer to help the clinician understand the individual's issues. They may also have different expectations from the clinician. Generally, whoever accompanies the individual to the office is the one whom the clinician expects to interact with in follow-up of any issues that are identified, but when a group home is called about a change in care or for updated information, a different staff person who knows nothing about the recent clinical visit may answer. The clinician needs to be aware that communication among group home staff (and other concerned parties) is often lacking.

Consent and Guardianship

Consent for medical care and procedures is an issue that is directly related to the communication issues discussed previously. In most states, once an individual reaches the age of 18, he or she is presumed competent to make informed decisions on his or her own behalf unless and until a court has ruled that he or she is not competent. In such situations, a legal guardian is assigned to make informed decisions for the individual. Many advocates for individuals with developmental disabilities promote the idea of avoiding guardianship assignments in order to allow an individual the dignity of making his or her own decisions. There may be times, however, when this practice is not in the individual's best interest.

Most clinicians recognize that even individuals with sophisticated intellectual capacities can be influenced to make medical decisions depending on how the clinician presents the issue. Individuals with significant intellectual disabilities may be more easily swayed to make less-than-optimal choices. In an urgent situation when there is no guardian to give or withhold consent, an individual's care may be determined solely by medical clinicians, who may be unfamiliar with the individual's comprehensive needs. To prevent this, the individual with cognitive disabilities should have a competency assessment during a nonurgent period to allow for the assignment of a suitable, permanent guardian (possibly limited to medical decisions, if appropriate) so that when a medical crisis occurs, the guardian will be able to make informed decisions on behalf of the individual.

Residential staff often will accompany an individual on an office visit without the presence of the guardian. One might think that by letting the individual attend the office visit with the residential staff, the guardian has effectively consented to the visit, including associated routine procedures, as well as to the clinician's communication with the residential staff. In those situations where communication between residential staff and the guardian is not consistent, however, these assumptions may be called into question.

EXAMINATION PROCEDURES

An individual who does not understand the purpose of the clinic visit may have a heightened level of anxiety and may attempt to prevent any physical contact between him- or herself and the examiner or the examining equipment. In pediatric offices, parents commonly physically restrain young, anxious children while the clinician performs relatively invasive procedures, such as ear exams or administration of immunizations. When the individual is a strong, full-grown adult, such restraint procedures are not always possible and may create a risk of injury to the individual and others. Furthermore, some advocates might question the extent to which such restraint should be allowed, especially when the legal guardian of the individual is not present.

Thus, performing even a simple ear exam, blood pressure measurement, or phlebotomy can present a logistic, ethical, and legal quandary. Such procedures may require an extremely gentle and careful (but not fearful) approach by the clinician, using techniques to help the individual feel more comfortable (e.g., having the individual hold hands with a familiar supporter) or to encourage compliance with procedures (e.g., lavishly praising any efforts the individual makes to attempt to comply). This process may require a significant time commitment—not only from the clinician but also from group home staff and/or other supporters who accompany the individual to the appointment—for even the most routine procedures.

Other techniques may help individuals be more comfortable with medical examinations and office procedures. During a period of months or years, an anxious individual may be able to be desensitized to common procedures by having the procedures presented repeatedly by familiar supporters at home in a gradual, nonthreatening manner until the experience becomes commonplace. Home visits (often performed by nurse practitioners rather than physicians) may be more comfortable for the individual, thereby enabling him or her to better tolerate and accept examinations and procedures. A home visit may also facilitate information gathering from multiple supporters, with multiple perspectives, who might not have been available to attend an appointment in the medical office.

Some disability advocates have raised concerns that home visits by clinicians interfere with the normalization of the individual's interaction with the community. For certain individuals, however, the benefit of ensuring adequate medical care in an environment that the individual appears to consider safe and comfortable seems to outweigh the questionable benefit of conforming to a strictly defined "normalization" protocol. Desensitization to the medical office may still be attempted in parallel with home visits.

Having a clinician travel to the individual's home may also free up time for several direct support staff, who, instead of spending hours accompanying one individual to and from the clinician's office, can stay home with the individual and spend those hours attending to the individual's housemates as well. Lack of available staff and transportation are the most frequent reasons given by group homes for office appointment cancellations and no-shows. Community systems that support home visits may alleviate these burdens.

Sometimes prescribing anxiolytic or sedative medication for an individual prior to an office or home visit is necessary, especially if the clinician is planning procedures known to be difficult for that individual. Generally, benzodiazepines (preferably short-acting for brief procedures), chloral hydrate, or antihistamines are used, alone or in combination. For some individuals, extraordinarily high doses are required, but these doses should only be used after lower doses have been previously attempted and incremental increases in dose have yielded no significant effect for that particular individual. Caution needs to be exercised as the same dose that previously was barely sedating for a particular individual may, in the presence of an acute illness or drug interaction, elicit a much more profound sedative effect. (If this occurs, usually the most important sign to monitor is the respiratory rate.) Rarely, an individual will not respond adequately to oral sedation with anything other than a neuroleptic medication. For some individuals, intramuscular and/or intravenous conscious sedation or general anesthesia might be necessary.

When performance of a procedure involves restraint or sedation techniques that increase the risk of injury to a particular individual, then the performance of the procedure itself may become more of a risk to that individual's health than the disease which the procedure is testing for and/or treating. Therefore, prior to performing any procedure, the clinician must consider the risk–benefit ratio for that individual. For example, if general anesthesia is required to perform a Pap smear of a non–sexually active woman, the risk of performing the test may be greater than the risk of the presence of disease for which the Pap smear is testing.

Sometimes the risk of sedation or general anesthesia can be "distributed" by performing multiple procedures at once. For example, if an individual will need to go under general anesthesia for dental rehabilitation, then other examinations might be able to be scheduled to be performed while the individual is under the same anesthesia. Optimally, routine exams of the ears, eyes (including fundi), genitals (including Pap smear in women), and rectum, as well as phlebotomy for routine labs, and other invasive examinations required for a particular individual could all be completed at the same time, thereby sparing the individual the risk (and cost) of additional episodes of sedation or general anesthesia. General anesthesia is usually reserved for a particular dental or surgical procedure, to which the routine exams are added, rather than imposing the risk of general anesthesia solely for routine screening exams.

Abbott, a muscular 27-year-old with a height of 6 feet, 3 inches, and a weight of 210 pounds, was seen for a routine tetanus-diphtheria vaccine booster. He had exhibited no appreciable response in the past to high doses of triazolam (up to 0.75 mg.), so he was given 1 mg. for this procedure. One hour after the dose, he was calm but not quite lethargic. Three group home staff members accompanied him and his mother to the office. His mother sat on a chair and held Abbott in her lap with her arms wrapped around his as the three staff members held Abbott's legs and head.

As Abbott's mother spoke soothing words, the clinician administered the vaccine injection in Abbott's upper arm. Abbott erupted, with the needle and syringe still stuck in his arm, and all six people landed on the floor. The clinician successfully completed the injection and removed the needle. No one was injured, but the overall risk of giving this injection may have been greater than the benefit. A better option might have been to delay the injection until the next time Abbott would be receiving intravenous conscious sedation or general anesthesia for dental rehabilitation.

UNDERSTANDING BEHAVIOR

Clinicians should recognize that many of the behaviors an individual may exhibit that appear to be maladaptive to the individual and perhaps disruptive to the evaluation usually serve some function for the individual and that in most cases, one of those functions is communication. Physical and/or emotional discomfort, either from internal disease or environmental influences (e.g., allergens, social stressors) may all manifest with self-injurious behavior and/or aggression. Seemingly maladaptive behaviors may be associated with an atypical seizure disorder, whereas seemingly epileptic seizures may actually be pseudoseizures, which function, in part, to call attention to the individual, perhaps because of some unresolved distress. Familiar supporters may be able to recognize subtle differences in an individual's behaviors that result from one etiology (e.g., epileptic seizures) as compared with another (e.g., pseudoseizures).

It also is important to recognize the potential interaction of two or more etiologies. For example, severe constipation can precipitate a true epileptic seizure, and it also can manifest in attempts to communicate distress (perhaps via pseudoseizures or self-injurious behavior). In this case, rather than adjusting antiepileptic medication or instituting a behavior support plan, the most effective therapy to decrease the seizures and/or self-injurious behavior may be a laxative. The most reliable method for discerning the multitude of possible interacting etiologies for a variety of behaviors and developing an effective therapeutic plan is an interdisciplinary approach by a variety of clinicians, all experienced in the care of adults with developmental disabilities, preferably with extensive input from supporters who have been closely acquainted with the individual for a long time.

COORDINATION OF MEDICAL CARE OUTSIDE THE OFFICE

Coordination of care outside the clinician's office (including off-hours interactions, hospitalizations, and specialty consultations) likewise presents unique challenges. Consider the example of a group home resident who becomes acutely ill on a weekend and unfamiliar staff covering the group home place a call to an unfamiliar clinician who is covering the medical practice. This clinician's ability to put the acute issue into context may be compromised. Institution of appropriate medical care may depend on the availability of familiar supporters, and/or the primary care clinician, even when these people would usually not be available. When more familiar supporters cannot be contacted, it may be appropriate to have an individual examined in the office or emergency room in order to obtain more objective information than can be obtained over the phone, to better ascertain the significance of the acute presentation.

Urgent Evaluation

Even with direct examination of the individual by a clinician covering the practice or the emergency room, it is often extremely helpful for the examining physician to communicate with the clinician most familiar with the individual (especially if the familiar clinician is experienced in managing the common problems of adults with developmental disabilities). In addition to offering historical background information, the familiar clinician can suggest the best approach for the acute presentation, can help interpret the individual's behaviors, can offer techniques to facilitate adequate performance of examinations and/or other procedures, and can help verify that appropriate consent has been obtained when necessary. Just as a pediatrician will often trust a mother to know what works for her child, clinicians would be well advised to seriously consider the information, concerns, and recommendations offered by familiar supporters, even those without health care training, about how best to approach and manage a particular individual's problems.

Ethyl was 45-year-old, 60-pound woman with microcephaly, severe intellectual disabilities, deafness, and kyphosis who communicated primarily by poking at and scratching herself or others. She had no recent pulmonary issues and was expected to live another 25–30 years (based on Table 6.6-1, which is discussed later). She was taken to the emergency room shortly after exhibiting acute distress during eating, with sudden onset, copious drooling, and choking—classic signs of acute, complete esophageal obstruction, a life-threatening

Table 6.6-1. Life expectancy (additional years) by age and cohort

	Cannot lift head			Lifts head			Rolls/sits			General population
Sex/age	TF	FBO	SF	TF	FBO	SF	TF	FBO	SF	
Female										
15 y	15.4	21.3	—	21.1	27.7	43.4	25.0	39.2	52.7	65.0
30 y	13.4	23.8	—	16.2	28.1	33.0	21.5	34.1	40.1	50.4
45 y	—	20.4	—	16.1	20.6	23.6	23.3	24.1	29.4	36.2
Male										
15 y	11.7	16.9	—	16.7	22.8	38.8	20.3	34.3	48.7	58.3
30 y	12.0	22.0	—	14.7	26.2	31.0	19.8	32.1	38.0	44.5
45 y	—	17.5	—	13.6	17.7	20.6	20.3	21.0	26.3	31.1

Key: y = years; TF = tube fed; FBO = fed by others, without a feeding tube; SF = self-fed; — = group too small for reliable computation of life expectancy or confidence interval.

From Strauss, D., & Shavelle, R. (1998). Life expectancy of adults with cerebral palsy. *Developmental Medicine and Child Neurology, 40,* 374; reprinted by permission.

emergency. Her inability to cooperate meant that an endoscopy would require physical restraint and sedation, probably even general anesthesia.

The emergency room and admitting physicians considered avoiding the invasive endoscopy, hoping that Ethyl's problem was a burn on her pharynx, which can be managed with intravenous antibiotics and steroids; however, given the presentation, a complete esophageal obstruction was a distinct possibility. Performing the endoscopy promptly on admission could mean the difference between life and death. The potential benefit of the invasive procedure outweighed the risk, even if general anesthesia was required. The recommendation was to proceed with sedation and endoscopy.

Acute Care Hospitalization

Due to communication difficulties, acute care hospitalizations similarly contain challenges. Like other clinicians, hospital staff generally will obtain information (e.g., about appetite and sleep) by an individual's self-report, and an individual is typically expected to call a nurse when necessary (e.g., when he or she is done using a bed pan). Furthermore, an individual may notice a change in medication color, dosage, or time and ask hospital staff to verify that the change is not an error. When an individual's means of communication are limited, however, few mechanisms exist for that individual and hospital staff to communicate many of these details to each other.

Probably the most optimal means for such observation and communication is to adopt the model used in many pediatric hospitals, which allows a family member to stay in the hospital room with the individual throughout the hospitalization. Aside from observation and communication, this practice also helps the individual to accommodate to the environment and to better cooperate with procedures. In the absence of family members, next best would be to allow the continued presence of familiar supporters, such as group home staff.

Unfortunately, even if the hospital welcomes them, many group home agencies do not have staff available to stay with an individual in the hospital. An ill individual left isolated in a hospital room day after day, unaware of where he or she is or why he or she is there is a disturbing thought. This individual might be restrained to the bed to maintain intravenous lines and enteric and urinary catheters, might never see a familiar face, and might not even have a television or radio left on for him or her. It is not so surprising, therefore, that hospital clinicians *un*familiar with individuals with developmental disabilities might observe this poor quality of life and wonder whether it is appropriate to perform aggressive and risky medical interventions. Hesitancy of clinicians to treat aggressively is further discussed later in the chapter. In order to avert some of these problems, Boston Medical Center has piloted a disability advocacy program for individuals with limited communication that utilizes volunteers during acute inpatient hospitalizations to facilitate communication between home and hospital and within the hospital.

Resuming Oral or Tube Feeding or Starting Tube Feeding

When individuals who can eat by mouth (PO) resume eating after a hiatus, and especially after abdominal surgery, physicians generally order clear liquids, then advance the diet as tolerated. Too rapid an advancement of diet can cause ileus and vomiting, perhaps with aspiration. Because individuals with developmental disabilities have a high risk of constipation or ileus and aspiration at baseline, when they switch from intravenous (IV) to PO hydration, starting with a clear liquid diet in small increments is even more important. IV hydration can be maintained while it is determined how well the individual is tolerating gradually increasing volumes PO.

Starting or resuming feeding through gastric or enteric tubes is no different: start with *clear* liquids at a low rate; gradually increase the rate of clear liquids, as tolerated, until the full target rate is achieved; then (and only then), advance the diet (i.e., begin frequent, brief infusions of formula alternating with long infusions of clear liquids, then gradually replace the clear liquids with increasing durations of formula feeding), as tolerated. Unfortunately, after an individual has had several days of IV hydration with no enteric intake, many clinicians directly order (or discharge the individual with an order for) a high volume of full-strength formula feeding; then, ileus may ensue. IV hydration may be maintained as enteric feeding is gradually (re)started with clear liquids, then advanced as described previously. The individual's status should continue to be closely monitored until the full diet has been documented to be well tolerated.

Specialty Consultation

Consultations to specialists (including physicians and/or other professionals) are often less complicated, especially when the consultations are elective and the primary care clinician has time to prepare materials that will facilitate communication about the issues and the context in which they are presenting. Also, there is often more opportunity to schedule the visits at a time when family members and/or more familiar group home staff can accompany the individual to the consultant's office. Although the best care is likely to be given by a specialist who has experience and a particular interest in the care of adults with developmental disabilities, singling out that specialist for a large volume of complex individuals may overwhelm his or her time constraints.

Referral to less-experienced specialists may have the societal advantage of exposing a larger number of clinicians to adults with developmental disabilities, but at the risk of less-than-optimal care for a particular individual. For example, a psychiatrist with little experience in the care of adults with severely limited cognitive and verbal abilities might attribute seemingly maladaptive behaviors to a chronic, irreversible organic brain syndrome rather than recognizing them as signs of an acute or subacute potentially treatable psychiatric illness, such as bipolar or obsessive-compulsive disorder, or as a manifestation of a medical illness, or as serving some other function for the individual, as noted previously. As with the acute, out-of-office visit discussed previously, an experienced, familiar clinician's input may help the consultant to adequately assess the individual and to clarify the diagnosis.

DIRECT SUPPORT RESPONSIBILITIES

Family members who live with individuals with severe developmental disabilities are generally assumed to accept various responsibilities, such as administration of medications and making assessments about an individual's health, including measurement of temperature, pulse, blood pressure, finger-stick glucose, or oxygen saturation. When necessary, families are expected to prepare certain food textures before feeding, to administer feeding and medications through a gastric or enteric feeding tube, and to inject insulin subcutaneously. Generally, all of these procedures are taught to one or two family members, who then consistently perform the procedures with the individual and can immediately recognize when there is a change in status.

Direct support staff are routinely assumed to take the place of family members and perform many of these tasks, but in a group home, several staff members may be responsible for these activities. Systems must be in place for training all of these supporters, monitoring their actions, recording their results, and communicating these results between staff and to the clinician, if necessary. Many states have addressed the issue of medication administration, with standard procedures for documentation and training of staff, but there often are no standards related to other procedures, such as measurement of blood pressure, finger-stick glucose, or oxygen saturation. Unfortunately, many group home agencies are not set up to train staff (and then train new staff) to perform such procedures, to maintain adequate documentation and communication of results, and to monitor staff performance.

In Massachusetts, as of 2005, the state's medication policy for clients of the Department of Mental Retardation prohibits direct support staff from administering parenteral injections, such as subcutaneous insulin. (Until recently, it prohibited them from administering medications given through a gastric or enteric feeding tube as well.) Authority to administer parenteral injections (and, formerly, medications via feeding tubes) rests only with licensed nurses or physicians. When such medication administration is acquired via twice daily visits from a member of the Visiting Nurse Association (VNA) 1) the individual's daily routine is disrupted by having to wait for the VNA member to arrive; 2) frequency of administration of these medications is limited to no more than twice daily; and 3) the cost would not be covered by Medicare beyond a few visits. Based on a standard Medicaid payment of $60 per VNA visit, for two visits per day, the cost solely for the VNA member *giving* the individual his or her medication, excluding the cost of all other residential, administrative, or medical care, is more than $40,000 per year.

APPROACH TO INDIVIDUALS WITH LIFE-THREATENING ILLNESSES

Life expectancy of adults with developmental disabilities is now generally significantly longer than most people, even clinicians, appreciate. Probably the most valuable study to date to address this issue was published in 1998 by Strauss and Shavelle. It is based on comprehensive data of more than 24,000 individuals with cerebral palsy. The most important outcome of this study is the recognition that among adults with cerebral palsy, just two clearly objective criteria were found to be the primary correlates of an individual's life expectancy: mobility and mode of feeding (see Table 6.6-1).

Presumably, severely impaired mobility per se is not a cause of death, but it increases the likelihood that the individual will have associated issues, such as gastroesophageal reflux and recurrent pneumonia as well as more significant central nervous system dysfunction, which would be correlated with an increased risk of seizures. Those adults with cerebral palsy who have full motor and feeding abilities, regardless of intellectual ability, have life expectancies approaching just 5 years less than those of the general population. Once a clinician appreciates this fact, he or she may be more comfortable with the imposition of aggressive medical interventions in order to treat an acute illness.

Clinicians unfamiliar with the care of adults with developmental disabilities often question the appropriateness of providing invasive therapy for individuals whom they perceive as having a "poor" quality of life. This problem is exacerbated when such clinicians observe an acutely ill individual and fail to recognize that this same individual may have a much higher level of functioning when he or she is not acutely ill. Even a clinician who would have been comfortable providing aggressive therapy for an individual with disabilities might withhold necessary therapy because of the clinician's misperception that the individual's lower level of functioning (observed during the acute illness) is his or her baseline. Communication between the individual's primary care clinician and the attending or consulting clinician can help clarify misunderstandings about the appropriateness of a particular management plan. Individuals with developmental disabilities, their supporters, and/or guardians might need to seek a second opinion when a clinician's recommendations seem unwarranted.

Rocco, a 35-year-old man with congenital rubella syndrome manifesting in severe intellectual disabilities, cerebral palsy, and blindness, was nonverbal and had a profound kyphoscoliosis. He was admitted to the hospital with signs of acute cholecystitis. The consulting surgeon observed him lying in a fetal position, apparently unresponsive, except for aggression directed at the surgeon during abdominal examination.

The surgeon expressed concern that given the man's body habitus, his anticipated inability to cooperate with postoperative care, and his overall poor quality of life at baseline, he was not a candidate for surgery. The surgeon recommended that efforts be made to keep the man as comfortable as possible and let nature take its course. The primary care team and guardian disagreed and convinced the surgeon to operate. Due to the individual's body habitus, the gall bladder could not be removed, even with an open procedure; however, the surgeon was able to place a drain, successfully relieving pressure and allowing for slow healing. The recovery period lasted months, but ultimately the individual returned to his former baseline, enjoying life as he did before.

When a clinician is caring for an individual with or without a prior disability but with a severe, progressive, irreversible illness, especially when it causes significant physical and/or cognitive impairment, then that clinician might approach the individual and/or family members regarding the avoidance of invasive, potentially uncomfortable interventions and shift the focus of care to keeping the individual's life as comfortable as possible, rather than as long as possible. In this author's opinion, the degree of disability or supports required should *not* drive that discussion. Rather, the decision to avoid aggressive interventions should be based on the anticipated irreversibility and unrelenting progression of a degenerative illness. Regardless of the intensity of supports an individual may require at baseline, pursuing medical interventions is usually appropriate if it is anticipated that such interventions may return the individual to a stable baseline.

Consider, for example, a woman with Down syndrome who develops pneumonia, requiring acute care hospitalization. Regardless of the severity of her disabilities, this woman would usually be hospitalized and provided every means necessary to support and sustain her, *unless* she has a progressive, irreversible, degenerative condition, such as Alzheimer dementia, in which case it *may* be appropriate, in the late stages, to consider shifting the focus of care from longevity to comfort and avoidance of aggressive intervention. In summary, having a developmental disability should not be a sole reason for limiting interventions, but it also should not preclude the option of limiting aggressive interventions when an irreversible, progressive, degenerative end-stage illness is superimposed. (Note that laws and regulations regarding end-of-life treatment vary considerably from one state to another and should be considered in relation to the previous guidelines.)

CONTINUOUS, COMPREHENSIVE CARE

One advantage to congregate living situations (residential institutions) is the ready availability of many experienced observers, including both direct support staff and multidisciplinary clinicians, who all interact with an individual resident. Because these staff members are all present in the same place, they can repeatedly discuss their ongoing observations and formulate and reformulate how best to understand and support an individual's medical issues, symptoms, emotions, thought processes, and motivations. In outpatient community settings, such a comprehensive and continuous approach is much more difficult and rarely, if ever, achieved. This may be a reason why Shavelle and Strauss (1999), Strauss and Kastner (1996), and Strauss, Shavelle, Baumeister, and Anderson (1998) found markedly increased mortality rates (by up to 88% overall) among adults with developmental disabilities living in the community compared with those with similar medical conditions living in institutions. This major challenge needs to be addressed by community support systems.

PAYMENT AND REIMBURSEMENT FOR MEDICAL CARE

Reimbursement issues continue to be a significant barrier to the provision of optimal care for adults with developmental disabilities in community settings. The majority (about 70%–85%) of adults with intellectual disabilities are covered primarily by Medicare, and secondarily by Medicaid. Most of the rest have only Medicaid. Very few are covered by private insurance. The amount of time it may take to perform even the simplest procedures and gather the necessary information during an office visit often makes it difficult to retrieve reimbursement (from any fee-for-service payer) that matches the time commitment involved to perform a quality evaluation. Third-party payer systems also tend to limit options for care in other ways. For example, Medicare will not reimburse for nurse practitioner home visits or for case management or health care coordination.

In Massachusetts, some agencies employ nurse practitioners as case managers or health care coordinators to help facilitate interactions between physicians and direct supporters. But often, their efforts are frustrated by limited communication with the prescribing physician or lack of opportunity to participate in the team managing an inpatient hospitalization. In the Boston area, a Medicaid-affiliated health maintenance organization, the Community Medical Alliance (CMA), gets a capitated (per member, per month) payment from Medicaid to supply medical services to people with severe physical disabilities, including a few adults who also have intellectual disabilities (Meyers, Glover, and Master, 1997). CMA provides cohesive teams of providers including physicians specifically qualified to care for people with severe disabilities and nurse practitioners with prescribing authority, who can perform home visits and coordinate comprehensive care among several providers, thus facilitating the practice described previously. Efforts are underway to establish similar services for Medicare-insured adults with severe intellectual disabilities.

CONCLUSION

Throughout the United States, some state agencies that are responsible for the care of adults with developmental disabilities finance medical clinics and/or systems that allow specifically qualified clinicians to spend the time necessary to provide quality care (Ziring et al., 1988), sometimes in familiar and comfortable home and/or day program settings. Every adult with developmental disabilities and limited means of reliable communication living in the community needs to have a wide variety of supporters (including medical personnel) and systems that 1) improve reliable communication and interpretation, 2) help the individual to safely and comfortably tolerate medical interventions, and 3) facilitate interactions with those health care personnel less familiar with the individual's needs. Each individual must be served by a health care system that affords the same quality, personalized, compassionate health care that anyone deserves, regardless of age or intellectual ability.

REFERENCES

Meyers, A.R., Glover, M., & Master, R.J. (1997). Primary care for persons with disabilities: The Boston, Massachusetts Model Program. *American Journal of Physical Medicine and Rehabilitation, 76*(3 Suppl.), S37–S42.

Minihan, P.M., Dean, D.H., & Lyons, C.M. (1993). Managing the care of patients with mental retardation: A survey of physicians. *Mental Retardation, 31* (4), 239–246.

Shavelle, R., & Strauss, D. (1999). Mortality of persons with developmental disabilities after transfer into community care: A 1996 update. *American Journal on Mental Retardation, 104*(2), 143–147.

Strauss, D., & Kastner, T.A. (1996). Comparative mortality of people with mental retardation in institutions and the community. *American Journal on Mental Retardation, 101*(1), 26–40.

Strauss, D., & Shavelle, R. (1998). Life expectancy of adults with cerebral palsy. *Developmental Medicine and Child Neurology, 40,* 369–375.

Strauss, D., Shavelle, R., Baumeister, A., & Anderson, T.W. (1998). Mortality in persons with developmental disabilities after transfer into community care. *American Journal on Mental Retardation, 102*(6), 569–581.

Ziring, P.R., Kastner, T., Friedman, D.L., Pond, W.S., Barnett, M.L., Sonnenberg, E.M., et al. (1988). Provision of health care for persons with developmental disabilities living in the community: The Morristown model. *Journal of the American Medical Association, 260*(10), 1439–1444.

6.7 THE ROLE OF THE NURSE PRACTITIONER IN CARE OF ADULTS

Adria Hodas

What does it take to live a life of happiness and pleasure, rich in experiences, with caring relationships? How can a person live to his or her fullest potential? Doing so can be challenging for anyone, but for a person with disabilities, especially developmental disabilities, the challenges can be daunting. Opportunities for growth can be stymied by lack of resources, negative attitudes, inadequate knowledge, and/or limited understanding of the disability and how best to help the person grow. But achievements can be exciting, and life can be fulfilling. So, what does it take to help the person with developmental disabilities fulfill his or her potential and goals?

First, clinicians have to develop an understanding of what it means to live a full life. Everyone shares the need to live in a safe and comfortable home, to have relationships with others, to be treated with dignity and respect, to have opportunities to be productive, and to receive health care and other therapeutic supports to maintain physical and emotional well-being. Each person has interests, strengths, a personal history, and desires that further define what quality of life means for him or her. Disabilities overlay and interplay with aspects of the lives of individuals with disabilities but should not dictate and dominate their lives.

Clinicians need to examine the supports that a person with disabilities needs and has available. What are the individual's goals, and what does it take to achieve these goals? Supports can be far reaching and complex and include family members and other advocates, health and mental health care providers, other therapeutic and behavioral specialists, teachers, vocational specialists, employers, clergy, and other members of the community. Clinicians also need to look at the environment in which the person lives, from the person's home to the broader community. Is it one with attitudes of caring and acceptance? Is it inclusive and fully accessible? Is it safe? Is it physically clean, comfortable, and appealing? Often the strengths and weaknesses of the supports and environment are a greater factor in the person's successes than are the qualities of the person him- or herself.

Professionals who work with individuals with developmental disabilities are charged with the job of looking holistically at the person, his or her supports, and the environment. They can enhance the person's quality of life and the quality of supports and the environment in which the person lives. Their work can often be focused as much on teaching and strengthening the supports and environment as on teaching and strengthening the individual. Successes in one area of life or supports will have a positive impact on many other areas, and failures in one area can likewise be detrimental to many other areas.

Bob was a 58-year-old man with Down syndrome and Alzheimer disease who lived in a group home and attended a day habilitation program. As Bob began to show cognitive decline due to Alzheimer disease, his nurse practitioner, Lesley, assisted with and monitored the ongoing functional assessments done by program staff, including assessments of personal care, household skills, social skills, vocational skills, communication, and behavior. Bob also experienced changes in his health status that were critical to monitor. Lesley checked Bob's nutrition and swallowing disorder. She especially watched for aspiration pneumonia because it is the most common cause of death in individuals with Down syndrome and Alzheimer disease.

Even before changes in Bob's health status were apparent, Lesley provided anticipatory guidance to assist program staff and family members in becoming flexible and making modifications in care and routines to avoid as many problems as possible. Appropriate evaluations were performed such as swallowing studies that led to changes in food and fluid textures. Lesley worked with the program staff, family members, and other health care providers to find creative solutions for Bob's resistance to medical evaluations and treatments. She also tried to find ways to readjust Bob's balance of activities, stimulation, and socialization to compensate for his declining health and cognitive status. Before and after Bob's passing, Lesley assisted staff, housemates, and family members through dying, death, and grieving stages.

Nurse practitioners who work in the community with individuals with developmental disabilities can have a variety of positions, including working for private vendors and state departments providing either consultative services or direct services. The role of a nurse practitioner can be a clinician performing assessments and care; a teacher of individuals with developmental disabilities, their staff, and their families; an advocate for the specific health needs of each individual and for the broader issues of health care of individuals with developmental disabilities; and a liaison with the generic health community. A clinician specializing in care of individuals with developmental disabilities can help others to understand the types of care that need to be provided, the rationale for the care, and the constraints to providing the care and can assist in negotiating for the most realistic and effective approach to management of the medical problem. All aspects of the role add up to providing health safeguards for individuals who need extra supports. The clinical role includes the following:

- Monitoring and managing chronic conditions
- Performing triage, monitoring, and managing acute illnesses and injuries
- Promoting wellness by integrating healthy activities and a nutritious diet into daily routines

- Assessing and managing changes in functional status and emerging medical conditions
- Interpreting recommendations by other health care providers to the individual, staff, and family and helping them to integrate the recommendations into daily routines
- Providing anticipatory guidance to prevent secondary disabilities
- Advocating for each individual

The approach to care utilizes accepted standards of nursing practice. The standards of practice developed by the Developmental Disabilities Nurse Association (DDNA) are particularly pertinent. In the introduction to the standards, the DDNA wrote that

> Activities include: providing a habilitative milieu concerned with assisting the development of a positive concept of self and achievement of optimum control of the environment by the individual; teaching positive health practices; preventing disease, maintaining health and well-being, and providing care during acute illnesses; participating with other disciplines in activities that increase the complexity of behavior patterns; advocating for people in the exercise of human and civil rights; and serving as a role model and resource person for individuals, families, other service providers, and the community. (1995, p. 1)

The essence of the nurse practitioner's role is knowing the individual beyond his or her health to include his or her preferences, behaviors, means of communication, hopes and dreams, and causes of pleasure and sadness. Combining knowledge of the person and understanding of clinical presentation of medical problems is critical to make sense of the manner in which a medical problem is demonstrated.

HEALTH CARE PLANS

The Health Care Plan is a comprehensive summary of the individual's health status and intervention plans that can be used for multiple purposes and with multiple audiences (e.g., other health care providers, program staff, representatives of the funding source, families). The content of the health care plan can include a profile of the individual, a current summary and history of the individual's health care problems, strategies for maintaining wellness, and strategies for management of chronic conditions. Descriptive information, such as details on how the individual expresses pain and illness; how the individual copes with medical exams and procedures; and communication and self-care skills, can be included in the profile.

The health care plan can be used to teach staff about the individual and the strategies to maintain optimal health. It can be used as a summary in emergency situations or with new health care providers and as a tool for review of the individual's overall health during the annual physical exam. When included in the individualized service plan (ISP), it can provide guidance for services, training, and daily supports. When updated annually, it can provide a long-term history of specific problem areas with information regarding which management approaches were successful. In essence, this valuable, portable medical record is maintained for the individual by the nurse practitioner.

An example of health strategies that might be included in the plan for an individual with cerebral palsy follows:

- Range of motion, use of orthotics, and good positioning to prevent contractures
- Safe mobility and accident prevention
- Modification of food and fluid textures for the management of dysphagia
- Interventions to prevent pressure sores including frequent skin checks, proper positioning, hygiene, nutrition, and hydration
- Bowel and bladder management
- Use of adaptive equipment to achieve optimal independence in self-care and other activities of daily living
- Referrals to the physiatrist, orthopedist, neurologist, and medical specialists
- Consultations with an occupational therapist, physical therapist, and speech therapist
- Management of related disorders such as seizures, mood disorders, and visual deficits

NEW ADMISSIONS

The success of an individual with disabilities who is placed in a new program relies on the program's preparation for the individual. When a referral is received, the nurse practitioner should review it before the individual is accepted into the program. Some of the initial questions to ask include

- Is the individual compatible with the other individuals in the program and with the physical layout of the program?

- Are there modifications in the physical layout of the program that will need to be made to accommodate this new individual, such as safety rails, ramps, or shower modifications?
- Is there equipment that will need to be obtained, such as a shower chair, bed side-rails, a food processor to puree food, a wheelchair scale, or adaptive equipment for activities of daily living?
- What are the status and management of any chronic medical conditions?
- Who are the current health care providers?
- What is the person's understanding of his or her health?
- How does the person communicate and seek out assistance when ill, in pain, or injured?
- What is the person's response to pain?
- What are the person's daily routines, including eating, sleeping, physical activity, bowel and bladder patterns, types of supports required for activities of daily living, and sexual activity?
- What are his or her self-medication skills?
- Are there diet modifications or restrictions?
- Are there safety concerns related to ambulation, pica, seizures, or inappropriate behaviors?
- Is the person able to cooperate with medical exams and procedures?
- What are the family's preferences for involvement in medical care?

Once the individual has been accepted into the program, the nurse practitioner works with the family or staff from the previous program to become as familiar with the individual as possible to ensure consistency of health care. Maintaining relationships with long-standing medical providers and not simply changing providers for the convenience of staff is helpful. The nurse practitioner also works with the program staff to provide any necessary training and to develop daily routines.

ONGOING INSTRUCTION

Almost everything the nurse practitioner says to individuals and staff is actually teaching. Instructions should be accompanied with a rationale that is geared to the level of the person receiving the instructions. Understanding the rationale means that the person is more likely to be motivated to follow the instructions, to feel empowered, and to learn and generalize the information. Formal training of staff is essential for providing daily care. Some of the topics that should be addressed include

- Recognition and management of seizures
- Nutrition, menu planning, hydration, and aspiration precautions
- Bowel management and prevention of constipation
- Bladder management
- Personal and oral hygiene, skin care, and prevention of skin breakdown
- Signs and symptoms of illness, including recognition of pain and changes in functioning (physical activity, bowel, bladder, eating, sleeping, alertness, social interactions)
- Effective communication with health care providers
- First aid and care of minor medical conditions
- Medication administration
- Safety, including injury-free lifting and hot and cold weather seasonal safety
- Infection control
- Care of diseases and disorders specific to each individual

Staff training should be competency based as much as possible. Posttests and demonstrations can be used to ensure competency. Staff attending a training may have a variety of backgrounds and may use English as a second language, which can make the training a challenge. Effective training is best accomplished by having staff actively participate in the training. Incorporating group activities and open discussions can help to engage staff, can make the information more relevant, and can help staff learn from each other through sharing experiences. Trainings usually need to be repeated periodically. The nurse practitioner should continually monitor for areas where it is apparent that staff need refreshers to prevent a decline in quality of care.

ONE NURSE PRACTITIONER'S WEEK

The following describes one week in the life of a developmental disabilities nurse practitioner working for a private vendor in community-based residential, day, and family supports.

Providing health care supports to individuals who reside in group homes and their staff means being available any time of the day or night. During the weekend, one individual was ill with gastroenteritis. Presenting symptoms included nausea, vomiting, and diarrhea that lasted throughout the weekend. Residential staff called for advice several times. Care was complicated because the man is Christian Scientist, so his medical interventions and use of medications are restricted. The residential staff and I worked with his mother to modify his diet and provide comfort and reasonable care while respecting their religious beliefs. Other weekend calls were more routine, such as consultation on respiratory congestion or constipation. Constipation is a serious problem that requires constant monitoring. In addition to the medical consequences of chronic constipation, many behavioral manifestations and significant quality-of-life problems can result from it.

A typical Monday morning starts with a review or follow-up of any concerns that arose over the weekend. The week will be a balance of visiting group homes, providing staff training, supervising nurses and other clinical staff, attending clinical meetings, reviewing new referrals, consulting with staff and families, and advocating for activities. As problems emerge, the priorities and activities are adjusted. In some cases, follow-up is passed on to other nurses or clinical staff for management.

Later on Monday, I attend the staff meeting in Bob's group home. Bob, as mentioned previously, is a man with Down syndrome and significant decline associated with Alzheimer's disease. Before the staff and I begin our more concentrated discussion of Bob's illness, we review the other individuals living in the residence. One lady has very recently moved in, and we are just getting to know her. We discuss basics such as her sleeping, eating, and toileting patterns. We then review medical appointments that have taken place over the past few weeks and those that are upcoming. Although staff contact me following each appointment with a report on the health care provider's findings and recommendations, this meeting is my opportunity to work with the staff in a more thorough manner. Often, staff follow the health care providers recommendations but don't actually understand the implications of the diagnoses or the treatments that have been prescribed. I use the staff meeting to provide teaching around the specific diagnosis and also to check on follow-up of the health care provider's recommendations to ensure that they are realistic and effective.

There are some upcoming medical appointments, including a psychiatry appointment. Before attending the appointment, the staff need to come to consensus on the individual's status and to decide on questions and possible recommendations for the psychiatrist to consider. We review the individual's behavioral data of the identified target behaviors to see trends since the last appointment; obtain data and concerns from the day program and family; and review any medical, environmental, or social factors that may have contributed to changes in behavior. Following the meeting, I spend some time with the individual to observe for medication adverse reactions. Later in the day, I confer with the behaviorist regarding the individual's upcoming psychiatric appointment.

Martin, another individual living in the residence, will be taken by staff tomorrow to his annual physical exam with his primary care physician. I assist the staff in preparing for the appointment by reviewing Martin's health status during the past year and recommending health screening tests that are due.

The staff meeting then turns to longer discussion of concerns about Bob's condition, the types of care he requires, and strategies for staff to manage his care. Staff ask questions about the progression of Bob's Alzheimer disease. We have an emotional discussion about end-of-life care. I want to be sure that the staff have the supports and resources needed to cope with this distressing situation. Before leaving the residence, I do a chart review on another individual in preparation for her annual ISP, and I ask questions of the staff about daily care (e.g., eating, sleeping, toileting, and menstrual patterns; activity levels) to help flesh out the paper review.

Tuesday is a staff training day in two different group homes. On this day, the trainings include seizure disorders and menu planning. At first, general information is presented, then the training is expanded to address specific issues that are relevant to the individuals living in the group home. The goals of the training are to help the staff understand the theory, apply it to the specific situations, and be able to use it later in new situations.

I am called on Tuesday by a parent regarding her daughter, Susan, who has cerebral palsy. Susan was recently started on Baclofen by her physiatrist. Her mother has concerns about the medication's efficacy and side effects. As a result of this discussion, I contact the occupational therapist at the day program to obtain feedback on upper motor range of motion. This conversation was the beginning of the coordination of care between the physiatrist, mother, the occupational therapist in the day program, and the occupational therapist who works with the physiatrist. Fragmented care with multiple health care providers is a large problem and results in inadequate care or duplicated services. Establishing connections and acting as a focal point to disseminate information can be a very important function of the nurse practitioner.

On Wednesday, I visit a day habilitation program with two purposes. The first one is to provide supervision to the nurse assigned to the program. We spend most of our time reviewing health concerns of the individuals who attend the program. Our discussion includes deciding to request a swallowing evaluation for an individual who has recently shown signs of dysphagia. We also discuss staff training needs in regard to a new referral and the man's seizure management that includes a vagal nerve stimulator and Diastat. Other subjects that are discussed are management of an individual with a new gastrostomy tube, concerns of medication side effects seen in another individual, the progress an individual has been making on a self-medication program, and interventions for an individual with recent unexplained weight loss.

The second purpose of the visit is to attend the monthly clinical meeting. The program manager, group leader, nurse, occupational therapist, physical therapist, physical therapy assistant, speech-language pathologist, and behaviorist gather to review one group of five individuals each month. We each give input based on our expertise, experience, and history with the individual. For example, when we discuss a cooking skills activity, the nurse may offer healthy alternatives to the food being prepared if the individual has a weight problem. We also discuss strategies to motivate an individual to increase participation in a gross motor program. Another individual is beginning to show some possible Alzheimer disease–related decline, so we discuss referrals for neurological evaluation and ways that we might need to modify his routines. When the meeting is over, each participant has a list of items that need follow-up. Throughout the discussion, I act as clinical supervisor by assessing the other clinical staff for areas in which I may need to provide resources for their growth and development.

On Thursday, I spend the morning visiting Jason, who has been referred to one of our group homes. He has cerebral palsy, a gastrostomy tube because of dysphagia, an active seizure disorder, and pica. Once I have met him, his family, and the nursing staff at his current program, I can begin the preparation for his move. We plan staff trainings on his seizure disorder and gastrostomy tube. Referrals are made to the physical therapist for a gait assessment and the behaviorist for management of the pica. I also contact Jason's current primary care physician to review his current medication orders.

One of the ways that the individuals in the group homes use to keep up their regular exercise is to participate in a track competition. They train weekly for 4 months prior to the big event. On this Thursday, I work with the program and recreation staff to evaluate the training programs for an individual who is overweight, an individual with cerebral palsy, a man who has insulin-dependent diabetes, and an older man with degenerative joint disease.

In the evening, I attend the quarterly human rights committee meeting where we review behavior and safety plans for several individuals. One woman with a weight problem is continually taking food from the refrigerator and cabinets, so we discuss the appropriateness of limiting her access to the kitchen. A man who has been a pipe smoker for more than 20 years has an oral lesion. His dentist is concerned about oral cancer and has indicated that it is imperative for the man to stop smoking. The committee reviews the situation and makes a variety of suggestions to help him quit.

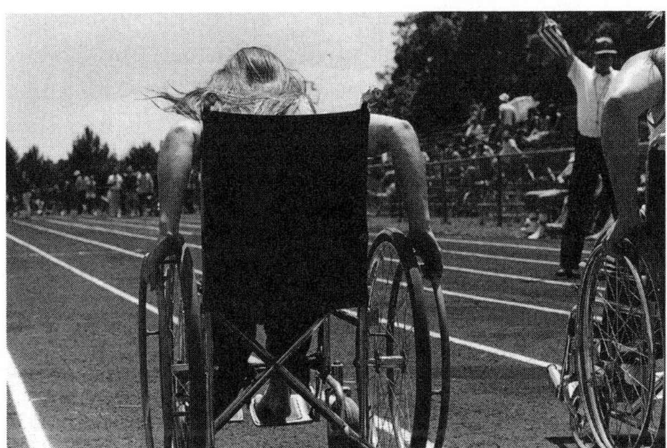

Figure 6.7–1. Individuals with disabilities can stay in shape by competing in track competitions. (© Digital Vision.)

On Friday, I attend a meeting of developmental disabilities nurses from around the state who work for private vendors and the state. Our purpose is to advocate for the health care needs of individuals with developmental disabilities. We discuss standards and practice issues, review policies and procedures, share experiences, and look for solutions to problems we face.

Throughout each day, a variety of problems need attention. Mary is ready for hospital discharge following an episode of gastrointestinal bleeding. She has new medications including an order for intravenous iron therapy. This requirement leads to a series of telephone calls to provide residential staff with information about the new medications and to make arrangements for the intravenous therapy.

During a seizure, John fell, received a head injury with a scalp laceration, and was referred to the emergency room for evaluation and care. I will notify the family and follow-up with staff to be sure that they understand and follow the emergency room instructions. I also plan to visit the group home in 10 days to remove John's sutures.

Peggy, a 50-year-old woman with Down syndrome, returns from her annual physical exam with a referral to a cardiologist for an echocardiogram because of a concern about a ventricular-septal defect. I have multiple discussions with staff and Peggy's mother about the problem and its management.

Tom is a man who is deaf, legally blind, and self-abusive. He has swelling and pain of his elbow. He is referred to the emergency room and found to have a fracture. The evaluation and treatment are complicated by his anxiety and resistance to medical exams and procedures.

Sandy has a dental abscess and needs an extraction. The dentist has given her antibiotics and pain medication, but the extraction cannot be done because she does not have a legal guardian. This situation prompts calls to initiate an emergency guardianship process.

Larry is a man with spina bifida who has no feeling below his waist. Although he is skilled at self-catherization, he has been having accidents, especially at night. As a result of his incontinence, he now has a stage 1 decubitus ulcer on his buttocks. He is a picky eater, so there are also concerns about his nutrition. A plan is put into place to improve his hygiene, nutrition, and positioning, and staff are trained in the daily treatment and routine. A referral is placed to the local visiting nurses agency to provide regular monitoring and treatment. Ongoing teaching is given to Larry because his understanding and participation in the care are crucial to successful healing.

Susan's seizure disorder has become worse during the past few months. She is spending an increasing number of days at home instead of going to her vocational training program because of her seizure activity. Her parents are not comfortable with the neurologist's approach to care, so we work together to explore other options.

Sam had a recent increase in his anticonvulsant medications and is now showing signs of toxicity. Blood levels need to be obtained and the neurologist consulted. David has been having recent episodes of urinary incontinence, which is unusual, so he is evaluated for and found to have a urinary tract infection. Staff report that Alan has been sent home from his day program with signs of conjunctivitis. Treatment and infection control procedures are reviewed with staff. Because it is summertime, the weather is humid and the temperature is nearing 90 degrees. I leave a message for all program managers reminding them to ensure that individuals increase fluid intake, stay in cool places, apply sunscreen when outside, and use insect repellant to prevent mosquito bites. On Saturday evening, Seth, who has recently started a new medication, has developed a facial rash and swelling; he is brought to the emergency room for evaluation.

Each day brings a new set of concerns and follow-up on the ongoing ones. Each concern may generate one or more of the following interventions: initiation of a treatment; referral to another medical provider for further evaluation and treatment; staff training; and consultation with family members, other clinical staff, or other health care providers.

CONCLUSION

Finding a role that provides more variety or challenges than being a nurse practitioner is difficult. Each new problem brings an opportunity to use a wide set of knowledge and skills. Clinical assessment and management, teaching, and advocacy are intertwined and are daily activities. Training of staff—not just in health care and medication issues, but in attitudes and understanding of the implications of the various disabilities and prevention of secondary disabilities—enhances their ability to provide care. Nurse practitioners can be employed by private vendors, can participate on a resource team, or can serve as consultants to add depth to the clinical team and enhance the health care safeguards. As they work with other health and mental health care providers and professional groups, they strive to provide adequate medical safeguards and to improve quality of care. The core of the role of the nurse practitioner is to help individuals with developmental disabilities, to direct care, and to help other clinical staff to learn and grow.

REFERENCES

Antonangeli, J.M. (1995). *Of two minds: A guide to the care of people with the dual diagnosis of Alzheimer's disease and mental retardation.* Boston: Fidelity Press.

Developmental Disabilities Nurses Association. (1995). *Standards of developmental disabilities nursing practice.* Eugene, OR: Aggen.

Martin, B.A. (1997). Primary care of adults with mental retardation living in the community. *American Family Physician, 56,* 485–494.

Marks, B.A., Brown, A., Hahn, J.E., & Heller, T. (2003, June). Nursing care resources for individuals with intellectual and developmental disabilities across the life span. *Nursing Clinics of North America, 38*(2), 373–393.

Nehring, W.M. (2003, June). History of the role of nurses caring for persons with mental retardation. *Nursing Clinics of North America, 38*(2), 351–372.

Ridenour, N., & Norton, D. (1995). Community-based persons with mental retardation: opportunities for health promotion. *Nurse Practitioner Forum, 6,* 19–23.

Roth, S.P., & Morse, J.S. (1994). *A life-span approach to nursing care for individuals with developmental disabilities.* Baltimore: Paul H. Brookes Publishing Co.

Service, K.P., & Hahn, J.E. (2003, June). Issues in aging: The role of the nurse in the care of older people with intellectual and developmental disabilities. *Nursing Clinics of North America, 38*(2), 291–312.

6.8 NURSING HOMES

Sandra L. Friedman

Thousands of individuals residing within the United States have ongoing medical and nursing needs that do not require hospitalizations in acute care facilities. Family members may assist in providing this care within the home environment. Nursing and other ancillary services may also be obtained within the community setting to assist people living at home. Sometimes, however, individuals are provided with needed nursing and medical services within a nursing home, or long-term care facility. In 1999, approximately 18,000 nursing homes, with 1.6 million residents, existed in the United States (Centers for Disease Control and Prevention, 2004).

The care provided in long-term care facilities has changed over the years. Social policy, laws, and regulatory standards have evolved and been developed in order to provide appropriate and comprehensive care. Instances of inadequate nursing home resources, as well as abuse and neglect, periodically come to the fore, particularly in cases of litigation. Despite these issues, many people receive needed, high-quality services in nursing home settings.

The appropriateness of nursing home placement, or lack thereof, for individuals with intellectual and other developmental disabilities has been questioned and continues to be addressed. Surely, nursing homes are not meant to be a substitute for community resources for people with disabilities who do not have chronic medical and nursing needs. Receiving services within a community setting is preferable even for individuals with ongoing medical problems and nursing requirements. A number of factors, however, may make this option impractical. In the mid-1990s, an estimated 1% of people with intellectual and developmental disabilities of all ages in the United States resided in nursing homes (Larson, 2004). This chapter reviews some of the historical, regulatory, social, and medical factors as they relate to individuals with intellectual and developmental disabilities who reside in long-term care facilities.

HISTORICAL PERSPECTIVE

The Social Security Act Amendments of 1965 (PL 89-97) established the Medicare and Medicaid programs. Nursing home benefits for extended care were included in Medicare, and eligibility for medical assistance by Medicaid was also expanded (Centers for Medicare & Medicaid Services, 2003). State Medicaid plans subsequently provided payments for skilled nursing facilities and intermediate care facilities. States also became responsible to license nursing homes, and systems were established to monitor the care provided in such settings (American Health Care Association, 2001; American Medical Directors Association, 2003; Department of Mental Retardation, 1989, 2000a, 2000b).

During this time period, a movement arose to deinstitutionalize people with intellectual disabilities. Individuals residing in large institutions who experienced significant issues with feeding, aspiration of oral secretions and food, infections, and other complicating medical problems often did not survive into adulthood. As institutions closed, a need arose to provide an array of essential services within the community (Speat & Conroy, 1998; Uehara, Silverstein, Davis, & Geron, 1991). Long waiting lists existed for community-based residential resources, as well as significant restrictions on the existing institutions (Mitchell & Braddock, 1990). Privately operated nursing homes became a placement option for thousands of individuals with intellectual and developmental disabilities. Initially, many of these facilities were more custodial in nature, without specific guidelines for intervention or goals for care.

Legislation, litigation, and changes in social policy began to pave the way for more individualized care and protection of civil rights. These changes resulted in supervision by state agencies and school systems to ensure that appropriate care be provided to individuals with developmental disabilities, with the goal of inclusion within the community. In 1977, the Health Care Financing Administration (HCFA), renamed in 2001 as the Centers for Medicare & Medicaid Services (CMS) was established. The role of HCFA, under the auspices of the Department of Health, Education, and Welfare, was to coordinate Medicare and Medicaid (American Medical Directors Association, 2003; CMS, 2003). In 1980, the Omnibus Reconciliation Act (PL 96-499) was enacted to provide oversight of Medicaid funded facilities, including skilled nursing facilities (Fogg, 1999). Surveys of the facilities through the years revealed that large numbers of people with intellectual and developmental disabilities who resided in nursing homes did not require the intensity of medical or nursing services provided in such settings (Lakin, Anderson, Prouty, & Polister, 1999; Lakin, Hill, & Anderson, 1991; Larson, Lakin, Anderson, Kwak, Lee, & Anderson, 2001).

In 1986, a report from the Institute of Medicine noted the need for more federal involvement in nursing home regulation, due to the lack of high-quality care. Regulations were therefore developed to ensure appropriate placement of individuals and to mandate level of care. As such, in 1987 the Nursing Home Reform Amendment, also referred as the Omnibus Budget Reconciliation Act (OBRA; PL 100-203), was passed, whereby the Department of Health and Human Services put forth revised standards for nursing homes and their administration (American Health Care Association, 2001; American Medical Directors Association, 2003). PL 100-203 became effective in 1989 and was revised in 1990. It addressed issues related to the care of residents in nursing homes, survey and certification of such facilities, and enforcement and sanctions related to these new regulations (Fogg, 1999; Mitchell & Braddock, 1990). The specifics of the regulations regarding nursing home care and operations are part of the Code of Federal Regulations and are published in the Federal Register. Changes in the regulations, along with interpretative guidelines, have occurred several times throughout the years.

The Americans with Disabilities Act (ADA) of 1990 (PL 101-336) provided antidiscriminatory statutes for individuals with disabilities. The ADA prevented discrimination of individuals based on their disabilities and mandated that appropriate accommodations be made to promote community integration. This law set the stage for the landmark *Olmstead* decision by the Supreme Court in 1999, which upheld the right of individuals with disabilities to receive integrated, community-based care appropriate to their needs (Fox-Grage, Folkerner, & Lewis, 2003). This ruling indicated that the cost of services could not be used as the determining factor regarding its appropriateness for an individual. The *Olmstead* decision underscored the need to provide more appropriate, community-based living arrangements for those who did not require nursing home services and desired to live in a less-restricted environment.

PL 100-203 set forth regulations to ensure that all nursing home residents are provided with high-quality care in order to maintain their physical, medical, and psychological well-being. All skilled nursing facilities that receive Medicaid and Medicare funding are mandated to provide assessments of the residents using the Minimum Data Set (American Medical Directors Association, 2003). This data is provided to the states and then submitted to CMS. As of March 1998, the Minimum Data Set has provided information on each resident relating to his or her developmental (e.g., cognition, communication, continence), emotional (e.g., behavior, psychosocial), medical (e.g., nutrition, medications, health condition, diseases), and rehabilitative (e.g., special therapies and procedures) functioning, as well as potential discharge status (Fogg, 1999).

The federally required Minimum Data Set drives the yearly care plan for each resident. Residents with intellectual and developmental disabilities who reside in a skilled nursing facility also have individualized service plans (ISPs), whereby goals are developed by an interdisciplinary team to ensure that residents' needs are being met in all domains of care. These goals are also reviewed quarterly and renewed annually.

Over the years, more individuals with intellectual and developmental disabilities have moved out of nursing homes and residential facilities into the community or to less restricted environmental settings (Coucouvanis, Polister, Prouty, & Lakin, 2003). There continues to be variability in the time frame by which different states move people out of institutions. Unfortunately, long waiting lists continue to exist for people to receive appropriate housing and services in a less restrictive community setting. Most states are also facing significant Medicaid budgetary constraints that affect their ability to provide needed supports for those with intellectual and developmental disabilities (Mahady & Pettey, 2003). The mandate to provide more appropriate placement to individuals with disabilities most likely will increase the regulatory burden for long-term care facilities.

PEDIATRICS

Most children and adolescents who reside in pediatric skilled nursing facilities, either long-term or temporarily, have severe to profound intellectual disabilities. These children and youth are generally nonambulatory or have limited ambulatory skills. Most are nonverbal, although a small group may use augmentative communication systems. They present with multiple medical problems that require 24-hour skilled nursing, with ongoing medication administration, treatments, and therapies. (Staub, 1989).

Abnormalities of muscle tone are frequent, requiring muscle relaxant medication, baclofen pumps, injections, orthotics, and sometimes surgery. Orthopedic problems, such as scoliosis, hip dislocation, and contraction deformities, are common. Chronic pulmonary problems are prevalent, such as reactive airway disease or pneumonia from infectious agents or aspiration of food or saliva. A resident may have difficulty clearing his or her own secretions, requiring chest percussion, vibration, and suctioning. Airway obstruction may occur due to anatomical or neurological causes, requiring tracheostomy tube placement and/or ventilatory assistance.

Feeding problems frequently occur, due to problems with chewing, swallowing, airway protection, aspiration, or gastroesophageal reflux. As such, most individuals have feeding difficulties and may require at least a portion of their nutrition be provided via a feeding tube. These residents are generally incontinent and may have neurogenic bladders, so they are at increased risk of urinary tract infections.

Children with intellectual and developmental disabilities are a heterogeneous group, with variable likelihood for developing seizure disorders. Individuals with severe intellectual disabilities in association with certain types of cerebral palsy, however, have been noted to be at higher risk of developing seizures compared with the general population (Alvarez, 1989). Anticonvulsant medications are generally used for treatment, although in many instances, total control of a child's seizure disorder may be impractical. Sometimes, less conventional types of medical management, such as ketogenic diets or vagal nerve stimulators, may also be necessary to improve control of seizures.

Given the multisystem medical problems of young people who reside in relatively closed quarters, good infection control must be in place. Pathogens that would be relatively benign in the general population can potentially result in significant morbidity and mortality in this group of individuals (Huskins et al., 2000).

Hospice and end-of-life care for children with intellectual and developmental disabilities may also be provided in a skilled nursing facility setting. In some situations, hospitalization is not appropriate or desired, and the family is not able to provide such care in their home.

Carly was a 2½-year-old girl with cerebral dysgenesis and severe hydrocephalus. She underwent a ventriculo-peritoneal shunt placement soon after birth and was hospitalized multiple times for shunt infections, malfunctions, and revisions. Nursing services were provided in her home in the evening, and a physical therapist provided home services on a weekly basis. Carly ate slowly and took all of her nutrition through a bottle. Her parents had decided that they did not want her to undergo gastrostomy tube placement as a means to supplement her nutritional intake.

Carly was visually alert and responded to sound. She smiled for pleasure and grimaced or cried for discomfort. She also produced occasional vowel sounds, although she did not babble. Carly was able to bat at objects and could roll over and sit with support.

Carly was considered to be near death during her last hospitalization for shunt-related problems. She developed skin breakdown over the shunt reservoir and leakage from the umbilical area. She was diagnosed with a low-grade peritonitis. Carly's physicians anticipated that, even with additional procedures, Carly would likely die in the near future. Her parents, therefore, decided to forego additional procedures and to redirect care from aggressive medical management to primarily comfort measures. They felt that the risk of additional procedures outweighed the benefit and would potentially cause undue suffering. The medical team caring for Carly concurred with the parents' wishes.

Carly went home and continued to be fed by her parents. She progressively lost weight because it took her a long time to feed orally. Her family had not expected her to be able to survive for an appreciable period of time, due to the fact that she no longer had a ventriculo-peritoneal shunt in place. Instead, Carly began to leak fluid, presumably cerebrospinal fluid, from a small wound in her scalp, although she did not develop any signs of significant infection. Over the following 5 months, the stress of caring for Carly became too great for her family. Carly needed to be held frequently for comfort, as she tended to otherwise be irritable. Nursing services were available only on a limited basis.

Carly's family decided to seek other options for her care. They ultimately decided on a pediatric long-term nursing facility that was approximately 20 minutes from their home. The family wanted her to be treated for medical conditions that would affect her comfort, although they did not want treatment that would extend her life. Surprisingly, Carly began to gain weight and grow, as there was staff available to spend more time feeding her. She developed a seizure disorder, for which her parents wanted her treated. Her family visited regularly, although they did not take her home for visits.

After residing approximately 1 year in the pediatric skilled nursing facility, Carly began to develop increasing irritability, particularly with movement. Her feeding decreased progressively, with decreased urinary output. She developed purulent drainage from an area on her scalp. She was provided with medication for comfort and soon thereafter passed away.

Indications for Placement

The concept of a medical home has been developed to promote coordinated, interdisciplinary care within the community setting, particularly for children with complex medical problems (American Academy of Pediatrics, 2004). Sometimes, however, families explore different options because their children's medical needs cannot easily be met in the home and community setting for a variety of reasons. Obtaining reliable home nursing services on a regular basis may be difficult, and limited options of community-based care may exist for medically fragile children. As children become older, lifting them and caring for their personal needs may become difficult. Parents may not be able to emotionally or physically deal with the demands of care. Their home may have inadequate space for the needed equipment, or the family may not live in accessible housing or be able to obtain a more desirable living situation.

Studies have looked at factors that may affect a family's decision to place their child outside of the home environment, as well as the emotional impact of such decisions. Outward appearances indicating disability, higher maternal socioeconomic status, larger number of other children in the home, and stress on the caregiver were factors associated with greater consideration of residential placement (Hanneman & Blacher, 1998). Other studies have indicated that family involvement and concern continues, regardless of placement (Blacher, Baker, & Feinkleid, 1999). Obviously, issues regarding placement decisions are complex and require an individualized approach.

Families also sometimes use pediatric skilled nursing facilities to obtain respite services for their child. The length of time requested for respite care may range from days to weeks, and occasionally several months. There may also be instances after an acute hospitalization whereby a child may require a temporary increase in nursing care, receiving it in a pediatric skilled nursing facility and then returning home. Children may also be admitted for a diagnostic assessment of medical, educational, and/or therapeutic services in the pediatric skilled nursing facility, with recommendations to ultimately be carried out in the community and home.

Despite federal guidelines for nursing home care, each state determines the eligibility guidelines for nursing home placement (Department of Mental Retardation, 2000a, 2000b). Children who are admitted to pediatric skilled nursing facilities in Massachusetts, for long-term or respite care, need to have a developmental level of 18 months or less and must require 24-hour skilled nursing care. The family completes a packet of supporting information, which is then reviewed for potential approval by the Medical Review Team through the Department of Public Health.

A child who has been placed in a pediatric skilled nursing facility may also display developmental and medical improvements that could be better served in a less restrictive setting. In those instances, alternative settings may be sought to more appropriately meet the needs of the child and family. Family supports and circumstances may also change, allowing a child to move back to his or her home. Provisions then need to be made to ensure smooth transition to the new living arrangement.

Change in Demographics

Chaney and Eyman (2000) have reported the patterns of mortality in residential facilities to have changed over the years. Individuals tend to die at older ages, with higher mortality rates noted for those with lower cognitive levels, presence of seizure disorders, and prenatal etiology for their intellectual disabilities. Similarly, the age of residents living in pediatric skilled nursing facilities has increased as life expectancy has increased.

Demographic changes, as noted in one of the four pediatric skilled nursing facilities in Massachusetts, revealed an older population, living longer with less resident turnover (Friedman, 1995). Children admitted to pediatric skilled nursing facilities also tend to have more complicated medical problems than previously, particularly for younger children. More individuals have undergone tracheostomy tube placements, as well as use ventilators, baclofen pumps, and gastrostomy and jejunostomy tubes.

Pediatric skilled nursing facilities were established to provide care for children from birth to age 22; however, facilities are faced with dilemmas regarding what type of placement is appropriate when an individual turns 22 years of age. Adult nursing homes, serving primarily geriatric residents, are generally not geared to the needs of young adults with significant medical issues and severe intellectual and developmental disabilities. Families often wish their children to remain in the familiar setting of the pediatric skilled nursing facility, with caregivers who know them well. Group homes are not readily available to medically fragile individuals, who require 24-hour skilled nursing. Parents of these young adults often are aging and not able to care for their children themselves. These young adults, therefore, may remain in the pediatric skilled nursing home setting, where young adult recreation and educational programs have been developed to meet their needs as best as possible. In Massachusetts, individuals with severe intellectual and developmental disabilities and complex medical problems cannot be admitted to pediatric skilled nursing facilities after the age of 22. Families may, therefore, request that their child be admitted to a pediatric skilled nursing facility prior to age 22 to assure placement on a long-term basis.

Ashton was an 18-year-old boy with an unusual chromosomal abnormality. He was nonambulatory, nonverbal, and incontinent and required assistance for all activities of daily living. Prior developmental assessment indicated that he was functioning at a level less than 1 year old and was diagnosed with profound intellectual disabilities. He seemed to respond positively to familiar caregivers and indicated when he was pleased or distressed. He had a history of gastroesophageal reflux, treated with medication. Several years ago, after recurrent episodes of pneumonia, a modified barium swallow had indicated significant aspiration with oral feeding. A fundoplication and gastrostomy tube were placed, and Ashton began to receive the majority of his nutrition via gastrostomy tube. He subsequently experienced a marked reduction in the development of significant pulmonary infections.

Ashton also had a seizure disorder that required the use of two anticonvulsants, with the occasional addition of another medication during times of poorly controlled seizure activity. He also had significant spasticity, requiring muscle relaxants and use of orthotic devices.

Ashton went to school in a neighboring community that housed a program for children with significant developmental disabilities. He was transported 1 hour each way in a school van. His parents provided the bulk of his medical treatments at home; however, as his medical needs increased, Ashton began to receive nursing services at home. Over time, lifting and moving Ashton from his bed became increasingly difficult. His father, who was responsible for much of the lifting and moving, became ill and required hospitalization. Ashton's mother requested additional nursing support, which was not reliably available.

Ashton's parents then began to explore other care options. They did not want to ask extended family members to assume ongoing responsibility for Ashton's care. No community-based options were available that were appropriate for Ashton's age and would also provide him with needed medical and nursing care. Ashton's parents considered temporary foster home placement but realized that they wanted something that would provide more comprehensive services on a long-term basis.

They were referred to the Medical Review Team through the Department of Public Health, where it was determined that Ashton was eligible for long-term placement in a pediatric skilled nursing facility, based on his need for 24-hour skilled nursing and his cognitive level of 18 months or less. Ashton's family toured the facility, which housed a school in addition to a young adult program, therapies, recreational, nursing, medical, and social work services.

The transition was quite difficult for the family, who continued to be very involved in Ashton's care. The skilled nursing facility was 45 minutes away from the family home; however, Ashton's parents participated in the parents' group and took Ashton home for holidays and special events.

Interdisciplinary Team

Pediatric skilled nursing facilities have evolved from custodial to goal-oriented care. As such, many disciplines are involved in the care of the child. Disciplines include medicine, nursing, therapies, education, psychology, social work, and administration. Within the disciplines are also professionals offering various levels of care, such as nurse practitioners, registered nurses, licensed practical nurses, and nurses' aides. Medical, behavioral, and social issues rarely affect only one discipline; therefore, an interdisciplinary team approach is generally implemented. Parents or guardians are also included as much as possible, particularly when significant issues require decision making or family involvement.

In addition to ISPs, federal laws have also addressed educational and therapeutic needs of children. All children are entitled to provision of medical, educational, and therapeutic services, regardless of their cognitive level, medical needs, or place of residence. The Rehabilitation Act of 1973 (PL 93-112) protected qualified individuals with disabilities from discrimination. This law provided for related services (e.g., speech therapy, physical therapy, psychological testing or counseling) in an educational setting for children with developmental disabilities or chronic medical conditions, regardless of whether they qualify for special education classroom placement (American Academy of Pediatrics, 2002).

The Education for All Handicapped Children Act of 1975 (PL 94-142) mandated a free appropriate public education for all children ages 5–18 in the least restrictive environment. Annual individualized education programs (IEPs) were established whereby educational assessments, objectives, and plans could be developed for each child with special needs. In 1990, the Individuals with Disabilities Education Act (IDEA; PL 101-476) reauthorized PL 94-142 and expanded the age of services to 22 years (Giangreco, 2001). The individualized family service plan (IFSP) was also introduced and addressed the needs of families and their children from birth to 3 years. In 1997, IDEA Amendments (PL 105-17) were signed into law, with the final regulations released in 1999. These amendments addressed issues related to identification, evaluation, services, and due process for all children with disabilities, including infants and toddlers.

Inconsistencies have been noted to exist between PL 105-17, Parts B and C, and Section 504 of the Rehabilitation Act of 1973 (American Academy of Pediatrics, 2002). These laws have been widely interpreted, and differences in provision of services exist both nationally and statewide. As schools are now caring for children with complex medical problems, what may be necessary medically may not be deemed necessary in the educational setting. In 1999, the Supreme Court ruled that complex nursing services can be considered as a related service. Controversies continue in the community setting about distinguishing educationally related services from rehabilitation services and determining financial responsibility to meet individual needs (American Academy of Pediatrics, 2002; Giangreco, 2001).

Children who reside in pediatric skilled nursing facilities, just as those living in the community, need to be provided with educational and related services mandated by federal law. IFSPs are provided for children younger than age 3, and IEPs are developed for each child between the ages of 3 and 22 years, with services provided to meet the established objectives. The IEPs are reviewed annually, with reevaluations occurring every 3 years.

Family and Surrogate Decision-Maker Roles

Placement of a child in a residential setting can be quite difficult for families. Families of children and adolescents placed in residential settings continue to be very connected and involved in the care of their children and have been noted to experience less guilt as time passes. In some instances, family life after placement has also been found to improve (Blacher et al., 1999).

Parents generally are the legal guardians for children until the age of 18 years. When parents are unavailable or unable to serve as the legal guardian or when the courts deem parents unfit to serve in that role, another person, such as another family member, a court-appointed designee, or a representative from an agency, such as the Department of Mental Retardation, would be appointed (Department of Mental Retardation, 1989). When an individual with severe or profound intellectual and developmental disabilities reaches adulthood, a determination is made regarding who is the legal decision-maker for that person. The courts appoint someone to be the legal guardian, which usually continues to be the parents or another family member.

The parent or guardian is responsible for providing for certain needs of the child in a pediatric skilled nursing facility, such as clothing or personal belongings. He or she provides consent for participation in certain activities, out-of-facility participation, treatments, transfer to acute care settings, and end-of-life decisions. When staff do not agree with the wishes of a parent and guardian and resolution cannot be reached with discussion of the involved parties, issues may be presented to an ethics committee for consideration.

ADULTS

An adult nursing home may be considered an option for care of adults with intellectual and developmental disabilities older than 22 who require 24-hour skilled nursing. The skilled nursing facility may also be used as an interim provision of care while a person completes recuperation from an acute illness, or on an ongoing basis to address chronic medical needs. These types of facilities care for various individuals, most of whom are elderly and more apt to have acquired, rather than developmental, cognitive disabilities. A person's previously identified cognitive level is not a primary determining factor for general nursing home admission, as may be the case in a pediatric skilled nursing home.

Admission to an adult nursing home is often based on the referral of a physician. An individual, his or her family, or the physician may determine that the nursing home setting would best be able to provide the needed nursing and therapeutic services. State agencies continue to play a part in the decision regarding appropriateness of placement. All available alternatives of care must be explored, and individuals must be provided with choices and support to make such decisions.

State Departments of Education are no longer responsible for the development and implementation of IEPs that establish goals and recommend needed services. In Massachusetts, the Department of Public Health oversees the development of ISPs, whereby goals, services, and monitoring systems are put in place. Representatives from the Department of Mental Retardation also attend annual meetings for adult residents. Periodic meetings are held that include service providers, family members, case coordinators, and other relevant individuals to review each person's status.

In 1999, litigation in Massachusetts resulted in the development of the Rolland Integrated Service Plan (RISP), addressing the needs of individuals with intellectual or developmental disabilities either residing in, or being admitted to, nursing facilities. RISP addressed the need to carry out the ISP goals, assuring that specialized services are carried over by the staff in all environments and settings. The emphasis is on an individual's personal preferences and aspirations, as opposed to focusing on his or her impairments (Commonwealth of Massachusetts, 2003).

Parents of adults with intellectual disabilities are often faced with the difficult task of determining the best residential setting for their children. McDermott, Valentine, Anderson, Gallup, and Thompson (1997) found that parents tend to worry and feel responsibility regardless of the type of residential placement. Pruchno and Patrick (1999), however, found that more caregiver burden was associated with extensive planning within the formal service system, and fewer burdens were associated with planning for residence with a family member. In general, individuals requiring more services also tended to require more planning for future residence within the formal system. After placing an adult with intellectual disabilities in a residential setting, mothers continue to be very involved and may even be less pessimistic about their child's situation. Improvements have also been reported in some family relationships over time (Baker, Blacher, & Pfeiffer, 1996; Seltzer, Krauss, Hong, & Osmond, 2001).

CONTROVERSIES REGARDING RESIDENTIAL PLACEMENT

The deinstitutionalization movement, the ADA, and the *Olmstead* decision have underscored the need to provide individuals with intellectual and developmental disabilities opportunities, resources, and support to live in the least restrictive environment. Although the nursing home setting provides an option of care to those with significant medical and nursing needs, individuals may not receive optimal care.

In November 2003, the Nursing Home Quality Initiative, a survey of 17,000 nursing homes in the United States, was released through the Department of Health and Human Services offices that oversee Medicare and Medicaid. Wide variation was found in the care that is provided in nursing homes nationwide (Viser, 2003). In general, residents whose families are more involved generally did better, presumably because the families provide some oversight of care (Speat, Conroy, & Rice, 1998).

Problems associated with residing in large facilities, compared with community settings, have been reported. Speat and Conroy (1998) noted that adults with intellectual disabilities residing in nursing homes were more apt to be treated with antipsychotic medications for behavioral issues than those who resided in group homes. Individuals who moved from nursing homes into the community displayed improved adaptive skills. In addition, adults who moved from nursing homes into the community experienced better health and improved adaptive functioning than those who remained in nursing home, regardless of age (Heller, Factor, Hsieh, & Hahn, 1998; Heller, Miller, & Factor, 1998).

Lack of Adequate Community Supports

Strauss and Kastner (1997) outlined concern regarding individuals who moved from large facilities in California to the community, noting an increase in mortality rate. When individuals have moved from an institutional to a smaller setting, adaptive skills and challenging behaviors have also been reported by some to initially worsen, although these negative behaviors appear to be self-limited over time (Stancliffe, Hayden, Larson, & Lakin, 2002). Certainly, if individuals are cared for in the community, adequate social, medical, and personal supports need to be in place to promote positive outcomes.

Overall, people with all levels of intellectual and developmental disabilities and medical needs do reside in the community and can be provided with needed services (Hayden & Kim, 2002). All age groups, however, experience difficulties with access to appropriate and needed medical care within the community. As of February 2004, lawsuits in 26 states have addressed the need to obtain better access to community services for individuals with developmental disabilities. These lawsuits address the broad categories of access to Medicaid home and community-based services, community placement of institutionalized individuals, and limitations on home and community benefits (Smith, 2004).

More than a half million adults with intellectual and developmental disabilities age 60 and older live in the United States (Massachusetts Developmental Disabilities Council, 2001). This number is expected to double by the year 2030. Janicki and Dalton (2000) reported an increase in dementia among adults with intellectual disabilities, particularly those with Down syndrome. For those individuals who have resided in a community setting, there will be a need to increase support services so that they can continue to reside in the least restrictive environment.

Financial Issues

Rhoades and Altman (2001) showed that people with the greatest number of limitations in activities of daily living and more severe levels of intellectual and developmental disabilities have the highest expenses. Some have noted that individuals who require significant care can have their needs met less expensively in a larger setting, where multiple supports and services are provided in a single location (Walsh, Kastner, & Green, 2003). Others, however, have reported that services could be provided at less expense in the community setting, with the added benefit of more favorable outcomes, such as community access and inclusion (Stancliffe & Lakin, 1998). Emerson et al. (2001) found that in the United Kingdom, there was no difference in costs when comparing expenses of people residing in small versus large settings. Those who remained in institutional settings after downsizing have also been reported to receive greater expenditure per person, although adaptive behaviors did not significantly change (Stancliffe & Hayden, 1998). Cost should not be the driving factor for determination of appropriate services and place of residence for an individual without respect for personal needs and civil rights (Eidelman, Pietrangelo, Garnder, Jesien, & Croser, 2003).

CONCLUSION

The social landscape of care for individuals with intellectual and developmental disabilities continues to change. Ongoing closing and downsizing of institutions and efforts to provide more appropriate placements for people who do not belong in nursing homes mean that more individuals with intellectual disabilities receive services within, and contribute to, the community. A subset of individuals continues to have significant medical and nursing needs. In fact, medical advances appear to have expanded the repertoire of medical treatments, affecting overall health, quality of life, and life expectancy. Individuals and their families themselves have different requirements and wishes, based on their own personal experiences and needs.

Further development of community resources is imperative so that families can make decisions regarding care based on what is best for each person, rather than what is necessary based on restricted options. If out-of-home placement is considered, either temporarily or longer term, ideally it should be at a location that promotes family involvement. The infrastructure within the community setting requires further development so that more resources are readily available. There should be realistic alternatives of care, such as smaller, age-appropriate facilities that can provide nursing services, yet in a more homelike atmosphere. Nursing homes will probably continue to be needed for some individuals with or without developmental disabilities, but services should be specifically geared toward an individual's medical and developmental requirements. The whole person should be considered, with efforts made to optimize functioning and provide individualized choices to improve quality of life.

Issues related to support staff, work force, and funding should also be addressed. Well-trained personnel must be available. To that end, competitive salaries and desirable work environments are needed. Despite living in an era of cost containment and financial constraints, adequate reimbursement must be provided for medical equipment, medications, and other necessary services to ensure high quality of care. The increased rate of nursing home litigation, which is affecting insurance rates and the ability of facilities to function, also warrants close attention and action. Funding for Medicare and Medicaid will become even more critical as the population in the United States ages.

Nursing homes can and do provide many necessary services and supports to those with ongoing medical needs. Individuals with intellectual and developmental disabilities have a wide array of needs. Although regulations and laws have been developed to end discrimination and past abuses, much variability exists in the quality of care and services provided in nursing home settings. Mechanisms are required to ensure greater consistency in the quality of care provided, without increasing the bureaucratic demands that interfere with service delivery. Nursing home care needs to improve for all people, including those with disabilities.

REFERENCES

Alvarez, N. (1989). Neurology. In I.L. Rubin & A.C. Crocker (Eds.), *Developmental disabilities: Delivery of medical care for children and adults* (pp. 130–159). Philadelphia: Lea & Febiger.

American Academy of Pediatrics. (2004). Policy statement: The medical home. *Pediatrics, 113*(5), 1545–1547.

American Academy of Pediatrics, Committee on Children with Disabilities. (2002). Provision of educationally related services for children and adolescents with chronic diseases and disabling conditions. *Pediatrics, 105*(2), 448–451.

American Health Care Association. (2001). *Long term care survey.* Washington, DC: Author.

American Medical Directors Association. (2003, January). *Synopsis of federal regulations in the nursing facility, implications for attending physicians and medical directors.* Retrieved from http://www.amda.com/federalaffairs.regulations_synposis.htm

Americans with Disabilities Act (ADA) of 1990, PL 101-336, 42 U.S.C. §§ 12101 *et seq.*

Baker, B.L., Blacher, J., & Pfeiffer, S.I. (1996). Family involvement in residential treatment. *American Journal on Mental Retardation, 101*(1), 1–14.

Blacher, J., Baker, B.L., & Feinkleid, K.A. (1999). Living or launching: continuing family involvement with children and adolescents in placement. *American Journal on Mental Retardation, 104*(5), 452–465.

Centers for Disease Control and Prevention, National Center for Health Statistics. (2004, March 25). *Nursing home care.* Retrieved from http://www.cdc.gov/nchs/fastats/nursingh.htm

Centers for Medicare & Medicaid Services. (2003, September 12). *Medicare information resource.* Retrieved from http://www.cms.hhs.gov/medicare/gov

Chaney, R.H., & Eyman, R.K. (2000). Patterns of mortality over 60 years among persons with mental retardation in a residential facility. *American Journal on Mental Retardation, 38*(3), 289–293.

Commonwealth of Massachusetts, Executive Office of Health and Human Services. (2003). *Rolland Integrated Service Plan (RISP).* Workshop by the Department of Mental Retardation, Department of Public Health, Department of Medical Assistance, and Massachusetts Rehabilitation Commission, Worchester, MA.

Coucouvanis, K., Polister, B., Prouty, R., & Lakin, K. (2003). Continuing reduction of population in large state residence facilities for persons with intellectual and developmental disabilities. In K.C. Lakin, D. Braddock, & G. Smith (Eds.), Trends and milestones. *Mental Retardation, 41*(1), 67–70.

Department of Mental Retardation. (1989). *Family/guardian monitoring process* (DMR Policy No. 89-10). Boston: Commonwealth of Massachusetts.

Department of Mental Retardation. (2000a). *Adults with mental retardation in nursing facilities* (DMR Policy No. 2000-4). Boston: Commonwealth of Massachusetts.

Department of Mental Retardation. (2000b). *Class members residing in nursing homes and rest homes* (DMR Policy 2000-2). Boston: Commonwealth of Massachusetts.

Education for All Handicapped Children Act of 1975, PL 94-142, 20 U.S.C. §§ 1400 *et seq.*

Eidelman, S.M., Pietrangelo, R., Gardner, J.F., Jesien, G., & Croser, M.D. (2003). Let's focus on the real issues. *Mental Retardation, 41*(1), 126–129.

Emerson, E., Robertson, J., Gregory, N., Hatton, C., Kessissuglou, S., Hallam, A., et al. (2001). Quality and costs of supported living residences and group homes in the United Kingdom. *American Journal on Mental Retardation, 106*(5), 401–415.

Fogg, R. (1999). *Nursing home regulation manual.* Washington, DC: Thompson Publishing.

Fox-Grage, W., Folkerner, D., & Lewis, J. (2003). *The states' response to the Olmstead decision: How are the states complying?* (Forum for State Health Policy Leadership). Washington, DC: National Conference of State Legislatures.

Friedman, S. (1995). Changing demographics in a pediatric skilled nursing facility: Are we seeing the impact of inclusion? *Abstracts from 119th Annual Meeting, Partnerships: Crossing the Bridge to the Future,* 161.

Giangreco, M.F. (2001). Interactions among program, placement, and services in educational planning for students with disabilities. *Mental Retardation, 39*(5), 341–350.

Hanneman, R., & Blacher, J. (1998). Predicting placement in families who have children with severe handicaps: A longitudinal analysis. *American Journal on Mental Retardation, 102*(4), 392–408.

Hayden, M.F., & Kim, S.H. (2002). Health status, health care utilization patterns, and health care outcomes of persons with intellectual disabilities: A review of the literature. *Policy Research Brief,* 13(1), 1–18.

Heller, T., Factor, A.R., Hsieh, K., & Hahn, J.E. (1998). Impact of age and transitions out of nursing homes for adults with developmental disabilities. *American Journal on Mental Retardation, 103*(3), 236–248.

Heller, T., Miller, A.B., & Factor, A. (1998). Environmental characteristics of nursing homes and community-based settings, and the well being of adults with intellectual disability. *Journal of Intellectual Disability Research, 42* (5), 418–428.

Huskins, W.C., Potter-Bynoe, G., Spencer, S., Erdman, D., Friedman, S.L., Sadeghi, L., et al. (2000). *An outbreak of rhinovirus respiratory tract facility infection associated with serious complications among residents of a pediatric long-term care facility.*

Fourth International Conference on Healthcare-Associated Infections, Atlanta.
Individuals with Disabilities Education Act Amendments of 1997of 1997, PL 105-17, 20 U.S.C. §§1400 *et seq.*
Individuals with Disabilities Education Act of 1990, PL 101-476, 20 U.S.C. 1400 *et seq.*
Janicki, M.P., & Dalton, A.J. (2000). Prevalence of dementia and impact on intellectual disability services. *Mental Retardation, 38*(3), 276–288.
Lakin, K.C., Anderson, L., Prouty, R., & Polister, B. (1999). Community residential services would require expansion of 72% to serve everyone in community settings. *Mental Retardation, 37*(3), 251–254.
Lakin, K.C., Hill, B.K., & Anderson, D.J. (1991). Persons with mental retardation in nursing homes in 1977 and 1985. *Mental Retardation, 29*(1), 25–33.
Larson, S. (2004). Access to health care: A research synthesis. *Health promotion for persons with intellectual/developmental disabilities: The state of scientific evidence.* Pre-conference workshop, American Association on Mental Retardation, Philadelphia.
Larson, S.A., Lakin, C., Anderson, L., Kwak, N., Lee, J.H., & Anderson, D. (2001). Prevalence of mental retardation and developmental disabilities: Estimates from the 1994/1995 national health interview disability supplements. *American Journal on Mental Retardation, 106*(3), 231–252.
Mahady, M., & Pettey, S.M. (2003). Impact of recent regulatory milestones on the long-term care industry. *Caring for the ages, Post-meeting reporter, 26th Annual Symposium, American Medical Directors Association,* pp. 22–23.
Massachusetts Developmental Disabilities Council. (2001). *Executive summary. FY 2001–2003 state plan.* Boston: Author.
Mitchell, D., & Braddock, D. (1990). Historical and contemporary issues in nursing homes reform. *Mental Retardation, 28*(4), 201–210.
McDermott, S., Valentine, D., Anderson, D., Gallup, D., & Thompson, S. (1997). Parents of adults with mental retardation in-home and out-of-home caregiving burdens and gratification. *Journal of Orthopsychiatry, 67*(2), 323–329.
Olmstead v. L.C. 527 U.S. 581; 119 S.Ct. 2176 (1999).
Omnibus Budget Reconciliation Act of 1987, PL 100-203, 101 Stat. 1330.
Omnibus Budget Reconciliation Act of 1980, PL 96-499, 94 Stat. 2599.
Pruchno, R.A., & Patrick, J.H. (1999). Effects of formal and familial residence plans for adults with mental retardation and aging mothers. *American Journal on Mental Retardation, 104*(1), 38–52.
Rehabilitation Act of 1973, PL 93-112, 29 U.S.C. §§ 701 *et seq.*
Rhoades, J.A., & Altman, B.M. (2001). Personal characteristics and contextual factors associated with residential expenditures for individuals with mental retardation. *Mental Retardation, 39*(2), 114–129.
Seltzer, M.M., Krauss, M.W., Hong, J., & Osmond, G.I. (2001). Continuity or discontinuity of family involvement following residential transfer of adults who have mental retardation. *Mental Retardation, 39*(3), 181–194.
Smith, G.A. (2004). *Status report: Litigation concerning home and community services for people with disabilities.* Tualatin, OR: Human Services Research Institute.
Social Security Act Amendments of 1965, PL 89-97, 42 U.S.C. §§ 301 *et seq.*
Speat, S., & Conroy, J. (1998). Use of psychotropic medications for persons with mental retardation who live in Oklahoma nursing homes. *Psychiatric Services, 49*(2), 510–512.
Speat, S., Conroy, J.W., & Rice, D.M. (1998). Improve quality in nursing homes or institute community placement? Implementation on OBRA for individuals with mental retardation. *Research in Developmental Disabilities, 19*(8), 507–518.
Stancliffe, R.J., & Hayden, M.F. (1998). Longitudinal study of institutional downsizing: Effects on individuals who remain in the institution. *American Journal on Mental Retardation, 102*(5), 500–510.
Stancliffe, R.J., Hayden, M.F., Larson, S.A., & Lakin, K.C. (2002). Longitudinal study of adaptive and challenging behaviors of institutionalized adults with mental retardation. *American Journal on Mental Retardation, 107*(4), 302–320.
Stancliffe, R.J., & Lakin R.C. (1998). Analysis of expenditures and outcomes of residential alternatives for persons with developmental disabilities. *American Journal on Mental Retardation, 102*(6), 552–568.
Staub, R. (1989). Pediatric nursing homes. In I.L. Rubin & A.C. Crocker (Eds.), *Developmental disabilities: Delivery of medical care for children and adults* (pp. 42–47). Philadelphia: Lea & Febiger.
Strauss, D., & Kastner, T.A. (1997). Comparative mortality of people with mental retardation in institutions and the community. *American Journal on Mental Retardation, 101*(4), 424–429.
Uehara, E.S., Silverstein, B.J., Davis, R., & Geron, S. (1991). Assessment of needs of adults with developmental disabilities in skilled nursing and intermediate care facilities in Illinois. *Mental Retardation, 29*(4), 223–231.
Viser, M. (2003, January 12). How nursing homes compare. *Boston Globe, Globe West,* pp. C1, C5–C6.
Walsh, K.K., Kastner, T.A., & Green, R.G. (2003). Cost comparisons of community and institutional residential setting: Historical review of selected research. *Mental Retardation, 41*(2), 103–122.

6.9 STATE RESIDENTIAL FACILITIES

Theodor Feigelman and
Norberto Alvarez

There is no question that living arrangements for individuals with intellectual disabilities should be determined by choices in the community. The medical care provided should be accepted by the general population, who are familiar with their own health and health care needs. This includes selection of providers of health care based on reputation, knowledge, and respectful attitude. The history and evolution of institutions, or large state residential facilities (SRFs), is a tortured one and chronicles the story from a spirit of hope to a situation of degradation and inhumanity that cannot easily be forgotten.

The process of dismantling the SRFs and shifting residential and health care services to the community has been one of the great achievements of American society. This process is by no means complete and still has a long way to go. The goal ahead is clear; there are processes and obstacles to overcome. In the last edition of this book, the section on SRFs was substantial, and in this edition, it is vestigial. It is hoped that in future editions it will be a footnote.

This chapter describes the history of institutional care for individuals with intellectual disabilities, marking the process of deinstitutionalization toward self-determination in the community, and reviews the history of provision of health care within SRFs. The description of Wrentham Developmental Center in Massachusetts illustrates the clinical characteristics of individuals who remain in SRFs and the organization of services required to provide optimal health care for them. Finally, the chapter outlines an example of how the resources within SRFs can be used to enhance the services being provided in the community.

EVOLUTION OF INSTITUTIONAL CARE

In the later part of the 19th century, there was a spirit of hope that children with intellectual disabilities would benefit from appropriate educational opportunities. The earliest attempts in Europe were celebrated as being successful, and in the early part of the 20th century, the United States made a commitment to the education of children in *state developmental centers*. These centers had schools, workshops, and agricultural programs for education and rehabilitation and an array of medical and therapeutic services.

The centers were the only programs organized to provide a comprehensive set of educational, social, and medical services for children with developmental disabilities. Therefore, pediatricians often referred families to the centers. Many families enrolled their children in these centers because they wanted them to have the best of what was available. Some families were urged to place their children away from home and forget about them; however, other families kept their children at home. Alternative developmental and educational programs for children with disabilities were limited, but some were started by families in need most often within religious centers.

Although the developmental centers were committed to improving the abilities of the children, they did not have the understanding, technology, and resources that providers have today, and the progress made by the children individually, and the schools in the centers collectively, did not meet their expectations. As a result, the children tended to remain in the centers rather than become more competent and able enough to return to society. Over the course of time, the children became older, and the centers, more crowded; the spirit of education faded. By the middle of the 20th century, the educational basis on which the centers were conceived had given way to custodial models administratively based on a hospital system—the so-called *medical models*.

In the United States in 1910, the total population in residential settings was about 200,000. It had doubled to about 400,000 by 1940 and reached over 550,000 by 1955. In 1926, an estimated one tenth of the entire group, or 55,000, were determined to have intellectual disabilities. By 1967, more than 194,000 individuals were in SRFs because of their intellectual disabilities. In addition to the large numbers of individuals in the centers, the services provided were less than optimal and the living conditions and basic human rights had deteriorated to unacceptable levels.

During the Civil Rights era in the United States in the 1960s, the conditions within the SRFs were revealed to the public. Outraged parents, citizens, professionals, and community and public leaders initiated a cascade of events including litigation against states, holding them responsible for the unacceptable levels of care. Successful litigation imposed two sets of requirements on states: 1) to improve the quality of care provided within the residential settings, and 2) to assist individuals with intellectual disabilities to move into safe and appropriate residential settings in the community with access to necessary services. This process not only represented a "paradigm shift" in conceptual thinking but a complete change in economics, service delivery, and societal standards and expectations.

In retrospect, one phase of the process was coming to fruition, another set of unanticipated challenges arose and prompted rethinking and redesign of services and the funds that went with them. Phases of the process followed hard on each other as families, professionals, and policy makers began to appreciate at each level of achievement that more could be done to reach the desired goals. Institutional reform, accompanied by the process of deinstitutionalization, was built on the concept of *normalization*; however, this concept soon proved inadequate to rectify the situation. The concepts of *inclusion* and *self-determination* gained ground and have become part of our current set of expectations (see Chapter 5).

A parallel set of changes initiated by the Developmental Disabilities Assistance and Bill of Rights Act of 1975 (PL 94-103) and the Education for All Handicapped Children Act of 1975 (PL 94-142) provided infrastructural elements for bringing young children

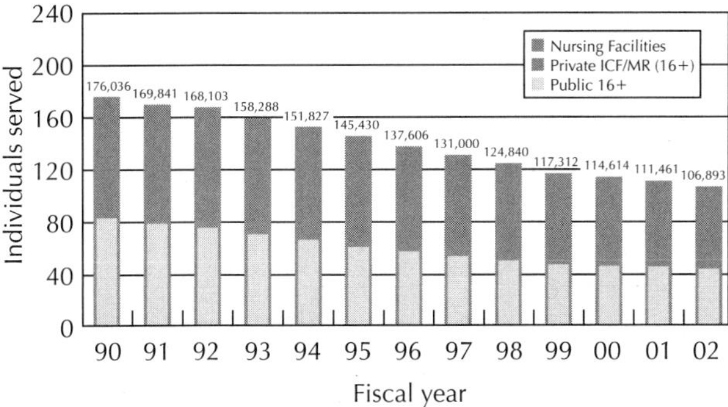

Figure 6.9-1. Individuals served in public and private institutions and nursing facilities in the United States fiscal years 1990–2002.

into the mainstream of educational and social opportunities. The hope and promise of a future quality of life based on opportunities for education and supports necessary for independent living arrangements and employment became available (see Chapter 2).

By 2000, the SRF populations in the United States had decreased to about 47,000 with evidence of ongoing decreases (see Figure 6.9-1). This approximated the SRF population back to where it was in the early 1920s, despite the fact that the U.S. population had more than tripled. Thus, the rate of institutionalization has decreased by approximately 67% in the past 80 years. In 1993, an estimated 13% of the entire population of individuals with intellectual disabilities were residing in SRFs. Indications point to a further decrease in this rate as institutions continue to downsize and close. Whereas prior to 1980 all 50 states had some form of SRF, by 2002 this number had decreased to 42 (i.e., 8 states decided to provide all services in community settings). There has been a similar phenomenon in Western Europe.

The decrease in SRF enrollment has resulted in a marked increase in the number of individuals living in community homes of one to six people. Between 1977 and 1998, these numbers increased from 20,000 to 263,000 (a thirteenfold increase), underscoring the reduction of significance of the SRFs and the gains in community residential living (Braddock, Hemp, & Rizzolo, 2004; Prouty, Smith, & Lakin, 2004). This shift in demographics can be traced to the actions of various advocacy groups, which continue to promote the support of community care.

QUALITY OF MEDICAL CARE

Some of the pioneers in the education of children with functional impairments—visual, hearing, intellectual, and physical—were physicians. Some of the earliest schools were named after the physicians (e.g., Perkins in Massachusetts). Indeed, the administration and management of the developmental centers was modeled on how hospitals were run at the time, and the administrators and superintendents were physicians. The staff consisted primarily of nurses, and the individuals residing in the centers were called *patients*. As the numbers of individuals in the centers increased and education and treatment modalities did not, the medical care for the individuals in the institutions became less current and sensitive, giving rise to a high mortality and morbidity as well as reduced quality of life.

The overcrowded living conditions and poor medical care, and consequently poor quality of life, led to litigation against the states and discrediting of the role of physicians in caring for people with developmental disabilities. The condemnation of the way in which people were cared for in institutional settings and the fact that they had been taken care of by physicians and nurses led to criticism of the medical model of care and the promotion of the *developmental model*, which was based on the promotion of programs that would enhance skill development and promote independence.

In response to the requirement to improve the quality of care for individuals living in the institutions and to help the individuals move into community settings, some states contracted with university-based teaching hospitals. They hired more competent physicians, provided more training for the physicians, promoted an interdisciplinary approach, and provided additional specialty and tertiary care services through the best hospitals in the area. This situation not only served to improve the quality of health care and quality of life for individuals with intellectual disabilities, but it also served to increase the exposure of primary care and specialty care physicians, nurses, hospital personnel, medical students, residents, and fellows in training to the health care needs of individuals with developmental disabilities; to develop improved understanding of the individuals and of their specific medical problems; and to develop strategies to improve the treatment and management of these individuals' conditions.

The results were multiple:

- Physicians and allied health professionals became more familiar and thus more competent in dealing with the health care needs of individuals with developmental disabilities.
- Systems were developed in communities to deal with these needs.
- Young professionals were trained in the care of individuals with developmental disabilities and could provide the care in the future.

Thus, medical care within institutions improved, and, in the process, there was improved care in community settings that had contractual or collaborative relationships with the providers of health care within the institutions.

What followed then was a shrinking of the population within institutions and a corresponding increase in individuals with intellectual disabilities in the community. The shrinking number of people who remained in SRFs thus had improved care, but the quality of care in the community was highly dependent on the availability and accessibility of services as well as the relationships that managers of community residences could arrange and develop with the community providers. This situation became more striking when individuals with the more severe disabilities were discharged from SRFs into the community. In the early days of deinstitutionalization, the most competent and healthy individuals left, and many of them blended into society. Over the course of time, however, individuals who were less able to be independent and those who had more medical problems were also discharged and some of the community settings into which they went to live were unequipped to deal with their medical problems (Crocker, 1987).

During the 1990s, there were reports that certain groups of individuals living in SRFs fared better than their counterparts in community settings (Strauss, Eyman, & Grossman, 1996). Critics of these studies should reflect that the comparison was not between the values of SRFs versus community living but on the quality of care provided in the comparative settings to individuals with varying degrees of intellectual disabilities in those settings at those times. Debates and discussions should not devolve on ideological grounds but should provide impetus to improve health care services and living conditions for all individuals with intellectual disabilities wherever they live. If adequate community services are available and accessible, individuals with intellectual disabilities will receive good quality health care (van Loon, Knibbe, & Van Hove, 2005).

Improvements in medical care for individuals with intellectual disabilities have resulted in improvements in life expectancies from an average of 19 years in the 1930s to 66 years in the 1990s (Braddock & Parish, 2001). The quality of care and the operational standards and oversights in SRFs are significantly improved and are managed very differently from how they were in the first half of the 20th century; nonetheless, the negative history of institutional care and the preference of community living over institutional care continues to reduce the populations in SRFs and to increase the number of individuals with intellectual disabilities living in community settings.

PROVISION OF MEDICAL CARE IN AN INSTITUTIONAL SETTING

Originally, states were responsible for managing all aspects of care in SRFs. As mentioned previously, however, the challenges of the 1970s to improve the conditions in SRFs resulted in relationships with academic medical centers that provided and monitored the health and habilitative care of individuals living in SRFs. This situation has evolved into business relationships between states and private corporations to provide the health care services. This model is acceptable as long as appropriate oversight ensures compliance with Federal standards.

This section describes the situation in a specific SRF to illustrate the characteristics of individuals still residing in SRFs as well as the make up of medical services to meet the heath care needs of the individuals being served. It serves to outline how the provision of health care is organized and structured to provide optimal care. In addition, attempts to extend services to individuals living in community settings are illustrated.

In the early 1970s, there were in excess of 1,300 individuals residing at the Wrentham Developmental Center in Massachusetts. In the late 1980s, there were approximately 1,000 individuals. At present, there are a total of 310 individuals. The group of people is older, with an average age of 59 years (30–91; see also Figure 6.9-2). There are 171 men and 139 women. Because the institution has been closed to new admissions since the late 1970s with few exceptions, individuals have been living there for many years. The average lifetime expended in the institution was 46 years (range 2–81 years).

Most of the individuals who remain in Wrentham Developmental Center are more significantly involved; the degree of intellectual disabilities is considered profound in 212, severe in 78, moderate in 23, and mild in only 7 individuals. For the most part, individuals who remain in Wrentham Developmental Center are more significantly involved medically or have behavior or psychiatric disorders that re-

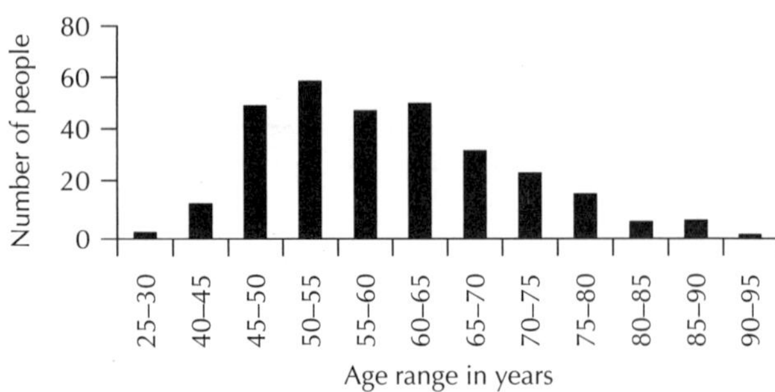

Figure 6.9-2. Age distribution of 310 individuals living at Wrentham Developmental Center. Most of the individuals are older, reflecting an aging population with limited new admissions.

quire more constant and complex management than can readily and reliably be provided in the community at present (see Table 6.9-1). The causes of death tend to be a result of end-stage conditions such as Alzheimer disease, renal failure, or acute on chronic pneumonia (see Table 6.9-2).

In order to provide adequate services for this population, it is necessary to have a high staff-to-resident ratio and an array of medical, psychiatric, psychological, and therapeutic services. The medical services are provided by a contract for services between a private corporation and the Commonwealth of Massachusetts. An in-house team consisting of one medical director/neurologist, three internists, and four nurse practitioners provides the medical services. There is also a respiratory therapist and a radiology technologist. The services are provided in house Monday through Friday from 8:30 A.M. to 5:00 P.M., and there is emergency coverage by telephone 24 hours per day, 7 days per week, by one of the physicians on the team. For emergency services that cannot be resolved within the institution, the individuals are referred to local hospitals.

There is an active outpatient program in the institution with specialists who visit the institution periodically. Depending on the needs, these clinics can be scheduled once per week to once every 2–3 months. The specialists also follow the residents if there is a need for any surgical procedures, which are performed at a specialized facility, usually a tertiary care hospital.

The provision of medical services employs a team approach in which the physician or nurse practitioner is one member of an interdisciplinary team that might include a nurse, occupational therapist, speech therapist, physical therapist, psychologist, social worker, nutritionist, and members of the staff who work daily with the individual. Every individual living in Wrentham Developmental Center has a complete reevaluation of medical conditions at least once per year.

ROLE OF STATE RESIDENTIAL FACILITIES IN COLLABORATION WITH THE COMMUNITY

The Office of the Surgeon General (2001) issued a report on health disparities for people with intellectual disabilities living in the community that catalogues the areas of need and areas of service and suggests a set of strategies for remedying the situation. At the same time, services in SRFs are more heavily funded and rigidly regulated, and the supervised environment in SRFs makes the provision of medical care more predictable and more comprehensive. For example, regulations from Medicare and Medicaid, the organizations that usually pay for the services provided in SRFs, require that individuals living in these institutions should receive, at least once per year, a complete evaluation of their medical condition. Even though some of these regulations might apply to the community, in general, they are much

Table 6.9-1. Medical conditions of the individuals residing at Wrentham Developmental Center

Condition	Number	Percent of total
Psychiatric disorders		
Individuals taking behavior modification medications	132	43%
Atypical psychosis	63	20%
Anxiety	28	9%
Pervasive developmental disorder	22	7%
Depression	11	4%
Bipolar disorder	14	5%
Pica	43	14%
Cerebral palsy	130	42%
Seizure disorder	125	40%
Eye conditions		
Cataracts	87	28%
Strabismus	61	20%
Severe visual impairment or blindness	58	19%
Refractory errors	35	11%
Glaucoma	18	6%
Keratoconus	17	5%
Corneal opacity	10	3%
Deafness	51	16%
Gastrointestinal (GI) disorders		
Esophagitis	63	20%
Gastritis, including upper GI bleeding	61	20%
Gallbladder disorders	56	18%
Gastroesophageal reflux	51	16%
Volvulus	28	9%
Feeding tubes	77	25%
Hemorrhoids	44	14%
Cardiovascular conditions		
Essential hypertension	52	17%
Heart conditions		
Conduction disorders and dysrhythmias	33	11%
Mitral valve lesions	16	5%
Lesions in other valves	7	2%
Cardiomyopathy	9	3%
Chronic heart failure	8	3%
Peripheral vascular system		
Phlebitis and varicose veins	17	5%
Aspiration pneumonia	48	15%
Dental problems		
Periodontal disease	161	52%
Edentulism	45	15%
Skin disorders		
Cellulitis	108	35%
Acne	52	17%
Seborrhea	85	27%
Skin abscess	41	13%
Osteoporosis	104	34%
Obesity	66	21%
Hepatitis A	30	10%
Hepatitis B	15	5%

Note: The multiplicity and complexity of the conditions reflects a population of individuals whose medical and/or psychiatric needs are significant and may well be an explanation for the fact that they a remain in the institutional setting.

Table 6.9-2. Mortality in Wrentham Developmental Center 2000–2004

Year	Number of deaths	Men	Women	Average age and range	Cause
2000	9	6	3	68 (49–90)	Respiratory (2 + 3) Alzheimer disease (4) Cardiorespiratory arrest (0 + 1) Myocardial infarction Chronic renal failure Melanoma
2001	7	2	5	63 (36–84)	Respiratory (2 + 4) Cardiorespiratory arrest (0 + 3) Alzheimer disease (2) Breast cancer (2) Renal failure
2002	8	6	2	69 (40–91)	Respiratory (4 + 2) Sepsis (0 + 4) Alzheimer disease (2) Acute myocardial infarction Plasmocytoma
2003	14	8	6	56 (39–82)	Respiratory (5 + 1) Sepsis (3) Congestive heart failure (2) Pancreatic cancer Intracranial bleeding Abdominal perforation Renal failure
2004	16	10	6	70 (49–91)	Respiratory (9) Sepsis (0 + 6) Carcinomas (4) • Non-Hogdkin lymphoma • Adenocarcinoma of esophagus • Rectal cancer with metastasis • Cancer of the sigmoid Cardiorespiratory arrest (3) Cerebrovascular stroke Renal failure Alzheimer disease
Total 2000–2004	54	32	22	65 (36–91)	Respiratory (25) Alzheimer disease (9) Cancers (9) Cardiorespiratory arrest (7) Cardiac (4) Renal failure (4) Cerebral vascular accident (2)

Note: For numbers that have a + sign, the first number is the primary diagnosis and the second number is secondary and associated with another diagnosis on the list.

more difficult to implement and quite often are not enforced. A study by van Loon et al. (2005) documented this point, showing that a mere 32% of adults with intellectual disabilities living in community settings received age-appropriate health screenings in areas such as cholesterol, blood pressure, vision, hearing, and dental care.

The situation in the community is dependent on generic medical care that is provided by local physicians who may have limited training, knowledge, and experience in the health care needs of individuals with intellectual disabilities. Although there are specific requirements to address health care needs, availability and access to quality services is variable and often lacking in one way or another (van Loon et al., 2005). In order to address this issue, community medical services programs have been established, which aim to provide enhancement of health care services from the SRF to the community (O'Donnell, 2003). These have been well described, often following the "Morristown Model," consisting of outpatient medical facilities that exclusively and expertly serve individuals with developmental disabilities (Ziring, 1988).

The Medical Safeguarding Program is not a primary care service, but its role is to complement and assist the primary care physician and other allied health care providers in delivering optimal health care for individuals with developmental disabilities living in the community. The goal is not to replace the community generic services but to complement and enrich them by these practices of supports and vigilance. Assisting primary care physicians means: preparing accurate, complete, and up-to-date medical information for a consultation; interpreting and explaining, if necessary, the presentation of symptoms; providing a past medical history; discussing diagnoses and treatment plans; offering access to medical specialists if necessary; assuring medical follow-ups with concerned parties; monitoring the results of the treatment plan; and being in contact on an as-needed basis with the primary care physician. Requests for services at the individual level come from a variety of sources: individuals with disabilities themselves, family members, guardians, service providers, service coordinators, primary care physicians, medical specialists, or other health professionals already involved with the individual.

Services offered by the Medical Safeguarding Program at the individual level for all individuals with developmental disabilities living in Southeastern Massachusetts are the following:

- Ad hoc consultations (e.g., a service coordinator may ask about the appropriateness of a given medication for an individual. The nurse would review the medication list and, after proper inquiries with the primary care physician if required, would advise the service coordinator that the medication as prescribed is either appropriate or needs to be changed.)
- Home visits for assessment and follow-up of an individual.
- Coordinatation of care among the individual, family, guardian, service provider staff, and physicians.
- Consultation with primary care physicians, specialists, nurses, occupational and physical therapists, and speech and language therapists.
- Training for support staff regarding the management of the individual's specific health issues.
- Contact with physicians and nurses assigned to the individual at admittance to an acute care hospital and monitoring throughout the hospitalization.

In addition to these services, detailed and continuous supports need to be in place. They consist of emergency protocols approved by primary care physicians and health care plans that describe, in language easily understood by direct care staff, the nature of the medical issues, their clear description, treatments given on a daily basis (e.g., medication, nutrition), information and training that staff need to get, contingency and emergency procedures, and a list of equipment required.

The program also provides support and advocacy during hospitalizations. These supports consist of an important, sometimes continuous, presence of a staff person, a member of the family, or a guardian at the person's bedside, which is organized and guided by the nurses. Extensive and continuous supports are provided during hospitalizations of vulnerable individuals, and training is provided for those who support individuals during hospital stays. The staff involved receive training on 1) the individual's health care needs, including the assistance needed for positioning or ambulation and on any other supportive devices routinely used, 2) assistance needed at mealtime, and 3) other special considerations, with the goal of informing and "guiding" hospital nursing staff.

The staff and family member or guardian will provide ongoing documentation by writing in a Hospital Journal developed for each hospitalized consumer. The Hospital Journal records visits by residential medical staff, visits by hospital staff and their purpose, medication administered, procedures and tests done and their results, nutrition and fluids taken if known, and any additional observations and comments. Also, a checklist for discharge planning and returning home from a hospital stay is provided. The nurses in the Medical Safeguarding Program visit the individual after he or she returns home and closely supervise the supports in place.

The Medical Safeguarding Program vigilantly applies the Department of Mental Retardation's policy regarding the withholding of life-sustaining treatment. Frequently, the nurses involved in the program, in collaboration with service coordinators, will discuss these issues with families, guardians, and primary care physicians. If conflicting views persist, pertinent administrative staff, the medical director, and other medical consultants will get involved. Sometimes, program staff provide a medical affidavit when a decision to go to court is made under the guidance of a Department of Mental Retardation attorney and will stay involved until the resolution of the case.

In collaboration with the primary care physicians and other health professionals (e.g., occupational and physical therapists, speech therapists) the nurses in the program provide recommendations regarding medical equipment and supplies. In the case of medically vulnerable people, the list of equipment appears in the health care plan written by the program nurses.

Medical Safeguarding Program staff participate regularly in the Regional Mortality Review Committee meetings. The nurses are also active participants in local health care committees. They organize training for staff and family members, are in communication with the hospitals in their respective areas, and help to resolve difficult issues regarding access to optimal care for the individuals in their area. Their role is to assist in developing better health care strategies (e.g., health care plans for highly vulnerable individuals, safeguarding during hospitalizations, clinical documentation for visits with primary care physicians, and risk management improvement) and to participate with the other committee members in the monitoring of these diverse strategies.

The Medical Safeguarding Program shows that the disproportionate financial investment in SRFs may be transferred to community settings in terms of training, technical assistance, and other supports, which is expected to not only result in providing needed services but also serve as a training vehicle for community providers and assist in the ongoing process of transferring all care to community settings.

CONCLUSION

Although SRFs started out as institutions for the promotion of education and development for children with developmental disabilities, they lost their original vision and mission and became the very antithesis of their original intent. The changes that have occurred during the second half of the 20th century in the process of transforming the SRFs into institutions that provide quality care and of improving the availability of health care to individuals with intellectual disabilities in community settings have gone far to improve the situation for many individuals with intellectual disabilities; however, there is still a long way to go to dismantle the existing institutions and what they have come to represent and to create within the community the necessary quality of health care to meet the most challenging and complex medical needs of individuals with developmental disabilities.

REFERENCES

Braddock, D., Hemp, R., & Rizzolo, M.C. (2004, October). State of the states in developmental disabilities: 2004. *Mental Retardation, 42*(5), 356–370.

Braddock, D., & Parish, S.L. (2001). An institutional history of disability. In G.L. Albrecht, K.D. Seelman & M. Bury (Eds.), *Handbook of disability studies* (pp. 11–68). Thousand Oaks, CA: Sage Publications.

Crocker, A.C. (1987). Monograph on health care for people with mental retardation. *Mental Retardation, 25*.

Developmental Disabilities Assistance and Bill of Rights Act of 1975, PL 94-103, 100 Stat. 840, 42 U.S.C. §§ 6000 *et seq.*

Education for All Handicapped Children Act of 1975, PL 94-142, 20 U.S.C. §§ 1400 *et seq.*

O'Donnell, C. (2003, July). *Community service contract with the Commonwealth of Massachusetts, Department of Mental Retardation, Southeast Region.* Boston: Shriver Clinical Services.

Office of the Surgeon General. (2001). *Closing the gap: A national blueprint for improving the health of individuals with mental retardation. Report of the Surgeon General's Conference on Health Disparities and Mental Retardation.* Washington, DC: U.S. Public Health Service.

Prouty, R.W., Smith, G., & Lakin, K.C. (Eds.). (2004). *Residential services for persons with developmental disabilities: Status and trends through 2003.* Minneapolis: University of Minnesota, Research and Training Center on Community Living, Institute on Community Integration.

Strauss, D., Eyman, R.K., & Grossman, H.J. (1996). The prediction of mortality in children with severe mental retardation: The effect of placement. *American Journal of Public Health, 86*, 1422–1429.

van Loon, J., Knibbe, J., & Van Hove, G. (2005, June). From institutional to community support: Consequences for medical care. *Journal of Applied Research in Intellectual Disabilities, 18*(2), 175.

Ziring, P., Kastner, T., Friedman, D.L., Pond, W., Barnett, M.L., Sonnenberg, E.M., et al. (1988). Provision of health care for persons with developmental disabilities living in the community—the Morristown Model. *Journal of the American Medical Association, 260*, 1439–1444.

Section II

Clinical Care

Chapter 7

Inborn Errors of Metabolism

7.1 Newborn Screening for Genetic Disorders

Paul M. Fernhoff

Parents' interaction with the largest genetic testing enterprise in the United States is often anxiety provoking. Geneticists are frequently asked whether universal genetic screening will ever become a reality. This author's response is that universal genetic screening has been ongoing since 1963, when a program began in Massachusetts. Other states established programs during the following decade. Programs go by several names. Most professionals call them newborn screening (NBS) programs. Some prefer to call them newborn metabolic screens, newborn heel sticks, or newborn filter paper card screening programs. Regardless of the name, screening programs have become an integral part of the evaluation of nearly all 4 million newborns per year in the United States and most newborns in industrialized countries. They have saved hundreds of thousands of children from disabilities and early death. These programs continue to grow because of innovative technology and because parents, health care professionals, and advocates understand the ability of NBS to prevent the effects of devastating disorders.

Sharon from the State Newborn Screening Follow-Up Service called Mrs. Lopez about her new daughter, Brianna. "Excuse me for disturbing you this late on a Friday evening," she said, "but Dr. Michaels said it would be all right if I called you directly. I'm calling to see how Brianna is doing."

Mrs. Lopez explained that Brianna was okay but was having more trouble breast feeding than her older brother had. "She's already 4 days old, and she doesn't suck well and is spitting up more," Mrs. Lopez said. "This morning I noticed that the whites of her eyes were turning yellow. Is there a problem?"

Sharon asked Mrs. Lopez if she remembered the heel stick test that was done before Brianna left the hospital. Brianna's test had indicated that she might have a problem with the way her body uses the sugar galactose, which is found in both mother's breast milk and in most regular baby formulas.

"Brianna needs to have further blood and urine tests run to see if she will need to be switched to a special galactose-free formula," Sharon said. "These tests will determine if Brianna has a condition called 'galactosemia.' Dr. Michaels has already arranged for you to bring her to the children's hospital so that the doctors there can look at her and obtain these studies. She may need to spend some time in the hospital."

"This sounds serious," Mrs. Lopez said. "Will she be okay?"

"Well, it can be serious," Sharon admitted, "but it would be best to bring her to the hospital as quickly as possible. I would like you to stop trying to breast-feed her and see if she will take some of the clear sugar water solution that they gave you when you left the hospital. When you get to the hospital, the doctors there will examine Brianna, run the tests, and if they are concerned, they will admit her to the hospital. If the tests are positive, the doctors and nutritionists will sit down with you and your family and be able to answer all your questions and give you a lot of information about the condition."

"Okay," Ms. Lopez said. "I'll call my husband at work and tell him to meet us at the hospital."

HISTORY OF NEWBORN SCREENING

The origins of the NBS are usually traced back to 1934 when Professor Asbjorn Fölling, a Norwegian biochemist, was asked by one his former students, Dr. Harry Egland and his wife to examine their two children with severe delays who had an unpleasant "wet fur-like" body odor and decreased skin pigment. After adding a compound called ferric chloride to each of their urines, Fölling found an unusual green color reaction (Fölling, 1934). This observation led him and others to recognize that the unusual color reaction in the urine was caused by excess amounts of phenylketones (i.e., byproducts of phenylalanine, an essential amino acid found in nearly all natural protein sources).

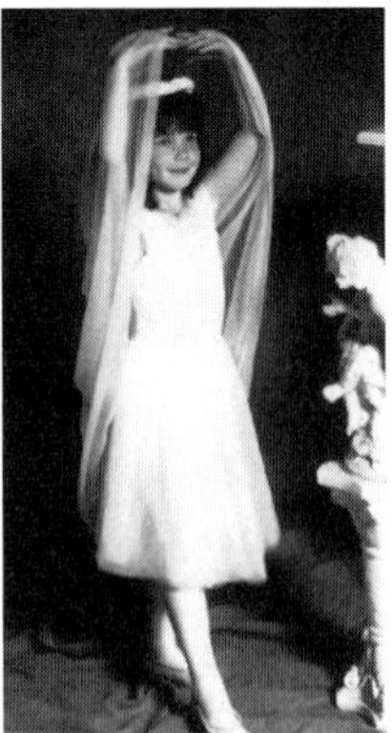

Figure 7.1-1. Child with treated phenylketonuria.

These initial observations confirmed that phenylketonuria (PKU) was a classical inborn error of metabolism and was caused by the inability of the affected individual's body to convert phenylalanine to another amino acid, tyrosine, because of the lack of function of the hepatic enzyme phenylalanine hydroxylase. Subsequent observations found that when individuals with PKU were given an artificial formula restricted in phenylalanine and enriched in tyrosine, their elevated blood phenylalanine levels could be reduced. If this formula was instituted within the first few weeks of life, most of the devastating effects of the PKU were prevented (see Figure 7.1-1).

Children with PKU who are untreated may appear normal for the first few months of life. As the metabolites of phenylalanine build up in the child's body, the parents may recognize a persistent, unpleasant musty or "wet-fur" odor. Children with untreated PKU develop severe eczema that is unresponsive to the usual therapy and usually have decreased skin and hair pigment compared with brothers or sisters, which is secondary to decreased production of tyrosine that is needed to produce melanin. By 6 months of age, children with untreated PKU will demonstrate poor growth of the head size reflecting failure of brain growth secondary to decreased myelin formation. Older children and adults with untreated PKU have irreversible severe cognitive impairments, seizures, and behavior problems. Therefore, individuals with PKU, as with nearly every metabolic disorder, must maintain lifelong dietary restrictions.

Nearly 25 years after Fölling's observation, a phenylalanine-restricted formula became commercially available. Once it was available, pediatricians and other primary care providers had to identify asymptomatic infants affected with PKU during the first few weeks of life before permanent brain damage was done. A solution to this public health problem and the technology that enabled NBS was the assay developed by Guthrie and Susi (1963). Robert Guthrie, who was the father of a child with intellectual disabilities and the uncle of a niece with PKU, recognized the need for a simple test that could be used on all infants to screen for this rare disorder. His solution was to use a card with a strip of filter paper that could be spotted with a few drops of blood obtained from a heel stick within the child's first 2 or 3 days of life. The blood spot could dry and then be sent to a laboratory for relatively rapid analysis for elevated amounts of phenylalanine. Guthrie's original filter paper card and bioassay for phenylalanine, along with the critical roles played by parents and advocates like Guthrie, helped establish and expand worldwide NBS programs.

After PKU screening programs began in the 1960s, continued technology spurred screening for other disorders that could be detected on the same filter paper card. As an example of the growth of NBS in one program, Table 7.1-1 displays the history of expansion in Georgia. An important aspect of NBS in the United States that has recently received significant attention has been the different disorders that are screened among states and regions. This issue is discussed more fully next.

NEWBORN SCREENING AS A CORE PUBLIC HEALTH PROGRAM

As mentioned previously, in 1963, Massachusetts became the first state to institute mandatory, universal NBS. Since then, considerable debate has occurred about whether NBS should be a core function of the public health system or be left to the responsibility of the primary care provider and family, as done for neonatal jaundice screening. Although some argue that the individual components of NBS are best provided by the private sector, the majority of health care professionals agree that NBS is best kept as a public health program to ensure that all infants are screened for a panel of disorders. Affected infants need to be quickly located and treated to prevent disability or death.

NBS is a five-part public health program: screening, short-term follow-up, long-term follow-up, diagnosis, management, and evaluation (Pass et al., 2000). In the United States, each state decides which disorders to include in its NBS panel and which laboratory will perform the screening tests. Each state is also responsible for evaluating its own NBS program. Screening, the first component of the program, begins in the hospital or

Table 7.1-1. History of disorders added to newborn filter paper card screening in Georgia

1969	Phenylketonuria (PKU)
1978	Maple syrup urine disease, homocystinuria, tyrosinemia, galactosemia, congenital hypothyroidism
1990	Congenital adrenal hyperplasia
1998	Sickle cell disease and hemoglobinopathies
2003	Biotinidase deficiency
2005	Medium chain acyl-CoA dehydrogenase deficiency
2006–2007	Full spectrum tandem mass spectrometry for fatty acid oxidation defects, organic acidemias, additional aminoacidopathies, and cystic fibrosis

birthing center after the child has had 24 or 48 hours of feeding. To ensure rapid delivery, the filter paper cards with the dried blood samples (see Figure 7.1-2) are best sent by a local or overnight courier to a centralized laboratory within the state or to a regional laboratory.

Too many NBS programs have experienced long delays and have been unable to track the filter paper cards using traditional mail services. Because every state public laboratory does not have the technical expertise to perform the increasing number of analytic procedures, several states now contract with either other state laboratories or commercial academic laboratories to perform the screening tests. Significant efforts and continuing education of the staff of the birthing hospital or center are needed to ensure that the blood specimens are properly obtained and that each card has accurate and fully completed demographic information. Electronic data entry at the birthing site will help improve accuracy and lessen the likelihood for insufficient or inaccurate demographic information that is needed to quickly locate a child with an abnormal screening result.

An unsatisfactory specimen results in the need to relocate the infant, repeat the heel stick, and risk delays in diagnosis and treatment of an affected child. If a screening test is unsatisfactory or abnormal, immediate follow-up is needed. The submitting facility and clinician of record must be notified as soon as possible about an unsatisfactory or abnormal test result. Short-term follow-up is often performed by personnel in the screening laboratory or under contract by the state with a tertiary care center.

Regardless of the day of the week or time of the day, the infant must be quickly located, and a decision must be made based on the degree of abnormality of the screening result and the child's clinical status as to whether to repeat the screen or immediately proceed to a diagnostic evaluation and treatment. Diagnosis usually involves consultation with specialists in metabolic genetic disorders, pediatric endocrinologists, pediatric hematologists, and/or metabolic nutritionists. After a diagnosis is confirmed, lifelong management is needed by or in consultation with these same specialists.

The final component of a NBS program is evaluation. The state Department of Health is usually responsible for ensuring that all infants are properly screened, that unsatisfactory specimens are kept to a minimum, that children with abnormal results are rapidly located and assessed for the disorder, and that children who are diagnosed and treated are properly followed and have their outcome monitored. Although NBS has been the responsibility of state public health programs, recently several concerns about NBS have

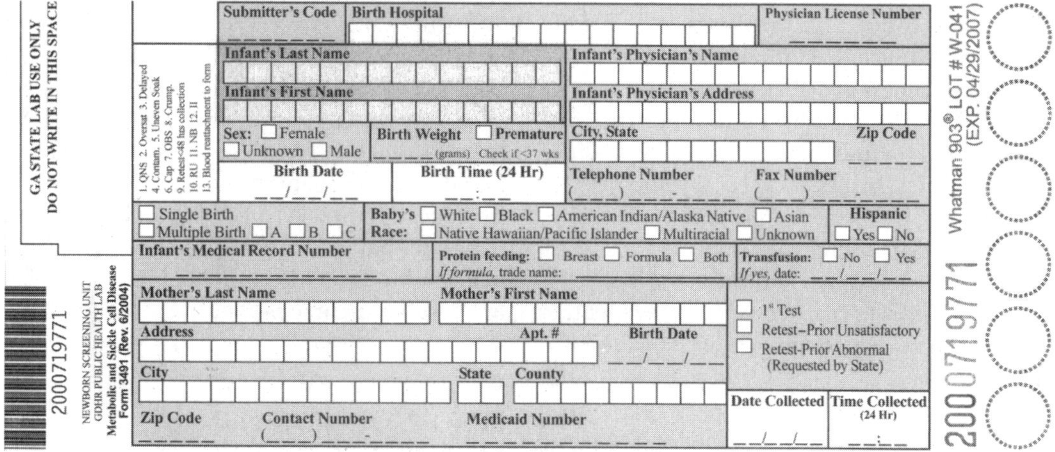

GA STATE LAB USE ONLY
DO NOT WRITE IN THIS SPACE

1. QNS 2. Oversat 3. Delayed 4. Contam. 5. Uneven Soak 6. Cap 7. OBS 8. Crump. 9. Retest<48 hrs collection 10. RU 11. NB 12. II 13. Blood reattachment to form

Submitter's Code | Birth Hospital | Physician License Number

Infant's Last Name | Infant's Physician's Name

Infant's First Name | Infant's Physician's Address

Sex: ☐ Female ☐ Unknown ☐ Male | Birth Weight (grams) ☐ Premature Check if <37 wks | City, State | Zip Code

Birth Date | Birth Time (24 Hr) | Telephone Number | Fax Number

☐ Single Birth ☐ Multiple Birth ☐ A ☐ B ☐ C | Baby's Race: ☐ White ☐ Black ☐ American Indian/Alaska Native ☐ Asian ☐ Native Hawaiian/Pacific Islander ☐ Multiracial ☐ Unknown | Hispanic ☐ Yes ☐ No

Infant's Medical Record Number | Protein feeding: ☐ Breast ☐ Formula ☐ Both; If formula, trade name: | Transfusion: ☐ No ☐ Yes; If yes, date:

Mother's Last Name | Mother's First Name | ☐ 1st Test ☐ Retest–Prior Unsatisfactory ☐ Retest–Prior Abnormal (Requested by State)

Address | Apt. # | Birth Date

City | State | County

Zip Code | Contact Number | Medicaid Number | Date Collected | Time Collected (24 Hr)

NEWBORN SCREENING UNIT
GDHR PUBLIC HEALTH LAB
Metabolic and Sickle Cell Disease
Form 3491 (Rev. 6/2004)

2000719771

Whatman 903® LOT # W-041 (EXP. 04/29/2007)

2000719771

Figure 7.1-2. Filter paper card used in Georgia. Demographic information about the child and health care providers is completed on the left side of the card and the blood spots from the heel stick will fill the six circles on the right. (Reprinted from the Georgia Department of Human Resources, Division of Publich Health.)

risen to national prominence. Because of the heterogeneity among states for which disorders are screened (Serving the Family, 2000), parents of affected children, medical specialists, and public health officials have begun discussions, in State NBS Advisory Boards and nationally through collaborative efforts of the Genetics Service Branch of the Maternal and Child Health Bureau, the Centers for Disease Control and Prevention, the National Institutes of Health, the American College of Medical Genetics, the March of Dimes Birth Defects Foundation, and the American Academy of Pediatrics.

A recent report prepared by the American College of Medical Genetics has proposed a uniform panel of tests that should be available to all infants. As new disorders are proposed to be added to the core NBS programs, a consensus hopefully will be reached based on data-driven decisions and expert opinions rather than historically individual preferences for which disorder to add to a screening panel in each state. Individual states must decide which disorders should be included on their screening panel and how to finance the entire NBS program.

LONG-TERM ASSESSMENT OF PROGRAMS AND CONSEQUENCES

Since the establishment of NBS programs, many attempts have been made to assess the long-term outcome of these programs both in human and in financial terms. Most economic studies have found significant cost-effectiveness/benefit from NBS programs in order to save dollars for health care and educational costs (Venditti et al., 2003). Although many studies have documented the incidence of specific disorders detected by NBS and relatively short-term outcomes in affected children, few population-based long-term studies have evaluated the effectiveness of NBS in preventing developmental disabilities. In order to determine whether NBS in Atlanta reduced the number of children with intellectual disabilities or less severe developmental delays from 1981 to 1991, three independent federal, state, and university data sources were linked. Of an estimated 147 infants who screened positive for a metabolic or endocrine disorder (i.e., were at risk for mental retardation if left untreated), only 3 children were identified with intellectual disabilities. Of an estimated 216 children who screened positive for a metabolic or endocrine disorder, 9 children were identified as having a developmental disability less severe than intellectual disabilities (e.g., speech-language impairments; Van Naarden, Yeargin-Allsopp, Schendel, & Fernhoff, 2003).

Despite the general successes of NBS programs, several unanticipated consequences have occurred. Initially, children with PKU were thought to only require a special diet during the first decade of life; however, as adolescents and young adults with PKU were removed from their phenylalanine-restricted diets or became less compliant with their diets, elevated blood phenylalanine levels proved deleterious to the structure and function of their mature brains. In addition, women with PKU who conceived and carried children while not controlling their own blood phenylalanine levels posed a significant risk for miscarriage or having babies with congenital heart disease, microcephaly, and developmental delays. This situation is called *maternal PKU* (Koch et al., 2003). Unfortunately, too many women with PKU were successfully treated as children but were unable to receive or stay on their PKU diet before and during their pregnancies. Many of these women have delivered multiple children with severe congenital impairments and long-term disabilities.

In a report of three states with well-organized metabolic services for care of individuals with PKU, only 8 (33%) of 24 women with PKU initiated the diet before pregnancy. Of 22 medical records reviewed, only 12 (55%) indicated control of blood phenylalanine levels before 10 weeks' gestation. Risk factors for late dietary control included young age and belief that treatment costs complicated the diet. Although all of the women expressed confidence in their Metabolic Clinic staff, few perceived that their obstetricians were knowledgeable about maternal PKU diet. Of 13 women enrolled in state-based assistance programs, 9 (69%) reported proof of pregnancy was required for eligibility. Many women using private insurance reported that their insurers were unwilling to pay for medical foods. When the data were stratified according to state of residence, differences were observed in the rate of live-born infants, prepregnancy medical food use, the average travel time to the Metabolic Clinic, and the gestational week when metabolic control was achieved. Studies that examined the long-term outcome of affected children found by NBS again emphasize the need to have lifetime access to experienced staff and resources and the ability to pay for expensive formula and low-protein medical foods, neither of which are routinely paid for by most third-party payers.

FUTURE OF NEWBORN SCREENING PROGRAMS

NBS programs grew slowly but progressively during their first 30 years of existence by adding a few selective tests to the screening panel. During the 1990s, however, the advent of new technologies, especially tandem mass spectrometry, made it possible to "multiplex" tests (i.e., run many analyses) on one filter paper card specimen. Although DNA technology is currently too expensive to use in a primary newborn screen, it is used to confirm a diagnosis from dried blood spots when a primary metabolic screen is abnormal, such as molecular confirmation of the diagnosis of cystic fibrosis on a blood spot with elevated concentrations of immunoreactive trypsin.

Several disorders that have been proposed to add to the screening panel, including fragile X syndrome, Duchenne muscular dystrophy, congenital immunodeficiencies, lysosomal storage disorders treatable by enzyme replacement therapy, congenital infections, cytomegalovirus, human immunodeficiency virus, and congenital hearing loss (Connexin 26 and 30 mutations). Several attempts have been made to agree on criteria for which disorders to add to a screening panel. Beginning with principles for screening for disease proposed by Wilson and Jungner (1968), these criteria have been modified for NBS to include those shown in Table 7.1-2. Surprisingly, the most difficult of the criterion to evaluate is whether there is an available and effective treatment for the disorder. For some disorders such as congenital hypothyroidism, early treatment with daily replacement doses of thyroid hormone prevents nearly all of the consequences of the mental and physical delays; however for other disorders, early identification may simply mean a better long-term outcome.

For example, early detection and treatment of cystic fibrosis with pancreatic enzyme replacement therapy significantly improves children's early growth and nutrition; however, evidence has yet to confirm that early detection improves pulmonary function and long-term survival. For other disorders, such as Duchenne muscular dystrophy and fragile X syndrome, early detection does not always lead to an improved outcome for the child and family. Parents have argued that early detection of their affected child would have helped them avoid a "diagnostic odyssey" to obtain a diagnosis and early intervention services. Also, early detection of these disorders gives parents and other members of the family important genetic information and reproductive options before having additional children with these disorders. Opponents, however, argue that identification through NBS could interfere with the family's ability to emotionally bond with the child years before he or she becomes symptomatic.

Table 7.1-2. Criteria for including disorders in newborn screening panels

Criteria
Significant morbidity and/or mortality
Available and effective treatment
Adequate time before onset of symptoms so that intervention can be effective
Clinical validity and clinical utility of the screen
Economically reasonable and cost beneficial/cost effective
Understanding of the natural history of the disease
Known and significant incidence in the population to be screened

Source: Wilson and Jungner (1968).

In order to evaluate when a disorder should be added to a NBS panel, the American College of Medical Genetics completed a project funded by the Genetic Disease Branch of the Bureau of Maternal and Child Health, which was the first attempt to achieve a mechanism for selecting disorders to include in a NBS panel. Whether this or any other system will work is yet to be seen; however, at least a national dialog has finally been established. As noted previously, each state remains sovereign in its ability to select which disorders to add to its screening panel, and, therefore, most states have established NBS advisory boards. Typically, these advisory boards consist of personnel from the state Department of Health, directors from the screening and diagnostic laboratories, follow-up personnel, health care professionals who diagnose and manage affected children, primary care providers, and parents and family members of affected children. These NBS advisory boards meet to discuss proposals to add or delete disorders to screening panels and to oversee the success and failures of their state's NBS program.

LEGAL, ETHICAL, AND FINANCIAL CONCERNS

NBS has always been enmeshed in ethical and legal issues. A child with a disorder that should have been detected but was missed on a NBS test raises many operational and legal concerns about whether and where the system failed. Table 7.1-3 shows several of the ethical concerns about NBS that have been extensively reviewed. Although very few programs require signed parental consent, most NBS programs use a policy of "informed dissent." Historically, parents have been given minimal information about the NBS test until shortly before their newborn is ready to be discharged from the hospital. They are told that their baby "will have a PKU test or a heel stick," and they are asked whether they have any objections. Most NBS programs allow parents to refuse the test for religious reasons. Fortunately, few parents refuse, but those who do place their child at risk for not being detected and treated early.

With the growth of the NBS advisory committees, a consensus has formed that the current education of parents about NBS is woefully inadequate and that more

Table 7.1-3. Ethical and legal concerns in newborn screening (NBS) programs

Should both parents give informed consent or informed dissent?
Should there be screening for disorders with no medical or nutritional therapy but for which early detection has psychosocial and reproductive benefits to the child and family?
Should newborns be screened for late-onset disorders?
Is ethnic and sex-specific screening appropriate?
Should all NBS programs screen for the same disorders?
Who has access to screening results?
Who has access to leftover dried blood spots, and how long should spots be stored?
Will results be linked with vital records and other newborn data systems?
How will the NBS program be financed?

information about NBS needs to be made available to parents during the last trimester of pregnancy. What does it means to be called back for a repeat study? How does a screening test differ from a diagnostic test, and how can parents obtain further information about the screening process and about specific disorders? Prospective parents need time to understand this important information about NBS, and the postpartum period is not optimal.

As discussed previously, NBS has been proposed for disorders such as Duchenne muscular dystrophy or fragile X syndrome for which there is no widely accepted medical or nutritional therapy but for which there may be psychosocial and reproductive benefits for the family and society. Inclusion of such disorders in a mandatory newborn screen is unlikely. An alternative approach would be to offer voluntary screening to parents of older, still presymptomatic infants. This screening, which would be done at 6 to 12 months of age, when most infants have a blood test for anemia, would still allow for earlier diagnosis, avoid the "diagnostic odyssey," and minimize interference with parent–infant bonding. Early diagnosis of these disorders will help these infants gain access to interventional services months or years before they normally would become eligible. With advances in molecular technology, NBS for disorders that do not become symptomatic until late childhood or adulthood will be technically feasible but unlikely to occur unless a compelling argument can be made that presymptomatic treatment during infancy will significantly benefit the course of the disorder.

Another ethical and legal issue is that parents are poorly, if at all, informed about the storage and use of their child's leftover dried blood spot. Some NBS programs store dried blood spots for a few months, whereas other NBS programs keep the dried spots for up to 21 years. Some dried blood spots are stored under ideal conditions; others are not. These spots are used for many purposes such as evaluation of new technologies, epidemiological, and forensic studies and for program quality control. Parents have the right to know what will happen to their infants' blood spots after the testing for the regular NBS is completed.

An important ethical concern is the ability to link demographic information and results of NBS with vital statistics such as birth and death records, referrals to early state developmental programs, and immunization records. Being able to link and track this information is extremely valuable to public health programs and primary care providers, but parents should have the right to know how this information on their child will be used, who will have access to the information, and how it will be kept confidential. Privacy advocates have raised important concerns about how this information will be stored, used, and retrieved.

Finally, as NBS programs have grown in scope, so have their costs. Most economic analyses of NBS programs have shown favorable cost–benefit/effectiveness ratios (Venditti et al., 2003). Continuing programs and adding new disorders to the screening panel, however, adds considerable burden to already financially strapped public health programs. Most state programs now obtain partial reimbursement from hospitals and third-party insurers not just to support the efforts of the screening laboratory, but also to help finance all segments of the entire 5-part NBS system. In general, this fee is the only one for the screening tests that is used to finance the system. Additional funds must come from state and federal programs.

Unlike countries with universal health care, the United States may be headed toward a two-tiered system of public and private NBS laboratories. Several commercial laboratories now offer core and "expanded" NBS tests and have challenged the public health laboratories' exclusivity in courts and state legislative bodies. In general, as new technology becomes available and additional disorders are proposed to be added to the screening panel, the commercial laboratories will offer these tests first directly to parents on a fee-for-service basis. Once screening for a disorder meets universal acceptance for inclusion in a core public health screening, it will then be included in panels along with the well-established disorders.

CONCLUSION

Newborn filter paper card screening has been in existence for more than 40 years. It is no longer just "the PKU test." NBS is an essential component of a comprehensive public health program that literally touches nearly every newborn. Fortunately, parents have many readily available on-line resources (see htttp://www.savebabies.com or http://www.genes-r-us.uthscsa.edu). Filter paper card NBS uses various technologies that have saved thousands of children from death and disability. With ongoing evaluation and input from a spectrum of health care professionals and families, NBS will continue as a public health program that benefits the vast majority of infants by protecting them from the consequences of an increasing number of devastating genetic and metabolic disorders.

REFERENCES

Brown, A.S., Fernhoff, P.M., Waisbren, S.E., Frazier, D.M., Singh, R., Rohr, F., Morris, J.M., Kenneson, A., MacDonald, P., Gwinn, M., Honein, M., & Rasmussen, S.A. (2002). Barriers to successful dietary control among pregnant women with phenylketonuria. *Genetics in Medicine, 4*(2), 84–89.

Fölling, A. (1934). Über Ausscheidung von Phenylbrenztraubensäure in den Harn als Stoffwecheselanomalie in Verbidung mit Imbezillitat. *Zeitschrift fur Physikalische Chemie, 277*, 169–176.

Guthrie, R., & Susi, A. (1963). A simple phenylalanine method for detecting phenylketonuria in large populations of newborn infants. *Pediatrics, 32*, 338–343.

Koch, R., Hanley, W., Levy, H., Matalon, K., Matalon, R., Rouse, B., et al. (2003). The maternal phenylketonuria international study: 1984–2002. *Pediatrics, 112*(6 Pt. 2), 1523–1529.

Pass, K.A., Lane, P.A., Fernhoff, P.M., Hinton, C.F., Panny, S.R., Parks, J.S., et al. (2000). Second U.S. newborn screening system guidelines II: Follow-up of children, diagnosis, management, and evaluation. Statement of the Council of Regional Networks for Genetic Services (CORN). *Journal of Pediatrics, 137*(4 Pt. 2), S1–S46.

Serving the family from birth to the medical home: A report from the Newborn Screening Task Force convened in Washington, D.C., May 10–11, 1999. (2000). *Pediatrics, 106*, S383–S426.

Van Naarden, B.K, Yeargin-Allsopp, M., Schendel, D., & Fernhoff, P. (2003). Long-term developmental outcomes of children identified through a newborn screening program with a metabolic or endocrine disorder: A population-based approach. *Journal of Pediatrics, 143*(2), 236–242.

Venditti, A.N., Venditti, C.P., Berry, G.T., Kaplan, P.B., Kaye, E.M., Glick, H., et al. (2003). Newborn screening by tandem mass spectrometry of medium-chain Acyl-CoA dehydrogenase deficiency: A cost-effectiveness analysis. *Pediatrics, 115*, 1005–1015.

Wilson, J.M.G., & Jungner, G. (1968). *Principles and practice of screening for disease.* (Public Health Paper No. 34). Geneva: World Health Organization.

7.2 MUCOPOLYSACCHARIDOSES

Frances Dougherty Kendall and Gerald Cox

Mr. and Mrs. Klein were devastated to learn that their two daughters, Hillary and Anya, had Hurler syndrome. Hillary had been a typical, healthy baby born full term after an uncomplicated pregnancy when Mrs. Klein (G1P0) was 29 years old. Hillary's skill attainment was normal, and she could walk, climb, and follow simple commands. Mrs. Klein became concerned, however, when Hillary's expressive language was limited to several single words. By 20 months old, Hillary had a history of unusual facial features, chronic congestion, and recurrent otitis media that required placement of bilateral myringotomy tubes.

A physical examination performed by a specialist revealed that Hillary had mild hirsuitism; macrocephaly; unusual facial features that included a prominent forehead, flattened nasal bridge, epicanthal folds, thickened lips, and an enlarged tongue; contracted fingers; a gibbus deformity (lumbar kyphosis); a small umbilical hernia; and hepatosplenomegaly. A skeletal X-ray survey noted dysostosis multiplex—a characteristic pattern of skeletal deformities, including a large skull with a deep and elongated sella, oar-shaped ribs, deformed and hook-shaped lower thoracic and lumbar vertebrae, pelvic dysplasia, and shortened tubular bones. Hillary's urine mucopolysaccharide profile was abnormal and noted dermatan sulfate and heparan sulfate. Her α-L-iduronidase activity was absent in leukocytes, confirming the diagnosis of mucopolysaccharidosis I (MPS I). The specialist informed Mr. and Mrs. Klein that Hillary's clinical features were consistent with the most severe form of MPS I, Hurler syndrome. Enzyme testing later confirmed that 6-month-old Anya also was affected.

Hillary underwent bone marrow transplantation from an unrelated donor and seemed to tolerate the procedure well. After a second transplant at 33 months of age, however, she contracted pneumonia and experienced acute renal failure. She passed away at 33 months of age. Mr. and Mrs. Klein were overwhelmed but tried to focus on Anya's treatment. At 11 months old, Anya underwent a successful transplant. By 19 months of age, she demonstrated good growth and development and minimal physical stigmata of Hurler syndrome.

The mucopolysaccharidoses (MPS) are a group of lysosomal storage disorders caused by the deficiency of enzymes that catalyze the stepwise degradation of glycosaminoglycans (previously called *mucopolysaccharides*). Glycosaminoglycans form the polysaccharide chains of proteoglycans, which are extracellular matrix macromolecules that are abundant in connective tissue and are important determinants of the viscoelastic properties of joints and other structures subjected to mechanical forces. The major glycosaminoglycans are chondroitin 6-sulfate, keratan sulfate, heparan sulfate, dermatan sulfate, and hyaluronate (Stryer, 1981).

Depending on the enzyme deficiency, the catabolism of one or more of the glycosaminoglycans is impaired. The lysosomal accumulation of glycosaminoglycan molecules results in cellular, and ultimately organ, dysfunction. Partially or nondegraded glycosaminoglycans are excreted in excess amounts in urine, which is the basis of screening tests. The clinical phenotype is dependent largely on the type and amount of storage material. For example, heparan sulfate is vital to neuronal cell membrane function, and its accumulation in the brain leads to severe neurological complications such as those seen in MPS III (Sanfilippo syndrome) and the severe forms of MPS I (Hurler syndrome) and MPS II (Hunter syndrome). Dermatan sulfate predominates in bone and soft tissues, which accounts for the somatic features seen in MPS I, II, and IV and its relative absence in MPS III. Keratan sulfate, which is even more bone-specific, accounts for the more predominant skeletal features seen in MPS IV.

Ten distinct enzyme deficiencies cause six distinct MPS disorders and their subtypes. Table 7.2-1 outlines the various disorders and their biochemical abnormalities (Beck, 2000).

Table 7.2-1. Biochemical classification of the mucopolysaccharide disorders

Number	Eponym	Enzyme deficiency	Glycosaminoglycan stored
MPS I (severe)	Hurler syndrome	α-L-iduronidase	Dermatan sulfate, heparan sulfate
MPS I (attenuated)	Hurler-Scheie syndrome	α-L-iduronidase	Dermatan sulfate, heparan sulfate
MPS I (attenuated)	Scheie syndrome	α-L-iduronidase	Dermatan sulfate, heparan sulfate
MPS II (severe)	Hunter (severe) syndrome	Iduronate-2-sulfatase	Dermatan sulfate, heparan sulfate
MPS II (attenuated)	Hunter (mild) syndrome	Iduronate-2-sulfatase	Dermatan sulfate, heparan sulfate
MPS IIIA	Sanfilippo A syndrome	Heparan-N-sulfatase	Heparan sulfate
MPS IIIB	Sanfilippo B syndrome	α-N-Acetylglucosaminidase	Heparan sulfate
MPS IIIC	Sanfilippo C syndrome	Acetyl-CoA: α-glucosaminide acetlytransferase	Heparan sulfate
MPS IIID	Sanfilippo D syndrome	N-Acetylglucosamine-6-sulfatase	Heparan sulfate
MPS IVA	Morquio syndrome, type A	Galactose-6-sulfatase	Keratan sulfate, chondroitin 6-sulfate
MPS IVB	Morquio syndrome, type B	β-galactosidase	Keratan sulfate
MPS VI	Maroteaux-Lamy syndrome	N-Acetylgalactosamine4-sulfatase (arylsulfatase B)	Dermatan sulfate
MPS VII	Sly syndrome	β-glucuronidase	Dermatan sulfate, heparan sulfate chondroitin 4-, 6-sulfates
MPS IX		Hyaluronidase	Hyaluronan

Note: MPS type designations V and VII are no longer used.

From Beck, M. (2000). Mucopolysaccharidoses and oligosaccharidoses. In J. Fernandes, J.M. Saudubray, & G. Van den Berghe (Eds.), *Inborn metabolic diseases: Diagnosis and treatment* (p. 419; Tables 36.1 and 36.2). New York: Springer; reprinted by permission. With kind permission of Springer Science and Business Media.

CLINICAL PRESENTATION

MPS I is caused by a deficiency of the lysosomal enzyme α-L-iduronidase and is the prototype of all MPS disorders. The spectrum of clinical phenotypes encompasses severe (Hurler disease), intermediate (Hurler-Scheie syndrome), and mild forms (Scheie disease), although it should be appreciated that the disease is a continuum and that "mild" is relative only with respect to the "severe" form, not the general population. *Severe* and *attenuated* are more recently introduced terms used to distinguish individuals with and without progressive cognitive impairment.

Although most babies with Hurler syndrome appear normal at birth, their first year of life is complicated by frequent ear, nose, and throat infections. Macrocephaly, macrosomia, hernias, and noisy breathing are often early features that go unnoticed. Children with severe MPS I subsequently develop unusual facial features (see Figure 7.2-1), thick skin, corneal clouding, hearing loss, hepatosplenomegaly, valvular heart disease, upper airway obstruction, skeletal deformities, joint stiffness, and secondary short stature. Skeletal survey reveals dysostosis multiplex (Figure 7.2-2). Children typically die within the first decade of life due to cardiopulmonary disease and/or neurologic decline.

Individuals with the milder variant (Scheie syndrome) are typically diagnosed in childhood to adulthood, have near-normal height and intelligence, and may have a normal life span. Somatic problems include stiff and painful joints, corneal opacities, carpal tunnel syndrome, and mild skeletal changes. Joint symptoms may be mistaken for arthritis. Chronic respiratory illnesses and mitral and aortic regurgitation due to valvular thickening affect most individuals with Scheie disease. Other individuals with the intermediate phenotype (Hurler-Scheie syndrome) develop somatic symptoms during childhood that can become debilitating and lead to death in the second to third decades but have little to no cognitive impairment.

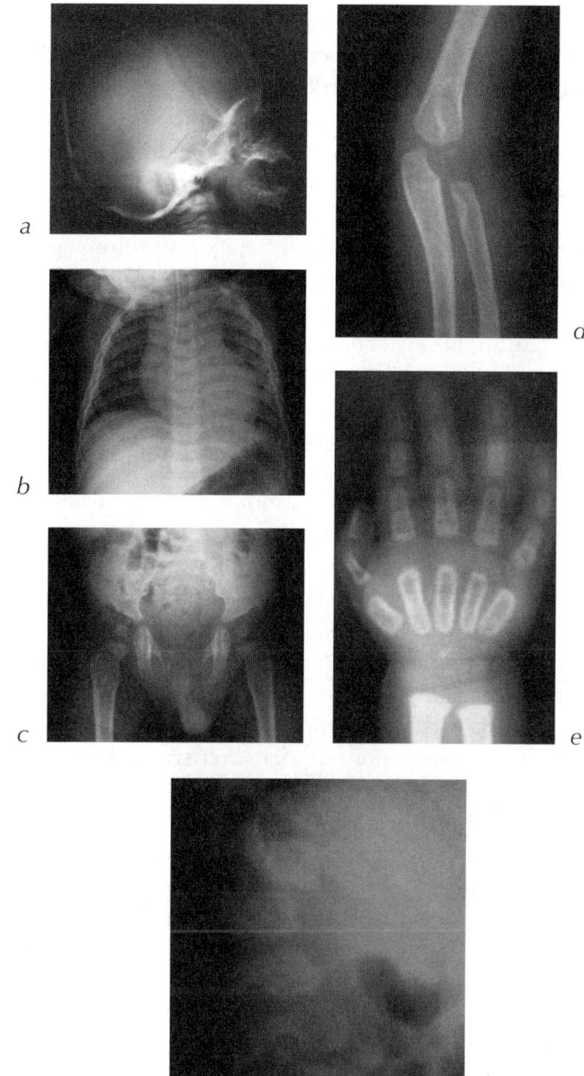

Figure 7.2-2. Multiple bony abnormalities in a 10-month-old boy with severe MPS I (Hurler syndrome). *(a)* skull x-ray showing a thickened calverium and a J-shaped sella tursica; *(b)* chest x-ray showing oar-shaped ribs and short, thickened clavicles; *(c)* pelvic x-ray showing shallow acetabulum and small capital femoral epiphyses; *(d)* upper limb x-ray showing widening and abnormal contours of the long bones; *(e)* hand x-ray showing short and broad metacarpal and phalangeal bones; *(f)* spine x-ray showing thoracolumbar gibbus deformity with anterioinferior beaking of vertebrae at the thoracolumbar junction.

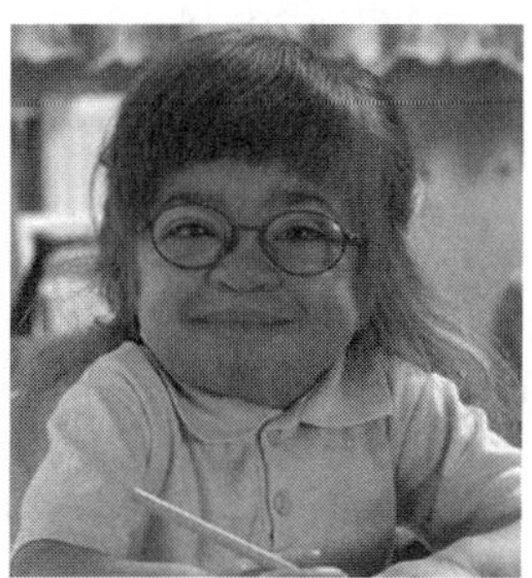
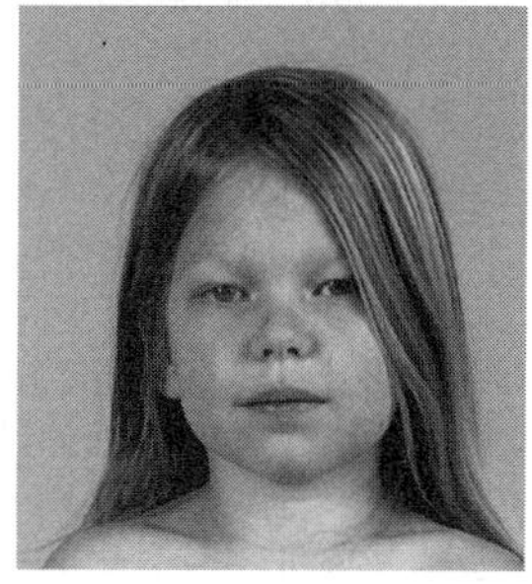

Figure 7.2-1. The clinical spectrum of MPS I. Microcephaly and unusual facial features in a girl with a more severe form (left photo) and lack of disinctive facial features in an attentuated patient (right photo). (Right photo courtesy of Professor F.A. Wijburg.)

Hunter syndrome, or MPS II, is the only X-linked MPS, and thus, almost exclusively affects boys. This disorder is caused by a deficiency of iduronate-2-sulfatase, which also leads to the accumulation of heparan sulfate and dermatan sulfate. MPS II can have severe or mild presentations. The severe form of MPS II is similar to MPS I, except for the lack of corneal clouding and slower progression of multisystem problems. The mild form of the disorder is associated with little to no cognitive impairment, a slow somatic course, and a prolonged life span (typically 40s or 50s, with the oldest survivor age 87; Neufeld & Muenzer, 2001).

Sanfilippo syndrome, or MPS III, has four subtypes caused by deficiencies of four different enzymes that all result in the impaired degradation and subsequent accumulation of heparan sulfate. All four subtypes of Sanfilippo syndrome result in severe central nervous system deterioration with minimal somatic problems, which makes this phenotype unique among the MPS disorders. Most individuals with this syndrome appear normal until 3–4 years of age, at which time developmental regression occurs, including loss of speech and gait abnormalities. As the disease progresses, hyperactivity and aggressive behavior usually occur.

Although bony changes are minimal and height growth is typically normal, characteristic somatic signs include coarse, often blond hair as well as hirsuitism. Unusual facial features and prominent hepatosplenomegaly are not typical. Individuals also can have seizures and hearing loss. Progressive neurological deterioration typically results in death from aspiration pneumonia during the first or second decade of life.

Two different enzyme defects result in Morquio syndrome, or MPS IV, and an accumulation of keratan sulfate. The disorder is characterized by short-trunked dwarfism, spondyloepiphyseal dysplasia on x-ray, fine corneal deposits, and normal intellect. Additional features include hepatomegaly, valvular heart disease, small teeth with thin enamel and frequent caries, unusual facial features, and hearing loss. The long-term prognosis is dependent on the development of skeletal-related complications, including atlanto-axial subluxation, cervical myelopathy with resulting paralysis, and restricted chest wall movement. The movie, *Simon Birch*, adapted John Irving's *A Prayer for Owen Meany*, recounts the life of a boy with Morquio syndrome.

Maroteaux-Lamy syndrome, or MPS VI, is caused by a deficiency of arylsulfatase B and accumulation of dermatan sulfate. This MPS disorder also has a clinical spectrum and similar somatic features as seen in MPS I but without cognitive impairment. The physical and visual complications, however, may affect development and result in psychomotor delays. In addition, the most severe form of MPS VI is associated with increased morbidity and mortality from cardiac and skeletal complications.

Sly syndrome, or MPS VII, results from a deficiency of β-glucuronidase and has an extremely variable phenotype ranging from hydrops fetalis to a Hurler-like presentation that includes dysostosis multiplex and hepatosplenomegaly and a later onset form (after age 4) with normal intelligence, mild skeletal changes, and minimal corneal clouding.

Hyaluronidase deficiency (MPS IX) is extremely rare, having been described in a single person with mild short stature, periarticular soft tissue masses, and hyaluronate accumulation.

DIAGNOSTIC TESTS

Typically, individuals with various forms of MPS disorders come to medical attention because of secondary complications arising from developmental delay, hepatosplenomegaly, and skeletal abnormalities. Table 7.2-2 summarizes most of the common presenting features. Many times, these features are so prominent that the diagnosis is obvious; however, differentiating between severe and milder subtypes, or between various MPS disorders with similar somatic but different neurological complications, is difficult. Therefore, definitive diagnosis requires confirmation by enzymatic assay in serum, leukocytes, and/or fibroblasts (Muenzer, 2004). In addition, the use of deoxyribonucleic acid (DNA) mutational analysis, particularly for individuals with MPS I and II, can provide information about possible outcome.

The first step in the biochemical diagnosis of a given MPS usually involves the measurement of urinary glycosaminoglycans. Because spot studies may produce false negatives and false positives, the use of a quantitative method such as the spectrophotometric assay using the dye dimethylene blue or one- or two-dimensional electrophoresis for the detection of glycosaminoglycans is recommended. Additional diagnostic adjuncts can include skeletal survey for dysostosis multiplex or other skeletal abnormalities; blood smears for the detection of abnormal cytoplasmic inclusions in lymphocytes; and histologic analysis of skin, liver, and bone marrow biopsies for the detection of enlarged lysosomes filled with abnormal storage material. Although readily available enzymatic assays negate the need for bone marrow biopsy in most cases, unusual clinical presentations may result in this procedure in some instances.

The differential diagnosis for a given MPS disorder includes other MPS types; oligosaccharidoses, in-

Table 7.2-2. Common presenting features of MPS disorders in infants and children

Physical appearance
Macrocephaly
Unusual facial features (prominent forehead, broad nose with flat nasal bridges, macroglossia, and thickened lips)
Protruding abdomen due to hepatosplenomegaly
Inguinal or umbilical hernias
Hirsutism
Neurologic, behavioral, and developmental features
Loss of development skills such as speech and learning
Mild mental deterioration
Behavioral problems
Hyperactivity (MPS III)
Hydrocephalus (communicating)
Ophthalmologic features
Corneal clouding (MPS I, IV, VI, and VII)
Photophobia
Ears, nose, and throat features
Recurrent otitis media
Chronic rhinitis
Enlarged tonsils and adenoids
Hearing loss
Abnormal teeth (spacing and shape)
Pulmonary features
Frequent pneumonias
Reactive airway disease
Noisy breathing and snoring
Obstructive sleep apnea
Cardiac features
Murmur caused by valvular disease (mitral, aortic)
Cardiomyopathy
Musculoskeletal features
Decreased joint range of motion
Bony abnormalities (dysostosis multiplex)
Decreased hand fine motor skills
Gibbus (lumbar kyphosis)
Stooped gait or stance

Note: These findings are collective. Individuals will have varied presentations, and absence of a particular finding or findings does not necessarily rule out an mucopolysaccharidosis disorder. Adapted from *Journal of Pediatrics, 144*(5 Suppl.), Muenzer, J., The mucopolysaccharidoses: A heterogeneous group of disorders with variable pediatric presentations, S32, Copyright 2004, with permission from Elsevier.

cluding Sialidosis; mucolipidoses (ML), in particular ML II or I-cell disease; the early infantile form of GM1 gangliosidosis; and genetic syndromes with unusual facial features (e.g., Coffin-Lowry, Fryns, and Costello syndromes). If an investigation for MPS disorders fails to diagnose an individual with a suspected MPS disorder, the addition of urinary oligosaccharides and disease-specific enzyme studies for other diagnostic possibilities, including ML II, are indicated.

GENETICS

When an individual is diagnosed with an MPS disorder, genetic counseling is recommended to inform couples of their recurrence risk and the availability of prenatal diagnosis as well as to offer testing to brothers and sisters. With the exception of MPS II, all MPS disorders are inherited in an autosomal recessive manner, meaning that a couple with a previously affected child has a 1 in 4, or 25%, recurrence risk for each subsequent pregnancy.

MPS II is X-linked and with rare exception (i.e., X-chromosome abnormalities) all affected individuals are boys. Both spontaneous new mutations in the iduronate-2-sulfatase gene causing this disorder and inheritance of a mutation from an asymptomatic carrier mother can result in MPS II. A woman found to be a carrier is faced with three possible future pregnancy outcomes: 25% chance of an affected son, 50% chance of an unaffected son or daughter, and 25% chance of a carrier daughter. Fathers with MPS II will pass on their altered iduronate-2-sulfatase gene to all of their daughters but none of their sons.

Couples who have had a child with an MPS disorder may be interested in prenatal diagnosis for subsequent pregnancies and should be informed of its availability. Enzymatic testing can be completed on amniocytes or tissue obtained by chorionic villus sampling; however, amniocytes are preferred by most testing laboratories. In addition, there have been some cases of false negative reports using chorionic villus sampling. Preimplantation genetic diagnosis of 8–16 cell stage blastomeres is theoretically possible if the mutation(s) are known.

At-risk siblings, particularly younger ones, should be tested to determine if they are affected. With recent advancements in treatment modalities, early diagnosis and treatment of an individual with an MPS disorder may improve functional status and slow disease progression. Older brothers and sisters may be interested in knowing their own carrier status because of concerns for having a child with an MPS disorder. Fortunately, DNA testing is now available to determine carrier status for all forms of MPS.

For autosomal recessive MPS disorders, healthy brothers and sisters should be counseled that they face a ⅔ risk of being a carrier. Because the incidence of individual MPS disorders (< 1 in 100,000) and their carrier frequencies (< 1 in 150) in the general population are low—much lower than the common genetic disorders such as cystic fibrosis (1 in 2,500 incidence and 1 in 25 carrier frequency)—the risk of a carrier having a child with an MPS disorder via a spouse who has no family history of MPS is very low (approximately 0.1%). Sisters of individuals with MPS II face the same recurrence risk as their mothers if they are found to carry the affected gene.

TREATMENT

Three types of treatment options are available for individuals with MPS: symptom-based or palliative care, hematopoietic stem cell transplantation (HSCT), and enzyme replacement therapy (ERT). Only HSCT and ERT address the underlying pathophysiology. The choice of therapeutic approach is dependent on the type of MPS, the neurological and medical status of the individual, and the availability of specific treatment options (e.g., ERT is available for MPS I and VI). Regardless of the treatment course taken, all individuals with an MPS disorder and their families should be offered counseling and psychosocial support to assist them in coping with the devastating, multifaceted effects of chronic illness. Such services can be provided by any number of groups, including local social work resources or national organizations such as the National MPS Society.

Palliative Care

A system-based approach to the complications seen with a given MPS disorder typically requires the coordination of care by a physician familiar with the widespread problems seen with these disorders, including the high risk of intubation difficulties and complications due to an enlarged tongue, redundant pharyngeal tissue, small airway, and unstable atlanto-axial joints. Ideally, a geneticist or metabolic specialist fills that role, but limitation of access to these specialists in many communities may dictate that a pediatrician, internist, or other specialist such as a developmental pediatrician assume that responsibility.

Most individuals with an MPS disorder will require care from many health care providers, including cardiologists, neurologists, otolaryngologists, pulmonologists, orthopedists, and physical and speech therapists. Ongoing treatment may require corrective surgeries for cardiac or orthopedic complications; the use of hearing aids and wheelchairs; institution of continuous positive airway pressure (CPAP) for obstructive sleep apnea; pain management; and various physical, occupational, and speech therapies. Managing physicians may use the MPS I Registry guidelines (see Table 7.2-3) developed by an International Board of Advisors to monitor individuals with MPS I (Genzyme Corp., 2005). These guidelines may be individualized for other MPS disorders and and are updated perodically on the MPS I Registry web site.

Hematopoietic Stem Cell Transplantation

HSCT provides individuals with an MPS disorder with normal donor stem cells that produce the missing or deficient enzyme and subsequently improves the secondary complications caused by the underlying disease. The high morbidity (e.g., graft-versus-host disease, infections) and mortality (greater than 15%–20%) associated with this procedure limits its use to severely affected individuals early in their disease course. Several studies have reviewed the outcomes of more than 200 children with MPS I who underwent HSCT (Neufeld & Muenzer, 2001; Wraith, 2001). Transplants performed before 24 months of age in children with developmental quotients greater than 70 were associated with better outcomes, including preservation of central nervous system function; reduced hepatosplenomegaly; and improved cardiac function, linear growth, and upper airway obstruction. Ophthalmologic and skeletal complications, however, were not significantly improved. Despite HSCT, many individuals with an MPS disorder still require orthopedic procedures to maintain quality of life.

Initial case reports have suggested that the use of ERT in individuals with MPS I prior to HSCT may improve their clinical status and ability to tolerate the transplant (Grewal et al., 2005). The use of HSCT for other MPS disorders, including most individuals with MPS II and all with MPS III, is not recommended because the procedure has not been associated with an appreciable improvement in neurological outcome. Some individuals with MPS VI and VII have received transplants.

Historically, bone marrow has been the source of donor cells, but increasingly umbilical cord blood is being used and appears to be more promising. Cord blood is more readily available than bone marrow, and it potentially has a higher rate of engraftment and lower rate of graft-versus-host disease (Staba et al., 2004).

Enzyme Replacement Therapy

Aldurazyme (laronidase or recombinant human α-L-iduronidase; BioMarin-Genzyme LLC) ERT was approved for the treatment of MPS I in the United States and European Union in 2003 and in several additional countries since. Aldurazyme (0.58 mg/kg or 100 Units/kg) provides individuals with an exogenous source of missing enzyme that is delivered as a weekly intravenous infusion over 4 hours. The Phase 3 clinical study was a

Table 7.2-3. Minimum schedule of assessments for MPS I

	Initial assessment	Every 6 months	Every 12 months	Every other year
General				
Demographics	X			
Patient diagnosis	X			
Medical history	X	X		
Physical exam	X	X		
General appearance	X	X		
MPS I disease clinical assessments				
Neurologic/central nervous system				
• Neurocognitive testing, including DQ-IQ	X		X	
• MRI of brian	X			X
• MRI of spine	X			X
• Nerve conduction studies (carpel tunnel syndrome)	X			X
Ophthalmologic				
• Visual acuity	X		X	
• Retinal exam	X		X	
• Corneal exam	X		X	
Auditory				
• Audiometry	X		X	
Cardiac				
• Echocardiogram	X			X
• Electrocardigram	X			X
Respiratory				
• Forced vital capacity/forced expiratory volume	X	X		
• Sleep study	X		X	
Gastrointestinal				
• Spleen volume	X			X
• Liver volume	X			X
Musculoskeletal				
• Skeletal survey by x-ray	X			X
Vitals and laboratory tests				
Height/weight	X	X		
Head circumference	X	X		
Blood pressure	X	X		
Enzyme activity level	X			
Urinary glycosaminoglycan level	X	X		
Urinalysis	X	X		
MPS health assessment				
MPS Health Assessment Questionnaire	X	X		

Key: DQ = developmental quotient; IQ = intelligence quotient; MPS = mucopolysaccharidosis; MRI = magnetic resonance imaging.

From Genzyme Corp. (2005). *Minumum schedule of assessments for monitoring patients with MPS I.* Retrieved February 28, 2005, from http://MPSI Registry.com; reprinted by permission.

double-blind, placebo-controlled study that demonstrated improvements in respiratory function (forced vital capacity) and mobility (6-minute walk test and joint range of motion) as well as reductions in urinary glycosaminoglycan excretion and hepatomegaly in patients treated for 26 weeks (Wraith et al., 2004). Sleep apnea and shoulder flexion improved in the most severely affected.

Although the effects of Aldurazyme on the central nervous system have not been evaluated, the most common reported adverse side effects were infusion reactions, including flushing, fever, headache, and rash. The most serious reaction was anaphylaxis in one individual. Although most individuals have developed IgG antibodies to the recombinant enzyme, their significance is unknown.

Enzyme replacement therapies also have been developed for MPS II and VI. Somatic changes and functional improvements similar to that following enzyme replacement therapy in MPS I have been reported in initial clinical trails (Staba et al., 2004, Harmatz et al., 2004). Double-blind, placebo-controlled Phase 3 clinical studies have recently been completed for both enzymes. Recombinant human iduronate-2-sulfatase for the treatment of MPS II is undergoing regulatory review. Naglazyme (galsulfase, recombinant human arylsulfatase B) has been shown to improve walking and stair-climbing capacity in individuals with MPS VI. Naglazyme was approved by the FDA for the treatment of individuals with MPS VI in 2005.

PROGNOSIS

All of the MPS disorders are chronic, progressive diseases, and most individuals die prematurely from associated complications involving cardiopulmonary disease. The life span of an individual with an MPS disorder depends on the phenotype, advancement of the disease process at the time of diagnosis, and available treatment modalities. Despite significant improvements in the care and treatment of individuals with an MPS disorder, morbidity and mortality remain high. For example, individuals with Hurler syndrome typically die by 10 years of age with a mean age of death of 5 years. Individuals with Hurler-Scheie syndrome typically die by 25 years of age (mean 15 years), and those with Scheie syndrome typically die by mid-adulthood.

CONCLUSION

MPS disorders are caused by specific deficiencies of lysosomal enzymes that catalyze the stepwise degradation of glycosaminoglycans. All MPS disorders share a chronic and progressive course, multisystem involvement, and result in significant disability and often premature death. Intellectual disabilities are seen in the severe forms of MPS I (Hurler syndrome) and MPS II (Hunter syndrome) and in all cases of MPS III (Sanfilippo syndrome). Normal intellect can be seen in the other types. Excess amounts of partially degraded glycosaminoglycan fragments are detected in the urine of individuals with the various forms of MPS. Definitive diagnosis of a specific disorder requires enzyme assays in serum, leukocytes, or fibroblasts. This group of disorders is inherited in an autosomal recessive fashion, with the exception of MPS type II (Hunter syndrome), which is X-linked. Prenatal diagnosis is available.

HSCT may improve the clinical course in some individuals with severe MPS I disease, but the procedure has high morbidity and mortality that limits its use to individuals early in the course of their illness. New breakthroughs in the use of ERT for MPS I, II, and VI, and the use of cord blood for HSCT offer new hope for individuals with an MPS disorder and their families.

REFERENCES

Beck, M. (2000). Mucopolysaccharidoses and oligosaccharidoses. In J. Fernandes, J.M. Saudubray, & G. Van den Berghe (Eds.), *Inborn metabolic diseases: Diagnosis and treatment* (pp. 415–421). New York: Springer.

Genzyme Corp. (2005). *Minimum schedule of assessments for monitoring patients with MPS I.* Retrieved February 28, 2005, from http://MPSIRegistry.com

Grewal, S.S., Wynn, R., Abdenur, J.E., Burton, B.K., Gharib, M., Haase, C., et al. (2005). Safety and efficiency of enzyme replacement in Hurler syndrome. *Genetics in Medicine*, 7(2), 143–146.

Harmatz, P., Whitley, C.B., Waber, L., Pais, R., Steiner, R., Plecko, B., et al. (2004). Enzyme replacement therapy in mucopolysaccharidosis VI (Maroteaux-Lamy syndrome). *Journal of Pediatrics, 144*(5), 574–580.

Muenzer, J. (2004). The mucopolysaccharidoses: A heterogeneous group of disorders with variable pediatric presentations. *Journal of Pediatrics, 144*(5 Suppl.), S27–S34.

Neufeld, E.J., & Muenzer, J. (2001). The mucopolysaccharidoses. In C.R. Scriver, A.L. Beaudet, W.S. Sly, & D. Valle (Eds.), *The metabolic and molecular bases of inherited disease* (8th ed., pp. 3421–3452). New York: McGraw Hill.

Staba, S.L., Escolar, M.L., Poe, M., Kim, Y., Martin, P.L., Szabries, P., et al. (2004). Cord-blood transplants from unrelated donors in patients with Hurler's syndrome. *New England Journal of Medicine, 350*(19), 1960–1969.

Stryler, L. (1981). *Biochemistry.* New York: W.H. Freeman.

Wraith, J.E. (2001). Advances in the treatment of lysosomal storage disease. *Developmental Medicine and Child Neurology, 43*, 639–646.

Wraith, J.E., Clarke, L.A., Beck, M., Kolodny, E.H., Pastores, G.M., Muenzer, J., et al. (2004). Enzyme replacement therapy for mucopolysaccharidoses I: A randomized, double-blinded, placebo-controlled, multinational study of recombinant human alpha-L iduronidase (Laronidase). *Journal of Pediatrics, 144*(5), 581–588.

7.3 SPHINGOLIPIDOSES

Deborah Marsden

Sphingolipids are components of lipid membranes involved in cellular signalling that are derived from ceramide and degraded by lysosomal hydrolases. They are divided into three classes: 1) cerebrosides, 2) sphingomyelins, and 3) gangliosides. Defects in the catabolic pathways of sphingolipids lead to storage of glycosphingolipids and phosphosphingolipids in the lysosomes of the central nervous system and/or viscera. There is some specificity for each enzyme and the tissue involved (e.g., macrophages in Gaucher disease, vascular endothelium in Fabry disease, neurons in the gangliosidoses).

Inheritance is autosomal recessive except for Fabry disease, which is X-linked. Population screening by mutation analysis for common mutations has been well established for Gaucher disease and Tay-Sachs disease and can be used for carrier screening in high-risk populations, such people of Ashkenazi Jewish ancestry. Newborn screening methodologies are currently being evaluated; they will likely be introduced in the near future and may allow for early, presymptomatic treatment where applicable. The different sphingolipidoses are listed in Table 7.3-1.

Table 7.3-1. Sphingolipidoses

Disorder	Deficient enzyme	Inheritance	Tissue involvement
Gaucher disease	Glucocerebrosidase	Autosomal recessive	Brain Liver Spleen
Fabry disease	α-Galactosidase	X-linked	Autonomic ganglia Central nervous system Glomeruli Myocardium Skin Vascular endothelium
Niemann-Pick disease Groups A and B	Sphingomyelinase	Autosomal recessive	Central nervous system Liver Lungs Spleen
Niemann-Pick disease Groups C and D	Cholesterol transport	Autosomal recessive	Central nervous system Liver Spleen
Krabbe disease	Galactocerebrosidase	Autosomal recessive	Central nervous system Liver Spleen
G_{M2}, Gangliosidosis			
Tay-Sachs disease	Hexosaminidase A	Autosomal recessive	Central nervous system
Sandhoff disease	Hexosaminidase A + B	Autosomal recessive	Central nervous system
G_{M1}, Gangliosidosis	β-Galactosidase	Autosomal recessive	Central nervous system Liver Skeleton Spleen
Farber disease	Ceramidase	Autosomal recessive	Central nervous system Granulomas Lymph nodes
Metachromatic leukodystrophy	Arylsulfatase A	Autosomal recessive	Central nervous system Peripheral nerves

GAUCHER DISEASE

Gaucher disease is caused by a defect of glucocerebrosidase. It is the most common lysosomal storage disease; the incidence is about 1/40,000 in the general population, with a much higher incidence in individuals of Ashkenazi Jewish descent (1/50 to 1/1,000). Diagnosis is confirmed by a leukocyte enzyme assay. The pathognomonic "Gaucher cell" is found in bone marrow. Deoxyribonucleic acid (DNA) mutation analysis shows prevalent mutations in the Ashkenazi population.

Gaucher disease has three clinical phenotypes—nonneuronopathic (Type I), neuronopathic (Type II), and intermediate or chronic neuronopathic (Type III)—which are outlined in Table 7.3-2. There is a wide clinical spectrum, with onset from infancy through adulthood. Typical features are hepatosplenomegaly (spleen more involved than liver), pancytopenia, bone pain crises, and neurodegeneration (Types II and III). Some individuals remain asymptomatic. The severity is largely due to the amount of residual enzyme activity. Carrier testing by enzyme assay, however, is unreliable due to overlapping of activity found in both affected and carrier individuals. Treatment with intravenous recombinant enzyme has been used very successfully for the nonneuronopathic variant (Type I). The enzyme does not cross the blood-brain barrier, so it is not effective in the other variants.

NIEMANN-PICK DISEASE

Niemann-Pick disease has four clinical phenotypes (see Table 7.3-3). Group A (infantile onset) and Group B (juvenile onset) are caused by a deficiency of sphingomyelinase that results in hepatosplenomegaly, progressive hypersplenism, pulmonary infiltration, and hyperlipidemia. Individuals with Group A experience rapidly progressive neurodegeneration. The severity and age of onset are usually, but not invariably, correlated with the residual enzyme activity. Individuals with Group B usually have little or no neurological involvement and survive into adulthood, at which time they may have complications from chronic infiltrative lung disease. Although Groups A and B are pan-ethnic, there is a higher frequency in individuals with Ashkenazi Jewish ancestry, with an incidence of about 1:40,000. Groups C and D are distinct disorders of intracellular cholesterol processing.

Diagnosis is confirmed for Groups A and B by leukocyte enzyme assay. Groups C and D are diagnosed by finding the characteristic filipin staining and deficient cholesterol uptake in cultured fibroblasts. Mutation analysis is available. Group D is clinically similar to Group C and is due to an allelic mutation in the same gene as Group C (*NPC1*). Due to a founder effect, the Group D mutation is common in the Nova Scotia region of Canada. Clinical trials of recombinant enzyme replacement treatment for Group B are underway.

FABRY DISEASE

Fabry disease is due to a deficiency of α-galactosidase, causing accumulation of globotriaosylceramide (GL3) in the vascular endothelium in many different tissues, including glomeruli, autonomic ganglia, myocardium, and the central nervous system. Clinical features are listed in Table 7.3-4. Women and girls who are carriers have variable symptoms due to random inactivation of the X chromosome (Lyonization), but they can be severely affected. The onset of symptoms in men and boys is usually in late childhood or adolescence with acroparesthesia (pain crises) and hypohidrosis (due to impaired vascular supply to nerve endings) that gradually ameliorate with time. Later, the characteristic skin

Table 7.3-2. Gaucher disease phenotypes

	Type I	Type II	Type III
Age of onset	Infancy to adulthood	Infancy	Childhood to adulthood
Symptoms/signs	Hepatosplenomegaly Growth retardation Anemia Thrombocytopenia Pathologic fractures Aseptic necrosis (hip) Painful bone crises Delayed puberty	Hepatosplenomegaly Oculomotor apraxia Spastic quadriparesis Seizures	Hepatosplenomegaly Lateral gaze palsy Ataxia Neurodegeneration Bone involvement
Life span	Variable—may be normal	Death by 2 years	Death by 2–60 years

Table 7.3-3. Niemann-Pick disease phenotypes

	Group A	Group B	Group C
Age of onset	3–6 months	Childhood	Infancy to adulthood
Symptoms/signs	Hepatomegaly Splenomegaly Hypotonia Spastic quadriparesis Cherry red spot Visual impairment Restrictive lung disease	Hepatomegaly Splenomegaly Pancytopenia Restrictive lung disease Short stature Hyperlipidemia	Cholestratic jaundice (neonatal) Hepatomegaly (may be mild) Splenomegaly (may be mild) Upward gaze palsy Seizures Dystonia Dementia
Life span	Death by age 3	Death occurs between late childhood and adulthood	Death in late adolescence or adulthood

lesions, *angiokeratomata*, that cluster in the area between the mid-abdomen to mid-thigh, particularly periumbilical, may be seen. Renal disease is progressive from about the third decade with end-stage renal failure by the fifth or sixth decade. Central nervous system disease (stroke, transient ischemic attacks) occurs later in men but may be the presenting factor in women. Other symptoms include abdominal pain, weight loss, and cardiomyopathy.

The diagnosis is confirmed in men by measuring the leukocyte enzyme activity. Because of variable tissue enzyme activity due to lyonization in women, measurement of enzyme activity may not be reliable, so mutation analysis is preferred. Recombinant enzyme therapy can reduce the accumulation of GL3 and may prevent progression of the disease if started before irreversible damage has occurred. Many individuals have been misdiagnosed or diagnosed with psychosomatic illness, particularly in adolescence, because of recurrent painful crises and gastrointestinal symptoms.

Table 7.3-4. Symptoms of Fabry disease

Age	Symptoms
Late childhood	Acroparesthesia Hypohydrosis
Adolescence	Abdominal pain Weight loss
Adulthood	Proteinuria Microalbuminuria End-stage renal failure Left ventricular hypertrophy Conduction defects Stroke or transient ischemic attack

KRABBE DISEASE (GLOBOID CELL LEUKODYSTROPHY)

Krabbe disease is caused by a deficiency of β-galactosidase with onset of symptoms by 6 months of age in the rapidly progressive infantile variant or later in infancy in the juvenile variant. Characteristic features are extreme irritability, tonic spasms, spasticity, extensor posturing, loss of bulbar functioning, blindness, and deafness. Cerebrospinal fluid protein levels are markedly elevated, and nerve conduction velocities are slowed. Magnetic resonance imaging of the brain shows evidence of demyelination. The diagnosis is confirmed by measuring the enzyme activity in leukocytes or fibroblasts. Some individuals with the more slowly progressive disease have been successfully treated with allogenic bone marrow transplantation.

TAY-SACHS DISEASE

Tay-Sachs disease, is a G_{M2} gangliosidosis due to a deficiency of hexosaminidase A. In the general population, the incidence is rare, but carrier frequency in individuals with Ashkenazi Jewish ancestry is approximately 1/30, with an incidence prior to the implementation of prenatal screening programs of approximately 1/3,600. There is also a higher frequency among individuals of French Canadian and Old Order Amish descent.

There are three clinical phenotypes, which are related to the residual enzyme activity. The classic infantile-onset variant is characterized by the appearance of symptoms before 3–6 months of age, with hypotonia, myoclonus, visual inattention, and hyperacuisis. Rapid progression of spasticity, loss of cognition, seizures, blindness, bulbar dysfunction, and extensor posturing result in death by about 4 years of age. The cherry red spot in the macular is universal. The juvenile-onset variant is more slowly progressive, usually starting in childhood with ataxia, cognitive decline, and progressive spasticity and death in adolescence. The cherry red spot is not always present; rather, there is optic atrophy and retinitis pigmentosa. The chronic or adult-onset variant is characterized by ataxia, dystonia, and choreothetosis beginning in the first decade. Cognitive decline is much later. Some individuals have neuropsychiatric symptoms. Treatment is supportive.

Sandhoff disease, which is pan-ethic, is due to a deficiency of both hexosaminidase A and B. Clinical symptoms are similar to Tay-Sachs disease.

CONCLUSION

Sphingolipidoses are diseases characterized by abnormal sphingolipid metabolism. These inherited disorders affect the central nervous system and viscera. Symptoms vary per person, and onset ranges from infancy to adulthood. Treatment varies, and genetic counseling is often helpful for parents of affected children.

REFERENCES

Barth, P.G. (2000). Disorders of sphingolipid metabolism. In J. Fernandes, J.-M. Saudubray, & G. van den Berghe (Eds.), *Inborn metabolic disease* (2nd ed.). Berlin: Springer-Verlag.

Crocker, A., & Farber, S. (1958). Niemann Pick disease: A review of eighteen patients. *Medicine (Baltimore), 37*, 1.

Eng, C.M., Guffon, N., & Wilcox, W.R. (2001). Safety and efficacy of recombinant human alpha-galactosidase A–replacement therapy in Fabry disease. *New England Journal of Medicine, 345*(1), 9.

Fried, K. (1973). Population study of chronic Gaucher's disease. *Israel Journal of Medical Sciences, 9*, 1396.

Greer, W.L., Riddell, D.C., Gillan, T.L., et al. (1997). The Nova Scotia (Type D) form of Niemann-Pick disease is caused by a G3097—>T transversion in NPC1. *American Journal of Human Genetics, 63*(1), 52.

Hagberg, B., Kollberg, H., Sourander, P., & Aleksson, O. (1970). Infantile globoid cell leucodystrophy (Krabbe's disease): A clinical and genetic study of 32 Swedish patients 1953–1967. *Neuropadiatrie, 1*, 74.

Johnson, W.G. (1981). The clinical spectrum of hexosaminidase deficiency disease. *Neurology, 31*, 1453.

Navon, R. (1991). The molecular and clinical heterogeneity of adult G_{M2} gangliosidosis. *Developmental Neuroscience, 13*, 295.

Pentchev, P.G., Comly, M.E., Kruth, H.S., et al. (1985). A defect in cholesterol esterification in Niemann-Pick disease (type CP patients). *Proceedings of the National Academy of Sciences of the United States of America, 82*, 8247.

Peterson, G.M., Rotter, J.I., Cantor, R.M., et al. (1983). The Tay-Sachs disease gene in North American Jewish populations: Geographic variations and origin. *American Journal of Human Genetics, 35*, 1258.

Scriver, C.R., Beaudet, A.L., Valle, D., Sly, W.S., Childs, B., Kinzler, K.W., & Vogelstein, B. (Eds.). (2001). *The metabolic and molecular bases of inherited disease* (8th ed., Vol. I–IV). New York: McGraw-Hill.

Weinreb, N.J., Charrow, J., Andersson, H., et al. (2002). Effectiveness of enzyme replacement therapy in 1,028 patients with Type I Gaucher disease after 2 to 5 years of treatment: A report from the Gaucher Registry. *Journal of the American Medical Association, 113*, 112.

7.4 MITOCHONDRIAL DISORDERS

John M. Shoffner

Leila was a 23-month-old girl with global developmental delay and a history of pseudo-obstruction of the gastrointestinal tract. Her expressive and receptive language were also delayed. Leila's mother, Maria, was surprised by Leila's delays because her pregnancy and Leila's birth were both unremarkable. Maria's two brothers, however, had learning disabilities, and she wondered if Leila's problems were somehow related.

Maria took Leila to the pediatrician, who observed that Leila had hypotonia, hyporeflexia, and motor and language delays. He was unable to diagnose anything, though, because of the nonspecific nature of her symptoms. In subsequent years, Maria had two more daughters who both had symptoms similar to Leila's.

Diagnosing mitochondrial disorders is a technically challenging and time-consuming process. The term *mitochondrial medicine* has emerged to encompass the complex synthesis of clinical, biochemical, pathological, and genetic information required for diagnosis. The multiorgan involvement and clinical heterogeneity of these diseases can make diagnosis difficult, which emphasizes the importance of a well-organized approach.

BIOCHEMISTRY

Mitochondria are cytoplasmic structures with an inner and outer membrane separated by an intermembrane space. The outer membrane is permeable to most small molecules and ions and contains a variety of proteins, such as monoamine oxidase, long-chain acyl-CoA synthetase, carnitine palmitoyl transferase 1 (CPT1), and mitochondrial protein import proteins. The inner mitochondrial membrane is impermeable to most metabolites. It has a convoluted structure with multiple folds called *cristae*. The inner membrane has a high content of protein and cardiolipin and contains oxidative phosphorylation (OXPHOS) enzymes as well as multiple classes of translocases. The space surrounded by the inner mitochondrial membrane, called the *mitochondrial matrix*, contains an array of enzymes, including those for the Krebs cycle (tricarboxylic acid cycle), the pyruvate dehydrogenase complex (PDC), b-oxidation of fatty acids, urea cycle, ketone metabolism, amino acid metabolism, heme metabolism, nucleotide metabolism, and the peptidases plus chaperonins necessary for mitochondrial protein import and OXPHOS enzyme assembly and maintenance. The matrix also contains mitochondrial deoxyribonucleic acid (mtDNA).

OXPHOS is an oxygen-dependent biochemical process localized to the mitochondrial inner membrane that produces most of the adenosine triphosphate (ATP) required by cells for normal function. A complex array of nuclear deoxyribonucleic acid (nDNA) and mtDNA genes operate coordinately to produce functional OXPHOS enzymes. The mtDNA is a 16,569-nucleotide pair, double-stranded, circular molecule that codes for two ribosomal ribonucleic acids (rRNAs), 22 transfer ribonucleic acids (tRNAs), and 13 of the 82 structural proteins of the mitochondrial electron transport chain.

Four highly complex enzymes referred to as the respiratory chain receive electrons from the catabolism of carbohydrates, fats, and proteins in order to generate a proton gradient across the inner mitochondrial membrane (see Figure 7.4-1). Complexes I and II (succinate dehydrogenase) collect electrons from the catabolism of fats, proteins, and carbohydrates and transfer them sequentially to coenzyme Q_{10}, complex III, and complex IV (cytochrome c oxidase). Complex II is also part of the tricarboxylic acid cycle (Krebs cycle). These four enzymes contain flavins, coenzyme Q_{10} (ubiquinone), iron–sulfur clusters, hemes, and protein-bound copper. Complexes I, III, and IV utilize the energy in electron transfer to pump protons across the inner mitochondrial membrane, producing a proton gradient that is used by complex V (adrenosine 5′-triphosphate [ATP]

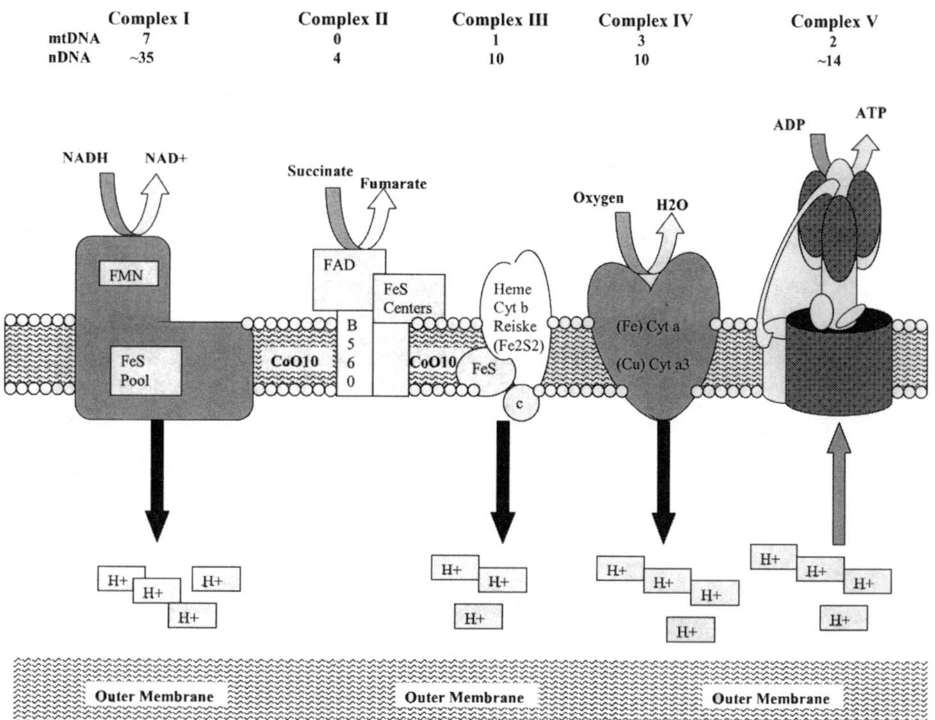

Figure 7.4-1. Oxidative phosphorylation. Electrons are collected from carbohydrate, fatty acid, and protein oxidation by oxidative phosphorylation. Complexes I, III, and IV pump protons into the space between the inner and outer mitochondrial membranes. This stored energy is used by complex V to generate ATP.

Key: mtDNA = mitochondrial DNA coded subunits; nDNA = nuclear DNA coded subunits, FeS and Reiske (Fe_2S_2) = iron sulfur groups; NADH and NAD+ = reduced and oxidized nicotinamide adenine nucleotide; B560, Cyt a, Cyt a3, Cyt b, and c = cytochromes; Q_{10} and CoQ_{10} = coenzyme; FMN = flavin mononucleotide; FAD = flavin adenine dinucleotide; ADP = adenosine diphosphate; ATP = adenosine triphosphate; H+ = protons.

synthase) to condense ADP and inorganic phosphate into ATP. The adenine nucleotide translocase (ANT) delivers ATP to the cytoplasm in exchange for ADP.

Mitochondrial disorders result from the deficiency of any of these proteins. Deficiencies are caused by genetic mutations in mtDNA or nDNA that are transmitted maternally or by Mendelian patterns (autosomal dominant, autosomal recessive, X-linked).

SYMPTOMS

Several hundred genes are estimated to control OXPHOS, accounting for the enormous phenotypic heterogeneity observed with mitochondrial disorders. Phenotype expression may be nonspecific, and recognition is difficult and may require assessment by an individual who specializes in mitochondrial disorders. Refer to Shoffner (2001) for a detailed discussion of mitochondrial disorder phenotypes. Symptoms can be confined to a single organ (monosymptomatic), can be present in a few organs (oligosymptomatic), or can be systemic. The course may be degenerative or relatively static over time. Clinical changes can occur slowly over several decades, making the course appear static to physicians who treat individuals with mitochondrial disorders.

Cognitive impairment is common in individuals with mitochondrial disorders and is most likely related to the high degree of reliance of the brain on OXPHOS for normal functioning. Like so many clinical manifestations of mitochondrial disorders, the cognitive impairments are extremely heterogenous. In infants and children, the cognitive features are often nonspecific, consisting primarily of developmental delays. Many individuals remain undiagnosed. Those who show developmental regression usually receive aggressive evaluations due to the dramatic nature of their symptoms. Many individuals with mitochondrial disorders have normal intelligence when they are initially evaluated. It is unclear whether normal intelligence is maintained throughout the lives of most of these individuals because long-term follow-up data is limited. Frequent neurologic manifestations include abnormal tone, seizures, extrapyramidal movements, and autonomic dysfunction. Isolated cognitive impairments in individuals with mitochondrial disorders is unusual.

As is found in a number of metabolic diseases, features resembling autism spectrum disorders can also be observed in rare individuals with mtDNA mutations (Graf et al., 2000; see Chapter 23.1). Although most individuals with autism spectrum disorders do not have mitochondrial disorders, those with multiorgan involvement, abnormal brain magnetic resonance images, or metabolic abnormalities should be carefully examined.

Adults with mitochondrial disorders also display a large array of cognitive symptoms that can include intellectual disabilities, psychosis, depression, and dementia (Amemiya et al., 2000). Like children with mitochondrial disorders, adults usually demonstrate a complex, multisystem disorder. The age of onset of cognitive symptoms is usually less than 50 years of age. Although mitochondrial impairments do not appear to play a primary role in most neurodegenerative diseases with onset after 50 years of age, secondary defects may be important contributors to disease pathogenesis. The most likely role of mitochondrial dysfunction in most late-onset neurodegenerative diseases (e.g., Alzheimer disease) is to predispose individuals to neurodegeneration or to accelerate cell dysfunction and loss (Byrne, 2002; Chinnery et al., 2000; de la Monte et al., 2003; Shoffner, 1997).

CLASSIFICATION

Mitochondrial diseases are characterized by several hundred phenotypes. The basic steps for diagnosis involve phenotype recognition, metabolic testing, muscle histology and immunohistochemistry, OXPHOS enzyme analysis, and, in some individuals, mtDNA or nuclear DNA analysis. The multiorgan involvement and clinical heterogeneity of these diseases can make diagnosis difficult (see Figure 7.4-2).

Maria was anxious to find out what was happening to her three girls. Leila underwent metabolic testing that revealed lactic aciduria. A specialist also recommended that a muscle biopsy be performed because of Leila's lactic aciduria, hypotonia, hyporeflexia, and family history. Leila's muscle histology showed significant myofiber size variation and scattered fibers with reduced complex IV (cytochrome c oxidase) activity. No ragged-red fibers were identified; however, ragged-red fibers are rare in children younger than 5 years of age. The findings were consistent with a mitochondrial myopathy.

Leila's OXPHOS enzymology showed a generalized defect that was characterized by reduced activity measurements in multiple OXPHOS enzyme complexes (complexes I–IV). The enzymology correlated with the cytochrome c oxidase deficient fibers observed in her muscle biopsy; however, complex I was the most significantly affected OXPHOS enzyme.

Based on the muscle biopsy changes and OXPHOS enzymology, the specialist recommended that more detailed genetic testing be performed. MtDNA deletions, duplications, and depletion were excluded in muscle by Southern blot analysis. MtDNA sequencing revealed a heteroplasmic mu-

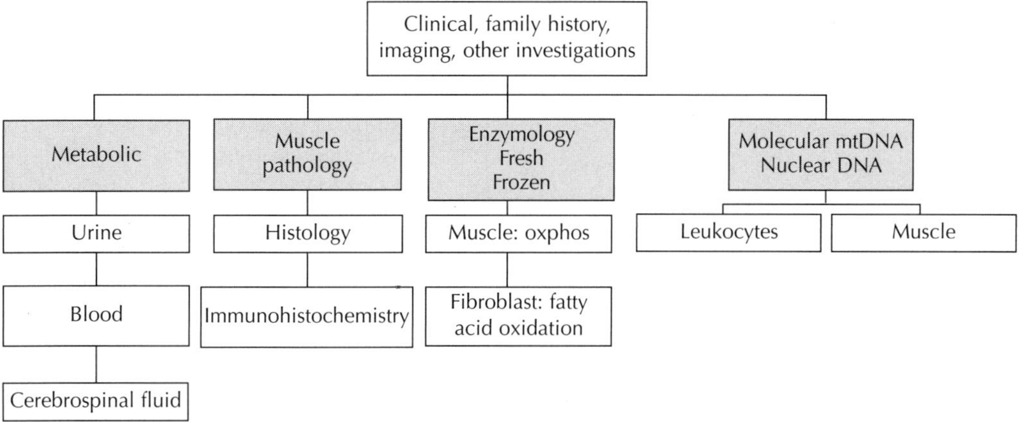

Figure 7.4-2. An algorithm for diagnosis of mitochondrial disorders. Proper diagnosis of mitochondrial disorders requires interpretation of data from clinical assessment, metabolic investigations, muscle pathology, muscle enzymology, and mtDNA or nuclear DNA testing. Assessment of b-oxidation (fatty acid oxidation) shows a secondary defect in about 25% of individuals with mitochondrial disorders.

tation (C5463T) that changed a leucine to a phenylalanine in the ND2 subunit of complex I (see Figure 7.4-3). Leila's family harbored a pathogenic mtDNA mutation (C5463T) that was heteroplasmic along the maternal lineage. All three of Maria's daughters had more than 90% mutant mtDNAs in the tissues tested.

Testing revealed that both of Maria's brothers were heteroplasmic for the mutation. Their learning disorders could have been due to the mutation, but this observation was difficult to establish. The family was counseled concerning the risks of maternally transmitted mtDNA mutations.

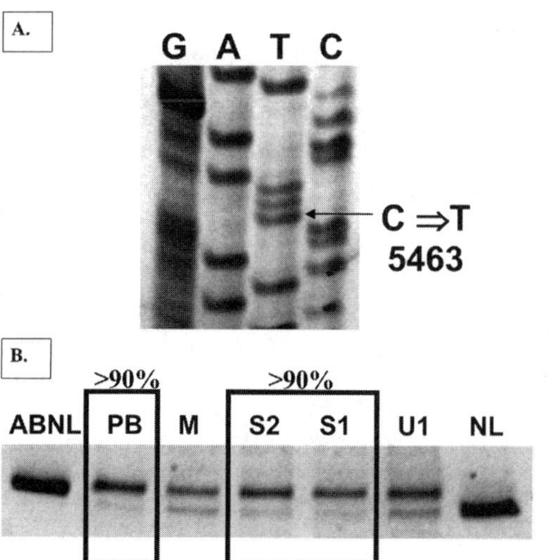

Figure 7.4-3. MtDNA sequencing for Leila, her sisters, and her maternal lineage family members. Item A shows the sequence of the ND2 subunit of complex I in mtDNA isolated from Leila's (i.e., proband, PB) skeletal muscle. A C5463T mutation was identified (arrow). In order to assess heteroplasmy, a restriction endonuclease digest was performed on Leila as well as on her maternal lineage family members, as shown in Item B. The upper band is produced by the presence of the C5463T mutation (ABNL = abnormal). The lower band is the normal sequence (NL). All of the maternal lineage family members who were tested were heteroplasmic for the C5463T mutation. Leila's muscle mtDNA and mtDNA from leukocytes from Leila's two symptomatic sisters (S1, S2) have more than 90% mutant mtDNAs. Higher percentages of normal mtDNAs are present in leukocyte mtDNA from Leila's mother (M) and from her maternal lineage uncle (U1), who has a learning disorder.

Most families who harbor mtDNA mutations will possess private or semiprivate mutations. Thus, mtDNA sequencing is required to identify most mtDNA mutations.

Due to the extreme clinical heterogeneity inherent in mitochondrial disorders, classification is based on the disease mechanism. MtDNA mutations produce defects in OXPHOS enzyme polypeptides or in mitochondrial protein synthesis. Nuclear gene mutations produce defects 1) in OXPHOS enzyme subunits, 2) in proteins responsible for OXPHOS enzyme assembly, 3) in proteins that incorporate metals into OXPHOS enzymes, 4) in proteins that regulate intergenomic communication, 5) in cofactors that transfer electrons between OXPHOS enzymes, 6) in proteins responsible for movement of mitochondria within cells, and 7) in proteins that deliver ATP to the cytoplasm. In order to diagnose individuals with mitochondrial disorders, manage their symptoms over time, and provide genetic counseling, an understanding of these mechanisms is important. Table 7.4-1 summarizes the major sites of cellular dysfunction that produce mitochondrial disorders. OXPHOS subunit immunohistochemistry is helpful in identifying individuals with mitochondrial disorders and assessing which individuals may harbor a mtDNA mutation (Hanson, Capaldi, Marusich, & Sherwood, 2002; Marusich et al., 1997; Rahman et al., 2000; Sparaco, Cavakkaro, Rossi, & Rizzuto, 2000; Sparaco, Schon, DiMauro, & Bonilla, 1999; Tanji, Vu, Schn, DiMauro, & Bonilla, 1999.

Table 7.4-1. Oxidative phosphorylation (OXPHOS) disease phenotypes

Mitochondrial deoxyribonuceic acid (mtDNA) mutations

1. MtDNA deletions and duplications
    - Kearns-Sayre syndrome
    - Chronic progressive external ophthalmoplegia syndromes
    - Pearson syndrome
    - Diabetes mellitus and deafness
    - Mitochondrial myopathy
    - Fahr syndrome variants (complex phenotypes with prominent cerebral calcifications)
2. Missense mutations (abnormal OXPHOS enzyme subunits)
    - Leber hereditary optic neuropathy
    - Leber hereditary optic neuropathy plus dystonia
    - Leigh disease
    - Pigmentary retinopathy, ataxia, and neuropathy syndromes
3. Transfer ribonucleic acids (tRNA) mutations (abnormal mitochondrial protein synthesis)
    - Myoclonic epilepsy and ragged-red fiber disease (MERRF)
    - Mitochondrial encephalomyopathy, lactic acidosis, and stroke-like episodes (MELAS)
    - Diabetes mellitus (usually with deafness)
    - Hypertrophic cardiomyopathy plus mitochondrial myopathy
    - Mitochondrial myopathy
4. Ribosomal RNA mutation (abnormal mitochondrial protein synthesis)
    - Maternally inherited deafness with aminoglycoside sensitivity

Nuclear DNA mutations

1. Nuclear DNA mutations in OXPHOS subunits
    - Complex I (NDUFV1 subunit)
    - Complex I (NDUFS1 subunit)
    - Complex I (NDUFS2 subunit)
    - Complex I (NDUFS4 subunit)
    - Complex I (NDUFS7 subunit)
    - Complex I (NDUFS8 subunit)
    - Complex II (SDHA subunit)
    - Complex II (SDHB subunit)
    - Complex II (SDHC subunit)
    - Complex II (SDHD subunit)
2. OXPHOS cofactor defects
    - Primary CoQ_{10} deficiency: myopathy, ataxia, encephalopathy
3. Defects in intergenomic communication
    - MtDNA depletion disease (often tissue specific)
        - Thymidine kinase deficiency: fatal skeletal myopathy
        - Deoxyguanosine kinase deficiency: hepatopathy, encephalopathy
    - Multiple mtDNA rearrangements
        - Thymidine phosphorylase: MNGIE
        - Mitochondrial DNA polymerase gamma: CPEO syndromes
        - Twinkle mutations: CPEO syndromes
        - Adenine nucleotide translocator 1: CPEO syndromes
4. Defects in OXPHOS enzyme assembly and processing
    - Complex IV assembly defects
        - SURF1 mutations: Leigh disease
        - COX10 mutations: renal tubulopathy, leukoencephalopathy, deafness, hypertrophic cardiomyopathy, Leigh disease, anemia
        - COX15 mutations: Fatal cardioencephalomyopathy
        - SCO1 mutations: hepatopathy, ketoacidosis, encephalopathy
        - SCO2 mutations: Fatal cardioencephalomyopathy
    - Complex III assembly defects
        - BCS1L mutations: GRACILE
    - Frataxin mutation: Freidreich ataxia
    - *ABC7* gene mutations: X-linked sideroblastic anemia and ataxia
    - Heat shock protein 60 deficiency: facial dysmorphism, hypotonia, cardiac failure
    - Paraplegin mutation: spastic paraparesis with ragged-red fiber myopathy
    - TIMM8A/*DDP1* mutations: Mohr-Tranebjaerg syndrome, Jensen syndrome
5. Defects in intracellular movement of mitochondria
    - Mitochondrial dynamin related guanosine triphosphatase (*OPA1*) mutations: Kjer type optic atrophy
6. Mitochondrial membrane defects
    - Tafazzin mutations: Barth syndrome

Fred was a 46-year-old man who was referred to a specialist due to his slowly progressive, lifelong neurologic disorder with multisystem features. As a teenager, he had experienced significant exercise intolerance. Lipomas developed on his neck and slowly increased in size with advancing age. By his thirties, Fred had clearly evident proximal muscle weakness. By 44 years of age, he had moderate proximal weakness, muscle wasting, and myalgias with creatine phosphokinase elevations of 700–800 IU/ml. Fred was treated for depression when he turned 46. He also developed difficulties with balance and intention tremors. A brain magnetic resonance image demonstrated areas of increased signal intensity (T2 weighted images) in subcortical white matter of the parietal-occipital region bilaterally.

Fred's family history did not reveal an identifiable transmission pattern. He had a healthy daughter, two healthy brothers, and two sisters with adult-onset diabetes mellitus (one insulin dependent and one diet controlled). His family history was otherwise noncontributory.

Fred's specialist noted that cervical lipomas that appear during adolescence or early adulthood are important clues to the presence of a mitochondrial disease, particularly when observed with neuromuscular symptoms. He ordered metabolic testing that showed increased cerebrospinal fluid lactate, increased blood lactate and pyruvate, and increased plasma alanine. These metabolic changes were consistent with a defect in cellular energetics.

A muscle biopsy was performed and showed a mitochondrial myopathy with cytochrome c oxidase (complex IV) deficient myofibers. OXPHOS subunit immunohistochemistry showed scattered myofibers with a decrease in the mtDNA coded subunits I and II of cytochrome c oxidase (complex IV) and a decrease in the closely associated nuclear DNA coded subunit VIc. In order to further clarify the disorder, OXPHOS enzymology was performed and showed a defect in cytochrome c oxidase (complex IV) function. Based on these findings, Fred underwent mtDNA point mutation testing that revealed a heteroplasmic G-to-A point mutation in the mtDNA at position 8344 within the transfer RNA Lysine gene at position (Shoffner et al., 1990).

GENETIC COUNSELING

In order to perform genetic counseling, the precise mutation that produces a mitochondrial disorder must be determined. The inheritance of mitochondrial disorders may occur by maternal or Mendelian patterns (autosomal dominant, autosomal recessive, X-linked). Sporadic mutations in either the mtDNA or the nuclear DNA may also produce mitochondrial disorders (Parvari et al., 2001). When considered as a group, the most common pattern of inheritance is autosomal recessive.

MtDNA mutations pose a significant complexity to genetic counseling. An enormous array of these mutations are known. The cytoplasmic location of the mtDNA within the mitochondria is associated with a unique inheritance pattern called *maternal inheritance*, which refers to the *nearly* exclusive transmission of mtDNAs from a mother to her children. Sperm mtDNA disappear in early embryogenesis by selective destruction, inactivation, or dilution by the approximately 150,000 oocyte mtDNAs (Cummins, Kishikawa, Mehmet, & Yanagimachi, 1999). Rarely, mtDNA can be passed paternally, as was observed in one individual with a mitochondrial myopathy associated with a 2 base pair deletion in the ND2 polypeptide of complex I. This mutation occurred on the paternal mtDNA background and was present in the individual as a mixture of maternal and paternal mtDNAs (Schwartz & Vissing, 2002, 2003). In addition to these cases, paternal mtDNA has been identified in abnormal embryos.

When a pathogenic mtDNA mutation is present, it is transmitted in a *homoplasmic* or *heteroplasmic* fashion. The mtDNAs within a cell or tissue are referred to as homoplasmic when all of the mtDNAs share the same sequence. They are referred to as heteroplasmic when mtDNAs with different sequences coexist. Normal and mutant mtDNA sequences differ only at the nucleotide or nucleotides that have been mutated. As a general rule, pathogenic mtDNA mutations can be either homoplasmic or heteroplasmic, whereas neutral polymorphisms are almost always homoplasmic.

Segregation of the normal and mutant mtDNAs with cell division is a complex process and is influenced by a number of variables including the specific mtDNA mutation present, the nuclear DNA background, and the specific cell type. Consequently, the precise ratio of mutant to normal mtDNA does not correlate well with the clinical phenotype or the severity of the biochemical defect. Three loci in the nuclear DNA on chromosomes 2, 5, and 6 of a mouse model appear to account for approximately 12%–36% of the variance in mtDNA segregation (Battersby, Loredo, Osti, & Shoubridge, 2003). Women with a heteroplasmic mutation in their mtDNA have as high as 60%–70% risk of transmission of mitochondrial disease to their children.

MANAGEMENT

Management of mitochondrial disorders is difficult. Frequently, multiple specialties must cooperatively manage the individual's care. Because many of the phenotypes display multiorgan involvement, early recognition and treatment is important. For example, screening of fasting blood glucose and glucose tolerance testing can detect diabetes mellitus. Once diabetes is detected, treatment can be instituted, thus decreasing risk of complications. Early recognition and treatment of many of the complications of mitochondrial disorders is an important measure for reducing the cost of health care for these individuals.

Avoidance of certain classes of medications that worsen the individual's OXPHOS defect can also be important. In many individuals with mitochondrial disorders, medication side effects are enhanced. Close follow-up of these individuals is necessary when new medications are instituted. For example, epileptic seizures are the first recognized symptom in about 53% of individuals with mitochondrial encephalomyopathies. Valproate is frequently considered a treatment option for individuals with epilepsy, but an important adverse effect of valproate treatment is impairment of fatty acid oxidation, which can further compromise mitochondrial ATP production. Mitochondrial diseases are considered to be a risk factor for valproate-induced liver failure and, in many cases, should be excluded before treatment with valproate (Krahenbuhl, Brandner, Kleinle, Liechti, & Straumann, 2000). Individuals with mitochondrial encephalomyopathies have experienced worsening of seizures on valproate (Lam, Lau, Williams, Chan, & Wong, 1997).

Metabolic therapies for mitochondrial disorders attempt to increase mitochondrial ATP and decrease free radical production. Metabolic therapies that have been reported to produce a positive therapeutic effect include coenzyme Q_{10}, uridine, idebenone, triacylglycerol, phylloquinone, menadione, succinate, ascorbate, and riboflavin. The assessment of the efficacy of these treatments, however, has been difficult, due to the clinical and genetic heterogeneity of mitochondrial disorders. The therapeutic efficacy of any reported compounds is limited. In this context, individuals should avoid alternative medicine approaches to disease management. Alternative medicine practitioners may prescribe numerous supplements and herbs without regard to the individual's disease process, and for some individuals, these substances can be dangerous.

Dicarboxylic aciduria and secondary impairment of long chain fatty acid oxidation occur in individuals with mitochondrial disorders. Cornstarch supplementation, avoidance of fasting, and decreased dietary intake of long-chain fatty acids may be helpful in selected individuals; however, the long-term benefits of dietary manipulations are unknown.

The effects of mild degrees of aerobic activity are a frequent concern voiced by individuals with mitochondrial disorders and their physicians. In 10 adults with mitochondrial myopathies, moderate treadmill training over 8 weeks resulted in a 30% improvement of aerobic capacity, a 30% drop in resting lactate and postexercise lactate levels, and a 60% improvement in adenosine triphosphate recovery as measured by P-NMR testing (Taivassalo et al., 2001). Physical therapy, mild exercise, and weight management are important aspects of the management of mitochondrial disorders.

CONCLUSION

Physicians in all specialties are becoming increasingly aware of mitochondrial disorders. Although the prevalence of mitochondrial disorders in the general population is unknown, the number of requests for pediatric and adult evaluations are increasing rapidly. A basic awareness of mitochondrial disorder phenotypes as well as the essential elements of medical evaluation are important for appropriate disorder management and referrals. Centers that specialize in mitochondrial disorder evaluations can be instrumental in working with referring physicians to develop a cost-effective diagnostic plan that is individualized to suit the person's needs.

MtDNA and nuclear DNA sequencing can be important in delineating the inheritance. After a complete evaluation, genetic counseling based on Mendelian principles or mtDNA principles of inheritance can be applied. Although approaches that assess individuals for mtDNA mutations are evolving rapidly, significant ambiguity in diagnosis often remains even after detailed testing is complete. Advances in the understanding of mutations in nuclear OXPHOS genes will powerfully improve diagnosis and management of mitochondrial disorders and counseling for individuals with these disorders.

REFERENCES

Amemiya, S., Hamamoto, M., Goto, Y., Komaki, H., Nishino, I., Nonaka, I., et al. (2000). Psychosis and progressing dementia: Presenting features of a mitochondriopathy. *Neurology, 55*(4), 600–601.

Battersby, B.J., Loredo-Osti, J.C., & Shoubridge, E.A. (2003). Nuclear genetic control of mitochondrial DNA segregation. *Nature Genetics, 33*(2), 183–186.

Byrne, E. (2002). Does mitochondrial respiratory chain dysfunction have a role in common neurodegenerative disorders? *Journal of Clinical Neuroscience, 9*(5), 497–501.

Canafoglia, L., Franceschetti, S., Antozzi, C., Carrara, F., Farina, L., Granata, T., et al. (2001). Epileptic phenotypes associated with mitochondrial disorders. *Neurology, 56*(10), 1340–1346.

Chinnery, P.F., Taylor, G.A., Howell, N., Andrews, R.M., Morris, C.M., Taylor, R.W., et al. (2000). Mitochondrial DNA haplogroups and susceptibility to AD and dementia with Lewy bodies. *Neurology, 55*(2), 302–304.

Cummins, J.M., Kishikawa, H., Mehmet, D., & Yanagimachi, R. (1999). Fate of genetically marked mitochondrial DNA from spermatocytes microinjected into mouse zygotes. *Zygote, 7*(2), 151–156.

de la Monte, S.M., Chiche, J., von dem Bussche, A., Sanyal, S., Lahousse, S.A., Janssens, S.P., et al. (2003). Nitric oxide synthase-3 overexpression causes apoptosis and impairs neuronal mitochondrial function: Relevance to Alzheimer's-type neurodegeneration. *Laboratory Investigation, 83*(2), 287–298.

Graf, W.D., Marin-Garcia, J., Gao, H.G., Pizzo, S., Naviaux, R.K., Markusic, D., et al. (2000). Autism associated with the mitochondrial DNA G8363A transfer RNA(Lys) mutation. *Journal of Child Neurology, 15*(6), 357–361.

Hanson, B.J., Capaldi, R.A., Marusich, M.F., & Sherwood, S.W. (2002). An immunocytochemical approach to detection of mitochondrial disorders. *Journal of Histochemistry and Cytochemistry, 50*(10), 1281–1288.

Krahenbuhl, S., Brandner, S., Kleinle, S., Liechti, S., & Straumann, D. (2000). Mitochondrial diseases represent a risk factor for valproate-induced fulminant liver failure. *Liver, 20*(4), 346–348.

Lam, C.W., Lau, C.H., Williams, J.C., Chan, Y.W., & Wong, L.J. (1997). Mitochondrial myopathy, encephalopathy, lactic acidosis and stroke-like episodes (MELAS) triggered by valproate therapy. *European Journal of Pediatrics, 156*(7), 562–564.

Marusich, M.F., Robinson, B.H., Taanman, J.W., Kim, S.J., Schillace, R., Smith, J.L., et al. (1997). Expression of mtDNA and nDNA encoded respiratory chain proteins in chemically and genetically-derived Rho0 human fibroblasts: A comparison of subunit proteins in normal fibroblasts treated with ethidium bromide and fibroblasts from a patient with mtDNA depletion syndrome. *Biochemica et Biophysica Acta, 1362*(2–3), 145–159.

Parvari, R., Brodyansky, I., Elpeleg, O., Moses, S., Landau, D., & Hershkovitz, E. (2001). A recessive contiguous gene deletion of chromosome 2p16 associated with cystinuria and a mitochondrial disease. *American Journal of Human Genetics, 69*(4), 869–875.

Rahman, S., Lake, B.D., Taanman, J.W., Hanna, M.G., Cooper, J.M., Schapira, A.H., et al. (2000). Cytochrome oxidase immunohistochemistry: Clues for genetic mechanisms. *Brain, 123*(3), 591–600.

Schwartz, M., & Vissing, J. (2002). Paternal inheritance of mitochondrial DNA. *New England Journal of Medicine, 347*(8), 576–580.

Schwartz, M., & Vissing, J. (2003). New patterns of inheritance in mitochondrial disease. *Biochemical and Biophysical Research Communications, 310*(2), 247–251.

Shoffner, J.M. (1997). Oxidative phosphorylation defects and Alzheimer's disease. *Neurogenetics, 1*(1), 13–19.

Shoffner, J.M. (2001). Oxidative phosphorylation disease. In C.R. Scriver et al. (Eds.), *The metabolic and molecular bases of inherited diseases.* (pp. 2367–2423) New York: McGraw-Hill.

Shoffner, J.M., Lott, M.T., Lezza, A.M., Seibel, P., Ballinger, S.W., & Wallace, D.C. (1990). Myoclonic epilepsy and ragged-red fiber disease (MERRF) is associated with a mitochondrial DNA tRNA(Lys) mutation. *Cell, 61*(6), 931–937.

Sparaco, M., Cavallaro, T., Rossi, G., & Rizzuto, N. (2000). Immunohistochemical demonstration of spinal ventral horn cells involvement in a case of "myoclonus epilepsy with ragged red fibers" (MERRF). *The Clinical Neuropathologist, 19*(4), 200–207.

Sparaco, M., Schon, E.A., DiMauro, S., & Bonilla, E. (1999). Myoclonic epilepsy with ragged-red fibers (MERRF): An immunohistochemical study of the brain. *Brain Pathology, 5*(2), 125–133.

St. John, J., Sakkas, D., Dimitriadi, K., Barnes, A., Maclin, V., Ramey, J., et al. (2000). Failure of elimination of paternal mitochondrial DNA in abnormal embryos. *Lancet, 355* (9199), 200.

Taivassalo, T., Shoubridge, E.A., Chen, J., Kennaway, N.G., DiMauro, S., Arnold, D.L., et al. (2001). Aerobic conditioning in patients with mitochondrial myopathies: Physiological, biochemical, and genetic effects. *Annals of Neurology, 50*(2), 133–141.

Tanji, K., Vu, T.H., Schon, E.A., DiMauro, S., & Bonilla, E. (1999). Kearns-Sayre syndrome: Unusual pattern of expression of subunits of the respiratory chain in the cerebellar system. *Annals of Neurology, 45*(3), 377–383.

CHAPTER 8

SYNDROMES OF MULTIPLE CONGENITAL ANOMALIES

8.1 SPINA BIFIDA

Robert A. Jacobs

Spina bifida is one of the most common and complex birth defects in the United States. It occurs with a birth prevalence rate of 3.0–7.8 per 10,000 live births. Clinical manifestations are diverse, resulting from anatomic anomalies of the spinal cord and brainstem. The former causes weakness, paralysis and loss of sensation in the lower extremities, and neurogenic bowel and bladder. The latter, Chiari II (also known as Arnold-Chiari Type II) malformation, may lead to hydrocephalus, and in a small number of infants, to symptoms of brainstem dysfunction with significant cranial nerve involvement. Swallowing incoordination, vocal cord paresis or paralysis, apnea, bradycardia, and/or central hypoventilation occur in these infants with significant clinical morbidity and frequent mortality. Major neurosurgical, orthopedic, and urological problems may be present at birth or develop later as secondary conditions. Behavioral, developmental, and educational problems associated with these anatomical and surgical conditions may develop as well.

Team care is optimal for children with spina bifida and has become the standard in most communities. These teams are multi- and/or interdisciplinary and involve routine participation by pediatricians, specialists in orthopedics, urology, and neurosurgery, nursing, social work, psychology, nutrition, physical and occupational therapy, and orthotics (see Figure 8.1-1). Consultation from neurology; psychiatry; genetics; ear, nose, and throat; pulmonary; ophthalmology; stoma therapy; dentistry; orthodontics; radiology; and renal may be required periodically, and these consultants need to be included in the overall team. Family involvement is also important for a successful treatment plan (Wolraich, 1983).

Marie was born to a 40-year-old mother, Rita, who had come to the United States late in her second trimester of pregnancy. Rita had received little prenatal care, but the pregnancy had been without problem, despite her previous miscarriages, and she was expecting an uneventful delivery and discharge from the newborn unit at the community hospital where she had gone to deliver. Shortly after the delivery, she saw the nurses talking near Marie. She felt something was wrong, but nothing was said to her, and Marie was taken to the nursery before Rita could see her. A short time later, a doctor from the nursery came and told Rita that Marie had spina bifida and would be taken to the regional neonatal intensive care unit (NICU) for surgery. Rita had many questions but was told that the doctors at the NICU would explain everything.

The terms used to describe spina bifida and its associated conditions are at times confusing. A practical classification for neural tube defects (NTD) has been proposed based on whether the spinal portion of the neural tube is visible (open spinal NTD) or not (closed spinal NTD), or is primarily cranial in location (cranial NTD). Open NTD result embryologically from a failure of primary neurulation, with involvement of the entire central nervous system. Closed NTD represent a failure of canalization and fusion of the end of the primary neural tube. This failure of secondary neurulation affects only the spinal cord and, in general, will not have associated Chiari II malformation or hydrocephalus (McComb, 1997).

EPIDEMIOLOGY

No single theory or mechanism accounts for all cases of NTD. These disorders are felt to be the result of a combination of environmental and genetic factors occurring

Grateful acknowledgement is given to Liz Dennon, Diantha Smith, Constance Nicholson of the USC University Center of Excellence in Developmental Disabilities at Childrens Hospital Los Angeles, USC Keck School of Medicine, for their assistance and patience in the preparation of this manuscript, to Christine Bottrell for assistance in final proofreading, and to Narine Galudzhyan for her assistance in the literature review.

The valuable advice of Dr. Barbara Korsch over a generation is gratefully acknowledged and appreciated.

Additional acknowledgment and thanks are given to Laurie Christman who painted the oil painting "Mother and Child with Spina Bifida" (1988) and donated it to the Spina Bifida Program at Childrens Hospital Los Angeles.

Preparation of this paper was partially supported by grant funding of the Maternal and Child Health Bureau (MCHB) #2T73-MC00008-10 and the Administration on Developmental Disabilities (ADD) #90DD0540.

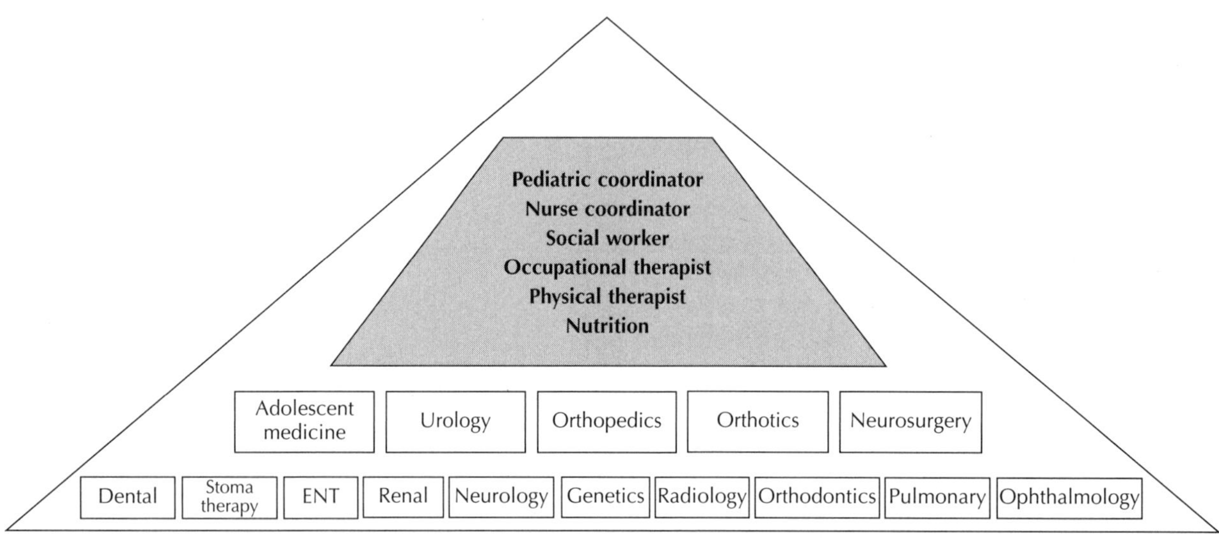

Figure 8.1-1. Team for a child with spina bifida.

at a critical point in fetal development. Diverse environmental factors—chemical, nutritional, and infectious—have been reported as possible etiologic causes of NTD. Chemical agents known to affect neurulation (e.g., valproic acid, carbamazepine), hyperthermia from both febrile illnesses and hot tub use in the first months of pregnancy, Trisomy 18 and triploidy, craniosynostosis, and families in which there have been other "schisis" birth defects (i.e., cleft palate, omphalocele, bladder extrophy, diaphragmatic hernia, and tracheoesophageal fistula) have been reported to have an etiologic association. Reports of myelomeningocele in association with complex congenital heart disease exist but have been infrequent. There is a higher incidence of neural tube defects in infants of mothers who are obese, have maternal diabetes, and have lower socioeconomic status. Dietary factors have been examined with recent focus on vitamin intake and levels of vitamin C and folate.

EMBRYOLOGY

Two major theories for the pathophysiology and development of the fetus with spina bifida are 1) primary neural tube defect involving failure of closure of the neural tube occurring during the fourth week of gestation; and 2) secondary neural tube defect, or reopening of the previously closed neural tube. Neurulation, thought to begin on day 17 postconception, occurs with formation of the neural plate followed by a folding over and then fusion of surface glycoproteins with cellular fusion to form the neural tube. The "zipper" model is thought to account for neural tube closure, with closure beginning at the cervico-medullary junction and proceeding in caudal and cephalic directions until fusion of the anterior and posterior neuropores occurs on days 24 and 26, respectively. Incomplete closure of the anterior and posterior neuropores results in anencephaly and lumbosacral myelomeningocele, respectively. Development of Chiari II (Arnold-Chiari type II) malformation may be due to cerebrospinal fluid (CSF) leakage from an open NTD, which results in inadequate fetal ventricle distention with resultant small posterior fossa and brain and skull anomaly (McComb, 1997; McLone & Knepper, 1989; Van Allen, Kalousek, Chernoff, & Hall, 1993).

SCREENING

At the end of the first trimester, alpha-fetoprotein is elevated in maternal serum when the fetus has an open NTD, abdominal wall defect or several less-common anomalies and decreased where the fetus has Down syndrome or trisomy 18. Elevated alpha-fetoprotein in amniotic fluid identifies 90%–95% of fetuses with open NTD. Acetylcholinesterase testing, which is not used as frequently, is more neural tissue specific, with reported 99%–100% accuracy and remains so after 20 weeks gestation when elevated alpha-fetoprotein has been found in amniotic fluid. Anencephaly and the intracranial signs of spina bifida—"lemon" sign deformity of the frontal bone, and/or cerebellar compression "banana" sign of the Chiari II malformation—are diagnosed by ultrasonography with great accuracy. Ultrasound alone, however, is inadequate to identify all cases of open NTD. In addition, small skin-covered and/or low sacrum lesions continue to be difficult to diagnose, regardless of the testing approach utilized (California AFP Screening Program, 1994; Platt et al., 1992).

At an estimated 17 weeks' gestation, Mrs. Jimenez had blood drawn at the Obstetrics Clinic for MSAFP testing. When she received a call from the clinic that the test was positive, she scheduled an appointment at the Prenatal Diagnostic Center to discuss her options. She was advised that more definitive testing, amniocentesis and high resolution ultrasonography, was recommended. She told the genetics counselor at the Prenatal Diagnostic Center that she would like to discuss the recommendations with her husband and perhaps her parish priest. She would get back to them with a decision in several days.

Three days later, she returned to the Prenatal Diagnostic Clinic having discussed her choices with her husband, other family members, and her parish priest. Mrs. Jimenez had amniocentesis and high definition ultrasonagraphy. The results were positive for both spina bifida and hydrocephalus. Based on discussions with her husband, other family members, and her parish priest, she decided to proceed with the pregnancy.

Identification of significant fetal abnormalities has allowed women and families the ability to choose whether to continue or terminate a pregnancy. Few topics have caused as much public debate in the United States and other countries as that surrounding therapeutic abortion; however, when pregnancy termination is not an option, identification may frequently be important to allow better management of the pregnancy and delivery.

FETAL REPAIR

Dramatic advances in prenatal diagnosis have led to the development of techniques for surgical intervention to correct fetal anatomic abnormalities. In fetuses with NTD, neurological damage resulting in paresis of the legs and bladder and bowel incontinence was felt to be the result of "two hits"—the initial embryologic abnormality and secondary exposure of the spinal cord tissue to the amniotic fluid. Fetal surgery for myelomeningocele was first proposed to protect the exposed spinal cord, but expected improvement in leg and bladder function did not occur (although hindbrain herniation of the Chiari II malformation is significantly reduced with decrease in the occurrence of hydrocephalus). Surgical intrauterine repair has been accomplished by endoscopic techniques at 22–24 weeks gestation and by standard neurosurgery closure through a hysterotomy at 28–29 weeks gestation. To date, several hundred fetuses with myelomeningocele have had surgical intrauterine repairs at three tertiary pediatric centers: University of California at San Francisco, Children's Hospital of Philadelphia, and Vanderbilt University.

NEONATAL CARE AND CONCERNS

For some parents of children with spina bifida, prenatal diagnosis provides them with several months to seek answers to their questions. Many parents, however, believe they will deliver a healthy baby and find that they have to face major decisions without any preparation. Parents and other family members or their friends will ask many questions about future ambulation, cognitive ability, and expectations for survival and life expectancy. Early provision of accurate information by well-informed practitioners in a caring manner is essential for parents. By the time of discharge from the NICU, ambulatory potential, based on motor and sensory examination, may be predicted with reasonable accuracy by the orthopedic surgeon and physical therapist. Caution, however, is important, as many changes may occur as the years progress with development of secondary conditions such as tethered cord, progressive scoliosis, or excessive weight gain that were unforeseen at the time of these early examinations. Cognitive potential is far more difficult to predict at this early age. Risk factors to consider include the presence of massive hydrocephalus as measured by head circumference and radiologic imaging, microcephaly, severe prematurity or very low birth weight, development of meningitis or ventriculitis, intraventricular hemorrhage, other major neonatal complications and/or other major congenital anomalies, and social circumstances. The presence of adverse risk factors, however, is not predictive.

NEUROSURGICAL MANAGEMENT

Back Closure

Most infants born with open NTD in the United States have surgical intervention within the first several days of life. Early closure (within 24 hours) is not necessary, and delayed (1–7 days) or late (after 1 week) closure cause no increase in infection or change in cord function if the lesion is kept clean and is covered with sterile nonadherent dressing and the infant is given broad spectrum intravenous antibiotic coverage at full therapeutic doses. Delay in closure allows time for parents to come to grips with their feelings and grief and to review intervention options with their physician without detriment to their infant. Large lesions may require delay in closure due to a two-stage procedure or skin grafting with assistance from a plastic surgeon to achieve optimal closure and repair. In many countries, closure may be significantly delayed due to resource limitations and problems with access to care (Charney, Sutton, Bruce, & Schut, 1983; McComb, 1997).

Closed NTD have minimal risk of infection, and primary repair is usually delayed for 3–6 months, allowing growth of the infant and better technical repair. These lesions are not associated with Chiari II malformation, which negates any risk of associated hydrocephalus or brainstem symptomatology from the anatomic deformity. Surgical repair of the back lesion does not result in improved cord function as dysplastic neural tissue is usually present, accompanied by varying degrees of poor muscle development and hypoplasia. Sporadic leg movements are frequently noted, and it is important that reflex movement not be mistaken for true function or strength. Parents must recognize that surgical repair of the back lesion will not result in recovery of normal neurological function.

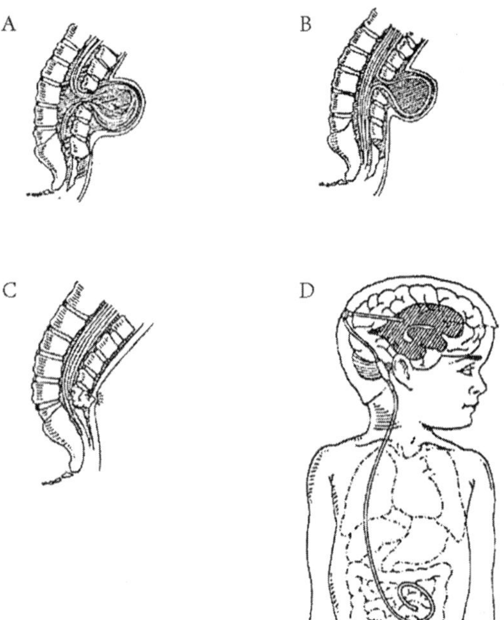

Figure 8.1-2. Myelomeningocele (a), meningocele (b), occult spinal dysgraphism (c), and hydrocephalus with ventriculoperitoneal shunt (d). (From Davoh, C.T., & Kinsman, S.L. [1995]. *Medical facts about spina bifida.* Baltimore: Kennedy Krieger Institute/Spina Bifida Association of America; reprinted by permission.)

Hydrocephalus and Shunt Placement

Hydrocephalus, resulting from the Chiari II malformation, occurs in more than 90% of infants with open NTD lesions. Ventriculoperitoneal (VP) shunt placement is usually performed 5–7 days after back closure, although some neurosurgeons may choose to place the shunt at the time of initial back closure, particularly if significant hydrocephalus is evident (see Figure 8.1-2). The availability of imaging studies, cranial ultrasound, computerized tomography (CT) scans, and magnetic resonance imaging (MRI) has allowed for early detection and diagnosis of hydrocephalus and timely shunt placement with shorter hospitalization.

The proximal end of the shunt is placed within the lateral ventricles, with care taken to avoid the choroid plexus and lateral walls, and attention is given to the number of patent holes and their location in the silastic shunt to assure adequate CSF drainage. The distal end of the shunt is placed in the peritoneal cavity. In some, VP shunts may become unsuitable, and an alternate site for the distal end of the shunt tubing must be sought. This situation occurs in children with recurrent shunt failure or infection risk related to peritonitis or pseudocyst formation, multiple abdominal surgeries, or necrotizing enterocolitis (NEC) as a neonate.

Ventriculopleural shunts are an alternate choice for shunt placement when VP shunt placement is no longer feasible. Ventriculopleural shunts require adequate space and serosal surface area for resorption of the CSF draining into the pleural cavity. Otherwise, pleural effusion may develop, causing respiratory compromise and/or infection and signs of increased intracranial pressure as adequate drainage is diminished. For these reasons, ventriculopleural shunts are not utilized in those younger than 5 years of age and are used with caution in those age 5–10 years. Current use of ventriculoatrial (VA) shunts is limited to clinical situations in which the peritoneal cavity is unsuitable for placement of the distal shunt tubing and when age or other pulmonary complications preclude placement in the pleural cavity. A small but significant number of adults remain with VA shunts, many placed years ago, and remain at risk for pulmonary hypertension and cor pulmonale despite many years of asymptomatic use. Periodic evaluation with electrocardiogram (EKG), chest x-ray, and/or cardiac echocardiogram for these individuals is necessary.

Shunt Malfunction

Shunt malfunction is a frequent and expected complication of ventricular shunt systems, regardless of the site of the distal tubing. Proximal catheter occlusion is the most common cause of shunt malfunction with accumulation of cellular debris from the choroid plexus, glial ependymal tissue, and/or blood elements. Distal catheter obstruction is the next most common cause. Other causes to be considered during evaluation of shunt function include valve dysfunction, fracture or disconnection of the shunt, improper placement or migration of the shunt catheter, or shunt infection.

Malfunction occurs in 30%–40% of infants younger than 1 year, 2 to 3 times over the first few years of life in many, and in 70% by age 10 years. Fussiness, irritability, lethargy, vomiting, or a bulging and tense fontanelle must be watched for in the young infant. Older children usually experience headache and vomiting, although adolescents and young adults may at times present with less obvious and atypical symptoms, such as neck pain or changes in upper extremity strength and hand function as the initial or only sign. Other less frequent presentations include changes in behavior or school performance; swelling around the shunt reservoir, valve, or tubing; changes in extraocular muscle function with recent eye deviation or downward gaze "sunset" sign; apnea; or seizure. The onset and duration of symptoms is usually sufficient to allow thorough evaluation of shunt function, although an occasional child with cardiovascular instability and/or apnea requires immediate relief of pressure. Seizures, an infrequent presentation of shunt malfunction, require thorough and appropriate evaluation.

Testing may include imaging studies utilizing cranial ultrasound, CT scan, or MRI, and/or aspiration of the shunt. Close inspection of the shunt for skin redness or palpation for swelling around the shunt is important and helpful, but pumping the shunt to assess function is no longer felt to be helpful. Continued improvement of digital imaging with storage and transmission, both within the medical center and to/from distant sites, will aid clinicians in the diagnosis of shunt dysfunction regardless of the location of the child.

Shunt Infection

Infection of ventricular shunts is a common complication of shunt placement, occurring in 2%–15% of shunt placement or revisions, with a rate of 2%–4% in major medical centers. Neonates with open myelomeningocele or poorly healing back wounds after initial back closure are particularly at risk for shunt infection, usually with organisms found in the vaginal and fecal flora. After the neonatal period, *S. epidermidis* (coagulase negative) is the most common organism found, followed by *S. aureus* (coagulase positive). Most shunt infections (70%) occur in the first 30–60 days after surgery, and 80% of infection occur within 6 months.

Infection of the shunt is treated with intravenous antibiotics appropriate to the specific organism isolated, and, in most instances, the infected shunt must be removed and replaced following antibiotic treatment. Intraventricular antibiotics do not seem to be beneficial for most individuals. Diagnosis of shunt infection is made through examination of CSF obtained from the shunt. CSF obtained from lumbar puncture yields positive results in only half of cases of shunt infection, and when attempting to diagnose bacterial meningitis, CSF obtained from the shunt is inadequate (Bayston, 1989).

Distal shunt infection may present with the clinical symptoms and signs of peritonitis—abdominal pain, vomiting, fever, and abdominal tenderness and guarding. Abdominal ultrasound examination is extremely helpful in evaluation for appendicitis or in differentiation from a CSF pseudocyst. Abdominal pseudocysts, seen in less than 1% of those with VP shunts, are an inflammatory response around the distal tip of the VP shunt. Symptoms of shunt malfunction are common in individuals with pseudocyst, abdominal symptoms in over half, and fever in one third. When spontaneous bacterial peritonitis (SBP) is suspected, care must be taken to prevent ascending infection of the shunt and ventriculitis. Recurrence of shunt infections is unfortunately common, with recurrence rates of 15%–52% reported (Kulkarni, Rabin, Lamberti-Pasculli, & Drake, 2001; Salomao & Leibinger, 1999).

Chiari II Malformation

Chiari Type II (Arnold-Chiari) malformation, present in more than 90% of infants with open myelomeningocele, is the predominant cause of hydrocephalus in these infants. Less frequently, in about 3%–5% of infants with Chiari II malformation, vocal cord paralysis and swallowing incoordination may develop and cause severe symptomatology of stridor, apnea, cyanotic spells, bradycardia, opisthotonus, upper extremity weakness, and dysphagia with aspiration. This condition frequently leads to significant morbidity and has made Chiari syndrome the most frequent cause of death for infants and children with an open NTD. Varying degrees of ana-

Table 8.1-1. Arnold-Chiari malformation

Types	Clinical	Pathology
Grade 1	Stridor	Brainstem compression Traction on vagal nerve
Grade 2	Stridor Apnea	Hemorrhage or ischemia Disruption of neurons/nuclei
Grade 3	Stridor Apnea Cyanotic Spells Dysphagia	Necrosis Dysgenesis

Reprint from *Journal of Pediatrics, 3,* Charney, E.B., Rorke, L.B., Sutton, L.N., & Schut, L., Management of Chiari II complication in infants with myelomeningocele, 364–371, Copyright 1987, with permission from Elsevier.

tomic and pathologic involvement allow classification into Grades 1, 2, and 3 (Charney, Rorke, Sutton, & Schut, 1987; see Table 8.1-1).

Infants with Chiari syndrome have abnormalities in control of ventilation during both sleep and wakefulness and impaired central chemosensitivity to both hypoxia and hypercapnea. Sleep disordered breathing (SDB) in children with myelomeningocele has been described by identification of three groups: central apnea, central hypoventilation (shallow or slow breathing with hypercapnea and hypoxemia), and obstructive apnea with airway blockage. As many as 20% of children with myelomeningocele have moderate to severe SDB with effects on weight gain and growth, school performance and behavioral problems, and cardiovascular function (Kirk, Morielli, & Brouillette, 1999). Symptoms in older children may present as swallowing difficulty with bulbar palsy, syrinx, and/or progressive scoliosis. Surgery, where symptoms are of late onset, is directed toward relief of specific pressure from the syrinx, cord tethering, or lesions of the fourth ventricle, and is more effective than that in the early onset syndrome.

Tethered Cord

Tethered cord may be either a primary defect, as frequently seen in closed NTD, primarily lipomyelomeningoceles with cord tethering and compression from a lipomatous mass, or dermoid cyst lesion, or a secondary condition occurring between age 6 to 15 years in 11%–27% of those with previously operated open lesions. Traction on the conus medullaris and cauda equina leads to stretching, ischemia, and loss of neurological function. MRI provides the best definition of the anatomical lesions but does not, however, allow differentiation of who would benefit from operative intervention.

In infants with a closed NTD, untethering surgery has been recommended while they are asymptomatic with minimal or absent deficit. The majority of these infants develop orthopedic problems and many develop neurogenic bladder. The natural history of those with closed NTD lesions is not well understood or fully described, raising questions by some as to whether routine prophylactic surgery is indicated for all infants. Secondary tethering in those with previous back surgery should only be operated on if individuals have significant clinical findings. These may include spasticity, weakness and decreased sensation in the lower extremities, changes in urinary or bowel function, urinary tract infections (UTIs), back and/or leg pain, progressive scoliosis, and/or development of foot deformity. Relief of back pain occurs in most following surgery, but results are variable, and improvement in ambulation is more likely than improvement of urinary symptoms (Banta, 1991; Sarwark, Weber, Gabrieli, McLone, & Dias, 1996; Shurtleff et al., 1997).

Syringomyelia

Syringomyelia, also known as syrinx, hydromyelia, or hydrosyringomyelia, is an anatomical dilatation of the central spinal canal due to alteration of CSF circulation, found in almost 20% of those with Chiari II malformation. Symptom presentations are diverse, with symptoms and signs of both upper and lower spinal cord, and have been classified into three groups: Group I has symptomatology of the Chiari syndrome and must be differentiated from other causes of this syndrome as well as shunt obstruction; Group II must be differentiated from tethered cord, which is easily done with MRI imaging; and Group III has a mixed presentation of Groups I and II, as well as rapidly progressive scoliosis. MRI studies may demonstrate a syrinx with either segmental or more generalized (holocord) dilatation and has good correlation with clinical symptoms. Prior to considering surgery for the syrinx, careful evaluation is required to ensure that the shunt is working and that a clinically significant tethered cord is not present. Intervention for syrinx is conservative and is only performed when signs of neurological deterioration are present (LaMarca, Herman, Grant, & McLone, 1997).

Chronic Headaches

Headaches are a frequent and significant symptom of shunt malfunction but also a common and frequent complaint in children and adolescents with and without myelomeningocele and hydrocephalus. Frequent nonmigraine headaches are present in 6%–8% of children, and migraines, in 4% of children. Nonmigraine headaches are experienced in 15.4% of children with shunted hydrocephalus, and migraines are experienced in 8.5% of these children. Combined child and parent report shows that 21.5% of children experience a "shunt migraine condition." In those with chronic headaches, significant difficulty in the evaluation of shunt function may result, particularly in the determination of overdrainage or slit-ventricle syndrome, which frequently presents with essentially normal ventricles on CT scans (Stellman-Ward, Bannister, Lewis, & Shaw, 1997).

Seizures

Seizures occur in 14%–29% of individuals with myelomeningocele and hydrocephalus, and 2%–8% of those without hydrocephalus. Seizures are more common in those with intellectual disability, history of meningitis/ventriculitis, intraventricular hemorrhage, or other CNS anomaly. Shunt malfunction may present with seizures in a small percentage of children, although rarely as the sole symptomatology (Stellman, Bannister, & Hillier, 1986).

UROLOGICAL MANAGEMENT

Significant urologic disability exists in more than 90% of children with spina bifida regardless of the level of lesion, and it is not unusual to care for a child with a low sacral lesion with minimal or absent orthopedic involvement but major problems related to his or her neurogenic bladder or bowel (see Figure 8.1-3). No clear correlation between the level of the child's spinal cord lesion and the type of neurogenic bladder exists. Prevention of UTIs, preservation of upper tract function to prevent chronic renal failure and end-stage renal disease (ERSD), and achievement of social continence are goals (see Chapter 21).

Marie had her first UTI at age 7 months, which was quickly followed by a second and third infection during the next 2 months. Her pediatrician was concerned because she had fevers with all of the episodes. Marie had a normal renal ultrasound and voiding cystourethrogram (VCUG) as a neonate, but she had missed an appointment for her follow-up renal ultrasound at age 6 months. The urologist in the Spina Bifida Clinic recommended new radiologic imaging studies.

Rita was told that Marie's renal ultrasound was abnormal, showing renal enlargement and dilatation of the renal pelvis bilaterally. VCUG showed bladder trabeculations and Grade 3 reflux. The urologist showed Rita how to do intermittent catheterization and advised her that surgery would become necessary if Marie did not experience clinical and radiologic improvement during the next 2–3 months. Marie continued to have recurrent UTIs, so a vesicostomy was performed. By age 3 years, Marie was doing significantly better, and the vesicostomy was undone. She did reasonably well during the next 3–4 years, and her annual radiologic imaging studies were stable.

Urinary Tract Infection

Residual urine and incomplete bladder emptying caused by the neurogenic bladder are the major reason for UTIs in children with spina bifida. UTIs are caused by

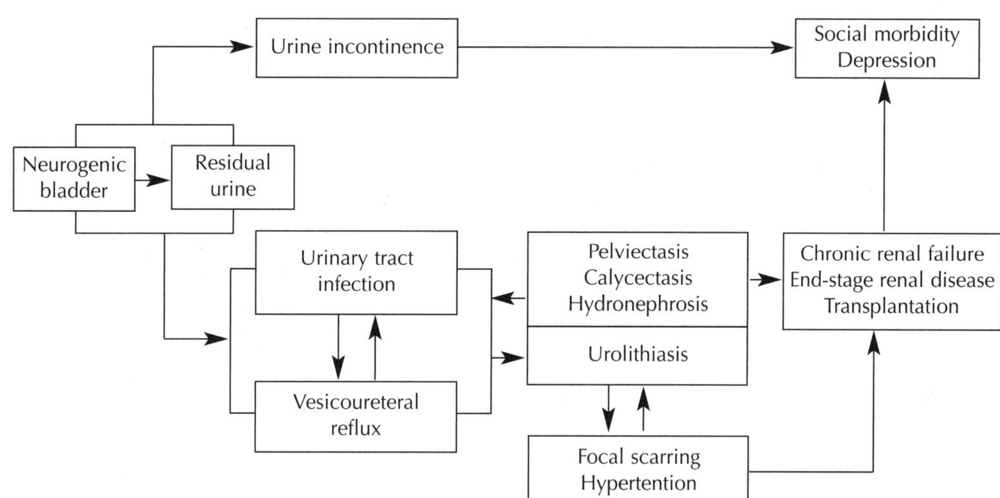

Figure 8.1-3. Neurogenic bladder—interrelation of pathological and social morbidity.

a large number of bacteria, although most are from gram negative organisms, with *Escherichia Coli* being the most common. Frequent infection of the urine, vesicoureteral reflux, hydronephrosis, and focal scarring may lead to systemic hypertension and chronic renal failure. Bladder and renal calculi are common and may lead to additional UTIs. Treatment for stones includes cystoscopy, ureteroscopy, renal pelvis tubes, and extracorporeal shock wave lithotripsy (ESWL), which has proven to be effective and safe. Vesicostomy may be utilized in infants to provide improved drainage when earlier treatment with intermittent catheterization, antibiotic prophylaxis and treatment of infection, and pharmacological management of bladder tonicity are unsuccessful in preventing UTIs and protecting upper urinary tract function. It is usually temporary and well tolerated, although prolapse and stenosis of the opening may occur, and urine leakage may cause skin irritation and rash.

Preservation of Renal Function

Prevention of UTI and routine monitoring of upper tract function with imaging studies have significantly decreased progression to ESRD in those with spina bifida. With appropriate care, ESRD is now infrequent, unless major problems with adherence to recommended regimens have arisen. If ESRD does occur, renal dialysis is indicated, and renal transplantation is a possibility. Despite significant improvements in care, renal parenchymal damage occurs in almost 20% of children with spina bifida and is twice as common in those older than age 10 years than in those younger than 5 years.

Most pediatric centers use a combination of renal ultrasound, VCUG, urodynamic evaluation, and/or radionucleotide imaging to periodically assess bladder and kidney status, and look for interval change. Renal ultrasound is noninvasive and has replaced use of intravenous pyelograms (IVP), whereas renal scans may provide useful information about parenchymal scarring and renal function. Initial testing is begun as a neonate, with reevaluation 3–6 months later as clinically indicated, and periodic annual evaluation is required beginning at age 1 year, even when previous studies have been negative.

Radiographic imaging has shown 85%–90% of newborns with myelomeningocele to have normal urinary tracts. Ten percent of abnormalities develop in utero from outlet obstruction, and three percent develop from spinal shock following surgical closure of the back. Urodynamic studies, if available, are recommended in the newborn period. Bladder contractility and external sphincter activity allow for three types of lower urinary tract function: synergic, dyssynergic (with and without detrusor hypertonicity), and complete denervation. In those with dyssynergy on newborn urodynamic evaluation, upper urinary tract changes are reported in 71% by age 3 years. These changes are significantly less in those who are synergic or have complete denervation (Bauer, 1992).

Outlet obstruction, frequently associated with dyssynergy, and a small, noncompliant, trabeculated bladder contribute to the likelihood of poor renal function. Significant changes may occur over time, necessitating periodic urodynamic testing. Identification of risk factors allows early initiation of clean intermittent catheterization (CIC), use of medication, and/or surgery when necessary. Early surgical intervention should be considered when there is poor adherence to recommendations and likelihood of satisfactory follow-up is of concern. Surgical goals are to increase bladder capacity and decrease bladder pressure and vesicoureteral reflux. Surgical procedures available to achieve these goals include ureteral reimplantation, bladder augmentation (enterocystoplasty), and detrusorectomy.

Social Continence

Incontinence of urine and feces is a significant cause of morbidity and can lead to significant social problems including depression and adjustment problems in the adolescent and young adult.

At age 14 years, Juan saw an adolescent medicine consultant at the Spina Bifida Clinic. He brought up his concerns about still being in a diaper despite his use of intermittent catheterization and asked whether anything else could be done for his urine leakage. Bowel management was also a concern for Juan. He was embarrassed at school because his slight fecal soiling made him smell bad. He dreaded the possibility that he would have an accident at school. Juan was now a senior in high school and was considering applying to a community college the following fall. The adolescent medicine consultant made an appointment for Juan with a urologist to discuss medication and to obtain urodynamic testing and asked the nurse coordinator to offer suggestions for bowel management.

Urine incontinence results from reflex emptying, overflow, or an incompetent urinary sphincter. CIC is used to remove residual urine, improve urinary drainage, and provide decompression of raised intravesical pressure. Intermittent catheterization is superior to indwelling catheters, which are socially unacceptable due to significant malodor, leakage, and frequent complications of UTI. The combination of CIC, medication for incontinence, and antibiotic therapy have proven effective both in the management and prevention of UTIs and upper urinary tract deterioration and in urinary control.

When used alone, CIC provides complete continence in only about one fourth of children and is not effective in those with small bladder capacity and low-outlet resistance. Anticholinergic medications such as oxybutynin (Ditropan) and propantheline (Probanthine) are used to inhibit bladder contractions and to increase capacity; and alpha-adrenergic agents such as phenylpropanolamine, ephedrine, and pseudoephedrine (Sudafed) can increase outlet resistance. Medication, in conjunction with CIC, allows half of these children to become completely continent, and almost all show improvement in continence status. With CIC, more than 80% of these children can be reasonably dry. Self-catheterization increases as age and experience improve. Poor hand function, blindness, cognitive deficit, visual perceptual problems, obesity, severe scoliosis, and inadequate space or privacy for adequate toileting make it difficult, but not impossible, to achieve self-catheterization. Complications are few but include epididymitis, urethral stricture, perforation with false passage formation, bleeding, and/or loss of catheter into the bladder.

A number of surgical procedures have been developed to provide social continence, including artificial urinary sphincter, creation of an artificial bladder or Koch pouch with intussuscepted nipple, bladder augmentation (enterocystoplasty), and use of the Mitrofanoff procedure. Bladder augmentation allows enlargement of the bladder with increase in volume capacity and lower intravesical pressure. Other procedures to achieve continence through increased outlet resistance include urethral lengthening and reimplantation; bladder neck reconstruction; and external urethral compression through use of an artificial urinary sphincter, fascial sling, or periurethral injections of collagen. External urethral sphincter dilatation has been reported to provide long-term help to those with high leak pressure and poor bladder compliance.

BOWEL MANAGEMENT

Constipation and bowel incontinence are common problems for those with spina bifida. Intervention to achieve an effective bowel continence program and avoid chronic constipation and impaction must begin in infancy, before physiological and behavioral patterns are established (see Chapter 14.2). Bowel continence requires normal external sphincter control, internal sphincter reflex relaxation, and rectal and perianal skin sensation, which are dependent on intact sacral nerve roots and normal colon motility. Bowel programs have several goals—avoidance of constipation, regular complete evacuation, and prevention of incontinence with achievement of accident-free days. Maintenance of a regular, soft, formed stool is important to prevent constipation, megacolon, and development of overflow incontinence.

Bowel management consists of regularly scheduled toileting, stool softeners to prevent constipation, and dietary measures such as additional fiber. Those with an inability to sit with stability or to utilize the Valsalva maneuver due to the high level of their lesion may frequently require regular suppository or enema, digital stimulation, or, in rare cases, manual removal. The Malone procedure, a cutaneous-appendicael conduit to the right colon, utilizes an antegrade continence enema (ACE) through the abdominal stoma for those with intractable constipation and fecal soiling. The skin opening is frequently at the umbilicus, convenient for those in a wheelchair or with high bracing. Complications of surgery include conduit stenosis, stricture, or perforation (Koyle, Kaji, Duque, Wild, & Galansky, 1995).

The Spina Bifida Association of America (SBAA) has developed a 13-point assessment program: 1) stool consistency, 2) frequency, 3) amount, 4) mobility, 5) paraplegia level, 6) diet, 7) medication, 8) anal/rectal canal tone, 9) previous regimen, 10) family routine, 11) age, 12) bathroom accessibility, and 13) learning/training issues. Based on this assessment, an individualized treatment program is developed using five approaches: behavioral (habit) training, digital stimulation, daily suppository, "cone enema," and ACE procedure (Leibold, Ekmark, & Adams, 2000). This program is adjusted as the child gets older and increases in maturity and independence.

ORTHOPEDIC MANAGEMENT

Good orthopedic management is essential to the development of a stable posture; ambulation when possible; maintenance of joints in a functional position; and prevention of decubitus ulcers, infection, and pathologic fractures (see Chapter 13). Knowledge of the level of spinal cord dysfunction allows planning of orthopedic management and prevention of further deformity and contracture. Ambulation groups based on function—community ambulators, household ambulators, nonfunctional ambulators, and nonambulators—have provided a useful framework for understanding the ambulatory and mobility capabilities of those with spina bifida. Children with functional quadriceps and lesions below L-3 will be functional ambulators, though they may require a wheelchair for longer trips. Those with no functional quadriceps or with lesions above L-3 are unlikely to be community ambulators. Children with lesions below S-1 are likely to ambulate without bracing (McDonald, Jaffe, Mosca, & Shurtleff, 1991).

Most children will lose the ability to walk if their weight is excessive. To improve their mobility, adolescents and young adults who ambulated as children may choose, or need, to use a wheelchair. Those who had thoracic and high lumbar lesions may become wheelchair dependent as their body mass increases during adolescence and adulthood. Children with midlumbar and lumbosacral lesions have a better prognosis for ambulation. Secondary neurological changes from tethered cord, syringomyelia, or foot ulceration and infection are additional factors that may undermine ambulation, even in those with sacral lesions.

Foot

Foot deformities or "clubfeet," affecting 75% of these children, are the most common orthopedic abnormality in children with spina bifida. Multiple forms of foot abnormalities occur, with 85% being paralytic from muscle imbalance. The goals of therapy are to have a plantigrade foot with muscle balance that can be braced to allow an upright stance (Drennan, 1999). General principles of care include use of manipulation (passive range of motion) or immobilization by serial casting in the infant, with soft tissue releases in the child younger than 4 years of age, and use of osteotomies after age 4 years. Cavus feet are usually not a problem until adolescence, and specific attention to prevent plantar ulcers under the metatarsal heads is important.

Hip

Subluxation or dislocation of the hip is present in 35%–50% of children with spina bifida, may be unilateral or bilateral, and may present at birth or develop later. The paralytic form of subluxation and dislocation associated with low lumbar level lesions is the most common, affecting 50%–75% of these children. Hip contractures, commonly present, make bracing and ambulation difficult. Change in neurologic condition with late onset of dislocation in those with low lumbar and sacral level lesions requires evaluation for cord tethering, syrinx, or other lesions. Treatment goals of hip reduction include improved ambulation and trunk alignment, decreased bracing needs, and reduced energy consumption for walking. Hip reduction and correction of pelvic obliquity without changing forces acting on it will result in redislocation of the hip. Surgical procedures include muscle transfers, pelvic procedures, and contracture release. Following surgery, seating must be reevaluated to avoid development of decubiti, prolonged casting avoided to prevent pathologic fracture, and bracing initiated to prevent recurrent contracture (Dias, 1991).

Knee

Congenital hyperextension of the knee and flexion contractures of the knee in children may develop. Knee problems among teenagers and young adults are common. Gait abnormalities place stress on the knee, causing instability and degenerative changes, with significant import for community ambulators. Forearm crutches decrease stress and weight bearing on the knees and may decrease or put off the onset of arthritic changes.

Scoliosis

Scoliosis is a significant and common problem for those with spina bifida and affects posture and ambulation. It may lead to difficulty with wheelchair seating, decubiti, and back pain, as well as more serious complications involving compromise of cardiac, pulmonary, and intra-abdominal organs. Serial evaluation clinically and radiographically is required. Scoliosis may be congenital or paralytic (developmental), with congenital scoliosis more progressive, and paralytic scoliosis more common. Almost 90% of children with T-12 or above lesions, 80% of children with high lumbar lesions, and 23% of children with low lumbar lesions have scoliosis. Scoliosis is infrequent with sacral lesions, and its presence should always raise suspicion of a tethered cord or other abnormality (Banta, Drummond, & Ferguson, 1999).

Scoliosis is treated by use of bracing and surgery. Use of a polypropylene thoracolumbosacral orthoses (TLSO) body jacket may slow or arrest progression of the scoliosis. A TLSO body jacket may be restrictive and interfere with respiration or sweating, resulting in problems of temperature control in hot climates or areas of poor ventilation. Surgery has consisted of anterior and posterior spinal fusion with many different approaches to instrumentation utilized. For paralytic scoliosis, the two-stage approach has significantly improved outcomes. Surgery has a high incidence of serious complications including superficial and deep wound infections, pseudoarthrosis and instrumentation loosening, decubuti, seating problems, and risk of intraoperative catastrophe with an operative mortality of 1%–2%.

Kyphosis

Kyphosis occurs in 6%–20% of children with myelomeningocele and is more common in infants with thoracic lesions. Present at birth, it is progressive and may make initial closure of the back lesion difficult. It responds poorly to bracing, and surgery becomes necessary to relieve pressure on the overlying skin, prevent shortening of the trunk, provide a stable sitting balance, and prevent compromise of respiration from crowding of abdominal and thoracic organs. Early initiation of therapy is essential, and surgery is difficult with a high complication rate for failure of fusion, infection, and/or skin breakdown.

Pathologic Fractures

Pathologic fractures occur in 10%–30% of children with spina bifida. Children with high-level lesions are more frequently affected. Fractures result from osteoporosis and sensory loss and occur more commonly when there is limited weight bearing due to prolonged casting, immobilization following surgery, or wheelchair dependence. The injury may seem insignificant and barely be noticed. Awareness of the insignificance of the traumatic event and the extreme fragility of these bones is essential, as it is common for protective services or a police report to be made following such an injury (Lock & Aronson, 1989). Fractures are frequently painless, despite significant swelling from hematoma formation. Some children may have fever, hypotension, and tachycardia, in addition to localized redness and swelling of the involved area. Sedimentation rate may be significantly elevated when this occurs and may be difficult to differentiate from cellulitis, osteomyelitis, and/or pyoarthritis.

Orthotic Principles

Bracing is performed to increase function and to prevent development and progression of deformity (see Table 8.1-2). Advances in brace manufacture—lightweight and adjustable construction—have revolutionized expectations for children using them. Bracing is used to stabilize a weight-bearing joint, improve daytime function, maintain position following surgery, permit use of shoes, prevent contractures, and allow successful ambulation. Level of lesion, weight and body mass, other physical limitations, and motivation are all factors that contribute to the success or failure of bracing efforts.

Table 8.1-2. Commonly used braces

Ankle–foot orthoses (AFO)	Stabilizes the ankle joint. Used by a child with L4 to S1 motor level. Child may need forearm crutches or a walker.
Knee–ankle–foot orthoses (KAFO)	Stabilizes the knee and compensates for weak quadriceps. Used by a child with L3 to L4 motor level. Child frequently needs forearm crutches.
Hip–knee–ankle–foot orthoses (HKAFO)	Allows upright posture with hips in extension. Used by a child with thoracic and L1 to L3 motor level.
Reciprocating gait orthoses (RGO)	Allows ambulation for those with high lesions. Is expensive and requires great motivation to use successfully.
Thoracic–hip–knee–ankle–foot orthoses (THKAFO)	Provides upright position for those with high lesions, thoracic to L2 motor level.
Thoracolumbosacral orthoses (TLSO)	Body jacket prevents progression of spinal curvature.
Parapodium	Allows young children age 1–2 years limited mobility through a swivel action. Provides an upright stance that allows the pursuit of age-appropriate developmental skills.

SKIN INTEGRITY

Paraplegia and sensory deficit, orthoses use, intellectual disabilities, macrocephaly, kyphosis, upper extremity impairment, incontinence, and/or poor adherence to medical recommendations are significant risk factors for skin breakdown and development of decubitus ulcers (see Chapter 20). Improvements in adaptive equipment and custom seating, training of parents to identify skin problems early, training of children to use a mirror for self-inspection, and use of pressure release techniques have all contributed to improvement in the prevention of decubiti. Breakdown is frequent in the perineal area and over a kyphotic deformity, both of which experience frequent rubbing and have poor protection. Unbalanced scoliosis, pelvic obliquity, and loss of lordosis following spinal fusion results in pressure over the ischium and/or sacrococcygeal area. Problems with seating and poorly fitting braces, aggravated by urine and fecal soiling, leads to skin breakdown in these areas. These problems are more common in those with L2 or above lesions. Decubitus ulcers are less frequent in the lower extremities, but when present, are seen in those who are physically active and have motor levels of L4–5 or below. Foot lesions are frequently found in those with sacral lesions. They can be difficult to heal and can lead to serious infection and possible need for amputation. Therapy for skin breakdown includes cleaning and debridement, hydrotherapy, antibiotics when infection is present, and surgery, particularly myocutaneous rotation flaps when appropriate to provide protective covering and to restore sensation.

OPERATIVE AND ANESTHESIA RISKS

Most individuals with spina bifida have multiple surgeries during their lifetime. An experienced anesthesiologist is required so that routine anesthesia precautions appropriate to age and condition are provided. For newborns, careful attention must be given to avoidance of hypothermia; provision of appropriate intravenous fluids; prevention of acidosis; and appropriate measures to minimize risk of infection, particularly sepsis, meningitis/ventriculitis, or UTI and urosepsis. Intubation is done in the decubitus position or with the back supported on a "head ring" to minimize danger to back lesions. Infants may have "short trachea syndrome," a reduction in the number of cartilage rings from a normal of 17 rings, to 15 or fewer, with tracheal bifurcation higher than normally expected. As a result, intubation of these infants may be difficult, with placement of the endotracheal tube in the right main stem bronchus. Support of the chest and pelvis needs to be provided with careful attention to avoiding pressure on the abdomen, as this can result in obstruction of the inferior vena cava or pressure on the diaphragm. There is an increased incidence of necrotizing enterocolitis, and the anesthesiologist and those assisting in the operative suite must minimize or avoid hypotension, hypoxia, and acidosis.

Operation involving the shunt requires specific attention to cardiovascular stability and the complications of increased intracranial pressure. Restrictive lung disease frequently accompanies severe scoliosis, and careful preparation for spinal fusion requires preoperative assessment of pulmonary function, cardiovascular evaluation, a coagulation panel, and arrangements for sufficient blood and blood products to be available.

The anesthesiologist and surgeon need to be alert to the risk of intraoperative catastrophe from anesthetic agents, anaphylactic reaction to latex, unsuspected cardiac arrhythmia, and/or reaction to blood or blood products. Hemodynamic instability from anaphylactic reaction to latex may present as hypotension, increased airway resistance, and circulatory collapse. Reactions are more likely in those who have undergone multiple prior surgeries and hospitalizations but may occur in those as young as 2 years, particularly during surgical procedures. Procedures of great length, such as anterior spinal fusion, are at higher risk of exposure to latex antigen and subsequent reaction. The reaction itself may be difficult to perceive until intraoperative catastrophe has occurred, due to the child's anesthetized condition (Banta, Bonanni, & Prebluda, 1993). Primary prevention in medical centers as a whole, and operating rooms specifically, is essential. Using nonlatex gloves and catheters and washing the powder off rubber gloves is important, as is using latex-free equipment in the operating room. This approach to primary prevention starts in the NICU with the infant's first hospitalization, as significant sensitization may occur with initial back closure, and then with all subsequent hospitalizations and surgical procedures.

Problems of respiration are common in those with Chiari syndrome and sleep disordered breathing, and particular attention to secretion control as well as ventilation and autonomic control when arousing from anesthesia is necessary. The risk of malignant hyperthermia may be increased, with a 1.5% incidence, and may be catastrophic in those with brainstem dysfunction and prolonged seizures. Blood and blood products may cause serious reaction in the operating room, or risk of hepatitis or human immunodeficiency virus acquisition, if appropriate blood preparation and screening for these entities is not performed.

LATEX (RUBBER) ALLERGY

Latex allergy is common in individuals with spina bifida and anomalies of the genitourinary system. In 1991, the Food and Drug Administration Medical Bulletin reported 18%–40% of individuals with spina bifida and 6% of medical personnel to be latex sensitive. This compares to latex sensitivity of approximately 1 in 3,000 in the general population. Environmental exposure to rubber products in both the community and hospital is widespread with exposure in toys (e.g., balloons, squash balls) or at medical sites where rubber catheters, gloves, enema catheters, latex adhesive tapes and bandages, components of intravenous infusion sets, anesthesia equipment, and dental bite blocks are common. Reactions are more common in rubber products with significant residual protein impurities, accounting for why reactions are more likely with some products than others. In addition, cross reactivity exists with many foods, including avocados, bananas, kiwi, passion fruit, and water chestnuts.

Possible reactions include skin rash, perioral tingling, rhinitis, conjunctivitis, a warm feeling, difficulty swallowing, and apprehension. In rare cases, catastrophic reactions with bronchospasm, angioedema, tachycardia, and hypotension may occur. Exposure may come from the skin, mucous or serosal membranes, inhalation, or intravenous routes. Reactions may be Type I IgE mediated or Type IV T-cell mediated delayed hypersensitivity reaction, which is the more common. The RAST, skin-prick, and intradermal tests are used in evaluation of possible latex allergy. Skin-prick tests are highly accurate, but reports of reactions including anaphylaxis have limited their use, while RAST testing has significant limitation due to variability (53%–100%) in sensitivity. Latex-specific IgE has been detected by ELISA 92% and RAST 94%, and although useful, does not replace a careful medical and environmental history and recognition by parents, school personnel, and health care providers that latex exposure is to be minimized and avoided whenever possible (Kwittken, Sweinberg, Campbell, & Pawlowski, 1995).

The best treatment is prevention through education of children and families about where latex may be found in the medical and community setting. A medical alert bracelet and autoinjectable epinephrine should be provided when latex sensitivity is suspected. Many medical centers have worked to create a latex-free environment, and for those with known latex sensitivity, prophylactic presurgical management with diphenhydramine, cimetidine or ranitidine, and corticosteroids is frequently used.

ADOLESCENTS AND YOUNG ADULTS

Adolescents and young adults with myelomeningocele have the same beliefs, dreams, goals, and expectations as typically developing adolescents (see Figure 8.1-4). These physical and psychosocial needs are important and must be addressed in the ambulatory care and community setting. When possible, a specialist in adolescent medicine should be included in the team. The HEADSS (Home and family relations; Education; Activities in or out of school; Drug, alcohol, or tobacco use; Sexuality and orientation; and Suicidal ideation or depression) assessment provides assistance in transition planning to adult health, social service, and education settings (Roland, Jacobs, Angone, Fallick, & MacKenzie, 1997). Adolescents with spina bifida may have concerns about weight gain and body image, ambulation and mobility, social and school problems, progression of scoliosis and other orthopedic problems, and their sexual development and sexuality.

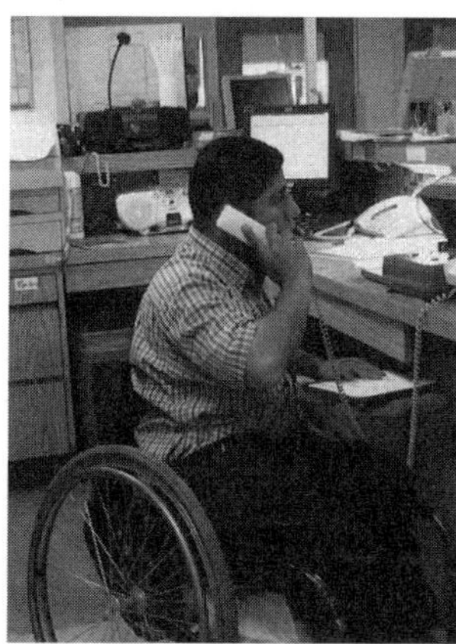

Figure 8.1-4. Eddie had his original surgery at Childrens Hospital Los Angeles and has been successful in achieving inclusion, independence, and employment.

In the past, individuals with spina bifida frequently reported being socially isolated and sexually inactive. This, along with limitations in mobility, urine and fecal incontinence, and low self-esteem, resulted in early and continued isolation and associated depression. Health providers and parents need to be sensitive to these social needs and attempt to foster social involvement whenever possible, including recognition of the young adult's sexual aspirations and hopes for long-term relationships and marriage.

Both men and women with spina bifida may have sexual intercourse and experience orgasm, although sensation in the genital area is diminished, necessitating erotic stimulation elsewhere to achieve sexual pleasure and orgasm. As many as 70% of women with spina bifida may conceive, and most have a relatively uneventful pregnancy and delivery. Urinary incontinence may be increased late in pregnancy, and cesarean section is commonly needed. Men with spina bifida have been able to father children, but problems with erection and ejaculation are common. Use of sildenafil (Viagra) has been reported to improve erectile function in 80% of those receiving the medication and provide improved sexual confidence. Infertility in males is common due to problems of ejaculation, and frequent history of high fevers from infection and undescended testicles, with resultant poor semen quality and abnormal testicular histology on biopsy. Despite this, advances in assisted reproduction technology should allow more men to achieve parenthood.

CONCLUSION

Prior to the provision of back closure and ventricular shunt placement, only 5%–10% of infants with spina bifida survived their first year of life. Currently, the most common cause of death is from Chiari II brainstem dysfunction in infancy and early childhood years. Survival expectations improve significantly after age 5 years, with an annual death rate between age 5–30 years of approximately 1% annually (McLaughlin et al., 1985). At least 75% of children born with spina bifida are expected to reach their early adult years. Ventriculitis, ESRD, and hydrocephalus have become the common causes of death after the early childhood years, with renal complications leading to ESRD being the leading cause of death in adults. Use of alcohol, drugs, tobacco, and dietary patterns leading to obesity are common and have significant importance for the health of those with spina bifida. Physical exercise, injury prevention measures at home, at work, and in the car, and strong social and psychological support systems are extremely important to minimize these risks. Families are urged to seek information and support from the organizations listed in Table 8.1-3.

Table 8.1-3. Advocacy, consumer, and professional organizations

American Academy for Cerebral Palsy and Developmental Medicine

6300 North River Road, Suite 727, Rosemont, IL 60018-4226; 847-698-1635; 847-823-0536 (fax); http://www.aacpdm.org

Mission: Encourages the study of cerebral palsy and other childhood-onset disabilities. Promotes professional education for the treatment and management of these conditions. Improves the quality of life of people with these disabilities.

Association of University Centers on Disabilities (formerly American Association of University Affiliated Programs)

1010 Wayne Avenue, Suite 920, Silver Spring, MD 20910; 301-588-8252; 301-588-2842 (fax); http://www.aucd.org

Mission: Advances policy and practice for and with people who have disabilities, their families, and their communities by supporting members to engage in research, education, and service that encourage independence, productivity, and satisfying quality of life.

California Birth Defects Monitoring Program

1917 Fifth Street, Berkeley, CA 94710; 510-549-4155; 510-549-4175 (fax); http://www.cbdmp.org

Mission: Promotes the discovery of causes of birth defects and communicates results.

Family Voices, Inc.

3411 Candelaria NE, Suite M, Albuquerque, NM 87107; 505-872-4774 or 888-835-5669; 505-872-4780 (fax); http://www.familyvoices.org

Mission: Advocates for health care services that are family-centered, community-based, comprehensive, coordinated, and culturally competent for all children and youth with special health care needs. Promotes the inclusion of all families as decision makers at all levels of health care. Supports essential partnerships between families and professionals.

Hydrocephalus Association

870 Market Street, Suite 705, San Francisco, CA 94102; 888-598-3789; http://www.hydroassoc.org

Mission: Provides support, education, and advocacy for individuals, families, and professionals.

International Federation for Spina Bifida and Hydrocephalus

http://www.ifglobal.org

Mission: Improves the quality of life of people with hydrocephalus and spina bifida throughout the world. Decreases the prevalence of hydrocephalus and spina bifida through primary prevention.

Society for Research into Hydrocephalus and Spina Bifida

http://www.srhsb.org

Mission: Advances education and promotes research into hydrocephalus and spina bifida. Brings together workers in different fields who have a common interest in hydrocephalus and spina bifida so that they may be aided in their joint endeavour to prevent, cure, or alleviate these conditions.

Spina Bifida Association of America

4590 MacArthur Blvd., NW, Suite 250, Washington, DC 20007-4226; 800-621-3141 or 202-944-3285; 202-944-3295 (fax); http://www.sbaa.org

Mission: Promotes the prevention of spina bifida. Addresses the specific needs of the spina bifida community. Serves as the national representative of its chapters.

REFERENCES

Banta, J.V. (1991). The tethered cord in myelomeningocele: Should it be untethered? *Developmental Medicine and Child Neurology, 33,* 173–176.

Banta, J.V., Bonanni, C., & Prebluda, J. (1993). Latex anaphylaxis during spinal surgery in children with myelomeningocele. *Developmental Medicine and Child Neurology, 35,* 540–548.

Banta, J.V., Drummond, D.S., & Ferguson, R.L. (1999). The treatment of neuromuscular scoliosis. *AAOS Instructional Course Lectures, 48,* 551–562.

Bauer, S.B. (1992). Neurogenic vesical dysfunction in children. In P.C. Walsh, A.B. Retik, T.A. Stamey, & E.D. Vaughn (Eds.), *Campbell's urology* (6th ed., pp. 1634–1668). Philadelphia: W.B. Saunders.

Bayston, R. (1989). *Hydrocephalus shunt infections.* London: Chapman and Hall.

California AFP Screening Program. (1994). *AFP update for prenatal care providers.* Berkeley, CA: Author.

Charney, E.B., Rorke, L.B., Sutton, L.N., & Schut, L. (1987). Management of Chiari II complication in infants with myelomeningocele. *Journal of Pediatrics, 111*(3), 364–371.

Charney, E.B., Sutton, L.N., Bruce, D.A., & Schut, L.B. (1983). Myelomeningocele newborn management: Time for parental decision. *Zeitschrift fur Kinderchirurgie, 38*(Suppl. II), 90–93.

Davoh, C.T., & Kinsman, S.L. (1995). *Medical facts about spina bifida.* Baltimore: Kennedy Krieger Institute/Spina Bifida Association of America.

Dias, L.S. (1991). Hip deformities in myelomeningocele. *AAOS Instructional Course Lectures, XL,* 281–286.

Drennan, J.C. (1999). Current concepts in myelomeningocele. *AAOS Instructional Course Lectures, 48,* 543–550.

Kirk, V.G., Morielli, A., & Brouillette, R.T. (1999). Sleep-disordered breathing in patients with myelomeningocele: The missed diagnosis. *Developmental Medicine and Child Neurology, 41,* 40–43.

Koyle, M.A., Kaji, D.M., Duque, M., Wild, J., & Galansky, S.H. (1995). The Malone antegrade continence enema for neurogenic and structural fecal incontinence and constipation. *Journal of Urology, 154,* 759–761.

Kulkarni, A.V., Rabin, D., Lamberti-Pasculli, M., & Drake, J.M. (2001). Repeat cerebrospinal fluid shunt infection in children. *Pediatric Neurosurgery, 35,* 66–71.

Kwittken, P.L., Sweinberg, S.K., Campbell, D.E., & Pawlowski, N.A. (1995). Latex hypersensitivity in children: Clinical presentation and detection of latex-specific immunoglobulin E. *Pediatrics,* 693–699.

LaMarca, F., Herman, M., Grant, J.A., & McLone, D.G. (1997). Presentation and management of hydromyelia in children with Chiari Type-II malformation. *Pediatric Neurosurgery, 26,* 57–67.

Leibold, S., Ekmark, E., & Adams, R.C. (2000). Decision-making for a successful bowel continence program. *European Journal of Pediatric Surgery, 10*(Suppl. I), 26–30

Lock, T.R., & Aronson, D.D. (1989). Fractures in patients who have myelomeningocele. *Journal of Bone and Joint Surgery. American Volume, 71*(8), 1153–1157.

McComb, J.G. (1997). Spinal and cranial neural tube defects. *Seminars in Pediatric Neurology, 4*(3), 156–166.

McDonald, C.M., Jaffe, K.M., Mosca, V.S., & Shurtleff, D.B. (1991). Ambulatory outcome of children with myelomeningocele: Effect of lower extremity muscle strength. *Developmental Medicine and Child Neurology, 33,* 482–490.

McLaughlin, J.F., Shurtleff, D.B., Lamers, J.Y., Stunts, J.T., Hayden, P.W., & Kropp, R.J. (1985). Influence of prognosis on decisions regarding the care of newborns with spina bifida cystica. *New England Journal of Medicine, 312,* 1589–1594.

McLone, D.G., & Knepper, P.A. (1989). The cause of Chiari II malformation: A unified theory. *Pediatric Neuroscience, 15,* 1–12.

Platt, L.D., Feuchtbamm, L., Filly, R., Lustig, L., Simon, M., & Cunningham, G.C. (1992). The California Maternal Serum Alpha-Fetoprotein Screening Program: The role of ultrasonography in the detection of spina bifida. *American Journal of Obstetrics and Gynecology, 166,* 1328–1329.

Roland, M., Jacobs, R., Angone, E., Fallick, B., & MacKenzie, R. (1997). Principles of management of adolescents with spina bifida in the ambulatory setting. *European Journal of Pediatric Surgery,* 7(Suppl. I), 57–58.

Salomao, J.F., & Leibinger, R.D. (1999). Abdominal pseudocysts complicating CSF shunting in infants and children. *Pediatric Neurosurgery, 31,* 274–278.

Sarwark, J.F., Weber, D.T., Gabrieli, A.P., McLone, D.G., & Dias, L. (1996). Tethered cord syndrome in low motor level children with myelomeningocele. *Pediatric Neurosurgery, 25,* 295–301.

Shurtleff, D.B., Duguay, S., Duguay, G., Moskowitz, D., Weinberger, E., Roberts, T., & Loeser, J. (1997). Epidemiology of tethered cord with meningomyelocele. *European Journal of Pediatric Surgery,* 7(Suppl. I), 7–11.

Stellman, G.R., Bannister, C.M., & Hillier, V. (1986). The incidence of seizure disorder in children with acquired and congenital hydrocephalus. *Zeitschrift fur Kinderchirurgie, 41*(Suppl. I), 38–41.

Stellman-Ward, G.R., Bannister, C.M., Lewis, M.A., & Shaw, J. (1997). The incidence of chronic headache in children with shunted hydrocephalus. *European Journal of Pediatric Surgery,* 7(Suppl. I), 12–14.

Van Allen, M.I., Kalousek, D.K., Chernoff, G.F., & Hall, J.G. (1993). Evidence for multisite closure of the neural tube in humans. *American Journal Medical Genetics, 47,* 723–743.

Wolraich, M.L. (1983). *The needs of children with spina bifida: A comprehensive view* [Monograph]. Iowa City: University of Iowa, Department of Pediatrics, Division of Developmental Disabilities.

8.2 CONGENITAL MULTISYSTEM DISORDERS, CRANIOFACIAL ANOMALIES, AND AN ARRAY OF GENETIC DISORDERS

Lawrence C. Kaplan

This chapter discusses the general identification and management of three categories of congenital developmental disabilities: 1) congenital *multisystem* disorders, exemplified by the VACTERL and CHARGE associations; 2) the broad group of conditions comprising *craniofacial anomalies;* and 3) the even broader group represented by children with alterations in *chromosome* structure and number. It offers, through representative examples, a useful approach to beginning the diagnostic process and coordinating specialty care of children with complex congenital multisystem disorders, with special emphasis on family-focused principles.

From the primary care perspective, a basic set of priorities should be considered when any child with a complex disability is evaluated:

1. Making the initial diagnosis
2. Anticipating outcome and planning care
3. Helping educators understand the child and his or her potential in school
4. Helping parents understand their child's condition

In the 1970s, David W. Smith proposed principles of dysmorphology that were intended to be used in the initial evaluation of children with congenital differences. Although molecular genetics has added considerable precision to this process, Smith's concepts continue to provide valuable guidance in the first moments of evaluation of young children as well as throughout their lives. The principles behind this approach are grounded in a basic understanding of normal embryogenesis and fetal growth and enable clinicians to see human development as a dynamic process between biological, biomechanical, and environmental effects (Jones, 1997).

Adverse biological forces that influence human development can derive from molecular, biomechanical, or environmental factors and result in three types of consequences on the human embryo, fetus, and infant: malformation, deformations, and disruptions (see Figure 8.2-1). An essential lesson from these three patterns of abnormal morphogenesis is that they are neither mutually exclusive or predictive of cognitive and neurodevelopmental potential. See Table 8.2-1 for common clinical examples.

An important outgrowth of the key principles of dysmorphology is the concept of "associations." Associations are two or more distinct features that have a higher than normal likelihood of occurring together. They differ from malformation syndromes in that their component features do not always occur together, whereas the cardinal features seen in malformation syndromes do. In some associations, abnormalities occur that are medically significant and potentially life threatening but not apparent. The clinician thus must always

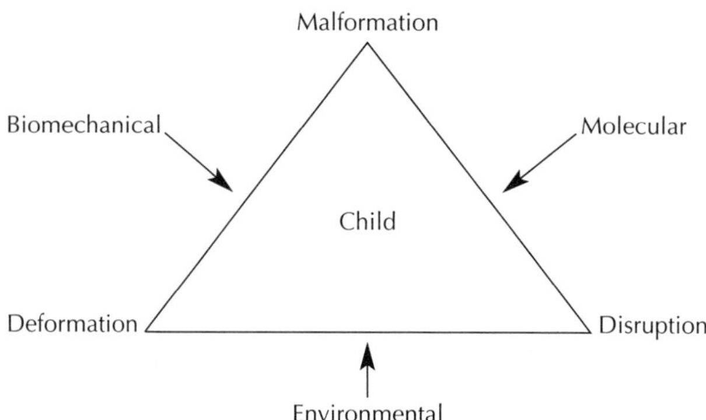

Figure 8.2-1. The relationship between pathoetiology of congenital disorders and alterations of morphogenesis.

attempt to rule out as many features of an association as possible, either by examination or by diagnostic testing. Unlike malformation syndromes, in which the diagnostic process can often involve all-or-nothing recognition, the clues may be subtle, as with VACTERL and CHARGE associations.

MULTISYSTEM DISORDERS

VATER (VACTERL) Association

VATER association describes the nonrandom occurrence of four congenital malformations that may be recalled mnemonically by the five-letter acronym (Quan & Smith, 1973). Elements of the first iteration of this association include:

1. Spectrum of *vertebral* defects
2. *Anal* atresia
3. *Tracheoesophageal* fistula with *esophageal* atresia
4. *Radial* dysplasia (upper extremities).

Since the association was first described in 1972, the acronym has been expanded to VA*C*TER*L* to include cardiac malformations, renal anomalies, and more extensive limb anomalies (Khoury, Cordero, Greenberg, James, & Erickson, 1983; Quan & Smith, 1973). *R* applies to both radial limb dyspasia (RL) and renal anomalies (R) (see Figure 8.2-2). The genetic/dysmorphology literature includes many descriptions of variants of both of these entitites, but for practical purposes—especially because of the importance of early identification of clinically significant congenital heart disease—VACTERL association most accurately characterizes what the careful clinician should remember when evaluating a child.

Table 8.2-1. Examples of errors of morphogenesis

	Anomalies	Syndromes	Associations
Malformation	Hemivertebrae	Down syndrome	CHARGE
	Preauricular skin tags	Prader-Willi syndrome	VACTERL
	Hemangioma	Angelman syndrome	MURCS
Deformation	Postural plagiocephaly	Torticollis-plagiocephaly	Occur as secondary effects
	Clubfoot deformity due to fetal constraint		
Disruption	Intercranial hemorrhage	Amnion rupture	Unknown
	Amnion rupture sequence	Congenital rubella syndrome	
	Meningoencephalitis	Fetal alcohol syndrome	

Source: Jones (1997).

Nearly every case reported thus far of VACTERL association has been sporadic, indicating no apparent genetic or chromosomal etiology, and, to date, no definitive teratogens have been associated with the condition. The incidence of VACTERL association is 1.6/10,000 live births, and in the large international epidemiologic study of 2,295 infants with multiple congenital anomalies, 286 (12.5%) had VACTERL association as defined by a minimum of three of the established defects (Botto et al., 1997). Another study, which analyzed data on 5,260 infants controlling for a number of putative confounding variables, confirmed that the clinical features represented in this "core" acronym are indeed distinct and that these features coincide more frequently than any other anomalies that may be also encountered on examination (Källén, Mastroiacovo, Castilla, & Källén, 2001).

The most coincident features include *anal*, *vertebral*, and *genitourinary tract* abnormalities. Beyond the occurrence of radial limb and cardiac abnormalities, anorectal, vertebral, and genitourinary have a relatively high probability of being discovered. For example, anorectal atresia is found in more than 80% of individuals with both congenital vertebral anomalies and genitourinary tract abnormalities and in more than 66% of those with vertebral anomalies when anal and genitourinary anomalies are present (Botto et al., 1997; Erkan, Lam, Yazici, & Magid, 2001). Although these data point to the nonrandom nature of this association, they indicate that the implications of missing any part of this important triad can have clinical consequences to the child. In addition, the nature of the limb anomalies is protean, including not only polydactyly, syndactyly, or limb reduction anomalies but also rheumatologic limb problems (e.g., arthropathy) that manifest later in life and may be due to subtle differences in bone, muscle, and soft-tissue anatomy (Erkan et al., 2001).

The tracheoesophageal fistula is commonly associated with esophageal atresia; however, the rare "H-type" fistula can also occur in VACTERL association (Haller, Berdon, Levin, & Iyer, 2004). The cardiac abnormalities can vary widely and include endocardial cushion defects (e.g., ventricular septal defects) and more complex conotruncal malformation patterns (e.g., transposition of the great vessels), or tetrology of Fallot (Temtamy & Miller, 1974). Renal abnormalities can include duplication of the collecting system; urethral atresia with hydronephrosis; renal aplasia; and a variety of kidney and bladder dysplasia patterns, as well as multicystic kidneys. This latter malformation has lead to the recent hypothesis that the mutant mitochondrial deoxyribonucleic acid (mtDNA) in multicystic kidney disease occurs 100% of the time in individuals with VACTERL, thereby pointing to a possible molecular basis for VACTERL (Damian, Seibel, Schachenmayr, Reichmann, & Dorndorf, 1996).

Vertebral anomalies are also varied and can include hemivertebrae, bifid vertebrae, vertebral fusion, butterfly and wedge vertebrae, and sacral dysgenesis and agenesis. The vertebral defects may also be seen with other congenital musculoskeletal malformations including the

V Vertebral anomalies (including hemi, "butterfly," fused vertebrae, Klippel-Feil anomaly, and Sprengel deformity)

A Anal atresia (with or without associated upper and lower gastrointestinal malformations)

C Cardiac malformations (including ventricular septal defect, atrial septal defect, pulmonary atresia, complex cyanotic heart disease)

T E Tracheoesophageal fistula with esophageal dysplasia (including "H-type" defect)

R L Radial limb and renal anomalies (including absent radius, missing thumbs, horseshoe kidneys, duplicated collecting systems, renal hypoplasia, bladder extrophy)

Figure 8.2-2. Features of VACTERL association.

Klippel-Feil anomaly (cervical fusion, short neck, low hairline) and the Sprengal deformity (elevation of the scapulae) (Erkan et al., 2001). Other less common abnormalities may be seen including laryngeal stenosis, rib anomalies, and external genital anomalies. The anal atresia may be associated with more complex anorectal anomalies such as rectovaginal, rectourethral, or rectovesical fistulae (Källén et al., 2001).

The key clinical guidance implied in the term "association" is to begin with the acronym, and, only after addressing its specific general components, systematically extend one's search for variants from there. With this general overview of VACTERL association in mind, one can consider essential points in the care of children with this condition.

Making the Initial Diagnosis The diagnosis of VACTERL association is typically made early in the child's life. In the delivery room, obvious morphologic features may be evident, if in fact prenatal diagnosis has not already alerted the obstetrician and pediatrician of potential differences (Table 8.2-2). In every case, attention to the infant's airway is the most important consideration. Respiratory distress may reflect tracheal airway malformation, and providing oxygen, even if by mask or "blow by," will provide a small amount of additional time and latitude to further consider the possibility of airway malformation, restrictive lung disease, or cyanotic heart disease.

Because some features of VACTERL association may also occur in CHARGE association (presented

Table 8.2-2. Diagnostic and treatment priorities by system of VACTERL association

Predominant feature	Diagnostic priorities	Essential anticipatory care and surveillance	Consultation priorities
Musculoskeletal abnormalities	Perform physical examination. Take x-ray skeletal survey. Take magnetic resonance imaging (MRI) of the spine and posterior fossa.	Determine functional capacity of spine and long bones. Monitor for scoliosis, leg length discrepancy, altered range of motion, arthritis, and arthralgia arthroses.	Orthopedic surgeon Hand surgeon Neurosurgeon Psychiatrist Physical therapist Occupational therapist
Genitourinary anomalies	Determine if bowel obstruction is present. Conduct an abdominal-renal ultrasound.	Anticipate early surgical management. Anticipate need for ostomy. Anticipate bowel and bladder incontinence. Check for ambiguous genitalia.	Pediatric general surgeon Urologist Visiting nurse Ostomy specialist
Airway and upper gastrointestinal abnormalities	Determine airway patency in the newborn period. Perform a bronchoscopy and/or endoscopy.	Check for gastroesophogeal reflux and aspiration. Determine the need for a gastrostomy or jejeunostomy tube. Determine the need for surgical repair of tracheoesophageal fistula. Consider the presence of laryngeal malformation.	Pediatric general surgeon Otolaryngologist Respiratory therapist
Other abnormalities or issues	Conduct a chest x-ray. Conduct an electrocardiogram. Conduct a head computerized axial tomography or MRI.	Monitor for evidence of congenital heart disease, central nervous system malformation, or eye abnormalities.	Geneticist Ophthalmologist

next), any child with obvious congenital malformations should raise the possibility of choanal atresia. If respiratory distress occurs and the clinical impression is poor movement of air through the nostrils, passage of a nasogastric tube will help to establish if the airway is patent. Being able to pass the tube into the stomach and aspirating stomach contents suggests no esophageal atresia but does not rule out H-type tracheoesophageal fistula, which may account for aspiration and respiratory distress.

Palpation of the entire length of the spine may uncover irregularities in one or more vertebrae, and careful examination of the location of the child's hairline can aid in identifying potential cervical spine abnormalities when the hairline appears unusually low. Renal abnormalities, unless imperforate anus or urogenital defects are obvious, may be difficult to diagnosis, even with careful palpation of the abdomen. Consider these possibilities in more than 50% of children who have imperforate anus (Denton, 1982).

Although x-ray, and cardiac imaging will provide more precise details in suspected cardiac, limb, or spine defects, the clinician should use the acronym in prioritizing further workup. This should prompt him or her to consider cardiac malformation, tracheoesophageal fistulae, and bowel obstruction (even if the anus is displaced or slightly abnormal) as the most critical concerns in the early postnatal period. Spine and limb anomalies can be evaluated once the child is stabilized.

Anticipating Outcome and Planning Care Care, counseling, and advocacy priorities are outlined in Table 8.2-2. Based on case literature and unreported clinical experience, VACTERL association should not be considered or portrayed to parents or professionals as a "mental retardation condition" because this is rarely the case. More often, children with VACTERL association have normal brain anatomy and can achieve normal cognitive, speech, and social developmental milestones (Jones, 1997).

Clinicians should anticipate, however, the potential for gross and fine motor delay if limb anomalies or limited postural support due to the vertebral abnormalities interfere with attainment of normal motor milestones. One proviso should be considered as well: the impact of multiple surgical procedures on the child's development. Clinicians should expect and be proactive about evaluating delay in any developmental milestone in the setting of stressful, painful, or chronically debilitating procedures, including even routine postoperative or well-child care.

The diagnosis of VACTERL, or documentation of most, if not all, of its components, will qualify the child for early intervention services as an "established condition." This diagnosis, along with pain- and stress-free treatment protocols and the constant availability of caring adults, will minimize the risk of anxiety, depression, or slower-than-expected recovery of lost developmental skills. Often, families become overly engaged in the logistics of medical management, so the primary care provider can remind them that *disability* is a relative term, and that typical experiences can complement normal development, strengthen a child's self-image and self-esteem, and reduce the family's sense that a disability exists (Lerner & Lerner, 1977). Children with VACTERL association may have visible congenital anomalies, so a "can-do" or "overly self-assured" attitude gleaned from trying typical activities and challenges will help them deal with potential teasing or social challenges when they get older.

Helping Educators Understand the Child and His or Her Potential in School Educator training focuses primarily on the theories and techniques of teaching, not on medical diagnosis and management. Even in the field of special education, educators need and appreciate similar anticipatory guidelines as families receive from health professionals, but they often have limited access or guidance to seek it. In the case of VACTERL association, the child's appearance may project inaccurate impressions of his or her health or potential, so a major priority of the family and primary care professionals is to familiarize teachers and therapists with the child (see Table 8.2-3).

Clinicians should outline the child's level of endurance and physical capabilities. Vertebral anomalies, with the exception of rare cases, are usually stable and do not fracture, and if a child wishes to, he or she should be encouraged to participate in the same school activities as his or her peers (Pillemer & Cook, 1989). Congenital heart disease, especially if cyanotic, will affect on a child's endurance, and it is helpful to point this out to dispel the concern that the child is coming to school "critically ill" or too fragile to partake in many, if not most, of the routines (Rosenthal & Jacobson, 1968). Once repaired, tracheoesophageal fistulae may be associated with gastroesophageal reflux. Clinical risk may include aspiration and pneumonia, which, from an educational standpoint, are treatable and have symptoms similar to any pulmonic respiratory infection.

Toileting may be challenge for the child with VACTERL if he or she requires colostomy for a gastrointestinal malformation because of potential problems with hygiene, access to a bathroom in school, embarrassment, and self-consciousness. Children with anorectal malformations may have difficulties with encopresis,

Table 8.2-3. Areas of educational support for children with multiple congenital conditions

Educational issue	Educational considerations	Possible actions
Understanding the diagnosis	Educational literature is generally deficient in information about rare childhood conditions. Development of an individualized educational program will be extremely difficult without a better understanding of the child's condition.	Conduct a parent–teacher meeting with the primary care provider present. Read functional ability-focused literature. Communicate unknown information about the intellectual abilities of the child.
Vision and hearing concerns	Separate "pull-out" sessions with occupational therapy, physical therapy, speech pathology, education, and nursing may reduce time for socialization and challenge academic learning. Schools often have shortages of teachers of blind and deaf children. Specialty schools should be included in educational planning discussions. Expect atypical behaviors seen in children with vision and hearing impairments that mimic social language disorders, including autism.	"Adaptive" therapies may be preferable. Early involvement of technology support is helpful. Place judicial emphasis on teaching techniques employing visual and auditory cues.
Socialization with peers	Developmental ages of typical children affect their capacity to support and accommodate children with congenital abnormalities.	Conduct an educational dialogue with peers and their parents if needed. Praise and encouragement will be copied and assimilated by classmates if witnessed. Support the child's right to discuss his or her differences with peers and adults.
Activities of daily living	Depending on the child, nursing may play a central role. Accessibility may be an issue.	Add special needs care protocols to the individualized education program. Have a private bathroom for children with incontinence. Use single-level schools or grades if possible.

soiling, and the tell-tale odor of leakage of stool and urine through an incompetent sphincter or rectourethral fistulae (Bulut & Tekant, 1991). The anatomic differences that cause these things to occur should be explained in detail to teachers, with drawings and diagrams if necessary. Most important, the family and, at some point early in the process, the *child* should convene with teachers to develop a plan to deal with incontinence that minimizes difficulty or embarrassment.

Helping Parents Understand Their Child's Condition Parents of a child with VACTERL association should insist on understanding the anatomic differences that constitute their child's condition. This information frequently overwhelms parents when initially presented. Diagrams, drawings, and analogies using common terms and concepts are especially helpful. Such analogies as "plumbing" to describe the renal system or differently shaped or asymmetric "building blocks" to describe vertebrae are rarely insulting to parents and often help demystify the child's dysplastic anatomy.

Parents of children undergoing spinal fusion or limb reconstruction often expect a surgical site to be fragile and tenuous throughout the child's life. Usually, uncomplicated bone fusions can be stronger than the initial anatomy, and a review of how bone callous reorganizes and reshapes can help families understand ultimate surgical outcomes.

Although not a consideration for all children with VACTERL, parents should understand that one long-term effect of bowel surgery is a change in bowel motility and peristalsis due both to interruption in intrinsic bowel wall nervous innervation and possible bowel diversion or reconstruction. Sometimes, these functions can return or be relearned by the child, so parents should pay attention to changing gastrointestinal function over time.

With respect to social-emotional development, parents should understand that preschool through approximately fourth grade is a period in which peers naturally want to be accepting of others and will include children with subtle or obvious disabilities into their world of play and friendship. A child with VACTERL association should be as full a participant with peers as possible and should try things that on first blush may seem difficult to do. Children who feel or who have been taught to feel vulnerable and fragile often struggle through periods of intense peer pressure in the later school years, especially if they encounter teasing. Parents can anticipate this common social challenge and help their children to carry confidence into adolescence (Kaufman, 1972, Pierce & Wardle, 1993).

CHARGE Association

Suzie was delivered at term via cesarean section to a 28-year-old mother of three. Prenatal ultrasound was suggestive of complex congenital heart disease. In the delivery room, Suzie was cyanotic and in significant respiratory distress. Passage of a nasopharyngeal catheter was unsuccessful through both nares, and she required immediate oropharyngeal intubation and mechanical ventilation.

Suzie's cyanosis persisted, consistent with cyanotic heart disease, and she was small for gestational age, with a head circumference appropriate for size. The physical examination was further notable for bilateral external ear deformities, bilateral choroids coloboma, and an asymmetrical cry. Further evaluation identified tetrology of Fallot, bilateral boney choanal atresia, and bilateral profound sensorineural deafness. Despite her coloboma, Suzie had functional vision with corrective lenses.

She underwent successful repair of her congenital heart malformation and choanal artesia, both by her third birthday and began to receive early intervention services before she was 6 months of age. In elementary school, with a special education program in place, she became an avid reader, could lip read, and could carry on clear conversations with effort. By early high school, she asked to attend a school for deaf children in order to learn and use sign language, and she remained at that school until graduation. Following graduation from secondary school, she continued in a prevocational program for 1 year, then attended a community college near her family's home. She is currently seeking employment in a telemarketing company.

Suzie is extremely proficient in computer use and has a large number of friends with whom she maintains close and regular ties via e-mail. Her family is close-knit, and have always encouraged her to try her best at everything she does. Her parents and brothers have all been strong disability rights advocates.

Perhaps more than many multiple congenital anomaly conditions, CHARGE association represents an example of concomitant abnormalities whose variability means the difference between significant impairment or remarkable achievement in overcoming disabilities. Each element of this nonrandom association can be essentially inconsequential or extremely complex. Many principles discussed for VACTERL apply to CHARGE association. CHARGE association, first suggested by Bryan Hall in 1979, consists of six mnemonic elements that correspond to the following clinical features (Hall, 1979):

1. Coloboma
2. Heart defects
3. Atresia choanae (choanal atresis)
4. Retarded growth and development
5. Genital anomalies
6. External ear and/or deafness

Unlike VACTERL association, the components of CHARGE association may be divided into potentially significant sensory abnormalities (external ear and/or deafness, and coloboma), constitutional or endocrine-metabolic differences (retarded growth, genital anomalies), and potentially life-threatening health conditions (heart defects, choanal atresia). These health-related problems may directly impact developmental outcome (Davenport, Hefner, & Mitchell, 1986; Källén, Robert, Mastroiacovo, Castilla, & Källén, 1999; Pagon, Graham, Zonana, & Yong, 1981; see also Figure 8.2-3). Table 8.2-4 outlines essential clinical considerations of CHARGE association.

Although the criteria for CHARGE are generally accepted, relationships between individual features will vary. Choanal atresia is most often used as the index finding, possibly because it presents most dramatically and correlates best with the other associated features (Harris & Källén, 1997). CHARGE association is often referred to as a syndrome because concomitant features tend to occur more predictably than other associations, and many clinicians feel that CHARGE association has a recognizable "facies."

C	Coloboma (may involve retina, choroid, and iris)
H	Congenital heart disease (includes endocardial cushion defects, valvular heart defects, transposition of the great vessels, heterotaxy, and complex cyanotic heart disease)
A	Atresia choanae, or choanal atresia (includes unilateral and/or bilateral bony or membranous choanal atresia as well as choanal stenosis)
R	Retarded growth and development (short stature, developmental delay, including mental retardation in children at highest risk)
G	Genital anomalies (originally described in boys)
E	External ear anomalies, conductive and/or sensorineural hearing loss or deafness, and inner ear malformations

Figure 8.2-3. Features of CHARGE association.

CHARGE association is a sporadic condition, but numerous familiar case reports exist, and deletions of the short arm of chromosome 3 or a balanced 6–8 translocation have been described. Estimated prevalence is 1:10,000 (Källén et al., 1999). The pathoetiology has been hypothesized as abnormal migration of embryonic cephalic neural crest to a number of target structures throughout the developing embryo. Destinations that give rise to elements of the branchial arches of the head; boney nasal choanae; retina, choroids, and iris; thymus; testes; ovaries; peripheral nerves; and the conotruncal cardiac midline are among those sites that subsequently lack normal populations of these neurectoderm precursors (Lin, Chin, Devine, Park, & Zackai, 1987; Siebert, Graham, & MacDonald, 1985).

Some evidence suggests that other central nervous system structures are usually normal and that significant cognitive impairments and intellectual disabilities result from catastrophic events associated with complete upper airway obstruction by choanal atresia or identifiable brain malformations (Harvey, Leaper, & Bankier, 1991; Kaplan, 1985; Lin, Siebert, & Graham, 1990). Growth retardation is rarely associated with any endocrinologic abnormalities, and the combination of increased calorie requirements due to heart disease and/or chronic airway insufficiency, may contribute to delayed growth. The reason for intrauterine growth retardation and postnatal growth delay is not understood (Davenport et al., 1986). Like other multiple malformation syndrome or associations, a number of other abnormalities may be seen in CHARGE association, including rib and spine anomalies, micrognathia, and craniofacial anomalies, prompting the clinician to complete a thorough initial assessment (Källén et al., 1999).

Making the Initial Diagnosis The initial diagnosis is based on the suspicion of uncovering specific obvious abnormalities, and on more careful testing of vision and hearing in this condition. Seven percent of children with CHARGE association have an asymmetric cry, but respiratory distress or evidence of cardiac disease provide the earliest clues for the diagnosis (Asher, McGill, Kaplan, Friedman, & Healy, 1990). In cases where bilateral boney choanal atresia are present, respiratory distress can be severe and encountered immediately at birth. Although computed tomography (CT) or magnetic resonance imaging (MRI) scanning will provide definitive diagnosis of choanal atresia, inability to pass a nasogastric tube through the nostrils or difficulty placing an endotracheal tube through the nares suggest choanal atresia. Because respiratory failure may be imminent, orotracheal intubation with mechanical ventilation is appropriate to prevent profound hypoxia (Blake, Russell-Eggitt, Morgan, Ratcliffe, & Wyse, 1990). Often, continuous positive airway pressure alone is adequate when upper airway obstruction is the cause of the respiratory distress.

Aside from features evident on physical exam, particularly microtia and microphallus in boys, the remainder of the diagnosis can be made more deliberately, utilizing more precisely brain stem auditory evoked responses to test hearing and consultation with an ophthalmologist for a thorough eye exam (Baer, Poulsen, Howard-Teplansky, & Harris, 1999). Although sometimes evident in the iris, coloboma are more commonly seen in CHARGE association in the choroid and retina and are often beyond the ability of a standard ophthalmoscope.

Making the diagnosis with fewer than four features can be difficult, and as in any congenital abnormality, the assessment by a geneticist/dysmorphologist is essential. In older children with microtia and coloboma, for example, finding sensorineural hearing loss strengthens the diagnosis; however, some geneticists may make this diagnosis based on fewer features. Because one or more features of CHARGE association can overlap with known chromosome abnormalities, one of them (i.e., Trisomy 18) being lethal, it is advisable to obtain a chromosome analysis that includes banding to look for the kinds of interstitial deletions, duplications, and rearrangements that are being identified with increasing frequency due to more thorough genetic testing of children with errors of morphogenesis (Blake et al., 1998; Oley, Baraitser, & Grant, 1988).

Anticipating Outcome and Planning Care CHARGE association presents unique challenges in terms of prioritizing care as outlined in Table 8.2-4. Health care priorities must be established for any child with significant cardiac disease as well as the pattern of

Table 8.2-4. Diagnostic and treatment priorities by system for the CHARGE association

Predominant feature	Diagnostic priorities	Essential anticipatory care and surveillance	Consultation priorities
Potential airway obstruction due to choanal malformation	Establish airway patency in the delivery room without waiting for imaging studies.	Plan a surgical strategy to minimize hospitalizations. Avoid chronic use of nasal stents and dilatation procedures.	Otolaryngology Plastic surgery
Cardiac malformation	Conduct a clinical exam with initial electrocardiogram and chest x-ray. Take blood pressure for four extremities.	Consider temporary placement of a tracheostomy if repeated anesthesia is anticipated for cardiac procedures and if child experiences restenosis of choanae after extubation.	Cardiology Cardiothoracic surgery
Genitourinary track abnormalities	Conduct a careful examination with an abdominal-renal ultrasound for newborns.	Urinary tract infections in boys or girls with CHARGE warrant further investigation.	Urology
Risk of deafness	Newborn hearing screening is helpful but not adequate.	Pattern of external ear anomalies do not predict if child will have sensorineural hearing loss or deafness.	Otolaryngology Audiology
Risk of blindness	Newborn eye exam is not definitive. Receive an ophthalmology consultation.	Coloboma may obscure the optic nerve and cause blindness. Microphthalmia may occur. A prosthetic eye will reduce orbit deformation over time.	Ophthalmology
Slow growth	Assess the child's ability to breathe and swallow by observation and possibly cinefluoroscopy.	Consider early placement of a gastrostomy or jejeunostomy tube if oromotor skills or surgery will interfere with the child's nutition and growth.	Gastroenterology
Developmental monitoring	Conduct a developmental evaluation beginning in the child's first 6 months.	Interdisciplinary assessment will provide the most useful and comprehensive data to the family and school. Recurrent illness and surgery may result in developmental setbacks that are not necessarily permanent.	Qualified child development specialty team

choanal atresia that creates significant upper airway obstruction. One clinician's experience caring for more than 100 children with CHARGE association is that otorhinolaryngologic management should be aggressive, and a key goal should be to establish through surgery, if necessary, as patent and as functional an upper airway as possible early in the child's life. The most frequent cause of hospitalization of children with CHARGE association is upper airway obstruction, aspiration pneumonia, and vomiting secondary to abnormal anatomy of the nasal airway (Kaplan, 2004).

Developmental priorities must include careful attention to the care of a child with potential multisensory disability including profound sensorineural deafness and/or visual impairment. A helpful developmental surveillance strategy is to anticipate and address the types of developmental complications of sensory disability, including 1) speech and language delay, 2) gross and fine motor planning and coordination difficulties, 3) limited or impaired access and assimilation of new information, and 4) patterns of inattentiveness that may reflect both attention deficit disorder, as well as the inattentiveness that occurs when sensory input is incomplete or diminished (Goldson, Smith, & Stewart, 1986). As a model for children with congenital sensorineural deafness, involving audiology early is advisable, especially because some of the inner ear malformations seen in CHARGE association can cause progressive hearing loss prompting adjustments in amplification aids or consideration of cochlear implants (Langman, Quiglet, & Souliere, 1996; Lin et al., 1990).

Although both VACTERL and CHARGE associations are not typically associated with significant cognitive disabilities, intellectual disabilities become more of a concern in the presence of microcephaly, significant motor findings (e.g., spasticity), profound hypotonia, or seizures. They can be diagnosed most accurately in children after age 6, but early developmental testing using such tools as the Bayley Scales for Infant Development (Bayley, 1993) can be used to guide in the discussion about significant delays appearing during infancy and in the toddler years. For any condition in which vision and auditory input is altered, however, tools that rely on these modalities for data may be less predictive of intellectual disabilities. An expert in the developmental evaluation of children with blindness and deafness can be a valuable resource in assessing children with CHARGE association (Davidson & Harrison, 1997; Moores, 1997).

Helping Educators Understand the Child and His or Her Potential in School Advising schools that the child has a sensory impairment and needs appropriate modifications is, in many ways, more important for educational planning than describing his or her medical needs (see Table 8.2-3). Like VACTERL association, CHARGE association involves both health and developmental risks and, as such, should meet the eligibility requirements for special education and other services for children with vision and hearing impairments. The child can be presented to teachers as someone who will require special services but who will also benefit greatly from the socialization that occurs in an inclusive classroom. Another important concept to share with teachers is the notion that "distractibility" may reflect the sensory impairment and not attention-deficit/hyperactivity disorder. Asking teachers to observe the child when he or she has close one-to-one teacher support and adequate access to the schoolwork may demonstrate that the child has good attentiveness and concentration, pointing away from an attention disorder.

Helping Parents Understand Their Child's Condition Parents of children with CHARGE association should be aware of the unusually strong family support resources throughout the world for CHARGE association. They should also know that much can be learned from what families and professionals already know about children who are deaf or blind. This will help them make informed decisions concerning such issues as total communication, signing, deaf education, cochlear implantation, and plastic surgery of the external ears. Finally, parents should constantly keep in mind that health and development are "equals" in terms of their importance to follow-up care. As early as the child is referred to appropriate medical-surgical specialists, he or she should be also referred to a strong child development evaluation team for initial assessment, follow-up care, and access to individuals who can assist with educational planning through late adolescence and possibly beyond.

CRANIOFACIAL ANOMALIES

Craniofacial anomalies may be categorized in a novel way by considering whether a particular abnormality (or group of abnormalities) represents a malformation, deformation, or disruption, *and* whether it involves elements of asymmetry, orofacial clefting, or abnormal vascularity (see Table 8.2-5). As in many congenital abnormalities, physical features are clues to etiology, and some of these features are key indicators of sporadic conditions, whereas others strongly suggest single-gene, chromosomal conditions. *Asymmetry* may be observed in paired organ structures in which one eye or orbit, for example, will be asymmetrically smaller than the other. It can also be observed on either side of the "anatomic midline." In genetic terms, this is an embryonic reference point with some compelling experimental evidence that balanced "sidedness" may be under some genetic control.

In physical examination terms, comparing and making note of any paired structure to its counterpart is helpful (Kaplan, 1985). In hemifacial microsomia, orbit, mandible, ear, facial nerve, and soft tissue are asymmetric in approximately 90% of cases, with right-sided predominance (Converse, Coccaro, Becker, & Wood-Smith, 1973; see Table 8.2-5). Asymmetric growth and development of the brancial arches is the presumed etiology. The underlying mechanism for this asymmetry, however, is thought to be unilateral vascular *disruption.* Treacher Collins syndrome involves *bilateral* malar hypoplasia, zygomatic clefts, lateral downslanting palpebral fissures, eyelid or corneal coloboma, absent eyelashes, dental malocclusion, and marked micrognathia and is a symmetrical disorder. Etiologically, Treacher Collins syndrome is a *malformation syndrome* believed to be due to mutations in the *TCOF1* gene located on chromosome 5 (Treacher Collins Syndrome Collaborative Group, 1996).

The Robin sequence, also referred to as Pierre-Robin syndrome, includes micrognathia, cleft palate, and glossoptosis with the tongue sitting posteriorly in the oropharynx (van den Elzen, Semmekrot, Bongers, Huygen, & Marres, 2001). This symmetrical craniofacial anomaly is thought in most cases to be the result of intrauterine constraint, in which a compressed growing mandible displaces the tongue in such a way that it is displaced upward, impeding normal closure of the palatal shelves and resulting in a "U-shaped" cleft palate. Robin sequence is an example of a *symmetric deformation*

Table 8.2-5. Diagnostic namogram for craniofacial anomalies with clinical examples

	Symmetry	Clefting	Vascular abnormality
Malformation	Hemifacial (craniofacial) (A) Treacher Collins syndrome (S) Binder syndrome (S)	Cleft lip Cleft palate	Sturge-Weber syndrome Proteus syndrome Klippel-Trenaunay-Weber syndrome Incontinentia pigmenti syndrome
Deformation	Twin crowding (A, S) Bicornuate uterus/fibroid (A) Postnatal positional plagiocephaly (A) Flattened occiput with supine sleep (S)	Dental malocussion in cleft palate Narrow-small palate secondary to midline cleft tongue	Webbing of the neck in cystic hygroma Tissue overgrowth with vascular malformation
Disruption	Intravenous stroke and secondary unilateral facial paralysis Microtia	Amnion rupture sequence Cleft lip Cleft palate	Hemifacial microsomia Intracranial stroke secondary to atrioventricular malformation

Key: A = asymmetric pattern; B = symmetric pattern

craniofacial syndrome. In cases where mandibular growth is abnormal due to a primary connective tissue, the mandibular defect can be considered a *symmetric malformation,* but the secondary effects will include *symmetric deformation* of the tongue and palate (Graham, 1988).

Orofacial *clefting* includes conditions in which the palate lip or portions of the superior midface have failed to close in a normal manner. The mechanisms and causes of this broad group of conditions include abnormalities in the migration, elaboration, and the differentiation of cells that populate the diverse structures that ultimately form the mature face (Young, Schneider, Hu, & Helms, 2000). Induction, expansion, and shaping of the midface also results from the forward growth of the brain. Therefore, brain malformations may result in deficiencies and underdevelopment of the midface, an important consideration in the assessment of newborns with neurologic or known neuroanatomic differences.

Genes involved in midface patterning, including genes that sequentially regulate and "orchestrate" embryonic growth, have been identified and include genes that control patterning, proliferation, differentiation, and maturation of extracellular stroma destined to become part of the head and neck. Mutations in these genes may create clear autosomal recessive and dominant patterns of craniofacial maldevelopment. The transforming growth factor (TGF) involved in facial cellular development is closely associated with this gene group (Stoll, Qian, Feingold, Sauvage, & May, 1993). These genes may be considered to cause *malformational clefting.*

Facial clefts, especially cleft lips and palate, can themselves be symmetric or asymmetric, complete or partial. Animal models and some human examples exist of facial clefting arising from compression with resultant necrosis of vascular supply and clefting along the necrotic margin. The most severe and often most dramatic clefting patterns occur as a result of disruption of normal developing midface structures including amniotic bands in which tethering and tearing of tissues occurs (Chen, Yang, Jacobson, & Sulik, 1996; Kaplan, Kurnit, & Welch, 1985; Kaplan, Matsuoka, Gilbert, Opitz, & Kurnit, 1985). Finally, prenatal exposure to known teratogenic agents, including cigarette smoking and alcohol, may cause cleft lip and palate.

Vascular craniofacial anomalies may either be malformations or disorders of vascular growth that result in distortion of the face, thus creating deformational changes in facial structures (Mulliken, Fishman, & Burrows, 2000). One example of the latter is the effect that lymphatic hypertrophy in cystic hygroma may have on the growth and stretching of overlying fetal neck skin (Saenger, 1993; Turner, 1938). In Turner and Noonan syndromes, which are associated with this vascular abnormality, children typically have deformations of the skin (redundant skin and webbed neck). Vascular malformations represent true dysplasia of vascular structures and are, therefore, also true malformations. When they occur in the head and neck, they can result in a variety of conditions including port-wine stains (Sturge-Weber syndrome), arterio-vascular malformations, and more extensive lesions as seen in various forms of the Proteus syndrome, which includes conditions that share a number of features with neurofibromatosis, Klippel-Trenauney-Weber syndrome, and others. Because they are malformations, they do not involute and disappear on their own, and, if extensive, they distort the face (Mulliken, Burrows, & Fishman, 2004).

Hemangioma are "tumors" of blood vessels bearing some resemblance to other rapidly dividing hyperplastic tumor cell types that involute spontaneously (Burns, Kaplan, & Mulliken, 1991). They can markedly distort facial structures, and craniofacial surgeons will usually wait for most of these to involute on their own by the child's second birthday before attempting to correct resultant facial deformity. Hemangiomata, while not malformations, cause *deformations* of normal facial integrity (Mulliken et al., 2004).

Prognosis is often very difficult to predict for many craniofacial anomalies, but in general, certain conditions are well understood, and surgical management is constantly being refined. Some examples include uncomplicated unilateral, and bilaterally symmetric cleft lip and palate, hemifacial microsomia, and Binder syndrome.

Diagnosis

The diagnosis of craniofacial anomalies is often made by recognizing distinct patterns that define a particular syndrome. This process is most common for distinct craniosynostosis syndromes such as Apert, Crouzon, and Pfeiffer syndromes, and for other conditions such as Treacher Collins syndrome (Cohen, 1986). Although definitive diagnosis is usually best made by an expert in craniofacial anomalies or genetics/dysmorphology, using the nomogram illustrated in Table 8.2-5 can be helpful.

The examiner should first determine if the predominant abnormality represents asymmetry, clefting, and/or vascular, then try, based on his or her level of confidence, to determine if the abnormality represents malformation, deformation, or disruption. Necessary interventions may lead one to identifying other abnormalities such as oral or oronasal malformation, but like most congenital conditions, trying to answer early if intracranial abnormalities are present is important. Clues to this answer may come from the presence of microcephaly, evidence of encephalocele or aplasia cutis, aberrant hair whorl patterns that may indicate abnormal *prenatal* brain growth, and abnormalities in the neurologic examination that point to central nervous system malformation (e.g., spasticity, seizures, paralysis, abnormal movements). All symptoms must be confirmed or further evaluated by cranial CT or MRI scanning.

Routine chromosome analysis with banding is controversial from a "cost–benefit" perspective but useful from a clinical standpoint. It is recommended especially when the examiner does not have immediate access to genetics-dysmorphology consultants or does not recognize a distinct nonchromosomal disorder. In addition, clinicians should expect that the child will have a definitive hearing and vision evaluation early in life.

Anticipating Outcome and Planning Care

Like VACTERL and CHARGE associations and a number of single-gene and chromosome syndromes, careful distinctions should be made between the craniofacial deformity and cognitive function, relying on developmental screening and a clear understanding of the child's central nervous system anatomy and function before making the conclusion of significant cognitive impairment. This distinction should always be communicated to the family, and, if necessary, to other health professionals and educators. Second, because many craniofacial abnormalities and syndromes involve the branchial arches, VIII cranial nerves, external ears, and inner ear, the child's capacity to hear at the frequency of conversational speech should be determined and followed by a qualified audiologist.

Helping Parents Understand Their Child's Condition

The primary care provider should help families become familiar with the child's craniofacial surgical plan, if one is necessary. Close attention should be paid to the age of the child when surgery is performed. Usually, craniofacial surgeons plan procedures taking into account the child's developmental and social stages and needs. For example, younger children generally handle the stresses of surgery and recovery more easily than older children, especially adolescents (Arndt, Travis, Lefebvre, & Munro, 1987). At the same time, children with some craniofacial anomalies are anxious to have corrective procedures completed because of their natural and developmentally appropriate need to feel included and accepted (Phillips & Whitaker, 1979). In this case, planning procedures based on this developmental need may be important. The primary care provider can take a proactive role in being sure the family is aware of these factors so that they can make sensible decisions for their children around the timing of surgery, recovery, and, if necessary, rehabilitation.

ALTERATIONS IN CYTOGENETIC, SINGLE GENE, AND MOLECULAR STRUCTURE AND NUMBER

For practical purposes, there are three principle domains within which the human genome is expressed and may be assessed in children. Each of these are characterized by separate methodologies and nomenclatures. These levels and their estimated contribution to birth disabilities include:

1. Chromosome (cytogenetic) expression—5%
2. Single gene (mendelian) expression—20%
3. Non-Mendelian expression including multifactoral and polygenic—75%

Chromosome Disorders

Chromosome disorders affect 1:200 newborns, yet more than 90% of embryos and fetuses with chromosome anomalies do not, in fact, survive pregnancy (Brent, 1986). Thus, although chromosome disorders are relatively frequent in living children, they still comprise a relatively small proportion of known *genetic* diseases (Hsu, 1998). Common subcategories of chromosome disorders include 1) *nondisjunction,* in which the copied chromosome pairs do not separate, leading to an imbalance in the final chromosome content of the embryo (see Table 8.2-6 for representative conditions); 2) *recombinations,* in which chromosome abnormalities occur as the result of unequal exchanges of "pieces" of different chromosomes; 3) *deletions/duplications,* in which either portions of a chromosome are missing or duplicated; and 4) *translocations,* in which breaks in two different chromosomes generate new rearrangements that may either produce new patterns of genetic information or simply result in rearrangement with no net change in information (Sutherland, 1996). Diagnosis may require both standard cytogenetic tests and the application of more sophisticated molecular analysis, such as special fluorescent in situ hybridization techniques (FISH) for specific conditions.

Single Gene Disorders

Single gene disorders derive from mutations in certain genes of one or both parents that alter normal morphogenesis or the function of enzymes that catalyze the production or degradation of important body proteins. Based on a detailed family history, specialists can often apply statistical techniques to determine if these particular disorders are autosomal dominant, recessive, or X-linked (Jones & Cahill, 1994). The family history in dominant conditions finds affected individuals in each generation, unless the child represents a first affected individual. In recessive conditions, affected individuals may "skip" generations. X-linked conditions imply that women are carriers and that men are affected.

One of the most striking aspects of single gene disorders is that they may manifest as significant malformation syndromes, or as small variations in cell function. They may cause minor difficulties, for example, in red-brown color discrimination, or result in the production of metabolic products that can cause progressive neurologic deterioration and death. A wide range of metabolic disorders, or inborn errors of metabolism, result from mutations in single genes or genes linked to one another (see Chapters 7.1–7.4). Among the best understood are Phenylketonuria, Hurler and Hunter syndromes, homocystinuria, and Tay-Sachs disease (Baer et al., 1999).

Non-Mendelian Disorders

Non-Mendelian disorders represent a growing group of conditions that do not follow the typical pattern seen in single-gene dominant, recessive, and X-linked inheritance and include novel expressions of DNA that cannot be easily predicted by Mendelian genetic statistical methods (e.g., fragile X syndrome). Multifactorial and polygenic disorders and traits fall within the group of the most common genetic conditions known in clinical practice and comprise a subset of non-Mendelian inheritance. These conditions result from the interaction of multiple genes with environmental factors (Hagerman, 1996; McKusick, 1998).

Making the Initial Diagnosis

Two clinical indications should prompt consideration of chromosome, single-gene, or non-Mendelian disorders. The first of these is the recognition of a loss of developmental milestones at any age, which is common enough in the single-gene metabolic disorders to warrant consultation (see Table 8.2-6). The second is the finding of two or more minor anomalies with or without necessarily suspecting a "named" clinical entity, or any pattern of multiple malformations. In this situation, chromosome analysis is always justified, although genetic consultation is essential to complete the evaluation (Jacobs, Browne, Gregson, Joyce, & White, 1992). "Minor anomalies" are unusual morphologic features that are of no serious medical or cosmetic consequence to the patient. They are important to consider and

Table 8.2-6. Cytogenetic, single-gene, and non-Mendelian disorders

	Condition	Pathoetiology	Clinical considerations
Cytogenetic (chromosomal)	Autosomal trisomies (e.g., Down syndrome, Trisomy 21)	1:730 live births; nondisjunction event Trisomy 21 (95%) Translocation (3%–4%) Mosaicism seen	Characteristic phenotype Hypotonia IQ score 25–50, occasionally > 50 Congenital heart disease in 40% Duodenal atresia and annular occur Incidence of Alzheimer-like dementia higher in later life
	Autosomal deletions 5p– (e.g., Cri du Chat syndrome)	Partial deletion of the short arm of chromosome number 5 1:20,000–1:50,000 Involves critical region 5p15.3	Low birth weight Failure to thrive Hypotonia High cry Intellectual disabilities Microcephaly Hypertelorism Malformed ears IQ score < 20 Potentially lethal condition
	Contiguous gene syndromes (e.g., Angelman syndrome)	Small maternally-derived interstitial deletion between 15q11 and 15q13 Genotype overlap with possible Prader-Willi syndrome	Microcephaly Maxillary hypoplasia prognathism Ataxia Severe to profound intellectual disabilities Loss of motor and sensory skills possible
	Sex chromosome anomalies (e.g., Turner syndrome, XO)	Aneuploidy, rearrangement, or mosaicism 1:400 live births 50% have monosomy 45X	Short stature Shield chest Wide-spaced nipples Webbed neck Lymphatic malformation of neck Cubitus valgus Nevi Streak ovaries and infertility Developmental delay or mild intellectual disabilities Verbal IQ performance higher than performance IQ score
Single gene	Autosomal dominant (e.g., Apert syndrome)	Single-gene mutation expressed equally in boys and girls Some variable expressivity	Craniosynostosis Syndactyly Brachycephaly Midface retrusion Occasional cleft palate Kleeblattschadel deformity of skull
	Autosomal recessive (e.g., phenylketonuria, PKU)	Single-gene mutation for enzyme phenylalanine Hydroxylase Altered phenylalanine metabolism resulting in elevation of neurotoxic metabolites	Included in newborn metabolic screening panel in all U.S. states Low phenylalanine diet to prevent intellectual disabilities and motor disability Special obstetrical care during pregnancy for mothers with PKU
	X-linked inheritance (e.g., incontinentia pigmenti—recessive form)	Deletion gene transmitted via the X chromosome No male–male transmission Dominant form lethal in males	Irregular pigmented lesions preceded by blisters Hypodontia Approximately 30% have developmental delay, microcephaly, spasticity, or seizures
Non-Mendelian inheritance	Unstable deoxyribonucleic acid (DNA; e.g., fragile X syndrome)	Fragile X mutation in the region of unstable CGG triplet repeats on the X chromosome	Most common form of familial intellectual disabilities in boys Mild to severe intellectual disabilities

Table 8.2-6. *(continued)*

Condition	Pathoetiology	Clinical considerations
	Incidence 1:1,000 in boys, 1:2,000 in girls	Speech and language delay Narrow face Large jaw Ears that appear long Postpubertal macroorchidism in boys in the differential diagnosis of pervasive developmental delay
Multifactorial inheritance (e.g., spina bifida)	Combined effects of multiple genes and environmental factors Increased recurrence risk with each affected family member 1–2:1,000 frequency	Clinical spectrum includes anencephaly, primary and secondary neural tube defects that are often associated with Arnold-Chiari II malformation Developmental and motor delay expected Intellectual disabilities not expected but are seen with more severe cases
Mitochondrial inheritance (e.g., Leigh syndrome)	Mutation of susceptible mitochondrial DNA (mtDNA) resulting in the dysfunction of electron transport chain	May present as delayed milestones, congenital global developmental delay, seizures, or white matter degeneration Visceromegaly rare in most conditions Some instances lethal

note because of the strong association between finding them and uncovering more complex major anomalies, including cardiac, renal, and central nervous system abnormalities.

Finally, like many other fields in medicine, the redundancy of physical findings between every category of abnormality, especially craniofacial and chromosomal disorders, should encourage, not dissuade, the clinician from requesting chromosome analysis, metabolite studies such as serum quantitative amino acids, or DNA-based analysis for specific conditions. Having these studies complete by the time a full genetic evaluation is planned helps both the geneticist and the family use their time more efficiently and may expedite final diagnosis.

Anticipating Outcomes and Planning Care

Every child with special needs benefits from a care plan based on the known natural history of his or her unique condition. Clinicians should recognize however, that the natural history of the individual clinical components of multisystem disorders is as much a contributor to the overall outcome as the condition itself. In other words, successful organ or system-specific care may not always be possible in some conditions, and these alone may result in death or significant disability.

Helping Educators Understand the Child and His or Her Potential in School

The approach to informing educators about genetic disorders should be similar to that described elsewhere in this chapter (see Table 8.2-3); however, there is a relative paucity of developmental data for this group of children. The growth of disorder-specific parent–professional partnerships that focus considerable attention on gathering this data has made some inroads for some conditions, notably, but not exclusively, organizations for Down, Williams, Prader-Willi, and Angelman syndromes; the myopathies; storage disorders; and conditions involving short stature. Parent–professional information from these organizations can provide a wealth of information to educators and parents about both the natural history of rare disorders, as well as educational, social, and support needs.

Helping Parents Understand Their Child's Condition

As is the case with many genetic disorders, some parents of children with single-gene disorders may find themselves to be the most up-to-date source of information about their children in their community—whether they choose to be or not. Therefore, primary care providers should ask them periodically if they are finding this responsibility overwhelming or undesirable. Many parents function in this extended role because they feel that there is no one else nearby who can help them, and this responsibility tires them. Exhaustion is usually a strong indicator of parents' need for care coordination or case management. Involving this resource should not be interpreted as taking informed parenting roles away from the child's parents. The primary care provider can also help in these situations by reminding parents that even experts need help and that their knowledge has made an impact on others responsible for their child's health and education.

CONCLUSION

Taking a coordinating role in the evaluation and care of children with multiple congenital anomalies and multiple medical problems is a rewarding experience for primary care providers. Although pediatric care of children with special needs will continue to benefit from the advances in basic research and clinical subspecialty care, primary care providers will always play a key advocacy role and should feel confident in applying these basic principles of dysmorphology and habilitation in the medical home setting.

REFERENCES

Arndt, E.M., Travis, F., Lefebvre, A., & Munro, I.R. (1987). Psychosocial adjustment of 20 patients with Treacher Collins syndrome before and after reconstructive surgery. *British Journal of Plastic Surgery, 40*(6), 605–609.

Asher, B.F., McGill, T.J., Kaplan, L., Friedman, E.M., & Healy, G.B. (1990). Airway complications in CHARGE association. *Archives of Otolaryngology—Head & Neck Surgery, 116*(5), 594–595.

Baer, M.T., Poulsen, M.K., Howard-Teplansky, R.B., & Harris, A.B. (1999). Effects of nutrition on development and behavior. In M.D. Levine, W.B. Carey, & A.C. Crocker (Eds.), *Developmental pediatrics* (3rd ed., pp. 294–309). Philadelphia: W.B. Saunders.

Bayley, N. (1993). *Bayley Scales of Infant Development—Second Edition.* San Antonio: The Psychological Corporation.

Blake, K.D., Davenport, S.L., Hall, B.D., Hefner, M.A., Pagon, R.A, Williams, M.S., et al. (1998). CHARGE association: An update and review for the primary pediatrician. *Clinical Pediatrics, 37*(3), 159–173.

Blake, K.D., Russell-Eggitt, I.M., Morgan, D.W., Ratcliffe, J.M., & Wyse, R.K. (1990). Who's in CHARGE? Multidisciplinary management of patients with CHARGE association. *Archives of Disease in Childhood, 65*(2), 217–223.

Botto, L.D., Khoury, M.J., Mastroiacovo, P., Castilla, E.E., Moore, C.A., Skjaerven, R., et al. (1997). The spectrum of congenital anomalies of the VATER association: An international study. *American Journal of Medical Genetics, 71*(1), 8–15.

Brent, R.L. (1986). The complexities of solving the problem of human malformations. *Clinics in Perinatology, 13*(3), 491–503.

Bulut, M., & Tekant, G. (1991). Encopretic children: Experience with fifty cases. *Turkish Journal of Pediatrics, 33,* 167.

Burns, A.J., Kaplan, L.C., & Mulliken, J.B. (1991). Is there an association between hemangioma and syndromes with dysmorphic features? *Pediatrics, 88*(6), 1257–1267.

Chen, S.Y., Yang, B., Jacobson, K., & Sulik, K.K. (1996). The membrane disordering effect of ethanol on neural crest cells in vitro and the protective role of GM1 ganglioside. *Alcohol, 13*(6), 589–595.

Cohen, M.M. (Ed.). (1986). *Craniosynostosis: Diagnosis, evaluation, and management.* New York: Raven Press.

Converse, J.M., Coccaro, P.J., Becker, M., & Wood-Smith, D. (1973). On hemifacial microsomia: The first and second branchial arch syndrome. *Plastic & Reconstructive Surgery, 51*(3), 268–279.

Damian, M.S., Seibel, P., Schachenmayr, W., Reichmann, H., & Dorndorf, W. (1996). VACTERL with the mitochondrial np 3243 point mutation. *American Journal of Medical Genetics, 62*(4), 398–403.

Davenport, S.L.H., Hefner, M.A., & Mitchell, J.A. (1986). The spectrum and clinical features in CHARGE syndrome. *Clinical Genetics, 29,* 298–310.

Davidson, P., & Harrison, G. (1997). The effectiveness of early intervention for children with visual impairment. In M. Guarlnick (Ed.), *The effectiveness of early intervention* (pp. 483–495). Baltimore: Paul H. Brookes Publishing Co.

Denton J.R. (1982). The association of congenital spinal anomalies with imperforate anus. *Clinical Orthopaedics & Related Research, 162,* 91–98.

Erkan, D., Lam, L.A., Yazici, Y., & Magid, S.K. (2001). VATER association: Is it recognised by rheumatologists? *Clinical Rheumatology, 20*(2), 128–131.

Goldson, E., Smith, A.C., & Stewart, J.M. (1986). The CHARGE association: How well can they do? *American Journal of Diseases of Children, 140*(9), 918–921.

Graham, J.M. (1988). *Smith's recognizable patterns of human deformation.* Philadelphia: W.B. Saunders.

Hagerman, R.J. (Ed.). (1996). *Fragile X syndrome: Diagnosis, treatment, and research* (2nd ed.). Baltimore: Johns Hopkins University Press.

Hall, B.D. (1979). Choanal atresia and associated multiple anomalies. *Journal of Pediatrics, 95*(3), 395–398.

Haller, J.O., Berdon, W.E., Levin, T.L., & Iyer, K.V. (2004). Tracheoesophageal fistula (H-type) in neonates with imperforate anus and the VATER association. *Pediatric Radiology, 34,* 83–85.

Harris, J.R.E., & Källén, B. (1997). Epidemiology of choanal atresia with special reference to the CHARGE association. *Pediatrics, 99*(3), 363–367.

Harvey, A.S., Leaper, P.M., & Bankier, A. (1991). CHARGE association: Clinical manifestations and developmental outcome. *American Journal of Medical Genetics, 39*(1), 48–55.

Hsu, L.Y.F. (1998). Prenatal diagnosis of chromosomal abnormalities through amniocentesis. In A. Milunsky (Ed.), *Genetic disorders and the fetus* (4th ed., pp. 179). Baltimore: Johns Hopkins University Press.

Jacobs, P.A., Browne, C., Gregson, N., Joyce, C., & White, H. (1992). Estimates of the frequency of chromosome abnormalities detectable in unselected newborns using moderate levels of banding. *Journal of Medical Genetics, 29*(2), 103–108.

Jones, K. (1997). *Smith's recognizable patterns of human malformation* (5th ed.). Philadelphia: W.B. Saunders.

Jones, O.W., & Cahill, T.C. (1994). Basic genetics and patterns of inheritance. In R.K. Creasy & R. Resnik (Eds.), *Maternal fetal medicine* (3rd ed., p. 35). Philadelphia: W.B. Saunders.

Källén, K., Mastroiacovo, P., Castilla, E.E., & Källén, B. (2001). VATER non-random association of congenital malformations: Study based on data from four malformation registers. *American Journal of Medical Genetics, 101*(1), 26–32.

Källén, K., Robert, E., Mastroiacovo, P,. Castilla, E.E., & Källén, B. (1999). CHARGE association in newborns: A registry-based study. *Teratology, 60*(6), 334–343.

Kaplan, L.C. (1985). Choanal atresia and its associated anomalies: Further support for the CHARGE association. *International Journal of Pediatric Otorhinolaryngology, 8*(3), 237–242.

Kaplan, L.C. (2004). *Personal observations.* Unpublished document.

Kaplan, L.C., Kurnit, D.M., & Welch, K.J. (1985). Anterior midline defects: Association with ectopia cordis or vascular dysplasia defines two distinct entities. *American Journal of Medical Genetics, 21*(1), 203–204.

Kaplan, L.C., Matsuoka, R., Gilbert, E.F., Opitz, J.M., & Kurnit, D.M. (1985). Ectopia cordis and cleft sternum: Evidence for mechanical teratogenesis following rupture of the chorion or yolk sac. *American Journal of Medical Genetics, 21*(1), 187–202.

Kaufman, R.V. (1972). Body image in physically ill teen-agers. *Journal of the American Academy of Child Psychiatry, 11,* 157.

Khoury, M.J., Cordero, J.F., Greenberg, F., James, L.M., & Erickson, J.D. (1983). A population study of the VACTERL association: Evidence for its etiologic heterogeneity. *Pediatrics, 71*(5), 815–820.

Langman, A.W., Quiglet, S.M., & Souliere, C.R. (1996). Cochlear implants in children. *Pediatric Clinics of North America, 43*(6), 1217.

Lerner, R.M., & Lerner, J. (1977). Effects of age, sex, and physical attractiveness on a child–peer relative, academic performance, and elementary school adjustment. *Developmental Psychology, 13,* 585.

Lin, A.E., Chin, A.J., Devine, W., Park, S.C., & Zackai, E. (1987). The pattern of cardiovascular malformation in the CHARGE association. *American Journal of Diseases of Children, 141*(9), 1010–1013.

Lin, A.E., Siebert, J.R., & Graham, J.M, Jr. (1990). Central nervous system malformations in the CHARGE association. *American Journal of Medical Genetics, 37*(3), 304–310.

McKusick, V.A. (1998). *Mendelian inheritance in man.* Baltimore: Johns Hopkins University Press.

Moores, D.F. (1997). Educating the deaf (3rd ed.). In National Institutes of Health, *Early identification of hearing loss in infants and young children: Consensus development conference of early identification of hearing loss in infants and young children.* Boston: Houghton Mifflin.

Mulliken, J.B., Burrows, P.E., & Fishman, S.J. (Eds.). (2004). *Vascular anomalies: Hemangiomas and malformations.* Oxford, England: Oxford University Press.

Mulliken, J.B., Fishman, S.J., & Burrows, P.E. (2000). Vascular anomalies: Review. *Current Problems in Surgery, 37*(8), 517–584.

Oley, C.A., Baraitser, M., & Grant, D.B. (1988). A reappraisal of the CHARGE association. *Journal of Medical Genetics, 25*(3), 147–156.

Pagon, R.A., Graham, J.M., Jr., Zonana, J., & Yong, S.L. (1981). Coloboma, congenital heart disease, and choanal atresia with multiple anomalies: CHARGE association. *Journal of Pediatrics, 99*(2), 223–227.

Phillips, J., & Whitaker, L.A. (1979). The social effects of craniofacial deformity and its correction. *Cleft Palate Journal, 16*(1), 7.

Pierce, J.W., & Wardle, J. (1993). Self-esteem, parental approval, and body size in children. *Journal of Child Psychology and Psychiatry, 34,* 1125–1136.

Pillemer, F.G., & Cook, K.V. (1989). The psychological adjustment of pediatric craniofacial patients after surgery. *Cleft Palate Journal, 26*(3), 201.

Quan, L., & Smith, D.W. (1973). The VATER association. Vertebral defects, Anal atresia, T-E fistula with esophageal atresia, radial and renal dysplasia: A spectrum of associated defects. *Journal of Pediatrics, 82*(1), 104–107.

Rosenthal, R., & Jacobson, L. (1968). *Pygmalian in the classroom.* New York: Holt, Rinehart, and Winston.

Saenger, P. (1993). Clinical review 48: The current status of diagnosis and therapeutic intervention in Turner's syndrome. *Journal of Clinical Endocrinology & Metabolism,* 77(2), 297–301.

Siebert, J.R., Graham, J.M., Jr., & MacDonald, C. (1985). Pathologic features of the CHARGE association: Support for involvement of the neural crest. *Teratology, 31*(3), 331–336.

Stoll, C., Qian, J.F., Feingold, J., Sauvage, P., & May, E. (1993). Genetic variation in transforming growth factor alpha: Possible association of BamHI polymorphism with bilateral sporadic cleft lip and palate. *Human Genetics, 92*(1), 81–82.

Sutherland, G.R.J.M. (1996). *Chromosome abnormalities and genetic counseling.* New York: Oxford University Press.

Temtamy, S.A., & Miller, J.D. (1974). Extending the scope of the VATER association: Definition of the VATER syndrome. *Journal of Pediatrics, 85*(3), 345–349.

Treacher Collins Syndrome Collaborative Group. (1996). Positional cloning of a gene involved in the pathogenesis of Treacher Collins syndrome. *Nature Genetics,* 7, 130.

Turner, H.H. (1938). A syndrome of infantilism, congenital webbed neck and cubitus valgus. *Endocrinology, 23,* 566.

van den Elzen, A.P., Semmekrot, B.A., Bongers, E.M., Huygen, P.L., & Marres, H.A. (2001). Diagnosis and treatment of the Pierre Robin sequence: Results of a retrospective clinical study and review of the literature. *European Journal of Pediatrics, 160*(1), 47–53.

Young, D.L., Schneider, R.A., Hu, D., & Helms, J.A. (2000). Genetic and teratogenic approaches to craniofacial development. *Critical Reviews in Oral Biology & Medicine, 11*(3), 304–317.

CHAPTER 9

OTHER GENETIC SYNDROMES

9.1 RETT SYNDROME

Alan K. Percy

Rett syndrome, a developmental disorder of young girls, was first recognized in the early 1960s by the Viennese developmental pediatrician Andreas Rett (1966b). Early published accounts of Rett syndrome were, however, brief and not widely circulated. About the same time, Bengt Hagberg identified girls in Sweden with similar clinical features. Following a chance meeting of Rett and Hagberg around 1980, new interest emerged in this unique disorder resulting in the first English language publication on Rett syndrome by Hagberg and colleagues in 1983 (Hagberg, Aicardi, Dias, & Ramos, 1983). Following that report, Rett syndrome was soon diagnosed in the United States, Japan, and throughout Western Europe (Percy, Zoghbi, & Riccardi, 1985). As a result, several epidemiologic studies (see Table 9.1-1) were conducted, indicating a prevalence of Rett syndrome ranging from 1:10,000 in Sweden (Hagberg, 1985) to 1:22,000 in Texas (Kozinetz et al., 1993). Thus, Rett syndrome is clearly a disorder that occurs throughout the world. More than 3,000 girls or women with Rett syndrome have been identified in the United States.

CLINICAL CHARACTERISTICS

Rett syndrome is characterized by profound cognitive impairment, communication dysfunction, stereotypic movements, and pervasive growth failure, all following a period of apparently normal development during the first 6–18 months of life (Hagberg, 1993). From the initial reports, intense efforts were made to establish a biologic marker for Rett syndrome. The studies of Rett and colleagues noted an association between Rett syndrome and hyperammonemia, although subsequent studies did not substantiate this finding (Rett, 1966). All other attempts to find a biologic marker have been unsuccessful until recently, when a gene for Rett syndrome was identified (Amir et al., 1999). Thus, diagnosis has to be based on clinical criteria, shown in Table 9.1-2, including normal pre- and perinatal periods and apparently normal development for the first several months of life (Hagberg, Hanefeld, Percy, & Skjeldal, 2002). Thereafter, purposeful hand skills are lost along with regression of psychomotor and communication functions.

Regression may begin as early as 9 months of age or as late as 2½ years. During this period, features similar to the autism spectrum disorders are typical in the sense that eye contact is poor and attempts at socialization and communication are severely limited. Also during this period, profound irritability without apparent explanation is common. Often the first clinical sign of Rett syndrome, as previously described by Rett, may be a deceleration in the rate of head growth. Beginning as early as 3 months of age, this may be profound, leading to microcephaly in some girls (Schultz et al., 1993).

Stereotypic hand movements consisting of hand-washing or hand-wringing movements or hand-clapping/hand-patting movements emerge between ages 1 and 3 years. In some instances, hand mouthing or picking at the hair or clothes is the predominant stereotypic movement. These hand stereotypies typically occur in the midline but occasionally involve one hand in the mouth and another pulling or picking at the clothes or consist of hand patting or hand wringing behind the back. Most girls with Rett syndrome are able to walk, but between 1 and 4 years truncal ataxia appears and gait becomes apraxic (i.e., has a broad-based, wandering, purposeless character). They often initiate walking by first stepping backwards (retropulsion). When standing, they tend to rock from side to side.

Mary Ellen is a 7-year-old girl who was born at term following an uneventful pregnancy. She developed appropriately through the first 9 months in motor and language skills; however, she was slow to walk (18 months) and lost midline play at 1 year. At the same time, she was noted to be inattentive to visual and auditory cues and lost all language and gesture play (waving and Pat-a-cake) at 18 months of age. Stereotypic hand movements (hand clapping/tapping including behind the back and hand mouthing) were noted at 18 months as well. Bruxism appeared shortly thereafter. Mary Ellen's breathing pattern at that time was normal, but irregular breathing while awake (both hyperventilation and breath

Table 9.1-1. Rett syndrome prevalence estimates

Location	Year	Number of individuals with Rett syndrome	Prevalence
Western Scotland	1982	19	1:15,000
Switzerland	1982	27	1:24,600
Western Sweden	1982	12	1:13,000
Japan	1988	24	1:25,000
Texas	1990	103	1:22,800
Australia	1995	79	1:22,000
Sweden	1996	69	1:13,000

holding) appeared around 3 years of age. She walked initially, but has had difficulty with balance for the past year and presently uses a walker (see Figure 9.1-1).

Mary Ellen's growth parameters followed a typical pattern for Rett syndrome. Her length and weight were in the 90th percentile throughout her first 18 months, but both declined subsequently. Her length is now near the 60th percentile, and her weight is at the 25th percentile. Mary Ellen's head circumference was initially at the 50th percentile, began decelerating rapidly by 9 months, and has been below the 2nd percentile since age 2. Her hand growth is near the 70th percentile, whereas her foot growth is at the 3rd percentile. She receives lamotrigine for seizures and has had intramuscular botulinum toxin for tight heel cords. She participates in a variety of interventions to improve motor and communication skills.

The diagnosis of Rett syndrome requires a detailed history, particularly a review of pre- and perinatal events and developmental progress and a neurological evaluation that includes growth parameters. The family can be critical to this process by recalling the temporal sequence of the child's abnormalities, such as delays in achieving developmental milestones, loss of motor or communicative skills, and appearance of hand stereotypies. The clinician should conduct several ancillary evaluations including audiologic and ophthalmologic assessments, chromosome analysis with high-resolution banding, and a molecular probe for Angelman syndrome if the

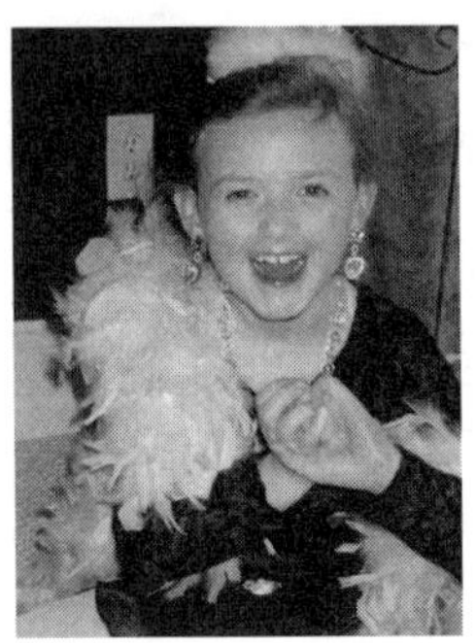

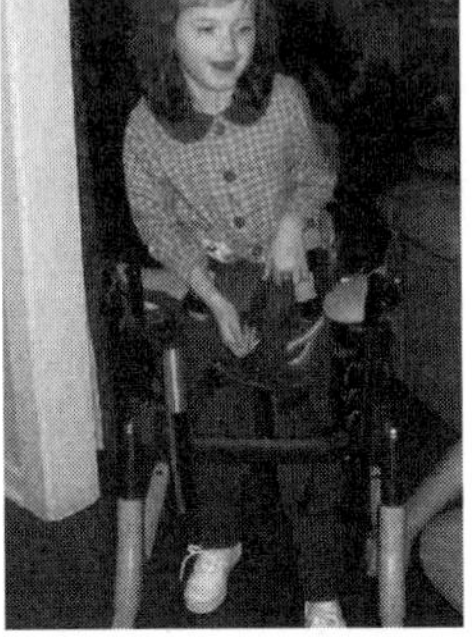

Figure 9.1-1. Mary Ellen is a 7-year-old girl with Rett syndrome.

Table 9.1-2. Rett syndrome obligate clinical criteria

Criteria	Onset
Normal at birth	—
Apparently normal early development • May be delayed from birth	6–8 months
Postnatal deceleration of head growth rate in most	3 months–4 years
Loss of achieved purposeful hand skills	6 months–2½ years
Psychomotor regression • Emerging social withdrawal, communication dysfunction, loss of learned words, and cognitive impairment	9 months–2½ years
Stereotypic movements • Hand washing/wringing/squeezing • Hand clapping/tapping/rubbing • Hand mouthing	1–3 years
Gait dysfunction • Impaired (dyspraxic) or failing locomotion	1–4 years
Absence of • Organomegaly, or other signs of storage disease • Optic atrophy or other retinal changes • Intrauterine growth retardation • Evidence of perinatal or postnatal damage • Acquired neurological disorders due to infections or head trauma • Existence of identifiable metabolic or other progressive neurological disorder	—

Adapted from *European Journal of Paediatric Neurology, 6*(5), Hagberg, B., Hanefeld, F., Percy, A., & Skjeldal, O. An update on clinically applicable diagnostic criteria in Rett syndrome: Comments to Rett Syndrome Clinical Criteria Consensus Panel Satellite to European Paediatric Neurology Society Meeting, Baden, Germany, 11 September 2001, 293–297, Copyright 2002, with permission from European Pediatric Neurology Society.

MECP2 gene test is normal. An electroencephalogram (EEG) is also recommended; however, many behavioral features associated with Rett Syndrome may resemble clinical seizures. Thus, video-EEG monitoring, if available, is preferable. At this time, a broad investigation for inherited metabolic disorders is not warranted. Definitive diagnosis is accomplished by performing mutation analysis on leukocyte deoxyribonucleic acid (DNA) for the gene *MECP2*, which encodes the methyl-CpG-binding protein 2 (MeCP2).

CLINICAL STAGING

Based on the careful studies of Hagberg and colleagues, Rett syndrome has been characterized in four clinical stages (Hagberg & Witt-Engerstrom, 1986). This system provides a format for plotting the clinical progression of Rett syndrome but also considers that transition from one stage to the next is generally along a continuum rather than an abrupt change. The first stage is the early onset stagnation period that occurs from age 6 to 18 months. Usually, this stage has a duration of weeks to months and consists of delay in developmental progress without clear evidence of regression.

The second stage is rapid developmental regression with an onset from age 1 to 3 or 4 years. During this period, previously acquired skills in motor and communication function are lost. In addition, impairment of cognitive performance becomes apparent. This stage may be relatively brief, lasting days to weeks or as long as a year. During this stage, Rett syndrome should be differentiated from autism spectrum disorders, infantile neuronal ceroid lipofuscinosis, Angelman syndrome, and an acute toxic or infectious encephalopathy. Infantile neuronal ceroid lipofuscinosis and Angelman syndrome, in particular, may present a Rett syndrome–like phenotype, including deceleration in the rate of head growth, seizures, and stereotypic movements. The natural history of these two disorders is quite different from Rett syndrome, and both can be differentiated from Rett syndrome by appropriate molecular genetic or biochemical testing.

The third stage, the pseudostationary period, may last for many years, perhaps as long as several decades. This stage is reserved for those girls with preserved ability to walk. During this stage, communication functions (e.g., socialization, eye contact) may improve remarkably, but a very slow decline in motor function is noted such that ambulation and the stereotypic hand movements decline in speed and frequency. Nevertheless, ambulation may persist into middle age. In Stage 3, Rett syndrome must be differentiated from the ataxic static encephalopathies, spinocerebellar degeneration, and neuronal ceroid lipofuscinosis. Angelman syndrome should be considered as well as idiopathic psychomotor retardation.

The fourth stage, late motor deterioration, is defined by the loss of ambulation, that is, when a wheelchair is required at all times. For those girls who never walk, staging moves directly from Stage 2 to Stage 4. Thus, Stage 4 is further subdivided to differentiate girls who lose ambulation (4A) from those who never ambulate (4B). Typically, girls in Stage 4B are remarkably hypotonic and develop severe motor disability with muscle wasting and skeletal deformities. Despite this transition to Stage 4, communication functions in the form of eye contact and socialization may be quite good and continue into adulthood. Even though motor skills may diminish over time, cognitive function is maintained.

VARIANT PHENOTYPIC EXPRESSION

Variant phenotypic expressions of Rett syndrome occur. The most common is the so-called *formes fruste*, which consists of delay in onset of Rett syndrome features until age 8–10 years. In addition, a preserved speech variant, a congenital form in which no period of developmental progress is noted, and an early onset seizure form have been recognized. Because of the relatively severe epileptic encephalopathy, the early onset seizure form is also characterized by little or no normal early development.

Criteria for delineating the variant phenotypes require fulfillment of at least 3 of 6 main criteria and at least 5 of 11 associated features for Rett syndrome (see Table 9.1-3) (Hagberg et al., 2002). In a cohort of girls with Rett syndrome in Sweden, Hagberg (1993) noted that of 130 girls or women, 82% fulfilled the classic criteria, 12% were formes fruste, and the remainder consisted of the late regression, preserved speech, or congenital forms.

Table 9.1-3. Rett syndrome variant phenotypes criteria

Inclusion criteria
- Meet at least 3 of 6 main criteria
- Meet at least 5 of 11 supportive criteria

Six main criteria
- Absence or reduction of hand skills
- Reduction or loss of babble/speech
- Reduction or loss of communication skills
- Deceleration of head growth from first years of life
- Monotonous pattern of hand stereotypies
- Rett syndrome disease profile: a regression stage followed by a recovery of interaction contrasting with slow neuromotor regression

Eleven supportive criteria
- Breathing irregularities
- Bloating/air swallowing
- Bruxism (harsh sound)
- Abnormal locomotion
- Scoliosis/kyphosis
- Lower limb amyotrophy
- Intense eye contact/eye pointing
- Diminished response to pain
- Laughing/screaming spells
- Cold, purplish feet that usually have growth impairments
- Sleep disturbances including night screaming outbursts

Adapted from *European Journal of Paediatric Neurology, 6*(5), Hagberg, B., Hanefeld, F., Percy, A., & Skjeldal, O. An update on clinically applicable diagnostic criteria in Rett syndrome: Comments to Rett Syndrome Clinical Criteria Consensus Panel Satellite to European Paediatric Neurology Society Meeting, Baden, Germany, 11 September 2001, 293–297; Copyright 2002, with permission from European Pediatric Neurology Society.

RETT SYNDROME IN BOYS AND MEN

Convincing descriptions of boys and men with Rett syndrome have been few. Boys with more than one X chromosome (Klinefelter syndrome–XXY) have been described with clinical features typical for Rett syndrome. Furthermore, with the identification of mutations in *MECP2*, other affected boys have been identified, including a boy with a rapidly progressively encephalopathy, his mother, and two girls with Rett syndrome, all sharing the same mutation in *MECP2*; several boys with developmental delays and cognitive impairments; and two boys with spastic paraparesis. Aside from boys with Klinefelter syndrome, however, boys with *MECP2* mutations do not have the clinical features of Rett syndrome.

SPECIFIC CLINICAL ISSUES IN RETT SYNDROME

Clinical expression and, therefore, the resulting functional level of Rett syndrome may be quite variable. Nevertheless, several specific clinical issues should be addressed including cognitive impairment, growth failure, breathing irregularities, seizures, scoliosis, gastrointestinal function, self-abuse, and life expectancy. In general, survival is quite prolonged, growth failure is pervasive, and no consistent metabolic abnormality has been identified despite intensive investigations of amino and organic acids, mitochondrial function, and urea cycle metabolism. Each of these clinical issues is considered in some detail next. These important issues should be discussed with the parents or principal caregivers. The International Rett Syndrome Association (IRSA) is an important resource for individuals and families. IRSA maintains an active web site (http://www.rettsyndrome.org) and has several very useful publications.

Cognitive Impairment

Assessing cognitive function in girls with Rett syndrome is extremely problematic. The absence of effective fine motor and communication skills severely limits the application of available standardized tests. Nonetheless, cognitive impairment is regarded as significant with mental developmental age at the 8- to 10-month level and gross motor function ranging from 12 to 18 months. Using assessments that depend only on visual response, cognitive levels still appear to be in the severe impairment range. Adaptive skills, including feeding, dressing, and toileting functions, are not acquired effectively, such that individuals with Rett syndrome will require support in these areas throughout life. Despite these difficulties, appropriate physical, occupational, and speech-language therapy, including augmentative communication, should be provided to individuals with Rett syndrome throughout their life span (Budden, 1997).

Growth Failure

Growth failure in Rett syndrome is pervasive; the first evidence is deceleration in the rate of head growth as early as 3 months of age (Schultz et al., 1993). Median head circumference values fall to the second percentile for typically developing individuals by age 4–5 years. Weight begins to decline from the normal value near the end of the first year of life with the median value falling below the 5th percentile for typically developing individuals by age 7 years. Height or length falls off around 15 months of age with the median values again declining to the 5th percentile for typically developing individuals around age 7 years. Hand and foot growth is also affected—more so for the feet than for the hands—with the reduction in rate of foot growth paralleling that of height (Schultz, Glaze, Motil, Hebert, & Percy, 1998). The rate of hand growth tends to be more preserved.

Breathing Irregularities

Irregular breathing during wakefulness was among the features noted by Rett in his initial reports (Glaze, Frost, Zoghbi, & Percy, 1987). In some girls, both hyperventilation or breath holding may occur. Breath holding may be prolonged and very impressive, if not frightening, occasionally exceeding 1 minute. In other girls, this symptom may be quite subtle and, hence, underrecognized. Parents and other caregivers should be advised to look for specific features of breath holding or hyperventilation, no matter how subtle, as well as evidence of brief oral expulsion of air or saliva. Air swallowing (aerophagia) may accompany these irregular breathing patterns. Air swallowing may be striking and produce marked abdominal distension; however, the distension will abate, particularly, during sleep.

Typically, the irregular breathing has its onset in early childhood (3–5 years) and is maximal during the early school-age period (5–10 years), during which time it may dominate much of the waking activities. Thereafter, breathing irregularities diminish in frequency and intensity. Efforts to modify breath holding or hyperventilation with medication have generally been unsuccessful. The opiate antagonist naltrexone has been reported to provide some benefit, but this response is not uniform and may be due, at least in part, to the sedating properties of this drug. Irregular breathing occurring during sleep is not a typical feature of Rett syndrome. Should it be noted, causes of obstructive apnea should be investigated.

Seizures

Reports of seizure frequency in Rett syndrome provide quite variable rates, ranging from 30% to 80% (Glaze, Schultz, & Frost, 1998; Steffenburg, Hagberg, & Hagberg, 2001). The EEG is invariably abnormal after age 2 years, featuring slowing in background activity, reduction or loss of posterior dominant rhythm, and recurrent spike and slow spike and wave activity. Despite the presence of epileptiform changes, clinical seizure activity may be minimal or absent in the majority of girls. A major challenge may be differentiating behavioral patterns from seizures and may often require video-EEG monitoring to resolve the question. Seizure control is typically not difficult in individuals with Rett syndrome. Seizures usually respond to carbamazepine or sodium valproate. Lamotrigine has also proved effective. Although generally well tolerated, carbamazepine or valproate may be associated with agitation or self-abusive behavior.

Ambulation

Ambulation is noted in 80% of girls with Rett syndrome, about ¼ of whom will lose their ability to walk during or after the period of regression. Thus, overall, about 60% of girls with Rett syndrome remain ambulatory. Ambulation should be encouraged as long as possible. Furthermore, weight-bearing should be encouraged in all girls with Rett syndrome who do not walk, including the use of standing frames. Bones tend to be undermineralized, and weight bearing may aid in improving this problem.

Scoliosis

The incidence of scoliosis in Rett syndrome increases with age (see Chapter 13). It is present in about 8% of preschoolers and in more than 80% of girls older than 16 years of age (Lindstrom, Stokland, & Hagberg, 1994). The overall incidence is about 50%. Onset is typically at age 8 or somewhat before, after which it may become clinically significant requiring medical or surgical attention. Progression is much more common in those girls who are nonambulatory. Bracing is considered with a 25° curvature although systematic studies have not established that bracing actually delays progression. Surgery is recommended strongly when curvature exceeds 40°.

Gastrointestinal Function

Nutrition is often a major problem in Rett syndrome that requires the guidance of a nutritionist with regard to dietary supplementation. Girls with Rett syndrome appear to have increased protein requirements. Ultimately, gastrostomy feeding may be necessary in some girls to preserve growth. Gastroesophageal reflux, esophagitis, and gall bladder disease may be problematic. Recurrent periods of unexplained irritability or apparent distress may result and require appropriate evaluation and treatment by a gastroenterologist.

Constipation is also a significant problem in Rett syndrome. Various strategies have been employed with variable success, including use of high-fiber foods, enemas, mineral oil, and milk of magnesia. The frequent use of enemas is discouraged as it may lead to dependency on this mode of treatment. Furthermore, prolonged use of mineral oil may interfere with proper absorption of the fat-soluble vitamins. Despite the availability of flavored milk of magnesia, many girls resist taking it. Most recently, Miralax (polyethylene glycol) has proved particularly effective. It is tasteless and odorless and may be dissolved in juice, making it more palatable and much better tolerated.

Self-Injurious Behavior

Self-injurious behavior is seen occasionally in the form of hair pulling; biting of the fingers, hands, or other parts of the upper extremities; and hitting about the face (see Chapter 23.5). Aggressive behavior toward others, consisting of hitting, biting, or hair pulling, may also occur. Before considering pharmacologic intervention, care should be taken to exclude other medical problems, particularly gastrointestinal dysfunction (gastroesophageal reflux or constipation) as noted previously, or as a side effect of medications already in use. After excluding such problems, low dose risperidone (0.5 mg twice a day) may be effective in reducing this behavior.

Longevity

Survival may be expected well into adulthood. In the only systematic study, survival followed that of all girls up to age 10; however, survival of the Rett syndrome study cohort to age 35 was about 70% compared with 98% for all women and 27% for individuals with profound cognitive and motor impairments (personal experience, unpublished data). Understanding the possibility of prolonged survival of individuals with Rett syndrome is important in order to guide parents and other caregivers about long-term care.

Other Associated Features

Other features associated with Rett syndrome include bruxism (teeth grinding), interrupted sleep patterns, and vasomotor disturbances comprised of cold feet and hands. Bruxism tends to be most prominent during early childhood. In general, attempts to treat medically have not been fruitful. Sleep is often fragmented (Glaze et al., 1987), and girls with Rett syndrome often do not sleep well for many nights in succession or are awake in the night, often playing quietly or laughing for no apparent reason, which may result in very disrupted sleep for parents. Occasionally, chloral hydrate, diphenhydramine, or hydroxyzine may be required to assist in sleep. Vasomotor disturbances appear to represent autonomic nervous system dysfunction. Sympathectomy occurring during the surgical management of scoliosis has been noted to reverse these findings on the operated side. No effective treatment is available otherwise.

NEUROPATHOLOGY

The principal morphologic features of the brain in Rett syndrome are reduced weight, reduced volume of frontal cortex and deep gray nuclei, reduced melanin deposition in the substantia nigra, smaller neurons, reduced dendritic arborizations, and the absence of any recognizable disease process suggestive of a neurodegenerative disorder (Armstrong, 1995; Armstrong, Dunn, & Antalffy, 1988; Jellinger, Armstrong, Zoghbi, & Percy, 1988). The fundamental neurobiologic problem in Rett syndrome appears to be an arrest in normal neural maturation. Thus, Rett syndrome has the profile of a developmental disorder, not that of a neurodegenerative condition. Solid neuropathologic evidence demonstrates no progressive neuropathologic features or any evidence of neuronal loss or extensive gliosis. The brain has a normal appearance but is small, typically being about 60%–70% of expected weight for age. Although brain weights are uniformly low, no pattern of progressive reduction with increasing age is noted. No evidence of migrational disruption is noted, but the neurons do appear to be small, to be too close together, and to have too few processes. Golgi studies reveal markedly shortened and relatively primitive dendritic arborizations, suggesting a failure in the proper development or maintenance of synaptic connections in Rett syndrome.

Although the mechanisms are probably quite different, other neurodevelopmental disorders have similar neuropathologic features. For example, in Down syndrome, dendritic branches are increased early in infancy but thereafter are reduced such that dendritic spines are deficient already by 4 months of age, remaining so into adulthood. In Angelman syndrome, decreased dendritic arborizations and dendritic spines are prominent findings. Finally, in autism spectrum disorders (see Chapter 23.1), increased packing density and decreased cell size are also noted.

GENETIC BASIS OF RETT SYNDROME

Rett syndrome is clearly established as a genetic disorder predominantly affecting girls. The proposed genetic mechanism is X-linked dominant, producing a much more aggressive phenotype in boys or even fetal demise. Rett syndrome is largely sporadic, much less than 1% representing recurrence within a family. As the number of familial recurrences is very small, most girls with Rett syndrome represent new mutations. Clinicians should advise parents that the risk for recurrence of Rett syndrome is very small. For those parents who may wish to have additional children, specific consultation with a genetic counselor is recommended. When a specific mutation is known in an individual with Rett syndrome, assessing the carrier status of the mother is possible by testing for the same mutation in her peripheral blood; however, the failure to identify the same mutation would not exclude the presence of a germline mutation. Recurrence of such a mutation would, however, be unlikely.

Prior to the identification of mutations in *MECP2*, several lines of evidence supported a genetic basis for Rett syndrome: 1) Rett syndrome had been described reliably only in girls; 2) in twin studies, monozygotic twins have been consistently concordant (i.e., if one twin has Rett Syndrome, the second also has Rett Syndrome); 3) several familial cases are known in which either sisters, half-sisters, or aunt/nieces have Rett syndrome; 4) vertical transmission has been reported, namely, a woman with Rett syndrome gave birth to a girl who also has Rett syndrome; and 5) recognition that in half sisters, the transmitting woman (i.e., their mother) demonstrated nonrandom X-inactivation such that she expressed the normal X-chromosome predominantly whereas random X-inactivation was present in the two affected half sisters.

MECP2, located at Xq28, encodes methyl-CpG-binding protein 2 (MeCP2), which is important in the regulation of gene transcription and is highly expressed in the brain (Amir et al., 1999). More than 200 different mutations have been defined in *MECP2* in girls or women with Rett syndrome, although eight specific mutations account for about two thirds of the mutations identified to date (Amir et al., 1999; Huppke, Held, Hanefeld, Engel, & Laccone, 2002; Laccone, Huppke, Hanefeld, & Meins, 2001). Most of the known mutations are truncating, that is, result in formation of an incomplete form of the MeCP2 protein. Missense mutations produce a full-length MeCP2 protein but one with reduced functional integrity.

Mutations in *MECP2* have been identified in 90%–95% of girls with classic Rett syndrome. This number is likely to increase as the gene is sequenced more completely. In the case of variant forms of Rett syndrome, the number with mutations in *MECP2* is considerably lower. Initial attempts to develop phenotype–genotype correlations in girls with classic Rett syndrome indicate that the most important determinant of clinical severity is variability in X-chromosome inactivation (Amir et al., 2000). The position of the mutation or whether it is truncating is also important (Cheadle et al., 2000), but the X-inactivation pattern appears to be the major determinant of severity. Namely, skewed inactivation of X-chromosomes bearing mutations in *MECP2* produces milder clinical involvement. The spectrum of clinical phenotypes associated with mutations in *MECP2* varies widely and includes autism spectrum disorders and nonsyndromic intellectual disabilities. As such, the clinical impact of *MECP2* mutations extends well beyond Rett syndrome.

LONG-TERM MANAGEMENT

Long-term management of girls and women with Rett syndrome involves appropriate physical and occupational therapy, speech-language therapy, nutritional support, orthopedic intervention, and seizure management (Budden, 1997; Hagberg, 1993). The principal orthopedic concern is monitoring of scoliosis and, when necessary, surgical intervention with stabilizing rods. Emphasis should be placed on establishing optimal communication by building on the improved social interaction and eye contact, which develop by school age. Augmentative communication strategies may be quite effective. Failure to maintain proper weight gain may reflect swallowing dysfunction or gastroesophageal reflux. These conditions may require referral to a gastroenterologist for appropriate evaluations. Physical activity should also be maintained as best possible.

As noted previously, long-term planning needs to be considered as well. Given the potential longevity of girls and women with Rett syndrome, other health issues must be considered. Women with Rett syndrome have the same medical and dental needs as other women, and these needs should be given proper attention. In particular, gallbladder disease has been described in many girls and women with Rett syndrome. Prolonged QT segment is present in many as well. An electrocardiogram should be performed annually. Gynecologic care should also be provided annually.

CONCLUSION

Rett syndrome is a genetic disorder that affects many girls and women throughout the world. Clinical expression is variable but includes cognitive impairments, breathing irregularities, pervasive growth failure, and stereotypic movements. Individuals with Rett syndrome can be expected to live well into middle age. Parents and caregivers must be guided in the provision of optimal care and health maintenance to promote both general health as well as those issues specific to Rett syndrome. Not the least of these is maintaining effective socialization and interaction with family and friends.

REFERENCES

Amir, R., Van den Veyver, I., Schultz, R., Malicki, D., Tran, C., Dahle, E., et al. (2000). Influence of mutation type and X chromosome inactivation on Rett syndrome phenotypes. *Annals of Neurology, 47*, 670–679.

Amir, R., Van den Veyver, I., Wan, M., Tran, C., Francke, U., & Zoghbi, H. (1999). Rett syndrome is caused by mutations in X-linked *MECP2*, encoding methyl-CpG-binding protein 2. *Nature Genetics, 23*, 185–188.

Armstrong, D. (1995). The neuropathology of Rett syndrome–overview 1994. *Neuropediatrics, 26*(2), 100–104.

Armstrong, D., Dunn, K., & Antalffy, B. (1998). Decreased dendritic branching in frontal, motor and limbic cortex in Rett syndrome compared with Trisomy 21. *Journal of Neuropathology and Experimental Neurology, 57*(11), 1013–1017.

Budden, S.S. (1997). Rett syndrome: Habilitation and management reviewed. *European Child & Adolescent Psychiatry, 6*(Suppl. 1), 103–107.

Cheadle, J., Gill, H., Fleming, N., Maynard, J., Kerr, A., Leonard, H., et al. (2000). Long-read sequence analysis of the *MECP2* gene in Rett syndrome patients: Correlation of disease severity with mutation type and location. *Human Molecular Genetics, 9*, 1119–1129.

Glaze, D., Frost, J., Zoghbi, H., & Percy, A. (1987). Rett's syndrome: Characterization of respiratory patterns and sleep. *Annals of Neurology, 21*, 377–382.

Glaze, D., Schultz, R., & Frost, J. (1998). Rett syndrome: Characterization of seizures and non-seizures. *Electroencephalography and Clinical Neurophysiology, 106*, 79–83.
Hagberg, B.A. (1985). Rett's syndrome: Prevalence and impact on progressive severe mental retardation in girls. *Acta Paediatrica Scandinavica, 74*, 405–408.
Hagberg, B. (Ed.). (1993). *Rett syndrome—Clinical and biological aspects.* London: MacKeith Press.
Hagberg, B., Aicardi, J., Dias, K., & Ramos, O. (1983). A progressive syndrome of autism, dementia, ataxia, and loss of purposeful hand use in girls: Rett's syndrome. Report of 35 cases. *Annals of Neurology, 14*, 471–479.
Hagberg, B., Hanefeld, F., Percy, A., & Skjeldal, O. (2002). An update on clinically applicable diagnostic criteria in Rett syndrome: Comments to Rett Syndrome Clinical Criteria Consensus Panel Satellite to European Paediatric Neurology Society Meeting, Baden Baden, Germany, 11 September 2001. *European Journal of Paediatric Neurology, 6*(5), 293–297.
Hagberg, B., & Witt-Engerstrom, I. (1986). Rett syndrome: A suggested staging system for describing impairment profile with increasing age towards adolescence. *American Journal of Medical Genetics, 24*(Suppl. 1), 47–59.
Huppke, P., Held, M., Hanefeld, F., Engel, W., & Laccone, F. (2002). Influence of mutation type and location on phenotype in 123 patients with Rett syndrome. *Neuropediatrics, 33*(2), 63–68.
Jellinger, K., Armstrong, D., Zoghbi, H.Y., & Percy, A.K. (1988). Neuropathology of Rett syndrome. *Acta Neuropathologica, 76*(2), 142–158.
Kozinetz, C.A., Skender, M.L., MacNaughton, N., Almes, M.J., Schultz, R.J., Percy, A.K., et al. (1993). Epidemiology of Rett syndrome: A population-based registry. *Pediatrics, 91*, 445–450.
Laccone, F., Jünemann, I, Whatley, S., Morgan, R., Butter, R., Huppke, P., et al. (2004). Large deletions of the *MECP2* gene detected by gene dosage analysis in patients with Rett syndrome. *Human Mutation, 23*, 234–244.
Lidstrom, J., Stokland, E., & Hagberg, B. (1994). Scoliosis in Rett syndrome: Clinical and biological aspects. *Spine, 19*(14), 1632–1635.
Percy, A.K., Zoghbi, H., & Riccardi, V.M. (1985). Rett syndrome: Initial experience with an emerging clinical entity. *Brain and Development, 7*(3), 300–304.
Rett, A. (1966). Uber ein eigenartiges hirnatrophisches Syndrom bei Hyperammonamie im Kindesalter. *Wiener Medizinische Wochenschrift, 116*, 723–726.
Schultz, R.J., Glaze, D.G., Motil, K.J., Armstrong, D.D., del Junco, D.J., Hubbard, C.R., et al. (1993). The pattern of growth failure in Rett syndrome. *American Journal of Diseases of Children, 147*, 633–637.
Schultz, R.J., Glaze, D.G., Motil, K.J., Hebert, D., & Percy, A. (1998). Hand and foot growth failure in Rett syndrome. *Journal of Child Neurology, 13*, 71–74.
Steffenburg, U., Hagberg, G., & Hagberg, B. (2001). Epilepsy in a representative series of Rett syndrome. *Acta Paediatrica, 90*(1), 34–39.

9.2 DOWN SYNDROME

Allen C. Crocker

Provision of health care for individuals with Down syndrome (children, adults, families) is a lively field. Numerous guides have been written about this topic (see the reference list for suggestions). Families have become experts now as they have joined societies, gone to conferences, attended workshops, and read books. Furthermore, there are dedicated clinical support centers, about 30 for children and about 10 for adults in the United States. A special health professional society (Down Syndrome Medical Interest Group) and journal (*Down Syndrome Quarterly*) located in the United States, and others are found elsewhere. Many of the conundrums about the disorder have been focused and explored.

Care for individuals with Down syndrome is usually straightforward, but some special challenges remain. Substantially drawn in are the cardiologist, neurologist, otolaryngologist, gastroenterologist, ophthalmologist, orthopedist, and psychiatrist. The birth incidence is relatively high (about 1 per 1,000 live births), the ascertainment is 100%, and the sense of familiarity is strong. Most community pediatricians have 3–6 such children in their practice; the penetration for internists is low but variable. Many physicians (and other health providers) will eventually develop a relationship with support groups for children with whom they relate, and they will come to know the drill at school and in recreation or employment circumstances. In so many pioneering ways, individuals with Down syndrome have come to be the prototype or pioneer for lives with special needs. See Table 3.2 for additional details.

PREGNANCY AND DELIVERY

A universal distribution exists in the world for births of infants with Down syndrome. The fetus is sturdy, with fewer losses than many others with chromosomal aberrations. There are no environmental correlations with genesis of the crucial trisomy 21 or translocation 21, except for the well-known one of advancing maternal age. This, of course, has been the origin of many study and screening efforts (which have had limited effect on birth incidence).

Obstetrics, fetal medicine physicians, and pediatricians come into action with the pregnant couple; very significant are the reports offered by specialized ultrasonographers. Resort to amniocentesis is obviously essential for actual diagnosis, though concerns persist in families' minds regarding the safety of this procedure. Pregnancy interruption after diagnosis is now at a lower rate, it is encouraging to note. Recent surveys have provided important information about the degree to which traditional counseling of parents by physicians regarding the new baby with Down syndrome fails to meet parental needs, both for those diagnosed prenatally and those postnatally (Skotko, 2005a, 2005b). Clearly, a more helpful, hopeful, and humanistic discussion should occur.

For involved fetuses, definitive prenatal cardiac studies, often including echocardiograms, are valuable and alert the delivery team. There is a mild increase in preterm births among infants with Down syndrome, and babies may be up to 400 g lighter than comparable sisters and brothers of the same family (Pueschel, Rothman, & Ogilvie, 1976). If it has not occurred up to that time, the diagnosis of Down syndrome is ordinarily suggested by the phenotype within minutes of birth, to the mother if not others. Significant delay in the speculation about the diagnosis (up to a month) is an extreme situation.

NEWBORN PERIOD

Three urgent considerations for the newborn infant with Down syndrome are 1) examination for congenital heart disease, 2) review for intestinal obstruction (duodenal atresia), and 3) inspection for cataracts. These items invoke the child's care needs (and destiny). All babies in concern for having Down syndrome require professional study by a pediatric cardiologist (see Chapters 18.1 and 18.2); the lesions may be elusive at first. Most of the babies can be cared for well in a regular newborn nursery; for others, the cardiac concerns require newborn intensive care unit assistance. Breast-feeding may be ineffective for a day or two, in part by oromotor hypotonia, but commonly succeeds.

A flurry of inquiry and adjustment will be generated by the new child, with family apprehension about his or her individual needs. (Much of this will have been accommodated if prenatal diagnosis occurred.) Kindly and accurate medical guidance has great value, and the time of discovery can be turned into an excited beginning. These are seminal moments for all parties.

The little person with Down syndrome shows in varying degrees the expected phenotypic pattern, with family traits contributing strongly. Typically, he or she is small and notably flexible (low muscle tone). The face is generally cheerful; the nose, small; and the nasal bridge (upper midface), flattened. Epicanthic folds are almost always visible. Ears are short and commonly folded over a bit. The face looks round, and the mandible, small. Hair is often thin, and chubbiness may be seen. The umbilicus is protruding. The anterior fontanelle stays patent for 2 years or so, and dentition is substantially delayed. Fingers tend to be short and fat. The fifth finger may curve, and a single palmar crease (four-finger line) is common. The first and second toes are separated. These little children are quite simply adorable.

THE SMALL CHILD

By present perceptions, five cautionary examinations are recommended for all children with Down syndrome in early life. Hearing screening should be carried out (visual reinforcement audiometry or behavioral testing audiometry) by 6 months of age, irrespective of the results of newborn hearing studies. A professional pediatric ophthalmologic exam is to be accomplished during first year of life (age 6–12 months). Thyroid function testing is done early if growth is poor, otherwise by the second or third birthday (usually TSH and T4 assays) as a reference frame. Later follow-up depends on the practitioner's concern (some do annual).

X-rays of the lateral cervical spine (three views: extension, neutral, flexion, in lateral projection) are also procured by age 3, though there is less confidence now in the capacity of this exam to predict clinically important atlanto-axial instability. Repeats are made in mid/late childhood and early adulthood (or possibly one waits until there might be asymmetry or limp).

A screen for celiac disease is advised for all children with Down syndrome, using first the tissue transglutaminase antibody and the total IgA level. There is the uncommon occurrence of deficiency of intestinal neurons, producing a crucial constipation and the need for surgical assistance (Hirschsprung bowel anomaly).

In this period begins the extraordinary countdown of early development, as crawling, creeping, sitting, standing, and then finally walking alone are achieved in partnership with early intervention. Hypotonia seems workable after all! In current times, congenital cardiac lesions are monitored with great care; surgical repair is undertaken in the early months if serious physiologic disadvantage is present. The mortality is low for operative intervention. Verbal language slowly moves forward, often on a parallel track with sign language. The family is only partially able to have their questions answered about developmental rate because of personal variations.

This is the period of otitis media and poor middle ear drainage, with hearing impairment and ventilation tubes. It is also the time of gastroesophageal reflux, with the implicit potential for aspiration. Obstructive sleep apnea can be a challenge. Otolaryngeologic help is needed again.

Strabismus is common, perhaps aided by glasses. A few children have seizures, some as infantile spasms (hypsarrhythmia). The latter have a favorable outlook but require assistance from a neurologic specialist. Very rarely, diabetes mellitus may develop, usually in the infant or toddler years.

At this point, personality is beginning to declare, and the preschool will get a chance to share it. The family (and child) have traveled far in these 3 years and usually are firm in their resolve. Important guides are available for parents (Pueschel, 2001; Stray-Gundersen, 1995).

THE REST OF CHILDHOOD

For the young person with Down syndrome, childhood is generally a healthy (and happy) time. The developmental gap is thoughtfully accommodated by an inclusive classroom with an aide in the local school. Personal traits are interesting and sometimes obstinate. Continuing work with language intelligibility is a must, and social skills need to be learned.

Ear infections, commonly prominent in the toddler period, decrease by the preschool years, especially if ventilation tubes have been used. One also expects reflux to diminish, and sleep to be more peaceful. Constipation may be stressful. Toilet training is characteristically complete by 4–5 years. Eating is a wonderful activity, and obesity can be starting.

Friendships are school-based and not always as fulfilling as is wanted. Family relations, however, are durable and rewarding. Sport activities and other community programs are real favorites. Immunizations are given in the pediatrician's office, on a typical schedule. It is sometimes commented that an average youth with Down syndrome going through neighborhood schools (inclusion) will, by the twelfth grade, be reading at about the fifth-grade level.

YOUNG ADULT AND ADULT

Growth continues at the usual sequence and timetable. Survey studies have shown that the average young man with Down syndrome, at the 50th percentile, completes his growth at 153 cm., or 61 inches, at age 18, and young women at 145 cm., or 57 inches (Cronk, Crocker, Pueschel, Shea, Zackai, Pickens, & Reed, 1988). Men can be regarded as not fertile, whereas women have considerably reduced fertility. Secondary sexual maturation is normal in schedule and degree for both.

Youth is a challenging time for many individuals with Down syndrome, in which social alliances are difficult and goals unclear. Concrete social programs are helpful, and guidance in vocational activities (see Figure 9.2-1). At the present time, postsecondary educational opportunities are limited, but these experiences are being sought by many families. Most make the move to community living arrangements in their 20s, with a change to adult-oriented medical care offices.

Marriage is sought by some young people and may indeed be feasible if a very thoughtful support system is established. Health care needs are usually modest. Heart disease rates are low, although aortic regurgitation may be left from earlier surgery, and mitral valve prolapse is increased. As adulthood proceeds, some visual or auditory impairments can develop. Dry skin is difficult, and arthritis may occur, as may hypothyroidism. Clinicians should check the cervical spine before giving anesthesia.

Mental health varies, sometimes with adjustment problems and depression in the earlier decades. Self-talk is common (and benign). Activities may become reduced; in fact it is commented that the middle years seem reduced. Periodontal infection is common. Malignant disease, however, is intriguingly reduced. Individuals with Down syndrome, many of whom had considerably older parents, are now found in almost all of the community program sites, sometimes with limited family companionship remaining. Daily functions grad-

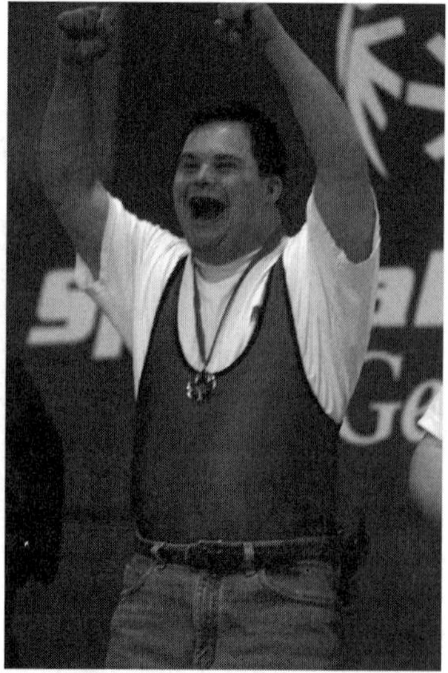

Figure 9.2-1. Evan celebrates winning a medal for powerlifting at the Special Olympics.

ually become reduced in the 40s, but only a moderate group (about 40%) develop full dementia of the Alzheimer type.

CONCLUSION

Most individuals with Down syndrome die in their 50s (see Chapter 26); however, some occasionally reach their 70s. Many stories have been told of the warmth, loyalty, and special vision of these older adults. The extra chromosome has a legacy.

REFERENCES

Cohen, W.I., Nadel, L., & Madnick, M.E. (Eds.). (2002). *Down syndrome: Visions for the 21st century.* New York: Wiley-Liss.

Cronk, C., Crocker, A.C., Pueschel, S.M., Shea, A.M., Zachai, E., Pickens, G., et al. (1988). Growth charts for children with Down syndrome: 1 month to 18 years of age. *Pediatrics, 81,* 102–110.

Pueschel, S.M. (2001). *A parent's guide to Down syndrome: Toward a brighter future* (Rev. ed.). Baltimore: Paul H. Brookes Publishing Co.

Pueschel, S.M., & Pueschel, J.K. (Eds.). (1992). *Biomedical concerns in persons with Down syndrome.* Baltimore: Paul H. Brookes Publishing Co.

Pueschel, S.M., Rothman, K.J., & Ogilvie, J.D. (1976). Birth weight of children with Down syndrome. *American Journal of Mental Deficiency, 80,* 442.

Pueschel, S.M., & Rynders, J.E. (Eds.). (1982). *Down syndrome: Advances in biomedicine and the behavioral sciences.* Cambridge, England: Ware Press.

Skotko, B. (2005a). Mothers of children with Down syndrome reflect in their postnatal support. *Pediatrics, 115,* 64–77.

Skotko, B. (2005b). Prenatally diagnosed Down syndrome: Mothers who continued their pregnancies evaluate their health care providers. *American Journal of Obstetrics and Gynecology, 192,* 670–677.

Stray-Gundersen, K. (1995). *Babies with Down syndrome: A new parent's guide* (2nd ed.). Bethesda, MD: Woodbine House.

Van Dyke, D.C., Mattheis, P., Eberly, S.S., & Williams, J. (Eds.). (1995). *Medical and surgical care for children with Down syndrome: A guide for parents.* Bethesda, MD: Woodbine House.

9.3 FRAGILE X SYNDROME

Jeannie Visootsak

Fragile X syndrome is the most common cause of inherited intellectual disability. The condition has sparked many important genetic and clinical findings. It is also one of the first known human diseases with a trinucleotide repeat expansion and has led to findings of trinucleotide repeat expansion in other conditions. For instance, CAG repeat is also responsible for an X-linked spinal and bulbar muscular atrophy (Kennedy disease), which is an adult-onset form of motorneuron disease associated with signs of androgen insensitivity (LaSpada, Wilson, Lubahn, Harding, & Fischbeck, 1991). Fragile X syndrome causes a wide array of cognitive and behavioral characteristics, ranging from mild problems to the severe end of the spectrum.

Josh was the third child in his family and weighed 8 lb, 4 oz at birth. His mother had a normal pregnancy and full-term gestation with spontaneous vaginal delivery. Prenatal ultrasound revealed that Josh had an enlarged right kidney that did not require treatment when he was a newborn. Josh later had a shunt inserted into his ureter for blockage at 1 ½ years of age. This shunt was maintained in place for 4 months. Otherwise, Josh's medical history was unremarkable.

At 2 years, 11 months old, Josh was taken by his mother to the Neurology Clinic due to his developmental delays. He rolled over at 1 year, crawled at 1 ½ years, and walked at 2 years. He knew 10 words but did not point to express his needs or wants. He also had poor eye contact, preferred to play by himself, and enjoyed spinning objects. Josh's mother noted that he lacked imaginary or interactive play. When he was excited, he would flap his hands and arms. He also made flicking movements of his fingers when agitated or excited. Josh's mother was overwhelmed because he was extremely hyperactive and usually did not follow commands. In addition, he was aggressive to his brother and sisters and frequently made loud, spontaneous vocalizations.

On physical examination, Josh weighed 16.3 kg (90th percentile) and measured 38 in (75th percentile) in height and 50 cm (50th percentile) in occipitofrontal circumference. No dysmorphic characteristics were noted. Josh's mother informed the neurologist that no family members had intellectual disabilities, developmental delays, autism, attention-deficit/hyperactivity disorder, or learning disabilities. Both parents completed high school. His 7-year-old brother and sisters, ages 5 and 1 year, were developing appropriately for their chronological age.

Josh was diagnosed as having an autism spectrum condition based on his impairment in socialization skills, excessive self-stimulatory and repetitive behaviors, and expressive and receptive language delay. He was given a trial ¼ tablet of 0.1mg. Clonidine to help with his hyperactivity and aggressiveness. He was also referred for fragile X study. The testing indicated that Josh had full mutation fragile X syndrome. As a result, his family received genetic counseling and screening.

Early studies of the demographics of intellectual disabilities have consistently shown an excess of boys with fragile X syndrome versus girls. The explanation for this excess of affected boys results from the understanding that the gene for the disorder resides on the X chromosome. Because boys have only one X chromosome, they are susceptible to many genetic conditions that rarely affect girls. X-linked, or sex-linked conditions were first noticed by Martin and Bell (1943), who reported a family with 11 boys with intellectual disabilities and a few girls with mild intellectual disabilities. They concluded that this family had a genetic form of intellectual disabilities as a result of an X-linked condition. Herbert Lubs (1969) later identified a family over three generations in which only boys had intellectual disabilities. He revealed that the boys had a constriction near the end of the long arm of the X chromosome. In 1977, Grant Sutherland reported that this marker X chromosome could be appreciated under certain laboratory conditions.

Folate-deficient media is needed for adequate expression of the fragile site on the bottom end of the X chromosome. The "fragile" X site or marker eventually gave rise to the syndrome name. Widespread advances in cytogenetic testing helped to provide identification of fragile X syndrome for more than a decade before the gene responsible for the syndrome was identified in 1991.

DIAGNOSTIC EVALUATION

Diagnosis of fragile X syndrome is based on the expression of a folate-sensitive fragile site at Xq27.3 (FRAXA) induced in a cell culture deficient in folic acid. The cytogenetic test, however, has limitations in yielding a high rate of false negative findings in women known to be carriers of fragile X. Direct deoxyribonucleic acid (DNA)–based testing is considered diagnostic in determining the size of the fragile X CGG repeat, and it is now utilized in place of cytogenetic technique.

In 1991, the fragile X gene (fragile X mental retardation gene 1, *FMR1*) was described. *FMR1* contains a tandemly repeated trinucleotide sequence (CGG) near its 5' end (Fu et al., 1991; Verkerk et al., 1991) The mutation causing fragile X syndrome involves expansion of this repeat segment. In an unaffected individual, the number of CGG repeats in the *FMR1* gene varies from 6 to approximately 50. Individuals with fragile X syndrome can have two types of mutation: premutations (approximately 50–200 CGG repeats) and full mutations (greater than 200 repeats). For mutations of more than 200 repeats, the CpG island upstream of *FMR1* becomes hypermethylated (Sutcliffe et al., 1992), causing transcriptional silencing of the gene. The lack of *FMR1* expression results in fragile X syndrome (Pieretti et al., 1991). All boys and men with full mutation show clinical features of fragile X syndrome; however, girls and women with more than 200 linear CGG repeats have a disparity in clinical effect, likely as a result of random X inactivation.

Boys and girls with a premutation are generally unaffected intellectually but are at risk for medical complications as they get older. Men with premutations transmit the repeat to all of their daughters as a premutation. These daughters are unaffected but are at risk of having offspring with fragile X syndrome. Men with full mutations transmit a premutation to all of their daughters because they have only premutation-sized repeats in their sperm (Reyniers et al., 1993). The male germline is not protected from expansion to the full mutation; rather, evidence suggests that the premutation-sized repeats (which are contractions of the full mutation) are preferentially copied in the rapidly dividing male germline (Malter et al., 1997). Men with premutations or full mutations transmit neither to their sons because they transmit their Y chromosome to their sons.

Women heterozygous for either a premutation or full mutation have a 50% chance of passing the mutation on to each child. Women with a premutation transmit to the next generation either as premutation or expanded into a full mutation, depending on the size of the premutation (Ashley-Koch et al., 1998; Nolin et al., 1996). As the number of repeats in the premutation increases, the likelihood is greater that the premutation will expand to full mutation in the female germline. Unlike the male germline, full mutations in the female germline rarely contract to the premutation size.

Methylation status is important in distinguishing between borderline premutation and full mutation. Molecular diagnostic techniques reveal the prevalence of fragile X syndrome to be 1 in 4,000 boys in most population studies (Crawford et al., 2001; Turner et al., 1996). The prevalence of the premutation is 1 in 259 girls in the general population (Rousseau, Rouillard, Morel, Khandjian, & Morgan, 1995).

PHYSICAL CHARACTERISTICS

The physical features of individuals with fragile X syndrome are subtle and may become more apparent with advancing age. In addition, the various levels of *FMR1* gene product, known as the fragile X mental retardation protein (FMRP) create a wide spectrum of phenotypic involvement. Among individuals with full mutations, the *FMR1* gene becomes methylated, preventing transcription and translation of the gene (Pieretti et. al., 1991; Sutcliffe et al., 1992). Lack of the FMRP is responsible for fragile X syndrome. The degree of cognitive impairments in fragile X syndrome appears to correlate with the amount of FMRP produced in each individual (Kaufmann et al., 1999). Full mutation boys and men have depleted FMRP levels and are more severely affected.

The condition is still underdiagnosed in young children because the fragile X phenotype is nonspecific. Despite the diverse information on the clinical features, unique pattern of inheritance, cytogenetic, and molecular diagnosis, the diagnosis of fragile X syndrome is still challenging (Stoll, 2001). Bailey, Skinner, and Sparkman (2003) revealed that parents are usually the first to become concerned with their child's developmental milestones at an average of 13 months. Professional confirmation of developmental delay did not occur until an average age of 21 months, and fragile X syndrome diagnosis occurred at an average age of nearly 32 months. Late diagnosis results in children missing out on early intervention services, and many families continue to have additional children without knowledge of reproductive risk.

Hagerman (1991) developed a 13-item fragile X checklist to assess physical and behavioral characteristics of boys whom they evaluated for fragile X syndrome. This study suggested that both physical and behavioral abnormalities are helpful in suspecting the diagnosis. They found that large or prominent ears, large testicles, perseverative speech, and tactile defensiveness were characteristics that differentiated fragile X syndrome from others. Prepubertal boys demonstrated hyperextensible finger joints, hyperactivity, and hand flapping.

Individuals with fragile X syndrome have elongated faces, prominent ears, and prognathism (Lachiewicz, Dawson, & Spiridigliozzi, 2000; Simko, Hornstein, Soukup, & Bagamery, 1989; see Figure 9.3-1). These classic features are more commonly seen after puberty. High arch palate with or without dental crowding is seen in most cases. Other characteristics include macrocephaly, broad forehead, epicanthal folds with hypertelorism, and flattening of the nasal bridge (Simko et al., 1989). Macroorchidism, or large testicles, is not a useful clinical sign because it is uncommon in prepubertal boys. Enlargement of testicles usually begins at 8 years of age (Lachiewicz et al., 2000). Individuals with fragile X syndrome have skin that is fine and velvety. Most have joint laxity with hyperextensible joints (Hagerman, 1991). Calluses from hand biting may be present.

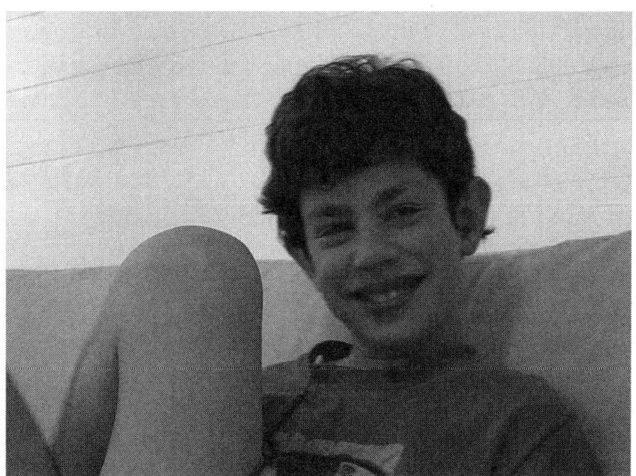

Figure 9.3-1. A boy with fragile X syndrome.

MEDICAL IMPLICATIONS

Individuals with fragile X syndrome have been reported to have chronic ear infections and recurrent sinusitis in childhood, mitral valve prolapse, and dilation of the ascending aorta. The most common neurological abnormality in fragile X syndrome is seizures. More recently, carriers of the fragile X premutation were found to be affected by a multisystem, progressive neurological disorder (Jacquemont et al., 2003). Men older than 50 with the fragile X premutation developed progressive intention tremors and cerebellar ataxia. Their symptoms also were accompanied by progressive cognitive and behavioral challenges, including memory loss, executive function impairments, anxiety, and reclusive behavior. Other features included Parkinsonism, peripheral neuropathy, lower limb proximal muscle weakness, and autonomic dysfunction (urinary and bowel incontinence and impotence). In addition, these men had hyperintensity on the T2 weighted magnetic resonance images in the cerebellar peduncles (MCP).

The radiological findings in men with tremor and ataxia serve as a diagnostic component for the fragile X–associated tremor/ataxia syndrome (FXTAS). These results suggest that the *FMR1* gene is responsible for a neurodegenerative disorder (FXTAS), and consideration for DNA testing for the *FMR1* premutation may reveal additional carriers among individuals with multisystem atrophy, essential tremor associated with late-onset cerebellar ataxia, or atypical Parkinson disease (Jacquemont et al., 2003).

A clinical finding in women with premutation is premature ovarian failure (POF), which is present in approximately 20% of women with premutation expansions (Sherman, 2000). POF does not occur in women with full mutation; therefore, the loss of FMRP is not believed to be responsible for POF (Schwartz et al., 1994).

COGNITIVE PROFILE

The level of cognitive function in individuals with fragile X syndrome varies widely depending on the degree of methylation of the *FMR1* gene (Merenstein et al., 1996). Merenstein and colleagues (1996) found that men and boys with fully methylated, full mutation alleles have mild to moderate intellectual disabilities, with a mean IQ score of 41. Men and boys with mosaic (some cells with premutation and some cells with the full mutation) have a mean IQ score of 60, whereas men and boys with a full CGG expansions and partial methylation have a mean IQ score of 88. In addition, men and boys with fragile X syndrome show weaknesses in auditory-verbal and visual-perceptual short-term memory (Dykens, Hodapp, & Leckman, 1987). They have great difficulties with sequential processing and sustaining attention and effort.

Men and boys with fragile X syndrome have strengths in verbal skills, especially tasks involving long-term memory (Dykens et al., 1987). Children with fragile X syndrome in general show a decline in IQ score over time (Fisch, Simensen, & Schroer, 2002). In addition, they show a decline in all domains of adaptive behavior—communication, daily living skills, and socialization. Declines in adaptive behavior scores reflect that these children acquire adaptive behavior skills at a slower rate than do other children of their age. Declines in IQ score and adaptive skills do not represent a regression. As a result, children fall further behind their peers as they grow older. Early intervention for these children is important to foster their independency with daily living skill activities.

The cognitive functioning in affected women and girls also relates to the amount of *FMR1* protein produced. Furthermore, it is also influenced by X activation in which one X chromosome is randomly inactivated in all cells. The level of involvement depends on the X activation ratio, the proportion of cells that have the normal X chromosome relative to the cells with the expanded CGG repeat. Women and girls with full mutations are less affected cognitively as compared with men and boys because they produce some *FMR1* protein from their normal X chromosome. In women and girls with full mutation, 71% had IQ scores below 85, suggesting borderline or mild/moderate intellectual disabilities (de Vries et al., 1996). When compared with their first-degree female relatives, full mutation women and girls had significantly lower mean Full Scale IQ, Performance IQ, and Verbal IQ scores, suggesting a dominant effect of the *FMR1* gene full mutation in the mental development of girls.

Women and girls with fragile X syndrome also demonstrate similar strengths and weaknesses to men and boys with fragile X syndrome. Strengths in verbal skills are often recognized with great difficulties in visual-perceptual and spatial construction (Mazzocco, Hagerman, & Pennington, 1992). Furthermore, these women and girls may have problems integrating information and sustaining attention and effort.

LANGUAGE

Young children with fragile X syndrome may initially come to medical attention for expressive language delay or perseverative speech. Boys with fragile X syndrome have delays in both the receptive and expressive language development. They gain expressive language skills more slowly than receptive language skills, and the discrepancy between expressive and receptive language skills increases as the children became older (Roberts, Mirrett, & Burchinal, 2001). Boys with fragile X syndrome also react to the socially demanding characteristics of conversation by becoming aroused and producing faster and more repetitive speech. They exhibit a greater incidence of repetitive speech when compared with individuals with other developmental disabilities matched for chronological age and language age (Belser & Sudhalter, 2001). These results suggest that the repetitive speech seen in individuals with fragile X syndrome is possibly caused by the effect of physiological arousal due to hypersensitivity to social and sensory stimuli.

BEHAVIORAL CHARACTERISTICS

Boys with fragile X syndrome often exhibit behavior consistent with those seen in boys with autism. These behaviors are often significant and persistent enough to result in a dual diagnosis of fragile X syndrome and autism or autistic-like tendencies. The explanation for this relationship is unknown. Bailey et al. (1998) reported that nearly 25% of the individuals with fragile X syndrome in the study's sample met the clinical criteria for autism based on the Childhood Autism Rating Scales (CARS; Schopler, Reichler, & Renner, 1988). Several autistic-like characteristics include gaze avoidance, tactile defensiveness or sensitivity to touch, hand biting, and hand flapping. In addition, boys with fragile X syndrome may also demonstrate perseveration or repetition in speech and behavior that are consistent with autism spectrum disorders (see Chapter 23.1). Some children with fragile X syndrome are shy and socially anxious but seem interested in social interactions and are more aware of their surroundings than children with autism.

Boys with fragile X syndrome also demonstrate social avoidance at a young age. They are likely to turn their head or move away from unfamiliar people or objects; however, they do not tend to remain withdrawn or avoid familiar people. They are often slow to warm up in social situations. Children with fragile X syndrome may or may not have hyperactivity or inattentiveness. When compared with other children with developmental disabilities, they show impairments in motor skills, impairments in attention, increased hyperactivity and avoidance of novel objects, decreased social withdrawal, and greater degrees of positive mood (Kau, Reider, Payne, Meyer, & Freund, 2000).

Girls with the fragile X mutation showed a greater frequency of avoidant disorder and mood disorder compared with a non–fragile X control group (Freund, Reiss, & Abrams, 1993). They also have a higher frequency of stereotypy and habit disorder. Furthermore, they have greater impairments in their interpersonal skills and are rated by their parents and teachers as significantly more withdrawn and depressed when compared with control subjects. Girls with fragile X syndrome are vulnerable to social anxiety, social avoidance, withdrawal, and depression.

MANAGEMENT AND INTERVENTION

Early recognition of the characteristics of fragile X syndrome has important implications for the affected individuals and their family members. Infants tend to have subtle physical features, but fragile X syndrome can be diagnosed during infancy in cases of known family history (Lachiewicz et al., 2000; Simko et al., 1989). Most infants are hypotonic and require early physical therapy. In addition, children with fragile X syndrome have developmental delays and a relative lack of speech. Toddlers may still have hypotonia and motor delays. Continuing physical therapy and occupational therapy with sensory approaches to address sensory integration deficits is important (see Table 9.3-1). Early speech and language intervention is recommended to help with receptive and expressive language delays. Oral motor exercise is also advised to help with coordination of the muscles of articulation.

School-age children may experience adverse response to touch on the skin (tactile defensiveness), difficulty touching tongue to lips (oral-motor incoordination), soft skin over the dorsum of the hands, and hallucal crease (Lachiewicz et al., 2000). These items are subjective but may be helpful to clinicians trying to diagnose these children. Furthermore, behavioral symptoms of gaze avoidance, hand flapping, hand biting, hyperactivity, impulsivity, and short attention span may be present. Physical characteristics of elongated face, ears longer than the 75th percentile, and head circumference greater than the 50th percentile should raise suspicion.

Behavior is often marked by hyperactivity, discipline challenges, and temper tantrums. Self-abusive behavior with hand biting, head banging, or pulling of hair may occur (see Chapter 23.5). Autistic-like behaviors, including rocking, spinning, poor eye contact, and difficulty with transitions may also be present (Simko et al., 1989). Every child with fragile X syndrome will need an individualized educational program that addresses the child's particular strengths and weaknesses, with emphasis on communication, daily living skills, and motor and cognitive development. School-age children also need to be in an optimal learning environment with special education support. They should continue to receive speech-language therapy and occupational and physical therapy.

Adolescents with fragile X syndrome should continue to receive educational and social support. Vocational training should be incorporated in individualized educational planning. Social skills training may be needed for those with social anxiety or avoidance. Adolescents with depression or mood disorders may need ongoing counseling and pharmacological intervention as well.

Adolescents with fragile X need to understand the nature of their condition and the risks of transmitting it to their offspring. Adolescent boys with full mutation rarely have children due to cognitive and social impairments. Adolescent girls with full mutation, however, can have normal relationships and reproduce; therefore, genetic counseling is important. Adolescents who are carriers of the premutation require genetic counseling to understand the complex inheritance pattern of the expanded CGG repeat. Psychological counseling may be needed for adolescents who have a challenging time dealing with this condition.

Because individuals with fragile X syndrome have a normal life expectancy, anticipatory guidance throughout childhood and adolescence is important to help them achieve an optimal life in adulthood. Vocational training is essential, and the level of support (ranging from as needed to constant) provided is based on the individual's cognitive and adaptive functioning. Consistent routines with few transitions are also essential in

Table 9.3-1. Management of fragile X syndrome

System	Concern	Evaluation	Management
Ear, nose, and throat (ENT)	Frequent otitis media	ENT consult	Screening hearing evaluation, antimicrobial therapy, tympanostomy tubes
Vision	Strabismus, nystagmus	Ophthalmology consult, visual acuity testing	Corrective surgery, patching, corrective lenses
Cardiovascular system	Mitral valve prolapse, aortic dilation	Cardiology consult	Echocardiogram, limited physical exercise
Gastrointestinal tract	Gastroesophageal reflux, feeding problems	Gastroenterology consult	Thickened foods, antireflux positioning, gastric motility agents
Musculoskeletal system	Hip dislocation, club feet, joint laxity, flat feet, pectus, scoliosis	Orthopedics consult	X-rays, early physical therapy, possible surgery
Genitourinary system	Inguinal hernia	Urology consult	Possible surgery
	Macro-orchidism	Check testis size	Regular evaluation
Central nervous system	Hypotonia, seizures, fragile X–associated tremor/ataxia syndrome	Neurology consult	Electroencephalogram, magnetic resonance imaging, seizure medication
Dental care	High palate, dental caries, dental anomalies	Dental consult	Regular dental screening, preventative care
Cognitive/behavioral systems	Developmental delay, intellectual disabilities, learning disabilities	Developmental evaluation/ psychoeducational assessment	Early intervention therapy, speech therapy, individualized education program/support
	Behavioral problems	Behavioral evaluation	Behavioral management and/or pharmacotherapy
	Sensory integration disorder	Occupational therapy evaluation	Occupational therapy addressing sensory issues

order for the individual to function on a daily basis without maladaptive behavior. Family support with educational and vocational domains is imperative.

SCREENING AND TESTING

Fragile X syndrome remains a challenge to diagnose because its physical characteristics are nonspecific and family history may be noncontributory. In 1994, the American College of Medical Genetics recommended the following guidelines to aid clinicians in making referrals for fragile X syndrome testing (Park, Howard-Peebles, Sherman, Taylor, & Wulfsberg, 1994):

1. Boys and girls with intellectual disabilities, developmental delay, or autism, especially if they have any physical or behavioral characteristics of fragile X syndrome, a family history of fragile X syndrome, or relatives (men or women) with undiagnosed intellectual disabilities.
2. Individuals seeking reproductive counseling who have family history of fragile X syndrome or a family history of underdiagnosed intellectual disabilities.
3. Fetuses of known carrier mothers
4. Individuals who have a cytogenetic fragile X test result that is discordant with their phenotype, including individuals with a strong indication (including risk of being a carrier) who have had a negative or ambiguous test result and individuals with an atypical phenotype who have had a positive test result.

Based on the American College of Medical Genetics policy statement (Maddalena et al., 2001), DNA analysis is the method of choice if one is testing specifically for fragile X syndrome and associated trinucleotide expansion in the *FMR1* gene. If the etiology of intellectual disabilities is unknown, DNA analysis for fragile X syndrome and chromosomal analysis should be performed as part of a comprehensive genetic evaluation. For individuals who are at risk due to an established family history of fragile X syndrome, DNA testing alone is sufficient.

CONCLUSION

Many immediate or extended family members of individuals with fragile X syndrome may carry the condition in the premutation or full mutation pattern.

Family members should understand the nature of the condition and receive updated information regarding genetic testing, preventive medical care, and issues relating to development, behavior, cognitive, and adaptive skills. Individuals with fragile X syndrome should receive early interventional therapy and educational support. They should also have sufficient parental and social supports to foster their growth and development into adulthood. The National Fragile X Foundation (http://www.fragilex.org) is an excellent resource for families of children with fragile X syndrome.

REFERENCES

Ashley-Koch, A.E., Robinson, H., Glickman, A.E., Nolin, S.L., Schwartz, C.E., Brown, W.T., et al. (1998). Examination of factors associated with instability of the *FMR1* CGG repeat. *American Journal of Human Genetics, 63*, 776–785.

Bailey, D.B., Mesibov, G.B., Hatton, D.D., Clark, R.D., Roberts, J.E., & Mayhew, L. (1998). Autistic behavior in young boys with fragile X syndrome. *Journal of Autism and Developmental Disorders, 28*, 499–508.

Bailey D.B., Skinner D., & Sparkman, K.L. (2003). Discovering fragile X syndrome: Family experience and perceptions. *Pediatrics, 111*, 407–416.

Belser, R.C., & Sudhalter, V. (2001). Conversational characteristics of children with fragile X syndrome: Repetitive speech. *American Journal of Mental Retardation, 106*, 28–38.

Crawford, D.C., Acuna, J.M., & Sherman, S.L. (2001). *FMR1* and fragile X syndrome: Human genome epidemiology review. *Genetics in Medicine, 3*, 359–371.

de Vries, B.B., Wiegers, A.M., Smits, A.P., Mohkamsing, S., Duivenvoorden, H.J., Fryns, J.P., et al. (1996). Mental status of females with an *FMR1* gene full mutation. *American Journal of Human Genetics, 58*, 1025–1032.

Dykens, E.M., Hodapp, R.M., & Leckman, J.F. (1987). Strengths and weaknesses in intellectual functioning of males with fragile X syndrome. *American Journal of Mental Deficiency, 92*, 234–236.

Fisch, G.S., Simensen, R.J., & Schroer, R.J. (2002). Longitudinal changes in cognitive and adaptive behavior scores in children and adolescents with the fragile X mutation or autism. *Journal of Autism and Developmental Disorders, 32*, 107–114.

Freund, L.S., Reiss, A.L., & Abrams, M.T. (1993). Psychiatric disorders associated with fragile X in the young female. *Pediatrics, 91*, 321–329.

Fu, Y.H., Kuhl, D.P., Pizutti, M., Sutcliffe, J.S., Richards, S., et al. (1991). Variation of the CGG repeat at the fragile X site results in genetic instability: Resolution of the Sherman paradox. *Cell, 67*, 1047–1057.

Hagerman, R.J. (1991). Fragile X checklist. *American Journal of Medical Genetics, 38*, 283–287.

Jacquemont, S., Hagerman, R.J., Leehey, M., Grigsby, J., Zhang, L., Brunberg, J.A., et al. (2003). Fragile X premutation tremor/ataxia syndrome: Molecular, clinical, and neuroimaging correlates. *American Journal of Human Genetics, 72*, 869–878.

Kau, A.S.M., Reider, E.E., Payne, L., Meyer, W.A., & Freund, L. (2000). Early behavior signs of psychiatric phenotypes in fragile X syndrome. *American Journal of Mental Retardation, 105*, 266–299.

Kaufman, W.E., Abrams, M.T., Chen, W., & Reiss, A.L. (1999). Genotype, molecular phenotype, and cognitive phenotype: Correlations in fragile X syndrome. *American Journal of Medical Genetics, 83*, 286–295.

La Spada, A.R., Wilson, E.M., Lubahn, D.B., Harding, A.E., & Fischbeck, K.H. (1991). Androgen receptor gene mutations in X-linked spinal and bulbar muscular atrophy. *Nature, 352*, 77–79.

Lachiewicz, A.M., Dawson, D.V., & Spiridigliozzi, G.A. (2000). Physical characteristics of young boys with fragile X syndrome: Reasons for difficulties in making a diagnosis in young males. *American Journal of Medical Genetics, 92*, 229–236.

Lubs, H.A. (1969). A marker X chromosome. *American Journal of Human Genetics, 21*, 231–244.

Maddalena, A., Richard, C.S., McGinniss, M.J., Brothman, A., Desnick, R.J., Grier, R.E., et al. (2001). Technical standards and guidelines for fragile X: The first of a series of disease-specific supplements to the Standards and Guidelines for Clinical Genetics Laboratories of the American College of Medical Genetics. Quality Assurance Subcommittee of the Laboratory Practice Committee. *Genetics in Medicine, 3*, 200–205.

Malter, H.E., Iber, J.C., Willemsen, R., de Graaff, E., Tarleton, J.C., Leisti, J., et al. (1997). Characterization of the full fragile X syndrome mutation in fetal gametes. *Nature Genetics, 15*, 165–169.

Martin, J.P., & Bell, J. (1943). A pedigree of mental defect showing sex-linkage. *Journal of Neurological Psychiatry, 6*, 154–157.

Mazzocco, M.M., Hagerman, R.J., & Pennington, B. (1992). Problem-solving limitations among cytogenetically expressing fragile X women. *American Journal of Medical Genetics, 43*, 78–86.

Merenstein, S.A., Sobesky, W.E., Taylor, A.K., Riddle, J.E., Tran, H.X., & Hagerman, R.J. (1996). Molecular-clinical correlations in males with an expanded *FMR1* mutation. *American Journal of Medical Genetics, 64*, 388–394.

Nolin, S.L., Lewis, F.A., Houck, G.E., Glickman, A.E., Limprasert, P., Li, S.Y., et al. (1996). Familiar transmission of the *FMR1* CGG repeat. *American Journal of Human Genetics, 59*, 1252–1261.

Park, V., Howard-Peebles, P., Sherman, S., Taylor, A., & Wulfsberg, E. (1994). Policy statement: American College of Medical Genetics. Fragile X syndrome: Diagnostic and carrier testing. *American Journal of Medical Genetics, 53*, 380–381.

Pieretti, M., Zhang, F.P., Fu, Y.H., Warren, S.T., Oostra, B.A., Caskey, C.T., et al. (1991). Absence of expression of the *FMR-1* gene in fragile X syndrome. *Cell, 66*, 817–822.

Reyniers, E., Vits, L., De Boulle, K., Van Roy, B., Vanvelzen, D., de Graaff, E., et al. (1993). The full mutation in the *FMR-1* gene of male fragile X patients is absent in their sperm. *Nature Genetics, 4*, 143–146.

Roberts, J.E., Mirrett, P., & Burchinal, M. (2001). Receptive and expressive communication development of young males with fragile X syndrome. *American Journal of Mental Retardation, 106*, 216–230.

Rousseau, F., Rouillard, P., Morel, M.L., Khandjian, E.W., & Morgan, K. (1995). Prevalence of carriers of premutation-size alleles of the *FMR-1* gene and implications for the population genetics of the fragile X syndrome. *American Journal of Human Genetics, 57,* 1006–1018.

Schopler, E., Reichler, R.J., & Renner, B.R. (1988). *The Childhood Autism Rating Scale.* Los Angeles: Western Psychological Services.

Schwartz, C.E., Dean, J., Howard-Peebles, P.N., Bugge, M., Mikkelsen, M., Tommerup, N., et al. (1994). Obstetrical and gynecological complications in fragile X carriers: A multicenter study. *American Journal of Medical Genetics, 51,* 400–402.

Sherman, S.L. (2000). Premature ovarian failure in the fragile X syndrome. *American Journal of Medical Genetics, 97,* 189–194.

Simko, A., Hornstein, L., Soukup, S., & Bagamery, N. (1989). Fragile X syndrome: Recognition in young children. *Pediatrics, 83,* 547–552.

Stoll C. (2001). Problems in the diagnosis of fragile X syndrome in young children are still present. *American Journal of Medical Genetics, 100,* 110–115.

Sutcliffe, J.S., Nelson, D.L., Zhang, F., Pieretti, M., Caskey, C.T., Saxe, D., et al. (1992). DNA methylation represses *FMR-1* transcription in fragile X syndrome. *Human Molecular Genetics, 1,* 397–400.

Sutherland, G.R. (1977). Fragile sites on human chromosomes: Demonstration of their dependence on the type of tissue culture medium. *Science, 197,* 265–266.

Turner, G., Webb, T., Wake, S., & Robinson, H. (1996). Prevalence of fragile X syndrome. *American Journal of Medical Genetics, 64,* 196–197.

Verkerk, A.J., Pieretti, M., Sutcliffe, J.S., Fu, Y.H., Kuhl, D.P., Pizzuti, A., et al. (1991). Identification of a gene *(FMR-1)* containing a CGG repeat coincident with a breakpoint cluster region exhibiting length variation in fragile X syndrome. *Cell, 65,* 905–914.

9.4 PRADER-WILLI SYNDROME

Randell Alexander

Prader-Willi syndrome was first described by Prader, Labhart, and Willi (1956). They noted an unusual syndrome in which individuals had poor feeding in infancy, underdeveloped sexual organs, short stature, poor muscle tone, a characteristic appearance (e.g., small hands and feet, facial features), and cognitive impairment. The most striking feature of the syndrome was onset of marked obesity after infancy. This seemingly insatiable appetite could lead to morbid obesity and death in the teens or 20s if unchecked. Since Prader and colleagues' initial report, considerable research and experience has helped to clarify the syndrome and has led to new concepts in genetics.

Various estimates place the incidence of Prader-Willi syndrome as between 1/10,000 to 1/15,000 births. Although such estimates might place the prevalence of Prader-Willi syndrome as between 17,000–28,000 in the general population, the shortened life expectancy of individuals with Prader-Willi syndrome probably cuts the true prevalence by as much as half. The implications are that Prader-Willi syndrome is only occasionally encountered by clinicians or school personnel and is, therefore, underdiagnosed. Consequently, parents often have difficulty obtaining professional expertise about this condition, even if their child is diagnosed correctly.

During Wendy's pregnancy with Joey, she noticed that Joey had decreased fetal movements. He was born full term with an average birth weight, but in the nursery he had difficulty feeding with an apparent weak suck. He was fed by a gavage tube for the next 2 weeks in the hospital. With frequent small feeds, he was discharged home, where he had problems gaining weight for the next 6 months. Wendy later described Joey during this period in his life as a somewhat floppy and underweight child with delayed motor milestones. The doctors had no diagnosis for this condition, presuming some sort of congenital hypotonia.

Joey first sat by himself at 12 months, crawled by 18 months, and walked independently at 25 months of age. By 12 months, his feeding had improved to the point that he achieved normal weight gain. Wendy thought that his feeding problems had resolved, and only some hypotonia and developmental delay remained.

Joey continued to eat well, and, at about 24 months of age, Wendy even noticed that he began to seem chubby. Neither she nor Joey's pediatrician were concerned at the time; however, the weight gain continued to accelerate until Joey was four standard deviations above the mean of weight for age when he was 4 years old. About that same time, he began to have some behavior problems with tantrums and refusals. Some of these were connected with food, but others seemed to occur with changes in routine. At this time, he also had surgery for undescended testicles. During this admission, pediatric consultation was obtained for his obesity. He subsequently was referred to genetics, where the clinical diagnosis of Prader-Willi syndrome was first made.

CLINICAL CHARACTERISTICS

Prader-Willi syndrome is often considered as having two phases. The first phase is marked by infant hypotonia and poor feeding. The second begins during the toddler years and continues for a lifetime. This phase is characterized by a seemingly insatiable appetite, morbid obesity if untreated, and behavior problems (Alexander & Greenswag, 1995). During pregnancy with a child with Prader-Willi syndrome, mothers may notice decreased fetal movements compared with other pregnancies. Children are full term and are essentially normal size at birth. Apgar scores are often low.

Typically, the earliest clues of Prader-Willi Syndrome emerge at birth. The newborn often has thermoregulation problems with low temperatures. This condition reflects dysfunction of the hypothalamus, which controls basic regulatory functions of the body. Most children are hypotonic—often to a considerable degree. As a result of their hypotonia, they feed very poorly with a poor sucking response. They also tend to take only small feeds and may be undernourished. They may need to be fed with a gavage tube, and overt failure to thrive is sometimes a problem. In some instances, the failure to feed well has led to concerns about neglect. During this period of life, parents typically are distressed about their hypotonic and poorly feeding child. The hypotonia and feeding problems in the newborn unit increasingly lead to diagnostic studies—including genetic testing that establishes the diagnosis.

By 1 year of age, most children with Prader-Willi syndrome eat well by themselves. From the parents' point of view, their formerly poor-feeding child now seems to be out of the woods and on a more normal path. The generalized hypotonia improves, and the child is more active. Developmental milestones are delayed, but the overall improvement leads to a false sense of security about how the child will later fare. By 2–3 years of age, overeating and obesity are apparent to most parents (see Figure 9.4-1). The onset of behavior problems is around 4 years of age (Greenswag & Alexander, 1990). Obesity and behavior problems dominate the rest of the individual's life.

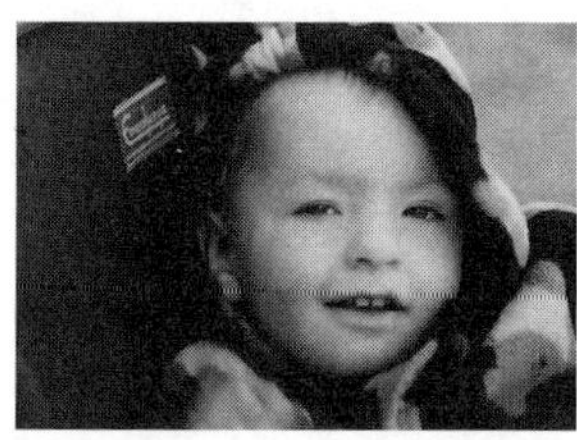

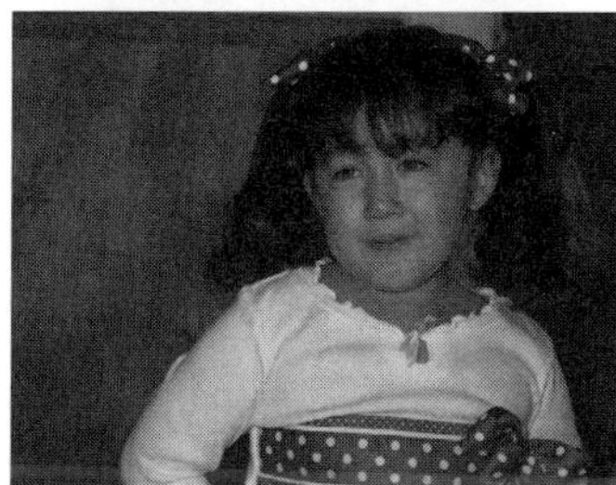

Figure 9.4-1. Children with Prader-Willi syndrome. Boy age 1 year (top photo); girl age 4 years (bottom photo).

Table 9.4-1. Clinical characteristics of Prader-Willi syndrome

Major criteria
Neonatal hypotonia
Hyperphagia (overeating) leading to obesity
Cognitive impairments (usually mild intellectual disabilties)
Lack of sexual development—hypogonadism (incapable of having children)
Other developmental disabilities
Behavior problems (e.g., stubborn)
Minor criteria
Short stature
Small hands and feet
Vision/eye problems
Skin picking
Sleep problems
Features of additional medical concern
High vomiting threshold (if vomiting, child may be sicker than thought)
High pain tolerance—may not report pain (even fractures) as readily
Seldom has fevers when ill, or may have low temperatures

Reproduced with permission from *Pediatrics*, Vol. 19, Pages 398–402, Copyright © 1993 by the AAP.

A number of specific clinical characteristics of Prader-Willi syndrome are listed in Table 9.4-1 (Holm et al., 1993). Some of the problems appear to be linked to problems with hypothalamic regulation (neonatal temperature control problems, alteration in the satiety set point, lack of sexual development), but a specific lesion or neurotransmitter abnormality has yet to be found. Physical characteristics are listed in Table 9.4-2, and typical developmental milestones are given in Table 9.4-3. Note that the developmental milestones are explained mostly by the usual mild intellectual disabilities and the mild hypotonia. The hypotonia persists at least in a mild form into adulthood and may be a component of problems with articulation skills, scoliosis, and occasionally respiratory problems (especially with illness).

GENETIC MECHANISMS

In the past, Prader-Willi syndrome was usually not diagnosed, developmental problems were poorly addressed, and morbid obesity developed by teenage or early adulthood, which led to death. Advances in genetic understanding and testing now enable a diagnosis based not only on clinical characteristics but also on laboratory confirmation. In turn, early diagnosis can lead to much more effective management to avoid or minimize some of the complications of the disorder.

Prader-Willi syndrome involves a portion of the long arm of the 15th chromosome. In about 70% of the cases, there is a deletion of a portion of this chromosome (15q11-q13). Often, the portion can be detected

Table 9.4-2. Physical characteristics of individuals with Prader-Willi syndrome

Almond-shaped eyes
Triangular-shaped mouth
Narrow bifrontal skull diameter
Small hands and feet
Central fat distribution (most prominent about the stomach, hips, and thighs)
Hypogonadism
Cryptorchidism and small testes (men and boys)
Hypoplastic labia (girls and women)
Short stature if untreated (men 5′0″; women 4′8″)
No adolescent growth spurt
Delayed bone closure
Eye problems
Myopia
Strabismus

From Alexander, R., & Greenswag, L. (1995). Medical and nursing interventions. In L. Greenswag & R. Alexander (Eds.), *Management of Prader-Willi syndrome* (pp. 66–80). New York: Springer-Verlag; adapted with kind permission of Springer Science and Business Media.

by so-called "stretched chromosome" testing (prometaphase banding). There are two portions to a chromosome, one derived from the mother and one from the father. Traditional notions of genetics for 100 years were that it did not matter whether the deleted portion was originally derived from the father or the mother—that the portions were equivalent (except for X and Y chromosomes)—however, research has demonstrated that if the deleted portion is from the father, the child will have Prader-Willi syndrome. If the deleted portion is from the mother, the child will have Angelman syndrome (a quite different genetic condition). This discovery led to a reconceptualization of genetic inheritance and the concept of "genomic imprinting," whereby it matters whether the mother's or the father's chromosome is being expressed.

In about 25% of the cases of Prader-Willi syndrome, the cause is maternal disomy. Rather than the key portion of the chromosome having only the mother's half (and none from the father), in disomy there are two halves in that area—both from the mother. (Note that paternal disomy would lead to Angelman syndrome.) Although the mechanism is not completely accepted, a leading hypothesis is that at one point there actually are two copies of the mother's chromosome in this key location and one of the father's. Presumably the father's copy is lost as embryonic development proceeds.

The remainder of the cases involve a more complicated genetic transmission but still result in the influence of the mother's genetics at the key site and not the father's. Overall, the odds of having another child with Prader-Willi syndrome are extremely low, about the odds of having a child with Prader-Willi syndome in the first place. In a few rare instances, however, there have been unusual chromosomal rearrangements such that the risk is higher. This scenario is one important reason for genetic testing of all suspected cases.

For cases suspected by clinical criteria (e.g., hypotonia in the newborn period), referral to a geneticist is appropriate. A number of geneticists also recommend that any child with unexplained intellectual disabilities should receive genetic evaluation. The specifics of the genetic testing are conducted by geneticists and include prometaphase banding (looking for deletions), fluorescent in situ hybridization (FISH; keying in on the portion where the deletion may occur), and more specialized tests for disomy.

An important concern with any genetic condition is the question of who is "at fault." Understandably families want to reflect on whether the condition came from one side of the family; however, this discussion is inappropriate with Prader-Willi syndrome in that the disorder is almost invariably caused by a random event in how the chromosomes separated and came together in creating the child. The parents could have done nothing to cause or prevent this disorder.

Table 9.4-3. Developmental milestones for individuals with Prader-Willi syndrome

Motor
Sits unsupported—1 year
Walks—2 years
Rides tricycle—4 years
Language
Says first words—21 months
Uses sentences—3.5 years
Reads—7.5 years
Knows basic math skills—8.5 years
Cognitive
Normal range (but not high)—12%
Borderline or mild intellectual disabilities—70%
Moderate/severe intellectual disabilities—18%

MANAGEMENT

Prader-Willi syndrome is one of the prime examples of a pervasive developmental disability in that it typically results in delays/impairments in nearly every area of professional inquiry. There is no cure, and management and prevention of complications is paramount.

Medical Management

In addition to a developmental pediatrician with knowledge of Prader-Willi syndrome, other key medical specialties include ophthalmology (vision problems), orthopedics (e.g., scoliosis), endocrinology (growth hormone issues, possibly diabetes), and dentistry (enamel problems, acid etching of teeth from rumination). Individuals with Prader-Willi syndrome are short during childhood and as adults. In the past, growth hormone levels were evaluated in children. Some individuals were found to have low levels, and some were not. Growth hormone was given accordingly (see Chapter 19). Further research showed that growth hormone per se was not always the issue. Serum levels of insulin growth hormone factor (IGF–1) were often low, which is not the case for other forms of obesity. Therefore, Prader-Willi syndrome can most correctly be characterized as an IGF axis deficiency (Lee et al., 2000).

Growth hormone improves IGF–1 and other growth factor levels. It increases the rate of growth and seems to improve final adult height. When given to individuals with Prader-Willi syndrome, it decreases fat mass by about 10%. It also increases muscle and bone mass, resulting in an improved fat to muscle ratio. The clinical result is a child who appears leaner and grows taller at a rate more comparable to typically developing peers; however, growth hormone is not a "cure" for obesity issues, and the appearance of a more central distribution of fat persists.

Side effects of growth hormone are few. Although behavior change is possible with growth hormone, anecdotally parents often report improved behavior (e.g., less opposition). Pulmonary function is sometimes improved, but it is not clear whether this result is a function of decreased fat or better weight. The net effect of growth hormone is also reported to help with sleep apnea, but again the mechanism may be through less fat/weight. Thus, experience shows that growth hormone seems to help with body composition, energy, and possibly behavior. Most experts in Prader-Willi syndrome recommend growth hormone during the growth years, and most families opt to use it. Since July 2000, the Food and Drug Administration has approved growth hormone for all children with Prader-Willi syndrome. Demonstrating a specific growth hormone deficiency is not necessary. Studies are underway to determine whether growth hormone would also be beneficial for adults with Prader-Willi syndrome.

Sex hormones (e.g., estrogen, testosterone) have been used to help with bone density for older individuals. Because boys have underdeveloped genitalia and may be self-conscious around peers, testosterone has been used to help with appearance. Estrogen to aid the appearance of girls has not been used as much. Sex hormones can be given as injections, patches, and gels.

The relative lack of activity, lack of puberty and its hormones, and the need for strict diets that are otherwise low in calcium means that children and young adults may not build sufficient bone density. Combined with hypotonia, insufficient bone density may lead to scoliosis and osteoporosis. Before starting compensatory hormone therapy, a dual-energy x-ray absorptiometry (DEXA) scan may be helpful. Norms in children and individuals with Prader-Willi syndrome are still being established but should prove to be a useful way to monitor bone density and may guide various interventions even more.

Children with Prader-Willi syndrome are prone to daytime sleepiness. Grade school children frequently fall asleep in class in the afternoon. Snoring is also a common complaint. Sleep apnea may be part of the reason for these symptoms. Although some children are extremely overweight, the sleepiness and apnea do not seem to be on the basis of a Pickwickian mechanism. Even small weight loss may have a significant effect on these symptoms. If weight loss alone does not work, referral to a sleep apnea clinic is necessary. Continuous positive airway pressure masks can be effective in reducing many of the symptoms and are generally well tolerated.

Dental examinations should be regularly scheduled and attention given to possible tooth damage from rumination or enamel deficits (Alexander, Greenswag, & Nowak, 1987; see Chapter 22). Some children have thickened saliva, which can lead to more frequent caries. Other possible medical interventions are listed in Table 9.4-4.

Nutrition Management

Eating problems are a major source of concern and must be constantly addressed when the child is old enough that obesity is a risk. The seemingly insatiable appetite exceeds that of even most obese children and adults and is a major threat to health and life. Individuals with Prader-Willi syndrome seek food from a wide variety of sources and may be seemingly more clever in obtaining it than would be suggested by their IQ scores. For example, some children have obtained their par-

Table 9.4-4. Additional medical interventions for individuals with Prader-Willi syndrome

Calcium and multivitamins
Annual examination for scoliosis
Fluoxetine to help with skin picking
Exercise
Annual flu shot
Prevnar and pneumococcal vaccines
Sunscreen to protect individuals with fair skin

ents' credit card and ordered food delivery while their parents were away or not paying attention. Food sources must be locked up in most cases, such as placing locks or chains on refrigerators, locks on cabinets, and motion detectors in the kitchen to catch food seeking at night. Unusual food sources must also be protected (e.g., garbage, dog food).

Individuals with Prader-Willi syndrome may be given or steal food from classmates or in other situations. Because school lunches have far more calories than a Prader-Willi syndrome diet allows, school teachers must constantly watch that only the appropriate food is consumed. Unfortunately, classmates and grandparents may not see the harm in even small amounts of food and literally contribute to killing the child with their "kindness." A problem in achieving adequate caloric consumption is when parents fail to adhere to the diet, perhaps hoping (erroneously) that the child will self-regulate his or her intake. Families in which the parents are themselves obese are likely to be less successful.

After high school graduation, Joey's obesity worsened. Despite attempts by the parents to regulate his diet, his obesity worsened dramatically, and he developed problems with breathing with exertion. A stomach stapling procedure was done as a last-ditch attempt to control his morbid obesity. [*Note:* Such surgery would not be advocated today because of the high failure rate.] His postoperative course was stormy, and he almost died. Over the course of the next 5 years, he was able to eat relatively normally, and his residual stomach pouch expanded such that his weight once again had to be watched.

Often, caloric intake for individuals with Prader-Willi syndrome is calculated as about 7 kcal/cm. For a young adult, the caloric need to maintain weight is about 1,000 cal/day. To lose weight, approximately 800 cal/day is needed. At all ages, children with Prader-Willi syndrome need much less food than caregivers usually think. Parents should watch the scale as a guide to what the child's actual caloric needs are. If the child gains weight with very few calories, then parents should assume that additional food is being obtained elsewhere.

Nutritionists often have the family furnish 3-day diet histories. From this history, a balanced diet can be constructed. Children with Prader-Willi syndrome will not be eating as much or necessarily the same types of food that others in the family may. This situation requires some management of mealtime so that squabbles do not arise.

Because the calories are so few, even a well-balanced diet is deficient in the total amount of certain nutrients. Supplemental iron, calcium, and vitamins are important (e.g., multivitamin, calcium supplement). Monitoring food intake from all sources is imperative. Food should be sent to school, and no other should be given or taken. Special arrangements for parties can be made. Food should never be used as a reward. If foraging is suspected, daily weights can be obtained to enable caloric adjustments. Physical exercise is encouraged, but is insufficient as a weight loss method.

Behavior Management

Along with the constant food seeking, behavior problems are the largest management concern of parents. The key behavior problem is usually referred to as "stubbornness," but that term is inadequate to fully describe the intensity and constancy of the problem. Refusals and inflexibility are customary, and tantrums may be expected to changes in routines. Some obsessive-compulsive behaviors are not uncommon. As children get older, these behaviors may worsen. If children get large enough, they may pose a physical risk to caregivers.

Medications seem to be of little value. Children with Prader-Willi often are given methylphenidate or antidepressants, but these medications are not very useful. In contrast, selective serotonin reuptake inhibitors (e.g., fluoxetine) seem to help, particularly with obsessive-compulsive symptoms. Doses at the low end of the normal range work best, and, if the treatment is not working, physicians should *reduce* the dose. Behavior strategies can be of considerable help, but it is best to think of the problem as one requiring management, not one with a "cure." A stable, predictable environment is key.

EDUCATION

Children with Prader-Willi syndrome should get special services to cover their multitude of health issues. Prader-Willi syndrome is a recognized disability and is covered by the Individuals with Disabilities Education Act of 1990 (PL 101-476) and other federal laws; however, professionals may need to help parents understand the need to advocate with the school (e.g., at the individualized education plan meeting). Because most children have mild intellectual disabilities, speech-language problems, and mild motor problems, they may be placed in special classrooms to more individually address their needs. Although most children with Prader-Willi syndrome have modest hypotonia and fine and gross motor skills, occupational and physical therapy can be of considerable value (see Chapters 24.1 and 24.2). Most children have speech-language impairments for which therapy is also useful.

ADULTHOOD

In his 20s, Joey was in relatively good health. He began to be followed by a Prader-Willi Syndrome Clinic, and his weight was kept in relatively good control. His behavior was occasionally problematic but better than most of his peers with Prader-Willi syndrome. His parents lived on a farm and wanted Joey to keep living with them rather than a group home. When Joey was in his mid 30s, his parents were appreciably older and began legal procedures to assume guardianship and make a will naming Joey's sister as guardian in the event of their death. Despite their earlier reluctance, Joey's parents began to see that being with his peers was the least restrictive placement versus living at home with them and having little contact with anyone else.

When Joey was 34 years old, he was placed in a group home with follow-up by clinic personnel to help the staff understand the food restrictions and behavior management necessary to make this placement successful. Joey began working in a sheltered workshop. He reported that he really enjoyed both his group home and workshop experiences, and his parents seemed very pleased as well. He continues to do well physically and behaviorally. He takes vitamins and calcium, gets an annual flu shot, and maintains a diet of 1,100 cal per day. His only exercise is a modest amount of walking, and he has the appearance and apparent energy level of someone older than his age.

If food intake is not carefully regulated for adults with Prader-Willi syndrome, morbid obesity and life-threatening complications will result. Because people with Prader-Willi syndrome have an innate food-seeking drive, they cannot realistically limit themselves. Hence, independent adult living leads to more obesity (Greenswag, 1987). Early intervention and regular management can be highly successful in avoiding the most extreme obesity, but few can maintain a "normal" weight range unless caloric intake is tightly controlled (see Figure 9.4-2).

In the past, individuals with Prader-Willi syndrome did not live long enough to develop age-related medical conditions nor did they suffer the consequences of their disorder's weaknesses; however, teenagers with Prader-Willi syndrome have an increased risk of obesity-related (Type II) diabetes. At an older age, the risk of osteoporosis is magnified by dietary and sedentary impairments. Sedentary lifestyle (and perhaps mild hypotonia) is probably responsible for poor tolerance of respiratory infections. Death from otherwise routine viral respiratory infections is a risk for those in their 20s or older. Even if individuals with Prader-Willi syndrome are not obese and are carefully managed, they will most likely die 10–20 years before their typically developing peers as a consequence of never being in good cardiovascular shape.

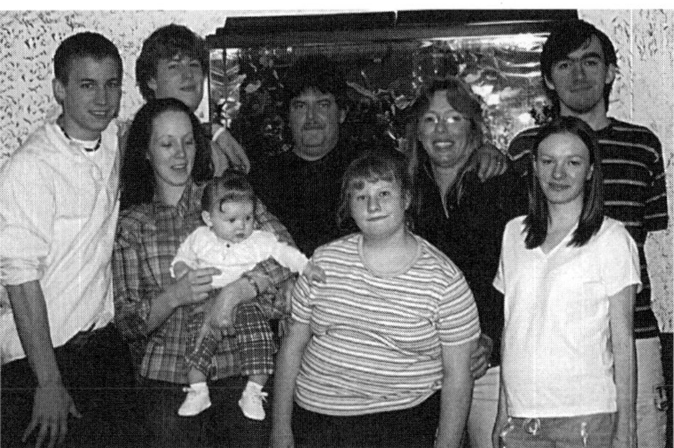

Figure 9.4-2. Family support is important to helping teenagers with Prader-Willi syndrome maintain a healthy weight.

Guardianship of individuals with Prader-Willi syndrome is important to obtain prior to the age of majority. Not only is it legally easier to do so, but it is important as part of a long-range management plan. People with Prader-Willi syndrome cannot function as well in the activities of daily living as their IQ scores indicate. They would overeat themselves to death if not in supervised living. As a result, many parents recognize the need for residential placement. Such placement may be the least restrictive living condition in that they would be living with peers (in age if not diagnosis), and there may be a degree of independence in non–food-related arenas. Often, a sheltered workshop is ideal. A major problem is the lack of good residential homes and particularly homes that control both food and behavior. The Prader-Willi Syndrome Association (see http://www.pwsaga.org) has appropriate residential care as one of its top priorities.

CONCLUSION

Prader-Willi syndrome is a genetic condition with many manifestations requiring the services of a wide variety of professionals. The incessant eating leads to morbid obesity and early death unless weight is strictly managed. Behavior problems are another major problem, often exhausting the parents and necessitating management in home and school situations. With proper attention to the myriad of developmental areas that need management, individuals with Prader-Willi syndrome live longer, have improved weight and behaviors, and have an improved quality of life.

REFERENCES

Alexander, R., & Greenswag, L. (1995). Medical and nursing interventions. In L. Greenswag & R. Alexander (Eds.), *Management of Prader Willi syndrome* (pp. 66–80). New York: Springer-Verlag.

Alexander, R., Greenswag, L., & Nowak, A. (1987). Rumination and vomiting in Prader-Willi syndrome. *American Journal of Medical Genetics, 28*, 889–895.

Greenswag, L. (1987). Adults with Prader-Willi syndrome: A survey of 232 cases. *Developmental Medicine and Child Neurology, 29*, 145–152.

Greenswag, L., & Alexander, R. (1990). Early diagnosis in Prader-Willi syndrome: Implications for managing weight and behavior. *Dysmorphology and Clinical Genetics, 4*, 8–12.

Holm, V., Cassidy, S., Butler, M., et al. (1993). Prader-Willi syndrome: Consensus diagnostic criteria. *Pediatrics, 19*, 398–402.

Individuals with Disabilities Education Act (IDEA) of 1990, PL 101-476, 20 U.S.C. §§ 1400 *et seq.*

Lee, P., Allen, D., Angulo, M., et al. (2000). Consensus statement—Prader Willi syndrome: Growth hormone (GH)/insulin-like growth factor axis deficiency and GH treatment. *The Endocrinologist, 10*, 71S–74S.

Prader, A., Labhart, A., & Willi, H. (1956). Ein syndrome von adipositas, kleinwuchs, kryptorchismus und oligophrenie nach myotonicartigem zustand in neugeborenalter. *Schweizerische Medizinische Wochenschrift, 86*, 1260–1261.

9.5 WILLIAMS SYNDROME

Jeannie Visootsak

Williams syndrome is an autosomal disorder resulting from a submicroscopic deletion of continguous genes on the long arm of chromosome 7. It is associated with a distinctive facial characteristic, cardiac abnormalities, infantile hypercalcemia, and growth and developmental delays. The condition also includes a well-delineated constellation of cognitive-linguistic profile and behavioral phenotype.

Manny, a 19-month-old boy, was referred to the developmental clinic for evaluation of developmental delay. The pregnancy was normal, and Manny was born at 37 weeks of gestation with a birth weight of 6 lb, 6 oz, and no perinatal complications. Manny had feeding difficulties and constipation during his infancy and had surgical repair of bilateral inguinal hernias. His developmental milestones were delayed. He sat independently at 10 months and cruised at 17 months. At 19 months, Manny did not walk independently. He babbled at 6 months and said "dada" nonspecifically at 12 months. Although he did not have any specific words at 19 months, he babbled throughout the day.

On physical examination, Manny appeared to be a small child with height of 30 in (10th percentile), weight of 21 lb (less than 5th percentile), and head circumference of 47 cm (25th percentile). Manny also had distinctive features of periorbital fullness, bright blue eyes with a stellate pattern to the iris, small upturned nose, and a large mouth with full lips. His parents also reported that Manny was outgoing and inappropriately friendly with strangers.

Manny's physical profile and past medical history were consistent with a diagnosis of Williams syndrome. Deoxyribonucleic acid (DNA) cytogenetic testing with fluorescent in situ hybridization (FISH) studies demonstrated a deletion on chromosome 7, consistent with Williams syndrome.

HISTORICAL BACKGROUND

Williams syndrome was independently described by Williams, Barrett-Boyes, and Lowe in 1961 and Beuren, Apitz, and Harmjanz in 1962. It is characterized by intellectual disabilities, growth deficiency, congenital cardiovascular anomaly (supravalvular aortic stenosis, or SVAS), and distinctive facial appearance (broad forehead, wide-set eyes, drooping cheeks, and wide mouth; see Figure 9.5-1). This condition became known as *Williams-Beuren syndrome*, but the common terminology in the United States is *Williams syndrome.*

In 1964, Garcia, Friedman, Kaback, and Rowe described the first case of SVAS with idiopathic infantile hypercalcemia. Subsequently, Bonham-Carter and Sutcliffe (1964) expanded on the cardiovascular manifestations in Williams syndrome by identifying that multiple arterial stenoses often occur at the bifurcations of major arteries, both in the pulmonary and systemic circulations. Although most of the early studies focused on the medical issues of Williams syndrome, unique cognitive and behavioral characteristics of individuals with Williams syndrome were also recognized by researchers. These individuals were highly verbal, overly friendly, outgoing, and loquacious.

GENETICS

Williams syndrome occurs with an estimated incidence of 1/20,000 live births (Morris, Demsey, Leonard, Dilts, & Blackburn, 1988). It is considered a contiguous gene deletion syndrome of the long arm of chromosome 7 at 7q11.23. Most cases occur sporadically, but there have been a few reported cases of parent-to-child transmission. These families showed an autosomal dominant in-

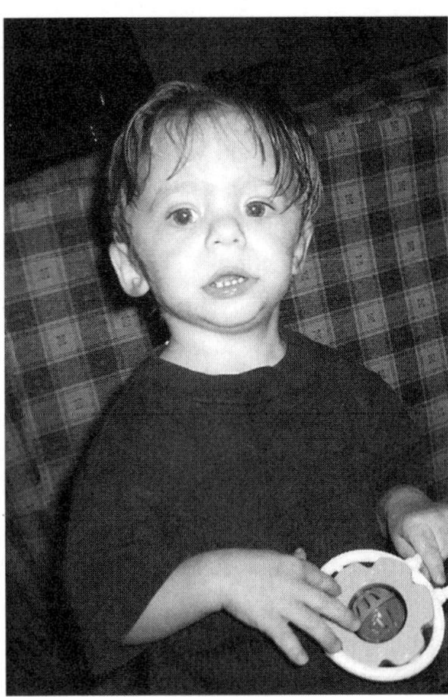

Figure 9.5-1. A child with Williams syndrome.

heritance pattern in which the parents had a 50% chance of transmitting the disorder to their offspring.

Elastin is a connective tissue protein that provides strength and elasticity to the skin, lungs, large blood vessels, and the walls of arteries and organs. Insufficiency of the gene for elastin, *ELN*, on chromosome 7 leads to SVAS, which can occur as an isolated autosomal dominant trait or as part of a broader pattern of clinical implications (Li et al., 1997). Furthermore, *ELN* deletion or mutation explains some of the features of Williams syndrome, such as some of the facial features, hoarse voice, bladder and bowel diverticula, cardiovascular disease, and orthopedic problems. Other characteristics such as hypercalcemia, intellectual disabilities, and distinctive personality remain unexplained.

Aside from *ELN*, researchers attempted to investigate other genes in the region that may be involved in the Williams syndrome genotype-phenotype relationships. One of these genes, LIM-kinase 1 *(LIMK1)*, encodes a protein kinase and is expressed in the developing brain (Tassabehji et al., 1999). *LIMK1* may be responsible for visual-spatial construction abilities. Based on several studies, researchers concluded that not all individuals with *LIMK1* deletion had Williams syndrome's cognitive profile. This area needs to be further redefined to solidify genotype-phenotype correlations.

FISH testing confirms the clinical diagnosis of Williams syndrome by detecting submicroscopic deletions of *ELN* at 7q11.23 (Lowery et al., 1995). The probe consists of fluorescently labeled DNA sequences that bind specifically to the DNA in the region that is commonly deleted in Williams syndrome. Although the diagnosis can be made on the basis of clinical criteria, 99% of individuals with Williams syndrome can be identified by FISH.

PHYSICAL CHARACTERISTICS

Although the facial appearance of individuals with Williams syndrome is distinctive, the features can be subtle and difficult to recognize. The facial characteristics evolve with age and are not apparent in infants and young children. Therefore, infants are typically identified as a result of classic findings such as SVAS and hypercalcemia, rather than their physical features.

In the first year of life, infants with Williams syndrome usually experience failure to thrive (81%), feeding difficulty (71%), colic (67%), constipation (43%), and vomiting (40%) (Morris et al., 1988). Some of these manifestations (vomiting, constipation, irritability) may be associated with hypercalcemia. Inguinal hernias and umbilical hernias are often diagnosed in the infancy period. Diagnosis of Williams syndrome may be delayed if physicians do not recognize that severe vomiting, excessive irritibility, and gastroesophageal reflux in the first year of life are patterns consistent with Williams syndrome. Because neonates or infants with Williams syndrome may have subtle physical features, physicians should be aware of the constellation of medical symptoms (severe vomiting, excessive irritability and colic, gastroesophageal reflux) of Williams syndrome.

In the childhood period, the facial and behavioral characteristics of Williams syndrome begin to evolve and raise clinical suspicion. Developmental delay is usually recognized, with walking independently at 21 months, talking at 21.6 months, and toilet training at 39 months (Morris et al., 1988). By the time they reach first grade, children with Williams syndrome may have academic difficulties. They also develop a hoarse or brassy voice. Older children are typically suspected of having Williams syndrome as a result of their behavioral characteristics and cognitive-linguistic profile.

Craniofacial Features

The typical Williams syndrome craniofacial dysmorphology becomes obvious at approximately 6 months of age, evolves fully during childhood, and assumes a coarser appearance by adolescence and adulthood (Morris et al., 1988). The facial appearance is characterized by several soft tissue variations, such as broad forehead with bitemporal narrowing, flat nasal bridge, anteverted nares, wide mouth with fleshy lips, long philtrum, full and drooping cheeks, curly hair, and prominent earlobes. Furthermore, ocular findings may include broad palpebral fissures, ocular hypertelorism, epicanthal folds, medial eyebrow flaring, and periorbital fullness. Eventually, the subcutaneous tissue is lost and results in graying of the hair and wrinkling of the skin, which causes individuals with Williams syndrome to appear older.

The craniofacial anomalies are often associated with unique phonation and oral abnormalities. Individuals with Williams syndrome often have a hoarse and brassy voice. The majority of individuals also have small teeth with wide spacing, malocclusion, occasional missing teeth, and high incidence of dental caries. Enamel hypoplasia is also common. Most of the common oral problems can be corrected with preventive dental care and orthodontic treatment (see Chapter 22).

MEDICAL IMPLICATIONS

Williams syndrome is a multisystem disorder. Medical issues may serve as an early diagnostic clue in cases of facial subtlety.

Cardiovascular Implications

The majority of children with Williams syndrome have cardiovascular anomalies. SVAS is the most common cardiac anomaly associated with Williams syndrome. It occurs in approximately 60% of individuals (Wessel, Pankou, Berdau, & Lons, 1997). SVAS may occur alone or in combination with other vascular stenoses, such as peripheral pulmonary stenosis or renal artery stenosis. The severity of peripheral pulmonary disease decreases during childhood and adulthood; however, the course of SVAS is variable. Stenoses of peripheral vessels, including the renal, carotid, coronary, subclavian, and mesenteric arteries, have been reported. The vascular stenoses can be congenital or develop over time. The consequences of progressive stenoses are myocardial ischemia, stroke, myocardial infarction, and sudden death. Hypertension is also observed frequently in adolescents and adults with Williams syndrome, even without vascular stenoses. Cardiologic surveillance is essential over the life span of an individual with Williams syndrome.

Vision Implications

The most common ocular abnormality for individuals with Williams syndrome is strabismus, predominantly the esotropia form (Winter, Pankau, Amm, Gosch, & Wessel, 1996). Other impairments include hyperopia, glaucoma, myopia, and amblyopia (see Chapter 16). Because visual-spatial tasks are difficult for individuals with Williams syndrome, how these ocular problems correlate to visual spatial tasks is unknown. Approximately 75% of individuals with Williams syndrome have a distinctive stellate iris pattern, involving a white lacy or prominent starbust pattern. This ocular finding does not affect vision, but it is one of the useful diagnostic features of Williams syndrome.

Auditory Implications

Hyperacusis, or oversensitivity to sound, occurs in over 90% of children with Williams syndrome (Van Borsel, Curfs, & Fryns, 1997). The etiology of hyperacusis is unknown. Children with hyperacusis tend to respond to loud or sudden sounds by covering their ears, hiding, or crying. The common offending sounds include vacuum cleaners, sirens, telephones, airplanes, or lawn mowers. Children may also experience anxiety in anticipation of such noises. In addition, otitis media is present in approximately 60% of children and may lead to hearing loss.

Gastrointestinal Implications

In the infancy period, gastroesophageal reflux, infantile colic, chronic constipation, excessive vomiting, and feeding difficulty may be present (Morris et al., 1988). The constellation of symptoms often result in failure to thrive, and chronic constipation may result in rectal prolapse. Hypercalcemia is seen in 15% of infants and young children with Williams syndrome. It is usually associated with constipation and abdominal pain. The etiology of hypercalcemia in Williams syndrome is unknown. Adults are often prone to abdominal pain, which may occur from diverticulitis, chronic constipation, or peptic ulcer disease.

Genitourinary Implications

Renal problems are seen in approximately 18% of individuals with Williams syndrome (Pober, Lacro, Rice, Mandell, & Teele, 1993). Common findings include renal aplasia, renal hypoplasia, horseshoe kidney, bladder diverticuli, and nephrocalcinosis. The most common impairment is bladder diverticula. Renal artery stenosis is more common in adults with William syndromes, and it is possibly caused by the deficiency of elastin in vascular tissue. This finding may correspond to the higher incidence of hypertension in adults with Williams syndrome. Because the prevalence of genitourinary abnormalities in Williams syndrome is significant, baseline renal and bladder ultrasound and urinalysis should be performed routinely.

Growth Implications

Infants with Williams syndrome typically have lower birth weights and smaller head circumferences than typically developing infants, but they often catch up to the low–normal range by late childhood. Short stature, however, is present in 50% of individuals with Williams syndrome (Pankau, Partsch, Gosch, Oppenmann, & Wessel, 1992). Growth disturbance with failure to thrive is commonly seen during infancy and childhood. The height of adults with Williams syndrome is in the lower percentiles of the normal range (Morris et al., 1988). Growth hormone deficiency does not appear to play a role in short stature.

Head and weight growth are also affected in Williams syndrome. Mean head circumference is at the 2nd percentile for the first 4 years of life and at the 25th percentile thereafter (Morris et al, 1988). Weight gain is low during the first year of life because of feeding and gastrointestinal issues. Both weight and length are below the 5th percentile for the first 4 years but increase during childhood. Weight remains within the normal ranges in adulthood, and the final height is in the low-normal or below normal range. Growth curves are now available exclusively for individuals with Williams syndrome.

Musculoskeletal Implications

Infants and young children with Williams syndrome have hyperextensible joints and decreased muscle tone (Morris et al., 1988). By childhood and adolescence, the hypotonia resolves, and joint contractures may arise. Contractures are common in the legs and result in ambulation difficulties with leg pain and cramping. In adulthood, joint contractures may occur with other common musculoskeletal anomalies, such as lordosis, scoliosis, kyphosis, and radioulnar synostosis (Chapman, De Plaiss, & Pober, 1996). These problems can lead to gait abnormalities and gross and fine motor coordination difficulties. Physical therapy evaluation should be included in children with Williams syndrome. Early recognition of joint contractures is essential to prevent complications.

Neurological Implications

In the infancy period, muscle hypotonia is present and causes delays in gross and fine motor skills. As muscle tone increases with age, children and adults may develop hypertonia (Chapman et al., 1996). Gait discoordination, abnormal balance, and increased deep tendon reflexes may also occur.

Cognitive Implications

Individuals with Williams syndrome function in the normal to severe spectrum of intellectual disabilities. Although there is a wide range of involvement in Williams syndrome, the majority of individuals have mild intellectual disabilities. Interestingly, the cognitive profile is not linear but consists of relative strengths and weaknesses. A full-scale IQ score can be misleading and lacks the overall cognitive profile in these individuals. Williams syndrome is associated with a relative strength in cognitive-linguistic profile and impairments in visuospatial components (Volterra, Capirci, Pezzini, Sabbadini, & Vicari, 1996).

Young children with Williams syndrome have language delays and may not begin to speak in sentences until the age of 3 (Morris et al., 1988). They then show language skills improvement over time to eventually excel linguistically. Relative to other individuals with intellectual disabilities, children with Williams syndrome speak more fluently and show advanced skills in language and communication skills, especially in syntax, vocabulary, and prosody (Volterra et al., 1996). Their language is well developed phonologically and syntactically. Their hyperverbal conversational style may play a role in their outgoing and social characteristics.

Other areas of strength are auditory short-term memory, facial recognition, and musicality. Many children and adults with Williams syndrome succeed in tasks involving auditory short-term memory. For instance, they can recall long strings of digits. They also have remarkable facial recognition and recall. Infants and toddlers with Williams syndrome tend to show particular interest in the faces of others (Wang, Doherty, Rourke, & Bellugi, 1995). Furthermore, researchers have also noted that individuals with Williams syndrome excel in musical tasks, including singing, playing musical instruments, and recognizing songs (Dykens, Hodapp, & Finucane, 2000). Musical interest in individuals with Williams syndrome needs to be explored further because it may serve as a leisure activity to improve self-esteem and social skills.

Despite these strengths, individuals with Williams syndrome also have relative weaknesses in areas of comprehension, visual-spatial skills, and fine motor coordination (Wang et al., 1995). Weaknesses are most prominent in visual-spatial tasks, especially in overall drawing or in processing visual information. Comprehension is suboptimal, and content of speech may lack spontaneity. Inappropriate use of stereotyped and scripted phrases may be present. Children also have difficulty understanding mathematical concepts. They also may have impairments in nonverbal tasks, such as visuospatial cognition, problem solving, eye–hand coordination, and motor planning. In regards to perceptual planning and fine motor control, individuals with Williams syndrome draw disorganized and disjointed depictions of objects.

Because individuals with Williams syndrome show strengths in language and facial recognition (left hemispheric process) and weakness in visuospatial ability (right hemispheric process), researchers began to perform neuroanatomical studies to shed light on the syndrome's unique cognitive-linguistic profile. These findings report that there are no distinct right and left hemisphere differences in the brains of individuals with Williams syndrome. The overall brain volume in individuals with Williams syndrome is on average 80% the size of brains of typically developing individuals. Individuals with Williams syndrome experience normal development in the frontal cortical region, limbic structures (e.g., amygdala, hippocampus), and neocerebellar volumes (Bellugi, Wang, & Jernigan, 1994). The linguistic competencies of individuals with Williams syndrome may relate to the sparing of the frontal cortex and neocerebellar structures from impairment. The limbic system and amygdala are also spared, and these structures are associated with facial processing and recognition skills.

Behavioral Implications

Individuals with Williams syndrome were described by Beuren et al. (1962) to be "friendly and charming." One of the distinctive personality traits of Williams syndrome is unusually talkative and outgoing nature. Individuals with Williams syndrome are overfriendly, loquacious, and empathetic, which sets them apart from their peers (Dykens et al., 2000). These positive traits also have negative consequences. Parents are often concerned that the great ability to form interpersonal contacts may lead to possible exploitation or false expectation of their child's mental and physical abilities. Furthermore, children with Williams syndrome are often insecure and anxious. Despite their socially uninhibited profile, they have problems making friends due to their low tolerance for frustration and teasing and their tendency toward excessive chatter and impulsivity. These individuals are so eager to have friends that they often become overbearing.

Several studies have revealed that individuals with Williams syndrome are at risk for externalizing maladaptive behaviors, such as hyperactivity, inattentiveness, impulsivity, attention seeking, and temper tantrums. Hyperactivity is observed in 63%–87% of children with Williams syndrome (Gosch & Pankau, 1994). Individuals also encounter many internalizing problems, including anxiety, obsessions and preoccupations, somatic complaints, and fears (Dykens & Rosner, 1999). Many have marked persistent anxiety-producing fears and avoid their fearful stimuli or endure them with tremendous distress (see Chapter 23.3). Fears include heights, being teased, and encountering medical procedures.

Many of the behavioral attributes of Williams syndrome seem to be less common in adults with Williams syndrome. As time evolves, adults and adolescents with Williams syndrome are less likely to demonstrate the salient features of overfriendliness, hyperactivity, anxiety, and disobedience; however, depression increases with advancing age (see Chapter 23.4). Symptoms of depression may be masked by the friendly and charming demeanors of adults with Williams syndrome (Dykens & Rosner, 1999). In addition, maladaptive behaviors are often overlooked in individuals with Williams syndrome because of their good verbal skills. In such cases, behavioral and emotional disturbances persist (Einfeld, Tonge, & Vaughan, 2001).

Recognition of problems and early intervention are important. Many children and adolescents with Williams syndrome seek music therapy and lessons early in their life to alleviate anxiety and improve attention span. Music lessons not only teach music skills but also improve confidence in social relationships, motor dexterity, and emotional well-being. Furthermore, social skills training is beneficial in teaching appropriate social cues, pragmatics, and conversational skills. With early intervention strategies, children with Williams syndrome children appear to adapt well to the transition to adolescence and adulthood.

MANAGEMENT AND INTERVENTION

Table 9.5-1 provides information on the management of Williams syndrome. Infants with Williams syndrome are typically hypotonic with joint laxity. Hypotonia and joint laxity improve in childhood; however, joint limitation can be progressive and interfere with coordination (Chapman et al., 1996; Morris et al., 1988). Early intervention with physical and occupational therapy are necessary. Infants with hypercalcemia must have their dietary intake of calcium and vitamin D limited. Low calcium formula or breast feeding should be recommended because human milk has lower levels of cal-

Table 9.5-1. Management of Williams syndrome

System	Concern	Evaluation	Management
Gastrointestinal tract	Colic, irritability, poor feeding	Serum total calcium level	Reduced calcium and vitamin D intake, no vitamin D supplements
	Gastroesophageal reflux	pH probe study	Thickened foods, antireflux positioning, gastric motility agents
	Constipation	Gastroenterology consult	Dietary modification, stool softeners
	Rectal prolapse, diverticulitis	Contrast studies, colonoscopy	Surgery in some cases
Ear, nose, and throat (ENT)	Frequent otitis media	ENT consult	Screening hearing evaluation, antimicrobial therapy
Vision	Strabismus, hyperopia	Ophthalmologic consult, visual acuity testing	Corrective surgery, patching, corrective lenses
Cardiovascular system	Cardiac murmur, supravalvular aortic stenosis, peripheral pulmonic stenosis	Cardiology consult	Echocardiogram If normal, echocardiogram every year in children younger than 5 years of age, then every 2–3 years through adult years, surgery in some cases
Genitourinary system	Bladder diverticuli	Baseline bladder urinalysis and ultasound	Urinalysis every 1–2 years in asymptomatic children younger than 10 years
	Nephrocalcinosis	Spot urine Ca/Cr ratio	Nephrology consult
	Renal structural anomalies (horseshoe kidney, renal cysts, renal hypoplasia)	Renal ultrasound, BUN/Cr to follow renal function	BUN/Cr followed annually, nephrology consult
Musculoskeletal system	Joint contractures	Physical examination	Screening by age 3, ongoing physical therapy
Cognitive/behavioral systems	Developmental delay, intellectual disabilities, attention-deficit/hyperactivity disorder	Developmental evaluation	Early interventional therapy, psychoeducational evaluation, individualized education planning, behavioral management, and/or pharmacotherapy

From Lashkari, A., Smith, A.K., & Graham, J.M. (1999). Williams-Beuren syndrome: An update and review for the primary pediatrician. *Clinical Pediatrics, 38,* 203; adapted by permission.

cium and vitamin D than most formulas. Usually the hypercalcemia is mild and resolves in the second year of life.

Narrowing of arteries, particularly SVAS and peripheral pulmonary stenosis, are potentially progressive lesions that increase the risk of morbidity and sudden death for individuals with Williams syndrome. Hypertension and cardiac hypertrophy are common in older children and adolescents due to narrowing of the great vessels and/or renal arteries (Pober et al., 1993; Wessel et al., 1997). Prompt intervention is important to prevent further complications.

Although individuals with Williams syndrome have impressive vocabulary, prosody, and social interactions, they often use inappropriate phrases. Speech and language therapy is particularly important in helping children understand and produce more complex language. Hyperacusis, hyperactivity, easy distractibility, anxiety, and uninhibited personality may interfere with learning and social judgment skills. Social skills training programs are recommended to improve interpersonal relationships and to prevent abuse or exploitation due to overfriendliness with strangers.

CONCLUSION

Health professionals need to help parents of children with Williams syndrome to understand the nature of their child's condition and provide anticipatory guidance regarding issues relating to development, behavior, and preventive medical care. Brothers and sisters of a child with Williams syndrome should also be involved in the care in order to gain a better appreciation of the child. They are often jealous of their brother or sister with Williams syndrome, who is more social and talkative. The child with Williams syndrome usually receives more attention and praise from teachers, family members, and strangers. For this reason, siblings may feel isolated, timid, or angry. By having sufficient parental and social supports, early involvement in speech therapy, access to specific educational curricula, and many other therapeutic interventions to manage specific communication, cognitive, and behavior issues, individuals with Williams syndrome can lead productive lives. Families are encouraged to contact the Williams Syndrome Association, a volunteer organization with chapters distributed throughout the United States (http://www.williams-syndrome.org), for support and information.

REFERENCES

Bellugi, U., Wang, P., & Jernigan, T.L. (1994). Williams syndrome: An unusual neuropsychological profile. In S.H. Browman & J. Grafram (Eds.), *Atypical cognitive deficits in developmental disorders: Implications for brain function* (pp. 23–56). Mahwah, NJ: Lawrence Erlbaum Associates.

Beuren, A.J., Apitz, J., & Harmjanz, D. (1962). Supravalvular aortic stenosis in association with mental retardation and certain facial appearance. *Circulation, 26*, 1235–1240.

Bonham-Carter, R.E., & Sutcliffe, J. (1964). A syndrome of multiple of arterial stenosis in association with the severe form of idiopathic hypercalcemia. *Archives of Disease in Childhood, 39*, 418–419.

Chapman, C.A., De Pleiss, A., & Pober, B.R. (1996). Neurologic findings in children and adults with Williams syndrome. *Journal of Child Neurology, 11*, 63–65.

Dykens, E.M., Hodapp, R.M., & Finucane, B.M. (2000). *Genetics and mental retardation syndromes: A new look at behavior and interventions.* Baltimore: Paul H. Brookes Publishing Co.

Dykens, E.M., & Rosner, B.A. (1999). Refining behavioral phenotypes: Personality-motivation in Williams and Prader-Willi syndromes. *American Journal on Mental Retardation, 104*, 158–169.

Einfeld, S.L., Tonge, B.J., & Vaughan, R.W. (2001). Longitudinal course of behavioral and emotional problems in Williams syndrome. *American Journal on Mental Retardation, 106*, 73–81.

Garcia, R.E., Friedman, W.F., Kaback, M.M., & Rowe, R.D. (1964). Idiopathic hypercalcemia and supravalvular aortic stenosis documentation of a new syndrome. *New England Journal of Medicine, 271*, 117–120.

Gosch, A., & Pankau, R. (1994). Social-emotional and behavioral adjustment in children with Williams-Beuren syndrome. *American Journal of Medical Genetics, 53*, 335–339.

Lashkari, A., Smith, A.K., & Graham, J.M. (1999). Williams-Beuren syndrome: An update and review for the primary pediatrician. *Clinical Pediatrics, 38*, 189–208.

Li, D.Y., Toland, A.E., Boak, B.B., Atkinson, D.L., Ensing, G.L., Morris, C.A., et al. (1997). Elastin point mutation causes an obstructive vascular disease, supravalvular aortic stenosis. *Human Molecular Genetics, 6*, 1021–1028.

Lowery, M.C., Morris, C.A., Ewart, A.K., Brothman, L.J., Zhu, X.L., Leonard, C.O., et al. (1995). Strong correlation of elastin deletions, detected by FISH, with Williams syndrome: Evaluation of 235 patients. *American Journal of Human Genetics, 57*, 49–53.

Morris, C.A., Demsey, S.A., Leonard, C.O., Dilts, C., & Blackburn, B.L. (1988). Natural history of Williams syndrome: Physical characteristics. *Journal of Pediatrics, 113*, 318–326.

Pankau, R., Partsch, C.J., Gosch, A., Oppenmann, H.C., & Wessel, A. (1992). Statural growth in Williams-Beuren syndrome. *European Journal of Pediatrics, 151*, 751–755.

Pober, B.R., Lacro, R.V., Rice, C., Mandell, V., & Teele, R.L. (1993). Renal findings in 40 individuals with Williams syndrome. *American Journal of Medical Genetics, 46*, 271–274.

Tassabehji, M., Metcalfe, K., Karmiloff-Smith, A., Carette, M.J., Grant, J., Dennis, N., et al. (1999). Williams syndrome: Use of chromosomal microdeletions as a tool to dissect cognitive and physical phenotypes. *American Journal of Human Genetics, 64*, 118–125.

Van Borsel, J., Curfs, L.M., & Fryns, J.P. (1997). Hyperacusis in Williams syndrome: A sample survey. *Genetic Counseling, 8*, 121–126.

Volterra, V., Capirci, O., Pezzini, G., Sabbadini, L., & Vicari, S. (1996). Linguistic abilities in Italian children with Williams syndrome. *Cortex, 32*, 663–677.

Wang, P.P., Doherty, S., Rourke, S.B., & Bellugi, U. (1995). Unique profile of visuo-perceptual skills in a genetic syndrome. *Brain and Cognition, 29*, 54–65.

Wessel, A., Pankau, R., Berdau, W., & Lons, P. (1997). Aortic stiffness with the Williams-Beuren syndrome. *Pediatric Cardiology, 18*, 244.

Williams, J.C., Barratt-Boyes, B.F., & Love, J.B. (1961). Supravalvular aortic stenosis. *Circulation, 24*, 1311–1318.

Winter, M., Pankau, R., Amm, M., Gosch, A., & Wessel, A. (1996). The spectrum of ocular features in the Williams-Beurenn syndrome. *Clinical Genetics, 49*, 28–31.

9.6 ANGELMAN SYNDROME

Joseph Wagstaff

Angelman syndrome is a hereditary neurodevelopmental disorder characterized by severe developmental delay with lack of speech, easily elicited smiling and laughter, seizure disorder, and characteristic gait. Most of the clinical manifestations of Angelman syndrome arise from lack of a functional maternal copy of the *UBE3A* gene, which encodes a ubiquitin-protein ligase. The incidence of Angelman syndrome has been estimated to be between 1 in 10,000 and 1 in 20,000 (Clayton-Smith & Laan, 2003; Williams, 2003). Often, the diagnosis of Angelman syndrome either is not considered or is rejected because most of the distinctive features of individuals with Angelman syndrome are behavioral rather than dysmorphic, and the phenotype is not easily described in words. In addition, genetic testing for Angelman syndrome is complex, and no single laboratory test can "rule out" the diagnosis of Angelman syndrome. Recurrence risk of the disorder in brothers and sisters of individuals with Angelman syndrome can range from less than 1% to as high as 50%, depending on the specific genetic etiology, so accurate diagnosis can have important clinical implications. Treatment for Angelman syndrome, however, remains symptomatic with no specific therapies.

CLINICAL CHARACTERISTICS

Consensus diagnostic criteria for Angelman syndrome were published in 1995 and are reproduced in Table 9.6-1. These criteria are useful in assessing the possibility of a diagnosis of Angelman syndrome but are not intended to be used on their own for either establishing or excluding the diagnosis of Angelman syndrome. Usually, pregnancy and delivery of children with Angelman syndrome are uncomplicated; fetal activity and size at birth (including head circumference) are normal. Feeding difficulties, especially difficulty with breastfeeding and gastroesophageal reflux, are often the first manifestations of Angelman syndrome but are very nonspecific and rarely lead to a diagnosis of Angelman syndrome in infancy.

During the first year of life, several distinctive characteristics become apparent in most children with Angelman syndrome. First, motor development is delayed. Most children with Angelman syndrome are able to sit independently after 12 months of age. Second, children with Angelman syndrome smile and laugh with minor or no provocation, and they show frequent tongue protrusion and drooling that are often associated with laughter. Third, their movements have a jerky and/or tremulous quality. Fourth, their slow cranial growth causes head circumference percentile to decrease with age. Fifth, many children with Angelman syndrome who have chromosome 15 deletions show hypopigmentation of hair, eyes, and skin by comparison with other family members. Each of these characteristics can show enormous variability among children with Angelman syndrome; some of this variability reflects different genetic etiologies, but even within a single etiologic category, there is a wide range of phenotypic expression.

During the second year of life, most children with Angelman syndrome learn to sit independently, but independent walking is delayed until 3–6 years of age. Some children with Angelman syndrome may learn one or even several words, but most experience no significant development of spoken language. Between the ages of 1 and 3 years, more than 90% of individuals with Angelman syndrome develop seizures (see Chapter 12.2). Almost every seizure type has been reported in individuals with Angelman syndrome. The most frequently observed seizure type is drop attacks, and generalized tonic-clonic seizures may also occur. Characteristic electroencephalogram (EEG) findings in individuals with Angelman syndrome include very high amplitude slow waves at 2–3 per second occurring in runs and more prominent anteriorly, as well as spikes or sharp waves, mixed with high-amplitude 3–4 per second components posteriorly that occur during passive eye closure.

Table 9.6-1. Clinical characteristics of Angelman syndrome

A. Consistent (100%)
- Developmental delay, functionally severe
- Speech impairment, no or minimal use of words; receptive and nonverbal communication skills higher than verbal ones
- Movement or balance disorder, usually ataxia of gait and/or tremulous movement of limbs
- Behavioral uniqueness: any combination of frequent laughter/smiling, apparent happy demeanor; easily excitable personality, often with hand flapping movements; hypermotoric behavior; short attention span

B. Frequent (more than 80%)
- Delayed, disproportionate growth in head circumference, usually resulting in microcephaly (absolute or relative) by age 2
- Seizures, onset usually < 3 years of age
- Abnormal EEG, characteristic pattern with large amplitude slow-spike waves (usually 2–3/s), facilitated by eye closure

C. Associated (20%–80%)
- Flat occiput
- Occipital groove
- Protruding tongue
- Tongue thrusting; suck/swallowing disorders
- Feeding problems during infancy
- Prognathia
- Wide mouth, wide-spaced teeth
- Frequent drooling
- Excessive chewing/mouthing behaviors
- Strabismus
- Hypopigmented skin, light hair and eye color (compared to family), seen only in deletion cases
- Hyperactive lower limb deep tendon reflexes
- Uplifted, flexed arm position especially during ambulation
- Increased sensitivity to heat
- Sleep disturbance
- Attraction to/fascination with water

From Williams, C.A., Angelman, H., Clayton-Smith, J., Driscoll, D.J., Hendrickson, J.E., Knoll, J.H.M., et al. (1995). Angelman syndrome: Consensus for diagnostic criteria. *American Journal of Medical Genetics, 56,* 237–238; reprinted by permission.

The overall developmental pattern in Angelman syndrome generally involves slow acquisition of new skills, without loss of preexisting skills. This pattern can, of course, be interrupted by poorly controlled seizures, and distinguishing true developmental regression from uncontrolled epilepsy as the cause of loss of skills is important. Individuals with Angelman syndrome often are very sociable and take pleasure in interactions with family members and friends. Most children with Angelman syndrome become toilet trained during the daytime. Individuals with Angelman syndrome have a definite predisposition to accidental injury and invariably require supervision and assistance in their living situations throughout their lives.

Physical appearance of individuals with Angelman syndrome tends to change gradually with age. Physical characteristics such as mandibular prognathism, appearance of large mouth, and widely separated teeth become more pronounced in older individuals with Angelman syndrome (see Figure 9.6-1). Separated teeth are probably related to constant tongue thrusting and pressure of the tongue behind the teeth.

Sleep disturbance is frequent among individuals with Angelman syndrome, with at least 90% of individuals with Angelman syndrome showing sleep problems at some period of their lives. Children with Angelman syndrome often fall asleep normally in the evening, then wake after 2–3 hours of sleep and are unable to fall back to sleep. The onset of sleep disturbance can be in infancy, but parents more commonly complain about sleep problems starting in the second year of life, often close to the time of onset of seizures. Zhdanova, Wurtman, and Wagstaff (1999) showed that some children with Angelman syndrome who exhibit sleep problems have circadian phase shifts, with onset of melatonin secretion delayed by 3–4 hours compared with the normal pattern.

The following story by Barbara, the mother of a son with Angelman syndrome, describes some of the symptoms experienced by children with Angelman syndrome.

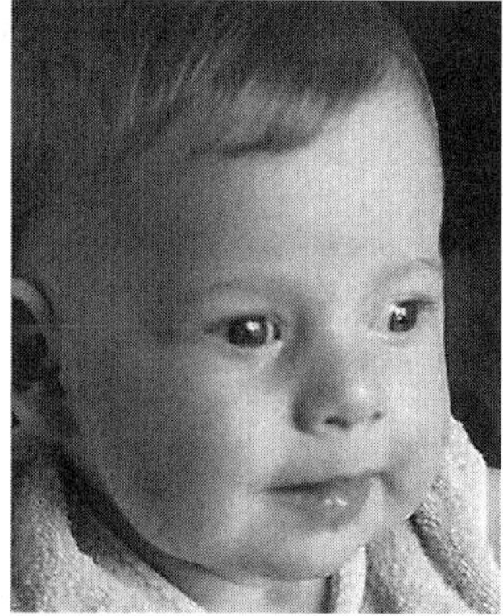

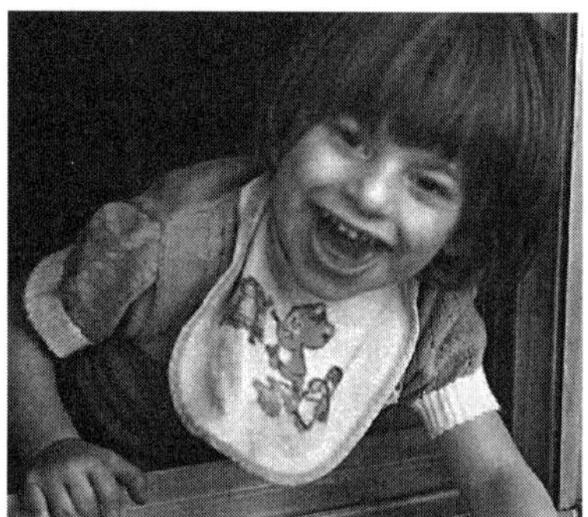

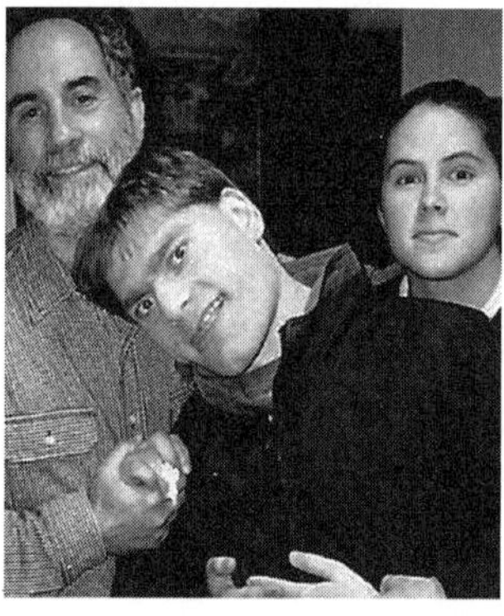

Figure 9.6-1. Jason at 6 months of age showed no distinctive features of Angelman syndrome (top photo). At age 14 months, a wide smile was apparent (middle photo). Mandibular prognathism was noticeable at age 25 years (bottom photo, Jason shown with his father and sister).

On the first day of spring, we drove 100 miles in a blizzard to pick up our 4-week-old healthy, normal baby boy. We had gotten a call from the adoption agency the day before, and they mentioned that the baby had been held for 4 weeks because the nurses in the newborn nursery noticed that he never cried, but "not to worry" because tests were done. He had an "epiglottal flap" and would be fine. We were thrilled, after waiting 3 years for an infant, and we spent the night talking about our excitement and how our lives would change forever. We had no idea!!!

Jason was beautiful, with a shock of reddish-blond hair and blue eyes. Once we were home with him, however, it seemed that he didn't "feel" like a healthy normal baby. He was very floppy—didn't seem to know where his body was in space. And he didn't seem to like being held—he banged his head painfully against my shoulder every time I tried to burp him. He seemed to have a tongue thrust and took 1½ hours to take 3 oz. of formula. And he never cried, never made any demands at all.

After 24 hours, I called the pediatrician, who said, "Barbara, I didn't expect you to be so anxious. Count your blessings that he doesn't cry." Feeling properly chastised, I went back to trying to feed and care for my baby. His entire first year of life, however, I noted that he could not hold his head up, he could not roll over, he could not sit up, he never "regarded a raisin" (on the Gesell Developmental Scale), and he never developed a pincer grasp. I was constantly being told by my pediatrician that I was "overprotective" and "anxious." After all, babies develop at their own rate, and, certainly, Jason was beautiful, precociously smiling and being social, to the delight of everyone wherever we went.

I tried to quell my fears until one afternoon when he seemed to be sleeping for an extraordinarily long time. I went to check on him, and he was stiff, unresponsive, and convulsing. I was home alone in an isolated rural area, without a car, and my husband was unavailable. There was no 911 to call. Jason's seizure was self-limiting, but when he stopped seizing, he was paralyzed on one side (Todd's paralysis, I believe).

I finally was able to contact the doctor, who said Jason probably had a seizure because he was febrile, and the doctor would see him the next day. The next day, Jason had no sign of fever or illness—and God knows I looked. By this time, I was practically seizing myself. I was so distraught. After more seizures, we were finally referred to a pediatric neurologist at the University of Vermont, and thus began my 29-year relationship with the branch of medicine called neurology. *(to be continued)*

GENETIC MECHANISMS

All known genetic mechanisms that cause Angelman syndrome involve the lack of a functional maternal copy of the *UBE3A* gene, which is located in 15q11-q13. Parental origin of mutations and chromosome rearrangements in this region plays a key role in Angelman syndrome pathogenesis because of the effects of genetic imprinting, a process that leads to differential expression of maternal versus paternal alleles of some human genes. In the brain, the maternal copy of *UBE3A* shows much higher transcriptional activity than the paternal allele so that loss of the maternal *UBE3A* allele causes Angelman syndrome while loss of the paternal *UBE3A* allele has no detectable phenotypic consequences. The known mechanisms causing Angelman syndrome, together with diagnostic test results, are shown in Table 9.6-2.

The most common genetic cause of Angelman syndrome is maternal deletion of the q11-q13 region of chromosome 15, found in approximately 70% of individuals with Angelman syndrome. These deletions encompass approximately 4 million base pairs of deoxyribonucleic acid (DNA), and almost all of these deletions occur de novo during oogenesis. Deletions of the same region are found in approximately 70% of individuals with a clinically distinct syndrome, Prader-Willi syndrome; however, in Prader-Willi syndrome, the deletions are always of paternal origin.

Standard or "high-resolution" karyotyping does not reliably demonstrate presence or absence of these deletions. The gold-standard method for detecting these deletions is fluorescence in situ hybridization (FISH) analysis with probes from the region commonly deleted in Angelman syndrome. Another diagnostic test that detects these deletions is methylation analysis using DNA probes such as SNRPN or PW71; this test is also positive in individuals with Angelman syndrome with either uniparental disomy or imprinting defect. Recurrence risk to brothers and sisters after parents have a child with an Angelman syndrome deletion is less than 1%.

The second cause of Angelman syndrome is point mutations within the *UBE3A* gene, found in 5%–10% of individuals with Angelman syndrome. More than 60 individuals with Angelman syndrome with *UBE3A* mutations have been reported since 1997, and most mutations are unique (see, e.g., Fang et al., 1999; Malzac et al., 1998). Most familial cases of Angelman syndrome involve *UBE3A* mutations, which show a remarkable pattern of inheritance: Maternal transmission of these mutations causes Angelman syndrome, while paternal transmission has no detectable phenotypic effect. Therefore, a woman who inherits a *UBE3A* mutation from her father will be phenotypically normal, but she will have a 50% chance at each pregnancy of transmitting the *UBE3A* mutation, and each child who inherits the *UBE3A* mutation will have Angelman syndrome.

Individuals with Angelman syndrome with *UBE3A* mutations show normal results from both FISH testing and methylation analysis; their *UBE3A* mutations can only be detected by direct DNA sequencing or other sequence-based approaches. This testing is available in a limited number of centers in the United States and around the world. Recurrence risk in brothers and sisters after a couple has a child with *UBE3A* mutation Angelman syndrome is 50% if the mother is a mutation heterozygote, and less than 1% if the mutation has occurred de novo and the mother is not a carrier.

The third cause of Angelman syndrome is imprinting defects, which cause the maternal copy of chromosome 15 to behave functionally as a paternal copy of the chromosome. These imprinting defects are found in 3%–5% of individuals with Angelman syndrome and presumably reflect disturbances in the processes that normally occur during oogenesis to establish maternal-specific patterns of imprinted gene activity. FISH testing is normal in these individuals because they do not have large deletions, but methylation analysis shows lack of a maternally-methylated allele. Polymorphism analysis shows both a maternal and a paternal contribu-

Table 9.6-2. Genetic causes and genetic testing in Angelman syndrome

		Test results				
Genetic category	Percent of total cases	FISH	Methylation	Polymorphism	*UBE3A*	Recurrence risk
Deletion 15q11-q13	70%	Deletion	Paternal only	Biparental	No mutation	< 1%
UBE3A mutation	5%–10%	No deletion	Biparental	Biparental	Mutation present	up to 50%
Imprinting defect	3%–5%	No deletion	Paternal only	Biparental	No mutation	up to 50%
UPD	2%–3%	No deletion	Paternal only	Paternal only	No mutation	< 1%
None of the above	15%–20%	No deletion	Biparental	Biparental	No mutation	Variable

Key: FISH = fluorescence in situ hybridization; UPD = uniparental disomy

tion for all markers on chromosome 15. Some individuals with Angelman syndrome imprinting defects have very small deletions in a region near the *SNRPN* gene, referred to as the imprinting center; if the same deletion is present in the mother, then the recurrence risk is 50%. Most individuals with Angelman syndrome imprinting defects have no detectable change in the imprinting center, and recurrence has not been reported in these cases (Buiting et al., 2003).

The fourth cause of Angelman syndrome is paternal uniparental disomy (UPD), where the individual with Angelman syndrome has inherited two normal copies of chromosome 15 from the father and no copy from the mother. UPD is found in 2%–3% of individuals with Angelman syndrome. As with deletion Angelman syndrome, these individuals have no maternal copy of 15q11-q13. FISH testing is normal, but methylation analysis shows lack of a maternally-methylated allele. Verification of UPD status requires analysis of DNA from the individual with Angelman syndrome together with DNA from both parents using polymorphic markers on chromosome 15; individuals with Angelman syndrome caused by UPD show no maternal contribution for any loci on chromosome 15. Recurrence risk after one child is born with UPD Angelman syndrome is less than 1%.

Between 15% and 20% of individuals with a clinical diagnosis of Angelman syndrome show normal results from FISH analysis, methylation analysis, and *UBE3A* mutation analysis. Other disorders in the differential diagnosis that should be considered in this group include Rett syndrome, X-linked alpha thalassemia and intellectual disabilities (ATR-X), and subtle chromosome rearrangements other than 15q11-q13 deletions. Genetic etiology and recurrence risks are probably very heterogeneous in this group.

A reasonable approach to laboratory diagnosis of Angelman syndrome involves, first, chromosome analysis to exclude visible chromosome rearrangements as the cause of the disorder, then FISH analysis and methylation analysis, either simultaneously or sequentially. If FISH testing is positive, then the diagnosis is deletion Angelman syndrome. If FISH is negative but methylation testing is positive, then polymorphism analysis will distinguish UPD from an imprinting defect. If an imprinting defect is found, clinical testing for presence of an imprinting center deletion is available and will provide important information regarding recurrence risk. If methylation studies are negative but the phenotype is clearly that of Angelman syndrome, then *UBE3A* mutation analysis should be pursued.

Although individuals with Angelman syndrome who have deletions, *UBE3A* mutations, UPD, and imprinting defects generally show a recognizably consistent set of distinctive behavioral and neurologic characteristics, there is enormous variability both within classes and between classes. Comparisons between individuals from different etiologic classes have shown that, in general, individuals with deletion Angelman syndrome are most severely affected whereas individuals with UPD and imprinting defect are most mildly affected. Individuals with *UBE3A* mutations tend to fall between the deletion and the UPD/imprinting defect groups in most measures of Angelman syndrome severity.

These rough correlations between phenotype and etiologic category can be explained based on the premise that absence of a functional maternal copy of *UBE3A* causes the "core" Angelman syndrome phenotype. Although hypoactive in the brain compared with the maternal copy, the paternal copy of *UBE3A* shows some transcriptional activity, and presence of two paternal alleles in UPD and imprinting defects seems to produce some amelioration of phenotype compared with one paternal allele in *UBE3A* mutation Angelman syndrome. Individuals with deletion Angelman syndrome, however, lack one copy of numerous other 15q11-q13 genes, in addition to lacking the maternal copy of *UBE3A*, and lack of these other genes appears to exacerbate the deletion phenotype.

MANAGEMENT

Most medical problems that affect individuals with Angelman syndrome are related to seizures and central nervous system function as a consequence of the brain-specific imprinting of *UBE3A*. Medications used most frequently for treatment of seizures in individuals with Angelman syndrome include valproic acid and clonazepam; other anticonvulsant agents, such as ethosuximide and topiramate, have also been effective in some individuals with Angelman syndrome. Some reports have been made of exacerbation of seizures in individuals with Angelman syndrome treated with carbamazepine or vigabatrin (Ostergaard & Balslev, 2001).

Jason spent almost a year at Children's Hospital Boston. At one point during the hospitalization, he ended up in intensive care on a ventilator for a month after becoming so sedated on nine anticonvulsants that he aspirated. Jason has tried every anticonvulsant that has come out of the pipeline.

We also tried the Ketogenic diet during that time. Jason lost so much weight that he looked like a concentration camp survivor, but he kept on seizing! Eventually, he stopped seizing, and we came home and slowly weaned him down to four anticonvulsants.

In March 2002, we received an invitation to the International Conference on Angelman Syndrome in Toronto, Canada. My husband and I decided to go in desperation. Maybe someone there would know what was happening to Jason. We went and met parents, researchers, neurologists, social workers—it was an incredible experience. There, we met a researcher from Stanford University (a molecular neuropharmacologist) who encouraged us to try an older drug used for infantile spasms—Zarontin—a calcium channel blocker, not a GABA receptor drug. He pointed out that children with chromosome 15 deleted Angelman syndrome lack GABA receptors (and most anticonvulsants are GABA drugs).

We came home. I went to a local neurologist to prescribe Zarontin for Jason, and within 3 days of reaching the therapeutic dose, Jason stopped seizing. A miracle! Gradually, he is regaining his former skills. He feeds himself finger foods. He's alert. He's mischievous. He's happy. He's walking with a walker. He's fun. He's interactive. He enjoys his former quality of life.

Sleep disorders in individuals with Angelman syndrome have been treated with diphenhydramine, clonidine, chloral hydrate, clonazepam, and melatonin. In some children with Angelman syndrome, diphenhydramine produces paradoxical stimulation. Many children with Angelman syndrome have longer duration of sleep and fewer movements during sleep when treated with a low dose (0.3 mg) of oral melatonin at bedtime (Zhdanova et al., 1999).

Gastroesophageal reflux in infants with Angelman syndrome is often treated with H2 blockers. Occasionally children with Angelman syndrome have severe enough gastroesophageal reflux to require gastrostomy with fundoplication. Constipation is often severe in children with Angelman syndrome and has been treated with increased dietary fiber, enemas, lactulose, Senokot, and Miralax (polyethylene glycol).

Many children with Angelman syndrome who show behaviors such as hair pulling and biting respond favorably to behavioral intervention and time-outs. Medical therapy with a number of agents to treat behavioral problems and hyperactivity has been tried in Angelman syndrome. In general, methylphenidate therapy has not proven to be very effective, whereas anecdotal reports describe better results with clonidine and risperidone.

Often, the major nonmedical concern of parents of children with Angelman syndrome is communication therapy for their nonverbal child. Because of the variability in cognitive levels and communication skills among individuals with Angelman syndrome, some of which is correlated with diagnostic category, communication therapy must be tailored to individual strengths and weaknesses. For most children with Angelman syndrome, speech is unlikely to progress past one or two words, so nonverbal means of communication should be emphasized. These means may involve photograph displays for choosing, or more stylized symbol displays; some individuals with Angelman syndrome are able to use sign language and communication boards. Receptive language skills also should be an emphasis of communication therapy.

EDUCATION

Early intervention programs should be made available to children with Angelman syndrome at the youngest age possible. Children with Angelman syndrome require communication therapy as described previously, as well as occupational therapy to help them to improve fine motor skills and oral-motor control (see Chapter 24.1). They need physical therapy to promote stability and ambulation (see Chapter 24.2). School programs for children with Angelman syndrome should be tailored to individual abilities. Children with Angelman syndrome are generally very sociable, and many learn very effectively from peers. Many educational settings work well for children with Angelman syndrome. Some children are in separate special education classes, others are in inclusive classes (usually with a one-on-one aide), and other children spend parts of each day in both settings. Coordination between school and home in providing consistent incentives for desirable behaviors is crucial. Areas of emphasis for most educational programs for children with Angelman syndrome are communication and self-help skills.

ADULTHOOD

Individuals with Angelman syndrome undergo pubertal changes at normal ages, and some women with Angelman syndrome have become pregnant. Facial features such as mandibular prognathism and large mouth tend to become more marked as individuals with Angelman syndrome grow into adulthood. Although some reports have suggested that seizures become less severe as individuals with Angelman syndrome reach adolescence and adulthood, adults with Angelman syndrome often continue to have significant seizures (Clayton-Smith & Laan, 2003). Adults with Angelman syndrome may become less mobile, and they may develop contractures as a consequence if physical therapy is not provided. General health in adults with Angelman syndrome, apart from seizures, is for the most part good, and some individuals with Angelman syndrome have lived into their 60s.

CONCLUSION

In spite of recent advances in the understanding of the genetics and pathogenesis of Angelman syndrome, diagnosis and management of individuals with Angelman syndrome remain challenging. Because of multiple genetic and epigenetic etiologies of Angelman syndrome, all of which lead to absence of a functional maternal allele of the *UBE3A* gene, diagnosis of Angelman syndrome may require several laboratory tests. In addition, 15%–20% of individuals with a clinical diagnosis of Angelman syndrome show normal results from all currently available diagnostic tests. Correct clinical and laboratory diagnosis of Angelman syndrome is important both for optimal seizure therapy and for accurate genetic counseling.

The role of medical professionals in the management of individuals with Angelman syndrome is complemented by an important role of parent support groups in providing information and support to families of individuals with Angelman syndrome. Many families of children with Angelman syndrome who have found it difficult to face their child's developmental delays, behavioral problems, seizures, and sleep disorders in isolation have found significant benefit from Angelman syndrome parent support groups, including the Angelman Syndrome Foundation (see http://www.angelman.org) and the International Angelman Syndrome Organization (http://www.asclepius.com/iaso). These organizations have helped parents of individuals with Angelman syndrome to make contact with each other through online listservs and through regional meetings, as well as to bring families into contact with professionals who have expertise in medical and developmental issues of individuals with Angelman syndrome.

REFERENCES

Buiting, K., Gross, S., Lich, C., Gillessen-Kaesbach, G., el-Maarri, O., & Horsthemke, B. (2003). Epimutations in Prader-Willi and Angelman syndromes: A molecular study of 136 patients with an imprinting defect. *American Journal of Human Genetics, 72*, 571–577.

Clayton-Smith, J., & Laan, L. (2003) Angelman syndrome: A review of the clinical and genetic aspects. *Journal of Medical Genetics, 40*, 87–95.

Fang, P., Lev-Lehman, E., Tsai, T.F., Matsuura, T., Benton, C.S., Sutcliffe, J.S., et al. (1999). The spectrum of mutations in *UBE3A* causing Angelman syndrome. *Human Molecular Genetics, 8*, 129–135.

Malzac, P., Webber, H., Moncla, A., Graham, J.M., Jr., Kukolich, M., Williams, C., et al. (1998). Mutation analysis of *UBE3A* in Angelman syndrome patients. *American Journal of Human Genetics, 62*, 1353–1360.

Ostergaard, J.R., &, Balslev, T. (2001). Efficacy of different antiepileptic drugs in children with Angelman syndrome associated with 15q11-q13 deletion: The Danish experience. *Developmental Medicine and Child Neurology, 43*, 718–719.

Wagstaff, J. (2004). *UBE3A* and the Angelman syndrome. In C.J. Epstein, R.P. Erickson, & A. Wynshaw-Boris (Eds.), *Inborn errors of development: The molecular basis of clinical disorders of morphogenesis* (p. 818). New York: Oxford University Press.

Williams, C. (2003). *How common is Angelman syndrome?* Retrieved December 12, 2003, from http://www.angelman.org/ASIncidenceStats.htm

Williams, C.A., Angelman, H., Clayton-Smith, J., Driscoll, D.J., Hendrickson, J.E., Knoll, J.H.M., et al. (1995). Angelman syndrome: Consensus for diagnostic criteria. *American Journal of Medical Genetics, 56*, 237–238.

Zhdanova, I.V., Wurtman, R.J., &, Wagstaff, J. (1999). Effects of a low dose of melatonin on sleep in children with Angelman syndrome. *Journal of Pediatric Endocrinology and Metabolism, 12*, 57–67.

9.7 PHAKOMATOSES

Bruce R. Korf and Elizabeth Thiele

The term *phakomatoses* encompasses a group of disorders characterized by the occurrence of patchy dysplastic, hamartomatous, and neoplastic lesions. The original disorders included in the term when it was coined by van der Hoeve were neurofibromatosis, tuberous sclerosis, and von Hippel-Lindau syndrome. Since that time, neurofibromatosis has been found to consist of at least two distinct disorders, now referred to as NF1 and NF2. Other disorders, such as basal cell nevus syndrome, might also legitimately be added to the classification (see Table 9.7-1). These disorders are sometimes referred to as *neurocutaneous disorders*, but this name may be misleading because not all of these conditions include manifestations in both the skin and the nervous system. Moreover, most of these disorders involve additional tissues. From the developmental point of view, the two most important phakomatoses are NF1 and tuberous sclerosis complex. This chapter will, therefore, focus on these two disorders.

NF1

Classification and Diagnosis

Five-year-old Liam was brought in for evaluation of slow speech development, hypotonia, and inability to maintain attention. He had attention-deficit disorder and both verbal and nonverbal learning disabilities. The examiner also noted multiple café-au-lait spots on Liam's skin and freckling in both his groin and axillary regions. Liam was short but had a large head circumference. His parents, Mr. and Mrs. McGee had not been concerned about the brown spots on his skin and knew of no family history of similar spots or of individuals diagnosed as having neurofibromatosis.

The term *neurofibromatosis* encompasses two distinct disorders, NF1 and NF2 (Stumpf et al., 1988), which are transmitted as autosomal dominant traits and involve the formation of tumors derived from cells of the nerve sheath. The tumors of NF1 are neurofibromas; however, those of NF2 are typically schwannomas. Individuals with NF1 also develop nontumor manifestations, including skeletal dysplasias, learning disabilities, and vascular stenosis and may develop malignancies such as glioma and sarcoma. The hallmark of NF2 is the occurrence of bilateral vestibular schwannomas, as well as schwannomas of other cranial, spinal, and peripheral nerves. Other tumors include meningiomas, ependymomas, and gliomas. The major nontumor manifestation of NF2 is cataract. Pigmentary changes in the skin are not reliably seen in individuals with NF2, and NF2 is not associated with learning disabilities. NF1 affects approximately 1 in 4,000 individuals, whereas NF2 is about ten-fold less common.

Diagnosis of NF1 is established by clinical criteria (see Table 9.7-2) (Gutmann et al., 1997). Features are often age dependent and may not be present in young children. Two diagnostic criteria are required to establish a definitive diagnosis. The most common presenting feature is multiple café-au-lait spots, defined as six or more spots larger than 5 mm before puberty or 15 mm after puberty. Although this sign is not sufficient to diagnose NF1 (there are rare individuals who have multiple café-au-lait spots without having NF1), the likelihood of NF1 is high in children who fulfill this criterion (Korf, 1990). Skin-fold freckling is usually the next sign to appear. Neurofibromas may not appear on the skin until puberty, but some children with NF1 have soft tissue overgrowth due to plexiform neurofibroma that is established at a young age. Skeletal dysplasia, most commonly involving the tibia, tends to occur within the first year of life.

The mainstay of diagnosis of NF1 has been clinical evaluation. Biopsy of a suspicious lesion might establish it to be a neurofibroma, but this step is not usually necessary. Biopsy of a café-au-lait spot does not provide important diagnostic information. The gene for NF1 has been identified, and mutation testing is possible (Messiaen et al., 2000). Molecular diagnosis requires exhaustive analysis of a wide variety of types of mutation, scattered across the 60 exons of the *NF1* gene. Testing may be done to resolve an uncertain diagnosis or to prepare for prenatal testing. With the exception of large *NF1* gene deletions that are associated with a severe phenotype (Kayes, Riccardi, Burke, Bennet, & Stephens, 1992), genetic testing does not predict the course of the disorder.

Liam's story represents a common scenario, in which a child presents with café-au-lait spots with no other signs of NF1. Such children may be identified by their pediatricians in the course of well child care or may come to attention because of learning disabilities. The presence of skin-fold freckling confirms the diagnosis (see Figure 9.7-1). Short stature is common in children with NF1 for unknown reasons. Macrocephaly is also a common sign with no specific neurological cor-

Table 9.7-1. Major phakomatoses

Disorder	Major features	Gene
NF1	Café-au-lait spots, neurofibromas, skeletal dysplasia, learning disabilities	*NF1*
NF2	Vestibular schwannomas, meningiomas, schwannomas, ependymomas, cataracts	*NF2*
Schwannomatosis	Schwannomas, without vestibular schwannomas	Unknown
Tuberous sclerosis complex	Cortical dysplasia, seizures, subependymal nodules, renal angiomyolipomas, cardiac rhabdomyomas, periungual fibromas, facial angiofibromas, hypopigmented macules	*TSC1;* gene product is tuberin protein *TSC2;* gene product is hamartin protein
von Hippel-Lindau syndrome	Hemangioblastomas, renal cell carcinoma, endolymphatic sac tumors	*VHL*
Basal cell nevus syndrome	Basal cell nevi, basal cell carcinoma, macrocephaly, medulloblastoma, jaw cysts	*PTCH*

relates. Approximately 50% of children with NF1 are affected sporadically, with no prior family history, due to apparent new mutation. If both parents are free of signs, their risk of having another affected child is very low (slightly above the population risk due to the possibility of gonadal mosaicism).

Natural History and Management

Mr. and Mrs. McGee were told of Liam's probable diagnosis of NF1. Liam was referred to a Neurofibromatosis Clinic. He was also started on stimulant medication for attention-deficit/hyperactivity disorder and was enrolled in a speech therapy program. The staff of the Neurofibromatosis Clinic confirmed the diagnosis and explained the natural history, management, and genetics of the disorder to Mr. and Mrs. McGee. An ophthalmological examination was done by a pediatric ophthalmologist, revealing iris Lisch nodules but normal vision.

NF1 is a progressive disorder that displays a wide range of variability, even among individuals in the same family. The progression of major features is noted in Table 9.7-3. Some features are congenital, such as large plexiform neurofibromas or skeletal dysplasias. Young children tend to have short stature but large head size. Café-au-lait spots begin to appear in the first few weeks of life and may continue to develop over the first 2 years. Skin-fold freckles usually appear between 3–5 years of age. Optic glioma, a tumor of the optic nerve or chiasm, occurs in approximately 15% of children with NF1 (Listernick, Louis, Packer, & Gutmann, 1997). These tumors can cause visual disturbance or hormonal imbalance (often presenting as precocious puberty), but also can remain indolent. Progression usually occurs by age 6 years if it is going to occur. Scoliosis may become apparent in later childhood or adolescence. Dermal neurofibromas usually begin after puberty and can continue to occur throughout life, causing significant cosmetic problems in some people. A lifelong risk of malignancy exists, especially malignant peripheral nerve sheath tumor, which is usually evidenced by sudden growth of a neurofibroma or unexplained pain. Malignancy usually occurs in deep plexiform or nodular neurofibromas, not dermal tumors.

Table 9.7-2. Diagnostic criteria for NF1

The diagnosis of NF1 is considered established in any individual displaying at least two of the following features:

- Café-au-lait spots—six or more larger than 5 mm prepubertally, or 15 mm postpubertally
- Skin-fold freckling—freckles in axillae, on groin, under breasts, and on neck
- Neurofibromas—two or more focal neurofibromas or one plexiform neurofibroma
- Lisch nodules—two or more Lisch nodules (iris hamartomas)
- Optic glioma
- Characteristic skeletal dysplasia—tibial or orbital dysplasia
- First-degree relative with the disorder who fulfills two or more of the above criteria

Source: Stumpf et al. (1988).

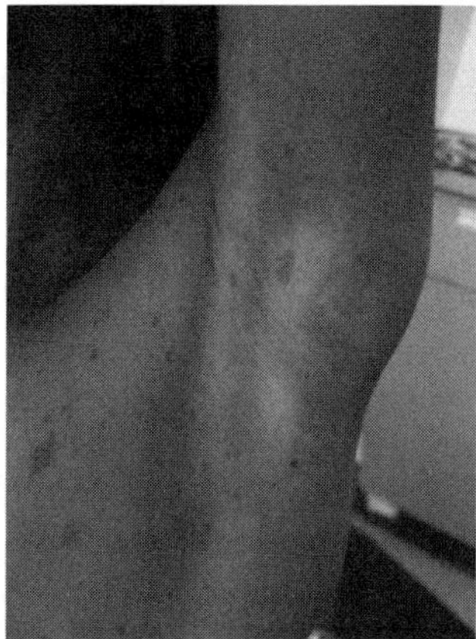

Figure 9.7-1. Neurofibromatosis axillary freckling.

No definitive treatment for NF1 exists, so management is limited to anticipatory guidance and symptomatic treatment. Life span is reduced on average, due to malignancy and vascular problems such as hypertension or hemorrhage. Neurofibromas may be removed by surgery, but larger plexiform neurofibromas are typically unresectable and may grow back after debulking. Optic gliomas are now treated with chemotherapy if the tumors are demonstrated to be symptomatic and progressive, but young children with asymptomatic tumors are best left untreated (Packer et al., 1988).

Individuals with NF1 are best followed annually by a clinician who is familiar with the disorder. Families should be alerted to the major signs of progression, such as development of neurofibromas, and the signs of malignant change. They should also be educated about the risk of learning disabilities. Controversy surrounds the use of routine neuroimaging in children with NF1. Brain magnetic resonance imaging (MRI) will detect optic gliomas, but, as noted previously, most of these do not require treatment. Current recommendations for management confine the use of MRI for clinical indications and do not endorse routine MRI of asymptomatic children (Gutmann et al., 1997).

For children referred to a specialty Neurofibromatosis Clinic, the first priority for clinic staff is to confirm the diagnosis, which is based on multiple café-au-lait spots and skin-fold freckling. Pursuing molecular diagnostic testing is unnecessary because the diagnosis is not in question and such testing does not predict the severity of the disorder. An ophthalmological examination should be arranged, principally to look for signs of optic glioma. Iris Lisch nodules are a common diagnostic marker of NF1, but they are of no significance with regard to visual function.

Although the prognosis of NF1 is always uncertain, clinic staff can provide reassurance with respect to some NF1 complications. Large plexiform neurofibromas that cause physical deformity, or skeletal dysplasia, are early-onset problems. Their absence at age 5 means that these complications will not occur. Follow-up in a Neurofibromatosis Clinic should be done on an annual basis. The goal is to detect treatable complications, provide the family with anticipatory guidance, and advise the family on new developments in diagnosis and management as these become available.

Developmental Manifestations

At 15 years old, Liam was in tenth grade and continued to use stimulant medication, with longstanding documentation of good effect with regard to his attention-deficit/hyperactivity disorder. Over the years, he had required tutoring in reading and math but had managed to remain in general education classes at his appropriate grade level. He enjoyed following sports but had never been particularly skillful in team sports. He swam uncompetitively. Clinically, Liam was in good health. About 4 years ago, though, he had developed small skin neurofibromas that sometimes itched but otherwise did not bother

Table 9.7-3. Natural history of NF1

Time of onset	Feature	Comment
Infancy	Café-au-lait macules	Begin in early days of life
	Plexiform neurofibroma	May grow during early childhood
	Tibial or orbital dysplasia	Orbital dysplasia associated with plexiform neurofibroma
Childhood	Skin-fold freckles	Highly specific to NF1
	Lisch nodules	Begin around 6 years
	Optic glioma	Usually noted between 3 and 6 years
	Developmental	May manifest hypotonia, learning disabilities, and/or developmental delay
	Scoliosis	Usually thoracic
Postpubertal	Dermal neurofibromas	May cause cosmetic problems
Lifelong	Malignancy	Gliomas and sarcomas

him. His vision remained normal, and his neurological examination was normal except for somewhat poor coordination. Liam's two sisters showed no signs of NF1.

NF1 is associated with a number of developmental features. More than 50% of individuals with NF1 have learning disabilities, including both verbal and nonverbal disabilities (North et al., 1997). No NF1-specific profile has been discerned. Children commonly display hypotonia during the early years of life, which may resolve, although poor coordination may persist. Attention-deficit disorder, with or without hyperactivity, is also common. Some children have slow cognitive development evident during the early years of life. Many of these have been found to have a distinct *NF1* gene mutation consisting of deletion of the entire gene and some surrounding DNA (Kayes et al., 1992; Wu, Austin, Schneider, Boles, & Korf, 1995).

Parents of children with NF1 should be informed about the risk of learning disabilities. Children suspected of having learning problems should be evaluated and provided appropriate support at home and at school. The cause of learning disabilities in children with NF1 is not known. Areas of increased T2 signal intensity are seen in the basal ganglia, internal capsule, cerebellum, and brainstem in children with NF1. Evidence also suggests that the number of such lesions may be correlated with the likelihood of learning disabilities (Denckla et al., 1996; North et al., 1994), but it is not helpful to document the presence of these lesions in predicting the cognitive outcome of a specific child.

Genetic Counseling

NF1 is inherited as an autosomal dominant trait with complete penetrance. An individual with NF1, therefore, has a 50% risk of transmitting NF1 to his or her children. Unaffected brothers and sisters of a person with NF1, however, are not at increased risk of having children with NF1. Due to the variable expression, the severity of the disorder cannot be predicted from generation to generation. Approximately 50% of cases occur sporadically, due to apparent new mutation of the *NF1* gene. Parents of a child with sporadic NF1 will not show signs of the disorder and face a minimal risk of having additional children with NF1. In rare instances, a parent may have additional germ cells with an *NF1* mutation (germline mosaicism) so that there is slight risk of recurrence even if the parents are not affected. Some individuals with NF1 exhibit segmental involvement, in which the signs of NF1 are restricted to a specific region of the body (Ruggieri & Polizzi, 2000). This condition is believed to be due to mosaicism for an *NF1* mutation acquired during early development. The features of NF1 may be ameliorated in some of these individuals, but they may face a risk of transmission of NF1 if the mutation is present in germ cells.

Pathogenesis

The gene for NF1 has been identified and is located on chromosome 17 (Cawthon et al., 1990; Wallace et al., 1990). It encodes a protein referred to as *neurofibromin.* Neurofibromin has the properties of a GTPase-activating protein, which regulates activity of the protein Ras (Xu et al., 1990). Ras is involved in transduction of signals from the cell membrane to the nucleus and binds GTP in its activated state. Loss of function of neurofibromin appears to leave Ras in its activated state, because neurofibromin ordinarily stimulates the conversion of active Ras-GTP to inactive Ras-GDP. Individuals with NF1 are heterozygous for a mutation in the *NF1* gene, but this condition does not appear to be sufficient to cause growth of a neurofibroma. Rather, these tumors arise when the remaining nonmutated copy of the *NF1* gene itself undergoes mutation in a Schwann cell, which leads to unregulated growth of that cell and recruitment of other nearby cells to proliferate as well (Cichowski & Jacks, 2001). What triggers this process to occur is unknown.

Knowledge of the importance of Ras to the pathogenesis of NF1 has led to the initiation of clinical trials with drugs known to function as Ras inhibitors. No definitive results have been obtained with these trials so far. A database of clinical trials for NF1 is maintained by the Children's Tumor Foundation (http://www.ctf.org/clinical_trials).

Final Comments on NF1

Liam's story is a common one for children with this disorder. Most do not experience major medical problems during the preadolescent years and begin to have neurofibromas during puberty. Morbidity in the first decade is most often due to skeletal dysplasia, growth of plexiform neurofibromas, or optic glioma. Those who do not have these complications usually do well during childhood. Their major challenges are usually due to learning disabilities and attention-deficit disorder. These conditions respond to the same interventions as are used in the general population. Attention-deficit/hyperactivity disorder in NF1 responds to stimulant medication in many cases. Early recognition of learning disabilities can lead to obtaining appropriate help at home and school, which will provide the child a chance to succeed. The learning problems do not become worse with age.

TUBEROUS SCLEROSIS COMPLEX

Classification and Diagnosis

Six-day-old Wendell developed respiratory distress and was seen by his pediatrician. The evaluation led to an echocardiogram, which revealed multiple intracardiac tumors, including a mass blocking his left ventricular outflow tract. The pediatrician also noticed several areas of skin hypopigmentation ranging in diameter up to 1.5 cm. Due to the intracardiac tumors and skin findings, Wendell had further testing, including a brain MRI. The MRI showed several regions of signal abnormality consistent with cortical tubers and subependymal nodules along the walls of the lateral ventricle, including the region of the foramen of Monro. Wendell had no family history of similar skin findings, heart tumors, or of tuberous sclerosis complex. Unfortunately, due to the degree of cardiac outflow obstruction, Wendell required cardiac surgery to remove the mass, which was confirmed to be a rhabdomyoma on pathological analysis.

Tuberous sclerosis complex is a genetic disorder in which the migration, proliferation, and differentiation of cells is disrupted in early fetal development (Crino & Henske, 1999). Tuberous sclerosis complex can affect any organ system with the growth of benign tumors but most commonly involves the brain, skin, heart, lungs, eyes, and kidneys. Disease expression is widely variable, with manifestations ranging from mild skin findings and asymptomatic brain lesions to seizures; intellectual disabilities; autism; and fatal kidney, cardiac, or pulmonary disease. Tuberous sclerosis complex is one of the more common single gene disorders, with an incidence of approximately 1 in 5,800 live births (Osborne, Fryer, & Webb, 1991). Approximately two thirds of individuals with tuberous sclerosis complex are affected sporadically, although evaluation of parents of children with tuberous sclerosis complex is recommended.

Two genes have been identified for tuberous sclerosis complex: *TSC1* and *TSC2*. *TSC1* is located on chromosome 9 (9q34) (Fryer et al., 1987), and *TSC2* is located on chromosome 16 (16p13.3) (Kandt et al., 1992). The protein products of both genes have been identified; the *TSC1* gene product is called *hamartin*, and the *TSC2* protein product *tuberin*.

Similar to NF1, tuberous sclerosis complex is inherited as an autosomal dominant trait with complete penetrance. An individual with tuberous sclerosis complex has a 50% risk of transmitting the disorder to each child. Within families, there is a wide variation in clinical manifestation among individuals with tuberous sclerosis complex and no known association between a particular mutation and phenotype. Mutational analysis has been performed on many individuals with tuberous sclerosis complex by different groups. Mutations in the *TSC2* gene appear to be five fold more common than *TSC1* mutations; however, the incidence of mutations is similar between the two genes in familial cases. Both somatic and germline mosaicism have been described in many individuals with *TSC1* or *TSC2* mutations, which has significant implications for genetic counseling and diagnosis.

The diagnosis is made by clinical criteria (Table 9.7-4) (Roach, Gomez, & Northrup, 1998), although genetic testing is available. Clinical criteria consist of major and minor features; major features are highly specific to tuberous sclerosis complex whereas minor features are seen frequently in tuberous sclerosis complex but also seen to a lesser degree in the general population. To be diagnosed with definite tuberous sclerosis complex, an individual must meet two major criteria or one major and two minor criteria. If an individual meets only one major criterion and one minor criterion, the individual has *probable tuberous sclerosis complex*. If an individual has one major feature or two or more minor features, he or she is classed as *possible tuberous sclerosis complex*. These distinctions are important as the individual should continue to be closely followed to allow for eventual diagnosis and to minimize the morbidity of involvement if the individual does indeed have tuberous sclerosis complex. In addition, the family can be aware of a possible genetic disorders.

The major criteria include findings in several different organ systems, including the brain, skin, kidneys, lungs, heart, and eyes. There are three different major criteria involving the brain and four involving the skin; therefore, an individual can be definitively diagnosed with tuberous sclerosis complex based on skin exam alone or on neuroimaging findings alone. A complete clinical evaluation is still recommended even for these individuals in order to document involvement and minimize morbidity from various manifestations.

As in Wendell's story, many children are diagnosed with tuberous sclerosis complex in infancy due either to the presence of cardiac rhabdomyomas (often identified on prenatal ultrasound), hypopigmented skin macules, or seizure activity.

Table 9.7-4. Revised diagnostic criteria for tuberous sclerosis complex

Major features
- Facial angiofibromas or forehead plaque
- Nontraumatic ungula or periungual fibroma
- Hypomelanotic macules (more than three)
- Shagreen patch (connective tissue nevus)
- Multiple retinal nodular hamartoma
- Cortical tuber
- Subependymal nodule
- Subependymal giant cell astrocytoma
- Cardiac rhabdomyoma, single or multiple
- Lymphangiomyomatosis
- Renal angiomyolipoma

Minor features
- Multiple randomly distributed pits in dental enamel
- Hamartomatous rectal polyps
- Bone cysts
- Cerebral white matter radial migration lines
- Gingival fibromas
- Nonrenal hamartoma
- Retinal achromic patch
- "Confetti" skin lesions
- Multiple renal cysts

Definite tuberous sclerosis complex—either two major features or one major feature plus two minor features

Probable tuberous sclerosis complex—one major plus one minor feature

Possible tuberous sclerosis complex—either one major feature or two or more minor features

From Roach, E.D.S., Gomez, M.R., & Northrup, H. (1998). Tuberous Sclerosis Complex Consensus Conference: Revised clinical diagnostic criteria. *Journal of Child Neurology, 13*, 624–628; reprinted by permission.

Natural History and Management

Wendell was diagnosed with tuberous sclerosis complex. Following cardiac surgery, he did very well until 5 months of age, when he developed clusters of stereotyped episodes characterized by his arms and legs extending briefly, then relaxing, then extending again. The clusters could last up to 15 min with multiple episodes per cluster and would typically occur after waking in the morning, or when he was going to sleep at night or at naptime. An electroencephalogram (EEG) done at the time was suggestive of hypsarrhythmia, and Wendell was diagnosed with infantile spasms and placed on seizure medications.

Tuberous sclerosis complex is a progressive disorder with wide phenotypic variability. Central nervous system involvement is a hallmark of the disorder, as the brain is affected in more than 95% of individuals with tuberous sclerosis complex (Gomez, 1988). Central nervous system pathologic features include cortical tubers, subependymal nodules, and subependymal giant cell astrocytoma, each of which is a major diagnostic criteria. White matter abnormalities are also frequently seen, including radial curvilinear bands.

Cortical tubers are located at the junction of gray and white matter and vary widely in size and distribution. Histologically, they are associated with marked disruption of the cortical lamination and are comprised of dysplastic, hypomyelinated aggregates of abnormal glial and neural elements with glial derived cells and astrocytes predominating. Tubers also contain "giant cells," which are enlarged, bizarre-appearing neurons or large cells with both neuronal and glial characteristics. Cortical tubers are thought to arise from mutated neural progenitor cells in the subependymal germinal matrix that give rise to abnormally migrating daughter cells, which in turn produce individual tubers. During life, they may undergo cystic degeneration or calcification.

Subependymal nodules occur either as discrete or roughly confluent areas of firm, hypertrophic tissue and are found most commonly at the caudothalamic groove in the vicinity of the foramen of Monro, although they can occur anywhere along the wall of the lateral ventricles. Histologically, subependymal nodules consist of astrocytes thought to arise from the subependymal zone. They typically calcify by puberty. Although generally asymptomatic, subependymal nodules can develop into subependymal giant cell astrocytomas in 5%–10% of individuals, who typically present with symptoms of increased intracranial pressure (head-ache, vomiting, papilledema) or increased seizure activity (Franz, 1998).

A variety of clinical issues are associated with these central nervous system pathologic features. First, epilepsy is the most common medical condition in individuals with tuberous sclerosis complex and occurs in 80%–90% of individuals during their lifetime (see Chapter 12.2). Epilepsy is also the most common presenting symptom in tuberous sclerosis complex, leading to diagnosis in up to 92% of individuals. The onset of seizure activity is typically in childhood, and approximately 69% of individuals have their first seizure at less than 1 year of age. Infantile spasms are also very common and occur in up to one third of children with tuberous sclerosis complex. Unfortunately, many children develop seizure disorders that prove intractable to anticonvulsant medications; epilepsy surgery has a very important role in helping control epilepsy in this population (Curatolo, 1996; Gomez, 1988; Franz, 1998).

Second, individuals with tuberous sclerosis complex are at risk for developmental delays and intellectual disabilities. Intellectual disabilities are seen in approximately 50%–80% of individuals with tuberous sclerosis complex (Franz, 1998) and are thought to be more likely in children with an earlier seizure onset, infantile spasms, or intractable epilepsy. Third, individuals with tuberous sclerosis complex are at risk of psychiatric and behavioral disorders and should be closely followed for evidence of difficulty. Fourth, autism is present in 17%–60% of individuals with tuberous sclerosis complex (Dowling & Curatolo, 2003; Harrison & Bolton, 1997) and is often seen in the absence of seizures, intellectual disabilities, or a high cortical tuber count (see Chapter 23.1). Some studies have suggested an association of autism with the presence of temporal tubers or cerebellar tubers (Bolton & Griffiths, 1997; Seri, Cerquiglini, Pisani, & Curatolo, 1999; Weber, Engelhoff, McKellop, & Franz, 2000). Finally, individuals with tuberous sclerosis complex may experience ophthalmologic involvement, which is characterized by retinal hamartomas that typically do not affect visual function.

Skin is the other most frequently involved organ system, and individuals with tuberous sclerosis complex may develop hypopigmented macules, angiofibroma, shagreen patch or periungal fibromas during their lifetime. In addition, renal involvement occurs in at least 50% of individuals with tuberous sclerosis complex and can include angiomyolipoma and renal cysts (Stillwell, Gomez, & Kelalis, 1987). Angiomyolipoma represents a major source of morbidity in adults with tuberous sclerosis complex, due to the presence of dysplastic blood vessels in the tumor growth, which are at risk for spontaneous hemorrhage. In addition, the presence of multiple angiomyolipoma can result in hypertension and affect kidney function.

Lung involvement, as lymphangiomyomatosis, occurs predominantly in women with tuberous sclerosis complex and is much more common than previously thought, now estimated to occur in as many as one third of women with tuberous sclerosis complex. Cardiac involvement, as illustrated in Wendell's story, occurs in approximately 50% of individuals with tuberous sclerosis complex and involves rhabdomyomas, which typically develop during late gestation, are most prominent during late fetal and early infancy, and then typically regress (Gomez, 1988). Occasionally, rhabdomyomas affect cardiac function and require resection, as in Wendell's case. In addition, hamartia can be seen in other organs, including the liver, pancreas, and intestines, although they typically do not affect functioning of these organs.

Specialty Tuberous Sclerosis Complex Clinics

Ideally, a Tuberous Sclerosis Complex Clinic will provide comprehensive diagnosis, surveillance, and management of various manifestations of tuberous sclerosis complex, as well as inform individuals and their families of new developments and treatment recommendations (see Table 9.7-5). A Tuberous Sclerosis Complex Clinic serves as a mechanism to coordinate care and information as well as a resource for primary care and specialty physicians. Individuals are typically seen on an annual basis and more frequently if seizure activity or other conditions require closer follow up. If evaluation in a Tuberous Sclerosis Complex Clinic is possible—not every center is able to develop such a program—the individual should be followed by a clinician familiar with the disorder and should be informed of national resources such as major medical centers in the area with specialized Tuberous Sclerosis Complex Clinics, the Tuberous Sclerosis Alliance, and other support and information resources.

Developmental Manifestations

At 13 years old, Wendell had been seizure free since infancy, although he continued to take anticonvulsant medications due to persistently abnormal EEGs. A recent neuropsychological evaluation showed his IQ score to be 120, although he did have some mild word-finding difficulties. He continued to have multiple hypopigmented macules and developed mild angiofibroma on his cheek surfaces. A recent renal ultrasound showed the presence of small angiomyolipoma bilaterally.

Table 9.7-5. Management of tuberous sclerosis complex

At diagnosis

- Brain magnetic resonance imaging (MRI)
- Echocardiogram (EKG)
- Renal ultrasound
- Ophthalmologic evaluation
- Genetic analysis
- Skin exam

At follow-up in childhood (annually)

- Neuropsychological evaluation at diagnosis of tubular sclerosis complex, on entering school, and as the occasion rises
- Brain MRI every 12 years to evaluate for possible subependymal giant cell astrocytomas (SEGA)
- Renal ultrasound every 1–3 years to evaluate for angiomyolipoma and cysts
- Echocardiogram if rhabdomyomas identified at diagnosis and as the occasion rises
- Skin exam

At follow-up in adolescence and adulthood

- Brain MRI every 1–2 years until approximately 22 years of age (to evaluate for possible SEGA)
- Renal ultrasound every 1–3 years throughout life and if renal manifestations are identified (to evaluate for angiomyolipoma and cysts)
- High resolution chest computed tomography during puberty and as the occasion arises (to evaluate for lymphangiomyomatosis)
- Skin exam

Many children with tuberous sclerosis complex may experience learning difficulties, including intellectual disabilities and autism spectrum disorders. Although roughly half of individuals with tuberous sclerosis complex are "on target" with regard to neurocognition, individuals who are "off target" may experience significant and profound developmental impairment and many exhibit autism spectrum disorders. Risk factors for neurocognitive and neurobehavioral impairment include early seizure onset, infantile spasms, and intractable seizure disorder. Correlation with tuber number and location is thought probable, although data are limited. Thus far, there is no known dependence of cognitive profiles on the locus mutated (*TSC1* or *TSC2*) or on specific mutations. Due to the risk of possible learning difficulties, all individuals diagnosed with tuberous sclerosis complex should undergo a neuropsychological evaluation at the time of diagnosis and, if they are diagnosed in early childhood, they should be reevaluated at school entrance age (Franz, 1998; Roach, DiMario, Kandt, & Northrup, 1999).

Final Comments on Tuberous Sclerosis Complex

Tuberous sclerosis complex is a multisystem disorder with significant variability in presentation and involvement among individuals diagnosed with the disorder. Individuals with the disorder should be monitored closely throughout their lives for possible manifestations of the disorder, as many symptoms occur during childhood and others during adulthood. Many children will be diagnosed with tuberous sclerosis complex after developing seizure activity, and as many as one third of children will experience infantile spasms. Due to seizure activity as well as the presence of cortical dysgenesis, children with tuberous sclerosis complex should be closely followed for the presence of learning disorders as well as behavioral difficulties. As for the child described, even children who develop infantile spasms can have a normal cognitive outcome, although developmental delays are more typical.

A 56-year-old woman named Margo was referred to a dermatologist due to growths on her fingernails and toenails. She was otherwise healthy, with normal neurocognitive development and no history of seizure activity. Margo lived with her husband and three children, all of whom were healthy. She had no family history of tuberous sclerosis complex. On examination, the dermatologist also identified mild facial angiofibroma and five hypopigmented macules on her trunk and extremities. Due to a concern for tuberous sclerosis complex, Margo was referred to a Tuberous Sclerosis Complex Clinic.

Although Margo met criteria for the diagnosis of tuberous sclerosis complex based on skin findings alone, she underwent a complete clinical and diagnostic testing in order to document organ involvement. Her brain MRI showed several cortical tubers and calcified subependymal nodules. Her renal ultrasound revealed a 8 cm mass, with signal characteristics consistent with angiomyolipoma. Her high-resolution chest computed tomography (CT) showed evidence of lymphangiomyomatosis. Due to the kidney mass, she was seen by the nephrologists in the clinic, and subsequently underwent selective embolization of the angiomyolipoma. Margo also had baseline pulmonary function testing done due to the chest CT findings, which were normal.

Because Margo had three children and many family members, she underwent deoxyribonucleic acid mutational analysis and was found to have a mutation in the *TSC2* gene. After her mutation was identified, her children were tested; one of the three was found to also carry the mutation and was diagnosed with tuberous sclerosis complex.

Although many individuals are diagnosed with tuberous sclerosis complex in early childhood due to seizure activity, skin findings, or heart tumors detected on prenatal ultrasound, many individuals are also diagnosed in late childhood, adolescence, or adulthood (e.g., Margo). In adults, renal and pulmonary manifestations are the greatest source of morbidity and mortality; therefore, individuals with tuberous sclerosis complex should have routine follow-up and surveillance studies of these organ systems. Many adults with tuberous sclerosis complex have some degree of cognitive impairment; support and assistance is often needed to help optimize job and living situations. Seizures do continue to occur in many adults with tuberous sclerosis complex, and some individuals are initially diagnosed with tuberous sclerosis complex after having a first seizure episode during adulthood.

CONCLUSION

This chapter describes the two most developmentally important phakomatoses, NF1 and tuberous sclerosis complex. Long-term outlook for individuals with NF1 remains uncertain. The major medical issues arise from internal plexiform neurofibromas that can grow or transform to malignancy and the possibility that large numbers of dermal tumors will appear over the years. No treatment is available that will prevent these symptoms from occurring, though active research is examining this area.

Due to the various organ involvement, individuals with tuberous sclerosis complex should be closely followed throughout their lives. Ideally, individuals can be followed through specialty multidisciplinary Tuberous Sclerosis Complex Clinics that allow coordination of testing and care and serve as a valuable source of information for individuals with tuberous sclerosis complex, their families, and health care professionals. Individuals with tuberous sclerosis complex should also be offered genetic counseling to discuss the implications of the diagnosis on family members as well as to allow prenatal counseling. In addition, treatments are available for many of the manifestations. With improved understanding of pathophysiologic mechanisms, specific pharmacologic treatments may be available in the future. Participation in a specialty Tuberous Sclerosis Complex Clinic may also allow an individual to participate in clinical trials of new medications and treatments for the various manifestations of tuberous sclerosis complex.

REFERENCES

Bolton, P.F., & Griffiths, P.D. (1997). Association of tuberous sclerosis of temporal lobes with autism and atypical autism. *Lancet, 349*, 392–395.

Cawthon, R.M., Weiss, R., Xu, G., Viskochil, D., Culver, M., Stevens, J., et al. (1990). A major segment of the neurofibromatosis type 1 gene: CDNA sequence, genomic structure, and point mutations. *Cell, 62*, 193–201.

Cichowski, K., & Jacks, T. (2001). NF1 tumor suppressor gene function: Narrowing the GAP. *Cell, 104*(4), 593–604.

Crino, P.B., & Henske, E.P. (1999). New developments in the neurobiology of tuberous sclerosis complex. *Neurology, 53*, 1384–1390.

Curatolo, P. (1996). Neurological manifestations of tuberous sclerosis complex. *Child's Nervous System, 12*, 515–521.

Denckla, M.B., Hofman, K., Mazzocco, M.M., Melhem, E., Reiss, A.L., Bryan, R.N., et al. (1996). Relationship between T2-weighted hyperintensities (unidentified bright objects) and lower IQs in children with neurofibromatosis-1. *American Journal of Medical Genetics, 67*, 98–102.

Dowling, M., & Curatolo, P. (2003). Autism. In P. Curatolo (Ed.), *Tuberous sclerosis complex: From basic science to clinical phenotypes* (pp. 91–108). New York: Mackeith Press.

Franz, D.N. (1998). Diagnosis and management of tuberous sclerosis complex. *Seminars in Pediatric Neurology, 5*, 253–268.

Fryer, A.E., Chalmers, A., Connor, J.M., Fraser, I., Povey, S., Yates, A.D., et al. (1987). Evidence that the gene for tuberous sclerosis is on chromosome 9. *Lancet, 1*, 659–661.

Gomez, M.R. (1988). Neurologic and psychiatric features. In M.R. Gomez (Ed.), *Tuberous sclerosis* (pp. 21–36). New York: Raven Press.

Gutmann, D.H., Aylsworth, A., Carey, J.C., Korf, B., Marks, J., Pyeritz, R.E., et al. (1997). The diagnostic evaluation and multidisciplinary management of neurofibromatosis 1 and neurofibromatosis 2. *Journal of the American Medical Association, 278*(1), 51–57.

Harrison, J.E., & Bolton, P.F. (1997). Annotation: Tuberous sclerosis. *Child Psychology/Psychiatry, 38*, 603–614.

Kandt, R.S., Haines, J.L., Smith, M., Northrup, H., Gardner, R.J.M., Shorr, M.P., et al. (1992). Linkage of an important gene locus for tuberous sclerosis to a chromosome 16 marker for polycystic kidney disease. *Nature Genetics, 2*, 37–41.

Kayes, L.M., Riccardi, V.M., Burke, W., Bennet, R.L., & Stephens, K. (1992). Sporadic neurofibromatosis 1, mental retardation, and dysmorphism. *Journal of Medical Genetics, 29*, 686–687.

Korf, B.R. (1990). *Diagnosis of neurofibromatosis and clinical overview*. New York: Thieme Medical Publishers.

Listernick, R., Louis, D.N., Packer, R.J., & Gutmann, D.H. (1997). Optic pathway gliomas. Children with neurofibromatosis 1: Consensus statement from the NF1 Optic Pathway Glioma Task Force. *Annals of Neurology, 41*(2), 143–149.

Messiaen, L.M., Callens, T., Mortier, G., Beysen, D., Vandenbroucke, I., Van Roy, N., et al. (2000). Exhaustive mutation analysis of the NF1 gene allows identification of 95% of mutations and reveals a high frequency of unusual splicing defects. *Human Mutation, 15*(6), 541–555.

North, K., Joy, P., Yuille, D., Cocks, N., Mobbs, E., Hutchins, P., et al. (1994). Specific learning disability in children with neurofibromatosis type 1: Significance of MRI abnormalities. *Neurology, 44*, 878–883.

North, K.N., Riccardi, V., Samango-Sprouse, C., Ferner, R., Moore, B., Legius, E., et al. (1997). Cognitive function and academic performance in neurofibromatosis 1: Consensus statement from the NF1 Cognitive Disorders Task Force. Neurology, 48(4), 1121–1127.

Osborne, J.P., Fryer, A., & Webb, D. (1991). Epidemiology of tuberous sclerosis. *Annals of the New York Academy of Sciences, 615*, 125–127.

Packer, R.J., Sutton, L.N., & Bilaniuk, L.T., et al. (1988). Treatment of chiasmatic/hypothalamic gliomas of childhood with chemotherapy: An update. *Annals of Neurology 23*, 79–85.

Roach, E.D.S., Dimario, F.J., Kandt, R.S., & Northrup, H. (1999). Tuberous Sclerosis Complex Consensus Conference: Recommendations for diagnostic evaluation. *Journal of Child Neurology, 14*, 401–407.

Roach, E.D.S., Gomez, M.R., & Northrup, H. (1998). Tuberous Sclerosis Complex Consensus Conference: Revised clinical diagnostic criteria. *Journal of Child Neurology, 13*, 624–628.

Ruggieri, M., & Polizzi, A. (2000). Segmental neurofibromatosis. *Journal of Neurosurgery, 93*(3), 530–532.

Seri, S., Cerquiglini, A., Pisani, F., & Curatolo, P. (1999). Autism in tuberous sclerosis: Evoked potential evidence of a deficit in auditory sensory processing. *Clinical Neurophysiology, 10*, 1825–1830.

Stillwell, T., Gomez, M., & Kelalis, P.P. (1987). Renal lesions in tuberous sclerosis. *Journal of Urology, 138*, 477–481.

Stumpf, D., Alksne, J.F., Aunegers, J.F., Brown, S.S., Conneally, P.M., Housman, D., et al. (1988). Consensus Development Conference on Neurofibromatosis. *Archives of Neurology, 45*, 575–578.

van der Hoeve, J. (1932). Eye symptoms in phakomatoses. *Transactions of the Ophthalmological Societies of the United Kingdom, 52*, 380–401.

Xu, G., Lin, B., Tanaka, K., Dunn, D., Wood, D., Gesteland, R., et al. (1990). The catalytic domain of the neurofibromatosis type 1 gene product stimulates: Ras Gtpase and complements Ira mutants of S. Cerevisiae. *Cell, 63*, 835–841.
Wallace, M.R., Marchuk, D.A., Andersen, L.B., Letcher, R., Odeh, H.M., Saulino, A.M., et al. (1990). Type 1 neurofibromatosis gene: Identification of a large transcript disrupted in three NF1 patients. *Science, 249*, 181–186.
Weber, A.M., Egelhoff, J.C., Mckellop, J.M., & Franz, D.N. (2000). Autism and the cerebellum: Evidence from tuberous sclerosis. *Journal of Autism and Developmental Disorders, 30*(6), 511–517.
Wu, B.L., Austin, M.A., Schneider, G.H., Boles, R.G., & Korf, B.R. (1995). Deletion of the entire *NF1* gene detected by FISH: Four deletion patients associated with severe manifestations. *American Journal of Medical Genetics, 59*(4), 528–535.

CHAPTER 10

PREMATURITY AND ITS CONSEQUENCES

I. Leslie Rubin

In July 1976, this author started a fellowship in Neonatology at the Rainbow Babies and Children's Hospital in Cleveland, Ohio. He was drawn to this emerging field of clinical activity because he was fascinated with the growing recognition that newborns had a variety of motor, cognitive, and social skills not previously realized. Also, there was a growing appreciation of the ability to assist the premature infants to survive the challenges of prematurity and grow up to be healthy and successful.

The author was particularly drawn to the Fellowship at Rainbow Babies and Children's Hospital because that program was promoting the new concept that if mothers and babies stayed in contact with each other immediately after birth, their relationship would be strengthened, and the baby would grow up to be healthier, happier, and more successful. The atmosphere in the newborn nurseries, and especially the neonatal intensive care units, was abuzz with the spirit of learning something new every day, of studying challenging questions, and of trying to make sure that every baby, no matter how premature or how small, would survive the challenges of breathing air, of acquiring adequate nutrition to grow and develop normally, and of being able to tolerate the environmental vicissitudes of extrauterine life.

At this time, one could appreciate four major areas in which emerging knowledge and understanding would change the landscape of clinical pediatrics and of society dramatically:

1. The clinical and academic rigor in trying to understand the physiology and pathophysiology of premature infants and what techniques and technologies could help to assure their healthy survival
2. The emerging technology of neuroimaging beginning with the computerized topographic (CT) scans of the head and brain and expanding to the use of ultrasound and magnetic resonance imaging (MRI).
3. The increasing appreciation of the fact that even if the infants could survive the neonatal period with all its stresses and insults, there was a likelihood that there would be physiological, medical, functional, and social consequences
4. The critical need to include and involve parents, especially mothers, in the entire process

At the time, it was felt that involving mothers would assure that there was a positive relationship between the mother and infant—captured in the term of those days, *mother–infant bonding*—that would improve the likelihood of health and well-being for the infants and their families.

BRIEF HISTORY OF PREMATURITY

Prematurity was originally defined using a birth weight of less than 2,500 g. Such infants were termed *low birth weight*, or LBW. By the 1970s, clinicians worked with infants of birth weights of less than 1,500 g, termed *very low birth weight*, or VLBW, infants. Seminal studies at the time of infants of low birth weight used the 1,500 g benchmark for their measurement of outcomes.

As the technology for managing breathing difficulties, nutritional needs, and other critical physiological parameters of organ function and cardiovascular stability improved, smaller and smaller newborn infants survived. The VLBW categorization soon gave way to the term *extremely low birth weight*, or ELBW, infant referring to an infant of 1,000 g or less, and rapidly thereafter, clinicians started to confront the reality that, as a result of what they had learned and what they were doing, they were able to rescue even smaller infants—weighing less than 750–800 g. As the infants of lower and lower birth weight were surviving, clinicians confronted babies born at earlier and earlier gestational ages all the way down to 23–24 weeks (Wilson-Costello, Friedman, Minich, Fanaroff, & Hack, 2005; see also Figure 10.1).

As the smaller and younger premature infants were surviving, clinicians became aware of significant complicating factors. Some of the necessary interventions

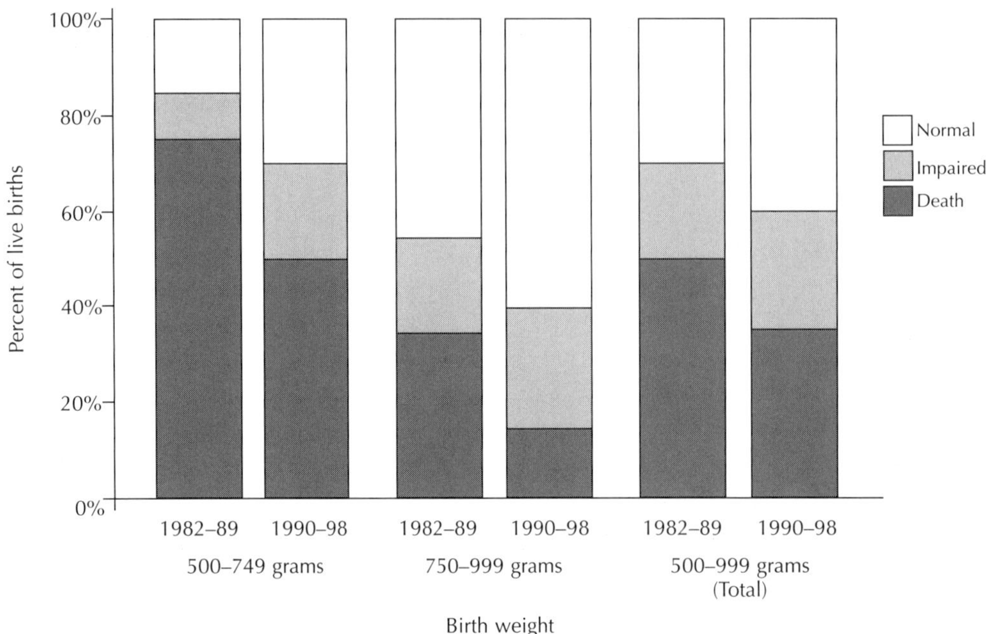

Figure 10.1. Percent of live births according to birth weight. (Reproduced with permission from *Pediatrics,* Vol. 115[4], Page 1001, Copyright © 2005 by the AAP.)

were causing serious side effects of their own (e.g., assisted ventilation could result in pneumothorax and perforation, high oxygen administration would result in retinopathy, nutritional supplements could cause unexpected metabolic disturbances). In addition, medical problems not previously appreciated to any degree began to arise, such as persistent patent ductus arteriosus (PDA) and nectrotizing enterocolitis (NEC), which posed threats to physiological homeostasis and survival. The treatment of NEC, if severe, might necessitate the resection of a segment of bowel, resulting in "short bowel syndrome," which also posed management problems and affected long-term outcome and quality of life (Hack, Taylor, Klein, & Mercuri-Minich, 2000; see Table 10.1).

Most significant for the long-term outcome was that central nervous system morbidity became more and more likely, resulting in developmental and functional difficulties in motor performance, cognition and learning, behavior, socialization, and sensory function. Last in this list, but not least, is the fact that the smaller, the younger, and the sicker the infants, the longer they would have to stay in the neonatal intensive care unit and in step-down nurseries to "feed and grow" and essentially become physiologically stable enough to go home.

This protracted length of time inevitably takes its toll on the family's resources—physical, emotional, social, and economic. Then, when the infants do eventually go home, the family has to deal with the reality of

Table 10.1. Continuum of pathology for prematurity

Organ system	Neonatal pathology	Long-term outcome
Brain	Hypoxic-ischemic encephalopathy, periventricular leukomalacia, intraventricular hemorrhage	Cerebral palsy, intellectual disabilities
Eyes	Retinopathy of prematurity	Visual impairment
Lungs	Respiratory distress syndrome/ ventilation	Bronchopulmonary dysplasia, reactive airway disease
Upper airway	Intubation	Feeding problems
Gastrointestinal tract	Necrotizing enterocolitis	Short bowel syndrome

taking care of an infant who had been in a sophisticated medical setting for months and now is in the family's home with comparatively little in the way of medical and nursing supports. As the medical problems are resolved, the families soon turn their attention to the developmental outcomes and the stresses that these also bring to bear on the family's resources (Taylor, Klein, Minich, & Hack, 2001).

Much of the knowledge and information available on optimal care of premature infants has come from data collection and research in the earlier years through the National Collaborative Perinatal Project and more recently through the National Institutes of Child Health and Development Neonatal Research Network. The Neonatal Research Network has been in operation since the mid 1980s and now consists of more than 16 academic neonatal centers around the country (Ehrenkranz & Wright, 2003).

This chapter addresses how to help premature infants develop optimally and to assist families in coping as best as possible. Obviously, the smaller and the younger the newborn, the higher the mortality and morbidity, the more complex the acute newborn presentation, and the more likely the infant will experience significant long-term sequelae.

FACTORS CONTRIBUTING TO PREMATURITY

Factors contributing to prematurity can be clear in some cases, whereas in others, the reasons are obscure. For simplicity, the factors can be divided into maternal, placental, and fetal, although in reality there is more often than not a combination of factors, and sorting out the primary factors is not easy. Be that as it may, exploring as many of the factors as possible that contribute to a serious medical problem is helpful as it may be beneficial in the acute and long-term management (see Figure 10.2).

Maternal Factors

Maternal factors relate primarily to the mother's health, well-being, and ability to support a healthy pregnancy. Physical factors include general health (any chronic medical conditions, including the need for medications),

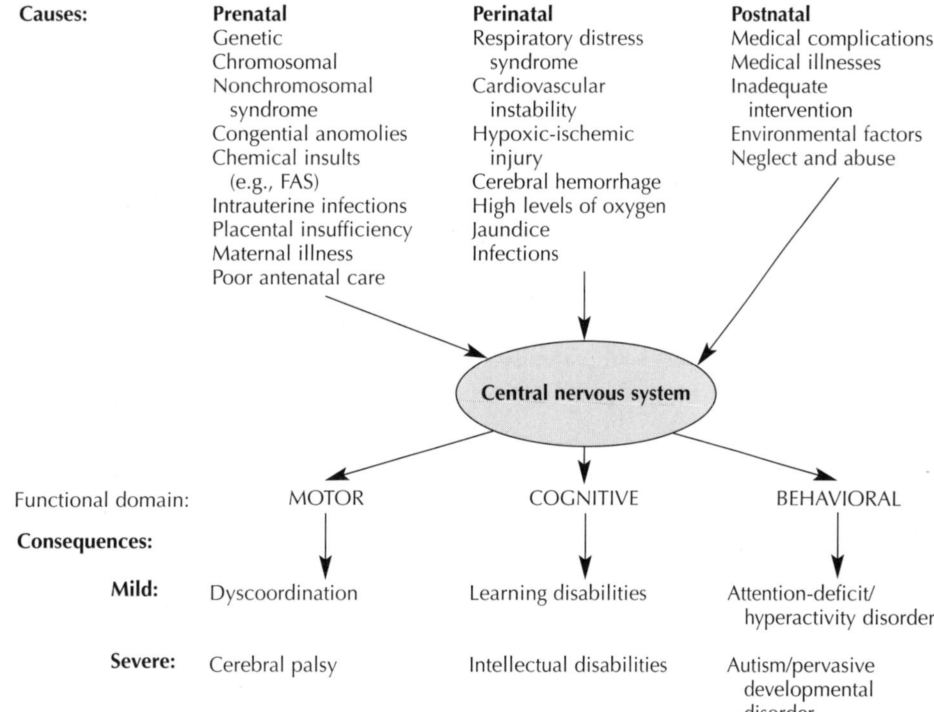

Figure 10.2. Central nervous system vulnerability and consequences due to prematurity (From Rubin, I.L. [1992]. Diagnosis and disabilities. *Journal of Intellectual Disability Research, 36,* 1–8; adapted by permission.)

previous obstetric history (especially previous premature infant or miscarriage), nutritional status (underweight or overweight), and general emotional and social well-being (whether the mother is smoking, drinking alcohol, or taking street drugs). Demographic factors such as educational achievement, socioeconomic status, marital status, and natural supports such as extended family or membership in community or religious organizations are important considerations and could be helpful in evaluating risk for prematurity. Maternal infections acquired during pregnancy like toxoplasmosis, other infections, rubella, cytomegalovirus infection, and herpes simplex (TORCH) and human immunodeficiency virus (HIV) are well known to be associated with serious effects on the fetus and newborn; however, more common infections may play a significant role in the etiology of prematurity and adverse neurodevelopmental outcomes than was previously realized (Neufeld, Frigon, Graham, & Mueller, 2005, Stoll et al., 2004).

Placental and Uterine Factors

Placental factors are intimately linked to mother's health, especially in relation to smoking, but also to maternal hypertension and the risk of preeclampsia. In addition, placental structural anomalies can jeopardize the pregnancy and result in early termination and prematurity. Placenta previa and abruption are major risk factors for prematurity and may present as obstetric emergencies. Congenital uterine anomalies can contribute to the unusual location of a placenta as well as to the premature onset of labor.

Cervical incompetence is another condition that can precipitously lead to early termination of pregnancy or later increase the risk for premature birth. Awareness of this condition and others in this category can help to inform preventive measures for the immediate as well as for later pregnancies.

The following story by Julie explains the complications she experienced during her pregnancy with her son Harrison, who was born prematurely.

Five years ago, I went in to have my ultrasound at 19 weeks pregnant to find out if we were having a boy or a girl. The specialist came back in, held my hand, and said, "I'm so sorry, but there is no fluid around your baby. It doesn't look good."

As I was sobbing my heart out in the specialist's office, his recommendation was that I terminate the pregnancy. He said he just wanted to see me get healthy and get on to my next pregnancy. He called it a failed pregnancy and sent me over to discuss my options with one of the doctors in the group I was seeing.

That doctor told me that he had never had a woman continue on with the pregnancy once she found out this information. At this point, there was less than a 1% chance for my baby to be born alive. Someone else told me that this condition was nothing to fool around with, that I could hemorrhage and die in 20 minutes.

I went home really scared, and I told my husband that I didn't want to die over this. If it was medically necessary, I should go ahead and do it, but the hospital had a 24-hour waiting period. That night, I couldn't sleep, and I went out on my deck and cried out to God. It was horrible enough that my baby wasn't going to make it, but having to make this decision was the worst part of all.

Everyone was telling me what to do at this point, but I realized that I was the one who would ultimately have to answer to God for my decision. I decided that as long as there was a heartbeat, I would continue on. My husband agreed, to my complete relief, because it's so important to have agreement with your spouse when you are both facing the bad complications the doctors were predicting.

I found out the next day that my life wasn't at risk at that point. I put myself on bed rest because my doctor said that he had no reasonable expectation of hospitalizing me. One of the specialists told me that out of 50 cases like mine, he had only had two babies survive.

Fetal Factors

The vitality of the embryo and fetus is obviously critically dependent on the mother's health and well-being as well as on the health of the placenta. Chromosomal and nonchromosomal syndromes as well as serious congenital anomalies can result in premature births, or the pregnancy may be interrupted by medical considerations for the health of the fetus. This situation is most significant for multiple births—not so much with twins, but increasingly with triplets and more.

NEONATAL COMPLICATIONS

Respiratory Distress Syndrome

The greatest challenge to the survival of a premature newborn infant is the ability to breathe. The deficiency of surfactant in the premature newborns prevents adequate and efficient breathing and oxygen exchange. The infant struggles to keep his or her lungs open, rapidly becomes exhausted, and enters into a serious metabolic debt. Rapid recognition of the situation is critical to optimal management and prevention of further complications.

Management with assisted ventilation and additional oxygen takes its toll. The pressures needed to adequately keep the lungs expanded and the blood oxygenated, if high, can cause the immediate effect of producing a pneumothorax and, if prolonged, seriously contributes to the development of long-term pulmonary complications of bronchopulmonary dysplasia. Advanced techniques, such as the use of extracorporeal membrane oxygenation (ECMO), have reduced the risk of lung damage and have improved the long-term outcome.

Bronchopulmonary dysplasia is the most common serious medical complication of prematurity and often delays discharge from nurseries. It may require prolonged use of assisted ventilation and oxygen administration and, in the long term, results in reactive airway disease with risks of frequent decompensation and infection, particularly with respiratory syncitial virus (see Chapter 15).

Cardiovascular Instability

The circulatory system of the premature newborn infant is not as well developed and certainly not able to maintain as steady homodynamic pressures as in the full-term infant, nor is it as resilient to dramatic changes. This condition is most evident in the effect of a sudden pneumothorax, which rapidly and dramatically changes the cardiopulmonary circulation and can have serious implications on cerebral blood flow.

The most common hemodynamic complication in premature newborns is the persistence of the patent ductus arteriosus (PDA), which results in significant effects on cardiorespiratory circulation; can compromise the management of the respiratory distress syndrome; and requires more forceful ventilator pressures, increased percentage of administered oxygen or more prolonged need for ventilator and oxygen support. Under these stressed circumstances, closure of the PDA with medication or surgical ligation will dramatically improve cardiovascular stability and management and resolution of lung disease. Obviously, surgical procedures in such small, sick, and vulnerable infants are not without complications, but the development of the thoracoscopic procedure is a dramatic improvement on the open thoracotomy procedures, with reduced morbidity and mortality.

Retinopathy of Prematurity

The vascularity of the newborn retina is very sensitive to variations in local oxygen concentration and responds with neovascularization. The new blood vessels are vulnerable to rupture and hemorrhage, and bleeding causes the serious complications of fibrosis, scarring, and retinal detachment. Obviously, knowledge of the causative factor (hyperoxia) and the serous complications results in close monitoring of the percentage of oxygen administered and regular surveillance of the retina by an experienced ophthalmologist through discharge and well into childhood (see Chapter 16).

Jaundice

Hyperbilirubinemia has long been known to result in brain damage through deposition of bilirubin in the nuclei of the brain. The most dramatic clinical picture is well known as kernicterus (*kern* = nuclei of the brain; *icterus* = jaundice); however, bilirubin levels lower than those causing kernicterus can result in brain damage. For that reason, bilirubin level is closely monitored in all newborns. Phototherapy is used for the milder levels, whereas exchange transfusions are used for more worrisome levels.

Premature newborns are more vulnerable to bilirubin deposition in the brain; therefore, much lower levels are tolerated. Also, more long-term sequelae of hyperbilirubinemia are evident in premature infants than had previously been realized. Whether bilirubin directly affects the outcome or whether associated clinical conditions predispose to the increased bilirubin levels will be answered in due course though appropriate research (Oh et al., 2003).

Necrotizing Enterocolitis

NEC is the most common serious gastrointestinal condition that affects premature infants and is associated with significant risk for morbidity and mortality. The etiology is felt to be multifactorial but primarily involves increased vulnerability of the gastrointestinal mucosa, which can be a result of cardiovascular disturbances and reduced blood flow to the gastrointestinal tract, and infection, which then aggravates the pathology. As with other medical conditions, smaller more premature infants are more vulnerable to the condition, and the condition is more likely to be severe in those infants.

Milder forms of NEC can be treated conservatively with bowel rest, antibiotics, and other supportive treatments whereas more severe stages may result in perforation and require surgical intervention and bowel resection. If the segment of bowel involved is long, then the risk of "short bowel syndrome" arises, which has its own long-term complications in management. Early recognition of the symptoms can reduce the likelihood of a more serious progressive stage and improve the long-term outcome. More severe forms of NEC that require surgery are associated with significant growth delay and adverse neurodevelopmental outcomes, as well (Hintz et al., 2005).

Other Medical Conditions

Dealing with all possible considerations is not within the scope of this chapter, but nutritional and metabolic factors; hematological complications; infections; and other physiological, pathophysiological, medical, therapeutic, pharmacological, and environmental factors can all play a part in the immediate neonatal period and, thus, can affect general health and well-being in the short- and long term.

NEUROPATHOLOGICAL CONSIDERATIONS

Ultimately, a major focus of the long-term outcome of very small premature infants is on functional measures. How well are these children doing academically and socially compared with their same age peers and are they keeping up physically in running, playing, or engaging in sports activities? Since Little's (1861) time, the relationship between the motor and mental development of children and their circumstances of birth have provided a causal connection to cerebral palsy. As seen in greater detail in Chapter 11, a causal connection exists and relates significantly to injuries to the central nervous system.

In the past, more infants were born at term and suffered from asphyxial injuries or traumatic hemorrhagic insults leading to cerebral palsy. Improvement in obstetric practice has resulted in a significant decrease in cerebral injuries in term infants, whereas the increase in survival of premature infants has contributed to the prevalence of cerebral palsy to the extent that the overall prevalence of cerebral palsy has not changed appreciably, only the demographics and relative proportion of term versus premature infants.

Advances in neuroimaging techniques, starting with the CT scan and progressing to the ultrasound and MRI, have helped significantly to locate the cerebral lesions associated with prematurity and to explain the pathophysiology of ischemic and hemorrhagic lesions of the premature brain (Volpe, 2001). Vascularity of the premature brain is highly vulnerable to both ischemic insults, particularly in the periventricular area because of the configuration of the arterial architecture, and hemorrhagic insults, particularly in and around the germinal matrix. At the core of the etiology is the cardiovascular circulation and the pressure and flow of blood through the brain. The cerebral blood flow is particularly vulnerable to sudden changes in blood pressure, such as can occur with a pneumothorax, and can increase the likelihood of cerebrovascular insults.

Ischemic Insults

Diffuse hypoxic ischemic events in premature newborns can cause damage at a variety of target areas in the brain, including the hippocampus, globus pallidus, and brain stem, affecting the pons and inferior olivary nuclei, the internal granule cells of the cerebellum, and the infarction of the spinal cord involving the anterior horn cells. This factor may explain why infants and children who were extremely premature and who suffered significant hypoxic ischemic insults have a complex and mixed picture of pyramidal tract signs as well as extrapyramidal tract features and even signs of spinal cord involvement. The most common site for ischemic insults in the premature brain, however, is in the periventricular region of the white matter. The cerebral arterial architecture in the white matter dorsal and lateral to the external angles of the lateral ventricles represents a vascular "border zone" that increases the likelihood of hypoxic ischemic insults in this region.

The term *periventricular leukomalacia* is a neuropathological diagnosis derived from the appearance of the lesions at autopsy. The affected areas have become necrotic, reflected in the liquefaction of the fatty tissue of the white matter. Increased survival of infants, and later improvement in technology, allowed clinicians to see the results of these lesions, often as cystic lesions in the periventricular area on neuroimaging studies that would later resolve. The finding of periventricular lesions is associated with an increased likelihood of later neurological impairment. Interestingly, the location of the lesions is in the pathways of the motor fibers to the legs (see Figure 10.3); hence, the most likely type of motor involvement is termed *spastic diplegia*, in which the legs are involved predominantly, though not exclusively. Because these lesions are primarily in the deep white matter and are localized to the periventricular areas, infants are less likely to have intellectual impairment and, if they do, the degree is likely to be more in the mild to moderate range compared with children with a more diffuse type of hypoxic ischemic injury.

Hemorrhagic Insults

Hemorrhagic insults to the premature brain occur predominantly in the germinal matrix and commonly extend into the ventricles. They can also extend into the sur-

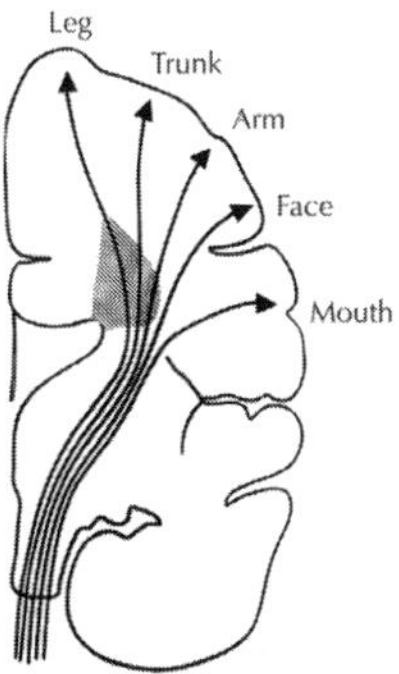

Figure 10.3. Schematic diagram of location of periventricular hemorrhagic infarction and descending corticospinal tract motor fibers. (Reprinted from *Neurology of the newborn* [4th ed.], Volpe, J.J., p. 455, Copyright 2001, with permission from Elsevier.)

rounding cerebral tissue. The pathology in these lesions is directly related to the richly vascularized and loosely supported connective tissue in the germinal matrix.

This region is the site of cellular proliferation during the early part of brain development and, therefore, requires rich nutrition that is brought by a plentiful supply of blood vessels. As the cells begin to migrate to the cortex and leave the germinal matrix, the blood supply remains rich for a period of time, and the connective tissue is no longer supported by the presence of proliferating cells—thus predisposing vessels to ready rupture with critical changes in blood flow and pressure. As the fetus matures, the germinal matrix is resorbed, and the likelihood of vascular rupture and resulting hemorrhage is greatly reduced.

The degree of hemodynamic change will result in a corresponding degree of hemorrhage that is divided into four "grades." Grades I–II are mild and tend to be more local to the subependymal germinal matrix (Grade I) or can extravasate into the ventricles (Grade II). Grade III is more severe and also by definition includes the dilatation of the ventricles, whereas Grade IV represents hemorrhage into the surrounding cortical white matter. Each degree is associated with comparable risks for adverse neurological outcomes.

Dilation of the ventricles with more severe forms of intraventricular hemorrhage can be acute and related to obstruction to cerebrospinal fluid flow by blood clots and obstructive or noncommunicating hydrocephalus, which can resolve. Later development of hydrocephalus as a result of an obliterative arachnoiditis, however, is a communicating type of hydrocephalus and will very likely require shunt placement for long-term management.

Pathogenesis of the ischemic and hemorrhagic lesions of the brain are similar, involving cerebral blood flow and pressure, vascular as well as extravascular, so that the lesions are often found together. The more severe the intraventricular hemorrhage, the more likely there will be an associated ischemic lesion, most likely in the periventricular area.

SPECIAL CASE OF MULTIPLE PREGNANCIES

Twin pregnancies pose a higher risk of prematurity and, therefore, risk for long-term sequelae. The problem appears to be greater if the twins are monochorionic rather than dichorionic. This situation is complicated by the risk of placental vascular anomalies and the possibility of intrauterine twin demise. Triplets and greater numbers of infants in one pregnancy are at even greater risk for prematurity and its consequences particularly the later-born infants (see Figure 10.4). The development of the infants may be further complicated by the limited attention that each infant can receive from the mother. For this reason, mothers of multiple births should receive extra support and attention (Feldman & Eidelman, 2005). The following story was written by a mother of triplets.

Babies so small they sounded like kittens when they were delivered, except the tiniest, which was too small to even cry. I was a new mother who was too mad and too scared to cry myself. Babies born at 28 weeks to the day and barely 2 lb—my body had failed to keep them safe . . . now it was up to the doctors and God.

The neonatal intensive care unit (NICU) is an amazing and horrible place. All the medical miracles saved my angels but broke my heart. Each of my three tiny babies would scream in pain, but no sound was heard because they had intubation tubes down their throats. There were three or four intravenous lines (some in the head), hourly blood draws, many meds, feeding tubes, heal pricks, and peripherally inserted central catheters.

The worst part of the NICU for me as "Mom" was the fact that I could not take away the pain, nor even comfort my tiny angels. I could not protect them from pain. I couldn't even hold them. As any Mom knows, there is nothing worse than watching your child suffer, and even worse, not be able to do anything about it.

Ahh, but a glorious gift the NICU gave us . . . my babies came home! Now, I was in control . . . finally. This was a wonderful gift and one of my biggest weaknesses as the mother of three 28-weekers. I was too scared to be flexible. I ran their schedule like a machine. Nothing would rock the boat on my watch. No babies would cry or want. This was quite a difficult and unrealistic plan. I just saw my three hurt so bad, and now I had control of their environment . . . or so I thought.

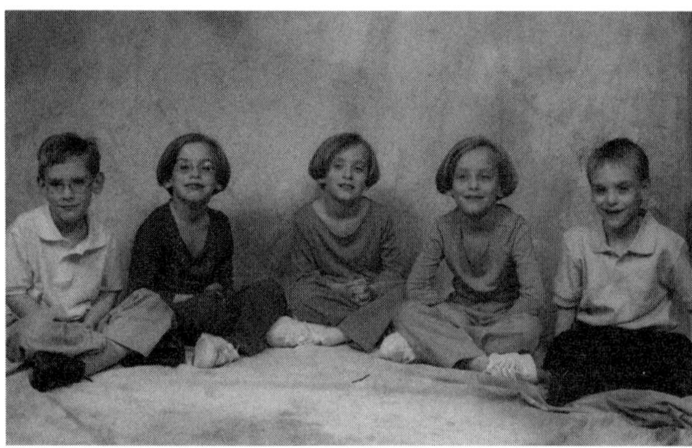

Figure 10.4. Of these quintuplets, who were born at 24 weeks' gestation, three have sequelae. To date, these children are the most premature and lightest total weight quintuplets (all surviving) ever born.

Between the meds and four or five doctors per baby, it took a flow chart and a journal just to keep up with their medical needs. The "alarms" were hourly. All three babies were on heart and breathing monitors; one was on oxygen. Someone always forgot to breathe or would aspirate after a feed or during the night. You know your life is not normal when you react quickly, but calmly to a blue baby on your lap.

On top of that, I insisted on feeding the two sickest exclusively, and I pumped for 7 months. (After all, Mom does it best, right?) Needless to say, I slept about 2 hours a night for the first 18 months. We never left the house for about 18 months unless it was to see a doctor, except for my awesome pediatrician, who drove across town to come to my house to examine my babies. He also called randomly to be sure I was not ready to be checked into the loony farm and slipped in a glass of wine now and then.

Well, we made it and not in a little way. All three of my miracles are "on the chart" and are healthy. You would never know they were tiny enough to wear my husband's wedding ring on their leg. Now at 4 years old, they are like every other 4-year-old. Tutus, earthworms, trains, mud, bikes, cake for breakfast, and three extra wiggly bodies in my bed during a thunderstorm have almost erased the memories of that early storm . . . almost.

As hard as our early years were, my family has a special gift that no "normal" family will ever understand. When you live day by day at the edge, it changes your perception of everything and everyone around you. It gives you a tiny glimpse of heaven that you will forever carry in your heart and share with everyone around you. I am so blessed to be my angels' mother.

DISCHARGE PLANNING

As mentioned earlier, one of the advances in the care of high-risk newborns, particularly those who are born prematurely, is the critical element of mother–infant bonding. During the 1950s and 1960s and well into the 1970s, full-term, healthy infants were separated from their mothers at birth by hospital protocol. Many infants were fed "sugar water" for their first feed, and, at that time, breast feeding was not encouraged. This practice was believed to be based on scientific fact, and time and proof were needed to demonstrate the value of early mother–infant contact.

In the mid-1970s, pioneers of neonatology, principally John Kennell and Marshall Klaus (1998), insisted that mothers of premature infants insert their arms into incubators and touch their premature and sick infants in order to feel a connection. They encouraged mothers to become intimately involved in the day-to-day care of their infants in order to prepare themselves for their infants' inevitable discharge. Previously, by the time mothers would take their infants home, they would be at a loss. They would not know how to take care of their infants, who had spent months in a hospital setting with all types of needed personnel and technology. Without medical and nursing support, mothers and fathers would have to adapt to a new and unfamiliar reality.

The discharge process is critical to ensuring optimal confidence in the mother for taking care of her fragile infant. It ideally and theoretically should begin with admission but should gain momentum as the infant moves from the life-threatening stages of the immediate neonatal period and dependence, to the intensive care unit, and then to a more stable and less-fragile state. The discharge process should not only make sure that all of the medical aspects of the child are considered (e.g., possible apnea monitor, breathing treatments, medications, feedings), but also that neurodevelopmental aspects are addressed (e.g., physical therapy) and that the family's emotional status is satisfactorily managed with appropriate supports built into the discharge process.

Follow-up appointments for medical attention, referrals for therapies and early intervention programs, and adequate support for families in the home are important aspects of the discharge process. At this time, parents ask many questions about the future of their children. Clinicians should obviously be supportive and encouraging, but they should also be realistic.

As one parent once said, "I have learned to wish for the best even as I fear and expect the worst." The rollercoaster emotional experiences during the critical newborn period take their emotional toll but also set the stage for the emotional reactions that will be associated with the anticipation of an optimal developmental pattern associated with the potential for success as the child grows. The critical element in the discharge planning process is to reassure the parents that the child is stable, that a good medical and social support system is in place, that appropriate referrals have been made to developmental services, that medical specialty follow-up clinics are available as needed, and that care will be coordinated.

The parents need to know and be reassured that they will be able to manage. Much of the care and coordination of services falls on the shoulders of the primary care pediatrician, but high-risk infant follow-up programs often provide this service particularly for the more medically complex infants. The following story by Julie about her son, Harrison, demonstrates the anxiety that parents feel during the discharge process and the need for adequate family supports to help parents manage caring for their premature infants.

Harrison was born at 27 weeks, weighing 1 lb, 10 oz, and measuring just 10¾ inches long. The doctor told us the baby was a boy, and we were elated. Then, the neonatologist came in and said that Harrison only had a 10% chance of making it through the first 24 hours.

At 4:30 A.M., the doctors came to my room and said, "You better come now to see your son." At 5:00 A.M., the neonatologist came to my room and said, "I'm sorry we've done all we can do . . . your son has about 2 hours left." So, I sat and watched the clock in my room as those 2 hours clicked away and prayed that my baby would survive.

The doctors were trying an experimental procedure utilizing nitric oxide, and my husband had to sign papers to give them permission. Harrison was still struggling for life on 100% oxygen. Then, the telephone rang, and Harrison's doctor said that Harrison had had the most incredible response to the experimental procedure.

Harrison was kept on the ventilator for 2 months. They would not let me even hold him until 5 weeks after he was born because of his extreme prematurity. When I finally did, it was so exciting. The entry in my journal reads, "I got to hold my precious Harrison, and he was so relaxed. He loves cuddling. He fell asleep right away in my arms, and I rocked him."

The most difficult part of his 3 months in the NICU was when they had to paralyze him due to a cyst on his lung. Then, he developed another cyst on his other lung. I really cried. Eventually both cysts were healed.

By the time Harrison was 4½ lb, he was ready to go home, finally! However, I had come down with bronchitis, so the doctors said that they would wait a few days. I had done the pumping of breast milk, but now I was sick and exhausted, and it was time for me to stop.

A few days later, the doctors let us take Harrison home, but we first had to take him directly across the street for a hernia operation at The Children's Hospital. They gave us a heart monitor in case his heart stopped beating and blow-by oxygen in case he stopped breathing. I was so scared by all of this. Over the next few years, he had two hernia surgeries, one hip surgery, a full body cast for 6 months, two ear surgeries, and several bouts with pneumonia.

After we got Harrison home from his hernia operation, I was still not feeling well at all. I was exhausted; my blood sugar seemed to be acting crazy. I had night sweats coming down from the hormones. He was eating every 3 hours, so I wasn't used to waking up all through the night.

I went to see an endocrinologist, and he put me on at least six different medicines at once . . . some for anxiety, panic, and depression. They made me worse. I felt like I was falling apart. I felt this "quaking" inside, sometimes feeling like I was going to jump out of my skin. I stopped taking those drugs.

This time was the scariest and darkest of my life. I had never felt this way before. I did not understand what was going on with my body. I kept thinking it should have been the happiest time for me now that Harrison was home, but I just felt so weak!

I then ended up in the emergency room, barely able to hold my head up. The emergency room doctors ran the tests on my blood, then got my doctor on the telephone. He said that I had posttraumatic stress syndrome. I had gotten through the hard part of the NICU, and now I had fallen apart.

Gradually, I felt better through alternative medicine and lots of naps. Today, Harrison is a happy little guy with an abundance of joy and a great sense of humor. He loves to entertain people with his jokes. He has become an expert on the solar system and the human body.

CONSEQUENCES OF PREMATURITY

There are multiple factors to consider in the health, growth, and development of premature infants once they are discharged from the hospital. Most important, there is an increased likelihood of sequelae in inverse proportion to birth weight (see Table 10.2).

Medical Conditions

Given the multiple medical problems that occur in the immediate neonatal period of very small premature infants, intermediate and long-term considerations are necessary in the management of these infants as they continue to grow and develop. Fortunately, as the infants grow and develop, their more acute and life-threatening problems become less of a concern, and attention becomes focused on the more chronic aspects of their health and development.

Respiratory Although the acute neonatal problems of hyaline membrane disease and the need for oxygen and assisted ventilation improve with time, many infants develop bronchopulmonary dysplasia and its clinical manifestation in reactive airway disease.

Table 10.2. Likelihood of sequelae based on gestation in weeks

	Gestation in weeks							
Estimates for	23	24	25	26	27	28	29	30+
Chances of survival	17%	44%	61%	72%	72%	88%	85%	> 94%
Percent of survivors with medical or developmental complications	~90%	~60%	50%	40%	30%	20%	10%	< 10%
Percent requiring assisted ventilation	100%	100%	100%	100%	89%	78%	80%	30%
Average number of days requiring ventilation and oxygen	125	120	90	80	60	30	11	8
Likelihood of chronic lung disease (needing extra oxygen for more than 1 month)	100%	100%	90.5%	67%	53%	40%	16.8%	8%
Probability of significant abnormal brain scans	27%	20%	14%	6%	8%	6%	8%	7%
Likelihood of jaundice requiring phototherapy	100%	100%	100%	100%	80%	50%	30%	20%
Likelihood of patent ductus arteriosus requiring treatment	80%	50%	32%	35%	25%	27%	26%	10%
Likelihood of infection	100%	100%	100%	100%	80%	70%	40%	30%
Average number of transfusions	9	7	7	6	5	4	2	1
Likelihood of feeding problems (requiring tube feedings for more than 8 weeks)	100%	100%	100%	70%	50%	20%	15%	0%
Likelihood of gastrointestinal problems (necrotizing enterocolotis requiring medical/surgical treatment)	100%	90%	50%	40%	30%	20%	10%	5%
Likelihood of long-term visual problems	23%	17%	10%	5%	5%	3%	0%	0%
Likely duration of apnea/ bradychardia (in weeks)	7	6	5	4	3	2	1	.5
Risk of family emotional stress	High	High	High	High	Mod.	Mod.	Low	Min.
Likelihood of IQ score less than 85	High	High	High	Mod.	Mod.	Low	Min.	Min.
Likelihood of having attention-deficit disorder	High	High	High	High	Mod.	Low	Low	Min.
Likelihood of being small in growth	100%	100%	100%	70%	50%	30%	10%	0%
Likelihood of future need for special education	100%	80%	50%	50%	30%	10%	5%	5%
Likelihood of need for follow-up eye and hearing at 4 months, 8 months, 18 months, and 3 years	100%	100%	80%	70%	50%	30%	20%	10%
Likelihood of need for early intervention requiring physical, occupational, and speech therapy	100%	100%	80%	70%	50%	30%	20%	10%

Key: Min. = minimal; Mod. = moderate.

Adapted by permission from Macmillan Publishers Ltd: Koh, T., Harrison, H., & Morley, C. (1999, Sept. 16). Gestation versus outcome table for parents of extremely premature infants. *Journal of Perinatology, 19,* 452–453, Copyright 1999.

Maintenance on bronchodilators and breathing treatments, with prompt attention to acute illness, and the use of respiratory syncytial virus (RSV) prophylaxis are critical in supporting infants and preventing serious and sometimes life-threatening decompensation requiring hospitalization.

Cardiac Generally, unless there is a complicating congenital heart lesion, besides the PDA, which has usually been closed in the neonatal period, the residual cardiac problems are secondary to the chronic lung disease of bronchopulmonary dysplasia. Prevention of fluid overload with the use of diuretics and possible need for cardiotonic drugs will be monitored by the cardiologist and, over the course of time as the infants grows and matures, this condition is also likely to improve.

Gastrointestinal and Nutrition More often than not, an infant will be feeding orally by the time of discharge and will be able to take enough fluid and nutrients to grow adequately. Some infants require gastrostomy feeding tubes (G tubes), but will use them less and less as they are able to tolerate oral feedings better. Often, infants can tolerate oral feedings under ordinary circumstances but, under the stress of illness or surgery, may not be able to take in enough to compensate for the increased loss or increased demand. In these situations, resorting to supplemental feedings by G tube may be necessary for limited periods of time. G tube feeding programs may also be necessary for infants with swallowing incoordination and infants who are at risk for aspiration (see Chapter 14.2).

Gastroesophageal reflux is very common in this group of infants and may be treated with medications that reduce acidity, reduce the risk of reflux, and promote more rapid gastric emptying. Constipation may also be a problem in some infants and may improve with dietary modification or laxatives. If the infant had NEC and required significant bowel resection, then the management is more complex; the infant may have an ostomy or may have short bowel syndrome, requiring delicate dietary management (see Chapter 14.1).

Growth Premature infants start off small. They have feeding and nutritional problems requiring significant modifications of diet to ensure adequate nutrition for health and growth, and they have multiple complicating factors that can compromise metabolism and growth. Statistics on long-term growth of premature infants suggests that their growth is unlikely to "catch up" to their same-age peers. They are more likely to remain in the lower percentiles on the growth charts (Dusick, Poindexter, Ehrenkranz, & Lemons, 2003).

Eye and Vision The use of high-concentration oxygen under high pressure in the treatment of repiratory distress syndrome in very small premature infants results in retinopathy of prematurity and can have serious complications that need to be closely monitored before discharge and regularly after discharge. Even if there is no obvious damage from the retinopathy of prematurity, regular checkups are important because relatively minor problems like refractory errors or opthalmoplegias can have a significant effect on vision.

Hearing The likelihood of central nervous system insults along with the use of aminoglycocide antibiotics increase the risk for hearing impairment. Although universal newborn screening should identify those infants who need attention or continued monitoring, clinicians should periodically check infants' hearing because the consequences of recurrent ear infections may also affect hearing (see Chapter 17.1).

Other Organ Systems Although this chapter has described the common organ systems affected during prematurity, other organ systems and body functions may be directly or indirectly affected. For this reason, bone metabolism resulting in a rickets of prematurity; liver function as complicated by some parenteral feeding formulas; kidney function; and endocrine function, especially thyroid, should be routinely monitored (see Chapter 19).

Neurodevelopmental Outcomes

The high risk for ischemic and/or hemorrhagic insults to the premature brain and nervous system increases with lower birth weight and gestational age until it becomes almost inevitable that there will be some manifestation of central nervous system dysfunction (see Figure 10.5). Although severe insults leave a clearly defined legacy of functional disabilities, such as cerebral palsy or intellectual disabilities, milder and more subtle insults may manifest in subtle features (e.g., learning disabilities, trouble paying attention) later in life when increased and more complex demands are placed on the child, as occurs commonly in the school setting. For simplicity, this chapter presents the potential outcomes in terms of motor, cognitive and intellectual, and social and behavioral expressions of central nervous system insults.

Motor Cerebral palsy is a well-known association with the central nervous system insults of prematurity and most commonly manifests as a spastic diplegia because of the location of the insults in the periventricular area and the fact that the long fibers from the cells in the motor cortex that go to the legs traverse this area. More extensive insults will obviously result in more severe and complex forms of cerebral palsy. What may not be fully appreciated are the more subtle manifestations.

Often, motor findings noted early on in life may seem to disappear, and the diagnosis of cerebral palsy is then no longer appropriate—as if the child has "grown out of" the cerebral palsy. The motor impairment is no longer obvious or significant enough to express itself, although coordination difficulties or "clumsiness" may be noted and may be expressed later in life when gross motor or fine motor coordination becomes a focal point of functional need. The simplest example may be handwriting, but running posture and participation in sports may also reveal subtle difficulties. Long-term monitor-

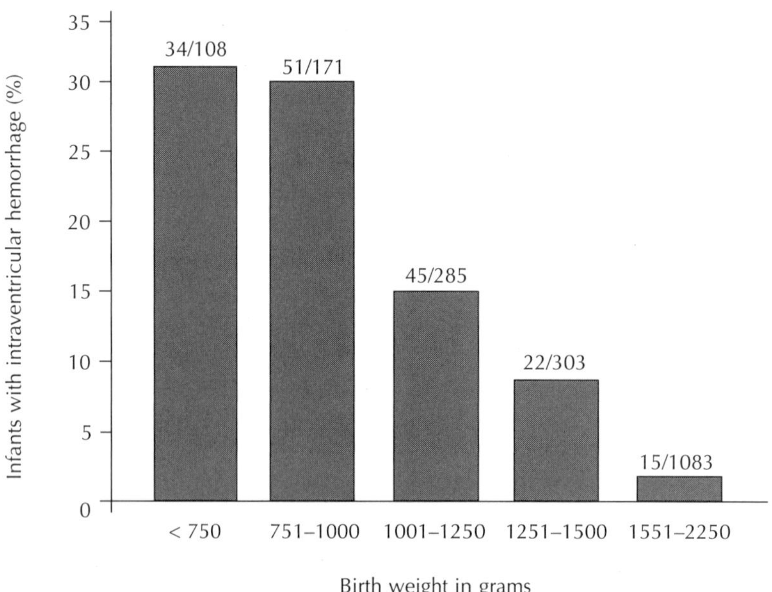

Figure 10.5. Percent of infants with intraventricular hemorrhage according to birth weight. (Adapted from *Neurology of the newborn* [4th ed.], Volpe, J.J., p. 429, Copyright 2001, with permission from Elsevier.)

ing with awareness of less-dramatic features of motor difficulties is necessary, as are appropriate therapies and support (see Chapter 11).

Cognitive and Intellectual Little (1861) noted that children who had adverse experiences around birth had "mental" as well as motor problems. Likewise, adverse outcomes of prematurity can result in intellectual impairment and disabilities; however, impairment or disability is not as clear-cut as clinicians had previously believed. Degrees and gradations of intellectual disability exist that in their mildest forms include difficulty learning at school and, at times, well-defined learning disabilities.

For this reason, as with motor manifestations, clinicians should appreciate the fact that if the child does not have a clearly defined intellectual disability, then subtle but significant expressions of difficulty with learning and complex intellectual challenges can manifest later in childhood when the demands of school become more complex. Anticipation of potential difficulties is not necessarily a burden to be placed on parents but should definitely be in the mind of the clinician (Hack et al., 2000).

Behavior and Social For many years, adverse outcomes of prematurity were thought to only be either motor or cognitive, but over time, clinicians have come to appreciate that children who were born prematurely and have had stressful neonatal courses also develop behavioral problems that most commonly have been identified in the attention-deficit/hyperactivity disorder (ADHD) spectrum (see Chapter 23.2). These manifestations are common and now constitute one of the features noted in long-term follow-up studies. Clinicians should be aware of the possibility of behavior problems, particularly ADHD, in growing infants and children who were born prematurely because of the complex emotional factors involved in the picture. The parents' stress about the premature infant; the many medical, developmental, social and emotional aspects surrounding the birth; the experience in the NICU; the eventual discharge home and the challenges of taking care of the fragile infant; and the infant's ongoing medical, neurodevelopmental, and social concerns all play a part in the psychodynamics of behavior and interaction.

Clinicians, however, need to be aware that apart from all the practical and emotional challenges described, children can have underlying neurological disturbances of perinatal origin in the expression of ADHD. What has not yet been described, but in due course is likely to become a real issue, is the expression of the neurobehavioral syndrome in the autism spectrum disorders (see Chapter 23.1). As clinicians look more closely and critically at the patterns of behavior of many growing and developing infants who were born prematurely, particularly those who were extremely premature, they will undoubtedly see more children who fit into this later category (Hack et al., 2000).

Combinations of Disabilities Neurodevelopmental consequences of prematurity relate to the vulnerability of the immature brain. In reality, the lesions are rarely as neat and focal as to have only one clearly defined manifestation but are more commonly manifested in a combination of degrees of motor, cognitive, and behavioral features, not to mention the complicating sensory impairments noted previously. In each child, these conditions express themselves to varying degrees and in varying patterns.

The important point to keep in mind is that all premature infants are at risk for central nervous system insults, and the expression should be viewed in functional terms that include all three major modalities—motor, cognitive/intellectual, and behavioral/social. Clinicians need to understand the growing and developing infant in these terms and to make sure that the child has appropriate attention to the obvious features. In addition, clinincians must be aware of the potential for more subtle—but nonetheless real and significant—features that can have serious impact on the child's performance and success in life. Consider Omar's situation, presented next.

Omar was born at 26 weeks, weighing 2 lb, 5 oz. He spent 2 months in the NICU on a ventilator, 3 months in the NICU without a ventilator, and 2 months in a step-down unit. He went home on oxygen.

Omar's neonatal course was complicated by multiple problems associated with extreme prematurity including respiratory distress, the need for assisted ventilation, complication of pneumothorax, patent ductus arteriosis that needed ligation, hyperbilirubinemia, retinopathy of prematurity, anemia, feeding problems, gastroesophageal reflux, bilateral inguinal hernia requiring surgical repair, and difficulty feeding that required a nasogastric tube and subsequently a G tube. At discharge, Omar's parents felt that he might not be ready to come home yet. Within 3 months, he needed to go back to the hospital due to a respiratory problem.

Omar's development was delayed in all areas. He sat at 1 year and walked at 2 years. His motor performance was notable for limping at times, and he also had poor handwriting. His parents reported that his coordination and difficulty walking resulted in his falling frequently, and he had even broken some teeth during falls.

Now 13 years old, Omar attends middle school in a self-contained classroom. He has difficulty with attention and focus and is not performing up to his IQ score of 75. When he is at home, he can be quite calm while playing with something that interests him; however, when he is in strange places, he tends to be very active and explorative. Omar does not understand personal space and often oversteps boundaries. He often annoys his peers and has pushed and hit children in the past.

Omar is easily frustrated and impatient. If there are any changes in his routine, he often has a "meltdown." His tantrums are less frequent than they used to be; however, when Omar becomes excited or distressed, he bites his finger or bangs his head on the television. He also is anxious about rain and storms and talks about them often.

Omar is dependent for bathing but can undress and dress himself except for buttons and shoelaces. He is not yet toilet trained and insists on having bowel movements in pull-up training pants. Omar has had a G tube all of his life. He is now eating more by himself, although his parents are still giving him medication through the tube. He is also drinking better.

When Omar was very young, he threw up a lot and was treated on Pepcid for reflux. At present, he does not have any features of reflux. Reportedly, he does occasionally have a problem with constipation, which is probably related to holding his stool.

Omar's vision is reasonable even though he experienced retinopathy of prematurity. His hearing is also normal, and he likes music and singing. Omar's parents enjoy his excellent singing voice.

On Omar's last visit to his pediatrician, he went directly into the doctor's office despite the fact that there was another patient in there. A little baby was in the office, and Omar was fascinated with the baby. He tried to play with the baby and tried to give her a toy, which he inadvertently tossed to her, not realizing that it could be harmful.

While the pediatrician talked to Omar's parents, Omar wandered about, came to speak to the doctor, dropped a toy into the doctor's lap, found a paper airplane, and tossed it around. After a while, he settled down and went to the corner and flipped through pages of a book. The doctor noted that Omar was relatively cooperative for the physical examination; however, he was quite distractible and needed to be redirected. The doctor concluded that Omar had residual neurodevelopmental features of mild intellectual disability, perhaps some learning disabilities, some motor coordination difficulties, behavioral features suggestive of ADHD, and social interactions suggestive of the autism spectrum disorder. The Childhood Autism Rating Scale (Schopler, Reichler, & Renner, 1988) score was 34.5, indicating that Omar could be diagnosed as having mild-moderate autism.

LONG-TERM OUTLOOK FOR PREMATURE INFANTS AND THEIR FAMILIES

Infant Follow-Up Programs

Most neonatal units have formal infant follow-up programs that intermittently check on infants' medical conditions and developmental progress as well as families' coping patterns. In addition, these follow-up clinics not only provide critical feedback to the neonatal units about how infants are doing, but also collectively provide data to guide clinical practice toward improving outcome.

Pediatricians and Specialty Providers

Most often families remain connected to their child's pediatrician and have a set of specialty visits with pulmonologists, ophthalmologists, neurologists, and other specialties as needed in addition to regular therapy visits in the home or in early intervention programs. Regular monitoring of various health-related problems such as reactive airway disease, including the need for RSV prophylaxis, and routine follow-up with an ophthalmologist is important as children may commonly experience refractory errors or ophthalmoplegias.

Developmental Progress and Early Intervention

Given the likelihood of neurodevelopmental disorders, infants must receive appropriate early intervention services. These services may be offered by infant follow-up programs, by the hospitals in which the NICUs and follow-up clinics are situated, or by community resources. All states are mandated to provide early intervention services to infants from birth to 3 years of age, and most of these services are provided in the family home.

The primary care pediatrician must be sure that the infant is receiving appropriate therapeutic services, as these services not only help with the infant's development but also provide the parents, particularly the mothers, with a set of elements that are extremely helpful. The parent is reassured that the infant is receiving necessary and appropriate therapies to assist in making good developmental progress. The mother also has a professional who will come into the home and is available to answer questions, provide information, and most importantly provide some support and reassurance. All these factors are especially important in the infant's early months. Early intervention can never be too early—unless the mother is not ready and is overwhelmed, in which case there needs to be more family support—and early intervention should never be ignored until it is too late.

Coordination of Care and Family Support

More than anything else, families who are under stress in caring for their infant, who have frequent visits to physicians' or therapists' offices, and who need to continue to hold their families' lives together must have someone who will help them to coordinate their infant's medical care and deal with the added stresses. Here, social workers or visiting nurses can be helpful, and parent support groups may be an emotional salvation to parents who unquestionably feel alone in their struggles. Groups for parents of multiple births are particularly active. It seems that the more the stress, the more the need for social support, and the more motivated the family is to become part of such a group.

Socioeconomic Status

The situation of socioeconomic status deserves special mention. Infant follow-up programs and studies of all sizes and from all places find a common thread in the long-term outcome of small premature infants. Not only are mothers of lower socioeconomic status more likely to have premature infants (see Table 10.3), but, controlling for physiological and pathological factors, infants born to mothers from social and economic circumstances that were less than optimal did less well than infants who came from families with good education, income, and social networks. The concept of *Social Capital,* as promoted by the American Academy of Pediatrics (2002, 2004) in their Medical Home Program, illustrates this situation very well. Even in the early days of NICUs caring for small premature infants, the follow-up data began to suggest that infants growing up in homes in which the mother's education, the father's employment, and the number of books in the home were better had more favorable outcomes.

Of interest, too, in this context is the finding that although mothers of extremely low birth weight infants worry more about their infants than mothers of infants born at term (which is understandable), mothers of higher socioeconomic status tended to worry more about their infants than mothers of lower socioeconomic status (Taylor et al., 2001). Although this statistic could be looked at in terms of emotional health and well-being, with acceptance being more of a characteristic of mothers of lower socioeconomic status, the mothers of lower socioeconomic status may have had more pressing day-to-day concerns and may have been satisfied that their infants had survived the newborn period and were in stable health. The mothers of higher socioeconomic status may have been concerned about whether they were doing their best for their infants and were getting the best services to make sure that their infants would grow up to be socially and economically successful. Although the findings and their interpretation are complex, they do help pediatricians, specialty providers, and therapists to be alert and make sure that each infant receives the best services necessary for optimal growth and development (Wood, 2003).

Cycle of Disadvantage and Disability The most challenging issues in dealing with prematurity, its causes, and its consequences are the sum of factors that are as-

Table 10.3. Pregnancy and birth outcomes

Indicator	Children who are impoverished	Children who are not impoverished	Ratio of impoverished to not impoverished
Low birth weight rate (< 2,500 g)	10/1,000 births	6/1,000 births	1.7
Infant mortality	14/1,000 births	8/1,000 births	1.7
Percent of adolescent girls who have newborns out of wedlock	11.0%	3.6%	2.1

Reproduced with permission from *Pediatrics*, Vol. 112[3], Page 710, Copyright © 2003 by the AAP.

sociated with circumstances of social and economic disadvantage. The causes of prematurity, such as young age, smoking, alcohol and other drugs, and risk for intrauterine infections are highly correlated with lower socioeconomic status and adverse social and environmental factors. Likewise, the long-term outcome of prematurity is associated with elements that prevail in families of lower socioeconomic status living in more stressed environments.

This case is particularly true for infants born to mothers who smoked and drank alcohol during pregnancy. The infants are likely to not only be premature but also to have consequences of intrauterine exposure to alcohol, a neurotoxin. The infants are likely to be more irritable (in association with the possibility of withdrawal symptoms as well as the neurobehavioral disregulation), which adds to the mothers' stress. In trying to cope with the stress, mothers may resort to drugs or alcohol, lose control, and inflict serious physical harm on the infants.

The abuse not only then can take its toll on the central nervous system from head injury or shaken baby syndrome, but also in the emotional consequences of

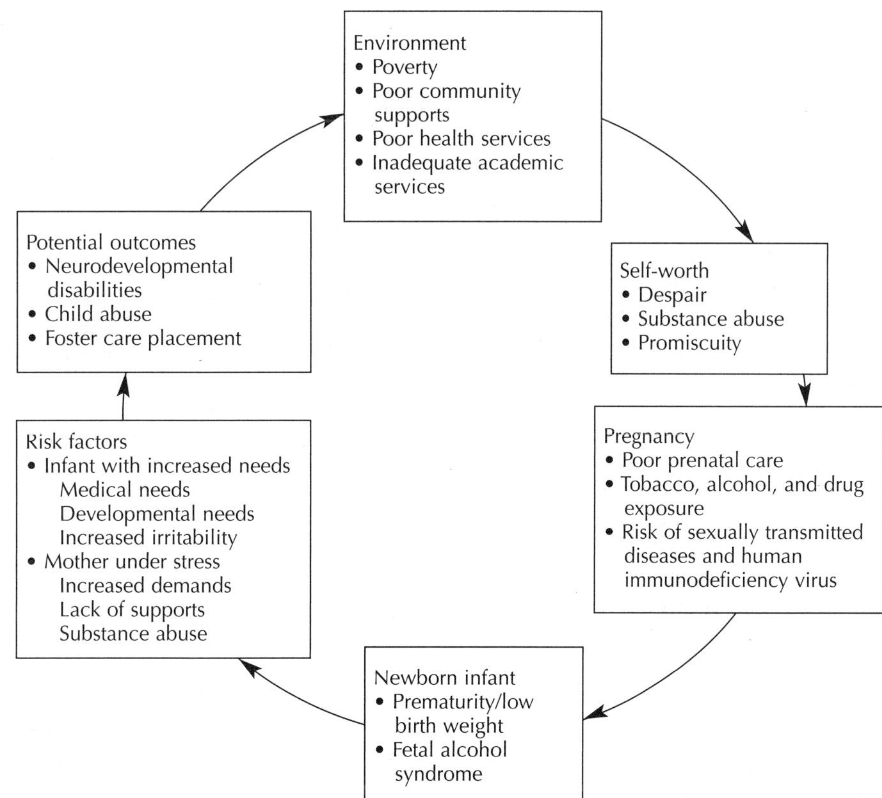

Figure 10.6. Cycle of disadvantage and disability. (From Rubin, I.L. [1990]. Etiology of developmental disabilities. *Infants and Young Children, 18,* 653–660; adapted by permission.)

neglect and abuse and the likelihood that the infant will be removed from the mother by the Department of Social Services (see Chapter 34). Infants and children who grow up in these circumstances are likely to have limited emotional and social stability, limited education, and limited social and vocational opportunities. Therefore, they are more likely to engage in substance abuse and gratification through casual and promiscuous sexual activities, resulting in an increased likelihood of sexually transmitted diseases and pregnancies that subject the fetus to an intrauterine environment that is hazardous to its embryonic and fetal health and development. The cycle then is repeated (see Figure 10.6).

For this group of infants and mothers, identifying risks as early as possible, providing strong early intervention programs, and offering programs that provide the mothers with rehabilitation and educational opportunities are critical. Because mothers who have had premature infants are likely to become pregnant again and are more likely to have additional premature infants, they need support on delaying further pregnancies. Mothers need to feel more secure in their role as parents and to appreciate the importance of caring for their infants. They need to know that someone cares about them and is encouraging their success.

CONCLUSION

Infants with extremely low birth weight who have been supported and sustained during their vulnerable neonatal periods by advances in knowledge and technology are more likely to have more complicated medical and neurodevelopmental consequences. Advances in the care of growing premature infants and of children with developmental disabilities have provided the necessary public and private medical, therapeutic, and educational services to promote optimal growth and development for these infants and their families. As a society, however, we need to be aware of the social, economic, and cultural circumstances that have created a cycle of disadvantage and disability. We need to break this cycle, not only to improve the outcomes of premature infants but also to reduce and prevent pregnancies that will unnecessarily result in premature infants.

REFERENCES

American Academy of Pediatrics. (2002, July). AAP policy statement: The medical home. *Pediatrics, 110*(1), 184–186.

American Academy of Pediatrics. (2004). *Social capital pre-conference sessions and faculty.* Retrieved from http://www.aap.org/catch/nationalconfSOCCAP.html

Dusick, A.M., Poindexter, B.B., Ehrenkranz, R.A., & Lemons, J.A. (2003). Growth failure in the preterm infant: Can we catch up? *Seminars in Perinatology, 27,* 302–310.

Ehrenkranz, R.A., & Wright, L.L. (2003, August). Highlights from the HICHD Neonatal Research Network. *Seminars in Perinatology, 27*(4), 302–310.

Feldman, R., & Eidelman, A. (2005). Does a triplet birth pose a special risk for infant development? Assessing cognitive development in relation to intrauterine growth and mother-infant interaction across the first 2 years. *Pediatrics, 115,* 443–452.

Hack, M., Taylor, H.G., Klein, N., & Mercuri-Minich, N. (2000). Functional limitations and special health care needs of 10- to 14-year-old children weighing less than 750 grams at birth. *Pediatrics, 106,* 554–560.

Hintz, S.R., Kendrick, D.E., Stoll, B.J., Vohr, B.R., Fanaroff, A., Donovan, KE.F., et al. (2005). Changes in neurodevelopmental outcomes at 18 to 22 months' corrected age among infants of less than 25 weeks' gestational age born in 1993–1999. *Pediatrics, 115*(6), 696–703.

Kennell, H., & Klaus, M.H. (1998, January). Bonding: Recent observations that alter perinatal care. *Pediatrics in Review, 19*(1), 4–12.

Koh, T., Harrison, H., & Morley, C. (1999, September 16). Gestation versus outcome table for parents of extremely premature infants. *Journal of Perinatology, 19,* 452–453.

Little, W.J. (1861). On the influence of abnormal parturition, difficult labor, premature birth and asphyxia neonatorum on mental and physical conditions of the child, especially in relation to deformities. *Transactions of the Obstetrical Society of London, 3,* 293–344.

Neufeld, M., Frigon, C., Graham, A.S., & Mueller, B. (2005). Maternal infection and risk of cerebral palsy in term and preterm infants. *Journal of Perinatology, 25,* 108–113.

Oh, W., Tyson, J.E., Fanaroff, A., Vohr, B., Perritt, R., Stoll, B.J., Ehrenkranz, R., Carlo, W.A., Shankaran, S., Poole, K., & Wright, L. (2003). Association between peak serum bilirubin and neurodevelopmental outcomes in extremely low birth weight infants. *Pediatrics, 112,* 773–779.

Rubin, I.L. (1990). Etiology of developmental disabilities. *Infants and Young Children, 18,* 653–660.

Rubin, I.L. (1992). Diagnosis and disabilities. *Journal of Intellectual Disability Research, 36,* 1–8.

Schopler, E., Reichler, R., & Renner, B.R. (1988). *The Childhood Autism Rating Scale (CARS).* Los Angeles: Western Psychological Services.

Stoll, B.J., et al. (2004). Neurodevelopmental and growth impairment among extremely low-birth weight infants with neonatal infection. *Journal of the American Medical Association, 292*(19), 2357–2365.

Taylor, H.G., Klein, N., Minich, N.M., & Hack, M. (2001). Long-term family outcomes for children with very low birth weights. *Archives of Pediatric and Adolescent Medicine, 155,* 155–161.

Volpe, J.J. (2001). *Neurology of the newborn* (4th ed.). New York: W.B. Saunders.

Wilson-Costello, D., Friedman, H., Minich, N., Fanaroff, A., & Hack, M. (2005). Improved survival with increased neurodevelopmental disability for extremely low birth weight infants in the 1990s. *Pediatrics, 115*(4), 997–1003.

Wood, D. (2003, September). Effect of child and family poverty on child health in the United States. *Pediatrics, 112*(3), 707–711.

CHAPTER 11

CEREBRAL PALSY

Sarah Winter and Michele Kiely

Stephen, a 12-month-old boy, is the first-born child of proud parents. His father notices his strong right-handed throw and dreams of watching his son's baseball games in the future. His mother notices that he always chooses to use his right hand, which she feels makes sense, as both of them are right handed. Stephen likes to keep his left hand out of the way by holding it up close to his body. His mother is pleased with his easy-going temperament and has often smiled at his determined nature. Her friends notice his unique way of crawling that she has always thought was cute. Stephen's mother and father have grown increasingly concerned that he has made few attempts at bearing weight on his legs when their friends' children have started to cruise along furniture and let go to take a few steps. Both parents decide to attend Stephen's next appointment with his pediatrician to ask about Stephen's developmental progress.

Melody is a 5-year-old girl who lights up any room she enters. Her mother has worked tirelessly with Melody and her therapists and teachers to achieve the goals she has accomplished thus far. Melody's mother puts no limitations on her daughter's future despite her diagnosis of cerebral palsy (CP). Her mother is thankful to have her daughter with her after she was born 3 months early. After 3 months in the neonatal intensive care unit, Melody arrived home on her anticipated birth date with a long list of medical problems, including bleeding into the brain, apnea, feeding problems, sepsis, jaundice, retinopathy of prematurity, seizures, and failure to thrive. Now, Melody is a small but strong girl who eats more than most children her age. She is doing very well in kindergarten, and everyone loves her. Melody gets around using ankle–foot braces and a walker.

At a parent–teacher conference, Melody's teacher shares two concerns. Melody falls more often, probably because her leg muscles are so tight that her braces hit each other and trip her. The teacher also feels that Melody has a winning way with adults and other children and will often get them to do things for her, including schoolwork. Melody's mother has worried about these things as well and is talking to Melody's therapists about how to address these concerns. She wishes she had more support. Melody's father left shortly after Melody's birth, and few relatives live nearby.

Sean is a happy 10-year-old boy who loves music and computer games. He has lived with his grandparents since his mother's death when he was 2. His grandparents are strong and capable people who realize that Sean comprehends things on a 4-year-old level. They have spent a great deal of time and money trying to find ways for Sean to communicate. Sean enjoys life most of the time despite muscles that are very tight, often writhing without control, occasional vomiting, difficulty growing, two recent episodes of pneumonia, and constipation.

His grandparents are extremely proud of his accomplishments. They remember that his physicians could not tell them what his future would be like given his very abnormal brain magnetic resonance imaging (MRI). They understood that Sean's brain was not injured but rather was always that way. Sean is now using a touch talker to answer simple questions, is sitting for brief periods of time independently, can help someone move him from his wheelchair, and is starting to drive a power chair. Some days his muscles are so tight that he cannot find the right level of control with the chair. He also gets frustrated and embarrassed by his drooling. His grandparents have faced more difficult things in the past. They feel that these problems can be solved as well.

CP is often described as a group of nonprogressive but often changing motor impairment syndromes secondary to lesions or anomalies of the brain arising at any time during brain development (Mutch, Alberman, Hagberg, Kodoma, & Perat, 1992). The description includes motor impairment syndromes, not simply spasticity. The tone abnormalities of CP can range from spasticity to hypotonicity. In addition, tone can be mixed and can vary in one child throughout the day. CP is nonprogressive. In fact, many children improve functionally over time, consistent with the nature of child development. CP is a also disorder of the brain and not of the musculoskeletal system. For example, the problem with Stephen's left hand and leg originates from the right side of his brain, not from his muscles. Understanding that CP is a neurodevelopmental disability with its primary impact on the motor system will assist families in understanding the impact of CP on the child's full functional abilities.

Little (1861) described CP as a condition that results from anoxia during labor and delivery. Decades of epidemiologic research refuting that conclusion have not changed the perception that CP is caused by a bad labor and delivery experience with anoxic damage to the brain. Although hypoxic ischemic encephalopathy does occur, it is only occasionally the cause of CP (Nelson & Grether, 1999).

Like the majority of developmental disabilities, a cure for CP is not available. The damage cannot be undone, and surgery cannot create new neuronal tissue. Nevertheless, medical professionals do provide assistance to individuals with CP and their families through diagnosis, management, and interventions that serve to minimize impairment and prevent secondary disabilities. Although preventing CP from ever happening in the first place would be ideal, the majority of research and clinical activities support maximizing each individual's potential to live life to its fullest.

EPIDEMIOLOGY

Long-term population-based data from Sweden and Australia show that the prevalence of CP has remained between 1.5 and 2.5 per 1,000 live births since the 1960s (Hagberg, Hagberg, Beckung, & Uvebrant, 2001; Hagberg, Hagberg, & Olow, 1975, 1993; Stanley, Blair, & Alberman, 2000), which is consistent with U.S. population-based studies (Boyle, Yeargin-Allsopp, Doernberg, Holmgreen, & Murphy, 1996). Knowing the prevalence of CP aids in the planning of appropriate and sufficient services. If there is an increase in the prevalence of the disorder, then more attention should be given to the development of services for individuals with CP. In addition, an analysis of trends over time may contribute to understanding of the causes of brain impairment, thereby increasing CP prevention.

Neonatal intensive care may lead to a decrease in the prevalence of neurological disabilities among premature, low birth weight infants; however, intensive care among infants with intrauterine growth retardation and increased survival in very preterm infants may actually cause the prevalence of CP to increase (Bhushan, Paneth, & Kiely, 1993; Kiely, Paneth, Stein, & Susser, 1981). Despite these speculations, overall prevalence rates and birth weight specific trends have remained stable over time (O'Shea, Klinepeter, Goldstain, Jackson, & Dillard, 1997; Winter, Autry, Yeargin-Allsopp, & Boyle, 2002). Likewise, the expected decrease in CP as a result of Caesarean section and fetal monitoring has not happened (Blair & Stanley, 1997). Given this stable trend in CP prevalence rates, the diagnosis and management of the concerns related to CP are skills that will be necessary for a long time.

CLASSIFICATION OF CEREBRAL PALSY

The classification system for CP serves to highlight the consistent differences in the variety of types of CP and associated conditions and to point out some similarities in etiology. CP is most often congenital, meaning that the cause is presumed as prenatal or perinatal (i.e., the time period beginning at the initiation of labor and ending at 30 days postdelivery). CP is less often acquired, such as through postnatal infection, trauma, and shaken baby syndrome.

CP is sometimes classified by degree of severity, such as mild, moderate, and severe; however, the assignation of this terminology is subjective, and this schema is not universally accepted. More often, CP is described by the terms *extrapyramidal* and *pyramidal*, or more commonly *spastic* CP. Within the spastic types, CP is described by topographical location of the body. The types of CP and frequency of distribution are outlined in Table 11.1.

Extrapyramidal versus Spastic Cerebral Palsy

Extrapyramidal versus *spastic* CP refers to the location of the abnormality or damage to the brain. Movement is initiated and regulated by the motor control system of the brain, including the pyramidal system, which carries the signal for muscle contraction, and the extrapyramidal system, which provides regulatory influences on that contraction.

Extrapyramidal Cerebral Palsy *Extrapyramidal CP* is a term used to describe movement patterns that are caused by damage to areas of the brain outside of the pyramidal tracts. It is often further divided into *dyskinetic* and *ataxic* types. Dyskinetic movement disorders include athetosis, chorea, dystonia, and hypotonicity. Many people with these disorders have more than one type. For example, individuals with choreoathetoid CP have the brief, jerking, purposeless movements of chorea and the long axial writhing movements of athetosis.

Table 11.1. Cerebral palsy by type and frequency of distribution

Types of cerebral palsy (CP)	Frequency of distribution
Nonspastic (extrapyramidal and mixed types)	23%
Spastic CP total	77%
Spastic diplegia	21%
Spastic hemiplegia	21%
Spastic quadriplegia	23%

Note: Data for 1986–1991 birth cohort MADDSP (Winter et al., 2002). Average of three birth weight cohorts rounded to nearest whole number.

Dystonic CP is characterized by involuntary sustained muscle contractions of agonist and antagonist muscles that cause twisting and abnormal postures. It can be present with wide fluctuations in tone. Many individuals with CP have both spasticity and dystonia. Identifying both movement disorders is essential when planning for interventions.

Hypotonic CP involves low resting muscle tone generalized throughout the body. It impairs function, is nonprogressive, is a result of damage to the developing brain, and is not known to be due to other causes. When this low muscle tone accompanies a condition such as Down syndrome or Prader-Willi syndrome, the term *hypotonic CP* is not added to the diagnosis. In these cases, hypotonia is understood to be a part of the underlying primary condition.

Ataxic CP results when damage occurs in the cerebellum. Ataxia is characterized by difficulties performing finely controlled movements and results in overshooting when reaching for objects and a wide-based unsteady gait.

Spastic Cerebral Palsy Approximately 75% of CP cases are primarily spastic CP. *Spasticity* is a movement disorder characterized by velocity-dependent increase in resistance to passive muscle stretch. Spasticity results when damage to the pyramidal tract occurs anywhere along its path. Attempts to localize the spasticity and describe spastic CP in terms of where it is expressed on the body, help to understand, in general, the etiology, the functional impairment, the associated conditions, and potential treatments for children with spastic CP. In practice, it is often difficult to differentiate some of the subtypes.

Diplegic CP describes spasticity in the lower extremities (e.g., Melody's condition). Older literature or literature from the British Isles may refer to this as paraplegia. Confusion sometimes occurs with using this term to describe the problems related to CP versus paraplegia secondary to a spinal cord injury. Although diplegic CP describes spasticity that occurs in the lower extremities, an individual with diplegic CP will often experience coordination difficulties of the upper extremities or even spasticity of the upper extremities even though the predominant impairment is in the lower extremities.

Hemiplegic CP occurs when the spasticity is on one side of the body (e.g., Stephen's condition). Typically, the arm is more affected than the leg and will assume a triple flexion posture, the classic position of the involved upper extremity with flexion of the wrist and elbow and adduction of the shoulder. *Quadriplegic CP* involves all four extremities. Generally, the legs are more involved than the arms. Individuals with quadriplegic CP frequently present with truncal hypotonia and hypertonicity of all four extremities. Rarely, a child may experience more spasticity in the upper extremities than the legs (i.e., double hemiplegia). *Monoplegic CP* is a term used to describe spasticity found in only one extremity. Practically, this situation may be the result of a hemiplegia in which the impairment of the leg is imperceptible, resulting in only functional impairment of the arm. *Triplegic CP* may also occur with involvement of both lower extremities and one upper extremity. This pattern may represent an injury causing a hemiplegic pattern in addition to an injury causing a diplegic pattern.

As with any classification system, extrapyramidal versus spastic CP does not completely describe what is seen in practice. Many individuals with CP (e.g., Sean) have a combination of the previously described movement abnormalities, which are referred to as mixed pattern CP. Because epidemiologic studies often use a primary diagnosis for classification, mixed pattern CP is likely underreported. As children grow and develop, their pattern of CP may change. An obvious spastic hemiplegia in a 2-year-old may appear to be monoplegia by the time the child reaches age 5. A spastic quadriplegic pattern may appear to be more consistent with spastic diplegia one day and spastic quadriplegia on another day, depending on the child's energy and state of health or level of anxiety during the examination.

DIAGNOSING CEREBRAL PALSY

Diagnosis presents a challenge to the many medical professionals involved in the care of children with CP. Many types of physicians are called on to make this diagnosis, including primary pediatricians, family practitioners, developmental pediatricians, pediatric neurologists, rehabilitation specialists, pediatric orthopedists, and geneticists. Diagnosing and imparting the diagnosis requires an understanding of the risk factors for CP, experience with neurologic examinations, use of the proper imaging studies, and delivering the news to the family and child in a compassionate, realistic, but hopeful manner. Physicians should keep in mind the good experiences the child may have in his or her lifetime (see Figure 11.1).

Understanding of the Risk Factors for Cerebral Palsy

In reviewing the history of an individual with CP, it is helpful to gather information about factors that are related to CP as an outcome. Oftentimes, it is easiest to consider these risk factors in three broad categories:

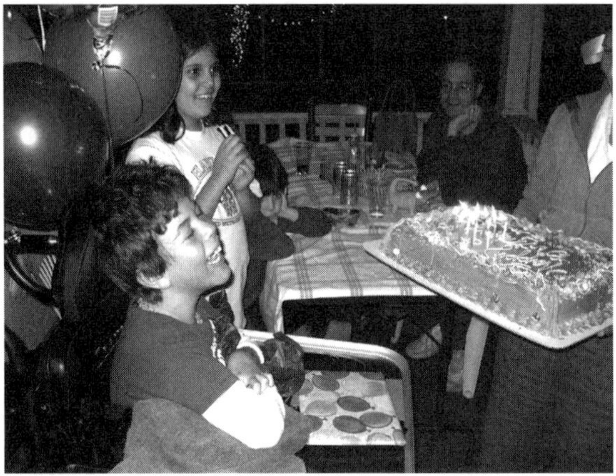

Figure 11.1. Liam shares a birthday celebration with family and friends.

prenatal, perinatal, and postnatal risk factors. The *prenatal period* includes that time prior to the onset of labor.

Many risk factors are interrelated. Infants born with intrauterine growth retardation are at risk for a variety of developmental disabilities including CP. The growth retardation may be a result of an injury or developmental abnormality of the brain or may be the result of a genetic defect. Recently, more genetic disorders are being identified as a cause for CP. Congenital malformations of the brain can be idiopathic, as is likely true in Sean's case, but a few of these disorders have been found to have specific chromosomal abnormalities. One exception is the deletion in the short arm of chromosome 17 in the Miller-Dieker form of lissencephaly (Dobyns et al., 1996). Ataxic CP represents a small percentage of these cases, but this type of CP is more likely to have a genetically determined origin. Children with ataxia are also more likely to have a slowly progressive neurologic disorder that is mistaken for CP.

Vascular events, such as stroke or hemorrhage, occur in the *prenatal* period. Sometimes the reasons for such events are known (e.g., maternal anticoagulation therapy resulting in fetal central nervous system hemorrhage; Factor V Leiden mutation that causes resistance to activated protein C and fetal stroke) (Thorarensen et al., 1997). Most often, evidence for the stroke is found on head imaging studies without a clear reason for the occurrence. The presence of calcifications on a head computerized tomography (CT) may point toward cytomegalovirus or toxoplasmosis. Other congenital infections may be diagnosed if laboratory testing is done at the appropriate time.

Because *perinatal* factors are related to CP, thorough investigation into the circumstances of the child's birth is important. The neonatal discharge record should be scanned for information on birth weight and gestational age, Apgar scores, head ultrasound results, and presence of neonatal seizures. Prematurity is a significant risk factor for CP. Because birth weight is more accurately determined, registries following the trends in CP have historically used birth weight as a proxy for gestational age. The risk of CP increases with decreasing birth weight (Stanley et al., 2000). Nevertheless, in one study of children born at extremely low birth weight < 1,000 g) only 17%, showed signs of CP at age 18 months (Vohr et al., 2000). Results of head ultrasound studies done in the neonatal period may offer additional information about the risk of CP. The presence of a grade III or IV intraventricular hemorrhage is often correlated with CP (Msall et al., 1994; Vohr et al., 1999).

Although the prevalence of neonatal asphyxia is low, it is devastating when it occurs. Sometimes the cause of the asphyxia is known such as prolonged hypoxia in the event of a placenta abruptio. In other cases, its onset is less defined, but the infant is clearly affected as evidenced by severely depressed Apgar scores. Neonatal seizures within the first 24 hours of life are correlated with poor developmental outcomes (McBride, Laroia, & Guillet, 2000). All of this information can usually be found by a brief review of the neonatal discharge summary.

Postnatal causes for CP tend to be more obvious and dramatic. Shaken baby syndrome or accidental trauma may result in significant motor impairment. The postnatal infections meningitis and encephalitis may result in CP. CP can also occur with central nervous system insults associated with sickle cell anemia, hypercoaguable states such as systemic lupus, or an intraoperative complication. Relatively small numbers of children have CP as a result of postnatal events (Murphy, Yeargin-Allsopp, Decoufle, & Drews, 1993).

Experience with Neurologic Examinations

Making the diagnosis of CP requires knowledge of the pediatric neurologic exam and its developmental progression. The diagnosis of CP consists of specific neurologic exam findings present in the developing child and a history that confirms the motor delay and/or deviance is not deteriorating. The neurologic findings include the following: 1) abnormality of muscular tone, 2) abnormalities of posture/movement, and 3) persistence of primitive reflexes. Findings consistent with central nervous system injury on head imaging studies are supportive but not necessary to the diagnosis of CP.

Motor delay in a child is most notable when a child fails to accomplish gross motor milestones. Normal gross and fine motor milestones are listed in Table 11.2. Walking is the most recognized developmental milestone and occurs in most children at 12 months, with the upper limit of normal being at 16 months. Crawling is not particularly helpful or uniform as many children will bypass crawling altogether.

Fine motor milestones receive less attention by both parents and medical personnel but can signal the presence of CP. Hand preference should not occur prior to 18 months. As in Stephen's case, hand preference at 6–12 months is often misinterpreted by parents as early hand preference rather than an abnormality of neurologic function in the nondominant hand. This condition is a frequent presentation of hemiplegic CP and should prompt a neurologic evaluation. The presence of persistent head lag, poor sitting balance, inability to bear weight on the legs, and the inability to walk by the appropriate time are other common triggers for an evaluation.

Assessing muscular tone in a child is a skill that requires experience and exposure to children and adults with abnormal tone. *Spasticity*, present in approximately 75% of children with CP, is described as the clasp knife response or as velocity-dependent increased resistance to passive muscle stretch. When severe, it is an obvious finding that is often accompanied by increased deep tendon reflexes. Spasticity can be worse when a child is anxious or ill. *Hypotonia* is low resting muscle tone and can also be present to a greater or lessor degree. It can often be elicited in the smaller child by noticing slip through on vertical suspension. Deep tendon reflexes are either decreased or increased with hypotonia. Muscular tone can change as a child develops, as commonly seen in infants with hypotonia who evolve to have spasticity by 12–18 months of age. This change is not due to a progression in the neuronal injury or abnormality but rather a maturation of the central nervous system.

Table 11.2. Motor milestones in normal child development

Milestone	Age
Gross motor	
Lifting head off table	1 month
Lifting chest up	2 months
Rolling	3–5 months
Sitting without support	7 months
Cruising	9–10 months
Walking alone	12 months
Jumping in place	24 months
Pedaling a tricycle	30 months
Fine motor	
Retaining a rattle	1 month
Holding hands unfisted	3–4 months
Transfering objects	5 months
Using immature pincer grasp	7–8 months
Releasing	12 months
Demonstrating hand preference	18 months

The diagnosis of CP also includes the presence of abnormalities of movement and posture. Observing movements and postural control is not typically noted in a neurologic exam. A neurodevelopmental exam of the gross and fine motor systems must be added, and abnormal movements should be noted. The "unique" way that Stephen crawls is likely to be him dragging his left side. Unless specific attention is paid to how this 12 month-old moves, this condition will be missed on the typical neurologic exam.

Movements to look for include athetotic movements, which are involuntary slow writhing of the wrist, fingers, and face, as experienced by Sean. These nonpurposeful movements get in the way of what Sean wants to do—drive his powered chair. In addition, chorea (dance-like movement) involves brief, jerking movements of the head, neck, arms, and legs. Ataxic movements include an unsteady-wide based gait and poor control of fine motor movements in the upper extremities. Finally, abnormal postural control is often present in children with CP.

In the infant exam, physicians should assess the infant's quality of head control, rolling, sitting balance, crawling, cruising, and walking. This exam will pick up on abnormalities even if the motor developmental milestones are intact. For example, a child may be perfectly capable of walking independently at 16 months of age, but he or she may walk toe to toe because of gastrocnemius spasticity. Attention to the fine motor exam through the evaluation of a child's grasp will pick up on the persistence of fisting or the presence of ataxic hand movements long before delays in walking are noticed. It is likely that, despite Melody's diagnosis of spastic diplegic CP, she has coordination difficulties with her hands that are more subtle than the findings in her legs.

Knowledge of the primitive reflex patterns is essential to the diagnosis of CP. Newborns have a repertoire of primitive reflexes that are normal and diminish over a period of approximately 6 months. A description of these reflexes is beyond the scope of this text but can be reviewed in other references (Capute & Accardo, 1996a, 1996b). Functionally, these reflexes must disappear to allow a child to attain normal postural and righting responses that are acquired at approximately 3–9 months. With CP, this normal evolution is disrupted. The persistence of a startle response or Moro reflex prohibits good sitting balance. The presence of a plantar grasp impedes an infant's ability to cruise. These abnormal patterns will be noticed when specific attention is paid to the neurodevelopmental exam.

Taken together, the presence of abnormal tone, movements, and postures and the persistence of primitive reflexes in an infant with motor delays that are nonprogressive constitutes the diagnosis of CP. The age at which CP can be diagnosed can be problematic. A balance must be struck between early and accurate diagnosis. In most cases, an accurate diagnosis can be made by 24 months. In many cases, a diagnosis of CP is clear by 12 months.

Use of the Proper Imaging Studies

As previously mentioned, imaging studies can be supportive to, but are not diagnostic of, CP. Significant changes are occurring in the realm of central nervous system imaging. MRI is the single most useful tool to enhance the history and physical exam in the diagnosis of CP. The majority of children with a major motor delay will have abnormalities on their MRIs (Candy, Hoon, Capute, & Bryan, 1993). In Sean's case, an MRI helped his grandparents to better understand the etiology for his CP. Congenital brain malformation can be identified and sometimes linked to an affected gene such as lissencephaly, as previously mentioned.

Knowledge of the specific brain malformation and possibly genetic substrate leads to more accurate diagnosis and prognosis. Localization of abnormality or damage on the MRI may allow for better prediction of type of CP and prognosis. A unilateral lesion is predictive of hemiplegic CP. The presence of hyperintense signal and atrophy of the putamen and thalamus predict extrapyramidal CP (Hoon et al., 1997).

Head ultrasound has the advantage of being widely available and safe. It is limited to neonates and young infants while the fontanels remain open. In preterm infants, the use of neonatal ultrasound can be very helpful in predicting CP (Hoon, 1995). After infancy, head CT is often the study of choice for any acute process, such as hemorrhage; however, MRI is the recommended study beyond infancy because it is superior in differentiating soft tissue differences (e.g., gray and white matter). Positron emission testing (PET) scans, functional MRI, and diffusion-weighted imaging may add to understanding of CP in the future, but currently they are not used as clinical tools (Chugani, 1993; Hoon & Melhem, 2000; Inder et al., 1999). Magnetic resonance spectroscopy (i.e., the observation of intracellular cerebral metabolites) is being used as an adjunct to the information provided by the MRI.

Delivering the News in a Compassionate, Realistic, But Hopeful Manner

Information of profound, serious impact regarding the health of a child should be presented in a private space without interruption, preferably in the company of both parents and any supportive person requested by the family. Ample time should be allotted so that family members can ask questions about any of the information the physician has presented. The diagnosis should be given in terms that can be understood by the parents, and written information should be given to supplement what is discussed in the clinical setting. A follow-up visit to review this information will reinforce the diagnosis.

"We were in shock and [had] a feeling of helplessness. It was not explained as to what CP really was [and] what we could do or if there was anything that could be done. We went home with helplessness and no hope." H.K., Lakeville, MN

"As a nonmedical person, it didn't really matter to me how it was explained. It was only some time after the injury when I could actually grasp—both emotionally and intellectually—what the doctors were even saying." J.B., Walton, KY

"When the doctors told us the news, I immediately pictured a child in a wheelchair." E.O., Cincinnati, OH

Although the basic principles surrounding the diagnosis of CP hold true, certain factors must be appreciated. Learning the description of CP and its functional implications, causes, and treatment may be secondary in the minds of parents who are also facing their child's diagnosis of profound intellectual disabilities or autism. Hearing that a child has CP and may limp when he or she walks may be hopeful news for a family faced with the possible death of their premature child. Physicians must try to understand how the diagnosis fits in the context of what the parents have experienced up to the moment of diagnosis.

Because CP has vastly different presentations, it is helpful to try to understand what experience parents have with individuals with CP or other disabilities. This action can be helpful when trying to gage the language and terminology that will be most helpful to a parent's understanding.

MULTIDISCIPLINARY INTERVENTIONS

Caring for children and adults with CP is a multimodal, multidisciplinary process that involves many professionals who support the individual with CP and the family's goals for the individual. No one provider or therapist can do it all. As with all developmental disabilities, facilitating the growth and development of people with CP requires an integration of family, medical, educational, therapeutic, and technological support systems.

Although every child and adult presents with a unique set of circumstances, common conditions occur within each type of CP. Broad generalizations about associated conditions can be made to help organize proactive planning regarding assessment of needs and services for individuals with CP. Table 11.3 presents frequently associated conditions occurring with the common subtypes of spastic CP. As a group, these conditions are associated with these types of CP, but in any individual person, all or none of these conditions may exist.

Medical Management

Every individual with CP should have a primary physician and medical home. The complexity of medical care is more easily navigated with the assistance of someone who oversees the medical care. Although this person need not be an expert in CP, an interest in the individual, a willingness to engage in long-term care, access to supportive services, and expertise in general medical health are necessary to provide the optimal medical home.

Growth Children with CP often experience abnormal growth and often struggle to maintain or gain weight. Many factors contribute to the common problem of failure to thrive; however, a solid understanding of the pediatric growth chart from the National Center for Health Statistics (NCHS) is necessary before diagnosing *failure to thrive.* The growth chart has two components: linear measurements and percentiles of weight and height. The reverse side of the chart includes the ponderal index or weight for height percentiles (the newer version includes the Body Mass Index chart; see http://www.cdc.gov/growthcharts/).

Clinical mistakes are often made when physicians assume that a child with CP is underweight and ignore information on height. Obtaining an accurate height may be difficult, especially for individuals with contractures of the hips, knees, and ankles. In such cases, arm span calculations may be used as a proxy for height. Failure to thrive is an appropriate diagnosis when weight is considered and compared with height and is still less than the 5th percentile. Although this method may not be the most accurate measure of nutritional status, the growth chart is readily available to all clinicians, clearly defines the need to consider both height and weight, and has been standardized on a large population (Ogden, et al, 2002). Experts in the field of CP and growth recommend the use of skin fold thickness as a measure of nutritional status because it is a more sensitive measure of failure to thrive (Samson-Fang & Stevenson, 2000).

Most often, the cause of failure to thrive in children with CP is organic. Weight gain is based on a larger number of calories ingested than being expended (see Chapter 14.1). Fortunately, Melody appears to be able to consume a large number of calories and has been healthy. Although small in stature, she is likely growing well. Sean's

Table 11.3. Multidisciplinary teams necessary to help each person with cerebral palsy

Child	Type of cerebral palsy	Etiology (pathophysiology)	Associated conditions (impairments)	Team members needed
Stephen	Spastic hemiplegia	In utero stroke	Spasticity, contractures, fine motor dysfunction, seizure, learning disability, gait disturbance	Nurse, developmental pediatrician, orthopedist, rehabilitation medicine specialist, physical therapist, occupational therapist, social worker, nurse, orthotic specialist
Melody	Spastic diplegia	Complications of prematurity	Spasticity, contractures, fine motor dysfunction, bone deformity, epilepsy, learning disability, gait disturbance	Nurse, developmental pediatrician, orthopedist, rehabilitation medicine specialist, physical therapist, occupational therapist, social worker, orthotic specialist, psychologist, neurologist
Sean	Mixed pattern quadriplegia	Congenital brain malformation	Contracture, bone deformity, intellectual disabilities, epilepsy, oromotor dysfunction, constipation, aspiration, respiratory compromise, poor weight gain, osteoporosis	Nurse, developmental pediatrician, orthopedist, rehabilitation medicine specialist, physical therapist, occupational therapist, social worker, orthotic specialist, neurologist, speech-language pathologist, dietitian, psychologist, pulmonologist

history is significant for possible problems in caloric intake. Children such as Sean have problems with both energy intake and energy expenditure. A child may be in constant motion or use a large amount of energy to move, expending a large number of kilocalories daily. In addition, problems with oromotor function may cause gagging, choking, and/or aspiration of food into the lungs, which prevents the ingestion of adequate calories.

Oftentimes, a combination of multiple factors such as oromotor dysfunction, muscle spasms with pain, poor sleep, constipation, and behavioral refusal all conspire to prevent adequate nutrition and subsequent growth. Addressing all of the factors contributing to poor growth will be more effective than concentrating on one single factor. Ultimately, if conservative measures don't work, a gastrostomy tube may be a necessary intervention on either a temporary or permanent basis. Parents will often express a sense of relief once a gastrostomy tube is placed.

Oromotor Dysfunction Oromotor dysfunction is often present in individuals with spastic quadriplegia and children with extrapyramidal CP. Children with spastic diplegia and hemiplegia rarely have difficulties with oromotor function. Language delay may indicate cognitive delays but may instead be a sign of oromotor dysfunction. In Sean's situation, his language is far more delayed than his cognitive functioning of 4 years. Expressive language delay with relatively higher receptive language skills may indicate significant oromotor dysfunction.

Drooling is another manifestation of poor oromotor control. Drooling may be worsened by poor head and neck control and decreased sensitivity to saliva in the mouth. The presence of a large amount of drooling can be very socially limiting, causing embarrassment to the individual with CP. In addition, excessive saliva will require multiple clothing changes and can damage reading materials and devices carried in the lap or wheelchair tray. It can also result in health problems such as skin breakdown on the face and neck and dehydration.

Multiple interventions are possible for this challenging problem, usually engaging multiple modalities (Blasco & Allaire, 1992). Speech-language therapists and occupational therapists may be able to facilitate oromotor skills and swallowing through feeding therapy as well as oromotor exercises. Behavior intervention to improve awareness of drooling will sometimes help. In addition, medications, such as glycopyrrolate have the advantage of being an effective intervention, but side effects can be prohibitive. Although it decreases the production of saliva, glycopyrrolate can dry the skin and increase constipation. Medications may lose efficacy over time. Surgical treatment is available but not usually considered until after conservative and medical management has failed. It involves ligation of the salivary and/or submandibular ducts or movement of the duct's point of entry into the mouth.

Oromotor dysfunction may result in aspiration of food or saliva into the lungs (see Chapter 15). The symptoms of aspiration may be obvious, such as choking and/or cyanosis with eating. Aspiration may also occur silently, causing no discomfort to the individual at all. In these situations, a child may experience failure to thrive, frequent pneumonia, or recurrent wheezing. Chronic aspiration should be a consideration in individuals with CP who experience oromotor dysfunction with recurrent wheezing.

Investigation of possible aspiration requires visualizing the food bolus pass from the mouth through the swallowing mechanism to the esophagus. This study is often called the video swallow study or oropharyngeal motility study. It is generally done by having the parent feed the child a variety of barium-containing foods in a radiology suite observed by the radiologist and speech-language therapist. Esophagram and upper gastrointestinal contrast study refer to the evaluation of the anatomy and function of the esophagus and stomach, respectively, but do not evaluate swallowing or the possibility of aspiration.

Gastrointestinal Dysmotility For reasons that are not clear, the smooth muscle of the gastrointestinal tract seems to be impaired in some children with CP. For example, Sean has significant difficulties with constipation. Problems with delayed gastric emptying, gastroesophageal reflux, and constipation are frequent in individuals with spastic quadriplegic CP (Del Guidice et al., 1999). These disorders are interrelated and compound one another. A child who has delayed gastric emptying is likely to reflux from the stomach, causing pain and discomfort. Thus, eating becomes more difficult, resulting in decreased intake of food and fluids. This decrease in turn causes constipation that, in turn, causes bloating and distension of the abdomen. Bloating and distension may then contribute to poor gastric emptying. This cycle of impairment is most often seen in children with poor mobility and poor nutritional status. It is rarely seen in children with spastic quadriplegia who are ambulatory or very active.

Interventions for this condition are also multiple. Improving the nutritional status through dietary supplements, feeding therapy, and or gastrostomy tube can break this cycle. Further information on constipation, its causes, and its treatment in children with disabilities can be found in Chapter 14.2.

Spasticity Management Although control of spasticity does not fix the primary pathology of CP that resides in the brain, it may decrease the sequelae of the increased tone. Problems such as musculoskeletal deformity, limitations of movement, and pain may be minimized by the use of interventions to reduce tone. Historically, diazepam and related medications were the only options for management of spasticity. Since the 1980s, selective medications and surgical interventions have become available. How to use these interventions, in what combinations, and at what time in the developmental progression of the individual patient are the questions being actively researched at this time.

At this point it may be helpful to look specifically at the tone-related problems of Stephen, Melody, and Sean.

At 12 months old, Stephen holds his left hand close to his body, which is likely due to spasticity in that extremity. He is not bearing weight on his legs. Perhaps this condition is due in part to weakness, in part to coordination difficulties, and in part to spasticity of the left leg.

Melody has spastic diplegia and is having trouble with scissoring of the lower extremities. For some reason, this condition now seems to be affecting her ability to maintain her balance. She likely has the equinus deformity of both feet (toe-to-toe gait) due to the spasticity in her gastrocnemius muscles.

Sean has an especially challenging combination of tone problems. He has difficulty with spasticity and choreoathetosis. The tightness in his hands makes it difficult for him to drive his wheelchair, which prevents him from getting to where he wants to go. Sean seems to be free of musculoskeletal pain at this time; however, at his age, he is likely to have musculoskeletal deformity such as spine curvature, possible hip dislocation, and contractures.

Treatment options for spasticity include oral medications, injection of medication into the affected muscle, intrathecal medication, and neurosurgical intervention. These interventions work on the level of spasticity. These cases bring out some principles of orthopedic management as well, but consideration of this topic is discussed in Chapter 13 on orthopedic management of individuals with disabilities. Table 11.4 provides possible clinical management plans for Stephen, Melody, and Sean.

Common oral medications used to decrease spasticity include diazepam, baclofen, and dantrolene. Dosing ranges and common side effects are listed in Table 11.5. (*Note:* Because doses change over time, verify doses before administering medication.) Valium is readily available, inexpensive, and has a long history of use. Unfortunately, it acts centrally, and the sedating side effects usually make this drug an undesirable choice for managing the problems of spasticity (Young, Robert, & Delwaide, 1981).

Baclofen acts primarily at the spinal cord level and is postulated to be gamma-aminobutyric inhibitory. In large doses, it may cause central nervous system sedation. Baclofen is used by starting at small doses and titrating to the desired effect over a period of weeks to months, usually ending with a dosing schedule of three times per day (Krach, 2001). Families must be educated that acute withdrawal from the drug may cause serious central nervous system effects such as hallucinations and/or seizures or acute increase in spasticity. Special consideration of how this drug is to be given around a surgical intervention is necessary, as there is no intravenous form available.

Dantrolene produces muscle relaxation by interfering with the release of calcium from the sarcoplasmic reticulum of the skeletal muscle. It does not directly affect the central nervous system. Dantrolene also requires titration to the desired effect and has the potential for fatal and nonfatal liver toxicity. The incidence of liver toxicity is much lower at doses less than 400 mg. per day (Gormley, 2001).

Intrathecal baclofen is made possible by the advent of technology allowing the drug to be delivered safely and consistently to the spinal canal. A small hockey puck–sized device is placed in the abdominal cavity in a lateral subcutaneous position (see Figure 11.2). A catheter is tunneled to an intrathecal catheter, usually positioned at the low thoracic area. This externally programmable device pumps very small amounts of baclofen on a continuous basis. This method has multiple advantages over oral medication. The amount of drug needed is smaller by ten-fold. In addition, the infusion is continuous, can be varied throughout the day by the programmable pump, and is relatively localized to the nerves at the site of the catheter placement. The complications may include mechanical failure; central nervous system side effects of lethargy and sedation; and operative complications including infection, disconnected tubing, catheter breakage, and cerebrospinal fluid leak (Albright, 1996). Despite these limitations, many centers report improvements in muscle tone, range of motion, and functional activities in individuals receiving intrathecal baclofen (Butler & Campbell, 2000).

Nerve blocks can be used to affect muscle tone in a very localized way. Two examples of chemical neuroly-

Table 11.4. Treatment considerations for three children with cerebral palsy

Child	Treatment of spasticity	Other options
Stephen (1-year-old with spastic hemiplegia)	He is young for any medical or surgical intervention. Physical therapy and possible bracing may be indicated now.	He may in the future benefit from botox on involved muscles of the hand and leg. Depending on the degree of spasticity, he may need surgical treatment of involved muscles.
Melody (5-year-old with spastic diplegia)	She may be an ideal candidate for selective dorsal rhizotomy as she is young, is motivated to participate in therapy, and has pure spasticity of lower extremities.	She may do well with oral baclofen. She also may do well with intrathecal baclofen after an oral dosing trial. She may need surgical correction of equinus deformity before or after the suggested interventions.
Sean (10-year-old with mixed pattern quadriplegia)	Physicians should consider no spasticity intervention as the spasticity may be useful to him because what is left is nonfunctional choreoathetosis.	He could take a low-dose oral medication such as baclofen or dantrolene. Physicians should consider baclofen pump placement because his spasticity is generalized and significantly affects his functioning. Physicians should address his contractures and deformity along with spasticity management.

sis are phenol blocks and botulism toxin A injections. Phenol alcohol and localized anesthetics have long been used to provide a local motor point block. Phenol denatures protein in the myelin sheath of the nerve, destroying the axon. As nerves are capable of regeneration within 3–6 months, this effect is temporary. Because phenol needs to be given very close to the nerve, electrical stimulation is needed to localize the nerve. Sedation and, in some cases, general anesthesia is needed because of discomfort with the procedure.

Botulism toxin acts to irreversibly block the cholinergic receptors of the neuromuscular junction, thus inhibiting the release of acetylcholine, which is required for muscle contraction. This effect, too, is temporary, usually lasting approximately 2–3 months. Botulism toxin can be rapidly administered without need for electrical stimulation, requires a much smaller volume and smaller needle for infusion, and causes less pain than the process of injecting phenol. The cost of botulism toxin, however, is quite high compared with other neurolytic agents. Botulism toxin injections have only been available for a little over a decade, so the efficacy of single or repeated botulism toxin injections on functional abilities in the long run is unknown. Its efficacy on short-term improvement in range of motion, muscle tone, and functional abilities has been described in several studies (Koman et al., 2001).

Finally, spasticity may be permanently addressed with a surgical intervention, the selective dorsal rhizotomy. This procedure involves the selective cutting of afferent nerves returning from the lower extremities to

Table 11.5. Common medications used for treatment of spasticity

Drug	Pediatric dosing range	Possible side effects
Diazepam (Valium)	0.2–0.8 mg/kg/d divided 6–8 hours	Central nervous system depression, acute withdrawal, habit forming
Baclofen (Lioresal)	Starting dose 2.5 mg per day titrated up to maximum of 20–60 mg, ending with a dosing schedule of three times per day	Acute withdrawal, central nervous system sedation
Dantrolene sodium (Dantrium)	0.5 mg/kg once a day for 7 days, increased weekly to 3 mg/kg; maximum of 400 mg.	Liver toxicity

Note: Because doses change over time, verify doses before administering any medications.

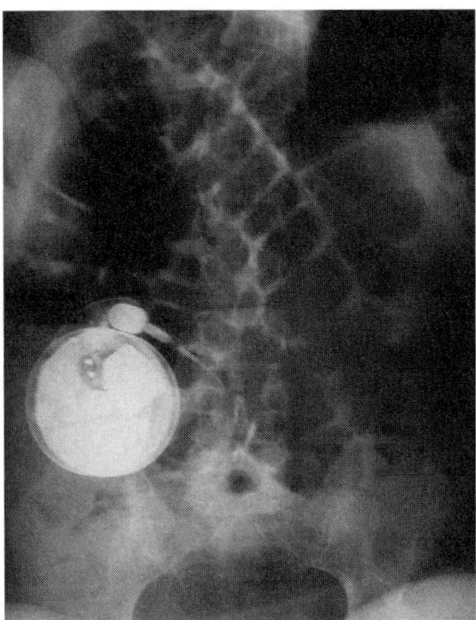

Figure 11.2. X-ray showing intrathecal baclofen device in place.

the lumbosacral spine. These nerves are identified using intraoperative electromyogram to determine which of the nerve rootlets carry the most abnormal response contributing to the spasticity. Following the surgery, an intensive rehabilitative program is undertaken by the child to relearn how to walk. An ideal candidate for this procedure is a child who has spastic diplegic, is 3–6 years of age, has no fixed contractures, has increased lower extremity tone, has been ambulating with devices for more than 6 months, has a supportive family, and can cooperate with rehabilitative therapy (Duhaime & Albinson-Scull, 1998). Outcomes of the selective dorsal rhizotomy show that it helps reduce spasticity and has a positive effect of gross motor function (McLaughlin et al., 2002).

Orthopedic Management Orthopedic intervention involves managing the sequelae of increased muscular tone, including treating and preventing skeletal deformity and addressing muscle, ligament, tendon, and surrounding soft tissue contracture (see Chapter 13). Orthopedic treatment and spasticity management are not mutually exclusive but rather are components of an appropriate medical intervention plan. The stories of Stephen, Melody, and Sean bring out some key concepts in orthopedic management of children with CP. First, the child and family must understand that surgical intervention to correct deformity or contracture does not equate with normalization of the gait pattern or curing the CP because the damage is to the brain, not the musculoskeletal system.

Second, orthopedic management of children with CP involves a complex decision algorithm integrating surgical skills, knowledge about the patterns of CP pathology, natural progression of the different subtypes of CP, and an understanding of child development. A gait analysis laboratory may add objective data to assist in these decisions (Schwartz, 2004). This type of surgery is best done by the surgeon with pediatric expertise and experience in CP. In Sean's case, he will require monitoring of the hip, knee, and ankle joints for risk of deformity. Orthopedic intervention may be necessary in addition to whatever tone-altering medications or surgeries are recommended. The timing and degree of intervention are challenging orthopedic decisions.

Finally, orthopedic management of CP takes time and consistent follow-up. There is no such thing as an emergent CP procedure. Perhaps many pediatric orthopedists enjoy this field, as there is opportunity to get to know these individuals and families over a long period of time. Stephen, Melody, and Sean will all benefit by a longitudinal relationship with a pediatric orthopedist. It may be, as in Stephen's case, that no specific orthopedic intervention is necessary.

Therapeutic Intervention

Therapeutic intervention is something that Melody, Sean, and Stephen will need at different levels at different times of their lives. The goal of therapy is to allow a child to participate as fully and developmentally appropriately as possible. This goal is accomplished in many ways but traditionally by initiating physical therapy, occupational therapy, and speech-language therapy. Therapy is provided in a variety of models. It can be done in a home-based model, a center-based program, a hospital outpatient model, and a multidisciplinary educational model. Therapy can be provided in the home, school, private office setting, hospital outpatient clinic, county facilities or at recreational centers. It can be provided in a group session or individual therapy. Finally, therapy can be provided as a direct service or in an indirect consultative fashion. It is sometimes difficult to know what the right intervention is for the right time.

In Stephen's case, his parents will likely want to be able to work with a therapist on Stephen's tightness of the muscles as well as his delayed motor skills. Stephen's development in other areas is not affected at this point. He will be best served by a physical therapist or occupational therapist to address his fine and gross motor skills and muscle tone. The physical therapist addresses problems related to gross motor functioning, including rolling, sitting, crawling, ambulation, muscle tone, and musculoskeletal problems such as range of motion and deformity. At this age, the functions of occupational therapy and physical therapy overlap quite a bit. Occupational therapists address issues of the child's "occupation," which is to learn skills of independence and to play (see Chapter 24.1). In a young child, these issues so often involve motor functioning that the occupational therapist's work seems very similar to that of the physical therapist (see Chapter 24.2); however, their goals are not the same, and they focus on different areas of function.

Stephen's parents will typically be very interested in every detail of the therapy, hoping for maximal change in his functional abilities. At this time, they are very interested in knowing everything there is to know about his condition. They want to know what the future holds for Stephen and what he will be able to do. His parents will rely heavily on what the therapist does and notices about their child's development. The therapist will be providing education as well as providing therapy. Oftentimes the therapist provides a great deal of emotional support to families at the time of initial diagnosis, although this support is rarely a specific written therapeutic goal. Stephen qualifies for early intervention services, which provide therapeutic interventions either in the home or at a county facility. In addition, Stephen's parents may wish to initiate therapy through a medical model at an outpatient or hospital-based facility.

Melody is a seasoned participant in therapy. She most likely receives therapy both at home and at school. Her school-based therapists are available to her due to the Individuals with Disabilities Education Act of 1990 (PL 101-476), which entitles her to therapy as an educationally related service. She attends therapy through her local hospital-based outpatient setting using a medical model of therapy. At this age, she probably enjoys going to therapy. These are people who know her well and give her lots of positive feedback. Her mother's relationship with the therapists appears to be quite good. Her mother is looking to Melody's therapists to help with the new problem of scissoring and falling down.

Melody probably has both a physical therapist and an occupational therapist working with her as the issues they are addressing can be quite different at this age. Melody's physical therapist has likely been involved in the decision for bracing her feet with ankle–foot orthotics, selecting the appropriate walker, and helping to decide whether a wheelchair is necessary for long-distance mobility. Her physical therapist has probably been doing range of motion exercises and evaluating any changes in her muscle tone. Her physical therapist at school has helped her to navigate the classroom and hallways of the school safely and has worked with Melody's teachers to make the classroom safe and accessible for her.

At Melody's age, the occupational therapist will concentrate on fine motor skills and activities of daily living. Melody has spasticity predominantly in the lower extremities but has trouble with her fine motor control of the hands as well. Coloring and cutting will be challenging for Melody. She may need adaptive equipment in the bathroom to take care of her toileting needs. Because Melody is a good eater, the occupational therapist doesn't have to focus on feeding. Melody is a social girl who is very talkative and has no communication difficulties and thus has not needed the input of speech-language therapy.

Sean is functioning at the developmental age of about 4 years. If he were developing typically, he would probably be tired of therapy and refusing to participate. Certainly, Sean has had his share of temper tantrums with the therapists. He has been working a long time to get where he is and still has a lot of frustrating problems to address. Sean likely sees physical therapy, occupational therapy, and speech-language therapy. Sean's grandparents should probably be thinking about episodes of therapy instead of continuous, no-end-in-sight, therapeutic relationships.

If asked, his grandparents would say that currently they are focusing their efforts on ways to communicate, which places the input of the speech-language therapist at the priority for them. Finding augmentative communication for Sean is an effort that involves all therapists as the mode of communication has to be mobile, perhaps fitting on his chair. It has to be functional for him despite his limited fine motor control. To find the best option for Sean, all disciplines will have to work together.

Although there are multiple concerns to address, Sean's grandparents, together with the therapists, are trying to identify the priorities (e.g., communication, comfort, ease of care for the family) and work on those accordingly. It may take the consultative services of therapists with very specific expertise (e.g., augmentative communication) to work with his primary therapist to find solutions to his problems with communication. There are only so many hours into the day to fit in learning, eating, socializing, relaxing, and sleeping. Sean and his grandparents need different things from the therapists now than they did when he was an infant.

Specific principles of therapy related to CP are beginning to emerge with new research on the efficacy and outcomes of therapeutic intervention. Physical therapists who work with individuals with CP often seek additional training in Neurodevelopmental Therapy. This therapeutic approach is founded on the principles outlined by Berta and Karel Bobath, a physical therapist and neuropsychiatrist, in the 1940s and has influenced therapeutic plans for children with CP for more than 50 years. Their goals were to establish normal motor development and function and to prevent contractures and deformity.

Beginning with the theory that children with CP should be placed in spasticity-reducing postures, the Bobaths evolved their practice and teaching to include a developmental sequence of acquiring skills. Then, they emphasized preparing children with tone abnormalities to do specific functional tasks in real-life settings. This philosophy or way of providing therapy is generally acquired through additional study beyond requirements for licensure in physical therapy. Multiple yet small sample size studies have yet to show a true advantage to this type of therapy over others when evaluating improvement in motor responses, prevention or reduction in the development of contractures, or the development of more functional motor activities (Butler & Darrah, 2001).

Another therapy that has received attention is the concept of force-used or constraint-induced therapy. This therapy forces the affected side to be used by restraining—tying back or casting the unaffected side of the body. This therapeutic approach is being tried in adults with hemiplegia resulting from a stroke (van der Lee, 1999). It is also being evaluated for efficacy in children with hemiplegic CP. Evidence exists that spastic muscles that are weak can improve in strength without increasing the spasticity (Dodd, Taylor, & Damiano, 2002).

MULTIDISCIPLINARY APPROACH

Table 11.3 outlines the need for a multidisciplinary approach to care for the needs of children and adults with CP. Each person with CP has his or her unique needs and goals for the future; however, there are common threads of care for all. In creating a system of optimal medical care for individuals with CP, one must consider how many areas of expertise are needed to provide early diagnosis, therapeutic intervention, treatment of primary and secondary conditions, and provision of supportive services (e.g., education, emotional support, links to financial and community supports).

Because no one person has this knowledge and expertise, many major urban areas have multidisciplinary clinics that include health care providers in some or all of the following fields: nursing, developmental pediatrics, orthopedics, physical therapy, occupational therapy, physical medicine and rehabilitation, neurology, social work, nutrition, psychology and speech-language therapy. Multiple other specialists are often drawn to a clinic for case-by-case needs. The availability in a singular clinic of these services depends on how the clinic is arranged and varies from site to site.

Families express a desire for this "one-stop shopping" but acknowledge some limitations. The appointments are long but often save extra visits. The clinics may be far away from home because these services are not available in every city. One of the major limitations at this time is the difficulty in finding this type of service for adults with CP. In the United States, centers that care for adults in this modality exist but are rare.

ISSUES IN ADULTHOOD

Many services are in place that families can use to plan for transitions. Early intervention programs plan the transition to special needs preschool programs and then on to primary and secondary education. Secondary education services are often linked with vocational assessment and training programs. Individuals with CP who are very dependent on others for care will require advanced planning for residential arrangements as adults. Some of these transitions require several months of advanced planning, such as the change from preschool to primary education. Some of the transitions require years of advanced planning. Legal expertise and financial advice will also be necessary. Fortunately, there are an increasing number of individuals who have interest and specialty training in these areas.

Adults with CP raise some common threads of concern. Families fear that life expectancy is shortened in individuals with CP. From a U.S. population-based study, the life expectancy of adults with CP can vary by 40 years or more depending on the functional level. High functioning adults with CP, as Stephen is likely to be, have a life expectancy close to that of the general population; however, life expectancy can be reduced by factors that impair an individual's functional level such as low cognitive level, all four extremity involvement, poor mobility, and dependent feeding (Strauss & Shavelle, 2001).

Adults with CP are concerned about pain, decline in mobility, fatigue, and loss of independence. In one survey of adults with CP, 35% reported decreased walking ability, 9% reported having stopped walking, and 18% of the respondents reported pain everyday (Andersson & Mattsson, 2001). Pain in individuals with CP is likely to come from the hips. Melody, for example, may experience overuse joint pain. In nonambulatory individuals, such as Sean, pain is very common. One survey of nonambulatory adults with a mean age of 27 years report hip pain present in 47% of respondents. Of that group, only 13.6% of those with pain had received medical treatment for the pain (Hodgkinson et al., 2001).

Osteoporosis is a concern that is not limited to individuals with CP; however, children and adolescents with moderate to severe CP have diminished bone densities and thus a propensity to fracture. In fact, osteopenia was found in 77% of a population-based cohort of children and adolescents with CP and 97% of the subgroup of children who were older than 9 and could not stand (Henderson et al., 2002). Given this knowledge and the known patterns of bone density loss in the general adult population, concern for increased bone fractures and subsequent pain and immobility is realistic. It raises many questions about the screening and treatment of osteoporosis.

Families of adults with CP and individuals with CP themselves raise concerns about competent primary and subspecialty medical care. The medical care and treatment of individuals with CP has usually been provided by pediatricians and pediatric subspecialists. The medical needs of the adults with CP may be left untreated, as few medical professionals caring for adults are familiar with CP and its related conditions. Oftentimes, unrelated conditions go untreated, as adults with CP find it difficult to find routine medical care. This is because the facility is not accessible or the medical care provider is not able or willing to accommodate a routine examination to a person with spasticity or continuous movements. Dental care is frequently hard to obtain for similar reasons (see Chapter 22). Routine care also may be limited by financial disincentives existing in some managed care organizations to care for individuals with disabilities.

"I need my primary care physician to interpret my medical concern in the context of my CP—neither ignoring that I have CP nor attributing every concern I have to CP." P.K., Cincinnati, OH

CONCLUSION

In the face of much frustration about the lack of knowledge and services for adults with CP, there are groups of people and national organizations trying to improve the knowledge and services for adults with CP. Private groups such as United Cerebral Palsy, professional groups such as the Academy of Cerebral Palsy and Developmental Medicine, and federal agencies such as the Administration of Developmental Disabilities and the Centers for Disease Control and Prevention are trying to address the concerns of these adults. In a conference on aging and CP supported by the Administration of Developmental Disabilities held in Washington, D.C., in 1997, participants identified specific areas of concern to target future research directives. These focused areas included general medical care, gastroesophageal reflux, dental care, nutrition, women's issues, sexuality, and communication. In addition, the round table discussion highlighted concerns about exercise and the lack of knowledge about how much, how intense, and what type of exercise will bring about the same benefits experienced by individuals without CP (see http://www.jik.com/awcp.html).

Perhaps by the time Stephen, Melody, and Sean reach adulthood, many answers to these questions about CP and aging will be known. As a result, their world will be accessible, they will have physicians who are comfortable and able to care for their medical needs, they will not fracture, they will have minimum pain on a day-to-day basis, and they will be able to communicate their unique experiences to their children and loved ones.

REFERENCES

Albright, A.L. (1996). Baclofen in the treatment of cerebral palsy. *Journal of Child Neurology, 11*(2), 77–83.

Andersson, C., & Mattsson, E. (2001). Adults with cerebral palsy: A survey describing problems, needs, and resources, with special emphasis on locomotion. *Developmental Medicine and Child Neurology, 43*(2), 76–82.

Bhushan, V., Paneth, N., & Kiely, J.L. (1993). Impact of improved survival of very low birth weight infants on recent secular trends in the prevalence of cerebral palsy. *Pediatrics, 91*, 1094–1100.

Blair, E., & Stanley, F.J. (1997). Issues in classification and epidemiology. *Mental Retardation in Developmental Disabilities Research Reviews, 3*, 184–193.

Blasco, P.A., & Allaire, J.H. (1992). Drooling in the developmentally disabled: Management practices and recommendations. Consortium on Drooling. *Developmental Medicine and Child Neurology, 34*(10), 849–862.

Boyle, C.A., Yeargin-Allsopp, M., Doernberg, N.S., Holmgreen, P., Murphy, C.C., & Schendel, D.E. (1996). Prevalence of selected developmental disabilities in children 3–10 years of age: The Metropolitan Atlanta Developmental Disabilities Surveillance Program, 1991. *Morbidity and Mortality Weekly Report CDC Surveill Summary, 45*, 1–14.

Butler, C., & Campbell, S. (2000). Evidence of the effects of intrathecal baclofen for spastic and dystonic cerebral palsy. *Developmental Medicine and Child Neurology, 42*, 634–645.

Butler, C., & Darrah, J. (2001). Effects of neurodevelopmental treatment (NDT) for cerebral palsy: An AACPDM evidence report. *Developmental Medicine and Child Neurology, 43*(11), 1–10.

Candy, E.J., Hoon, A.H., Capute, A.J., & Bryan, R.N. (1993). MRI in motor delay: Important adjunct to classification of cerebral palsy. *Pediatric Neurology, 9*(6), 421–429.

Capute, A.J., & Accardo, P.J. (Eds.). (1996a). *Developmental disabilities in infancy and childhood: Vol. I. Neurodevelopmental diagnosis and treatment* (2nd ed.). Baltimore: Paul H. Brookes Publishing Co.

Capute, A.J., & Accardo, P.J. (Eds.). (1996b). *Developmental disabilities in infancy and childhood: Vol. II. The spectrum of developmental disabilities* (2nd ed.). Baltimore: Paul H. Brookes Publishing Co.

Chugani, H. (1993). Position emission tomography scanning: Applications in newborns. *Clinics in Perinatology, 20*(2), 395–409.

Del Giudice, E., Staiano, A., Capano, G., et al., (1999). Gastrointestinal manifestations on children with cerebral palsy. *Brain & Development, 21*(5), 307–311.

Dobyns, W.B., Andermann, E., et al. (1996). X-linked malformations of neuronal migration. *Neurology, 47*(2), 331–339.

Dodd, K.J., Taylor, N.F., & Damiano, D.L. (2002). A systematic review of the effectiveness of strength-training programs for people with cerebral palsy. *Archives of Physical Medicine and Rehabilitation, 83*(8), 1157–1164.

Duhaime, A.C., & Albinson-Scull, S. (1998). Neurosurgical treatment of spasticity. In J.P. Dormans & L. Pellegrino (Eds.), *Caring for children with cerebral palsy: A team approach* (pp. 225–241). Baltimore: Paul Brookes Publishing Co.

Gormley, M.E. (2001). Treatment of neuromuscular and musculoskeletal problems in cerebral palsy. *Pediatric Rehabilitation, 4*(1), 5–16.

Hagberg, B., Hagberg, G., Beckung, E., & Uvebrant, P. (2001). Changing panorama of cerebral palsy in Sweden: VIII. Prevalence and origin in the birth year 1991/94. *Acta Paediatrica, 90*, 271–277.

Haberg, B., Hagberg, G., & Olow, I. (1975). The changing panorama of cerebral palsy in Sweden, 1954–1970: I. Analysis of general changes. *Acta Paediatrica, 64*, 187–192.

Hagberg, B., Hagberg, G., & Olow, I. (1993). The changing panorama of cerebral palsy in Sweden: VI. Prevalence and origin during the birth year period 1983–1986. *Acta Paediatrica, 82*, 387–393.

Henderson, R.C., Lark, R.K., Gurka, M.J., Worley, G., Fung, E.B., Conaway, M., et al. (2002). Bone density and metabolism in children and adolescents with moderate to severe cerebral palsy [Electronic version]. *Pediatrics, 110*(1), e5.

Hodgkinson, I., Jindrich, M.L., et al. (2001). Hip pain in 234 non-ambulatory adolescents and young adults with cerebral palsy: A cross-sectional multicentre study. *Developmental Medicine and Child Neurology, 43*(12), 806–808.

Hoon, A.H. (1995). Neuroimaging in the high-risk infant: Relationship to outcome. *Journal of Perinatology, 15*(5), 389–394.

Hoon, A.H., & Melhem, E.R. (2000). Neuroimaging: Application in disorders of early brain development. *Journal of Developmental & Behavioral Pediatrics, 21*(4), 291–302.

Hoon, A.H., Reinhaardt, E.M., Kelley, R.I., Breiter, S.N., Morton, D.H., Naidu, S.B., et al. (1997). Brain magnetic resonance imaging in suspected extrapyramidal cerebral palsy: Observations in distinguishing genetic-metabolic from acquired causes. *Journal of Pediatrics, 131*(2), 240–245.

Inder, T., Hyppi, P.S., et al. (1999). Early detection of periventricular leucomalacia by diffusion-weighted magnetic resonance imaging techniques. *Journal of Pediatrics, 134*, 631–634.

Kiely, J.L., Paneth, N., Stein, Z., & Susser, M. (1981). Cerebral palsy and newborn care: I. Secular trends in cerebral palsy. *Developmental Medicine and Child Neurology, 23*, 533–538.

Koman, L.A, Brashear, A., et al. (2001). Botulism toxin type a neuromuscular blockade in the treatment of equinus foot deformity in cerebral palsy: A multicenter, open-label clinical trial. *Pediatrics, 108*(5), 1062–1071.

Krach, L. (2001) Pharmacotherapy of spasticity. *Journal of Child Neurology, 16*(1), 31–36.

Little, W.J. (1861). On the influence of abnormal parturition, difficult labours, premature birth, and asphyxia neonatorum on the mental and physical condition of the child, especially in relation to deformities. *Transactions of the Obstetrical Society of London, 3*, 243–344.

McBride, M.C., Laroia, N., & Guillet, R. (2000). Electrographic seizures in neonates correlate with poor neurodevelopmental outcome. *Neurology, 55*(4), 506–513.

McLaughlin, J., Bjornson, K., Temkin, N., Steinbok, P., Wright, V., Reiner, A., et al. (2002). Selective dorsal rhizotomy: Meta-analysis of three randomized controlled trials. *Developmental Medicine and Child Neurology, 44*, 17–25.

Msall, M.E., Buck, G.M., Rogers, B.T., Merke, D.P., Wan, C.C., Catanzara, N.L., et al. (1994). Multivariate risks among extremely premature infants. *Journal of Perinatology, 14*(1), 41–47.

Murphy, C.C., Yeargin-Allsopp, M., Decoufle, P., & Drews, C.D. (1993). Prevalence of cerebral palsy among ten-year-old children in metropolitan Atlanta, 1985–1987. *Journal of Pediatrics, 123*, S13–S20.

Mutch, L., Alberman, E., Hagberg, B., Kodama, K., & Perat, M.V. (1992). Cerebral palsy epidemiology: Where are we now and where are we going? *Developmental Medicine and Child Neurology, 34*, 547–551.

Nelson, K.B., & Grether, J.K. (1999). Causes of cerebral palsy. *Current Opinion in Pediatrics, 11*, 487–491.

Ogden, C.L., Kuczmarski, R.J., Flegal, K.M., Mei, Z., Guo, S., Wei, R., et al. (2002). Centers for Disease Control and Prevention 2000 growth charts for the United States: Improvements to the 1977 National Center for Health Statistics Version. *Pediatrics, 109*, 45–60.

O'Shea, T.M., Klinepeter, K.L., Goldstein, D.J., Jackson, B.W., & Dillard, R.G. (1997). Survival and developmental disability in infants with birth weights of 501 and 800 grams, born between 1979 and 1994. *Pediatrics, 100*, 982–986.

Samson-Fang, L., & Stevenson, R. (2000). Identification of malnutrition in children with cerebral palsy: Poor performance of weight-for height centiles. *Developmental Medicine and Child Neurology, 42*, 162–168.

Schwartz, M.H. (2004). Comprehensive treatment of ambulatory children with cerebral palsy: An outcome assessment. *Journal of Pediatric Orthopedics, 24*(1), 45–53.

Stanley, F., Blair, E., & Alberman, E. (2000). *Cerebral palsies: Epidemiology and causal pathways.* London: Mac Keith Press.

Strauss, D., & Shavellem, R. (2001). Life expectancy in cerebral palsy. *Archives in Disease in Children, 85*(5), 76–82.

Thorarensen, O., Ryan, S., et al. (1997). Factor V Leiden mutation: An unrecognized cause of hemiplegic cerebral palsy, neonatal stroke, and placental thrombosis. *Annals of Neurology, 42*(3), 372–375.

van der Lee, J.H. (1999). Forced use of the upper extremity in chronic stroke patients: Results from a single-blind randomized clinical trial. *Stroke, 31*(4), 69–75.

Vohr, B., Allan, W.C., Scott, D.T., Katz, K.H., Schneider, K.C., Makuch, R.W., et al. (1999, June). Early-onset intraventricular hemorrhage in preterm neonates: Incidence of neurodevelopmental handicap. *Seminars in Perinatology, 23*(3), 212–217.

Vohr, B., Wright, L., Dusick, A., Mele, L., Verter, J., Steichen, J., et al. (2000). Neurodevelopmental and functional outcomes of extremely low birth weight infants in the national institute of child health and human development neonatal research network. *Pediatrics, 105*, 1216–1226.

Winter, S., Autry, A., Yeargin-Allsopp, M., & Boyle, C. (2002). Prevalence of cerebral palsy in a population based study. *Pediatrics, 110*(6), 1220–1225.

Young, R.R., & Delwaide, P.J. (1981). Drug therapy: Spasticity. *New England Journal of Medicine, 304*(2), 96–99.

CHAPTER 12

NEUROLOGY

12.1 CONGENITAL ANOMALIES OF THE BRAIN

Norberto Alvarez

Congenital anomalies of the brain may be macroscopic or microscopic, but the outcome is impairment of neurological function to a greater or lesser degree. Both internal and external factors can interfere with the normal development of the brain and spinal cord before birth, resulting in congenital malformation. The resulting malformation varies and is related to the stage in the development of the brain at the time of the injury. Tables 12.1-1 and 12.1-2 present a list of teratogens and conditions that can result in congenital malformations and how they relate to the time that the injury occurred.

New developments in neuroradiology and genetics have resulted in a marked increase in the knowledge of these malformations, as well as the ability to diagnose them (Leventar et al., 1999). Given the explosion in the number of genes associated with brain malformations, physicians should be familiar with databases such as Online Mendelian Inheritance in Man (OMIM) for current information (http://www3.ncbi.nlm.nih.gov/Omim/). In many situations, the malformations are not seen as isolated events but in association with other congenital malformations, quite often in well-recognized syndromes. Examples of these associations are presented in Table 12.1-3.

As mentioned previously, congenital anomalies of the brain are determined in part by the stage at which brain formation is interrupted. Anomalies of neurulation and formation of the neural tube can occur from the caudal most part of neurulation to the cranial part. The anomalies in the caudal area are represented by the spina bifida/myelomenigocele group of conditions discussed in Chapter 8.1. Anomalies in the cranial area are seen in the group of conditions that have encephaloceles, which are herniations of brain tissue through a bone defect most commonly in the occipital areas. The clinical features depend on the architectural intactness of the remaining cerebral tissue, and, again, these features may be dramatic and isolated or mild and associated with other anomalies.

ANENCEPHALY

Anencephaly is the most dramatic of the congential anomalies. The brain fails to develop, and infants do not survive the newborn period. The Medical Task Force on Anencephaly considered these children permanently unconscious, which raised many ethical issues, including the use of organs for transplants. Regulations in the United States do not permit children with anencephaly to be organ donors (Peabody, Emery, & Ashwal, 1989).

HYDRANENCEPHALY

Hydranencephaly, represents an almost complete absence of the cerebral hemispheres, which are reduced to only small portions of the cortex. There is no suggestion of a normal ventricular system, and only one unique sac with cerebrospinal fluid exists. The diagnosis can be made during pregnancy with an ultrasound. At birth, transillumination of the skull can also make the diagnosis. Some newborn infants may appear to develop normally for a few weeks, but in general most infant do not survive their first year of life.

HOLOPROSENCEPHALY

Holoprosencephaly occurs when the forebrain does not develop. There is no sagital division of the brain by the interhemispheric fissure, and the ventricle is limited to only one undivided structure (Leech & Shuman, 1986). The three main forms are the alobar, the semilobar, and the lobar. The first two are more severe, with the lobar form having only some minor changes. The condition is more frequent in diabetic mothers, and there are several chromosomal abnormalities and familial forms. In most instances, developmental delay is present. Also, children with holoprosencephaly have cerebral palsy (mostly spastic quadriplegia), many sensory impairments, and seizures. A few children might have normal development. Midline facial malformations, affecting the eyes or the nose or the maxillary areas, are associated dysmorphic features in some of the individuals. Some children with the lobar form of holoprosencephaly might be mildly affected and present with mild spasticity.

Table 12.1-1. Teratogen agents that cause brain and spinal cord malformations

Intrauterine infections
Toxoplasmosis
Rubella
Herpes virus types 1 and 2
Cytomegalovirus
Varicella virus
Mumps virus
Syphilis
Toxins and drug exposure during the intrauterine life
Alcohol
Tobacco
Carbon monoxide
Cocaine
Heavy metals (mercury, lead)
Medications (antiepileptic drugs: phenobarbital, phenytoin, valproic acid; antimetabolites)
Folate deficiency
Physical agents
Radiation
Trauma
Maternal diseases
Phenylketonuria
Toxemia gravidorum
Malnutrition
Diabetes mellitus

Adapted from *Pediatric Neurology: Principles and Practice* (3rd ed.), F.S. Swaiman & S. Ashwal (Eds.), Congenital Heart Defects, p. 318, Copyright 1999, with permission from Elsevier.

Table 12.1-2. Congenital malformations and fetal development

Neural tube defects
Chiari malformation*
Meningocele and myelomeningocele*
Spina bifida occulta*
Anencephaly
Encephalocele
Diastematomelia
Diplomyelia
Sacral agenesis
Defects in segmentation and cleavage
Holoprosencephaly
Defects in sulcation, proliferation, neuronal migration, and proliferatrion
Agenesis of the corpus callosum
Cerebellar abnormalities
Agenesis of the cerebellum
Agenesis of the vermis
Cerebellar hyperplasia
Dandy-Walker syndrome
Neuronal heterotopias
Periventricular
Subcortical white matter
Cortical or leptomeningeal
Lissencephaly
Pachygyria/macrogyria
Macro- and microgyria
Neuronal migration defects
Schizencephaly
Porencephaly
Megalencephaly
Microcephaly
Postneuronal migration disorders
Hydrocephalus
Hydranencephaly

*See Chapter 8.1

Adapted from *Pediatric Neurology: Principles and Practice* (3rd ed.), F.S. Swaiman & S. Ashwal (Eds.), Congenital Heart Defects, p. 318, Copyright 1999, with permission from Elsevier.

AGENESIS OF THE CORPUS CALLOSUM

The corpus callosum is composed of white matter fibers that connect both hemispheres. The total or partial absence of the corpus callosum might be an isolated finding; however, in most instances it is associated with other malformations, such as heterotopias, microgyria, hydrocephalus, and porencephalic cysts. Agenesis of the corpus callosum (see Figure 12.1-1) has been associated with numerous genetic disorders (Ashwal, 1999). Many children with agenesis of the corpus callosum have cognitive impairments; however, normal development is not unusual depending on the associated malformations.

CEREBELLAR ABNORMALITIES

Congenital cerebellar abnormalities are most commonly seen with a variety of malformations and syndromes. Clinical manifestations of cerebellar disorders might be subtle in some cases. Ataxia, hypotonia, incoordination, tremor, and delayed fine and gross motor development are neurological signs related to the cerebellar abnormality. The Dandy-Walker set of anomalies is predominantly that of cerebellar dysgenesis (see Figure 12.1-2).

NEURONAL HETEROTOPIAS

Neuronal heterotopias as a group probably represent the single most common set of conditions associated with cerebral dysgenesis. They may be mild and unidentifiable with existing neuroimaging studies or they may be obvious, in which case they are likely to have dramatic symptomatology with extremely challenging seizures. The conditions consist of clusters of abnormal gray matter, most often lacking any cortical lamination,

Table 12.1-3. Examples of congenital malformations of the brain and or the spinal cord associated with other conditions or syndromes

Syndrome	Associated malformations
Dandy-Walker syndrome	Hydrocephalus, partial or complete agenesis of the cerebellar vermis, posterior fossae cyst extending into the fourth ventricle, cranial nerve palsies
Aicardi syndrome (sex-linked, seen only in girls)	Agenesis of the corpus callosum, chorioretinal anomalies, infantile spasms, gray matter heterotopias, vertebral anomalies, intellectual disabilities
Trisomy 13 (Patau syndrome)	Holoprosencephaly, hypoplasia optic nerve and chiasma, cerebellar hypoplasia, Arnold-Chiari malformation, craniofacial abnormalities, anomalies in most major organs systems
Trisomy 18 (Edwards syndrome)	Microcephaly, heterotopias, agenesis of the corpus callosum, Dandy-Walker malformation, Arnold-Chiari malformation, prominent occiput, hands tight with fourth and fifth fingers overlapping the first and second, congenital heart defects, renal anomalies
Miller-Dieker syndrome (17p13.3 deletion)	Lissencephaly, microcephaly, craniofacial anomalies, seizures, developmental delays
Walker-Warburg syndrome (2p11.2 deletion)	Lissencephaly, hydrocephalus, occipital encephalocele, microcephaly, absent cerebellar vermis, skeletal and genital abnormalities
X-linked lissencephaly/subcortical band heterotopias	Lissencephaly, subcortical band heterotopias, agenesis of corpus callosum
Joubert syndrome	Agenesis of the cerebellar vermis, hyperpnea and apneas, ataxia, hypotonia, eye movement disorder, intellectual disabilities
Meckel syndrome (linked to 17q21-24)	Occipital encephalocele, microcephaly, renal dysplasia (polycystic kidney), polydactyly

that might be seen around the ventricles, in the subcortical white matter, or in the leptomeninges.

The causes of these arrested migrations are multiple. Heterotopias are seen in a variety of genetic and metabolic disorders. They can also result from viral infections as well as environmental factors (e.g., alcohol ingestion during pregnancy). The clinical picture varies but intellectual disabilities, intractable epileptic disorders, and cerebral palsy are frequently seen. Magnetic resonance imaging (MRI) is very useful for the identification of the different types of neuronal heterotopias (Leventer et al., 1999; Velez-Dominguez, 1998).

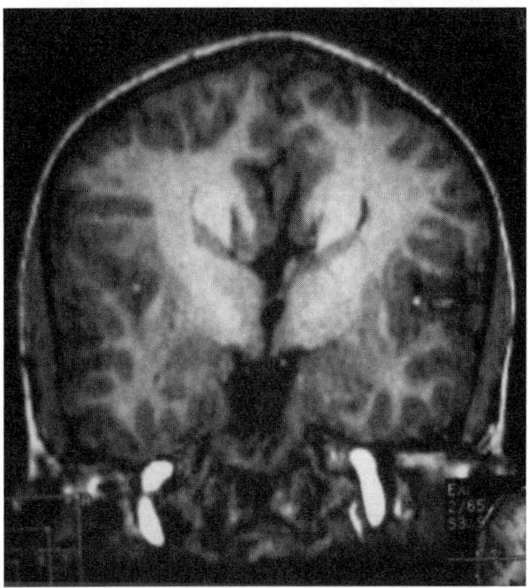

Figure 12.1-1. Computed tomography scan of an individuals with agenesis of the corpus callosum.

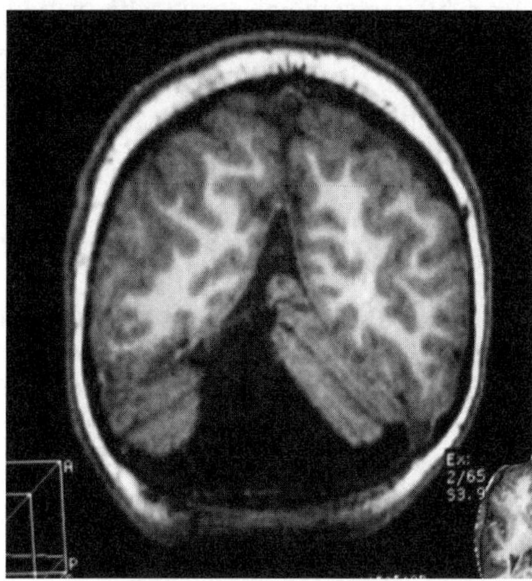

Figure 12.1-2. Computed tomography scan of an individuals with Dandy-Walker syndrome.

LISSENCEPHALY

With lissencephaly, the normal gyral pattern of the brain is absent and is replaced by a smooth cerebral surface. The cortical mantle is thick, and children experience associated neuronal migration disorders, including heterotopias. Several types of lissencephaly occur, and lissencephaly can be associated with many different syndromes (Dobyns & Truwit, 1995). Children with lissencephaly might be small for gestational age. Polyhydramnios might be a complication during pregnancy, and the neonatal period might be complicated by apneas. Microcephaly is common; however, some syndromes are associated with congenital hydrocephalus. Epileptic seizures are very frequent, and infantile spasms might be seen in early infancy. Developmental delays are almost always present. Determining the syndrome associated with the lissencephaly is important because the risk of recurrence varies with the etiology of the lissencephaly.

SCHIZENCEPHALY

Schizencephaly involves clefts in the cerebral hemispheres, mostly in the sylvian fissures. In addition, cortical areas near the schizencephaly might have an abnormal gyral pattern. The malformation could be unilateral or bilateral. Schizencephaly is thought to be the result of vascular accidents in the middle cerebral artery (Mancini, Lethel, Hugonenq, & Chabrol, 2001). In some cases, there is a family incidence, and genetic mutations have been described in some individuals. Many children with schizencephaly have other associated anomalies. Children with unilateral malformations have milder clinical manifestations than those with bilateral malformations. Developmental delays, epileptic seizures, and motor disorders are some of the manifestations seen in children with schizencephaly.

PACHYGYRIA/MACROGYRIA

Pachygyria/macrogyria refers to a decreased number of gyral formations in the cortex. Gray matter is thicker than usual, and the gyral might be bigger in size. The malformation might be diffuse involving the whole brain or might be limited to some areas. The degree of developmental delay varies and might be limited as presented in Heather's story.

Heather was born after a pregnancy that lasted 9 months. Her mother, Claire, had two prior miscarriages. She was in early labor almost weekly and had to be on bed rest for most of her pregnancy. Claire was on antidepressants during pregnancy. Her labor with Heather was induced and normal. Heather looked normal at birth and cried immediately.

Heather's development was normal in the social and language areas, but she experienced motor delays. At the age of 15 months, she was able to sit and stay in the sitting position; however, she could not get up to the standing position unless she was holding on to something. She had no muscle atrophies, but she did have generalized hypotonia, normal deep tendon reflexes, and no Babinski sign. In addition, Heather had no dysmorphic features.

Heather was started in an early stimulation program. At the age of 22 months, she showed marked improvements. Her social and language development were age appropriate, and her motor development was almost at age level. She was able to walk independently. MRI showed abnormal development of Heather's brain with diffuse thickening of the cerebral cortex, abnormal gyral pattern with pachygyria in almost the whole cortex.

Heather's situation presents several interesting questions regarding the etiology of pachygyria/macrogyria and the minimal delay in the presence of an extensive brain malformation. Claire was on antidepressive medication for the whole pregnancy; also, she had a history of prior spontaneous abortions that might be suggestive of a genetic disorder. One of the most striking features of Heather's condition is almost normal development in the presence of such a severe and diffuse malformation. In children with pachygyria/macrogyria, MRI is always useful. Genetic evaluation is also indicated because these malformations might be associated with genetic disorders.

PORENCEPHALY

Porencephaly, a cystic lesion in the brain, might be a complication of direct intrauterine trauma to the brain (e.g., after amniocentesis, traumatic breech delivery, intracerebral bleeding), or it might be congenital. The clinical picture is characterized by developmental delay, epileptic seizures, hemiparesis (when the brain lesion involved the motor areas), and athetosis (if the basal ganglia are affected) (Prayson & Hannahoe, 2004). In some instances, the cyst increases in size, and a shunt is needed. If the epileptic disorder is resistant to medications, children with porencephaly might be candidates for surgery. In most instances (e.g., Pedro's story), observation is enough, and most of the cysts do not need treatment.

Pedro was born after a normal pregnancy and delivery. At birth, he had right side hemiparesis. As he got older, his hemiparesis, which mostly affected his leg, became more obvious, and he experienced mild atrophy of the right leg. He

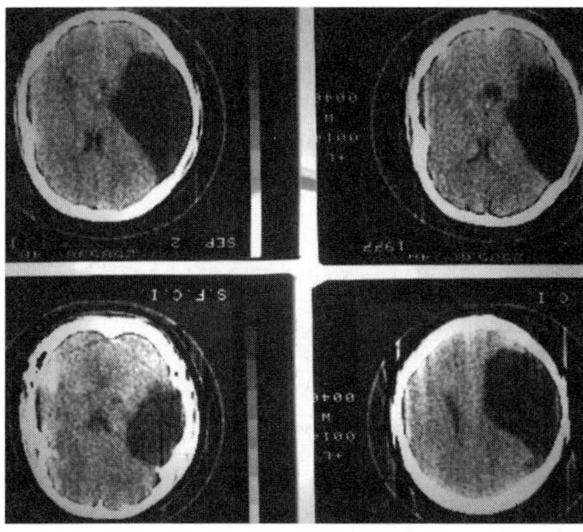

Figure 12.1-3. Computed tomography scan that was obtained when Pedro was 20 years old. Note the porencephalic cyst in the distribution of the left middle cerebral artery.

also had self-injurious behavior and never developed speech. In spite of abnormal electroencephalograms, he had no reported seizures. At 20 years old, Pedro had a computed tomography (CT) scan (see Figure 12.1-3), which showed a porencephalic cyst in the distribution of the left middle cerebral artery—clearly a vascular accident that occurred during intrauterine life. His condition remained stable, and his physicians believed that the cyst would remain the same for the rest of his life without need for surgery.

MEGALENCEPHALY/MACROCEPHALY

Megalencephaly refers to a brain whose size is two standard deviations larger than normal. This condition is usually associated with macrocephaly, which refers to the presence of a head circumference that is more than two standard deviations larger than normal. The most common type of megalencephaly is the asymptomatic familial form, in which the brain is normal, the head circumference is above 98% of the norm, neurological examination and development are normal, and one close relative (usually one of the parents, brothers, or sisters) has megalencephaly. This condition is transmitted as autosomal dominant and affects boys more than girls. In the familiar symptomatic form, children experience neurological impairments that might vary from mild learning disabilities to more severe disorders. A list of conditions associated with megalencephaly/macrocephaly is presented in Table 12.1-4.

The differential diagnosis is very complex, and an MRI of the head is always indicated. Because megalencephaly might be associated with neurodermatosis, clinicians should look for the presence of skin lesions such as café-au-lait spots and ashleaves. In the presence of progressive neurological symptoms, metabolic studies should be conducted to rule out inborn errors of metabolism and endocrinopathies.

Table 12.1-4. Common causes and syndromes associated with megalencephaly/macrocephaly

Asymptomatic familial anatomic megalencephaly (AFAM)
Symptomatic familial anatomic megalencephaly (SFAM)
Symptomatic (sporadic) anatomic megalencephaly (nonfamilial)
Bilateral megalencephaly associated with gigantism
Soto syndrome
Bilateral megalencephaly associated with dwarfism or short stature
Achondroplastic dwarf
Robinow syndrome
Multiple endocrinopathies
Bilateral megalencephaly associated with neurocutaneous syndromes
Tuberous sclerosis
Neurofibromatosis
Hypomelanosis of Ito
Linear nevus sebaceous
Multiple hemangiomatosis (e.g., Bannayan-Riley-Ruvacaba syndrome)
Megalencephaly secondary to metabolic encephalopathies
Tay-Sachs disease
Mucopolysaccaridosis
Gangliosidosis
Canavan disease
Alexander disease
Aminoacidurias/organic acidurias

Source: DeMyer (1999).

Rex was born after a normal pregnancy, but he had severe anoxia at birth. Rex also had hypertelorism, slanted eyelids, a frontal bossing with mild depression in the midline over the metopic suture, spastic quadriparesis, profound intellectual disabilities, cortical blindness, profound deafness, and epileptic seizures that were resistant to treatment. An electroencephalogram showed poorly formed activity and voltage depression over the posterior quadrants. Epileptiform activity consisted of multifocal spike and wave discharges in both frontal areas, some of them associated with subtle seizures (e.g., staring spells).

A CT scan taken when Rex was 24 years old (see Figure 12.1-4) showed marked dilatation of the ventricular system, almost no encephalic mass in the occipital and parietal areas, and some preservation of the frontal and temporal lobes. The remaining frontal areas might have had some other congenital malformations that were beyond the resolution of the CT scan. The ventricular dilatation was not associated with increased intracranial pressure. His condition was expected to remain the same in the coming years.

MICROCEPHALY/MICRENCEPHALY

Microcephaly refers to a head circumference that is less than two standard deviations from the normal, whereas micrencephaly refers to a brain whose size is less than two standard deviations from the normal. Microcephaly might be a normal variant, as seen in asymptomatic familiar microcephaly, whereas micrencephaly is more

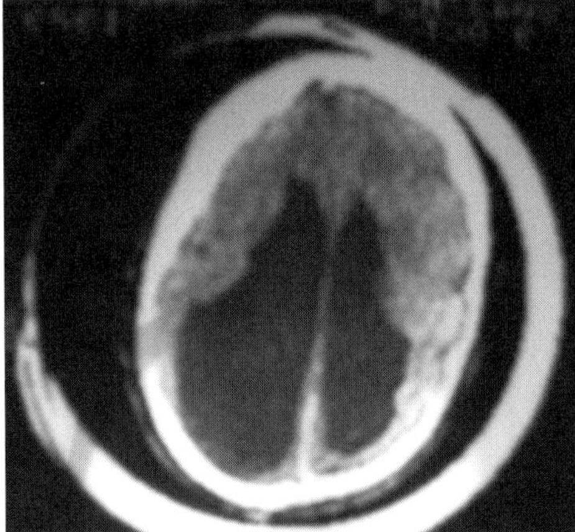

Figure 12.1-4. Computed tomography scan that was obtained when Rex was 24 years old. Note the marked dilatation of the ventricular system, almost no encephalic mass in the occipital and parietal areas, and some preservation of the frontal and temporal lobes.

often associated with brain malformations and some neurological impairments. In the symptomatic forms, the small brain may reveal extensive malformations, such as micro- or macrogyria, neuronal migration disorders, heterotopias, and lissencephaly. Micrencephaly can also be the result of prenatal or perinatal insult in an otherwise normal brain. Table 12.1-5 presents a list of medical conditions associated with microcephaly/micrencephaly.

Table 12.1-5. Common conditions associated with microcephaly/micrencephaly

Normal asymptomatic variation
Familial form (autosomal dominant, recessive, or X-linked)
Down syndrome
Maternal infections
Cytomegalovirus
Herpes
Toxoplasmosis
Syphilis
Rubella
Exposure to drugs during gestation
Alcohol
Tobacco
Marijuana
Cocaine
Antiepileptic drugs
Anoxia/ischemia
Maternal diseases
Diabetes
Phenylketonuria
Radiation exposure
Renal insufficiency
Very low birth weight

Adapted from *Pediatric neurology: Principles and practice* (3rd ed.)., F.S. Swaiman & S. Ashwal, Microcephaly, microencephaly, megalocephaly, and megalencephaly, p. 303, Copyright 1999, with permission from Elsevier.

HYDROCEPHALUS

Hydrocephalus refers to conditions in which there is enlargement of the ventricular system. Impairment of the normal egress and flow of the cerebrospinal fluid (noncommunicating), excessive production, and/or limited absorption of cerebrospinal fluid (communicating) are the causes that lead to hydrocephalus. In the noncommunicating type, the obstruction is the result of abnormalities in areas where the pathway is narrow and the enlargement of the ventricles is rostral to the point of obstruction. In the communicating type, the flow of cerebrospinal fluid is normal; however, there is an imbalance between the production and the absorption of cerebrospinal fluid, resulting in the accumulation of cerebrospinal fluid. Table 12.1-6 presents common causes of hydrocephalus.

Hydrocephalus could be acute or insidious. Both types are dangerous; however, acute hydrocephalus is an emergency condition that in most instances requires surgical treatment. In subacute forms, continuous accumulation of cerebrospinal fluid leads to enlargement of the head.

In some instances of communicating hydrocephalus, an eventual balance is reached between absorption and production, and the hydrocephalus arrests. Surgical treatment in these cases may not be necessary. If the condition occurred before the cranial commissures are closed, the increased intracranial pressure results in separation of the commissures, and, in the early stages, there is less pressure over the brain structures. Increased head circumference and bulging fontanels are the main signs. These signs will not be seen in older children or adults; instead, the clinical picture might consist of vomiting, headaches, visual problems, papilledema, behavioral changes, and/or acute cognitive deficits. If the commis-

Table 12.1-6. Common causes associated with hydrocephalus

Noncommunicating
Acqueductal abnormalities: stenosis, forking, gliosis
Obstructions due to: mass lesions, hemorrhages, parasites, exhudates
Obstruction of the fourth ventricle outlets: Dandy-Walker syndrome, Arnold-Chiari malformation
Communicating
Postinfectious: cytomegalic inclusion, disease, congenital syphilis, toxoplasmosis, meningitis, encephalitis
Increased intracranial venous pressure secondary to sinus thrombosis
Excessive production of cerebrospinal fluid
Choroid plexus papilloma

sures are closed, then there is pressure on the brain structures, and the symptoms reflect this pressure.

In arrested hydrocephalus, the symptoms might be more insidious, characterized by chronic headaches, gait difficulties, and behavior changes. Because the balance that resulted in the arrested hydrocephalus might be broken at any time, these children deserve close follow-up to determine if they need a shunt. MRI is the test of choice in the presence of enlarged head. Surgery is indicated in any individual who shows progression of symptoms. In some cases, acetazolamide or diuretics might control the hydrocephalus.

CONCLUSION

This chapter presents a variety of developmental anomalies of the brain. Medical history, combined with ultrasound and serological tests for infections, might in some instances help to determine the cause of the malformation even before birth. Given the variety of the causes that can result in brain malfunctions, however, it is not surprising that the etiology of brain malformations is often unknown. Children with congenital anomalies of the brain have different needs, treatments, and prognosis depending on the degree of impairment to neurological function.

REFERENCES

Ashwal, S. (1999). Congenital structural defects. In F.S. Swaiman & S. Ashwal (Eds.), *Pediatric neurology: Principles and practice* (3rd ed., pp. 234–300). St. Louis: Mosby.

DeMyer, W. (1999). Microcephaly, microencephaly, megalocephaly, and megalencephaly. In F.S. Swaiman & S. Ashwal (Eds.), *Pediatric neurology: Principles and practice* (3rd ed., pp. 303–306). St. Louis: Mosby.

Dobyns, W.B., & Truwit, C.L. (1995). Lissencephaly and other malformations of cortical development: 1995 update. *Neuropediatrics, 26*(3), 132–147.

Leech, R.W., & Shuman, R.M. (1986). Holoprosencephaly and related midline cerebral anomalies: A review. *Journal of Child Neurology, 1*(1), 3–18.

Leventer, R.J., Phelan, E.M., Coleman, L.T., Kean, M.J., Jackson, G.D., & Harvey, A.S. (1999). Clinical and imaging features of cortical malformations in childhood. *Neurology, 53*(4), 715–722.

Mancini, J., Lethel, V., Hugonenq, C., & Chabrol, B. (2001). Brain injuries in early fetal life: Consequences for brain development. *Developmental Medicine & Child Neurology, 43*(1), 52–55.

Medical Task Force on Anencephaly. (1990). The infant with anencephaly. *New England Journal of Medicine, 322*(10), 669–674.

Peabody, J.L., Emery, J.R., & Ashwal, S. (1989). Experience with anencephalic infants as prospective organ donors. *New England Journal of Medicine, 321*(6), 344–350.

Prayson, R.A., & Hannahoe, B.M. (2004). Clinicopathologic findings in patients with infantile hemiparesis and epilepsy. *Human Pathology, 35*(6), 734–738.

Velez-Dominguez, L.C. (1998). [Neuronal migration disorders]. [Spanish]. *Gaceta Medica de Mexico, 134*(2), 207–215.

12.2 EPILEPSY

Norberto Alvarez

Epilepsy is a condition characterized by recurrent clinical events (i.e., epileptic seizures) that are the result of abnormal activity of cortical neurons (Fisher et al., 2005). The protean signs and symptoms that conform the epileptic seizure are related to the particular neurons that are involved in the paroxysmal activity, mostly their primary function, and propagation within the central nervous system. An epileptic seizure occurs when there is a break in the balance between the different excitatory and inhibitory forces that are continuously active over the neurons. It is a manifestation of brain injury, but the injury that leads to epilepsy could be the result of multiple etiologies.

In the general population, the prevalence of active epilepsy is 0.7%–1% (Cowan, Bodensteiner, Leviton, & Doherty, 1989; Sidenvall, Forsgren, & Heijbel, 1996; Sillanpaa, 1992). Hauser and Hesdorfffer (1990) found that 5%–10% of children with IQ scores less than 70 had epilepsy; however, the incidence increased up to 50% in those children who had indications of neurological impairments such as cerebral palsy, and in these children the incidence as well as the prognosis of the

Table 12.2-1. Frequency of epilepsy and type of cerebral palsy

Type of cerebral palsy	Crowthers and Paine (1959)	Hilliard and Kirman (1957)	Ingram et al. (1964)	Stephens and Hawks (1975)
Hemiplegia				
Congenital	55	17	51	17
Acquired	72	—	—	—
Quadriplegia, diplegia	33	50	31	50
Extrapyramidal	23	4	25	4
Other forms	—	29	15	29

epileptic disorder was directly related to the type of cerebral palsy as seen in Table 12.2-1.

The International League Against Epilepsy (ILAE) has been a leading force in the attempt to classify epileptic seizures and syndromes. Tables 12.2-2, 12.2-3, 12.2-4, and 12.2-5 present definitions of terms that are frequently used as well as types and description of the seizures (Blume et al., 2001; ILEA, 1981, 1989). This classification is continuously under revision by a special task force; therefore, some of the definitions may be changed in the future.

EPILEPTIC SEIZURES

The early manifestation of the epileptic disorder is related to the severity of the brain damage. Steffenburg, Hagberg, and Kyllerman, (1996) found that in a group of 98 children with intellectual disabilities age 6–13 years, the average age of first seizures was 1.3 years for the whole group, but 0.8 years for children with profound intellectual disabilities and 3.1 years for children with mild intellectual disabilities. In addition, the risk of developing epilepsy remains high during the second decade of life (Brodtkorb, 1994). Multiple seizure types are more often seen in children with brain damage than in those who do not have any neurological impairments.

The remission rate is much lower in children with intellectual disabilities and even lower if they do have concomitant cerebral palsy. Although the possibility of reaching total remission and being off medication is very high for the general population, the presence of intellectual disabilities determines a poor prognosis for both remission and discontinuance of antiepileptic drugs

Table 12.2-2. Definition of terms and concepts related to epilepsy

Benign epilepsy syndrome—a syndrome characterized by epileptic seizures that are easily treated, or require no treatment, and remits without sequelae.

Epilepsy syndrome—a combination of signs and symptoms that defines a unique epileptic condition.

Epileptic disease—a condition with a single specific well-defined etiology.

Epileptic encephalopathy—a condition in which the epileptiform abnormalities themselves are believed to contribute to the progressive disturbance in cerebral function.

Epileptic seizure—An ictal event believed to represent a unique pathophisiologic mechanism and anatomic substrate. This diagnostic entity has etiologic, therapeutic, and prognostic implications.

Focal seizures and syndromes—conditions in which certain areas of the brain are involved in the epileptic event.

Idiopathic epilepsy syndrome—when there is no underlying structural brain lesions or other neurological condition to explain the condition. These types of epilepsies are presumed to be genetic. This type of epilepsy is seen in individuals with developmental disabilities but not as frequently as the symptomatic epilepsies.

Probable symptomatic epilepsy syndrome—term used when an organic etiology is suspected but cannot be demonstrated. The word criptogenic was used to refer to this condition in the past.

Reflex epilepsy syndrome—when all epileptic seizures are precipitated by sensory stimulation.

Simple and complex partial epileptic seizures—terms applied to conditions that originate in focal areas of the brain. There might be associated loss of consciousness (complex) or not (simple). These terms were used for many years, but the use of them is no longer recommended.

Symptomatic epilepsy syndrome—cases in which the epileptic disorder is the result of structural lesions of the brain. This type of syndrome is the most commonly observed in individuals with developmental disabilities.

From Blume, W.T., Luders, H.D., Mizrahi, E., Tassinari, C.A., van Emde Boas, W., & Engel, J. (2001). Glossary of descriptive terminology for ictal semiology. *Epilepsia, 42*(9), 1212–1218; adapted by permission of the International League Against Epilepsy.

Table 12.2-3. Epileptic seizure types

Self limited seizure types
Generalized seizures
- Tonic-clonic seizures
- Clonic seizures
- Typical absence seizures
- Atypical absence seizures
- Myoclonic absence seizures
- Tonic seizures
- Spasms
- Myoclonic seizures
- Eyelid myoclonias
- Myoclonic atonic seizures
- Negative myoclonus
- Atonic seizures
- Reflex seizures in generalized epilepsy syndromes

Focal seizures
- Focal sensory seizures
- Focal motor seizures
- Gelastic seizures
- Hemiclonic seizures
- Secondarily generalized seizures
- Reflex seizures in focal epilepsy syndromes

Continuous seizure types
Generalized status epilepticus
- Generalized tonic-clonic status epilepticus
- Clonic status epilepticus
- Absence status epilepticus
- Tonic status epilepticus
- Myoclonic status epilepticus

Focal status epilepticus
- Epilepsia partialis continua of Kojelnikov
- Aura continua
- Limbic status epilepticus
- Hemiconvulsive status with hemiparesis

Note: The term *focal* does not mean the epileptogenic region is a small, well-delineated focus of neuronal pathology; focal seizures, as well as focal syndromes, are almost always due to diffuse, and at times widespread, areas of cerebral dysfunction.

From Blume, W.T., Luders, H.D., Mizrahi, E., Tassinari, C.A., van Emde Boas, W., & Engel, J. (2001). Glossary of descriptive terminology for ictal semiology. *Epilepsia, 42*(9), 1212–1218; adapted by permission of the International League Against Epilepsy.

Table 12.2-4. Description of seizures

The epileptic seizure event often consists of two or more phenomena occurring simultaneously or sequentially and should be described accordingly

Astatic—loss of erect posture that results from an atonic, myoclonic, or tonic mechanism. This seizure is also called a drop attack and is frequently seen in persons with Lennox-Gastaut Syndrome. It is responsible for many accidental injuries.

Atonic—sudden loss or diminution of muscle tone lasting 1–2 s or more, involving head, trunk, jaw, or limb musculature.

Atypical absences—onset and termination of the impairment of consciousness is not as abrupt as in typical absences, and changes in tone are more pronounced. These seizures occur mostly in the context of more severe forms of epilepsies and frequently in association with other types, such as atonic, tonic, and myoclonic seizures.

Aura—a subjective ictal phenomenon that, in a given individual, may precede an observable seizure. If this phenomenon is not followed by an observable seizure, it constitutes a sensory seizure.

Clonic—myoclonus that is regularly repetitive, involving the same muscle groups, at a frequency of about 2–3 c/s, and is prolonged.

Dystonic—Sustained contractions of both agonist and antagonist muscles producing athetoid or twisting movements, which when prolonged may produce abnormal postures.

Epileptic spasm—a sudden flexion, extension, or mixed extension-flexion of predominantly proximal and truncal muscles that is usually more sustained than a myoclonic movement but not as sustained as a tonic seizure (i.e., about 1 s). These seizures are typically observed in infantile spasm syndrome.

Generalized tonic-clonic seizure—bilateral symmetrical tonic contraction then bilateral clonic contractions of somatic muscles. This seizure is usually associated with autonomic phenomena and is also known as a "grand mal" seizure.

Jacksonian march—traditional term indicating spread of clonic movements through contiguous body parts unilaterally.

Myoclonic—sudden, brief (< 100 ms) involuntary single or multiple contraction(s) of muscles(s) or muscle groups of variable topography (axial, proximal limb, distal).

Reflex seizure—seizure evoked by a specific afferent stimulus or by an activity. Afferent stimuli can be elementary (unstructured; e.g., light flashes, startle, a monotone) or elaborate (structured; e.g., a symphony). A preceding activity may be 1) elementary (motor), such as a movement; 2) elaborate (cognitive), such as reading or chess playing; or 3) both, such as reading aloud.

Tonic—a sustained increase in muscle contraction lasting a few seconds to minutes.

Tonic-clonic—a sequence consisting of a tonic followed by a clonic phase. Variants such as clonic-tonic-clonic may be seen.

Typical absences—brief impairment of consciousness of sudden onset and termination. In most instances, the absences are associated with other subtle symptoms such as eye blinking, myoclonic jerkings, changes in muscle tone, and automatism.

Versive—A sustained, forced conjugate ocular, cephalic, and/or truncal rotation or lateral deviation from the midline.

From Blume, W.T., Luders, H.D., Mizrahi, E., Tassinari, C.A., van Emde Boas, W., & Engel, J. (2001). Glossary of descriptive terminology for ictal semiology. *Epilepsia, 42*(9), 1212–1218; adapted by permission of the International League Against Epilepsy.

(AEDs). Also, these individuals are more likely to develop intractable seizures.

Infantile Spasms

Certain syndromes such as infantile spasms (West syndrome) and the Lennox-Gastaut syndrome (LGS) are more frequent in individuals with intellectual disabilities. Infantile spasms is an age-specific syndrome. In most children, the first signs are seen at 4–6 months, and spasms rarely begin after 18 months. Some seizures are characterized by brief head nods; however, the more common ones are brief generalized tonic seizures involving both arms and legs. The spasms are usually seen in clusters. The electroencephalogram (EEG) has a distinctive pattern: hypsarrhythmia, which is characterized by poorly organized background activities; frequent generalized discharges of spikes; polyspikes; and spike and slow waves complexes. There are also frequent episodes of attenuation with almost total suppression of the EEG activity.

Besides the seizures, most of the infants with infantile spasms have developmental delays, even if their development was normal before having seizures. Aggressive treatment is recommended; some recent research suggests that seizures in early life, by themselves, may produce more brain damage. Around 50% of children with infantile spasms developed LGS (Trevathan, 2002). The best treatment for infantile spasms still is controversial. Main therapies for the control of the seizures

Table 12.2-5. Common recognized epileptic syndromes

Benign familial neonatal seizures
Early myoclonic encephalopathy
Ohtahara syndrome
West syndrome (infantile spasms)
Bening myoclonic epilepsy of infancy
Dravet's syndrome
Benign chidlhood epilepsy with centrotemporal spikes
Early onset benign childhood occipital epilepsy (Panayatopoulus type)
Late onset childhood occipital epilepsy (Gastaut type)
Epilepsy with myclonic absence
Epilepsy with myoclonic-astatic seizures
Lennox-Gastaut syndrome (LGS)
Landau-Kleffner syndrome (LKS)
Epilepsy with continuous spike-and-wave during slow-wave sleep (other than LKS)
Childhood absence epilepsy
Progressive myoclonus epilepsies
Idiopathic generalized epilepsies with variable phenotypes
Juvenile absence epilepsy
Juvenile myoclonic epilepsy
Epilepsy with generalized tonic-clonic seizures only
Reflex epilepsies
Autosomal dominant nocturnal frontal lobe epilepsy
Familial temporal lobe epilepsies
Symptomatic (or probably symptomatic) focal epilepsies
Limbic epilepsies
Mesial temporal lobe epilepsy with hippocampal sclerosis
Mesial temporal lobe epilepsy defined by specific etiologies
Other types defined by location and etiology
Neocortical epilepsies
Rasmussen syndrome
Other types defined by location and etiology

From Blume, W.T., Luders, H.D., Mizrahi, E., Tassinari, C.A., van Emde Boas, W., & Engel, J. (2001). Glossary of descriptive terminology for ictal semiology. *Epilepsia, 42*(9), 1212–1218; adapted by permission of the International League Against Epilepsy.

are adrenocorticotropic hormones (ACTH), steroids, valproic acid, vigabatrine (especially for children with tuberous sclerosis), topiramate, and lamotrigine. In a few instances, surgery may be an option.

Dennis was born after a normal pregnancy and delivery. At birth, he was diagnosed with craniosinostosis in the coronal and sagittal sutures. He had corrective surgery at the age of 6 weeks. Two weeks after the surgery, he developed infantile spasms. At that time, he had jackknife seizures, with forward flexion of the torso and tonic stiffening of the body lasting a few seconds. Hundreds of these seizures were observed per day. He was initially treated with ACTH/prednisone. The seizures improved; however, he developed hypertension, and the steroids were discontinued. Eventually, the infantile spasm subsided, but he developed generalized tonic, generalized tonic-clonic, and myoclonic seizures.

Through the years, Dennis tried different combinations of carbamazepine, valproic acid, phenytoin, felbamate, vigabatrine, clorazepate, topiramate, and ketogenic diet with minimal or no effect on the epileptic seizures. EEGs were consistently abnormal due to the presence of multifocal epileptiform discharges and generalized voltage attenuation. Because of his poor response to the AEDs, Dennis had a vagal nerve stimulator implanted at the age of 6 with minimal response.

At the age of 11 years, Dennis was admitted to a local hospital for somnolence and seizures. The EEG on admission showed frequent epileptiform discharges. The somnolence improved when clorazepate was discontinued. He was discharged with a combination of levetiracetam 1,000 mg/D; phenobarbital 105 mg/D, and lamotrigine 200 mg/D With these medications, Dennis still has short-lasting generalized tonic seizures every day.

Lennox-Gastaut Syndrome

Approximately 1%–4% of childhood epilepsies and 10% of the cases of epilepsy starting in the first 5 years of life belong to the epileptic syndrome of childhood epileptic encephalopathy with diffused slow spike and waves (i.e., LGS) (Trevathan, 2002). Because the remittance rate is small, LGS is common in adults with brain damage. This syndrome is characterized by the presence of slow spike waves and poorly organized background activities in the EEG. The EEG abnormalities are often multifocal. Multiple seizure types characterize the clinical activity; the most frequent being akinetic-atonic seizures (drop attacks), myoclonic seizures, atypical absences, and generalized tonic seizures. Tonic-clonic seizures as well as status epilepticus are not unusual. The epileptic activity is usually activated by sleep, which shows bursts of generalized spikes frequently associated with generalized tonic seizures.

The first manifestations of the syndrome are seen in children age 1–8 years. Usually, these children have developmental delays. The drop attacks may lead to falls and frequent accidents. Aggressive attempts to control the seizures with high doses of AEDs or with polytherapy may lead to cognitive side effects. Somnolence, a common side effect of AED, may lead to more seizures. In association with the seizures, children with LGS also have cognitive impairments, challenging behavior, and different degrees of cerebral palsy.

Lucas is a 50 year-old man with moderate to severe intellectual disabilities, developmental delays, and spastic quadriparesis. He was able to walk independently but experienced deterioration in his gait at age 36. He now moves using a wheelchair. Lucas had his first seizure at the age of 10 months—a generalized tonic-clonic seizure lasting for 1 hour. He now has many types of seizures at least every 2 days, and seizures have been observed both while he is asleep and while he is awake. His EEG showed spike and slow wave complexes, isolated spikes and waves, and bursts of polyspikes. Both the EEG and the clinical pictures are suggestive of LGS.

Lucas has been on many AEDs through the years with some improvement in the frequency and the type of seizures but never with full control. Valproic acid was very effective in reducing the number of akinetic-atonic seizures. It also reduced the myoclonic seizures; however, Lucas still has frequent generalized tonic and tonic-clonic seizures. Episodes of severe status epilepticus decreased in frequency and intensity after the introduction of valproic acid. At the present time, he is on valproic acid 3,500 mg/D, phenytoin 330 mg/D, and topiramate 400 mg/D With these medications, the seizures have been reduced to one generalized tonic-clonic seizure every 3–4 days.

LGS is relatively frequent in individuals with intellectual disabilities and is very difficult to treat. In most instances, individuals need to be on AEDs for the rest of their lives and may be overmedicated because the seizures are frequent and often life threatening. Sudden falls during akinetic seizures frequently cause facial injuries. Some devices, such as helmets, may help to protect from injuries. Some of the new AEDs have been useful in this condition (De Los Reyes, Sharp, Williams, & Hale, 2004; Kelly, Stephen, & Brodie, 2004).

EPILEPSY AND NEUROCUTANEOUS SYNDROMES

Eighty percent or more of individuals with tuberous sclerosis experience epileptic seizures, and more than 60% of children with this syndrome have intellectual disabilities. (Gomez, 1988; Maria, Deidrick, Roach, & Gutmann, 2004; Pampiglione & Pugh, 1975; see also Chapter 9.7) The most common clinical presentation of seizures in tuberous sclerosis is infantile spasms. Other types of seizures, such as generalized tonic-clonic, atypical absences, and focal seizures, are also seen. The prognosis is better when seizures start after the second year of life, when infantile spasms are not seen, and when complex partial and secondary generalized seizures are predominant (Curatolo, Cusmai, Cortesi, Chiron, Jambaque, & Dulac, 1991; Jambaque, Cusmai, Curatolo, Cortesi, Perrot, & Dulac, 1991).

EEGs for individuals with tuberous sclerosis and infantile spasms show epileptiform discharges in most instances and slowing in a minority. The epileptic discharges are of the multifocal type, focal with temporal lobe predominance, hypsarrhythmia, and generalized spike and wave. Surgery is an option to be considered for individuals with persistent focal seizures resistant to medications (Maria et al., 2004; Romanelli, Verdecchia, Rodas, Seri, & Curatolo, 2004). Bebin and Gomez (1998) found a marked improvement and even total control of the seizures in 8 out of 9 individuals who underwent surgery.

Epileptic seizures are seen in 70% of children with Sturge-Weber syndrome in the first year of life, most frequently contralateral focal motor seizures that may or may not be followed by generalized seizures. EEGs show spike and wave abnormalities. The prognosis varies; as many as 50% may go into remission or have the number and the intensity of the seizures improve with medication. Surgery, either hemispherectomy or focal resections, is indicated in those individuals resistant to medication. One study showed that 13 of 20 individuals with Sturge-Weber syndrome, followed for at least 4 years after surgery, became seizure free (Arzimanoglou et al., 2000). In children with hemiparesis, hemispherectomy was particularly effective.

Three to five percent of individuals with Neurofibromatosis I have epilepsy, usually mild. Because epilepsy is not frequent, the presence of a convulsive disorder in these individuals requires a complete evaluation to rule out intracranial tumors (Rubinstein & Korinthenberg, 1990).

EPILEPSY IN THE CONTEXT OF SPECIFIC DISORDERS

Even though *neuronal migration disorders* are rare, they are frequently seen among individuals with epilepsy and developmental disorders, mostly in those instances when the epileptic disorder is resistant to AEDs.

Children with *congenital bilateral perysilvian syndrome* experience typical and atypical absences, atonic, and generalized tonic and tonic-clonic seizures. In general, the seizures are resistant to AEDs, and, in some instances, improvement was observed after splitting the corpus callosum (Kuzniecky, Andermann, & Guerrini, 1993).

The *syndrome of double cortex* consists in the presence of a heterotopic band of gray matter under the cortex. Most of these individuals have intellectual disabilities and epilepsy, which are related to the severity of the malformation. The epileptic disorder may be resistant to AEDs and is characterized by hypsarrhythmia, LGS, or focal or generalized seizures. Callosotomy may be useful for the treatment of atonic-akinetic seizures (Palmini et al., 1991).

Epilepsy has been reported in 14% of children with *pervasive developmental disorder* or *autism*, and the incidence may increase up to one third by the time the children reach adolescence (Pavone et al., 2004; Rapin, & Katzman, 1998; see Chapter 23.1). The presence of severe intellectual disabilities and/or motor impairments increases the incidence of epilepsy (Tuchman, Rapin, & Shinnar, 1991; Pavone et al., 2004). Approximately one third of individuals with autism experience a regression in language and socialization skills in the second year of life, which, in a small number of individuals, is associated with the development of epilepsy or EEG abnormalities (Hrdlicka et al., 2004). Some children improve after treatment with steroids and/or AEDs (Rapin & Katzman, 1998). Whether these subtle epileptic disorders originate in the amygdala, hippocampus, or cerebral cortex is unknown.

During childhood, many individuals with *fragile X syndrome* develop an epileptic syndrome characterized by focal epileptic seizures with clinical and EEG features very similar to the Benign Rolandic epilepsy (see Chapter 9.3). These seizures remit in adulthood (Montero, Puig, Toral, Martinez, & Rato, 1995; Musumeci et al., 1991). Epileptic seizures have been reported in 30%–80% of girls with *Rett syndrome* (see Chapter 9.1). The first epileptic crises are seen between 30 and 53 months and rarely after the age of 10 years. Seizures could be generalized tonic, tonic-clonic, focal, or myoclonic. In some cases, photic-induced seizures have occurred (Nieto-Barrera et al., 1999). EEG findings show poor background activity, and epileptiform activity is characterized by spike and slow spike and wave activity. Given the frequency of stereotyped behaviors in many girls with Rett syndrome, it is difficult to differentiate epileptic seizures from nonepileptic events. Medications such as carbamazepine, sodium valproate, topiramate, and lamotrigine are effective in the treatment of the seizure disorder. The repiratory dysrhythmia may also improve with topiramate (Goyal, O'Riordan, Wiznitzer, 2004).

Children with *Angelman syndrome* may also have epilepsy (see Chapter 9.6). Epileptic disorder is much more severe in individuals with class I type Angelman syndrome. Most of these children present with epileptic seizures before age 3 that may be resistant to medications. EEGs present runs of high-voltage spike and slow wave complexes as well as rhythmic theta activity in wide areas. The discharges might be facilitated by eye closure. Different seizure types that occur include atypical absences and LGS. EEG abnormalities may persist even when the seizures are well controlled. Valproic acid, benzodiazepines, and ethosuximide might be more effective than other AEDs. The presence of a trembling movement disorder can be mistaken for myoclonic seizures and can result in unnecessary medication and toxicity.

In the absence of other congenital malformations, epilepsy is not an important medical problem in children with *Down syndrome*, even in those with profound intellectual disabilities (see Chapter 9.2). Children with Down syndrome, however, experience infantile spasm–like disorders in early life that arrest. Epileptic seizures, generalized tonic-clonic, and myoclonic seizures are frequently seen in adults with Down syndrome concomitant with Alzheimer disease.

Landau-Kleffner syndrome (acquired epileptic aphasia) is seen in healthy children who acutely or progressively lose receptive and expressive language skills. In some of them, the aphasia coincides with the beginning of an epileptic disorder. In the progression of the disorder, children also developed cognitive impairment. This syndrome can be confused with pervasive developmental disorder. There is no specific treatment, and the disorder arrests at one point, but usually the children are left with sequelae.

An estimated 10%–60% of individuals with developmental disabilities have *psychiatric disorders*, and many of these individuals also have epilepsy (Kanner, 2002; Espie et al., 2003). Whether the presence of epileptic seizures is a predisposing factor for the comorbid psychiatric condition is unclear. Any AED can produce somnolence and depression when used in high doses, and there have been reports of serious behavior changes with gabapentin, lamotrigine, barbiturates, vigabatrine, and topiramate, among others, when taken at the recommended dose. Similarly, most psychotropic medications can induce seizure disorders in individuals who do not have epilepsy. The risk of epileptic seizures is related to several factors, including the total dose of the medication, rapid titration, the presence of central nervous system abnormalities, and the concomitant use of other proconvulsant drugs.

DIAGNOSIS

Diagnosing epilepsy in individuals with intellectual disabilities presents several difficulties. Obtaining valid information from individuals with moderate to severe intellectual disabilities is typically not possible. In a few instances, trained professionals might see the epileptic crisis; however, most often relatives, teachers, and caregivers, who are usually not familiar with epileptic disorders, are more likely to be present during an attack and are the main source of information. Educating these individuals in the recognition and description of epileptic disorders is very important (Mayville & Matson, 2004). The descriptions of seizures presented in Table 12.2-4 are very useful for this purpose.

Individuals with intellectual disabilities also have a high incidence of movement disorders, behavior disorders, and/or psychiatric disorders that may resemble epileptic seizures. For example, children with generalized spasticity may present generalized tonic crisis resembling seizures as a result of massive reflex reactions secondary to bladder distension, constipation, or pain. Frequently, individuals with intellectual disabilities look "absent," do not respond, or are slow to respond to stimulation. These episodes are frequently confused with absence seizures or with complex partial seizures. Sudden episodes of self-injurious behavior or aggression toward others are frequently confused with epileptic disorders originated in the temporal or frontal lobes.

Psychiatric medications, even when properly used, may induce abnormal movements that may resemble epileptic disorders. Withdrawal reactions can be seen when an individual refuses to take medications or when medications are discontinued. They may consist of behavioral changes, hallucinations, and muscle contractions (chorea or tic-like) that resemble myoclonic epilepsy or generalized tonic seizures. In addition, taking excess medication may be associated with an absent look.

Gastroesophageal reflux may result in generalized tonic extension of extremities and bending of the trunk (Sandifer syndrome), which may or may not be related to meals. The tonic crisis may be very difficult to differentiate from generalized tonic convulsions.

Few studies address the issue of the differential diagnosis between epileptic seizures and nonepileptic behaviors (pseudoseizures) in individuals with intellectual disabilities (Holmes, McKeever, & Russman, 1983; Neill & Alvarez, 1986). Approximately 20% of individuals with intellectual disabilities referred for epilepsy have had nonepileptic events. Episodes of absences, temper tantrums, and myoclonus are the most frequent nonepileptic events. Many individuals also have both epileptic and nonepileptic events. Nonepileptic events should be ruled out in any individuals with seizures resistant to AEDs, mostly if the behaviors do not fit into recognizable epileptic seizures.

Obtaining a good medical history is very important in these situations. Signs that can be elicited through the medical history and that may help to suspect the nonepileptic nature of the event include 1) the presence of precipitants; 2) the presence of very complex and prolonged motor activity (e.g., throwing chairs or objects with good coordination and aim); 3) the individual looking upset but not confused; 4) a rapid return to normalcy, without any period of confusion, mostly after long complex seizures; and 5) similar behaviors observed when the individual is not seizing. The presence of serious behavior disorders of epileptic origin in the absence of other sign of epileptic seizures is unusual but possible.

Routine Electroencephalograms

Diagnostic methods include routine and long-term EEGs and neuroimaging of the central nervous system. EEGs, combined with the clinical history, are still at the core of the diagnosis of epilepsy. A routine EEG is obtained as an outpatient procedure. In a few exceptions, admission to the hospital may be necessary. The EEG is a noninvasive procedure; however, most individuals with intellectual disabilities may need presedation plus sleep deprivation to obtain a complete recording. Even though EEG is the leading technique for the diagnosis of epilepsy, it can have false positives as well as false negative results. For that reason, the recording should be obtained and interpreted by qualified personnel. EEGs should be obtained while the individual is awake, drowsy, and sleeping. Whenever possible photic stimulation and hyperventilation should be obtained.

The routine EEG is relatively brief, lasting approximately 45 minutes to 1 hour. In most instances, the EEG is obtained in the interictal state while the individual is not having seizures. In few instances, the individual will have the clinical event during the recording. Even though clinical events are not observed, the presence of certain EEG patterns is suggestive of low seizure threshold. Interictal abnormalities may be enough in many instances to document the diagnosis and treat the individual; however, the diagnostic value of the EEG obtained at the time of the seizures is far superior. The presence of false negatives requires that the EEG be repeated when there is strong suspicion of epilepsy; however, having more than two normal EEGs in a suspicious case of epilepsy most likely indicates that the individual does not have epileptic seizures.

The EEG is also helpful when deciding what medication to select. For example, in the presence of generalized 3 cycles per second spike and wave discharges (the typical EEG in absence seizures), ethosuximide or valproic acid may be the medication of choice. EEGs with clear focal seizures are suggestive of a focal pathology; these individuals deserve a presurgical evaluation. Medications such as carbamazepine, valproic acid, and topiramate may be good choices in these cases.

Long-Term Electroencephalograms

Due to the short recording time of routine EEGs—usually no more than 1 hour—recording a clinical event is unusual. In addition, repeated interictal EEGs may be normal in individuals with epilepsy because electrodes in the scalp may not be good enough to record epileptiform activity originating in the deepest areas of the brain (e.g., amygdala, mesial frontal lobe areas).

EEGs may show nonspecific paroxysmal activities during hyperventilation, for example, or benign EEG variants that may be confused with epileptic activity. Several techniques have been developed to avoid the shortcomings of the routine EEG. They all require long-term EEG recording that may or may not be simultaneously obtained with video recordings. In some instances, individuals need to be admitted to a special unit for several days.

Long-term monitoring is time consuming, more expensive, and more disruptive of everyday activities than routine EEGs and, therefore, should be used in special circumstances. It is indicated in individuals with intractable seizures when nonepileptic events are suspected or when these individuals are considered for surgery. Long-term recording techniques are also useful for the quantification of seizures, the evaluation of triggers that may induce seizures, and the definition of seizure disorders. For example, individuals with grand mal seizures upon awakening or with juvenile myoclonic epilepsy present EEG abnormalities characterized by generalized spike and wave discharges activated by arousal after sleeping.

Cassette ambulatory EEG recording can be performed for several days. The individual carries a cassette that records a continuous EEG 24 hours a day. It has the advantage of recording the individual during routine activities and can be combined with video recording; however, because the individual is involved in his or her usual activities, video recording may not be practical. Individuals (or someone else) need to keep a log of the time in which clinical events are suspected. The recorders have an input signal that can be activated at the time of the suspicious events.

Video and simultaneous EEG recording offers the best option for the diagnosis of epilepsy. This procedure can be done as a short outpatient evaluation or the individual can be admitted to a special unit for several days of continuous monitoring. Digital equipment makes it easy to review many hours of recording. Video and simultaneous EEG recording facilitates the correlation between behaviors and EEG changes. This type of evaluation is indicated in every person with intractable seizures, especially when nonepileptic events are suspected. Long-term monitoring is almost always indicated prior to epilepsy surgery. In some cases, extracranial evaluation alone may be enough to localize the lesion responsible for the epileptic seizures.

Intracranial EEG recording is a very specialized technique indicated only in those individuals who are candidates for surgery and in whom the focal lesion could not be determined by the use of less-invasive methods. This method is different from the EEG techniques already discussed because the electrodes are placed inside the cranium in contact with the meninges or are positioned using special needles that are inserted directly in the brain tissue.

Neuroimaging of the Central Nervous System

The introduction of computerized axial tomography (CAT) scan and MRI techniques led to a dramatic improvement in the diagnosis of organic lesions in the central nervous system. These techniques were specifically beneficial for individuals with intellectual disabilities and epilepsy. In general, a conventional MRI or CAT scan is the minimum test to request for individuals with new onset seizure disorder. For individuals with seizures resistant to AEDs, more complex tests can be performed. Neuroimaging studies are very important in the identification of epileptic lesions that can be treated surgically. In many instances, the evaluation will show congenital lesions that may not be surgical, and it is not unusual to have normal neuroimaging studies even in individuals with profound intellectual disabilities.

The use of CAT scan is rather limited mostly because the MRI has a higher yield in terms of detecting brain abnormalities (Bronen et al., 1996). Conventional MRI is a very sensitive and specific test for the diagnosis of most of the structural lesions that are associated with developmental disabilities. Neuronal migration disorders, tumors, venous and arterial malformations, and hydrocephalus are some of the conditions in which MRI can be particularly useful. New advances in MRI technology allow for noninvasive vascular imaging. Magnetic resonance angiography and magnetic resonance venography are techniques that are particularly useful in the evaluation of vascular malformations, aneurysm, and intracranial dural venous thrombosis.

Positron emission tomography (PET) generates images using a radioactive tracer (i.e., fluorodeoxyglucose), which is taken up by the brain in proportion of the metabolic activity. Areas of the brain that are damaged take less glucose whereas the focal areas that result in seizure activity are hyperactive after an ictal event. PET scanning is more useful in temporal lobe epilepsy. It is not specific of any particular etiology because areas of poor metabolism are seen in many destructive pathologies of the brain.

Single photon emission computed tomography (SPECT) uses a radioactive tracer that is directly related to blood flow. The blood flow of a particular region of the brain is related to the metabolic demands of the region. When the individual is given the tracer near the time of the seizure, SPECT scanning helps to localize the epileptogenic area.

Magnetoelectroencephalography

Magnetoelectroencephalography (MEG) is the mapping of the magnetic activity produced by the brain. This technique is not as frequently used as the EEG. Some of the information provided by MEG is similar to the information provided by the EEG, but in some cases, it may provide better localizing information than the EEG.

THERAPEUTIC INDICATIONS

Unless the first event is a status epilepticus, starting treatment with AEDs after the first epileptic seizure is not necessary. In many children with normal neurological examination, unprovoked attacks are not followed by more seizures; however, the incidence of recurrence is higher in individuals with brain damage (Annegers, Shirts, Hauser, & Kurland, 1986). Most neurologists will recommend treatment after the second seizure. The ultimate goal is to use the least possible amount of medication to avoid side effects.

When medications are indicated, starting with one medication in a dose that is one third to one half of the total dose and increasing the medication slowly until the appropriate dose is reached is recommended. This approach limits the intensity and the frequency of the side effects. If the first medication chosen fails, then a second medication is added. If this medication proves to be effective, then the first medication should be discontinued. Otherwise, the added medication is changed for another one. The simultaneous use of more than two AEDs is, in general, not indicated. It is associated with improvement of seizure control in a few cases; however, the possibility of side effects increases with the number of AEDs. Studies performed in individuals with intellectual disabilities showed that in most instances polypharmacy is not necessary (Alvarez, 1989; Sivenius, Savolainen, Kaski, & Riekkinen, 1990), and in many individuals, seizure freedom can be achieved without unacceptable toxicity (Kelly et al., 2004).

Few prospective studies address the issue of how long antiepileptic treatment should be maintained. This author's personal experience is that it is possible to discontinue AEDs in certain individuals. In a group of 50 adults with brain damage and intellectual disabilities who completed a period of 2 years or more without any documented clinical seizure, the AEDs were slowly discontinued, and the individuals were followed for 8 years (Alvarez, 1989; Alvarez & Hazlett, 1983). At the end of the follow-up, 24 individuals remained seizure free. Seizures recurred in 11 individuals while the medications were in the process of being discontinued, and, in another 14, after the medications were completely discontinued.

Predictors of a seizure-free status at the end of 8 years of follow-up were: few documented seizures in lifetime, no gross neurological abnormalities, medication below therapeutic levels at time of discontinuance, and persistent normal EEGs before and after discontinuance of the medications. Recurrences were more frequent in those individuals with more severe degrees of intellectual disabilities and motor impairments and in those with persistent abnormalities in their EEGs. Similar findings were reported in a group of 65 children with cerebral palsy in whom the AED was discontinued after a 2-year seizure-free period. After 2 years of follow-up, there were recurrences in 41% of the children. In relation to the type of cerebral palsy, 61% of children with spastic hemiparesis and only 14% of children with diplegia showed recurrences (Delgado, Riela, Mills, Pitt, & Browne, 1996).

These studies showed that it is possible to identify groups of individuals in whom AEDs can successfully be decreased and even discontinued. In general, epileptic seizures will be controlled in most individuals with the available AEDs; however, approximately 20%–30% of children and adults will be resistant to drug treatment. This percentage can even be higher in individuals with multiple disabilities. In these individuals, surgery as well as vagal nerve stimulation are options to be considered (Bjornaes, Stabell, Heminghyt, Roste, & Bakke, 2004).

ANTIEPILEPTIC DRUGS

Several types of AEDs are available. Table 12.2-6 lists AEDs as well as their common side effects, drug-to-drug interactions, and relevant information. Table 12.2-7 provides guidelines on doses. (*Note:* Because doses change over time, verify doses before administering medication.) This section provides indications for specific AED use; however, there are no well-established guidelines for choosing one medication over another. Knowledge about the type of seizure, comorbidities, and prior toxicity are important in deciding what medication to use (Helmers & LaRoche, 2004a, 2004b).

New antiepileptic drugs have been introduced in the last few years, and several studies have shown that

Table 12.2-6. Antiepileptic drugs and their side effects and interactions

Drug	Common side effects	Common drug-to-drug interactions	Other relevant information
Benzodiazepines	Sedation, drowsiness, ataxia, cognitive impairment, increased oral secretions	Increases sedative effect when used in combination with other drugs with central nervous system depressant effect	Possible withdrawal seizures with sudden withdrawal of the medications
Carbamazepine (Tegretol, Tegretol-XR, Carbatrol)	Vertigo, ataxia, diplopia, drowsiness, skin reactions, hyponatremia	Induces its own metabolism and the metabolism of other drugs metabolized in the liver; do not coadminister with monoamine oxidase inhibitors.	Contraindicated in individuals with bone marrow depression
Ethosuximide (Zarontin)	Sedation, dizziness, anorexia, nausea, vomiting	Increases ethosuximide clearance in the presence of enzymes inducing drugs	Caution needed when used in individuals with hepatic or renal disease
Felbamate (Felbatol)	Bone marrow depression, liver toxicity	Inhibits liver enzymes and increases blood levels of phenobarbital, phenytoin; increases blood levels of valproic acid.	Indicated in only a few cases due to the severity of the side effects
Gabapentin (Neurontin)	Sedation, somnolence	Has no interaction with hepatic enzymes; has no interaction with other AEDs.	Might be useful in psychiatric disorders as well as in pain disorders
Lamotrigine (Lamictal)	Serious skin rashes including Steven Johnson syndrome and toxic epidermal necrolysis	Does not alter the protein bounding of other AEDs; is metabolized in the liver and the half life is affected by enzyme inducing drugs; increases the elimination of valproate.	Fewer behavior problems or other side effects with slow titration
Levetiracetam (Keppra)	Somnolence, infection (primarily common cold), dizziness, coordination difficulties, behavior problems	Has no known significant interactions	Majority eliminated unchanged in the urine; reduced dose for individuals with renal impairment.
Oxcarbazepine (Trileptal)	Clinically significant hyponatremia; may interfere with oral contraceptives.	Metabolizes through the P450 system, so drugs that induce this system decrease the plasma concentration of oxcarbazepine.	Neurologial complications more frequent when used in combination with other AEDs
Phenobarbital (Luminal)	Drowsiness, somnolence, reduced cognition, hyperactivity in children	Induces liver enzymes resulting in decreased blood levels of many other medications	Contraindicated in porphyria
Phenytoin (Dilantin)	Drowsiness, sleepiness, ataxia, skin rashes, gum hyperplasia; also irsutism, acne, unusual facial features	Metabolizes in the liver; is an inducer of hepatic metabolism; can reduce the blood levels of other AEDs as well as contraceptives among other drugs.	90% bound to albumin; conditions that lead to hypoalbuminemia increase non-bound fraction and may result in toxicity.
Primidone (Mysoline)	Central nervous system depression; contraindicted in porphyria.	Has similar interactions as phenobarbital	Has phenobarbital as a metabolite
Tiagabine (Gabitril)	Dizziness, somnolence, tremors, poor concentration; more common in polytherapy.	Metabolizes in the liver, so enzyme-inducing drugs accelerate the metabolism and shorten the half life of tiagabine	Rapid onset of action; withdrawal reactions less when slowly reduced; 96% bound to plasma proteins.
Topiramate (Topamax)	Decreased appetite and weight loss, renal stones, cognitive slowing, behavioral effects, glaucoma	May increase the blood levels of phenytoin; may reduce the efficacy of oral contraceptives.	Reduced dosage of 50% for individuals with renal dysfunction

Drug	Common side effects	Common drug-to-drug interactions	Other relevant information
Valproic acid, divalproex sodium (Depakene, Depakote)	Skin reactions, mood and behavior disturbances, thrombocytopenia, polycistic ovarian disease, weight gain	Increases the levels of phenobarbital and lamotrigine; is protein bound so displaced phenytoin can lead to high free-plasma levels and toxicity.	Prolonged coagulation time; better to discontinue before surgical procedures; contraindicated in pregnancy; use with precaution in sexually active women.
Vigabatrin (Sabril)	Risk of irreversible visual field defects, depression, psychosis		
Zonisamide (Zonegran)	Serious skin reactions including Steven Johnson and toxic epidermal necrolysis, increased body temperature (especially on hot days), anorexia, cognitive effects, somnolence	Is not an inducer of liver enzymes, so drugs that induce or inhibit hepatic enzymes decrease or increase the half life of zonisamide	Majority excreted unchanged in the urine; is a sulfonamide; contraindicated in individuals who show reactivity to sulfonamides.

individuals with developmental disabilities might benefit from the use of these drugs. However, a meta-analysis involving long-term use of lamotrigine, gabapentin, and vigabatrin in patients with chronic epilepsy showed a retention rate of less than 40% at the 6-year follow-up, and only 4% of the individuals became seizure free (Wong, Chadwick, Fenwick, Mawer, & Sander, 1999). Also, the mortality, the frequency of the seizure-related injuries, and the admissions to hospitals did not decrease as a result of the new antiepileptic medications evaluated in this study.

Benzodiazepines—diazepam (Valium); clonazepam (Klonopin); lorazepam (Ativan); midazolam (Versed)—are effective in the treatment of several seizure types including myoclonic, absences, and atonic seizures, but with limited use in chronic disorders because of the frequent side effects and the development of tolerance. Diazepam, lorazepam, and midazolam are very effective in the treatment of status epilepticus. Rectal administration of diazepam as well as oral sublingual administration of lorazepam are effective in the case of prolongued or repetitive seizures (Dreifuss et al., 1998).

Carbamazepine (Tegretol, Tegretol XR, Carbatrol) is very effective for the treatment of simple partial, complex partial, and generalized tonic-clonic seizures. It is not the drug of choice for generalized epilepsies and might even increase the number of absence seizures and atonic-akinetic seizures. It is rarely a good choice for LGS.

Gabapentin (Neurontin) is indicated in partial seizures and in generalized tonic-clonic seizures. It is also indicated in neuropathic pain.

Ethosuximide (Zarontin) is effective in the treatment of absence seizures in individuals with primary generalized epilepsy. It is also effective as co-adjuvant in myoclonic and atonic-akinetic seizures.

Felbamate (Felbatol) is effective against different types of seizures, especially in LGS and in intractable partial epilepsy. At the present time, felbamate has been virtually withdrawn from the market because of severe bone marrow depression and liver toxicity that resulted in death in some cases; however, it might be the drug of last resort in some individuals with very resistant seizures.

Lamotrigine (Lamictal) is effective against partial onset and generalized seizures, including LGS (Motte et al., 1997). Several reports suggest positive therapeutic interactions between lamotrigine and valproic acid.

Levetiracetem (Keppra) is effective as add-on therapy in individuals with partial epilepsy. It is also effective in generalized epilepsy.

Oxcarbazepine (Trileptal), used in monotherapy or as an add-on medication, is indicated in the treatment of partial epilepsy with or without secondary generalization. Oxcarbazepine and its active metabolite 10-monohydroxiderivate (MHD) have an antiepileptic activity similar to carbamazepine.

Phenobarbital (Luminal) is effective in generalized tonic-clonic seizures and partial seizures but not in primary generalized epilepsies. It is not effective in myoclonic, akinetic-atonic, myoclonic, or absence seizures. It is used in the treatment of seizures in the neonatal period and in status epilepticus.

Phenytoin (Dilantin) is indicated in the treatment of both simple and complex partial seizures and in generalized tonic-clonic seizures. It is not effective for myoclonic, atonic-akinetic seizures. The parenteral form, phosphenytoin (Cerebyx), is indicated in the treatment of status epilepticus.

Primidone (Mysoline) is closely related to phenobarbital and with almost the same indications except that it may be useful in juvenile myoclonic epilepsy. It is not effective in absence seizures.

Tiagabine (Gabitril) is effective for refractory partial seizures in adults. There are some indications that children may also benefit.

Table 12.2-7. Guidelines for antiepileptic drug dosing.

Drug name	Adult dose		Children's doses	
	Starting	Maintenance	Starting	Maintenance
Carbamazepine	200 mg twice daily	800–1200 mg/d divided three times daily or twice daily if extended release formulation is used	5–10 mg/kg/d divided twice daily	15–45 mg/kg/d divided twice daily to three times daily (depending on age and formulation)
Ethosuximide	500 mg/d divided twice daily	1,000–2,000 mg/d divided twice daily to three times daily	10 mg/kg/d divided twice daily	15–40 mg/kg/d divided twice daily to three times daily
Felbamate	400 mg three times daily	1,200 mg three times daily	15 mg/kg/d divided three times daily	45–60 mg/kg/d divided three times daily
Gabapentin	300 mg three times daily	900–3,600 mg/d divided three times daily	10 mg/kg/d divided twice daily	30–100 mg/kg/d divided three times daily
Levetiracetam	500 mg twice daily	1,500 mg twice daily	10 mg/kg/d divided twice daily	40–60 mg/kg/d divided twice daily
Methsuximide	300 mg/d once daily	600–1,200 mg/d divided twice daily	5–10 mg/kg/d once daily or divided twice daily	10–30 mg/kg/d divided twice daily or three times daily
Oxcarbazepine	300 mg twice daily	1,200 mg twice daily	4–5 mg/kg/d divided twice daily	20–45 mg/kg/d divided twice daily
Phenobarbital	60–90 mg at night	60–120 mg divided once daily or twice daily	2–3 mg/kg/d once daily or divided twice daily	2–6 mg/kg/d divided twice daily
Phenytoin	300 mg/d divided three times daily or twice daily	200–600 mg/d once daily or twice daily	4 mg/kg/d divided twice daily	4–8 mg/kg/d divided twice daily
Primidone	125 mg at night	1,000–1,500 mg/kg/d divided two or three times daily	1–2 mg/kg/d for 4–5 days	5–20 mg/kg/d divided two or three times daily
Tiagabine	4 mg/d	32–56 mg/d divided twice daily or three times daily	0.1 mg/kg/d	0.6–1 mg/d divided three times daily
Topiramate	25–50 mg/d divided twice daily	200–400 mg/d divided twice daily	0.5–1 mg/kg/d divided twice daily or every night	5–9 mg/kg/d divided twice daily
Valproic acid	500–1,000 mg/d divided twice daily	1,000–3,000 mg/d divided twice daily or three times daily	10–15 mg/kg/d divided twice daily	30–60 mg/kg/d divided twice daily or three times daily
Zonisamide	100 mg/d once daily or divided twice daily	200–400 mg/d once daily or divided twice daily	1–2 mg/kg/d once daily or divided twice daily	4–8 mg/kg/d once daily or divided twice daily
	Patients older than 12 years of age		**Children younger than 12 years of age**	
Lamotrigine and enzyme inducing AEDs without valproic acid	50 mg once daily for 2 weeks	300–500 mg/d divided twice daily	0.6 mg/kg/d divided twice daily for 2 weeks	5–15 mg/kg/d divided twice daily
Lamotrigine with valproic acid	25 mg every other day for 2 weeks	100–400 mg/d divided twice daily	0.15 mg/kg/d once daily for 2 weeks	1–5 mg/kg/d divided twice daily

Note: Because doses change over time, verify doses before administering medication.

Topiramate (Topamax) is effective in most seizure types, including LGS. In general, it is considered a safe medication. Cognitive slowing and behavioral changes are the most common cause of discontinuance of the medication.

Valporic acid, divalproex sodium (Depakene, Depakote), is effective against different types of seizures, including both focal and generalized seizures. It is especially useful in the treatment of absence, atonic-akinetic, and myoclonic seizures and is indicted in the treatment of infantile spasms and LGS.

Vigabatrin (Sabril), is not approved in the United States but has been in use since 1989 in many other countries. It is effective as add-on in the treatment of individuals with refractory partial epilepsy. It is also effective in the treatment of infantile spasms.

Zonisamide (Zonegram) is effective for the control of refractory focal epilepsy and also in generalized epilepsy. It has been reported as effective in infantile spasms in progressive myoclonic epilepsies and in juvenile myoclonic epilepsy (Kothare, Khurana, Hardison, & Legido, 2004).

In most individuals receiving AEDs, both the desirable therapeutic effect and toxic effects are related to the amount of medication in the blood. *Therapeutic range* is the range in which the individual should be in order to achieve maximal therapeutic effect with minimal side effects. In clinical practice, great variability among individuals and a rigid approach to the concept of the "therapeutic range" may lead to poor use of AEDs. Using blood levels to determine the "optimal range" (i.e., the level in which seizures are better controlled without side effects) is more useful. Obtaining blood levels of the AED at the time in which the individual is well controlled may serve as a baseline. A common mistake is treating the "blood level" instead of treating the individual. In this situation, physicians obtain blood levels and adjust the medication in an attempt to match a predetermined blood level. Blood levels, however, are indicated when poor compliance is suspected; when individuals are taking multiple medications; when there are indications of toxicity; and when the physician wishes to evaluate potential loss of efficacy.

Sixty-two-year-old Pam was evaluated because of epileptic seizures. She was taking valproic acid 500 mg three times a day; oxcarbazepine 600 mg twice day, and levetiracetam 500 mg twice a day. Pam's neurologist was concerned that Pam was being overmedicated and reviewed her history to find out how she had ended up taking three AEDs.

Pam had a well-documented history of short-lasting epileptic seizures, mostly generalized tonic-clonic, and a few episodes of status epilepticus that required her to be transferred to the emergency room. The first trip to the emergency room happened when Pam experienced a cluster of short seizures consisting of blank stares, unresponsiveness, and twitching of the left side of her face and her left extremities. This cluster of seizures lasted for 1 hour and was controlled with lorazepam. In the emergency room, Pam was started on oxcarbazepine 450 mg twice a day.

Pam had another seizure and a cluster of seizures 2 months later, which were controlled with lorazepam IV. She was febrile at the time, and her workup showed a urinary tract infection. Her blood level of valproic acid at the time was 94 mcg/mL.

Two months later, Pam again had seizures. As before, she was febrile and had a urinary tract infection. In the emergency room, levetiracetam 500 mcg twice a day was added to her therapeutic regime. Three months later, after a short seizure, oxcarbazepine was increased to 600 mg twice a day. Pam continued to have seizures every few months.

Pam had a low seizure threshold and a long-lasting history of well-documented epileptic seizures that were well controlled with one antiepileptic medication with no side effects. The increase in seizures she experienced was associated with febrile episodes. In these circumstances, not much was gained by increasing the AED, except maybe during the acute febrile phase. Oxcarbazepine did not decrease the frequency of the seizures, which recurred with another febrile episode. Adding levetiracetam to the other two medications at this point was not the best choice.

Pam is an example of the risk involved when the care of individuals with epilepsy is fragmented. Emergency room doctors who were not involved in Pam's chronic care added antiepileptic medications to her therapeutic regimen. In this case, it led to unnecessary polypharmacy.

Physical Side Effects In addition to the positive effects, AEDs have many undesirable adverse effects. Some of these side effects are related to the dose of the medication. Measuring blood levels may help; however, dose-related effects are cumulative in individuals taking more than one medication. In these circumstances, the blood level of an individual medication may be misleading because it might not be in the recognized toxic range. In these cases, discontinuance of the AED may not be necessary because adjustment of the dose may be enough. If dose-related side effects are present with doses that are not effectively controlling the seizures, then physicians should consider changing the medication. In most instances, dose-related effects are the result of the depressive effects of these medications on the central nervous system and consist of somnolence, drowsiness, excessive sleep, decreased cognitive abilities, and impairment in motor functions. Some dose-related effects such as decreased blood counts, decreased platelets count, low albumin, and hyponatremia can be detected only through blood tests during routine follow up.

Idiosyncratic reactions are side effects that are not related to the pharmacologic properties of the drug, and, in that sense, they are not predictable. They are not dose dependent but host dependent, and they can be life threatening. These side effects are rare. Skin reactions are the most commonly observed, followed by blood dyscrasias and liver dysfunction. Cutaneous reactions, usually a rash, are mild and improve when the drug is removed. Severe Stevens-Johnson syndrome and toxic epidermal necrosis are the more severe forms of cutaneous idiosyncratic reactions and may require admission to a hospital.

Long-term therapy, as is usually the case with AEDs, can result in toxic effects even if the medications are used in proper doses. For example, phenobarbital and phenytoin may result in cosmetic changes in the face, and phenytoin may produce gum hyperplasia. Osteoporosis and predisposition to fractures have been described with several AEDs. The first reports indicated that phenytoin, phenobarbital, and carbamazepine—all inducers of the P450 system—were associated with decreased bone density; however, this mechanism might not be the only one because valproic acid—an inhibitor of the P450 system—is also associated with decreased bone density. These drugs interfere with the metabolism of vitamin D, and, for that reason, it is recommended that all individuals using these medications receive enough vitamin D and calcium. The effect of the new AEDs on bone metabolism is not known yet (Pack & Morrell, 2004; Sheth, 2004).

Cognitive and Behavioral Side Effects All AEDs exert their therapeutic action through the central nervous system and thus have some effect on behavior. Most information on side effects of new AEDs is from unblinded studies or anecdotal reports; however, when these drugs are indicated in monotherapy within the accepted standards, the cognitive effects are modest. The most recent information is provided next.

Phenobarbital, even in therapeutic doses, can result in hyperactivity. This effect is mostly seen in children with a tendency or prior history of hyperactivity. It can also be seen in adults. Drowsiness, sleepiness, and some degree of slow down in cognitive functions have also been described. The behavioral effects of phenobarbital have been one of the limiting factors in the use of these medications.

The side effects produced by carbamazepine, phenytoin, and valproic acid are modest and found to be very similar among drugs in short- and in long-lasting studies, but they might have a negative impact in the performance of complex tasks.

Psychoses have been described in less than 1% of individuals taking *lamotrigine*. In a group of 37 children with intellectual disabilities and epilepsy, one developed psychosis-like symptoms that improved when lamotrigine was discontinued. Two developed insomnia and/or hyperactivity (Coppola & Pascotto, 1997). Aggressive behavior, irritability, and hyperactivity have also been reported. In some cases, the behavior was severe enough that lamotrigine had to be discontinued (Beran & Gibson, 1998). Other studies did not show any negative impact (Motte et al., 1997) or showed positive behavioral effects with improvement in bipolar disorders, depression, and mania. Improvement in mood and social skills was observed in individuals with LGS. The incidence of negative behavioral effects is higher in individuals with intellectual disabilities.

Adverse behavioral effects have been described when *gabapentin* was added to the therapeutic regime in several children and adults with developmental disabilities and some preexisting behavioral disturbances. The behavioral effects were more frequent in children younger than 10 years and mostly in those who had a baseline attention-deficit/hyperactivity disorder. In general, effects were mild, characterized by irritability, agitation, and aggression, but in some cases the medication had to be discontinued (Mikati et al., 1998). Gabapentin is effective in the treatment of mood disorders and is potentially effective in the treatment of pain. It may be useful in the treatment of some movement disorders such as bruxism and tardive dyskinesia.

A few instances of psychotic episodes and cognitive impairments were reported to have been induced by *topiramate*, with total improvement and return to baseline after the topiramate was discontinued. Some of the side effects may be related to the high doses recommended to initiate the treatment; starting with low doses minimizes side effects. Whether individuals with intellectual disabilities are particularly prone to have more complications is unclear.

Not much information is available on the effect of *tiagabine* in individuals with developmental disabilities. Tiagabine can result in some behavioral changes such as aggression, irritability, and lethargy. Because tiagabine can precipitate nonconvulsive status epilepticus, some of the behavioral disturbances may be the result of nonconvulsive status epilepticus.

The use of *felbamate* is limited because it results in aplastic anemia and severe hepatotoxicity; however, it may be indicated in the treatment of the LGS. In this particular syndrome, felbamate resulted in behavioral improvement, but whether the improvement is due to a pure behavioral effect or due to the improvement in seizure activity is uncertain.

A few instances of psychosis and depression are related to *zonisamide* use, although not much information is available regarding behavior problems in individuals with developmental disabilities. Behavior problems are more frequent in individuals with developmental disabilities taking *levetiracetam* (Brodtkorb, Kless, Nakken, Lossius, & Johannessen, 2004). In a small study involving four children with cognitive impairments and in some cases behavior problems, levetiracetam induced a reversible psychotic disorder.

SURGERY

The surgical treatment of epileptic seizures should be considered in any person with seizures resistant to AEDs. The presence of intellectual disabilities, even though it presents a special challenge, is not a contraindication for surgery when this is indicated. In general, when two or more appropriate AEDs are tried alone or in combination and have not resulted in good control of the seizures, surgery should be considered. The goal of the surgery is to reach a seizure-free condition or at least an important reduction of the number or the severity of the epileptic seizures.

When surgery is considered, the individual should go through a complete reevalution of the seizure disorder. Of most importance is to document without doubt the presence and the type of seizures. This procedure might be challenging in individuals with developmental disabilities who experience many nonepileptic events such as behavior problems, stereotyped behaviors, and abnormalities of muscle tone that may be confused with epileptic seizures. The evaluation would also include EEG with video monitoring, MRI with special techniques to localized potential lesions, and possibly PET and SPECT scanning.

The best candidates for surgery are those with focal lesions whereas those with diffuse or multifocal epileptogenic areas are the less desirable candidates. In most instances, individuals with developmental disabilities have more than one epileptogenic area and are not good candidates for surgery. In selected cases, surgery is a good option for the treatment of epilepsy in individuals with brain damage (Bjornaes et al., 2004).

Hemispherectomy have been practiced with good results in children with severe epileptic disorders and Sturge-Weber syndrome limited to one hemisphere, or children with congenital hemiparesis due to focal lesions. Removal of tubers has been indicated in children and adults with tuberous sclerosis. Even when several tubers are present, one of them might be responsible for the epileptic seizures; in that case, removal of the active lesion might be enough to improve the epileptic disorder. In some instances of infantile spasms, the seizures are secondary to focal lesions in the cortex (tuberous sclerosis, prenatal ischemic infarction, focal malformations in the cortex) that may be amenable to surgery. Splitting the corpus callosum (callosotomy) has been indicated in some individuals with LGS and frequent drop attacks due to intractable atonic-akinetic seizures.

The presence of intellectual disabilities should not be a contraindication for surgery; however, the ultimate prognosis may be related to the degree of intellectual disabilities, as seen in a group of individuals who had surgery due to temporal lobe epilepsy. In this group, 75% of the individuals with IQ scores between 70%–79% remained seizure free after the surgery, whereas only half of those with IQ scores between 50%–69% were seizure free (Chelene et al., 1998).

VAGAL NERVE STIMULATION

Vagal nerve stimulation (VNS) is a fairly novel treatment that was approved in the United States in 1997 as an adjunctive treatment for medically refractory epilepsy in adults and adolescents older than 12 years. Evidence suggests that this method is also safe and effective in younger children. The system consists of a programmable stimulator that is implanted subcutaneously in the chest. The stimulator is connected through wires to the left vagal nerve, which is electrically stimulated by a magnet activated on command or by a set program. The mechanism of action is not totally clear, but it is speculated that through the vagal nerve the impulses reach higher levels in the brain stem, which leads to the decrease in the number of seizures.

From the therapeutic viewpoint, VNS has a broad spectrum and seems to be effective in a variety of seizure disorders and syndromes. It has proved to be effective in LGS and in other epileptic encephalopathies that are usually resistant to pharmaceutical treatment (Frost et al., 2001). It is particularly useful in the treatment of the akinetic-atonic seizures (drop attacks) that are so common in the LGS. The implantation implies a surgical procedure, which can be done as an outpatient.

Complications and side effects include hoarseness of the voice, cough, shortness of breathe, and paresthesia. Because the stimulation can be preprogrammed and does not require any input from the individual, compliance is always good. The stimulator can be activated at any time if needed and could be useful in shortening long-lasting seizures and preventing status epilepticus. Because activation of the magnet is not associated with drowsiness, seizures can be aborted without this side effect. VNS is not associated with behavior deterioration and may even improve certain behaviors in some individuals. Intellectual disabilities are not a contraindication for this procedure (Gates, Roger, & Frost, 2001; Wilfong, 2002).

CONCLUSION

Individuals with higher degrees of intellectual disabilities tend to have a higher incidence of epilepsy. In some conditions (e.g., some forms of cerebral palsy), epilepsy and intellectual disabilities are strongly associated, whereas in other conditions, they are not. This chapter explains the classification of seizures, as well as diagnosis and treatment of epilepsy. In some instances, individuals may become seizure free. For many individual with intellectual disabilities, however, continued monitoring and medication are necessary to manage epilepsy.

REFERENCES

Alvarez, N. (1989). Discontinuance of antiepileptic medications in patients with developmental disability and diagnosis of epilepsy. *American Journal of Mental Retardation, 93,* 593–599.

Alvarez, N., & Hazlett, J. (1983). Seizure management with minimal medications in institutionalized mentally retarded epileptics. A prospective study. First report after 4½ years of follow up. *Clinical Electroencephalography, 14,* 164–172.

Annegers, J.F., Shirts, S.B., Hauser, W.A., & Kurland, L.T. (1986). Risk of recurrence after an initial unprovoked seizure. *Epilepsia, 27,* 43–50.

Arzimanoglou, A.A., Andermann, F., Aicardi, J., Sainte-Rose, C., Beaulieu, M.A., Villemure, J.G., Olivier, A., & Rasmussen, T. (2000). Sturge-Weber syndrome: Indications and results of surgery in 20 patients. *Neurology, 55,* 1472–1479.

Bebin, E.M., & Gomez, M.R. (1988). Prognosis in Sturge-Weber disease: Comparison of unihemispheric and bihemispheric involvement. *Journal of Child Neurology, 3,* 181–184.

Beran, R.G., & Gibson, R.J. (1998). Aggressive behaviour in intellectually challenged patients with epilepsy treated with lamotrigine. *Epilepsia, 39,* 280–282.

Bjornaes, H., Stabell, K.E., Heminghyt, E., Roste, G.K., & Bakke, S.J. (2004). Resective surgery for intractable focal epilepsy in patients with low IQ: Predictors for seizure control and outcome with respect of seizures and neuropsychological and psychosocial functioning. *Epilepsia, 45,* 131–139.

Blume, W.T., Luders, H.D., Mizrahi, E., Tassinari, C.A., van Emde Boas, W., & Engel, J. (2001). Glossary of descriptive terminology for ictal semiology. *Epilepsia, 42*(9), 1212–1218. Retrieved from http://www.epilepsy.org/ctf

Brodtkorb, E. (1994). The diversity of epilepsy in adults with severe developmental disabilities: Age at seizure onset and other prognostic factors. *Seizure, 3,* 277–285.

Brodtkorb, E., Kless, T.M., Nakken, K.O., Lossius, R., & Johannessen, S.I. (2004, April). Levetiracetam in adult patients with and without learning disability: Focus on behavioral adverse effects. *Epilepsy Behavior, 5*(2), 231–235.

Bronen, R.A., Fulbright, R.K., Spencer, D.D., Spencer, S.S., Kim, J.H., Lange, R.C., & Sutilla, C. (1996). Refractory epilepsy: Comparison of MR imaging, CT, and histopathologic findings in 117 patients. *Radiology, 201,* 97–105.

Chelune, G.J., Naugle, R.I., Hermann, B.P., Barr, W.B., Trenerry, M.R., Loring, D.W., Perrine, K., Strauss, E., & Westerveld, M. (1998). Does presurgical IQ predict seizure outcome after temporal lobectomy? Evidence from the Bozeman Epilepsy Consortium. *Epilepsia, 39,* 314–318.

Coppola, G., & Pascotto, A. (1997). Lamotrigine as add-on drug in children and adolescents with refractory epilepsy and mental delay: An open trial. *Brain & Development, 19,* 398–402.

Cowan, L.D., Bodensteiner, J.B., Leviton, A., & Doherty, L. (1989). Prevalence of the epilepsies in children and adolescents. *Epilepsia, 30,* 94–106.

Crothers, B., & Paine, R.S. (1959). Seizures and electroencephaly: The incidence of seizures among patients with cerebral palsy. In B. Crothers & R.S. Paine (Eds.), *The natural history and cerebral palsy.* Cambridge, MA: Harvard University Press.

Curatolo, P., Cusmai, R., Cortesi, F., Chiron, C., Jambaque, I., & Dulac, O. (1991). Neuropsychiatric aspects of tuberous sclerosis. *Annals of the New York Academy of Sciences, 615,* 8–16.

De Los Reyes, E.C., Sharp, G.B., Williams, J.P., & Hale, S.E. (2004). Levetiracetam in the treatment of Lennox-Gastaut syndrome. *Pediatric Neurology, 30,* 254–256.

Delgado, M.R., Riela, A.R., Mills, J., Pitt, A., & Browne, R. (1996). Discontinuation of antiepileptic drug treatment after two seizure-free years in children with cerebral palsy. *Pediatrics, 97,* 192–197.

Dreifuss, F.E., Rosman, N.P., Cloyd, J.C., Pellock, J.M., Kuzniecky, R.I., Lo, W.D., Matsuo, F., Sharp, G.B., Conry, J.A., Bergen, D.C., & Bell, W.E. (1998). A comparison of rectal diazepam gel and placebo for acute repetitive seizures. *New England Journal of Medicine, 338,* 1869–1875.

Espie, C.A., Watkins, J., Curtice, L., Espie, A., Duncan, R., Ryan, J.A., Brodie, M., Mantala, K., & Sterrick, M. (2003). Psychopathology in people with epilepsy and intellectual disability: An investigation of potential explanatory variables. *Journal of Neurology, Neurosurgery and Psychiatry, 74,* 1485–1492.

Fisher, R.S., van Emde Boas, W., Blume, W., Elger, C., Gentor, P., Lee, P., & Engel., J. (2005). Epileptic seizing and epilepsy: Definitions proposed by the International League Against Epilepsy (ILAE) and the International Bureau for Epilepsy (IBE). *Epilepsia, 46,* 470–472.

Frost, M., Gates, J., Helmers, S.L., Wheless, J.W., Levisohn, P., Tardo, C., & Conry, J.A. (2001). Vagus nerve stimulation in children with refractory seizures associated with Lennox-Gastaut syndrome. *Epilepsia, 42,* 1148–1152.

Gates, J., Roger, H., & Frost, M. (2001). Vagus nerve stimulation for patients in residential treatment facilities. *Epilepsy & Behavior, 2,* 563–567.

Gomez, M.R. (1988). *Tuberous sclerosis* (2nd ed.). New York: Raven Press.

Goyal, M., O'Riordan, M.A., & Wiznitzer, M. (2004). Effects of topiramate on seizures and respiratory dysrythmia in Rett syndrome. *Journal of Child Neurology, 19*(8), 588–591.

Hauser, W.A., & Hesdorffer, D.C. (1990). *Epilepsy: Frequency, causes and consequences.* Landover, MD: Epilepsy Foundation of America.

Helmers, S.L., & LaRoche, S.M. (2004a). The new antiepileptic drugs: Clinical applications. *Journal of the American Medical Association, 291,* 615–620.

Helmers, S.L., & LaRoche, S.M. (2004b). The new antiepileptic drugs: Scientific review. *Journal of the American Medical Association, 291,* 605–614.

Hilliard, L.T., & Kirman, B.H. (1957). *Mental deficiency.* London: Churchill Livingstone.

Holmes, G.L., McKeever, M., & Russman, B.S. (1983). Abnormal behavior or epilepsy? Use of long-term EEG and video monitoring with severely to profoundly mentally retarded patients with seizures. *American Journal of Mental Deficiency, 87,* 456–458.

Hrdlicka, M., Komarez, V., Propper, L., Kusilek, R., Zumrova, A., Faladova, I., Havlovicova, M., Sedlacek, Z., Blatny, M., & Urbanek, T. (2004). Not EEG abnormalities but epilepsy is associated with autistic regression and mental functioning in childhood autism. *European Child and Adolescent Psychiatry, 13,* 209–213.

Ingram, T.T.S., Jameson, S., Errington, J., & Mitchell, R.G. (1964). Living with cerebral palsy. In *Clinics in developmental medicine* (Vol. 14). London: Heinemann.

International League Against Epilepsy. (ILAE). (1981). Proposal for revised clinical and electroencephalographic classification of epileptic seizures. From the Commission on Classification and Terminology of the International League Against Epilepsy. *Epilepsia, 22*, 489–501.

International League Against Epilepsy. (ILAE). (1989). Proposal for revised classification of epilepsies and epileptic syndromes. Commission on Classification and Terminology of the International League Against Epilepsy. *Epilepsia, 30*, 389–399.

Jambaque, I., Cusmai, R., Curatolo, P., Cortesi, F., Perrot, C., & Dulac, O. (1991). Neuropsychological aspects of tuberous sclerosis in relation to epilepsy and MRI findings. *Developmental Medicine and Child Neurology, 33*, 698–705.

Kanner, A.M. (2002, Dec.), Psychiatric comorbidity in patients with developmental disorders and epilepsy: A practical approach to its diagnosis and treatment. *Epilepsy Behavior, 3* (6 Suppl. 1), 7–13.

Kelly, K., Stephen, L.J., & Brodie, M.J. (2004). Levetiracetam for people with mental retardation and refractory epilepsy. *Epilepsy and Behavior, 5*, 878–883.

Kothare, S.V., Khurana, V.I., Hardison, H., & Legido, M.J.J. (2004). Efficacy and tolerability of zonisamide in juvenile myoclonic epilepsy. *Epileptic Disorders, 6*, 267–270.

Kuzniecky, R., Andermann, F., & Guerrini, R. (1993). Congenital bilateral perisylvian syndrome: Study of 31 patients. The CBPS Multicenter Collaborative Study. *Lancet, 341*, 608–612.

Maria, B.L., Deidrick, K.M., Roach, E.S., & Gutmann, D.H. (2004). Tuberous sclerosis complex: Pathogenesis, diagnosis, strategies, therapies, and future research. *Journal of Child Neurology, 19*, 632–642.

Mayville, E.A., & Matson, J.L. (2004). Assessment of seizures and related symptomatology in persons with mental retardation. *Behavior Modification, 28*, 678–693.

Mikati, M.A., Choueri, R., Khurana, D.S., Riviello, J., Helmers, S., & Holmes, G. (1998). Gabapentin in the treatment of refractory partial epilepsy in children with intellectual disability. *Journal of Intellectual Disability Research, 42* (Suppl. 1), 57–62.

Montero, R.R., Puig, S.J., Toral, F.J., Martinez, F.J.M., & Rato, M.M. (1995). Sindrome X fragil y epilepsia. *Neurologia, 10*, 70–75.

Motte, J., Trevathan, E., Arvidsson, J.F., Barrera, M.N., Mullens, E.L., & Manasco, P. (1997). Lamotrigine for generalized seizures associated with the Lennox-Gastaut syndrome. Lamictal Lennox-Gastaut Study Group. *New England Journal of Medicine, 337*, 1807–1812.

Musumeci, S.A., Ferri, R., Elia, M., Colognola, R.M., Bergonzi, P., & Tassinari, C.A. (1991). Epilepsy and fragile X syndrome: A follow-up study. *American Journal of Medical Genetics, 38*, 511–513.

Neill, J.C., & Alvarez, N. (1986). Differential diagnosis of epileptic versus pseudoepileptic seizures in developmentally disabled persons. *Applied Research in Mental Retardation*, 7, 285–298.

Nieto-Barrera, M., Nieto-Jimenez, M., Diaz, F., Campana, C., Sanchez, M.L., Ruiz, D.P., et al. (1999). [Clinical course of epileptic seizures in Rett's syndrome]. [Spanish]. *Revista de Neurologia, 28*, 449–453.

Pack, A.M., & Morrell, M.J. (2004). Epilepsy and bone health in adults. *Epilepsy & Behavior, 5*(Suppl. 2), S24–S29.

Palmini, A., Andermann, F., Aicardi, J., Dulac, O., Chaves, F., Ponsot, G., et al. (1991). Diffuse cortical dysplasia, or the "double cortex" syndrome: The clinical and epileptic spectrum in 10 patients. *Neurology, 41*, 1656–1662.

Pampiglione, G., & Pugh, E. (1975). Letter: Infantile spasms and subsequent appearance of tuberous sclerosis syndrome. *Lancet, 2*, 1046.

Pavone, P., Incorpora, G., Fiumara, A., Parano, E., Trifiletti, R.R., & Ruggieri, M. (2004). Epilepsy is not a prominent feature of primary autism. *Neuropediatrics, 35*, 207–210.

Rapin, I., & Katzman, R. (1998). Neurobiology of autism. *Annals of Neurology, 43*, 7–14.

Romanelli, P., Verdecchia, M., Rodas, R., Seri, S., & Curatolo, P. (2004). Epilepsy surgery for tuberous sclerosis. *Pediatric Neurology, 31*, 239–247.

Rubinstein, A.E., & Korinthenberg, R. (1990). *Neurofibromatosis: A handbook for patients, families, and health-care professionals*. New York: Thieme Medical Publishers.

Sheth, R.D. (2004). Bone health in pediatric epilepsy. *Epilepsy & Behavior, 5* (Suppl. 2), S30–S35.

Sidenvall, R., Forsgren, L., & Heijbel, J. (1996). Prevalence and characteristics of epilepsy in children in northern Sweden. *Seizure, 5*, 139–146.

Sillanpaa, M. (1992). Epilepsy in children: Prevalence, disability, and handicap. *Epilepsia, 33*, 444–449.

Sivenius, J., Savolainen, S., Kaski, M., & Riekkinen, P.J. (1990). Therapeutic intervention in mentally retarded adult epileptics. *Acta Neurologica Scandinavica, 81*, 165–167.

Steffenburg, U., Hagberg, G., & Kyllerman, M. (1996). Characteristics of seizures in a population-based series of mentally retarded children with active epilepsy. *Epilepsia, 37*, 850–856.

Stephen, E., & Hawks, G. (1975). Cerebral palsy and mental subnormality. In A.M Clarke & D.B. Clarke (Eds.), *Mental deficiency: The changing outlook*. New York: Macmillan.

Trevathan, E. (2002). Infantile spasms and Lennox-Gastaut syndrome. *Journal of Child Neurology, 17*(Suppl. 2), 2S9–2S22.

Tuchman, R.F., Rapin, I., & Shinnar, S. (1991). Autistic and dysphasic children. II: Epilepsy. *Pediatrics, 88*, 1219–1225.

Wilfong, A.A. (2002). Treatment considerations: Role of vagus nerve stimulator. *Epilepsy & Behavior, 3*(6), 41–44.

Wong, I.C., Chadwick, D.W., Fenwick, P.B., Mawer, G.E., & Sander, J.W. (1999). The long-term use of gabapentin, lamotrigine and vigabatrin in patients with chronic epilepsy. *Epilepsia, 40*, 1439–1445.

12.3 OTHER NEUROLOGICAL CONDITIONS

Norberto Alvarez

Children and adults with developmental disabilities may have a variety of other neurological conditions. Three major factors determine the prevalence, character, and clinical expression of these conditions. First, the individual's *underlying neurological condition* may manifest itself in motor, cognitive, or behavioral features and may predispose the individual to a greater likelihood of seizures and sensory, motor, and other neurophysiological disturbances. Second, the individual's *underlying chromosomal or nonchromosomal genetic disorder* may have associated central nervous system dysfunction to varying degrees. In addition, some neurodegenerative conditions have specific metabolic disturbances with characteristic clinical presentation and well-known patterns of progressive impairment and organ system dysfunction. Third, individuals with developmental disabilities have an increased likelihood of using *medications that can have a negative effect on the central nervous system.* These medications include anticonvulsant medications, especially if multiple medications are used at the same time, and psychoactive medications. These factors may not only result in specific neurological conditions and syndromes but also may present in unusual ways that challenge diagnostic formulation.

This chapter reviews the experiences of a neurology referral clinic for adults with developmental disabilities and examines common conditions, including dementia, movement disorders, gait disorders, behavior disorders, and sleep disorders. Table 12.3-1 is a summary of 145 consecutive referrals to an outpatient Neurology Clinic for adults with intellectual disabilities. Individuals referred for epilepsy or cerebral palsy were not included in the table. This Neurology Clinic functions mostly to give a second opinion, and, in most instances, individuals have been evaluated by other physicians or have been screened by a multidisciplinary team before referral.

Table 12.3-1. One hundred forty-six consecutive referrals to an outpatient Neurology Clinic

Diagnosis	Number of people
Down syndrome	39
Early dementia	30
Atlanto-axial instability	9
Movement disorders	24
Tremors	9
Medication-related	9
Parkinson disease	4
Dystonia	2
Gait disorders	18
Behavior disorders	21
Peripheral nerve disorders	10
Compressive neuropathies	6
Peripheral neuropathies	3
Traumatic neuropathies	1
Cerebrovascular accidents	5
Stroke	3
Transient ischemic attacks	1
Intraventricular bleeding	1
Sleep disorders	6
Syncopal attacks	4
Visual problems	3
Ventriculo peritoneal shunt malfunctions	2
Headaches	2
Miscellaneous	13

Note: Epileptic disorders and cerebral palsy are not included in this table. Some individuals have more than one diagnosis.

Most of the consultations dealt with diagnoses that are common in any Neurology Clinic; however, some interesting differences exist. For example, few individuals with migraine headaches or pain syndromes are seen. The subjective nature of these disorders and the ability to describe the symptoms may serve to explain why there are so few referrals for these conditions. Although migraines and other headaches may occur as frequently, the presenting features may be more nonspecific and are more likely to express themselves as "behavior disorders." Some medications that are effective in the treatment of behavior problems (e.g., propranolol, tricyclic antidepressants) and some antiepileptics (e.g., valproic acid) are also effective in the treatment of migraine. This experience suggests that some frequent conditions that are rarely diagnosed in individuals with intellectual disabilities should be reevaluated. The most common cause of referral was in relation to individuals with Down syndrome and most notably for dementia of the Alzheimer type and atlanto-axial instability (AAI).

DEMENTIA

Dementia is an age-related disorder, but it should not be considered a natural event of aging. Rather, it is a pathological condition of the brain. The prevalence is approximately 1% among individuals in their 60s and 40% among individuals 85 years old. Dementia is the end result of different etiologies that share some common clinical features: continuous progressive deterioration of intellectual function, personality changes, and a marked decline in activities of daily living (see Table 12.3-2).

Vascular dementias are characterized by a stepwise but continuous deterioration. In these conditions, events such as strokes or transient ischemic attacks are an important clinical feature. New neurological signs such as paralysis of one side of the body or loss of vision are seen after the acute events. The presence of a progressive Parkinson syndrome, in the absence of the use of psychotropic medications, might suggest Lewy bodies disease, Parkinson dementia syndrome, or progressive supranuclear palsy.

A particular form of dementias that affect the frontal and temporal areas of the brain (i.e., frontotrempolal de-

Table 12.3-2. Useful test indicated in the workup of a person with suspected dementia

In all cases	Optional
Psychometric evaluation	
Imaging studies	
Magnetic resonance imaging of the head (preferred)	Positron emission tomography (PET) scan
Computed tomography (CT) scan of the head	Magnetic resonance angiography
Duplex scanning of carotid or vertebal arteries	
Blood studies	
Complete blood count	Lipid profile
Liver function tests	Paraneoplastic antibodies
Electrolytes	Apolipoprotein E genotype
Thyroid function tests	Drug screening
Serum B_{12} and folates	Tests for syphilis and human immunodeficiency virus
Other studies	
Electroencephalogram	Spinal tap
Electrocardiogram	Genetic studies for Alzheimer and Hungtington diseases
Chest X-ray	

mentias) are characterized by episodes of disinhibition, poor social judgment, and other behavior and psychiatric disorders in the early stages of the disease. Systemic diseases such as cancer or connective tissue disorders might also be associated with dementing illness.

Psychiatric disorders are seen with high frequency in individuals with developmental disabilities and dementia. Cooper (1996b) evaluated 134 individuals with developmental disabilities older than 65 years who were living in a community in the United Kingdom and found that psychiatric symptoms (e.g., onset or increase in aggression, loss of concentration, poor sleep, speech deterioration) were frequently seen as part of the dementia syndrome. Also, the prevalence of psychiatric disorders was 68% in those older than 65 years and 47% for those younger than 65 (Cooper, 1997a, 1997b).

Common causes of dementia include the use of multiple medications, which causes pseudodementia in older adults, and endocrine disorders, particularly hypothyroidism. Because the diagnosis of dementia requires the documentation of a progressive deterioration in activities of daily living (e.g., grooming, dressing, eating, drinking, travel skills), a simple battery of tests that can be performed by caregivers is more appropriate. The Reiss Screen for Maladaptive Behavior (Reiss & Valenti-Hein, 1994), the Down Syndrome Dementia Scale (DSDS; Gedye, 1995), and the WDC Tool (Alvarez, 2005) are examples of tools that can help in documenting the progression of dementia. The serial administration of any of these tests and comparison with baseline observations in the same individual is probably the most valid way to establish a diagnosis of dementia in one particular person. Information obtained through the medical history might lead to identify certain etiologies and help to institute the appropriate treatment. Dementias of rapid progression are more commonly the result of toxic or metabolic disturbances.

Although memory impairment is one of the early clinical symptoms of dementia in the general population, individuals with a severe to profound degree of intellectual disabilities show behavioral symptoms (e.g., apathy, irritability, emotional instability, psychiatric disorders). Documenting progressive decline in areas such as reasoning, thinking, planning, and organization is difficult. These changes are usually suspected through direct observations by caregivers. Inability to select appropriate clothing, to prepare food, or to set the table might be an early indication of dementia.

General physical examination will help to rule out treatable conditions as well as to document sensory impairments or other disorders that might mimic dementia. Some clinical conditions that are more common in individuals with developmental disabilities, such as hypothyroidism, psychiatric disorders, depression, multiple medications, sleep disorders, and sleep apnea, should be especially documented. Also, hearing and vision screening is indicated. Neurological examination is very important; however, abnormal neurological signs could be the result of prior medical conditions. In general and with few exceptions, in the absence of another valid explanation, the presence of progressive loss of functions should be considered to be an indication of dementia.

ALZHEIMER DISEASE

Alzheimer disease is the most common form of dementia, and it has particular importance in individuals with Down syndrome. The higher risk for Alzheimer disease in individuals with Down syndrome might be related to the extra copy of chromosome 21, the extra production of amyloid precursor protein, and subsequent increase of the toxic factor $Aß_{42}$ (Beach, 1999). The definitive diagnosis of Alzheimer disease is done only by the presence of specific changes found in the brain at the time of autopsy (see Table 12.3-3); however, in many instances, young individuals with Down syndrome had the histopathological changes found in Alzheimer disease and were asymptomatic.

Treatment

Cholinesterase inhibitors, such as donepezil, rivastigmine, and galantamine, demonstrated some benefits for the amelioration of the cognitive decline in Alzheimer

Table 12.3-3. Criteria for the clinical diagnosis of dementia of the Alzheimer type

Definite
Clinical features of probable Alzheimer dementia
Brain biopsy or autopsy with the neuropathological findings diagnostic of Alzheimer dementia
Probable (for individuals without histological confirmation but typical clinical picture)
Diagnosis of the dementia documented by changes in mental status and confirmed by neuropsychological tests
Impairments in two or more areas of cognition
Progressive worsening of memory and other cognitive functions
Consciousness is not altered
No brain or systemic disorder that could explain the clinical impairments
Onset between the ages of 40 and 90 years
Possible (proposed for individuals with atypical course)
Presence of the clinical syndrome of dementia with no other neurologic or psychiatric or systemic disorder to explain the symptoms and in the presence of variations in the onset, in the presentation, and in the clinical course
May be made when there is a second systemic or brain disorder that might produce dementia but is not considered to be the cause of the dementia

From McKann, G., Drachman, D., Folstein, M., Katzman, R., Price, D., & Stadlan, E. (1984). Clinical diagnosis of Alzheimer's disease: Report of the NINCDS–ADRDA Work Group under the auspices of the Department of Health and Human Services Task Force on Alzheimer's disease. *Neurology, 34*(7), 939–944; adapted by permission.

disease; however, they do not arrest the progression of the disease. Both rivastigmine and galantamine resulted in a significant decrease in body weight, a side effect that can be a limiting factor in the use of these medications (Prasher, 2004).

There are a few studies involving individuals with developmental disabilities taking these medications, and these studies mostly deal with individuals with Down syndrome. One of the studies involved three individuals with Down syndrome and showed that donepezil treatment resulted in urinary incontinency in two individuals (Hemingway-Eltomey & Lerner, 1999). Improvement in cognitive functions with donepezil was reported in another study involving four individuals with Down syndrome (Kishnani et al., 1999). The benefit that these drugs produce in people with Alzheimer disease is still modest and is mostly seen in the early stages of the disease (Prasher, 2004).

Evolution of Alzheimer Disease in Individuals with Down Syndrome

Individuals with Down syndrome develop a clinical and neuropathological picture similar to Alzheimer disease at an earlier age (Beach, 1999). Prospective studies showed that the prevalence of clinical dementia in individuals with Down syndrome is around 10% in those younger than 49 years; 50%–60% in those between 50–59 years; and almost 100% between the ages of 65–70 years (Evenhuis, 1997; Lai & Williams, 1989). The common clinical picture that emerges from these and other studies is characterized by subtle signs and symptoms in the early stages of the disease, most often changes in the behavioral sphere, personality changes, and irritability.

In those individuals who function at a high level, subtle but persistent deterioration in acquired skills and difficulties in learning new skills are apparent. In individuals with more profound intellectual disabilities, behavior changes might be limited to apathy and less social interaction. Continuous deterioration of activities of daily living takes place, and the individual becomes more and more dependent on others. Motor coordination also deteriorates, with loss of gait and other functions heavily dependent on muscle coordination (e.g., swallowing). Parkinson syndrome develops in some individuals. Epileptic seizures, most commonly myoclonic seizures, are also a frequent event.

Dan's story presents the clinical evolution of a person with Down syndrome who develops Alzheimer-like dementia and whose autopsy shows clear neuropathological features of Alzheimer disease. Even though the clinical condition in the advanced stages is very similar, the course of the progression of the symptoms varies among individuals.

Before developing dementia, Dan was a pleasant and congenial man with no behavior problems. He followed simple commands and understood simple orders. He walked independently and was independent in activities of daily living. He also had an active social life. The first symptoms Dan began to show, at the age of 51, were disorientation and confusion. For example, after a dance program, he refused to accept that the program was over and would not return to his residence. He was later found wandering outside, crying, and yelling in a state of confusion.

The next year, when Dan was 52 years old, he showed increased forgetfulness and periods of agitation in which he threw objects. At 54, he needed constant prompting to accomplish activities of daily living, but he still showered and changed his clothes daily. Dan developed poor participation due to frequent sleeping. By age 55, Dan was experiencing a steady rate of regression, including increased disorientation, confusion, wandering, and forgetfulness. He also developed difficulties in gait and myoclonic seizures.

By age 57, Dan had become assaultive. He occassionally used a wheelchair and started having toileting accidents. He became lethargic and displayed frequent inappropriate behavior. By the next year, Dan could no longer feed himself and could not tolerate bus rides to the community. Despite these challenges, Dan enjoyed music and expressed pleasure by smiling and laughing.

By age 59 years, Dan was incontinent of urine, totally dependent on others to perform activities of daily living, and no longer walked. A year later, he slept almost continuously and had minimal social interactions. He occasionally conveyed pleasure and displeasure by laughing or crying but was troubled by frequent pneumonias. Eventually, Dan was no longer able to swallow, and nasogastric and percutaneous endoscopic gastrostomy tubes were placed.

At the Neurology Clinic, this author had the opportunity to closely follow 11 individuals from the early stage to the time of death. Alzheimer disease was confirmed by autopsy in 10 of them. The mean age at the time of the first symptom was 50 years (36–62 years), and diagnosis of the disease was confirmed by a mean age of 52 years (37–62 years). Therefore, a gap of approximately 2 years existed between early indications of the disease and diagnosis. These individuals had sensory deficiencies that interfered with the interpretation of some of the presenting symptoms. Ten of the eleven individuals had visual disturbances before the beginning of the symptoms. Two were legally blind. One was blind in the right eye due to a congenital lesion and had very compromised vision in the left eye due to an advance cataract. Another had poor vision due to bilateral cataracts and became blind 4 years after the diagnosis was made. Another person had poor vision due to earlier retinal detachment. The other five individuals had cataracts, two of them with keratoconus, a disease of the cornea that produces a progressive impairment of vision. Marked hearing loss was demonstrated in two individuals and moderate in another two. Similar sensory impairments were reported in other series.

Intermittent periods of confusion and disorientation were, in most instances, the earliest signs of the disease. In many individuals, these episodes were seen almost 2 years before the first evaluation; however, in most instances individuals were sent for consultation 2–3 months after the first behavioral changes were observed. Simultaneously with the behavior changes, gait impairment, speech or communication disorders, and decreased participation in leisure activities were also commonly seen in the very early stages of the disease. Continuous deterioration in mental status was present, and an average of 4.4 years (2.5–6.11 years) after the diagnosis was made, these individuals were totally unaware of their surroundings.

Associated Conditions

Depression was diagnosed in eight individuals after the symptoms of Alzheimer disease were obvious. Seven of these individuals used Trazodone for treatment of the depression. Some short-term improvement was experienced, but in some individuals, Trazodone seemed to increase the severity of myoclonus. Depression should always be considered in the differential diagnosis of Alzheimer disease because severe depression might result in pseudodementias. In these individuals, depression was considered another symptom of the dementing disorder.

Injuries, resulting from poor balance, unsteady gait, poor visual-spatial perception and/or seizures, were frequently seen. For example, a person standing in front of a chair, looked at the chair and attempted to sit on it, misjudged its position, and fell to the floor. Another person who was walking suddenly stiffened and fell backward, hitting her head on the floor. Decubitus ulcers were observed in the advanced stage of the disorder. In general, they were difficult to treat, and, in some cases, the ulcers lasted for several weeks before they were fully healed.

Hypothyroidism was diagnosed in four individuals before diagnosis of Alzheimer disease was made, and in three more individuals during the follow-up. High incidence of autoimmune thyroiditis with hypothyroidism is common in individuals with Down syndrome, and in a few instances the treatment of hypothyroidism can reverse the clinical dementia. In this particular group of individuals, however, no lasting effect could be demonstrated when they become euthyroid.

As Alzheimer disease progresses, other medical issues emerge that require intervention. The development of epileptic seizures (either generalized tonic-clonic seizures or, more often, myoclonic seizures) is a common occurrence. Generalized tonic-clonic seizures were not very frequent, most often lasting for a few minutes, and status epilepticus was exceptional. Myoclonic seizures were more of a problem. Usually, the first episodes were poorly documented and, in many instances, not recognized as such. Myoclonic seizures were frequently observed in the early stages of the disease, when the individuals were mobile and still independent. Increased frequency of injuries and falls in individuals who had never had accidents were an indirect indication of the early myoclonic seizures.

These myoclonic seizures had the characteristics of being very sensitive to external stimulation. For example, noises in the environment could induce the seizures, especially when the individual was getting dressed, bathed, or fed. Also, touching or moving the individual was enough to induce clusters of myoclonic seizures. In the advanced stages, these seizures were almost a constant event. Myoclonic seizures are very resistant to treatment; also medications that might be relatively useful, such as benzodiazepines, might produce marked sedation. In general, small amounts of medications might be needed that can be reinforced with more medication at certain times, such as before meals. Because the tolerance for antiepiletic medication is, in general, very low, it is not beneficial to be very aggressive in controlling these seizures.

Eating disorders became a problem for individuals with Alzheimer disease as a consequence of impairment of the higher cortical functions and muscles needed for the normal act of swallowing and deglution. Choking, vomiting, and coughing became serious problems. In four cases, nasogastric tubes were used an average of 6.9 years (4.9–8.2 years), and in three, gastrostomy tubes were placed an average of 7.4 years (5.10–9.2 years) after the diagnosis was made to facilitate feeding. In most of the individuals, aspiration pneumonia was a complication frequently seen in the advanced stages.

Electroencephalograms (EEGs) obtained before the beginning of the disease were normal. As the disease progressed, EEG activity deteriorated. Computed tomography (CT) scanning showed diffuse brain atrophy with decreased brain matter and enlargement of the ventricles (see Figure 12.3-1). These CT scan changes are not diagnostic of Alzheimer disease, but, when present, there is a high correlation with Alzheimer disease, mostly if temporal lobe atrophy is present. Progressive regional enlargement of the temporal and occipital horns are linearly related to the duration of the dementia, and this focal enlargement is not seen in individuals with or without Down syndrome who do not have dementia.

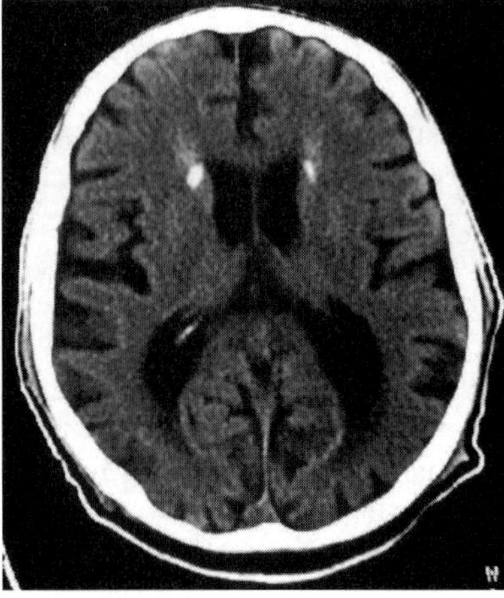

Figure 12.3-1. Computed tomography (CT) scan of a 60-year-old with Down syndrome who showed marked advanced clinical signs and symptoms of Alzheimer disease. The CT scan shows marked ventricular dilation, diffuse cortical atrophy, and bilateral symmetrical calcifications of the basal ganglia.

Ethical Issues

Several ethical issues emerge as the disease progresses and need to be addressed with the participation of the legal guardian. The most relevant are the use of tubes to feed individuals, resorting to hospice care when the disease is considered in the terminal stages, and deciding weather a Do Not Resuscitate order is indicated.

ATLANTO-AXIAL INSTABILITY

AAI is commonly seen in children and adults with skeletal dysplasias and can also be seen in individuals with generalized ligamentous laxicity such as the Ehlers-Danlos or Marfan syndromes. The incidence of AAI in Down syndrome varies between 10% and 30% (Alvarez & Rubin, 1986). The cause is not clear but it is probably related to generalized ligament laxity, in some instances associated with malformations of the odontoid bone. Trauma or manipulations to the neck, as seen in positioning of the neck for anesthesia, and acute upper respiratory infections can also be involved in some cases.

Due to the instability of the atlanto-axial joint, there is excessive posterior excursion of the odontoid bone that can result in spinal cord compression. In most instances, the AAI is a radiological finding. In a few individuals, it becomes symptomatic. Subtle signs and symptoms usually precede the severe symptoms resulting from the spinal cord compression. The presence of neck pain or torticollis in a person with Down syndrome is an indication to rule out AAI. When spinal compression occurs, the progression of the symptoms is gradual. When not treated, the symptoms might slowly progress to spastic quadriplegia.

The diagnosis can be done with lateral cervical x-ray of the neck in neutral, flexion, and extension. These x-rays show the anterior atlanto odontoid distance and the movement related to the changes in position. Distances less than 3 mm in flexion in adults and 4 mm in children are considered normal, with measurements more than 5–6 mm serving as an indication of high risk. The measurement of the posterior atlanto odontoid distance might also be of interest in deciding the degree of risk, and there is agreement that distances less than 14 mm are associated with high risk of spinal cord compression. CT scan and, in most cases, MRI of the cervical spine are also very useful when spinal cord compression is suspected. Lateral cervical x-ray is the preferred screening method for the evaluation of asymptomatic individuals and is required by the Special Olympics Committee in all children with Down syndrome who want to participate in the event.

The Neurology Clinic followed 152 adults with Down syndrome (average age 38 years, range 18–67 years). In 127, successive cervical x-rays were obtained during a span of time that varied between a few months to several years and found that, in most instances, successive x-rays did not show any change. When changes occurred, they were not significant. In some instances, increased anterior atlanto-odontoid distance was found, whereas in other instances, the distance was decreased. Also, in some individuals, both increases and decreases in the measurement of the AAI were found, going from measurements that suggest high risk to measurements that suggest no risk for complications.

One set of x-rays in asymptomatic children might be justified, but the question remains whether there is any real need to repeat the test in asymptomatic individuals. Preoperative screening, however, is indicated in individuals who are in need of anesthesia that requires manipulation of the neck. The treatment for the symptomatic AAI is the fusion of C1 to C2. In the case of asymptomatic AAI, the management is not clear, and clinical monitoring is advised.

MOVEMENT DISORDERS

Individuals with brain damage may be at a higher risk of developing a movement disorder when exposed to medications. For example, phenobarbital increases hyperactive behavior in children who are previously hyperactive. Behavior changes were also described in association with several antiepileptic medications (Kalachnik, Hanzel, Harder, Bauernfeind, & Engstrom, 1995). Phenytoin induced choreoathotic movement disorder in individuals with brain damage; gabapentin was found to produce facial dyskinesia in a 37-year-old man with severe intellectual disabilities (Buetefisch, Gutierrez, & Gutmann, 1996) and in 3 out of 28 individuals with severe neurological impairments and chronic epilepsy treated with additional gabapentin. Facial dyskinesia may be the result of the medication's direct effect on the brain or it may be the individual's expression of disturbing sensations that are often reported by sensitive and articulate individuals.

Movement disorders are also common among individuals with developmental disabilities. In a study on the prevalence of movement disorder in 1,227 individuals with developmental disabilities living in an institution, Stone, May, Alvarez, and Ellman (1989) found dyskinesia in 48%, dystonia in 29%, akathisia in 13%, Parkinsonism in 3%, and other paroxysmal movement disorders in 4% of the individuals surveyed. Seventy-two percent had at least one movement disorder, but some individuals had more than one.

Tardive dyskinesia is a well-recognized complication due to the chronic use of psychotropic medications. Individuals with developmental disabilities may also have psychiatric disorders and may be required to take neuroleptic medication. A survey of 1,101 adults with intellectual disabilities living in group homes found that 27% of them received one or more psychotropic drugs for the treatment of behavioral or emotional disorders (Aman, Sarphare, & Burrow, 1995). Neuroleptic drugs, the drugs most frequently associated with tardive dyskinesia, were prescribed in 21% of the cases. Other surveys in the United States found an incidence between 18% and 49% (Aman, Van Bourgondien, Wolford, Sarphare, 1995). The prevalence is much higher in individuals living in institutions, where the mean is reported at 57.4% with a range of 36.9%–85.9% (Baumeister, Todd, & Sevin, 1993). Due to the growing concern about the widespread use of neuroleptics in individuals with intellectual disabilities, a trend to use other medications instead of antipsychotics has been observed.

There are several scales useful in the evaluation of movement disorders, specifically tardive dyskinesia, such as the Abnormal Involuntary Movement Scale (AIMS; Munetz & Benjamin, 1988), the Dyskinesia Monitoring System: Condensed User Scale (DISCUS; Sprague & Kalachnik, 1991), and the Rockland-Simpson Dyskinesia Rating Scale (RSDRS; Simpson, Lee, Zoubak, & Gardos, 1979). The level of cooperation of the individual is also an important factor. Evaluation of the DISCUS in 344 individuals living in an institution showed very poor cooperation among individuals with a profound degree of intellectual disabilities (Granger, Yurkunski, Miller, Swanson, & Crinella, 1987). Another complicating factor is the presence of Parkinsonism, also a side effect of the neuroleptics, which can mask tardive dyskinesia, especially in older adults. Rao et al. (1987) found a significant association of tardive dyskinesia and Parkinsonism; however, a major problem is the high frequency of abnormal movements observed in these individuals that are similar but probably not related to the use of neuroleptics.

In a study involving 236 individuals with intellectual disabilities living in an institution, a significant amount of motor disorders were experienced by most individuals (Rogers, Karki, Bartlett, & Pocock, 1991). Of interest was the presence of orofacial movements in 71% of those treated with neuroleptics at the time of the study, 70% of those treated in the past but not on medications at the time of the study, and 52% of those who were never exposed to neuroleptics. Movements of the head, trunk, and limbs were found in 53% of those currently on medication, in 52% of those previously exposed, and in 32% of individuals who were never exposed to neuroleptics. Perioral movements of the face were present in 34% of those receiving neuroleptics, 20% of those previously on neuroleptics, and 27% of those who were never on neuroleptics. The quality of the movement disorder was similar in the different groups. Youssef and Waddington (1988) also found orofacial dyskinesia in individuals with intellectual disabilities who were never exposed to neuroleptics. Even though these movements were always more frequent in the treated group, these studies highlight the importance of a good medical history before accepting the diagnosis of tardive dyskinesia.

Farren and Dinan (1994) evaluated 61 women with intellectual disabilities using the AIMS and found that 64% had dyskinesia, predominantly orofacial, and 33% had lumbar or trunk dyskinesias. A significant increase in movement disorders occurred when the degree of disability increased but did not correlate with diagnosis, age, or exposure to neuroleptics. An evaluation of a large cohort of individuals older than 65 with no prior brain damage showed a low prevalence of akathisia (1.5%) and tardive dyskinesia (0.22%), which were usually associated with organic mental disorders and not necessarily to antipsychotic medications (Green et al., 1993). These findings suggest that cerebral damage by itself might be a factor in the presence of involuntary movement disorders. Degree of disability also increases the incidence of movement disorder (Farren & Dinan, 1994).

Neuroleptic malignant syndrome, a severe and potentially fatal complication of the use of psychotropic medications, has also been reported in individuals with developmental disabilities. The mortality has deceased from 20%–30% in early reports to almost 0% due to more awareness, early diagnosis, and better acute treatment. A review by Boyd (1993), however, found 29 cases of neuroleptic malignant syndrome in individuals with intellectual disabilities and a fatality rate of 21%, approximately twice that found in individuals without mental retardation. Neuroleptic polypharmacy was present in 55% of the individuals.

Stereotypies and Self-Injurious Behavior

Stereotypies are repetitive, patterned, involuntary, purposeless movements; they have some rhythmicity and might also have a ritualistic quality. They occur frequently among individuals with autism spectrum disorders. Self-injurious behavior (see Chapter 23.5) might be considered as extreme cases of stereotypies, in which the harmful consequences of the behavior and not necessarily the topography, is the basis for the label (Rojahn, 1986).

The organic basis of these behaviors is not well known. Some syndromes have specific behavioral phenotypes. Rett syndrome, for example, is characterized by a peculiar "hand washing" movement (Perry, 1991; see Chapter 9.1).

BEHAVIOR DISORDERS

Determining the organic versus nonorganic nature of the behavior disorder was a frequent cause of referral motivated by the concern that new structural lesions might be responsible for behavior deterioration. In most instances, behavior deterioration in individuals without dementia is not related to new neurological problems. Medical conditions that may be associated with pain or other conditions (e.g., menstrual pain, menopause, hypothyroidism) were often the reason for behavior deterioration. In addition, undiagnosed fractures, gastroesophageal reflux, abnormal reactions to medications, and sleep disorders were also factors. Two individuals had shunt malfunctions, and one had intracranial bleeding following head trauma. The most common reason found for changes in behavior, however, was related to changes in the environment.

PERIPHERAL NERVE DISORDERS

Peripheral nerve disorders are underdiagnosed in individuals with developmental disabilities. Given the high incidence of orthopedic disorders, joint deformities, osteoporosis, and scoliosis in these individuals, physicians should expect to diagnose more pain syndromes. Again, it is likely that a number of unexplained behavioral changes may be related to pain originating in root compressions, or nerve entrapments, or other musculoskeletal structures in individuals who are unable to identify or express their symptoms. Radiculo-myelopathy (Hirose & Kadoya, 1984) and carpal tunnel syndrome (Alvarez, Larkin, & Roxborough, 1982) have been described in individuals with long-standing choreoathetotic cerebral palsy. Long-standing movement disorder with intense flexion, extension, and mostly rotation of the neck is probably the main factor in this condition. The dystonia accelerates the development of cervical spondylosis and, with other local factors (e.g., spinal instability, congenital malformations of the spine), contributes to the cervical myelopathies and root compressions observed.

The spondylitic changes in individuals with dystonic cerebral palsy are more often at the C3–C4 levels (i.e., joints more involved in the rotation of the head) than at the C4–C5, C5–C6 level (i.e., joints more involved with flexion extension movement) (Hirose & Kadoya, 1984). Mechanical factors are also responsible for carpal tunnel syndrome and ulnar nerve compression (Alvarez et al., 1982). In these cases, a "double crush" syndrome can also be postulated. In case of entrapment neuropathies, surgery is indicated to prevent further damage and also to relieve the pain. Surgery for root compression in the cervical spine might be more difficult mostly due to postoperative complications. The critical element in this situation is an accurate diagnosis.

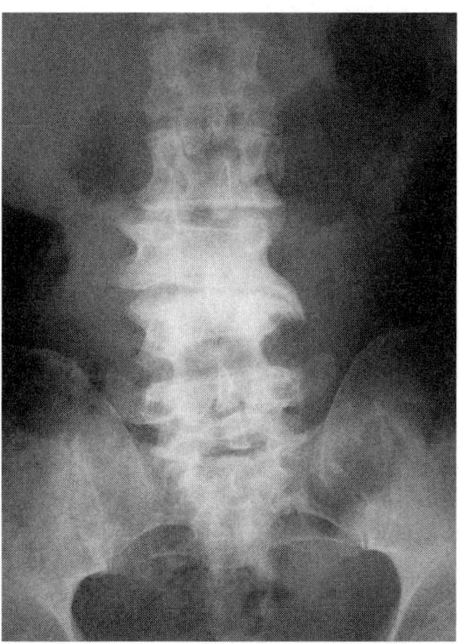

Figure 12.3-2. X-ray showing marked degenerative disease in several discs in the lumbar area and a subluxation between L1 and L2, and almost no disc space between L2 and L3.

Jorge was a 52-year-old man with a choreoathetoid form of cerebral palsy with dystonic posturing that affected almost all his muscles but was more intense in the muscles of his neck and his upper extremities. He did not have intellectual disabilities. Jorge began to complain of shooting pain in both arms, but the left arm more than right. The pain was almost constant and followed the lower cervical roots. He also experienced numbness in the distribution of the ulnar nerve in the left side. He had no muscle atrophies. Jorge had some pain in his lumbar area that, at times, extended to his legs.

Electromyography in the left arm showed that there was widespread chronic denervation involving multiple cervical roots. The denervation was more severe in the C8-T1 distribution. Even though there was denervation in the higher levels, it was less dramatic. The diagnosis was compatible with thoracic outlet syndrome. The cervical x-rays showed the advanced degenerative changes in the cervical spine (see Figure 12.3-2) and in the lower lumbar area (see Figure 12.3-3), which are related to the signs and symptoms presented. Jorge was not a candidate for surgery, and remained on analgesic medication. After several years of follow-up, his condition remained stable.

SLEEP DISORDERS

Epileptiform activity with or without clinical symptoms is commonly seen and results in marked destruction of the sleep cycle. Sleep apnea, more often the obstructive type, is also frequently observed. The anatomical changes in the neck, related to malformations, or orthopedic problems might be a predisposing factor. In an evaluation of 23 individuals with sleep disorder at the Neurologic Clinic, sleep patterns disrupted by frequent epileptiform discharges were observed in 12 individuals; obstructive or central sleep apnea were found in 6 individuals; and poorly organized sleep patterns and unexplained frequent arousal were found in 3 individuals (an avid consumer of coffee, a person with restless leg syndrome, and an individual with night terrors). Because many of these conditions have specific treatments, polysomnographic evaluations should be done when sleep disorders are suspected.

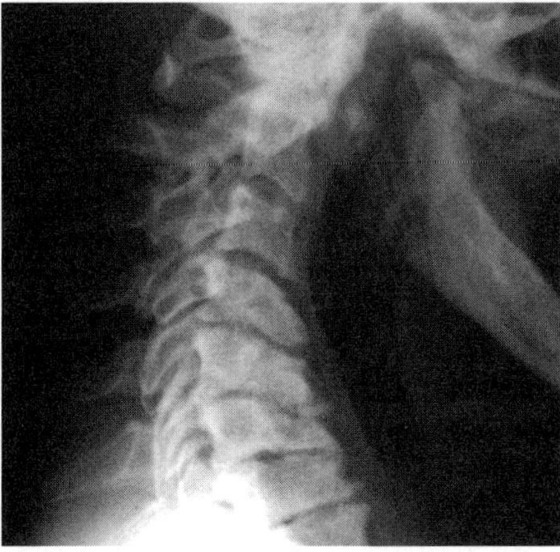

Figure 12.3-3. This lateral view of Jorge's neck shows a marked degree of osteoarthritic degeneration of the cervical vertebra. There are degenerative changes in almost all of the bodies, which are maximal in C4 and C8. Also, there is almost total occlusion of the disc spaces in the affected areas.

CONCLUSION

Children and adults with developmental disabilities may experience a variety of other neurological conditions, including dementia, AAI, movement disorders, peripheral nerve disorders, and sleep disorders. Individuals with Down syndrome are especially prone to Alzheimer disease. Physicians should keep these conditions in mind when monitoring the care of individuals with developmental disabilities.

REFERENCES

Alvarez, N. (2005). *Alzheimer disease in individuals with Down syndrome.* Retrieved from http://emedicine.com/neuro/topic552.htm

Alvarez, N., Larkin, C., & Roxborough, J. (1982). Carpal tunnel syndrome in athetoid-dystonic cerebral palsy. *Archives of Neurology, 39,* 311–312.

Alvarez, N., & Rubin, L. (1986). Atlantoaxial instability in adults with Down syndrome: A clinical and radiological survey. *Applied Research in Mental Retardation, 7,* 67–78.

Aman, M.G., Sarphare, G., & Burrow, W.H. (1995). Psychotropic drugs in group homes: prevalence and relation to demographic/psychiatric variables. *American Journal of Mental Retardation, 99*(5), 500–509.

Aman, M.G., Van Bourgondien, M.E., Wolford, P.L., & Sarphare, G. (1995). Psychotropic and anticonvulsant drugs in subjects with autism: Prevalence and patterns of use. *Journal of the American Academy of Child & Adolescent Psychiatry, 34*(12), 1672–1681.

Baumeister, A.A., Todd, M.E., & Sevin, J.A. (1993). Efficacy and specificity of pharmacological therapies for behavioral disorders in persons with mental retardation. *Clinical Neuropharmacology, 16*(4), 271–294.

Beach, T.G. (1999). Alzheimer disease and Down syndrome: Scientific symbiosis. A historical commentary. In J.M. Berg, H. Karlinsky, & A.J. Holland (Eds.), *Alzheimer disease, Down syndrome and their relationship* (pp. 37–52). New York: Oxford University Press.

Boyd, R.D. (1993). Neuroleptic malignant syndrome and mental retardation: Review and analysis of 29 cases. *American Journal of Mental Retardation, 98*(1), 143–155.

Buetefisch, C.M., Gutierrez, A., & Gutmann, L. (1996). Choreoathetotic movements: A possible side effect of gabapentin. *Neurology, 46*(3), 851–852.

Cooper, S.A. (1997a). Epidemiology of psychiatric disorders in elderly compared with younger adults with learning disabilities. *British Journal of Psychiatry, 170,* 375–380.

Cooper, S.A. (1997b). Psychiatric symptoms of dementia among elderly people with learning disabilities. *International Journal of Geriatric Psychiatry, 12,* 662–666.

Evenhuis, H.M. (1997). The natural history of dementia in ageing people with intellectual disability. *Journal of Intellectual Disability Research, 41,* 92–96.

Farren, C.K., & Dinan, T.G. (1994). Dyskinesia in mentally handicapped women: Relationship to level of handicap, age and neuroleptic exposure. *Acta Psychiatrica Scandinavica, 90* (3), 210–213.

Gedye, A. (1995) *Manual for the Dementia Scale for Down Syndrome.* Vancouver, Canada: Gedye Research and Consulting.

Granger, D.A., Yurkunski, J.M., Miller, N.H., Swanson, J.M., & Crinella, F.C. (1987). Systematic dyskinesia examination of profoundly mentally retarded persons: Cooperation and assessment. *American Journal of Mental Deficiency, 92*(2), 155–160.

Green, B.H., Dewey, M.E., Copeland, J.R., Saunders, P.A., Sharma, V., Larkin, B., et al. (1993). Prospective data on the prevalence of abnormal involuntary movements among elderly people living in the community. *Acta Psychiatrica Scandinavica, 87*(6), 418–421.

Hemingway-Eltomey, J.M., & Lerner, A.J. (1999). Adverse effects of donepezil in treating Alzheimer's disease associated with Down syndrome. *American Journal of Psychiatry, 156,* 1470.

Hirose, G., & Kadoya, S. (1984). Cervical spondylotic radiculo-myelopathy in patients with athetoid-dystonic cerebral palsy: Clinical evaluation and surgical treatment. *Journal of Neurology, Neurosurgery & Psychiatry, 47*(8), 775–780.

Kalachnik, J.E., Hanzel, T.E., Harder, S.R., Bauernfeind, J.D., & Engstrom, E.A. (1995). Antiepileptic drug behavioral side effects in individuals with mental retardation and the use of behavioral measurement techniques. *Mental Retardation, 33*(6), 374–382.

Kishnani, P.S., Sullivan, J.A., Walter, B.K., Spiridigliozzi, G.A., Doraiswamy, P.M., & Krishnan, K.R.R. (1999). Cholinergic therapy for Down's syndrome. *American Journal of Epidemiology, 145,* 134–147.

Lai, F., & Williams, R.S. (1989). A prospective study of Alzheimer's disease in Down syndrome. *Archives of Neurology, 46,* 849–853.

McKann, G., Drachman, D., Folstein, M., Katzman, R., Price, D., & Stadlan, E. (1984). Clinical diagnosis of Alzheimer's disease: Report of the NINCDS–ADRDA Work Group under the auspices of the Department of Health and Human Services Task Force on Alzheimer's disease. *Neurology, 34*(7), 939–944.

Munetz, M.R., & Benjamin, S. (1988, Nov.). How to examine patients using the Abnormal Involuntary Movement Scale. *Hospital and Community Psychiatry, 39*(11), 1172–1177.

Perry, A. (1991). Rett syndrome: A comprehensive review of the literature. *American Journal of Mental Retardation, 96,* 275–290.

Prasher, V.P. (2004). Review of donepezil, rivastigmine, galantamine and nemantine for the treatment of dementia in Alzheimer's disease in adults with Down syndrome: Implications for the intellectual disability population. *International Journal of Geriatric Psychiatry, 19,* 509–515.

Rao, J.M., Cowie, V.A., & Mathew, B. (1987). Tardive dyskinesia in neuroleptic medicated mentally handicapped subjects. *Acta Psychiatrica Scandinavica, 76*(5), 507–513.

Reiss, S., & Valenti-Hein, D. (1994, Feb.). Development of a psychopathological rating scale for children with mental retardation. *Journal of Consulting and Clinical Psychology, 62*(1), 28–33.

Rogers, D., Karki, C., Bartlett, C., & Pocock, P. (1991). The motor disorders of mental handicap: An overlap with the motor disorders of severe psychiatric illness. *British Journal of Psychiatry, 158,* 97–102.

Rojahn, J. (1986). Self-injurious and stereotypic behavior of noninstitutionalized mentally retarded people: Prevalence and classification. *American Journal of Mental Deficiency, 91*(3), 268–276.

Simpson, G.M., Lee, J.H., Zoubak, B., & Gardos, G. (1979, Aug. 8). A rating scale for tardive dyskinesia. *Psychopharmacology, 64*(2), 171–179.

Sprague, R.L., & Kalachnik, J.E. (1991). Reliability, validity, and a total score cutoff for the Dyskinesia Identification System: Condensed User Scale (DISCUS) with mentally ill and mentally retarded populations. *Psychopharmacology Bulletin, 27,* 51–58.

Stone, R.K., May, J.E., Alvarez, W.F., & Ellman, G. (1989). Prevalence of dyskinesia and related movement disorders in a developmentally disabled population. *Journal of Mental Deficiency Research, 33*(1), 41–53.

Youssef, H.A., & Waddington, J.L. (1988). Involuntary orofacial movements in hospitalised patients with mental handicap or epilepsy: Relationship to developmental/intellectual deficit and presence or absence of long-term exposure to neuroleptics. *Journal Neurology, Neurosurgery, and Psychiatry, 51,* 863–865.

12.4 TOURETTE SYNDROME

Howard S. Schub

Tourette syndrome is a clinically distinctive neurodevelopmental tic disorder first described by George Gilles de la Tourette in his famous publication of 1885. He described nine patients with a variety of distinct motor and vocal tics. For many decades, Tourette syndrome was regarded as a rare disability with unusual symptoms and no known etiology, but with the availability of a new medication, haloperidol, in the late 1960s and the pioneering work of Drs. Arthur and Elaine Shapiro (1988), new attention was focused on Tourette syndrome as a more common, easily diagnosed neurological disorder. The formation of the Tourette Syndrome Association increased public awareness of the disorder and the frequency of diagnosis.

Nine-year-old Ted was in third grade when he was brought in for evaluation of eye blinking, shoulder shrugging, and throat clearing. Although his motor and vocal tics had been present for 2 years, they had waxed and waned in severity during that time. Ted's throat hurt from the constant clearing, and he cried because other children teased him about his eye blinking. Ted's father had experienced facial grimaces when he was a child. The examiner noted that Ted was restless and fidgety and demonstrated frequent eye blinking, occasional shoulder shrugging, and occasional throat clearing. Ted could suppress the movements for a few minutes when concentrating.

DIAGNOSIS

Tics are involuntary, regularly repeated, simple contractions of a muscle(s) causing movements or sounds. Tourette syndrome is a clinically diagnosed multifocal motor/vocal tic disorder at one end of the "tic spectrum" disorders. These entities include transient tic disorder, chronic motor or vocal tic disorder, and Tourette syndrome. The official *Diagnostic and Statistical Manual of Mental Disorders, Fourth Edition* (DSM–IV; American Psychiatric Association, 1994) classification of Tourette syndrome is outlined in Table 12.4-1. Ted's symptoms represent a common clinical presentation of Tourette syndrome. Ted suffers from multiple motor tics and a vocal tic that have been present for 2 years and cause him marked distress.

Tics wax and wane in severity. In fact, a specific tic may disappear and be replaced by another one (Erenberg, Cruse, & Rothner, 1987). Stress and fatigue often make them worse, and generally, they do not occur during sleep. The urge to tic can be suppressed temporarily, but the accompanying buildup of internal tension is relieved only by producing a tic.

Although there are a great variety of simple and complex motor and vocal tics (see Table 12.4-2), common motor tics seen in clinical practice include eye blinking, facial grimacing, shoulder shrugging, head jerking, or arm thrusting. Common vocal tics include throat clearing, sniffing, barking, and coughing. Echolalia (repeating the words of others), palialia (repeating one's own words), and coprolalia (obscene words) are more complex but uncommon vocal tics. Although coprolalia is the symptom often associated with the notoriety of Tourette syndrome, it is actually uncommon and often transient. Most cases of Tourette syndrome

Table 12.4-1. DSM–IV Tourette syndrome classification

1. Diagnostic criteria for Tourette's syndrome (307.23)
   A. Both multiple motor and one or more vocal tics have been present at some time during the illness, although not necessarily currently.
   B. The tics occur many times a day (usually in bouts), nearly every day or intermittently throughout a period of more than a year; and during this period, there was never a tic-free period of more than three consecutive months.
   C. The disturbance causes marked distress or significant impairment in social, occupational, or other areas of functioning.
   D. Onset before age 18 years.
   E. The disturbance is not due to the direct physiological effects of a substance (e.g., stimulants) or a general medical condition (e.g., Huntington's chorea or post-viral encephalitis).

Table 12.4-2. Examples of simple and complex motor and vocal tics

Tic symptom dimensions	Examples
Simple motor tics	Eye blinking; eye movements; grimacing; sudden, brief, meaningless movements; nose twitching; mouth movements; lip pouting; head jerks; shoulder shrugs; arm jerks; abdominal tensing; kicks; finger movements; jaw snaps; tooth clicking; rapid jerking of any part of the body
Complex motor tics	Sustained looks; facial gestures; biting; slower, longer, more purposeful movements; touching objects or self; throwing; banging; thrusting arms; gestures with hands; gyrating and bending; dystonic postures; copropraxia (obscene gestures)
Simple phonic tics	Throat clearing; coughing; sniffing; spitting; sudden, meaningless sounds or noises; screeching; barking; grunting; gurgling; clacking; hissing; sucking; innumerable other sounds
Complex phonic tics	Syllables; words; phrases; statements such as sudden, more meaningful utterances ("Shut up," "Stop that," "Oh, okay," "I've got to," "Okay, honey," "What makes me do this?" "How about it," "Now you've seen it"); speech atypicalities (usually rhythms, tone, accents, intensity of speech); echo phenomenon (immediate repetition of one's own or another's words or phrases); coprolalia (obscene, inappropriate, and aggressive words and statements)

From Leckman, J., & Cohen, D. *Tourette's syndrome: Tics, obsessions, compulsions* (p. 25). Copyright © 1999 by John Wiley & Sons. Reprinted with permission of John Wiley & Sons, Inc.

are mild and often do not come to medical attention or require medication.

EPIDEMIOLOGY AND GENETICS

Prevalence estimates in most epidemiological studies suggest a rate of 5–10 individuals with Tourette syndrome per 10,000 births. A 3:1 male predominance is present, and tics usually begin in the first decade of life. Most studies report a median onset of simple motor tics at 5 or 6 years of age. Figure 12.4-1 reports Leckman and Cohen's (1999) age of onset data for 221 individuals with Tourette syndrome at the Yale Child Study Clinic. The period of worst tic severity is between 7 and 15 years, with a steady decline in variety, frequency, and severity after that age. Complete remission of tics may occur during later adolescence or adulthood, but estimates vary considerably as to how often this situation occurs. Predicting in which situations complete remission will occur is difficult. Often, adults have a limited number of tics that are predictably increased with stress or fatigue.

Since the late 1970s, investigators have demonstrated Tourette syndrome's familial concentration and tendency for vertical transmission from generation to generation (Pauls, 1992). Twin studies have confirmed a genetic role (Price et al., 1985). Single major-locus, polygenic, and multifactorial patterns of transmission have been proposed. Pauls and Leckman's (1986) segregation analysis study of 30 families suggested an autosomal dominant pattern with incomplete and sex-specific penetrances (boys more than girls) and variable clinical expression (Tourette syndrome, chronic tics, obsessive-compulsive disorder). Further studies are necessary to clarify the pattern of genetic transmission.

NEUROBIOLOGY

The molecular and cellular pathogenesis of Tourette syndrome is still unknown. An excellent review by Hoekstra et al. (2004) discussed anatomic and neuroimaging studies and provided support for the involvement of the basal ganglia and related cortico-striato-thalamo-cortical circuits as the site of Tourette syndrome symptoms. The possible involvement of these structures is supported by magnetic resonance imaging (MRI) studies that have identified basal ganglia and cortical volume differences between individuals with Tourette syndrome and individuals in a control group (Peterson & Skudlerski, 1998; Peterson et al., 2001; Peterson et al., 2003). The volume of the caudate nucleus has been found to

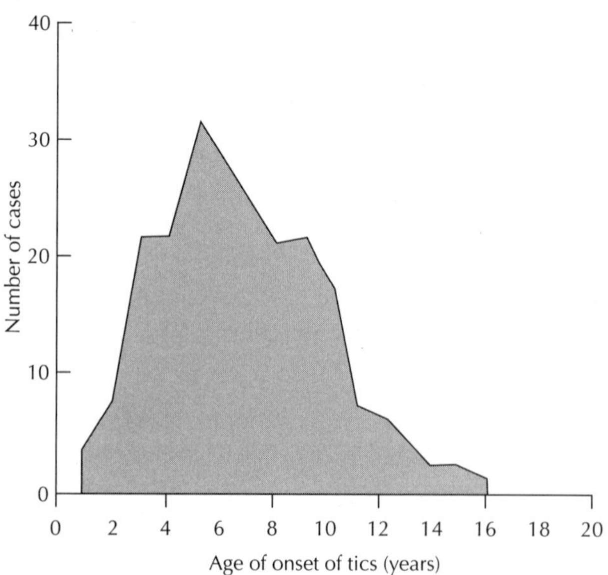

Figure 12.4-1. Age of onset of tics in a series of 221 individuals with Tourette syndrome evaluated at the Yale Child Study Clinic (unpublished data). These data were influential in resetting the age of onset criteria in the DSM–IV for Tourette's disorder from 21 years of age to 18 years of age (From Leckman, J., & Cohen, D. *Tourette's syndrome: Tics, obsessions, compulsions* [p. 39]. Copyright © 1999 by John Wiley & Sons. Reprinted with permission of John Wiley & Sons, Inc.)

be significantly reduced in children and adults with Tourette syndrome. Prefrontal and orbital frontal volumes are enlarged in children with Tourette syndrome but decreased in adults compared with individuals in a control group. In an interesting functional MRI study in which adults with Tourette syndrome suppressed tics, frontal cortical areas were activated. Finally, findings of positron emission tomography (PET) and single photon emission computed tomography (SPECT) suggest a role of the basal ganglia (Riddle et al., 1992; Stoetter et al., 1992). Reduced blood flow in the putamen and globus pallidus and reduced glucose utilization in the ventral striatum have been reported. The meaning of these studies and observations remains speculative but certainly allows for further anatomic and neuroimaging studies.

Further history revealed that Ted was diagnosed with attention-deficit/hyperactivity disorder (ADHD) when he was 6 years old. Approximately 2 years ago, he had taken methylphenidate briefly. He had stopped the medication when eye blinking began, but the tic did not disappear completely. Ted received special education help at school because of nonverbal learning disabilities. He had obsessive thoughts about cleanliness and compulsively engaged in repeated hand washing.

After evaluation, Ted's doctor prescribed pimozide 2 mg. at bedtime, which helped to control his tics. Ted's problems with attention span were not severe enough to warrant medication. His obsessive-compulsive disorder was treated for about 1 year with a selective serotonin reuptake inhibitor (SSRI) antidepressant. By late adolescence, Ted had only occasional eye blinking and took no medication.

ASSOCIATED CONDITIONS

The tics of Tourette syndrome are often accompanied by a variety of behavioral and learning disturbances. These issues are often more of a problem clinically and may indeed be the "target symptoms" requiring primary treatment. Obsessive-compulsive disorder occurs in approximately 50% of individuals with Tourette syndrome (Como, 1995). Common symptoms include obsessive worries and fears and compulsive counting, hand washing, gait patterns, and perfectionism. ADHD occurs in about 50% of individuals with Tourette syndrome. The task of treating attention problems without exacerbating tics is often a challenge. The symptoms of ADHD often precede the appearance of tics by an average of 2–5 years. Learning disabilities also occur in 50% of individuals with Tourette syndrome. Problems in reading, writing, and math are often encountered.

Neuropsychological studies have identified visuomotor integration and executive functioning as the domains most impaired (Coming & Coming, 1985). Psychologists that treat the behavioral manifestations of Tourette syndrome describe a characteristic pattern of "emotional storms." Argumentativeness, defensiveness, impulsivity, and negativism are common traits. Other socially inappropriate behavior can be seen as well, such as verbalizing insults or destroying property.

MANAGEMENT

The management of Tourette syndrome should be approached in a comprehensive manner that involves a balance of medical, psychological, and educational interventions. The first step is to educate the child and his or her parents about the definition of *Tourette syndrome*, the spectrum of tic disorders, and the disorder's natural history. Most families are reassured by knowing that tics wax and wane and that they are not intrinsically harmful or life threatening. Many families also find comfort in knowing that tics may improve or resolve with age. Providing families with resources to educate the school and peers about Tourette syndrome and to provide emotional support to the child is helpful. The Tourette Syndrome Association (http:///www.tsa-usa.org) is an excellent source of such information.

For some, education is the only necessary intervention, as the tics and associated neurobehavioral problems are not severe enough to warrant further treatment. Psychotherapy and/or environmental changes in the school, workplace, or home may be helpful. For others, more active treatment is necessary. The initial step is to identify the "target" symptom that is most interfering with daily functioning. This symptom is not always tics; it may be ADHD, obsessive-compulsive disorder, or other behavioral or learning problems.

Medication

Most patients with mild tics can adapt to their tics and avoid medication. When the tics are more severe and interfere significantly with function, pharmacotherapy may be advisable. The goal in treating tics is to achieve suppression rather than necessarily a tic-free state. Antidopaminergic agents and alpha2-adrenergic receptor agonists are the mainstay of monotherapy for tic disorders. Alternative drugs, including atypical neuroleptics, and combination pharmacotherapy are used in more complicated situations.

For individuals with mild or moderate tics, treatment is usually initiated with clonidine (Catapres), an alpha2-adrenergic agonist. Typical treatment begins with 0.05 mg at bedtime and is increased every few days until satisfactory control of tics or unacceptable side effects occur. Pulse, blood pressure, and electrocardiogram should be obtained prior to beginning treatment, and pulse and blood pressure should be monitored during treatment. Most individuals respond to 0.2–0.3 mg per day divided in 2 or 3 daily doses. Sedation is the most common limiting side effect but often abates after several weeks on the medication. Irritability, insomnia, headaches, hypotension, dizziness, and clinically insignificant electrocardiogram changes are less common side effects. Tolerance occurs on occasion, and dosage adjustments need to be made.

Guanfacine (Tenex) is a newer alpha2-adrenergic agonist. It has activity in the prefrontal cortex, affecting areas associated with attention and working memory. Guanfacine does not cause as much sedation or hypotension as clonidine. It is begun with a bedtime dose of 0.5 mg and increased to every few days to 0.75–3 mg in 2–3 divided doses.

For more severe tics or tics that require quicker treatment, a neuroleptic can be added or used instead. Haloperidol (Haldol) was the first approved treatment for Tourette syndrome (for adults in 1969 and for children in 1978). It is a D2 dopamine antagonist and also acts as an antagonist at alpha1-adrenergic receptors. Haloperidol was used widely with reported 70%–80% efficacy; however, frequent side effects, even at low doses, include sedation, weight gain, acute dystonic reactions, cognitive dulling, dysphoria, and akathesia. Another problem associated with its use is the difficulty faced in coming off the medication, with a worsening of tics in the month or two following discontinuation. As a result, haloperidol is rarely used today. Fluphenazine (Prolixin) is an occasionally used alternative.

Pimozide (Orap) is the most commonly used typical neuroleptic. It blocks D2 dopamine receptors but has no alpha-adrenergic activity. It is as effective as haloperidol in reducing tics but at low doses has much fewer side effects. At higher doses, electrocardiogram changes and tracings should be monitored at regular intervals during pimozide's use. Pimozide is started at 0.5–1 mg daily and increased weekly to a usual dose of 2–4 mg/day.

Atypical neuroleptics have been used in the treatment of moderate to severe tics. At low doses, these agents are potent serotonin (5-HT2) receptor antagonists, and at higher doses, they are dopamine D2-receptor antagonists. Risperidone (Risperdal) is the most commonly used medication in this class. The dose ranges from 1–2.5 mg per day. Weight gain is a frequent and problematic side effect. Extra pyramidal side effects, however, have typically not been a problem. Other atypical neuroleptics, such as ziprasidone and apriprazole, may have potential in the treatment of Tourette syndrome, but further studies are necessary.

Other medications that have been reported to improve tics include tetrabenazine, clonazapam, nicotine, baclofen, and calcium channel blockers. Botulinum toxin has been used in the treatment of refractory focal tics.

Treatment of Attention-Deficit/Hyperactivity Disorder

When ADHD is the target symptom alone, the child can be placed on atomoxetine (Strattera), a nonstimulant norepinephrine reuptake inhibitor and milder dopamine reuptake inhibitor. This medication is useful in the treatment of ADHD. It does not exacerbate tics and must be given on a daily basis to be effective. It is begun at 1.2 mg/kg/day and increased to 1.8–2.0 mg/kg/day as tolerated. The major side effect is dyspepsia, which is often transient. The efficacy of atomoxetine ranges from 30%–50%.

Clonidine may also be a useful medication, especially in the more "agitated" individual with Tourette syndrome in whom the improvement of tics would be a benefit. If symptoms are not adequately controlled, a trial of stimulant medications (methylphenidate or dextroamphetamine) may be warranted. Although stimulants may exacerbate tics in some individuals, this worsening may be acceptable if the target symptom of ADHD is much improved. There is no evidence that stimulant medications actually cause tics. On occasion, clonidine or a neuroleptic can be added to the stimulant to control the tic yet maintain the benefits of psychostimulant treatment. Tricyclic antidepressants are rarely used in the treatment of ADHD, especially when there is comorbid depression. See Chapter 23.2 for more information on ADHD management.

Treatment of Obsessive-Compulsive Disorder

Treatment of obsessive-compulsive disorder should include psychotherapy and, in some cases, antidepressant drugs such as the SSRIs. These medications include fluoxetine, sertraline, fluvoxamine, escitalopram, and citalopram. At the present time, clinicians should be cautious in the use of these medications because of recent data suggesting an increased risk of suicide among adolescents taking some SSRI antidepressants. This issue is presently under investigation by the Food and Drug Administration.

As a 38-year-old with Tourette syndrome, my tics have become milder—I think it is because I am happy with my life. I have a wonderful job. I have a wonderful and very supportive wife, and I have a great support system of family and friends. I believe that all of these positive factors have contributed to less tics. I work in a very good and positive environment for me—everyone has been sensitized to my syndrome so my work environment is very pleasant. Having Tourette syndrome has actually made my job more effective because I work with children and adults with disabilities, so I have first-hand experience in knowing what it is like to be different. I also have the attitude and strive to do the most for myself, so I like to do all the fun stuff that we all like to do.

Sometimes when I feel myself exhibiting more tics, I try to stop them with such actions as putting a pen in my mouth or sitting on my hands, or sometimes I will take a time-out and just try to be by myself to calm down. The events that get my syndrome active are more stressful situations, times that are very quiet, and very crowded and loud places, which I am sure most people with Tourette syndrome get more agitated in.

—S.R., October 2004

CONCLUSION

Tourette syndrome is a clinically diagnosed multifocal motor/vocal tic disorder. Although it is defined by unique and varied involuntary tics, the condition is often accompanied by neurobehavioral features including ADHD, obsessive-compulsive disorder, learning disabilities, and behavior disorders. The genetics and neurobiology of the disorder are still incompletely understood. Treatment is directed at the target symptom(s), whether it is the tic or one of the associated conditions. Finally, an understanding of the natural history of Tourette syndrome will allow the physician to treat the symptoms and support the individual and family throughout the course of this chronic disorder.

REFERENCES

American Psychiatric Association. (1994). *Diagnostic and statistical manual of mental disorders* (4th ed.). Washington, DC: Author.

Coming, D.E., & Comings, B.G. (1985). Tourette syndrome: Clinical and psychological aspects of 250 cases. *American Journal of Human Genetics, 37*, 435–450.

Como, P.G. (1995). Obsessive-compulsive disorder in Tourette's syndrome. *Advances in Neurology, 65*, 281–291.

Erenberg, G., Cruse, R.P., & Rothner, A.D. (1987). The natural history of Tourette syndrome: A follow up study. *Annals of Neurology, 22*, 383–385.

Hoekstra, P.J., Anderson, G.M., et al. (2004). Neurology and neuroimmunology of Tourette's syndrome: An update. *Cellular and Molecular Life Sciences, 61*, 886–898.

Leckman, J., & Cohen, D. (1999). *Tourette's syndrome: Tics, obsessions, compulsions.* New York: John Wiley and Sons.

Pauls, D. (1992). Issues in genetic linkage studies of Tourette syndrome: Phenotypic spectrum and genetic model parameters. *Advances in Neurology, 58*, 151–157.

Pauls, D., & Leckman, J.F. (1986). The inheritance of Gilles de la Tourette's syndrome and associated behaviors: Evidence for autosomal dominant transmission. *New England Journal of Medicine, 315*, 993–997.

Peterson, B.S., & Skudlerski, P. (1998). A functional magnetic resonance imaging study of tic suppression in Tourette syndrome. *Archives of General Psychiatry, 55*, 326–333.

Peterson, B.S., Stdlb, L., et al. (2001). Regional brain and ventricular volumes in Tourette syndrome. *Archives of General Psychiatry, 58*, 427–440.

Peterson, B.S., Thomas, P., et al. (2003). Baral gangliu volumes in patients with Gilles de la Tourette syndrome. *Archives of General Psychiatry, 60*, 415–424.

Price, R.A., Kidd, K.K., Cohen, D., et al. (1985). A twin study of Tourette's syndrome. *Archives of General Psychiatry, 42*, 815–820.

Riddle, M.A., Rasmusson, A.M., et al. (1992). SPECT imaging of cerebral blood flow in Tourette syndrome. *Advances in Neurology, 58*, 207–211.

Shapiro, A.K., Shapiro, E.S., et al. (1988). *Gilles de la Tourette syndrome.* New York: Raven Press.

Stoetter, B., Braun, A.R., et al. (1992). Functional neurocuratomy of Tourette syndrome: Limbic-motor interaction studied with FDG PET. *Advances in Neurology, 58*, 213–226.

CHAPTER 13

ORTHOPEDICS

Daniel J. Hedequist and Michael Millis

Orthopedics is a specialty that deals with disorders of muscles, tendons, bones, and joints. These disorders are diverse in their origin and may be as a result of congenital anomalies, metabolic processes, genetic disorders, or disorders arising from insults to the brain or spinal cord. The neurological system controls muscle movement; as a result, any disorder of the brain or spinal cord will cause an imbalance of muscle strength and function with resultant effects on the position and use of the individual's axial and appendicular skeleton. These effects are diverse and may range from a mild gait abnormality in an individual with hemiplegia to a severe spinal deformity in an individual with myelomeningocele. All of these effects may be seen by orthopedists as a functional problem and may be classified by their anatomical distribution and functional impairment.

Juliette had a seizure disorder and psychomotor delay. She was quite late with her developmental milestones and did not roll spontaneously until about 2 years of age. She never developed the ability to pull herself to a sitting position or to sit without support. Spasticity in all four extremities became apparent during her second year of life, and she received occupational therapy and physiotherapy. Bracing with ankle-foot-orthosis (AFO) was begun at 20 months of age.

When Juliette was 5, an increasing flexion-adduction deformity of her left hip was noted, at which point she also became uncomfortable sitting. Her discomfort and deformity progressed despite aggressive physiotherapy. Radiographs at this time documented a change from two well-reduced hips to a subluxed condition of the left hip, with secondary acetabular dysplasia (see Figures 13.1). Orthopaedic surgery was considered at this point to improve her comfort and to maintain her sitting function with the goal of avoiding a painful dislocation of the left hip that would have further compromised her sitting. To improve her condition for surgery, an aggressive nutritional program was begun, anticipating the metabolic challenge that a major orthopaedic operation would involve.

After 3 months of careful hypernutrition, Juliette underwent a left varus shortening intertrochanteric osteotomy and left pelvic osteotomy, with simultaneous adductor releases and psoas lengthening. Her antiseizure medications were carefully maintained perioperatively. She was immobilized for 2 months postoperatively in a bivalved spica cast, which she tolerated well. After release from the spica, with her osteotomies well-healed radiographically, she was much more comfortable. Her hip range of motion and her sitting posture were improved.

Approximately 1 year after her left hip surgery, an adduction deformity of her right hip began to develop with pain and limitation of motion. Radiographs documented a new subluxation of the right hip. After another period of supplemental nutritional support, she underwent right varus intertrochanteric osteotomy and shelf procedure with tendon releases to stabilize her right hip. Following another 2-month period in a spica cast, her clinical exam was greatly improved, with increased pain-free range of motion about the right hip and restoration of a comfortable symmetric sitting posture.

Orthopedic treatment goals for all individuals should be improvement in function, prevention of secondary physical impairments, and increase of developmental capabilities. These goals must be met by a combination of treatment modalities (medical, surgical, physical and occupational therapy, orthotic treatment). This chapter provides a basic overview of orthopedic treatment of anatomical and functional disorders seen in children with developmental disorders. An overview of non-surgical treatment modalities is discussed, followed by a discussion of specific anatomical regions and stories.

MULTIDISCIPLINARY CARE

Children with developmental disabilities have brought to the forefront of medicine the idea that a team-oriented approach is much better for patient care. They provide a great challenge to any one clinician because they require time and resources to obtain appropriate services. Generally, these children have many medical problems that require frequent visits to the hospital. The concept of multidisciplinary care has arisen in order to address the multifaceted aspects of these children's health issues (Gormley, 2001).

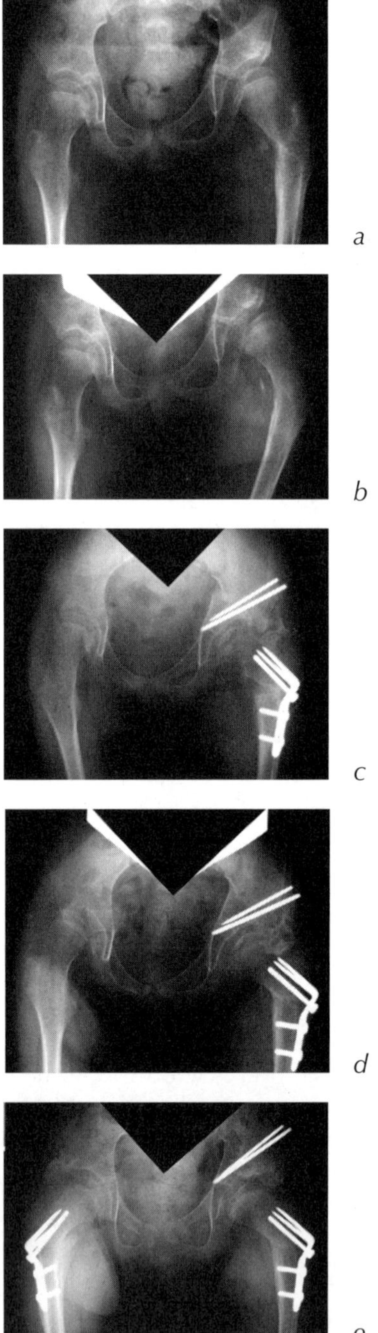

Figure 13.1. Changes to Juliette's hips. (*a*) AP radiograph of Juliette's hips at age 4. The range of motion of her hips was painless and symmetrical at this point. No hip subluxation was noted. (*b*) Age 5. Discomfort with sitting was noted, and flexion-adduction contracture of left hip was present. The radiograph shows superior and lateral subluxation of the left femoral head, with associated acetabular dysplasia. (*c*) Age 5.5, following varus intertrochanteric osteotomy and left Chiari pelvic osteotomy. Excellent postoperative healing was noted, with great improvement in the position of the femoral head. Juliette's clinical hip range of motion was pain free and symmetrical. (*d*) Age 6.5. Juliette has new onset of right hip pain with sitting due to a flexion-adduction contracture of her right hip. The radiograph documents new subluxation of her right hip. The stable position of her previously operated left hip was maintained. (*e*) Age 7, following healing from a right-sided hip stabilization procedure. A shelf procedure and varus shortening osteotomy were done with appropriate tendon releases. Excellent postoperative position was achieved.

Benito was a 10-year-old boy who immigrated to the United States with his mother and father. He had a history of neonatal hypoxia secondary to prematurity and had resultant spastic quadraparesis and mild intellectual disabilities. Benito's family had never been able to have any treatment rendered for him. Benito did not have a wheelchair and had not seen a pediatrician in 2 years, although his family stated that he was healthy. Benito's family wanted to know if they could obtain a wheelchair for him and were wondering if he would be able to attend school.

A general evaluation of Benito's health and socioeconomic situation was conducted by a coordinated care physician. This evaluation found Benito to be medically healthy and, more important, helped the process of getting Benito enrolled in a school program that would include many types of therapy. A social worker was consulted to help Benito's family obtain these services. The orthopedist evaluated Benito and, with the help of physical therapists, started a program of therapy and fit Benito for a wheelchair. The social worker also helped find funding for Benito's new wheelchair.

In a team approach, the child and his or her family lie at the center. Physical, occupational, and speech therapists are usually at the forefront of the clinical decision making. Although physicians play an important part in the child's life, therapists have a much greater grasp on the day-to-day living and pertinent physical issues for the child given that they have weekly interaction with the child and family.

Although Benito's scenario is not a common one, it does give an example of the importance of a team approach. Frequently, in a multidisciplinary clinic, the orthopedist and therapist will have a discussion with the family and may or may not use the orthotist. Given the multitude of medical problems, the primary care physician or coordinate care physician frequently becomes the team leader of these children's care.

We run a multidisciplinary Cerebral Palsy Clinic at our institution that includes multiple physical therapists, an orthopedist, a physiatrist, an orthotist, and a coordinated care clinical specialist. This set-up allows us to be prepared and to have greater physician and therapist interactions with the families when it comes to decision making regarding the need for further therapy, surgery, botox injections, or orthotic support. Many of these children also need the support of nutritional services, social services, and other medical services. These services can be coordinated with the visits to the multidisciplinary clinic in order to improve the individual's care and minimize multiple visits to the hospital.

PHARMACOLOGIC MANAGEMENT

The use of pharmacologic agents has greatly enhanced the orthopedic treatment of children with developmental disabilities. These agents are designed to specifically treat the presence of spasticity. Baclofen works to decrease spasticity by effecting gamma-amino butyric acid (GABA) receptor affinity (Tilton, 2003). Baclofen may be administered either orally or intrathecally via a pump (see Chapter 11). The spasticity is reduced by way of GABA receptors that inhibit monosynaptic extensor and polysynaptic flexor activity. Baclofen also works to limit nocioception by way of decreasing substance P levels.

Oral baclofen tends to cause somnolence and other side effects and thus sometimes is not tolerated. Intrathecal baclofen is administered by way of a pump that is inserted surgically under the rectus fascia and connected under the shin to a catheter that goes into the intrathecal space via the lumbar spine. Intrathecal baclofen has been shown to reduce spasticity and improve function in select individuals. Valium is another oral agent that potentiates GABA effects and acts to decrease spasticity. It is habit forming, and the doses needed to affect spasticity frequently cause an undesirable sedative effect.

Botulinum neurotoxins, although potent lethal toxins, clinically provide aid by decreasing the release of acetycholine at the neuromuscular junction (Delgado, 2003). This blockage leads to a diminishment of muscular hypertonia and its resultant deleterious effect on joint motion and extremity function. At a microscopic level, the effects of Botox on the neuromuscular junction last up to 3 months in animal studies; however, at the macroscopic level, in conjunction with therapy, the effects may last even longer. Clinically, an individual will usually experience a measurable improvement in passive joint range of motion and a measurable decrease in regional hypertonia following injections. Injections must be used in conjunction with intensive physical therapy and orthotics in order to maximize the clinical benefit.

In general, these injections are safe and are performed either in an office setting or as an outpatient procedure. The beneficial effects may start as early as 24–72 hours postinjection. Although there are limits on the amount of Botox that may be injected at one setting, the injections may be repeated as early as 4 months later. The adverse effects are minimal, transient, and rare and may include generalized weakness, pain, and transient low-grade fevers.

PHYSICAL THERAPY AND ORTHOTIC MANAGEMENT

Physical therapists aim to maximize function, improve skills, and minimize contractures and deformity. Although many philosophies deal with treatment methods, in general, the physical therapist's interventions focus on maintaining muscle length, improving muscle strength, and improving function (Hartley, 2002). Physical therapy also works to support other treatment modalities such as surgery, orthotics, and pharmacologic therapy. The therapist also acts as a facilitator between the child, family, and physicians.

Although most physical therapy revolves around the basic principles of joint range of motion and muscle strengthening and stretching, physical therapists frequently are involved in the decision-making processes with regard to orthotics and sitting appliances. The scope of orthotics reaches far beyond this chapter; however, a basic understanding of orthotics and seating appliances is necessary in order to care for children with developmental disabilities. The goals of any seating appliance are many fold and include ease of mobility, supportive sitting to allow for maximization of respiratory function, optimal positioning of the individual to facilitate interaction with his or her surroundings, and comfortable sitting position. Seating appliance options include headrests, side-sitting posts, adjustable footplates, and occasionally electric-driven controls. Modifications may be made for each individual in order to improve his or her function and interactions (Medhat & Redford, 1985).

Orthotics may be classified into upper extremity, lower extremity, and spinal orthotics. The use of spinal orthotics in order to halt progression of spinal deformity has not been shown to be effective in individuals with global involvement; however, individuals frequently have truncal hypotonia, and the addition of a soft spinal orthosis may greatly enhance their sitting ability and lead to better interactions with their environment, improved ability to clear secretions, and more comfortable sitting. Any spinal orthosis should be lightweight and breathable, easily applied, and used when the individual is sitting in a wheelchair. Spinal orthosis are not routinely used in a nonsupportive way (e.g., for control of large curvatures for sleep).

Upper extremity orthotics are best used when dealing with nonfixed deformities of the hand and wrist. These orthotics are used either to control hypertonicity and their resultant contractures or to facilitate hand motion and dexterity. They may be used as static devices to position the limb in a fixed place or dynamic devices that help facilitate underlying function. Regardless of their form, orthotics should be lightweight, easily applied, and used in conjunction with a hand therapist (Wilton, 2003).

Finally, bracing the lower extremity should focus on placing the feet in a plantigrade position and preventing deformity and contracture. The stalwarts in treatment are the AFO and the custom-molded foot orthotics (Renshaw, Green, Griffin, & Root, 1996). A prerequisite for using these orthoses are minimal preexisting deformity so that the foot can be placed into the brace and the ability to keep the individual's foot in the brace (i.e., minimal underlying spasticity). All orthotics are used in conjunction with many other modalities such as physical therapy, pharmacologic therapy, and surgical therapy in order to improve function and daily living.

SURGICAL MANAGEMENT

Jamal was a 15-year-old boy with spastic quadraparesis secondary to neonatal sepsis. He was nonambulatory and lived at home with his parents. He attended school and received weekly physical therapy and occupational therapy. In the past, Jamal had been able to use his power wheelchair, but his parents noticed that this activity was becoming increasingly difficult because of the position of Jamal's right upper extremity, which had changed during a recent growth spurt. Jamal's occupational therapist believed that any use of orthotics at this point would be difficult given Jamal's progressive contractures and limb spasticity.

Upper Extremities

The upper extremities of individuals with developmental disabilities usually become problematic with spasticity. The function, dressing ability, hygiene, and appearance of individuals can drastically be affected by hypertonic muscle forces acting across joints from the shoulder to the small joints of the hand. In general, hypertonicity of the upper extremity flexor groups creates the dominant position of the extremity. The position of the shoulder may create an adducted and internally rotated upper extremity. The elbow is usually held in a position of flexion given the hypertonicity of the biceps and weakness of the extensor musculature. The forearm position will help determine the position of the hand in space, which is usually one of forearm probation leading to a palm down position of the hand. Wrist flexor and finger flexor overactivity produce difficulty in obtaining extension of the wrist to a neutral position and the ability to grasp objects given the inability to open the hand.

Operations of the upper extremity must be aimed toward improvement in function, ease of dressing, ability to clean the limb, and cosmesis. Individuals with higher levels of voluntary control, better sensibility, and less-fixed contractures do the best with surgical management. Operations around the shoulder tend to focus on release or lengthening of the spastic muscles in order to improve motion. In general, elbow motion is improved by addressing the overactive biceps muscles and releasing any fixed contracture (Landi et al., 2003). The position of the wrist and hand in space first starts with the surgical management of the pronated forearm if present. Active supination of the forearm and thus wrist greatly enhances upper extremity function and is accomplished by procedures that either release the flexor-pronator mechanism or transfer these muscles to produce their antagonistic effect. Overall grasp and release function necessitates addressing finger and wrist deformities.

As mentioned previously, the most common wrist deformity is flexion. This deformity may be addressed by tendon lengthening or transfers in those individuals with some voluntary control of the wrist with an overactive wrist flexor mass. In individuals with severe fixed deformities, the position of the wrist in a functioning position may necessitate wrist fusion (Van Heest, 2003). The most common finger deformity seen in these individuals is a flexion deformity with a clenched fist posture. Tendon lengthening in concert with procedures addressing the wrist are needed to improve the individual's function and hand position.

Jamal was taken to the Orthopedic Clinic with a functional problem. Upon examination, he was noted to have significant spasticity of his biceps with spasticity of both his wrist flexors and finger flexors. His inability to extend his wrist and subsequently open his hand has affected his ability to power his wheelchair. In the past, Jamal had been managed with splints that had positioned his hand in a functional position; however, his occupational therapist felt that he had become too contracted to benefit from a splint treatment. The goal in treating Jamal was vocalized by his parents as returning him to the independent use of his power chair. He was managed by tendon lengthening of his wrist flexors and digital flexors in order to open Jamal's hand in space and allow for control of his power wheelchair.

Hips

Twelve-year-old Elise had severe intellectual disabilities and spastic quadraparesis. She resided in a pediatric long-term nursing facility and was a ward of the state. Elise's primary caregivers, the nursing facility staff, had voiced concerns over the continued difficulty that Elise was having with sitting in her wheelchair as a result of the position of her right leg. Staff members were also concerned about the difficulty that they were having in cleaning her perineal region given that her legs could not be spread apart. Elise was nonvocal and was unable to voice any complaints. Her physical therapist stated that contractures of Elise's hips had not responded to daily physical therapy during the last 6 months.

Individuals with global involvement have abnormal muscle forces across their hips that predispose them to subluxations and dislocations of the hips (Flynn & Miller, 2002). Incongruity of the hips leads to stiffness and resultant pain. Individuals with spastic cerebral palsy, however, are predisposed to adductor spasticity and gluteal weakness that leads to pulling of the limb medially with superior and lateral migration of the hip out of the acetabulum. These individuals have some sensibility around the hip, and an incongruent joint leads to both stiffness and pain. The stiffness associated with muscle imbalance around the hip leads to resultant pelvic obliquity as well as sitting difficulties. The obliquity of the pelvis can coincide with scoliosis and make sitting upright an even greater challenge. Pelvic obliquity and contractures about the hip also make personal hygiene in the perineal region difficult.

The goal of any operation around the hip is to obtain a joint that is pain free and has sufficient motion to allow for comfortable sitting, appropriate hygiene, and smooth transfers. In individuals with spasticity, the two forces acting on the hip that have the potential to cause problems are the hip flexors and the hip adductors. These muscles may lead to secondary problems with the hip joint (proximal femur and bony acetabulum). In individuals with concentric joints and limited abduction of the hip, tendon lengthening procedures will restore motion and lead to a prevention of subluxation and dislocation. Usually, release of the adductors is performed in concert with release of the hip flexors (iliopsoas).

With prolonged abnormal muscle forces acting across the hip joint, the individual will develop subluxation of the hip joint followed by dislocation of the hip joint. Usually, abnormal muscle forces and nonambulation will lead to a valgus deformity of the proximal femur and shallow acetabulum (hip socket). These deformities are treated with realignment of the bony structures through osteotomies of the proximal femur and/or acetabulum (Flynn & Miller, 2002).

Prolonged untreated muscle imbalance will lead to dislocation of the hip joint. The complete dislocation brought about by these abnormal muscle forces leads to a proximal femur that is stiff and occasionally painful. These fixed dislocations make it difficult for individuals to sit comfortably in a wheelchair and spread their legs apart in order have appropriate perineal care performed. The dislocations also increase the development of pelvic obliquity and resultant scoliosis. Once the hip becomes fixed and painful, the salvage operation is usually a resection of the proximal portion of hip joint in order to obtain a mobile, painfree, fibrous joint.

Although Elise was nonambulatory and nonvocal, she had caregivers who voiced two functional problems: sitting in a wheelchair and perineal care. Examination of Elise was extremely difficult given her severe spasticity; however, her right leg was clearly severely abducted and could not be brought into any abduction. This condition made getting her legs apart impossible. Examination showed that her hip on the right was fixed and had created an obliquity of the pelvis such that sitting with even pressure on the buttocks was impossible. Radiographs showed a fixed dislocation of the right hip with arthritic changes. The treatment goals for Elise were to create a mobile hip such that sitting and perineal care would be possible. Resection arthroplasty of the right hip might result in a much greater range of motion and significantly improved sitting.

Spine

Disorders of the spine are common in individuals with global involvement. In general, these deformities will evolve into either a lateral curvature of the spine (scoliosis), a forward bend of the spine (kyphosis), a backward bend of the spine (lordosis), or a combination (kyphoscoliosis or lordoscoliosis). The function of the bony spine is to protect the spinal cord and to help support the upright position of the body. Generally, spine deformities are not painful, but the sequela of large deformities are well known. In general, large deformities prevent these individuals from sitting upright. The ability to sit upright allows these individuals to interact with their environment, to sit comfortably in their wheelchairs, to help caregivers with hygiene and transfers, and to help clear secretions and the upper airway in order to prevent respiratory difficulties. All of these things may be compromised with deformities of large magnitude.

Individuals with hypotonia and spasticity alike have a tendency to develop significant spinal deformities. In general, once these deformities become large enough to require surgery, they have already created a difficulty with sitting, hygiene, comfort, and daily function. Not all individuals with deformities of the spine require an operation, but individuals who do have an operation have a significant medical and surgical complication rate. With that being said, the ability to obtain a balanced spine allows for improved sitting, improved interaction, and improved pulmonary status. Correction of spinal deformities is performed by fusing the bony spinal column and achieving correction of the individual's deformity by spinal implants. Posterior surgery or anterior-posterior surgery may be performed depending on the individual's age, curve type, and curve magnitude. In a recent study, the vast majority of parents and caregivers of individuals with cerebral palsy who underwent spinal fusion felt that the benefits from surgical correction clearly outweighed the increased risks of surgical complications (Tsirikos, Chang, Dabney, & Miller, 2004).

When Juliette was 7, her spine was free of scoliosis. She used a soft spinal othosis for sitting because of a tendency for her spine to collapse anteriorly into kyphosis (see Figure 13.2). When Juliette was 9, however, radiographs noted the onset of a right thoraco-lumbar scoliosis that progressed gradually despite aggressive bracing over the next 2 years (see Figure 13.3) until spinal fusion was decided on. Unfortunately, Juliette's medical condition was compromised for 24 months due to recurrent aspiration pneumonias, delaying her surgery for a year and a half. At this point, Juliette's scoliosis had increased from a moderate to severe degree (see Figure 13.4). Finally, through the combined effort of her developmental pediatrician, her neurologist, her gastroenterologist, her physiotherapist, her orthopedist, and her parents, her condition was felt optimal to undergo correction and stabilization of her spinal deformity. The goal of the surgery was to prevent aggressive deterioration in her ability to sit and, more importantly, to maintain her ability to breathe well.

Juliette underwent a posterior spinal fusion with instrumentation from T-4 to L-4, with satisfying correction achieved. Juliette was able to sit comfortably in her seating system, free of her soft spinal orthosis, by postoperative week 12 (see Figure 13.5). Clinical follow-up revealed maintenance of excellent sitting posture, reduced requirements for a seating system, improved respiratory function, and improved gastrointestinal function.

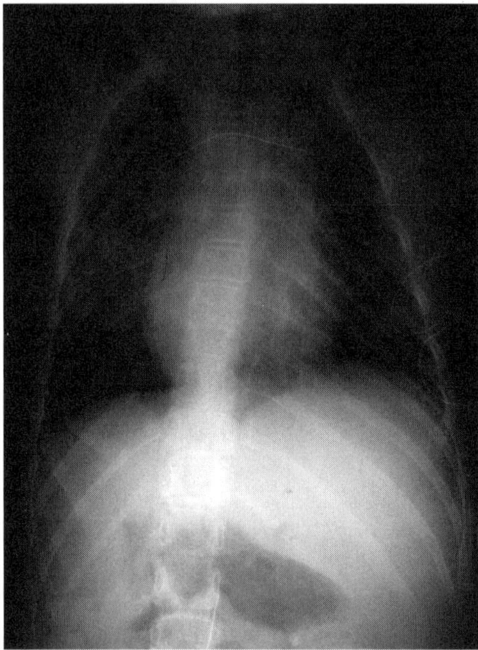

Figure 13.2. AP radiograph of Juliette's spine at age 7. Minimal scoliosis was present.

Feet

Disorders of the feet result from abnormal muscle forces across multiple joints of the feet. The resulting deformities can cause pressure points with shoe or brace wear and resulting skin breakdown. Individuals with global involvement frequently have sensory impairments that lead to a diminished protective effect and predispose them to ulcerations. The surgical options for treating individuals with feet deformities depend on the specific deformity present. In general, the goal of any operation around the foot is to obtain a plantigrade foot that has any weight-bearing forces or bracing forces evenly distributed.

Even force distribution with a neutral position of the foot will help prevent the breakdown of skin with its resultant soft tissue infections and ulcerations which may occur. This condition may be accomplished by means of tendon lengthening, tendon transfers, bony procedures, or a combination of all three (Renshaw et al., 1996). The end result of surgery may also result in a foot that requires bracing; however, if the foot is in a reasonable position with equal forces acting on it preventing any breakdown in the skin, then surgical treatment has been effective.

Thirteen-year-old Bessie had spastic diplegia. She was communicative and independently ambulatory at home and in the community. Bessie had had braces for her feet since she began walking at 2 years of age. Over the past year, however, she had experienced progressive difficulty with her braces and blistering on the inside of her feet. She had missed multiple days of school during the past 3 months given the pain associated with her feet and ambulation. Although Bessie did not mind wearing braces, she was frustrated by her continued difficulties and pain. Her father was concerned about the worsening appearance and function of her feet and about her long-term prognosis.

Physical examination revealed that Bessie had significant breakdown over the medial aspect of her feet. Her underlying spastic heel cord and peroneals had led to the progressive flattening of the arch and prominence of the medial aspect of the feet. Functional goals for Bess included returning to her baseline activity, pain relief, and improving the weight-bearing mechanics of her feet. Bessie was treated by a combination of tendon lengthening and bony surgery in order to meet her goals. She continued to wear braces, which improved her ambulatory status, and did not have any skin breakdown after surgery.

CONCLUSION

The treatment of children with developmental disabilities is both challenging and rewarding. The decisions regarding any treatment modality should be under-

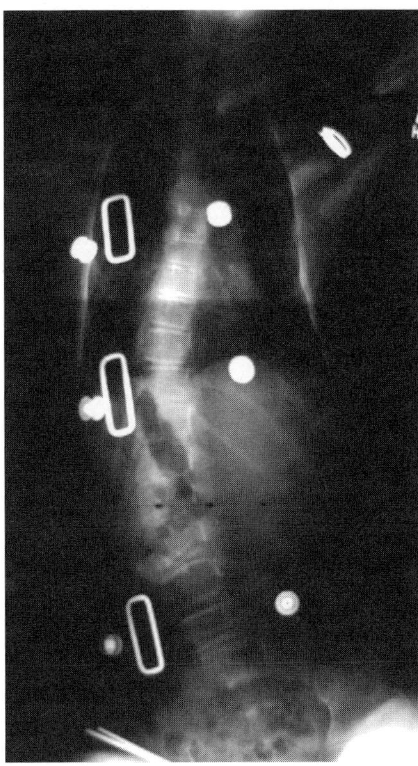

Figure 13.3. AP radiograph showing further progression of Juliette's thoracolumbar scoliosis despite bracing.

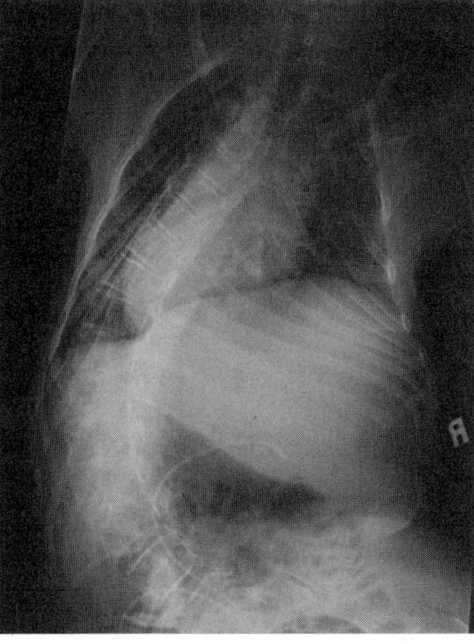

Figure 13.4. AP radiography showing a severe increase in Juliette's thoracolumbar scoliosis from age 9.5 to age 12.5. A delay in surgical treatment was needed due to Juliette's compromised medical condition.

If the family states that perineal care is difficult secondary to hip spasticity in a child with severe involvement, then the surgeon needs to exhaust all efforts to improve the hip range of motion regardless of the individual's cognitive ability. The art of medicine is de-taken with what is best for the child and the parents. Using a multidisciplinary team will help optimize the treatment regimen for these families. Although the surgical management of many orthopedic disorders is clear cut, management may be difficult for children with severe disabilities. The technical aspects of surgery are usually straightforward, but the decision regarding when to operate occasionally becomes difficult.

The most important step is listening to the family: What concerns do family members have? What difficulties are they encountering? Has any issue in particular brought them to the clinic? If a child has moderate scoliosis that has been present for years and is easily managed by wheelchair modifications, is there any clear benefit to surgery? Is a foot that is deformed but has no skin breakdown and is not painful to a child who uses a wheelchair better off with surgery to make it look better? Likewise, the inability of individuals with severe cognitive involvement to relay their complaints does not mean that they do meet the criteria for any surgical intervention. In these cases, the families and caregivers who live and take care of these children need to be considered their strong advocates and voice.

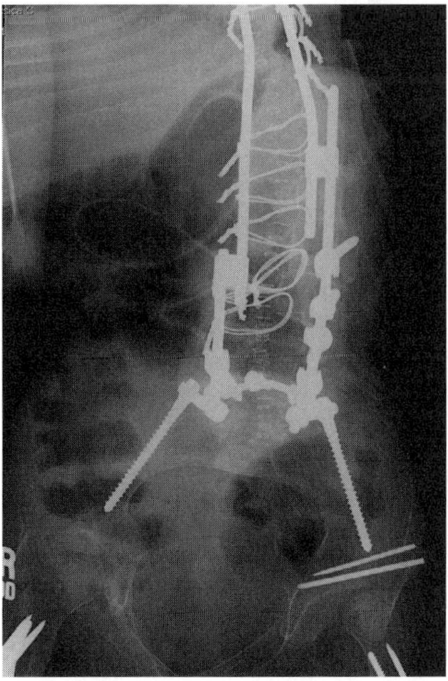

Figure 13.5. Supine AP radiograph of Juliette's thoracolumbar spine, documenting correction of her scoliosis with posterior spinal fusion from her upper thoracic spine to her pelvis.

ciding what is best for the individual. For children with developmental disabilities, using the team approach leads to better decision making and management. Above all, listening to the families and primary caregivers will lead to more realistic management of these children's orthopedic issues.

REFERENCES

Delgado, M.R. (2003). Botulinum neurotoxin type A. *Journal of the American Academy of Orthopaedic Surgeons, 11*(5), 291–294.

Flynn, J.M., & Miller, F. (2002). Management of hip disorders in patients with cerebral palsy. *Journal of the American Academy of Orthopaedic Surgeons, 10*(3), 198–209.

Gormley, M.E., Jr. (2001). Treatment of neuromuscular and musculoskeletal problems in cerebral palsy. *Pediatric Rehabilitation, 4*(1), 5–16.

Hartley, J. (2002). Physiotherapy in the management of cerebral palsy. *Hospital Medicine, 63*(10), 590–592.

Landi, A., Cavazza, S., Caserta, G., Leti Acciaro, A., Sartini, S., Gagliano, M.C., et al. (2003). The upper limb in cerebral palsy: Surgical management of shoulder and elbow deformities. *Hand Clinics, 19*(4), 631–648.

Medhat, M.A., & Redford, J.B. (1985). Experience of a seating clinic. *International Orthopedics, 9*(4), 279–285.

Renshaw, T.S., Green, N.E., Griffin, P.P., & Root, L. (1996). Cerebral palsy: Orthopaedic management. *Instructional Course Lectures, 45*, 475–490.

Tilton, A.H. (2004). Management of spasticity in children with cerebral palsy. *Seminars in Pediatric Neurology, 11*(1), 58–65.

Tsirikos, A.I., Chang, W.N., Dabney, K.W., & Miller, F. (2004). Comparison of parents' and caregivers' satisfaction after spinal fusion in children with cerebral palsy. *Journal of Pediatric Orthopedics, 24*(1), 54–58.

Van Heest, A.E. (2003). Surgical management of wrist and finger deformity. *Hand Clinics, 19*(4), 657–665.

Wilton, J. (2003). Casting, splinting, and physical and occupational therapy of hand deformity and dysfunction in cerebral palsy. *Hand Clinics, 19*(4), 573–584.

CHAPTER 14

GASTROENTEROLOGY

14.1 FEEDING AND NUTRITION

Stanley A. Cohen, Cathleen C. Piazza, and Aruna Navathe

Individuals with developmental disabilities are likely to have problems with feeding and nutrition. As many as 60%–90% of children with developmental disabilities have feeding problems based on parent report and observation (Reilly, Skuse, & Poblete, 1996) and videofluoroscopy (Griggs, Jones, & Lee, 1989). Often, feeding difficulties precede—and in fact herald—the diagnosis of cerebral palsy in 60% of children with mothers noting poor suck, vomiting, and choking (Reilly & Skuse, 1992). Many individuals with developmental disabilities may have significant oral motor dysfunction with medical sequelae (e.g., retching, choking, aspiration) and subsequent behavioral factors (Burklow et al., 1998; Crist & Napier-Phillips, 2001) that further affect their nutritional status.

The nutritional goals for individuals with developmental disabilities are obvious and implicit: 1) adequate nutritional substrates to maintain the individual's metabolic and fluid requirements, 2) sufficient energy intake to perform those metabolic tasks, 3) additional energy stores to withstand stress (e.g., infections) and optimize growth, 4) rehabilitation of malnutrition, and 5) correction and prevention of nutrient deficiencies. Poor nutritional state was often marked by linear growth failure, decreased lean body mass, and diminished fat stores (Stallings, Cronk, Zemel, & Charney, 1995). Aspiration pneumonia was often the expected mode of demise (Rogers et al., 1994).

Since the 1970s, however, enteral feedings and surgical intervention to protect the airways of individuals with severe disabilities have significantly improved outcomes for these individuals (Brant, Stanich, & Ferrari, 1990). In addition, the recognition of the complex interplay of gastroesophageal, oropharyngeal, and neurobehavioral factors have driven the development of multidisciplinary feeding programs that provide comprehensive evaluation and treatment of feeding disorders in children with developmental disabilities to improve their nutritional status and reduce their hospitalization rate (Schwartz et al., 2001).

The periods of greatest nutritional risk are 1) early infancy during the phase of rapid physical growth and brain development and 2) the second decade of life when nutritional needs increase as a result of increasing size—with feeding time needing to increase concomitantly to meet caloric and nutritional needs. Oral feeding difficulties can result in decreased feeding efficiency and can become more problematic as the child grows, requiring increased oral intake and skill as variously textured solids and cupped liquids are presented (Mirrett, Riski, Glascott, & Johnson, 1994). Moreover, children seem to have a slow convalescence from illnesses because of their inability to increase their energy consumption during or following illness.

Studies on small groups of children with developmental disabilities have demonstrated that increased nutrient intake can improve weight for height, muscle mass, subcutaneous energy stores, peripheral circulation, the healing of decubitus ulcers, and general well-being while decreasing irritability and spasticity (Rempel, Colwell, & Nelson, 1988; Sanders et al., 1990). The weight gain is both lean body mass (15%) and body fat (85%). Earlier initiation of nutritional intervention leads to significantly improved outcome, but this improved nutritional status may not translate into an increase in height or improved function. Even those receiving improved nutrition do not attain commensurate linear growth (Chad et al., 2000).

Data on adults is limited, despite the fact that increased survival of low birth weight infants and increased longevity results in 65%–90% of children with developmental disabilities surviving into adulthood, depending on the age at which survival is calculated (Rapp & Torres, 2000). In a study of 86 adult men and women recruited through a Cerebral Palsy Center or participating in regional games sponsored by the U.S. Cerebral Palsy Association, 40% had heights below the 5th percentile although their body mass indices and mean body fat were within normal range compared with healthy individuals (Ferrano, Johnson, & Ferrara, 1992). In a comparative study of 14 adults and 8 adolescents receiving enteral feedings, both groups had decreased body weight and height, although the adolescents were statistically lighter and shorter than the adults (body weight of 26.9 ± 4.9 kg vs. 37.8 ± 10.5 kg, and heights of 120 ± 12 cm vs. 149 ± 11 cm). The calculated percentage of body fat and measured resting energy expenditures, however, were similar for both groups (Dickerson, Brown, Gervasio, Hak, & Hak, 1999). These data suggest that individuals do not necessarily "grow out of" their feeding problems. That is, caloric intake may not improve with time, and intervention may be necessary to achieve adequate nutritional status if feeding problems are manifested early.

ETIOLOGY

Multiple factors complicate the ability of individuals with developmental disabilities to eat normally and obtain nutritional sufficiency by mouth (Cohen & Navathe, 1999). Recent classification recognizes the complex overlap of socioenvironmental and organic causes with physical features and concurrent, often consequential behavioral elements. Gastrointestinal abnormalities, neurological conditions, structural/oromotor disorders, and behavioral issues often contribute to aberrant eating dysfunctions (Rudolf & Link, 2002; Zangen et al., 2003). A model to evaluate undernutrition (see Table 14.1-1) can assist in understanding the issues involved in order to direct the assessment and approach the treatment of individuals with developmental disabilities who have feeding problems and/or potential nutritional deficiency/impairment.

Table 14.1-1. Etiologies of feeding disorders and undernutrition for children and adults with developmental disabilities

Historical perspectives	Genetic endowment Underlying illness Neurodevelopmental status
Current state	Oral motor competence Intercurrent illness Behavioral resistance Food medication interaction
Nutriture	Caregiver involvement Food availability Nutrient adequacy Appetite/alternative sources Energy requirements Activities, expenditures, losses Iatrogenic
Metabolic adaptation	Digestion, absorption Uptake, utilization Storage, excretion Hormonal homeostasis

From Cohen, S.A., & Navathe, A.S. (1999). Feeding the developmentally delayed child. *Journal of the Medical Association of Georgia, 88,* 71–76; adapted by permission.

Historical perspectives on etiology include inheritance as well as any genetic anomalies that may modify the inherent potential growth of the individual. The model then accounts for the individual's underlying condition. For example, a cardiorespiratory problem with tachypnea may not only increase caloric expenditure and need, but the rate of breathing may also complicate the issue of oral coordination and ability. Metabolic dysfunctions, such as phenylketonuria or fructose intolerance, may cause growth disturbances and vomiting if not recognized and appropriately treated. A multicenter study of 14 children with lifelong feeding aversion, retching, or vomiting (11 of the children had cerebral palsy) demonstrated motility and sensory abnormalities of the gastrointestinal abnormalities that responded to treatment in 80% of the children involved (Zangen et al., 2003).

Neurodevelopmental status logically has the largest affect on children and adults with neurological impairments. The natural history of the specific disease involvement is imperative in order to understand whether the individual's condition is degenerative, static, or temporary because this knowledge will guide therapy and nutritional counseling with the family. Lower nutrient levels are associated more with the degree of intellectual disabilities and learning of self-help skills than the motor disabilities imposed by cerebral palsy (Hammond, Lewis, & Johnson, 1996).

As indicated previously, *oral motor dysfunction* is a frequent concomitant and often one of the first signs of neuromuscular impairment. In addition, anatomic abnormalities such as cleft palate, laryngeal, clefts and tracheoesophageal fistula may accompany neurological impairments as part of a congenital or genetic syndrome. These problems often manifest with difficult or unsuccessful feeding, nasopharyngeal regurgitation, aspiration, choking, persistent drooling, recurrent respiratory tract infections, and/or poor weight gain (Griggs et al., 1989; Reilly et al., 1996).

Intercurrent illnesses as mundane as an upper respiratory infection may temporarily affect feeding function, and more prolonged infections (e.g., Rous sarcoma virus bronchiolitis) interfere with nutrition for a longer time period by increasing caloric needs and impairing efficient and effective feeding. Children with feeding impairments have a slower convalescence from illness because of their inability to increase their energy consumption (Patrick & Gisel, 1990).

Concurrent, acute, and chronic disorders such as food allergies, malabsorption, gastroesophageal reflux

(GER), delayed gastric emptying, metabolic anomalies, or congenital defects of the gastrointestinal tract may add another layer of complexity on assuring nutritional adequacy for those with neurological impairments. These medical problems may cause eating to be painful either directly (as in the case of GER) or indirectly (when illness causes general malaise or nausea, which becomes associated with eating). Again, the association of the presentation of food with pain may produce aversions to food. Temperature of food and texture sensitivity can play a big role in acceptance of food.

Nausea in particular plays an important role in the development of aversions to food (Schafe & Bernstein, 1997). When nausea is paired with eating, aversions to tastes may develop after only one or a few trials and may generalize to many foods. In addition, studies on conditioned food aversions show that when these aversions develop, they can be long lasting. Children with complex medical histories also miss early critical experiences with feeding. These early opportunities to feed are important for the development of appropriate oral motor skills such as tongue lateralization and elevation.

Infants with complex medical histories are subjected to numerous invasive diagnostic tests and procedures that may involve manipulation of the face and mouth (e.g., laryngoscope, nasogastric [NG] tube). *Negative behaviors* such as crying are likely to carry over into the feeding situation in children with a history of hospitalization (Gisel & Patrick, 1988). From the child's perspective, a spoon may not appear to be substantially different from a laryngoscope or other devices that are used during invasive tests and procedures. Therefore, the child may associate the presentation of objects to the face and mouth (e.g., a spoon) with these early negative experiences and exhibit behaviors such as crying, batting, and head turning when objects are presented to the face and mouth. Parents of hospitalized and medically fragile children often report "oral aversions" that affect feeding and other behaviors associated with the face and mouth (e.g., toothbrushing, face washing).

Although these food aversions and biobehavioral resistances to feeding may result from underlying medical problems, their presence can evolve into a dominant issue. In a study of 103 children referred to an interdisciplinary feeding team, 85% had a behavioral component to their feeding dysfunction irrespective of their underlying medical disorder whereas only 12% had an isolated behavioral issue (Burklow et al., 1998).

The parents' or caregiver's involvement is important throughout the entire range of events surrounding feeding. This obvious statement expands beyond a parent's normal expectation of parenthood. Unless ultrasound or amniocentesis indicates a problem with the fetus prenatally, parents are often ill prepared to raise a child with health problems. Feeding often becomes the quintessential embodiment of their parenting and nurturing. In addition to learning the basics of infant feeding, parents need to recognize problems quickly and carry out a plan to solve or ameliorate any problems. The caregiver's active involvement and competence is absolutely necessary but may require considerable support and education.

Problems for teenagers with developmental disabilities emanate from the increased quantity of nutrients and calories needed because of increased body size. The same may be true of adults depending on their feeding skills and their access to repletional fluids and calories. Decreased feeding efficiency occurs in individuals with cerebral palsy; chewing and swallowing takes 12–15 times longer than normal controls, which translates into extended mealtimes. Even then, longer feeding times may not be sufficient to compensate for caloric and nutritional needs (Gisel & Patrick, 1988), with caregivers often overestimating the individual's caloric intake and the time spent feeding their child with developmental disabilities (Stallings, Zemel, Davies, Cronk, & Charney, 1996). For a child who is not a self-feeder, feeding can be further compromised by an oral aversion that develops because of the times when the caregiver must approach the child's mouth with distasteful medications and foods that are difficult for the child to handle because of delayed oral motor skills.

The combined issues of nutriture become complex because most individuals with developmental disabilities have somewhat *different nutritional requirements.* Physical activity, intake, and often energy needs are less (Azcue, Zello, Levy, & Pencharz, 1996; Fried & Pencharz, 1991). In addition, their decreased ability to communicate can make it difficult for their caregivers to appreciate their hunger or satiety. When oral feedings are supplemented or replaced by nasogastric or gastrostomy feedings, the issues of oral resistance, interpretation of hunger signals, and feeding time are largely obviated, with rapid and sustained weight gain and small increments of height growth achieved (Patrick, Boland, Stoski, & Murry, 1994; Rempel et al., 1988; Sanders et al., 1990; Shapiro et al., 1986). (Please refer to the sections on physical assessment and enteral feedings for a more detailed discussion.)

Proper nutriture assumes that nutritious foods are available and provided and that nutrient needs are adequately met; however, nutrient sufficiency cannot be assumed for any given person due to limited knowledge of specific nutrient needs for individuals with neurological impairments and the high costs and low insurance reimbursements for medically necessary nutrition. Indeed, individual metabolic variation and physical activity may be different from one person to another and even at different points in time (with increased seizure activity or change in neurological status with an intercurrent or concurrent illness. Feeding time may also need to change for a particular child or adult based on oral consumption or the schedule for enteral feedings.

Each of the etiologic factors in Table 14.1-1 can be seen with its own dynamic continuum affecting and interrelating to the other factors. For example, a child's oral aversion may at times be greater than at others, perhaps as affected by, and then further affecting, the parent or caregiver's efforts and abilities (in a bidirectional biofeedback loop). Underlying this situation could be the degree to which the child's gastroesophageal reflux is active, which might be exacerbated by a meal containing acidic or spicy food (e.g., tomato sauce) or the position in which the child was fed. Thus, an understanding of the nutritional consequences of feeding for children or adults with developmental disabilities requires a broad understanding of the numerous factors that inform each other and continue to change.

PRESENTATION AND EVALUATION

The complex etiology of feeding problems necessitates an interdisciplinary approach to assessment and treatment. The intent of a thorough medical and nutritional evaluation is

- To recognize individuals with, or at risk for, chronic malnutrition and/or specific nutrient deficiencies
- To assess the extent of those problems or potential issues
- To identify underlying, contributory, or resultant conditions and behaviors
- To determine the sufficiency of current intake

This information then will allow the medial and therapeutic team to recommend continuation or modifications in the nutritional approach (including the food to be offered, the mechanics of delivery, and any therapies/behavioral changes that may improve both) with a plan for ongoing reassessment.

Thus, the medical evaluation (see Table 14.1-2) should document the full context and evolving history of the underlying illness, its resulting impairments, and its associated conditions. The child's medications should be noted in detail because as many as 25% of children who receive anticonvulsants and are nonambulatory have rickets (Crosley, Chee, & Berman, 1975). Impairments or associated conditions should be noted because these conditions may require specific medical, nutritional, or other types of intervention (e.g., a child with VACTERL association may have a ventriculoseptal defect requiring fluid limitations or additional calories; a child who had

Table 14.1-2. Medical evaluation for nutritional abnormalities

History
Illness and level of function
Development and acquisition of oral motor skills
Medications and associated conditions
Bowel habits
Dietary/feeding history
- Appetite, intake, and schedule
- Allergies, intolerances, and preferences
- Nutritional, vitamin, and mineral supplements
- Changes in activity, weight, appetite, or function
- Dysfunction with feeding, swallowing, or reflux

Physical (in addition to routine)
Height, weight, triceps skinfold thickness, and vital signs
Observation and general impression
Abdomen for constipation
Spine for kyphoscoliosis and sacral anomalies
Neurological for tone and level of function
Mouth for gag, swallow, seal, drooling, and mucosal problems
Signs of deficiency state or chronic illness
- Clubbing or ridging of nails
- Skin turgor and texture
- Bruises
- Decubiti

Laboratory (when indicated)
Complete blood count
- Hemoglobin
- Red blood count indices
- Lymphocyte population

Electrolytes with urea nitrogen
Proteins
- Albumin
- Prealbumin
- Transferrin

Calcium
Phosphorus
Alkaline phosphatase
Vitamin and mineral levels (rarely needed)
Anticonvulsant levels
Thyroid function
Radiography
- X-ray of hand for osteomalacia and bone age
- Ultrasound or scan of head for hydrocephalus
- Technitium 99 milk scan
- Upper gastrointestinal series
- Oropharyngeal motility study (modified barium swallow)

Videofluoroscopy
pH esophagram

anorectal surgery needs nutritional attention to bowel habits and delayed oropharyngeal skills and tracheo-esophageal fistulae that would dictate the amount, texture, and delivery of foods needed). Furthermore, the presence of feeding problems may be significant diagnostically, as indicated previously (Reilly et al., 1996).

Krystal weighed 6 lb, 5 oz, when she was born at 35 weeks gestation with labor induced because of polyhydramnios. She left the hospital nursing but began choking at home. Within 3 months, she had decreased her interest in eating. She was hospitalized a month later for bronchiolitis and was recognized to have clinical GER, which was later documented with pH esophagram that also demonstrated episodes of decreased esophageal clearance. A modified barium swallow study was performed because of Krystal's difficulty swallowing and revealed silent aspiration during initial swallow with good pharyngeal clearing and no aspiration using thickened feedings.

Krystal, however, continued to have difficulty even with appropriately tailored feedings and medications for GER and reactive airway disease. Hypotonia was noted, as were slightly delayed milestones (Krystal sat alone at 9 months) and poor oral motor skills. Testing revealed a 22q microdeletion, and sleep study showed persistent hypoxemia. An upper endoscopy was attempted but was unable to be accomplished because of esophageal obstruction with apparent cricopharyngeal spasm, which was seen on repeat modified swallow. Attempts to understand this condition further with x-ray, swallowing laryngoscopy, and repeat endoscopy were unrevealing.

A gastrostomy tube was placed and was eventually converted to a gastrojejeunostomy tube for feedings until fundoplication could be performed. Once Krystal was stable without further events and was gaining weight well, a repeat endoscopy revealed tight cricopharyngeal muscle and esophageal narrowing. An esophageal impedence study showed no further gastroesophageal reflux. Cervical spine films and magnetic resonance imaging (MRI) of the brain were normal with no evidence of Chiari malformation. Chest CT scan showed mild bronchiectasis and findings consistent with multiple episodes of recurrent aspiration or infection. A cricopharyngeus myotomy was subsequently performed.

Once Krystal's oral skills improve sufficiently and a repeat modified swallow indicates that the risk of aspiration has diminished, active oral feeding trials will resume. In the interim, Krystal will be actively followed in the Feeding Clinic as well as by her cadre of physicians and therapists. She is starting to actively taste foods, is drinking up to 6 ounces of water slowly for the first time without gagging, and no longer needs nightly suctioning.

Specific focus on the development of oral motor skills helps to determine if feeding dysfunction is an issue. The acquisition of feedings skills seem to parallel speech abilities as concurrent oral motor activities, with delayed or anomalous speech patterns often indicative of pervasive oral dysfunction (Croft, 1992). Refusal to eat contributes further to failure to develop appropriate oral motor skills and failure to gain weight. The individual's level of function and oral motor skill should be assessed carefully. Parents should be queried about the time required to feed the child, their own desire and ability to continue, and the quality of the interaction. If there are other caregivers at home or school who feed the child, the success of those feedings should be discussed as well. The less skilled the child is in terms of oral competency, the more likely the child is to refuse food and fail to gain weight. A circle then develops in which the child refuses food, fails to learn that eating is no longer painful, misses opportunities to practice and develop oral motor skills, and fails to gain weight, which may reduce the child's motivation to eat even further.

Dietary history, including a 3-day food record, should document the child's actual food and fluid intake and schedule, any food intolerances, preferences, and supplements. Past and current medications should be noted in detail. The individual or his or her parents also should be asked about any herbal, nutraceutical, or other formulations being administered and whether those treatments were recommended by a physician or self-prescribed. Parents may be reluctant initially to admit to alternative therapies, but the use of these therapies may alert the physician to the degree of the parents' frustration with their child's medical progress and to possible interactions of these substances with other foods or medications. Any changes in appetite, intake, oral function, weight, or activity should be addressed as part of an expanded systems review. The individual's bowel habits and urine output may have an important relation to the feedings and should be noted as well. This family-centered history should also include

- Degree of self-feeding and tube feedings as well as the timing and duration of each
- Textures, types, and amounts of foods offered and consumed
- Presentation of food including the setting and circumstances
- Individual's position
- Troublesome aspects of the feedings (e.g., choking, gagging, change in respiration, regurgitation, feeding refusal) and when they occur
- Interaction with the different caregivers and the amounts consumed with each

Anthropometrics will corroborate and amplify the physician's general clinical impression about the individual's nutritional status. Height and weight should be measured when possible. Specific growth charts are available for individuals with Down syndrome and cerebral palsy (Spender, Cronk, Charney, & Stallings, 1989). The latter uses single leg lengths to achieve better approximation of expected growth because children and adults with developmental disabilities often have contractures or severe spasticity countering any attempts at obtaining an accurate measurement of height or length. An estimate to use for standard growth charts, however, can be calculated by multiplying the tibial length (measured from the medial popliteal line to the bottom of the medial malleolus) by a constant of 3.26 and adding 30.8 cm. (stature = 3.26 × tibial length + 30.8 cm.) Similarly, upper arm measures can be utilized in individuals with myelomeningocoele to assess their growth on normalized curves (Belt, Ekvall, Cook, Oppenheimer, & Wessel, 1986).

Height and weight measurements in former premature infants must be adjusted for the months of prematurity in the first 3 years of life, with the expectation that infants with 32 week gestations will catch up by 2 years of age and infants with gestations of shorter duration may take 3 years to achieve their genetic growth potential. Body mass index (BMI) establishes a ratio between weight and height with comparative percentiles for the general population. Although easily calculated, this measure has not been tested adequately yet in those at different ages and levels of developmental disabilities. A single study in adults evaluated 44 men and 33 women with cerebral palsy. At a mean age of 27, they had a BMI of 22.6 ± 3.6 and 23.6 ± 7.2, respectively, with the percentage of body fat at 13.5 ± 6.0 and 23.2 ± 7.4, respectively (mean ± standard deviation) (Ferrano et al., 2002).

A weight for height should be obtained by first finding the individual's height age (the age at which the individual's current length would be at the 50th percentile on the appropriate National Center for Health Statistics [NCHS] growth chart). The ideal weight is traditionally the 50th percentile weight at that height; however, this practice may overestimate the ideal weight for those with neurodevelopmental impairment. The 25th percentile or lower perhaps is more appropriate. The individual's actual weight as a percentage of the ideal weight for height then can be used to assess the stage of wasting from malnutrition according to Waterlow Criteria (Waterlow, 1972). Divide the person's actual weight by his or her ideal weight for height. Mild malnutrition is less than 90% of the ideal weight. Moderate malnutrition is less than 80% of the ideal weight, and less than 70% of the ideal weight is severe malnutrition.

The limitations of this calculation due to genetic and ethnic background must be recognized. Discrepancies within the height age that may not have been reflected by the previous NCHS editions should now be corrected by the more heterogeneous populations that were used to standardize the current version; however, attempts to use height measures as a valid measure of stunting are fraught with difficulty in that individuals with developmental disabilities often have contractures and scoliosis. More sophisticated measurements, using mid-arm circumference and triceps or subscapular skinfold thickness may be worthwhile as a measure of muscle mass and energy stores, especially if they are used to monitor an individual's progress. A study of 69 children with cerebral palsy demonstrated that body fat (derived from skinfold thickness) and percentage weight compared with height age (calculated from upper arm length) differentiated children with malnutrition from those with seemingly sufficient energy stores and better growth (Davies, Antonucci, Charney, & Stallings, 1989).

Physical examination is useful in detecting dehydration, malnutrition, or specific nutritional deficiencies. Thus, as part of a comprehensive evaluation, the examiner should document the individual's skin turgor, subcutaneous tissue, and muscle mass carefully, noting any bruising, clubbing, edema, or rashes (these conditions may be the result of specific nutrient deficiency states). If a feeding tube is in place, the site should be examined for erythema, edema, granulomas, herniation, or the satellite lesions of a cutaneous yeast infection.

The physical examination also should focus on the sufficiency of oral motor skills as well as posture, tone, and neurodevelopmental function. Arching, spasticity, and neck position should be noted. Respiratory signs including stridor or wheezing are important indicators of the potential for aspiration. The characteristic of an infant's cry may allude to intrinsic laryngeal abnormalities or those that are secondary to gastroesophageal reflux. Specific anomalies may cause disordered swallowing, which may preclude safe oral feeding. Particular attention to swallowing dysfunction is necessary in muscular dystrophy and similar myopathic disorders. Drooling, mouth closure, and pocketing of food in the mouth during meals are all factors that require careful consideration as feeding therapy is planned, as these may be indicators of oral motor dysfunction. Any evidence of regurgitation, choking, or possible aspiration should be evaluated. Well-trained members of the team may observe the individual eating for a better understanding of his or her oral motor competencies.

Biochemical studies, such as serum zinc or Vitamin B_{12} levels, have limited use for nutritional evaluation, unless individuals have concomitant problems with malabsorption. Blood tests primarily measure the quality of the diet, whereas they are insensitive to quantitative insufficiencies, which are more frequent problems for these individuals (Gisel & Patrick, 1988). Protein status is usually normal when reflected by albumin, transferring, or prealbumin levels (i.e., their half-lives reflect protein status in the last month, 2 weeks, and week, respectively). Hemoglobin can screen for iron deficiency anemia, which is common. A hand or limb x-ray may indicate the presence of osteopenia or osteomalacia, particularly in individuals who are non–weight-bearing, as a more sensitive measure than chemical analysis for calcium, phosphorus, or alkaline phosphatase levels. The x-ray also can approximate a child's bone age. Anticonvulsant levels and liver/renal function tests also can be obtained when indicated.

Bone densitometry may not be cost effective because many individuals who are non–weight-bearing can be presumed to develop osteopenia eventually. Bone mineral content and density are reduced in nutritionally adequate children with spastic cerebral palsy with an even greater reduction in nonindependent ambulators. (Chad et al., 2000).

INTERVENTION

A regimen for feeding children and adults with developmental disabilities must provide adequate nutritional substrates and sufficient energy intake to maintain the individual's metabolic and fluid requirements with additional energy and micronutrient stores to withstand stressful events (e.g., infections). Malnutrition and nutrient deficiencies should be corrected and prevented, and children should be able to optimize their growth. In the context of achievable height, children with neurological impairment historically have been smaller (Chad et al., 2000; Stallings et al., 1995). Short-term studies with aggressive nutritional regimens have been able to increase weight, though not height (Brant et al., 1990; Rempel et al., 1988; Sanders et al., 1990). Normal weight for height is at the 50th percentile for those with normal activity; the 25th percentile for those able to perform independent transfers; and at the 10th percentile for those who are bedridden, with the exception that those younger than 3 years of age should be maintained at the 25th to 50th percentiles to assure sufficient growth (Krick, Murphy, Markham, & Shapiro, 1992).

Because nutrient requirements generally parallel energy needs, focus usually is directed toward caloric requirements. The disproportion between weight and height mean that calculations are usually conceived in terms of body surface area or height. These calculations can be modified for activity level and weight repletion. Normally growing children with spastic quadriplegic cerebral palsy have an energy intake of 60 ± 15% of the recommended daily allowance (RDA) for gender and age and 103 ± 32 % of that for weight, when exclusively gastrostomy fed (Azcue et al., 1996). Individuals who are nonambulatory require an average of 75% of the calories needed by individuals of comparable height who are ambulatory (Fried & Pencharz, 1991).

Resting energy expenditure (REE) is correlated poorly with body cell mass in individuals with spastic quadriplegia. Accretion of fat free mass is significantly reduced in these individuals. Moreover, the range of resting energy expenditure in adults extends from 16 to 39 kcal./kg./day when measured and significantly less than would be predicted by Harris Benedict and World Health Organization (WHO) equations (Dickerson et al., 1999). Total energy needs for children with spastic quadriplegic cerebral palsy (1.1 x measured REE) are considerably less than the 1.5 to 1.6 times calculated REE suggested by WHO standards (Hammond et al., 1996; Patrick et al., 1994). If resting energy expenditure is used to calculate an individual's needs, then it also must be modified by factors that address muscle tone (increasing 10% for hypertonicity; decreasing 10% for hypotonicity); activity (increasing 15% for those bedridden and 30% for those ambulating); and growth (Bandini, Schoeller, Fukagawa, Wykes, & Dietz, 1991).

Even though measurement of each individual's resting energy expenditure by indirect calorimetry or bioelectrical impedance might be optimal, repeated measurements might be impractical or at least difficult. Initially, at least, the primary physician or practitioner can calculate caloric needs based on centimeters of height (Banini et al., 1991; see Table 14.1-3) and add 5 kcal per gram of weight repletion needed (5,000 kcal/kg) divided by the time of acceptable accretion (e.g., 30–90 days). Another technique (Culley & Middleton, 1969) employs a calculation based on height with modifications: 11.1 kcal/cm for children with motor dysfunction who are nonambulatory; 13.9 kcal/cm in those who are ambulatory without motor dysfunction; and 14.7 kcal/cm for children without motor dysfunction. Estimations can also encompass basal metabolic rate and growth with variations applied for muscle tone and activity (Davies et al., 1989).

Jordan suffered encephalitis at 2 weeks of age and subsequently developed a seizure disorder and spastic quadriple-

Table 14.1-3. Caloric requirements for specific disabilities

Disability	Caloric requirement (kcal/cm height)	Comment
Cerebral palsy (5–11 years)	13.9	Mild-moderate activity
	11.1	Severely restricted activity
Down syndrome (1–3 years)	16.1	Boys
	14.3	Girls
Myelomeningocoele (older than 8 years)	7	For weight loss*
Prader-Willi syndrome	10–11	For maintenance
	8.5	For weight loss

*50% of normal recommended daily allowance for age/gender for maintenance.

gia with neurodevelopmental delay. At 5 years of age, he was noted to have precocious puberty with axillary hair, and at 10 years of age, he was recognized to have the secretion of inappropriate antidiuretic hormone managed with free water and furosemide. He had mitral valve prolapse, retinal detachment, and reactive airway disease as well. Jordan's long-standing GER with aspiration prompted conversion of his gastrostomy tube into a gastrojejeunostomy tube because he was not felt to be a surgical candidate.

Physicians had difficulty determining Jordan's appropriate feeding volume. He had progressive scoliosis and limb contractures, so standard calculations of caloric calculations based on body length were impossible. He also gained increased weight on even amounts that would be calculated based on single limb length. Oxygen consumption tests performed indicated that because of his negligible activity during the day, his actual needs were less than half of those calculated by any formula. At 16 years of age and 33.8 kg, Jordan had maintained a stable weight on 500 kcal. of a whey-based feeding per day that was supplemented with additional free water, vitamins, and minerals to attempt to attain nutritional sufficiency.

Oral Feeding

The technique of feeding and the food provided are interrelated. Standard, grocery shelved foodstuffs are the cheapest and simplest means of providing oral feedings. Moreover, the social and emotional pleasures and the expectations of mealtimes often are important for the caregiver, even if only a portion of the individual's nutrient needs can be delivered by mouth. Taste and texture can be varied if the child or adult is identified as a safe oral feeder. Children and adults who can swallow safely but cannot chew effectively may be able to receive the same foods in a puree or acceptable consistency created using a blender. Those who can tolerate solids but not liquids can have commercial thickeners added to their fluids. These children and adults should have optimal feeding posture and appropriate food temperature because these subtle nuances can make a real difference in feeding tolerance and the prevention of aspiration.

For infants, breast feeding should be encouraged for its various benefits. Human milk fortifier or proprietary formulae can be added to increase calories. Infant formulae can be concentrated an additional 10%–50% by decreasing free water for children whose nutritional status is compromised (see Table 14.1-4). This action allows feedings to lessen critical feeding rates and volumes with some infants and children unable to sustain growth on standard 20 kcal/oz products because of their volume sensitivity. Small quantities of carbohydrate polymers, cereal, or lipids (long or medium chain triglycerides) may be added progressively to either breast milk or formula (see Table 14.1-5), titrating to increase caloric density to 30 kcal while carefully monitoring the child for tolerance to assure adequate urination and to avoid diarrhea, vomiting, and/or feeding refusal.

Numerous proprietary products are now available as liquids or puddings to supplement calories, protein, and various nutrients. A particular product can be chosen based on the individual's need for fiber in regulating bowel movements and the person's tolerance of the product's components and taste. Other methods of calorie loading include modification of the foods added to a milk or soy base, which can be adapted for calories, fluid and fiber content, vitamin and mineral requirements, and allergy restrictions according to the child's needs. Potentially, these modular feedings or "homebrews" are

Table 14.1-4. Increased calorie concentrations of standard 20 kcal/oz infant formulas

	20 kcal/oz	22 kcal/oz*	24 kcal/oz	26 kcal/oz
Powder**	4 scoops	4½ scoops	4¾ scoops	5¼ scoops
Water to make	8 oz	8 oz	8 oz	8 oz
Powder**	1 cup	1 cup	1 cup	1 cup
Add	29 oz	26 oz	24 oz	21.5 oz
Concentrate	13 oz	13 oz	13 oz	13 oz
Water	13 oz	10½ oz	8½ oz	7 oz

*Concentrations are approximate and are useful for parental instruction.

** Scoops (equivalent to 1 Tbs) and cups should be level, not pressed or packed.

Table 14.1-5. Modular high calorie additions

	kcal/g	kcal/Tbs	Nutrient source
Human milk fortifier	—	3.5/packet	Whey, Na caseinate, corn syrup solids, lactose
Promod (protein)	4.7	18	Whey
Casec	3.8	17	Calcium caseinate, soy lecithin
Formula powder*	—	40	Variable
Nonfat dry milk	8.7	27	Milk
Medium chain triglycerides (MCT) oil	8.2	115	Triglycerides
Vegetable oil	8.9	124	Variable
Polycose	3.8	23	Glucose polymer
Moducal	3.7	30	Glucose polymer
Duocal	4.9	42	Hydrolyzed corn starch, refined vegetable oils, fractionated coconut oil
Additions	5.2	43	Sodium caseinate, whey, protein
Benecalorie (liquid)	1/mL	110	High oleic sunflower oil, calcium caseinates, sodium ascorbate, polysorbate, zinc
Rice cereal	4.2	15	Rice flour, soy oil, barley malt

*20 cal/oz infant formula

less expensive and offer the caregiver the perception of providing their child "real food" and "hands-on care." Because homebrew feedings may be thicker than commercial formulas, a large size feeding tube may be necessary. Bolus feedings may work better for homebrew tube feedings than a continuous drip because of the thicker consistency and increased risk of bacterial contamination without refrigeration.

If a currently available proprietary formula is used, the physician must recognize that these have fixed nutrient/energy ratios so that reducing the prescribed calories proportionate to the individual's needs based on height also may reduce that individual's intake of all other nutrients significantly below the recommended daily allowance for age. The potential reduction in calcium, phosphorus, and vitamin D poses risks of bone disease in individuals with other vitamin and mineral deficiencies, but many vitamin and mineral needs do parallel caloric requirements. In a study of children with cerebral palsy, most nutrient levels exceeded two thirds of the recommended daily allowances, but the serum level for calcium was decreased below normal levels (Hammond, Lewis, & Johnson, 1996). Thus, intervention with maintenance doses of vitamin D and calcium may be prudent as the individual ages, if he or she is not at particular risk for nephrolithiasis.

Children with food refusal have a different history or experience with food than typically eating children. Their problems often persist and worsen over time (Lindberg, Bohlin, & Hagekull, 1991). Therefore, the techniques or recommendations that are used for typically eating children may not apply to children with food refusal. Effective, empirically supported interventions in the treatment of complex feeding problems are those contingency management treatments that include positive reinforcement of appropriate feeding responses and ignoring or guiding inappropriate responses (Kerwin, 1999). The main goals of oral feeding are increasing oral intake and meeting the child's nutritional needs. The other major goals are to 1) decrease gastric tube dependence, 2) increase food texture, 3) increase food variety, 4) decrease bottle dependence, 5) increase self-feeding, 6) decrease inappropriate behaviors, and 7) support parental nurturance. (J. Fagan & A. Navathe, personal communication).

Initially, treatment for children with total food refusal and inappropriate mealtime behavior (e.g., crying, head turning, batting at the spoon, refusal to open the mouth) should focus on reducing these inappropriate mealtime behaviors and increasing more appropriate eating-related behaviors (e.g., opening the mouth) to establish that eating is no longer painful (Piazza, Patel, Gulotta, Sevin, & Layer, in press). Meals should be time limited and focus on a short-term, specific end goal. Caregivers also need to understand what secondary gains the child may achieve by avoiding food or engaging in inappropriate mealtime behavior.

Strategies used by the caregivers to get their children to eat (i.e., distraction, coaxing, allowing breaks from eating, or providing toys or preferred food) actually worsened behavior for 10 out of the 15 participants (67%) in one study (Piazza, Fisher, et al., in press). From a parental perspective, strategies such as terminating the meal or coaxing may produce the immediate effect of temporarily stopping the undesirable child behavior; however, problem behavior and food refusal appear to produce a favorable outcome from the child's perspective (e.g., avoidance of eating, increased parental attention, preferred foods or toys), and these refusal behaviors are likely to be repeated during subsequent meals. Eighty-nine percent of the children studied had earlier medical conditions (e.g., GER), which probably caused eating to be painful. Even though these medical conditions were resolved at the time of the study, the children had continued feeding refusal.

Often, the texture of presented food needs to be reduced when the child has limited experiences with oral intake because the child's oral motor skills are not sufficiently well developed to consume age-appropriate textures successfully (i.e., without choking, gagging, or fatiguing; Patel, Piazza, Santana, & Volkert, 2002). Some less complex textures should be presented to prevent fatigue and frustration. Small amounts of higher textures should continue to be presented to enable the child to maintain and advance his or her oral motor skills.

Because the etiology of the feeding problem is multidetermined, treatment should focus on all of the components (i.e., physiological, oral motor, and psychological) that contribute to feeding problems. A multidisciplined approach combining the services of a psychologist, occupational therapist, speech therapist, dietitian, and pediatric gastroenterologist is the most effective means for successful treatment, particularly for difficult feeding problems. Often, the programs provide a continuum of services (evaluation, outpatient therapy, day treatment, hospitalization) based on the individual's needs (Byars, et al., 2003; Schwartz et al., 2001).

Successful treatment of feeding problems should include measurable goals for each child's feeding behaviors that are developed by the interdisciplinary team and caregivers. Feeding behaviors (e.g., amounts consumed, acceptance of bites of food) should be measured objectively, and treatment decisions should be data based. Outcomes should be assessed regularly throughout the duration of treatment. A primary goal should be to establish feeding patterns that can be maintained by the caregivers in the home and in other environments. Thus, caregiver training should be an essential component to the success of the program.

Preliminary analysis of the outcome measures for one program with approximately 50 children, half of whom have been diagnosed with developmental disabilities (Blackman & Nelson, 1987), indicated that more than 87% of the goals for treatment were met by the time of discharge. All of the children met their goals for increasing texture, decreasing bottle dependence, increasing self-feeding skills, and increasing variety of foods consumed. When increases in oral calories were the goal of treatment, 70% of the children reached their goal for caloric intake. When increases in liquid intake (for children who did not consume liquids by mouth) were the goal of treatment, 80% of the children reached their goal for oral liquid intake. All others increased solid or liquid intake over baseline levels but did not reach their final goal during the day treatment admission. Even though all of the children did not reach their goal for oral intake, the mean percentage of the oral intake goal met was 82% for all, suggesting that even when children did not reach 100% of their oral intake goal, their levels of oral intake were increased substantially and within 20% of the goal. Progress toward increasing oral intake continued during outpatient follow-up.

Levels of enteral feedings were decreased for all children who entered the program receiving nutritional supplementation via tube, and 70% of children met their goals for decreases in enteral feedings. Children who entered the program with an NG tube either left the program without the tube (75%) or the NG tube was removed shortly after discharge (100%). Thus, surgical placement of a gastrostomy tube was avoided for 100% of children who entered the program as candidates for gastrostomy tubes as a result of the presence of failure to thrive and a NG tube at admission. The goals for decreasing inappropriate mealtime behaviors were met for 97% of the children. Eighty-eight percent of caregivers were trained to implement the treatment protocols with greater than 90% accuracy, and the treatment was transferred successfully to the home and community in 100% of cases.

Preliminary analysis of follow-up data indicates that the majority of children (87%) continue to be followed postdischarge from the day treatment program. Of those who are currently followed, 85% continue to make progress toward age-typical feeding, which includes further volume increases, further gastrostomy tube decreases and gastrostomy tube removal, increases in the variety of foods consumed, texture advances, initiation of cup drinking, and initiation of self-feeding. In addition, structured diagnosis specific treatment has resulted in increased tissue stores and decreased hospitalization (Schwartz et al., 2001). When combined with pharmacotherapy to treat esophageal spasm, duodenal dysmotility, reduced gastric pain threshold, and/or to increase appetite, 80% had improved emotional health, with 43% able to eat orally (Zangen et al., 2003).

When necessary, proprietary and homemade supplemental formulas can be delivered via nonoral means. Physiologically designed formulas of increased caloric and protein density can be used for gastric and nasogastric infusion because palatability is not an issue. The choice of formula may be less of an issue than the volume delivered for children and adults with developmental disabilities with these assistive feedings. The amount ingested is no longer defined by appetite but determined by caregivers and medical providers. Long-term overnutrition presents as much risk as undernutrition. Hypertension and obesity can increase cardiovascular concerns, especially in individuals with neuromuscular disorders. Moreover, overweight and obese children or adults with developmental disabilities present increased problems for caregivers who have to risk their own health in lifting or assisting movement. Therefore, calculations must approximate a child's need for calories and nutrients. Because these prescriptions for volume may over- or underestimate actual requirements and because growing children increase their nutritional needs as they age and grow, reevaluation at appropriate intervals for serial examination and measurement with the calculations revisited is perhaps more important than any individual prescription.

When safety of oral feeding is not an issue, these enteral techniques can merely supplement the child's own nutrition with the caregivers continuing to feed the child actively. Often, nocturnal drip feedings can provide 30%–50% of the child's nutrient needs so that day time meals can be offered orally without the pressure and large blocks of time that have to be devoted if all requirements had to be met by 3 or 4 daily meals. This dual feeding method often provides great satisfaction to parents and caregivers because the mealtime interaction is improved when there is no longer any need for force feeding of medication or nourishment. The risk of satiation (i.e., that the child will not be motivated to feed orally), however, must be considered in conjunction with the schedule of feedings. Even overnight tube feedings may produce satiation and unwillingness of the child to eat concomitant with NG or gastrostomy tube feedings.

Many parents are apprehensive about feeding and assuring adequate nutrition for their children. Understandably, caregivers for children with developmental disabilities may be even more so. Based on the method of delivery, the caregivers should be trained carefully in the preparation and delivery of the feeding. Parents should be reassured and provided with medical, nutritional, and home care agencies that can serve as resources. They should be informed that success may be most dependent on appropriate follow-up visits to assess the child's progress and adjust the feeding regimens. Moreover, social service agencies and/or medical care facilities should be encouraged to facilitate these efforts. In one study (Johnson & Maeda, 1989), a hospital providing high-calorie, ready-to-feed nutritional supplementation at cost improved compliance with dietary recommendations. Such a policy has the potential to increase the effectiveness of nutrition intervention.

CONCLUSION

Children with chronic illnesses often are compromised further as the result of secondary nutritional problems that require the attention of their primary care physicians and subspecialists. Recent advancements in understanding and meeting the nutritional needs of children and adults with developmental disabilities have resulted in an improved quality and length of life. Small studies have demonstrated improved weight for height, muscle mass, subcutaneous energy stores, peripheral circulation, healing of decubitus ulcers, and general well-being with enteral feedings with decreased irritability and spasticity.

These children, however, do not follow the same patterns for linear growth as other children. The goals for weight accretion must be considered in determining the actual caloric needs for each child. Alternative methods using height or, preferably, single limb length to calculate caloric needs are recommended.

The delivery of nutrient and energy sources should be based on the child's neurological function, oral motor skills, the presence of GER, or other superimposed conditions. The use of proprietary formulas with fixed nutrient/energy ratios may provide sufficient calories but also have the potential for specific nutrient deficiencies—most notably calcium, phosphorus, and vitamin D. In addition, the placement of a gastrostomy device is not without controversy because there is an increased mortality rate in adults with developmental disabilities who do not have tracheostomy tubes, which may be related to the underlying condition of these individuals or their increased risk of aspiration.

The complex etiology of feeding problems requires a multidisciplinary approach for successful treatment. Goals for treatment should be specified in measurable terms and outcomes should be tracked during treatment and over time. An intensive, data-based, multidisciplinary approach is successful for more than 85% of children. The highest levels of success (95% or better) are achieved in avoiding gastrostomy tube placement in individuals with failure to thrive and NG tubes and for individuals (e.g., those with food selectivity, texture inadequacies, skill deficits, or bottle dependence) with some preliminary oral intake.

Even though the outcomes for gastrostomy tube dependence are *slightly* lower over the short-term, progress continues during follow-up with caregiver cooperation. Most individuals continue to make significant progress toward their goals. Caregiver training and generalization to the home and community environments also can be achieved with high levels of success (more than 90%) and is critical to long-term maintenance of program gains. Two of the most important long-term aspects of the feeding program are to assure that once the ethical and technical issues are addressed: 1) the caregivers are adequately instructed, trained, and reassured; and 2) appropriate follow-up is arranged to assess the patients' progress and adjust the regimen to achieve an optimal outcome. Clinical research trials and critical analysis, however, are needed in many areas in order to determine and then disseminate best practices and optimal nutrition.

REFERENCES

Azcue, M.P., Zello, G.A., Levy, L.D., & Pencharz, P.B. (1996). Energy expenditure and body composition in children with spastic quadriplegic cerebral palsy. *Journal of Pediatrics, 129,* 870–876.

Bandini, L.G., Schoeller, D.A., Fukagawa, N.K., Wykes, L.J., & Dietz, W.H. (1991). Body composition and energy expenditure in adolescents with cerebral palsy or myelodysplasia. *Pediatric Research, 29,* 70–77.

Belt, B., Ekvall, S., Cook, C., Oppenheimer, S., & Wessel, J. (1986). Linear growth measurements: A comparison of single arm lengths and arm span. *Developmental Medicine and Child Neurology, 28,* 319.

Blackman, J.A., & Nelson, C.L.A. (1987). Rapid introduction of oral feedings to tube-fed patients. *Developmental and Behavioral Pediatrics, 8,* 63–66.

Brant, C.Q., Stanich, P., & Ferrari, A.P., Jr. (1990). Improvement in children's nutritional status after enteral feeding by PEG: An interim report. *Gastrointestinal Endoscopy, 50,* 183–188.

Burklow, K.A., Phelps, A.N., Schultz, J.R., et al. (1998). Classifying complex pediatric feeding disorders. *Journal of Pediatric Gastroenterology and Nutrition, 27,* 143–147.

Byars, K.C., Burklow, K.A., Ferguson, K., O'Flaherty, T., Santoro, K., & Kaul, A. (2003). A multicomponent behavioral program for oral aversion in children dependent on gastrostomy feedings. *Journal of Pediatric Gastroenterology and Nutrition, 37,* 473–480.

Chad, K.E., McKay, H.A., Zello, G.A., Bailey, D.A., Failkener, R.A., & Snyder, R.E. (2000). Body composition in nutritionally adequate ambulatory and nonambulatory children with cerebral palsy and a healthy reference group. *Developmental Medicine and Child Neurology, 42,* 334–339.

Cohen, S.A., & Navathe, A.S. (1999). Feeding the developmentally delayed child. *Journal of the Medical Association of Georgia, 88,* 71–76.

Crist, W., & Napier-Phillips, A. (2001). Mealtime behaviors of young children: A comparison of normative and clinical data. *Journal of Developmental and Behavioral Pediatrics, 22,* 279–286.

Croft, R.D. (1992). What consistency of food is best for children with cerebral palsy who cannot chew? *Archives in Disease in Childhood, 67,* 269–271.

Crosley, C.J., Chee, C., & Berman, P.H. (1975). Rickets associated with long term anticonvulsant therapy in a pediatric outpatient population. *Pediatrics, 56,* 52–57.

Culley, W.J., & Middleton, T.O. (1969). Caloric requirements of mentally retarded children with and without motor dysfunction. *Journal of Pediatrics, 75,* 380–384.

Davies, J.C., Antonucci, D.L., Charney, E.B., & Stallings, V.A. (1989). Use of upper-arm length and per cent body fat for nutritional assessment of children with cerebral palsy. *Developmental Medicine and Child Neurology, 31*(Suppl. 59), 39–40.

Dickerson, R.N., Brown, R.O., Gervasio, J.G., Hak, E.B., & Hak, L.J. (1999). Measured energy expenditure of tube-fed patients with severe neurodevelopmental disabilities. *Journal of the American College of Nutrition, 18,* 61–68.

Ferrano, T.M., Johnson, R.K., & Ferrara, M.S. (1992). Dietary and anthropometric assessment of adults with cerebral palsy. *Journal of the American Dietetic Association, 92,* 1083–1086.

Fried, M.D., & Pencharz, P.B. (1991). Energy and nutrient intakes of children with spastic quadriplegia. *Journal of Pediatrics, 119,* 947–949.

Gisel, E.G., & Patrick, J. (1988). Identification of children with cerebral palsy unable to maintain a normal nutritional state. *Lancet, 1,* 283–286.

Griggs, C.A., Jones, P.M., & Lee, R.E. (1989). Videofluoroscopic investigation of feeding disorders of children with multiple handicaps. *Developmental Medicine and Child Neurology, 31,* 303–308.

Hammond, M.I., Lewis, M.N., & Johnson, E.W. (1996). A nutritional study of cerebral palsied children. *Journal of the American Dietetic Association, 49,* 196–201

Johnson, R.K., & Maeda, M. (1989). Establishing outpatient nutrition services for children with cerebral palsy. *Journal of the American Dietetic Association, 89,* 1504–1506.

Kerwin, M.E. (1999). Empirically supported treatments in pediatric psychology: Severe feeding problems. *Journal of Pediatric Psychology, 24,* 193–214.

Krick, J., Murphy, P.E., Markham, J.F., & Shapiro, B.K. (1992). A proposed formula for calculating energy needs of children with cerebral palsy. *Developmental Medicine and Child Neurology, 6,* 481–487.

Lindberg, L., Bohlin, G., & Hagekull, B. (1991). Early feeding problems in a normal population. *International Journal of Eating Disorders, 10,* 395–405.

Mirrett, P.L., Riski, J.E., Glascott, J., & Johnson, V. (1994, Summer). Videofluoroscopic assessment of dysphagia in children with severe spastic cerebral palsy. *Dysphagia, 9*(3), 174–179.

Navathe, A.S. (2003). *Formulary nutrient content.* Atlanta, GA: Children's Healthcare of Atlanta.

Patel, M.R., Piazza, C.C., Santana, C.M., & Volkert, V.M. (2002). An evaluation of food type and texture in the treatment of a feeding problem. *Journal of Applied Behavioral Analysis, 35*, 183–186.
Patrick, J., Boland, M., Stoski, D., & Murry, G.E. (1994). Rapid correction of wasting in children with cerebral palsy. *Developmental Medicine and Child Neurology, 36*, 135–142.
Patrick, J., & Gisel, E. (1990). Nutrition for the feeding impaired child. *Journal of Neurological Rehabilitation, 4*, 115–119.
Piazza, C.C., Fisher, W.W., Brown, K.A., Shore, B.A., Patel, M.R., Katz, R.M., et al. (in press). Functional analysis of inappropriate mealtime behaviors. *Journal of Applied Behavioral Analysis.*
Piazza, C.C., Patel, M.R., Gulotta, C.S., Sevin, B.S., & Layer, S.A. (in press). On the relative contribution of positive reinforcement and escape extinction in the treatment of food refusal. *Journal of Applied Behavioral Analysis.*
Rapp, C.E., & Torres, M.M. (2000). The adult with cerebral palsy. *Archives of Family Medicine, 9*, 466–472.
Reilly, S., & Skuse, D. (1992). Characteristics and management of feeding problems of young children with cerebral palsy. *Developmental Medicine and Child Neurology, 34*, 379–388.
Reilly, S., Skuse, D., & Poblete, X. (1996). Prevalence of feeding problems and oral motor dysfunction in children with cerebral palsy: A community survey. *Journal of Pediatrics, 129*, 877–882.
Rempel, G.R., Colwell, S., & Nelson, R.P. (1988). Growth in children with cerebral palsy fed via gastrostomy. *Pediatrics, 82*, 857–862.
Rogers, B., Stratton, P., Msall, M., et al. (1994). Long-term morbidity and management strategies of tracheal aspiration in adults with severe developmental disabilities. *American Journal of Mental Retardation, 98*, 490–498.
Rudolph, C.D., & Link, D.T. (2002). Feeding disorders in infants and children. *Pediatric Clinics of North America, 49*(1), 97–112.
Sanders, K.D., Cox, K., Cannon, R., Blanchard, D., Pilcher, J., Papathakis, P., et al. (1990). Growth response to enteral feeding by children with cerebral palsy. *Journal of Parenteral and Enteral Nutrition, 14*, 23–26.
Schafe, G.E., & Bernstein, I.L. (1997). Taste aversion learning. In Capaldi, E.D. (Ed.), *Why we eat what we eat: The psychology of eating* (pp. 31–51). Washington, DC: American Psychological Association.
Schwartz, S.M., Corredor, J., Fisher-Medina, J., Cohen, J., & Rabinowitz, S. (2001). Diagnosis and treatment of feeding disorders in children with developmental disabilities. *Pediatrics, 108*, 671–676.
Shapiro, B.K., Green, P., Krick, J., Allen, D., & Capute, A.J. (1986). Growth of severely impaired children: Neurological versus nutritional factors. *Developmental Medicine and Child Neurology, 28*, 729–733.
Spender, Q.W., Cronk, C.E., Charney, E.B., & Stallings, V.A. (1989). Assessment of linear growth of children with cerebral palsy: Use of alternative measures to height or length. *Developmental Medicine and Child Neurology, 31*, 206–214.
Stallings, V.A., Cronk, C.E., Zemel, B.S., & Charney, E.B. (1995). Body composition in children with spastic quadriplegic cerebral palsy. *Journal of Pediatrics, 126*, 833–839.
Stallings, V.A., Zemel, B.S., Davies, J.C., Cronk, C.E., & Charney, E.B. (1996). Energy expenditure of children and adolescents with severe disabilities: A cerebral palsy model. *American Journal of Clinical Nutrition, 64*, 627–634.
Waterlow, J.C. (1972). Classification and definition of protein-calorie malnutrition. *British Medical Journal, 3*, 356.
Zangen, T., Ciarla, C., Zangen, S., DiLorenzo, C., et al. (2003). Gastrointestinal motility and sensory abnormalities may contribute to food refusal in medically fragile toddlers. *Journal of Pediatric Gastroenterology and Nutrition, 37*, 287–293.

14.2 GASTROINTESTINAL ISSUES

Laurie N. Fishman and Athos Bousvaros

Individuals with neurodevelopmental disabilities commonly have gastrointestinal illnesses complicating their underlying condition. Some of these problems are the direct result of the underlying neurological or neurodevelopmental disorder. For example, impaired oral motor coordination results in difficulty swallowing, and slow gastrointestinal motility predisposes to constipation. Other problems result from the chronic effects of impaired gastrointestinal function. Abnormal swallowing can lead to malnutrition or aspiration pneumonia, gastroesophageal reflux (GER) can lead to erosive esophagitis, and constipation can lead to megacolon and difficulty with urination.

Children and adults with developmental disabilities may not be able to express or localize gastrointestinal conditions. Thus, health care providers must be aggressive in establishing or ruling out gastrointestinal diagnoses. Failure to diagnose cholelithiasis may lead to gallbladder perforation and pyogenic liver abscess, and failure to diagnose severe constipation may even lead to intestinal volvulus. Caregivers must also consider the adverse effects of medication on the gastrointestinal system. Iatrogenic complications of therapies include altered liver function from anticonvulsants and diminished intestinal motility from the anticholinergic effects of psychotropic medications.

Gastrointestinal conditions can have a significant impact on health, quality of life, and quality of the child–caregiver relationship. Therefore, familiarity with the diagnosis and treatment of gastrointestinal conditions is important for any practitioner caring for individuals with developmental disabilities. This chapter reviews the diagnosis and treatment of oropharyngeal dysphagia, GER, gastritis, hepatitis, and constipation.

DYSPHAGIA

June is a quiet 4-month-old baby. Her mother does not mind spending 90 minutes feeding her a bottle. Occasionally, June will seem to sputter, but she has had no real choking. Now that June's mother is starting to introduce cereal, she is noticing that almost all the cereal ends up on June's face or body. June seems to stick her tongue out at the spoon. June's pediatrician is worried about June's slow weight gain.

The pediatrician has evaluated June to ensure that she does not have cardiac or respiratory disease. June has a normal palate and jaw. When the pediatrician watched June feed, she noted a prominent tongue thrust and occasional coughing. June arches away from the spoon when she is fed. The pediatrician thought the arching may have been caused by either hypertonia and persistent primitive reflexes, or by GER. Empiric treatment for GER did not change the symptom. Although June did not have prominent symptoms of coughing, sputtering, and choking, the pediatrician remembered hearing that aspiration can be completely "silent" and ordered a modified videoflouroscopic swallow study. The study demonstrated nasopharyngeal reflux, laryngeal "penetration," and occasional aspiration of barium into the lungs with thin liquids. June's liquid feeds were thickened by the addition of rice cereal, and she exhibited decreased sputtering and improved weight gain.

The term *dysphagia* refers to a disorder of swallowing, which may involve problems with any of the phases of a swallow, the reception and oral preparation of a bolus, the initiation of the reflexive swallow, and the pharyngeal phase, or the esophageal phase. Dysphagia may be the first sign of a neurodevelopmental condition because sucking, chewing, and swallowing are the earliest important functional expression of organized motor activity. Adults often continue to have dysphagia, and the following discussion is relevant for their care as well.

Dysphagia affects the majority of children with severe cerebral palsy and occurs because the neurologic control of motor functions by the cranial nerves involved in swallowing (V, VII, IX–XII) is impaired, resulting in poorly coordinated jaw and tongue movements, tongue weakness, delay in swallow initiation, and prominent oral reflexes. The incidence of dysphagia tends to correlate significantly with the severity of motor impairment. In children with severe cerebral palsy, the incidence of oral motor dysfunction is 76% compared with 21% of children with mild or moderate cerebral palsy (Reilly & Skuse, 1992).

Clinical Signs and Symptoms

Dysphagia may present with very slow feeding, inability to handle textures or solids, pocketing food, or feeding refusal. Feeding may be accompanied by coughing, sputtering, gagging, gurgling, or pocketing food. Inability to handle oral secretions can result in drooling, which may cause maceration of the skin.

The clinical consequences of dysphagia are significant, including inability to handle textures or solids; feeding refusal; color changes when feeding; and failure to thrive or poor weight gain. Children or adults with dysphagia often cannot adequately protect their airway while feeding. This aspiration may result in recurrent pneumonia or chronic lung disease. Dysphagia also results in long mealtimes, depriving children of time for other activities and causing stress for the parents and caregivers. A child with cerebral palsy can take 2–12 times longer to manipulate and swallow a pureed food bolus and up to 15 times longer to swallow a solid food bolus (Gisel & Patrick, 1988). Food spillage from the mouth can further decrease the efficiency of oral intake. Thus, mealtimes can become exceedingly long. In one report, parents described mealtimes that typically lasted more than 45 minutes each (Dahl et al., 1996). It may be impossible to administer an adequate caloric intake orally even if most waking hours are used.

Dysphagia may simply present as malnutrition. Malnutrition can manifest at different ages and stages, depending on the child's level of eating impairment. Children with severe dysphagia are unable to coordinate swallowing and breathing and thus exhibit severe failure to thrive in infancy. Others can maintain adequate nutrition until faced with a growth spurt or a setback due to illness or surgery.

Evaluation

A detailed feeding history is imperative. Long feeding times indicate problematic feeding, but this condition should be further quantified.

- Does the child seem to stop and tire?
- Does the child seem to have trouble catching his or her breath?
- Does the child cry after a few sips?
- Does the child have trouble with only thin liquids or only solids?
- Does the child chew and then spit out food, or pocket it in his cheek?

Observation of a mealtime by an experienced feeding specialist is crucial.

A physical and neurological examination should be performed to identify etiologies and consequences of dysphagia. Detailed examination of the oral cavity, palate, teeth, and tongue may indicate anatomic defects. Presence of a gag reflex is important. Drooling indicates poor lip closure and may indicate a disinclination for swallowing thin liquids. Overall muscular tone affects the ability to ingest, chew, and swallow and even to be placed in correct positions for meals. Abnormal lung examination may suggest recurrent aspiration. Epigastric pain to deep palpation suggests gastritis or esophagitis.

A chest radiograph may demonstrate whether longstanding aspiration is present. A modified videoflouroscopic swallow study (VFSS) will delineate the function of the oral, pharyngeal, and upper esophageal phases and how the swallow changes with posture and various food textures. A speech-language therapist usually performs this study in conjunction with a radiologist. The VFSS may be the only way to demonstrate silent aspiration.

Treatment

Treatment is aimed at increasing the child's capacity to eat while preventing the complications of malnutrition and aspiration. Improving oral feeds involves finding the optimal posture for the meal and cups or spoons that optimize the intake (Larnert & Ekberg, 1995). Desensitizing the oral area is important if defensiveness occurs. Some children may need brushing or other organizing interventions prior to feeds. Permitting play with food allows children to develop comfort with the process. Exercises that strengthen oral skills may involve nonfood toys, feeder bags, and strips of food.

Varying the type, taste, and texture of foods that are presented to a child is also helpful. Children with diminished oral sensitivity may enjoy spicy foods or drinks with carbonation. Very cold foods may also increase awareness of the position in the mouth. Children who fatigue quickly may need to alternate solid and liquids or take frequent breaks. Some children handle thick liquids well but aspirate on thin liquids. In these situations, all liquids can be thickened with yogurt, cereal, pureed fruits, or a commercial thickener.

An abnormal swallow may improve slowly or may not improve over time. Predicting the time course and natural history of dysphagia is often difficult. Individuals who have a known diagnosis associated with worsening muscular control or weakness may have deterioration of the swallow over time. In individuals who are expected to have prolonged oral motor dysfunction, the placement of a gastrostomy for supplemental feeding will improve quality of life.

Enteral Feeding Tubes Selection of the proper supplemental feeding system needs to take into account whether the child or adult can tolerate bolus feeds into the stomach, the degree of reflux present, and the risk of aspiration for this individual. Table 14.2-1 outlines some of the aspects associated with various types of feeding tubes. Tubes can be placed through the nose and are usually considered temporary, whereas tubes that enter the stomach or intestine directly through the skin are considered relatively permanent. A more detailed discussion of each tube and its indications follows.

Nasogastric Tubes Nasogastric (NG) tubes are often the first step in supplementing feeding and may be used to achieve "catch-up" growth or to temporarily support an individual until the underlying situation changes. In other cases, an NG tube is used as a trial prior to gastrostomy placement, or as a temporizing measure until a gastrostomy (G) tube can be placed. Although clinicians think of the NG tube as "less invasive" than a G tube, it is far more visible. For some families, this public image of their child with a tube coming out of his or her nostril can be very difficult.

Placement is accomplished by passing a small caliber flexible tube into one nostril and advancing it to the level of the stomach. A rough estimate of the length required is obtained by previously measuring from the nose to the ear and then to the epigastric region. Most institutions confirm placement by auscultation over the

Table 14.2-1. Clinical considerations about tube selection

Nasogastric tubes
Are very visible
Cause skin irritation on cheek
Allow for bolus or continuous feeds
Can cause septal erosion or sinusitis
Are useful as a temporary supplement or trial for gastrostomy
Gastrostomy tubes
May be placed surgically, endoscopically, or radiographically
May be done separately from fundoplication (before or after)
Allow for bolus or continuous feeds
Vent gastric air and formula well
Have adjustable lengths that minimize leaking
Gastrostomy skin-level devices ("buttons")
May be the initial device (if surgically placed) or may replace gastrostomy tube later
Have balloon anchor that may burst or lose volume and cause tube to fall out
Have antireflux valves that wear out quickly
Do not vent well
May leak if shaft length is too long
Jejunal tubes
Have skin-level device balloon that can obstruct lumen
Allow for continuous feeds only
Commonly clog or kink
Dislodge often
Are difficult to replace—cannot be done at home
May cause intussusception
Need a separate gastostomy port to vent the stomach
Are useful as a temporary diagnostic or therapeutic intervention

abdomen, listening for the "pop" of 3–5 cc of air sent through the NG tube by syringe. Supplemental confirmation may occur by aspirating gastric juices and documenting an acidic pH. These methods, although reliable, are imperfect. A child who is coughing, gagging, or distressed by the tube placement should either have it replaced or have the tube placement confirmed by radiographic means. Similarly, vomiting or vigorous coughing can displace the tube, and care should be taken to ensure its proper placement before feeds resume. Children with anatomic abnormalities of the esophagus, such as a repaired tracheoesophageal fistula, should have radiographic confirmation. Individuals with narrow nares or choanal atresia may not be candidates for these tubes as the tube may interfere with their breathing.

NG tubes should be replaced every 10–21 days. Clinicians should alternate the nostril in which the tube is placed to avoid alar erosion and eventual tissue destruction. Long-term use of an NG tube can cause sinusitis. The tape can cause significant skin irritation or breakdown, prevented by placement of an adhesive pad on the cheek and having the tube taped to the pad. NG tubes are generally used for a matter of weeks to a few months. If longer term supplementation is required, a gastrostomy should be placed.

Gastrostomy Tubes G tubes may be placed endoscopically, known as percutaneous endoscopic gastrostomy (PEG; Mamel, 1989). An endoscopist and assistant visualize the place in which the stomach and abdominal wall approximate each other. A wire is poked into the stomach and brought up and out through the mouth. The G tube is attached to the wire and is drawn back into the stomach by going down the esophagus. The procedure is relatively brief and is less invasive in that no sutures are placed. Recovery time is 1–2 days as compared with 5 days for a standard surgically placed tube. It is usually performed under general anesthesia for children, but some institutions perform PEG under sedation for older individuals.

This procedure, however, is not appropriate for all candidates. Very small infants and children with micrognathia or esophageal strictures may not be able to have the G tube pass down the esophagus. Prior abdominal surgery, VP shunts, or severe scoliosis may preclude the visualization or actual ability of the stomach to lie right next to the abdominal wall. Each institution or practice develops its own guidelines for absolute or relative contraindications for PEG placement.

Percutaneous G tube placement is performed without sutures, so time must elapse for maturation of the tract to withstand tube changes without disruption. In the authors' institution, the interval from placement to first change of the gastrostomy is 6 months. The authors typically use radiographic confirmation of correct placement after the first tube change as well.

Surgically placed G tubes require an incision, so the procedure is longer and more invasive, and the recovery time reflects this fact. A skin-level device may be placed initially rather than the traditional G tubes; however, most other aspects of the surgical tubes are comparable with those of the PEG tubes.

Once the tube is placed, it can leak, bleed, clog, fall out, or become infected (see Table 14.2-2). A tube that has fallen out is a serious problem. The stoma can close exceedingly quickly, so parents and caregivers should be prepared to handle this situation at home if at all possible. If the tube was placed more than 6 months prior, the tract should be mature. In those cases, the original or same size tube should be gently placed back in the tract. If resistance is met, a smaller diameter tube should be used. If no tube is available, a similar shaped object can be used and taped into place until the individual can be assessed. The replacement tube does not need to be sterile. If the tube was placed recently, it is best to check whether it is safe to replace. Most surgically placed tubes are fine to replace as the stomach is sutured to the anterior abdominal wall; however, tubes that were placed endoscopically or radiographically do not have sutures. Adhesions or scar tissue eventually form to keep the stomach and abdominal wall approximated. In these cases, early replacement of the tube can cause separation; the tube is then in the peritoneum rather than the stomach.

Foley catheters, sometimes used as primary or replacement tubes, do not have external bolsters and often migrate inward to cause a gastric outlet obstruction. The obstruction occurs because the internal balloon blocks the pylorus and causes vomiting. In this case, deflation of the balloon and gentle withdrawal of the Foley catheter promptly resolves the problem.

Tubes usually have an internal balloon or bolster inside as well as a bolster on the outside. For example, gastrostomies made by Corpak have a flat disc, G tubes made by Medical Innovations Corporation (MIC tubes) have a balloon, and Malencot and Bard tubes have a mushroom shaped bolster. Each tube has its own types of extension tubing, ports, and valves. Institutions tend to stock one or two types of tubing for efficiency, and practitioners usually become familiar with the peculiarities of those systems.

Jejunostomy Tubes If the individual cannot tolerate gastric feeds, a decision must be made to use a nasojejunal (NJ) tube, use a gastrojejeunal (GJ) tube, or perform a fundoplication. Having a GJ tube, as compared with a NJ tube or jejunal (J) tube alone, allows venting of the stomach and increased ease of adminis-

Table 14.2-2. Solving common gastrostomy tube complications

Problem	Reason	Intervention	Prevention
Leakage of stomach contents	Internal bolster is not snug against anterior stomach wall	Pull gently on the tube until resistance is met.	Mark or note where the external bolster is at the skin (i.e., 2 cm).
	Balloon has deflated or broken	Deflate and refill the balloon. If it is still loose, change the tube.	Periodically check the amount of water in the balloon.
	Poor fit of skin-level device	If device leaves pressure marks on the skin, use a longer size. If more than a dime's width of space is between the tube and the skin, add a pad or get a shorter tube.	DO NOT change to a larger diameter tube; it will only enlarge the stoma.
Obstruction of tube	Using blenderized foods rather than formulas	Milk the tube to loosen the obstruction. Flush the tube with warm water or cranberry juice.	Flush the tube with water after medication and bolus feeds. Flush the tube every 8 hours during continuous feeds.
	Using crushed tablet medicines or granules	Same as above	Same as above
Granulation tissue at the site	Friction at site	Stabilize the tube. Cauterize it with silver nitrate sticks or melt granulation tissue with 0.1% triamcinalone ointment	Ensure that the tube is not sliding in and out or side to side.
Bleeding around tube	Granulation tissue	Same as above	Same as above
	Erosion from pressure	Place an absorbent pad between the skin and the tube until the wound has healed.	Avoid leaving the extension tube in place all of the time.
Bleeding through the tube	Gastritis/ulcer or erosion caused by the tube	Use an acid blockade and/or carafate.	Treat bleeding early.
Erythema around tube	Cellulitis	Apply a topical antibiotic. If the condition worsens, administer an oral antibiotic.	Minimize skin breakdown by stabilizing the tube.
	Yeast infection	Apply a topical antifungal.	Avoid gauze as it holds in moisture.
Tube falling out	Accidental pulling	If site is mature, IMMEDIATELY place some tube (even if it is not sterile) in the stoma to keep it from closing.	Keep extra tubes (one the same size and one smaller) available at home.

tration of some medications. J tubes are usually placed fluoroscopically and are difficult to replace on an emergent basis. They are very slender and are likely to clog or kink. Some medications that are granular may be difficult to administer through this tube.

An important consideration with J tube feeds is that continuous feeds must be given rather than bolus feeds. This process may entail transporting a small pump throughout the day if the individual is active. Because the tube is placed in a part of the intestine that is not fixed in location, it can be dislodged or become the lead point for intussusceptions. A child who experiences repeated intussusceptions with one length of J tube may improve with a change to a different length of tube.

The authors encourage the use of J tubes only for short-term use, due to the difficulties involved in placing and maintaining these tubes. J tubes are most useful as a diagnostic trial, for example, when the role of reflux in causing pulmonary disease is unclear despite pH probe and milk scan studies. A 2-month trial of J feeds made a clear difference in several of the authors' patients, and the individuals went on to have successful outcomes after fundoplication. A caveat to this trial is that the children can still aspirate gastric secretions and should continue on maximal acid blockade during the trial.

GASTROESOPHAGEAL REFLUX

Katrina is a 15-year-old girl with hypotonia and significant developmental delays of unclear etiology. Her father is single and has done very well in caring for her at home. Katrina has always eaten pureed foods by mouth. She initially gained weight well, but her father has noted that her weight has leveled off over the past few years. Katrina has always had some choking with feeds, but her father is concerned that the choking has increased recently. Katrina has never had any respiratory difficulties, nor does she vomit. She does not ever appear to be in distress, but her father notes that her very limited communication and easy temperament make it difficult to tell if she is in pain.

Katrina's pediatrician is concerned about her unexplained anemia. Katrina was admitted to the hospital last year with a hematocrit of 17% and hemoglobin of 4.5 g/dL. She responded partially to iron administration but has remained persistently anemic.

Katrina was sent to a gastroenterologist who noted occult blood in her stools. The gastroenterologist decided that endoscopy would be the best test to evaluate the occult bleeding, and Katrina's father was comfortable with this plan. At the time of the first endoscopy, a tight stricture was found high in the esophagus. It was too tight to allow even the smallest endoscope to go through. The stricture was presumed to be from peptic esophagitis, so acid suppression was started (ranitidine 2 mg/kg/dose twice a day).

Katrina seemed more comfortable and gained a few pounds. A repeat endoscopy 2 months later demonstrated improvement in that the scope could pass through the stricture. Below the stricture was a long area of erythematous, friable esophagus with exudate. Katrina was switched to a stronger medication (omeprazole at 1 mg/kg/dose twice a day). Her anemia resolved, she gained 18 lb in the next 4 months, and her choking episodes stopped. Her father felt that she was happier than she had ever been.

GER is defined as the involuntary entry of gastric contents into the esophagus. In healthy children and adults, the most common mechanism of GER is the transient inappropriate relaxation of the lower esophageal sphincter. Hiatal hernia, low esophageal sphincter tone, and delayed gastric emptying are other predisposing conditions. The prevalence of GER is quite high in children with neurodevelopmental delays. Although the actual numbers vary with the population studied and the methods used for diagnosis, the prevalence of GER seems to be 70%–75% in these children (Guidice et al., 1999; Ravelli & Milla, 1998). Contributing factors include prolonged supine positioning, liquid feeds, and increased abdominal pressure from spasticity or seizures. Placement of G tubes were initially reported to increase GER (Berezin et al., 1986); however, larger prospective studies do not confirm G tube placement as a cause of reflux (Launey et al., 1996; Razwghi, Lang, & Behrens, 2002; Samuel & Holmes, 2002; Wheatley et al., 1991). Central nervous system disorders may also predispose to foregut dysmotility, as some investigators have found a higher incidence of delayed gastric emptying and gastric dysrhythmias in children with central nervous system disorders.

Signs and Symptoms

Symptoms that result from the GER itself may be difficult to distinguish from the symptoms secondary to complications of GER, which are varied and can be quite severe. Typically children will vomit and/or experience discomfort with feeds. Children without overt vomiting may arch, cry, or pull away from feeds due to discomfort. Rarely, infants or young children will develop Sandifer syndrome, a tonic posture consisting of head cocking and extension of the neck. Failure to thrive and malnutrition are common consequences of GER and may occur from feeding aversion or from direct volume losses as a result of vomiting.

Esophagitis is a common complication, and symptoms range from irritability, texture aversion, and dysphagia to hemetemesis or anemia from chronic bleeding (see Figure 14.2-1a). Chronic esophagitis may lead to strictures or the intestinal metaplasia known as Barrett's esophagus (see Figures 14.2-1b and 14.2-1c). This latter condition is considered at high risk for malignant transformation. Cognitive delay is considered a risk factor for Barrett's because the prevalence of Barrett's is higher in individuals with developmental delays (Hassall, 1997; Snyder & Goldman, 1990). The high rate of GER and inability to communicate well can lead to long delays in treatment of severe esophagitis in these individuals. Respiratory complications of GER include recurrent pneumonia, wheezing, apnea, cyanosis, or hoarseness. Wheezing and apnea can occur from the direct aspiration of gastric contents or from vagally mediated bronchospasm. Sinusitis and poor sleeping may also be experienced.

Differential Diagnosis and Evaluation

Evaluation in a relatively healthy child with typical symptoms may consist of a careful history; however, vomiting can occur from a variety of other causes in these children, including ventriculoperitoneal (VP) shunt failure, metabolic disturbance, food or medication allergy, intestinal malrotation, ureteropelvic junction obstruction, or various infections.

The best initial test to perform in most individuals with vomiting is a barium study of the upper intestinal tract (UGI series). The UGI series can identify a number of anatomic abnormalities that can cause vomiting such as antral web, malrotation, or superior mesenteric

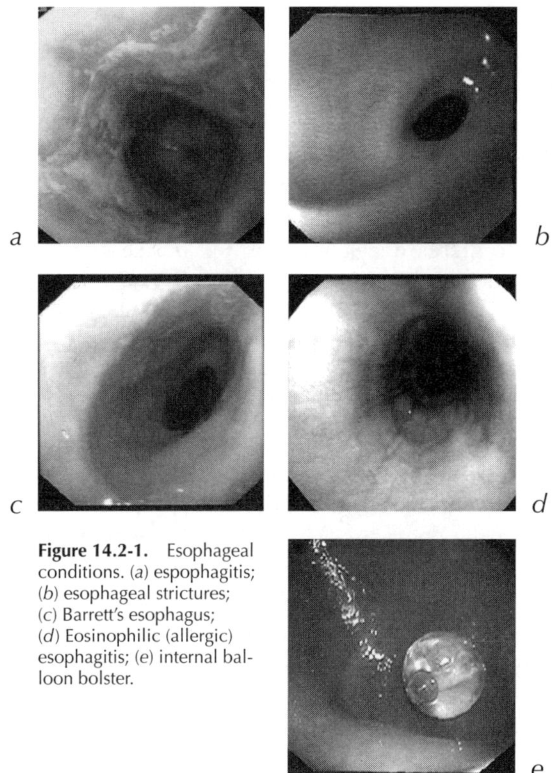

Figure 14.2-1. Esophageal conditions. (*a*) espophagitis; (*b*) esophageal strictures; (*c*) Barrett's esophagus; (*d*) Eosinophilic (allergic) esophagitis; (*e*) internal balloon bolster.

artery syndrome. In addition, the UGI series may identify ingested foreign bodies, lactobezoars (solidified curdled milk), or trichobezoars (ingested hairballs). The UGI series is an excellent test to identify anatomic problems but is inaccurate in the diagnosis of gastritis, esophagitis, or GER.

Although radiologists may be able to induce reflux with provocative maneuvers to increase abdominal pressure, such reflux may be an artifact. Most reflux occurs as the result of transient relaxations of the LES rather than increased abdominal pressure. Furthermore, a small amount of physiologic reflux occurs in most people. Unless massive reflux is seen on the barium study, there is poor correlation with other measures such as pH probe (Aksglaede, Funch-Jensen, & Thommesen, 1999; Al-Khawari, Sinan, & Seymour, 2002; Pan et al., 2003). For these reasons, the authors do not use the UGI series to diagnose reflux.

Overnight pH monitoring (pH probe) has been considered the gold standard in the diagnosis of reflux. In this study, a small catheter is passed through the nose into the esophagus and left for 12–24 hours. A small pH meter in the tip of the probe should be located at 5 cm. above the junction of the esophagus and stomach, and the location is often confirmed radiographically. During the study, the individual should not be taking any acid-suppressing medication. Continuous feeds cannot be run, as formula will buffer the acid and create a false-negative reading. In all other respects, the home regimen is followed during the time of the study.

The results reveal how many episodes of reflux occur, how long they last, and the total time that acid is in the esophagus. If these numbers are above the physiologic norms, the study is considered "positive" for pathologic reflux. The pH probe is particularly useful for documenting whether acid reflux is temporally related to events, such as coughing, apnea, or arching. If GER is associated with a symptom, the GER episode and the symptom occur at the same time.

A variation on the pH probe is the multichannel impedance study, which records the flux of acidic and nonacid material in the esophagus (Shay, Bomeli, & Richter, 2002; Tutuian et al., 2003). Although not widely available, it may be of great value in the future as it can demonstrate the height of the reflux as well as the number and duration of the episodes. Demonstrating that refluxate (whether acidic or nonacidic) comes to the posterior pharynx can be the deciding factor on whether to continue with medical therapy or move to surgical therapy for a child with respiratory complications.

Other tests reveal complications or predisposing factors for GER. Endoscopy with biopsies will reveal the extent of esophagitis or Barrett's esophagus by visual inspection. Biopsies can also determine if eosinophilic (allergic) or infectious esophagitis is present (see Figure 14.2-1d). An individual can have completely normal esophageal mucosa with uncomplicated reflux. Endoscopy can also be used to evaluate and treat strictures. Scintigraphy (gastric emptying scan and milk scan) can document gastroparesis and often can show aspiration.

Treatment

Tommy is a 4-year-old boy with severe cerebral palsy from perinatal anoxia. He has a history of GER, and his symptoms of reflux have dramatically increased since he began wearing a body jacket for his scoliosis and kyphosis. He has been spitting up 10–30 times per day and has been treated with antireflux medications. Tommy's mother is the principal caregiver. She has been overwhelmed with so many medical issues that she has not wanted to investigate the 2–3 pneumonias he gets each year; however, the pediatrician is very worried that these may represent aspiration and has convinced her to have some tests.

The first modified barium swallow test showed a very uncoordinated oral phase with delayed initiation of the swallow and large amounts of residue after the swallow. Although no aspiration was seen, the speech therapist was worried that Tommy would be at risk for aspiration and asked his mother to only give him thickened liquids.

The next year, Tommy only had one aspiration pneumonia. His mother admitted that she was not completely consistent with thickening his feeds. The next modified swallow study had to be terminated quickly because it demonstrated that Tommy had silent aspiration of thin liquids. He did cough and protect his airway better with thicker liquids.

Over the next several years, Tommy continued to have bronchitis and pneumonia, despite his mother's now determined efforts to thicken all feeds. The gastroenterologist involved in Tommy's care asked to have him undergo a pH probe while on the prokinetic agent to see how well the reflux was being addressed. The study demonstrated an abnormal amount of acid reflux into the esophagus. The gastroenterologist explained to Tommy's mother that the refluxate that enters the esophagus and pharynx from the stomach may be aspirated and lead to pneumonia. A fundoplication was recommended. Tommy's mother had many long conversations with the surgeon, gastroenterologist, and pulmonologist and finally agreed to the surgery.

Tommy did extremely well after the fundoplication. He did not have any further pneumonias, and many of his pulmonary medicines could be discontinued. He did not have a G tube placed because he could handle pureed foods and thickened liquids well; however, 2 years later, his mother contacted the gastroenterologist to say that hydration was becoming a problem. A percutaneous gastrostomy was placed for hydration only, and Tommy continues to eat solid foods.

Treatment of GER can start with conservative measures such as providing smaller, more frequent feeds; thickening feeds; and proper positioning. Medical management consists of acid-suppressing agents and prokinetic agents. Table 14.2-3 details dosing and side effects. (*Note:* Because doses change over time, verify doses before administering medication.) Most children respond well to initial acid suppression with a histamine-2 receptor antagonist such as ranitidine or cimetidine. If a child does not respond or has severe esophagitis, treatment should consist of a proton-pump inhibitor such as omeprazole or lansoprazole.

Both cimetidine and omeprazole are metabolized via the cytochrome P450 pathway and, thus, can potentially raise serum levels of certain anticonvulsant medications by inhibiting their metabolism. If a child or adult with well-controlled seizures suddenly has increased seizure activity after starting one of these medications, the level of anticonvulsant should be checked. The level does not need to be routinely checked after starting these acid-blocking medicines as this interaction is rarely of clinical significance.

Acid suppression will allow healing of the esophagitis in 2–3 weeks and should improve dysphagia. It may not change the volume of the refluxate, in which case a prokinetic agent may be required. These agents increase gastric emptying and may increase lower esophageal sphincter pressure. The medication cisapride was a very effective prokinetic but was removed from the market due to the cardiac side effects. Metoclopramide is an effective agent but may cause irritability, sleepiness, or dystonia. Erythromycin at low doses has been used to increase gastric emptying but should be carefully evaluated for potential drug interactions.

Surgical treatment of GER is available for children who fail medical management. A fundoplication involves wrapping the gastric cardia around the esophagus, which causes increased pressure at the lower esophageal sphincter and decreases the transient relaxations It can be performed with different kinds of wraps, (e.g. Nissen fundoplication, Thal fundoplication). These operations vary in the degree to which the cardia is wrapped and the specifics of the suturing. Many centers perform laproscopic fundoplications. If the surgeon is experienced and the child does not have multiple previous abdominal surgeries or other confounding factors, this type of surgery may be an excellent option.

In general, the outcome of any fundoplication is highly dependent on the skill and experience of the surgeon. The degree of preoperative evaluation varies from surgeon to surgeon. Some will perform the fundoplication based on clinical history alone, whereas others require careful documentation of GER by pH probe, gastric emptying scan, endoscopy, and esophageal manometry.

Prophylactic fundoplication, performed at the time of the gastrostomy placement in anticipation of increased GER, is not recommended in most children (Hament et al., 2001; Sullivan, 1999). In children with a normal pH probe prior to gastrostomy placement, a fundoplication is rarely required later. In children with an abnormal pH probe prior to gastrostomy, a fundoplication is only later required in less than one third of children (Sulaeman et al., 1998). The threshold to send a child with current symptoms for an antireflux procedure varies from center to center and has not been fully evaluated in a prospective standardized way.

Although a fundoplication relieves the symptoms in the vast majority of individuals, it is a major surgery and has a number of potential complications. If the wrap is too tight, it will cause esophageal obstruction. If it is too loose, GER will continue. Other anatomic problems include gas–bloat syndrome, retching, bowel obstruction from adhesions, dumping syndrome after pyloromyotomy, and recurrent GER with unwrapping or slipping of the fundoplication.

Table 14.2-3. Medications for gastroesophageal reflux

Drug	Pediatric dose	Adult dose	Side effects
Prokinetics			
Metoclopramide—1 mg/mL, 5 mg tablet, 10 mg tablet	0.1–0.2 mg/kg/dose three times a day	10 mg three times a day	Irritability, dystonia, sleepiness
Erythromycin—compound varies with pharmacy	5 mg/kg/dose three to four times a day	5 mg/kg/dose three to four times a day	Change to other medicine levels (affects P450)
H2 antagonists			
Ranitidine—15/mL, 75 mg, 150 mg	2–3 mg/kg/dose twice a day	150 mg twice a day	Diarrhea, headache (both rare)
Cimetidine—60/mL, 300 mg	10 mg/kg/dose three times a day	300 mg twice a day	Diarrhea, increased anticonvulsant levels (affects P450)
Famotidine—10 mg, 20 mg, 40 mg	0.5–1 mg/kg/dose twice a day	40 mg twice a day	Diarrhea, headache
Proton pump inhibitors			
Omeprazole 20 mg/5mg susp* 10 mg/5 mg 20 mg caps	1 mg/kg every day	20 mg once or twice a day	Diarrhea, headache, change to other medicine levels (affects P450 but less than other medicines)
Lansoprazole—15 mg/2 T, 15 mg, 30 mg	1–2 mg/kg every day	30 mg once or twice a day	Proteinuria, increased transaminases

*Compounded by pharmacy

Note: Because doses may change over time, verify doses before administering medication.

The frequency of complications varies, from 26% to 59% according to inclusion criteria, but is consistently reported to be higher in children with neurodevelopmental delay than in neurologically normal children. Despite these potential complications, the fundoplication can be a very useful procedure in some individuals with neurodevelopmental impairments. The vast majority have a dramatically improved quality of life after fundoplication.

Innovations include a variety of endoscopic or endoluminal antireflux procedures (Galmiche & Bruley des Varannes, 2003). The mucosa is pinched and sutured or altered with radio/heat frequencies. The net result is a tighter or smaller sphincter. Although these procedures hold great promise, it is still too early to know all the potential side effects or to judge the long-term efficacy. Given that individuals with developmental disabilities are at high risk for severe reflux and complications, the authors recommend that endoscopic procedures still be considered investigational for these individuals.

GASTRITIS AND PEPTIC ULCER DISEASE

Harriet is a 20-year-old woman with intellectual disabilities who resides in a residential home. Over the past 3 months, her mother has been concerned because Harriet seems pale and tired. Her only two medications are phenytoin for a well-controlled seizure disorder and intermittent ibuprofen for menstrual discomfort. Examination by her primary care physician demonstrated a pale woman in no distress with a nontender abdomen; however, her stool was dark and strongly positive for occult blood on three separate occasions.

Harriet's hematocrit was 24%, and serum iron was 15 mcg./dL. She underwent upper endoscopy under anesthesia, and a nodular gastritis was identified (see Figure 14.2-1e). Gastric biopsies showed *Helicobacter pylori.* The *H. pylori* was treated with a combination of amoxicillin, clarithromycin, and lansoprazole for 2 weeks. The anemia was treated with iron and did not recur during a 2-year period of follow-up.

Gastritis is defined as macroscopic or microscopic inflammation of the mucosal layer of the stomach. In contrast, gastric or duodenal peptic ulcers are deeper erosions that may penetrate into the deeper muscular layers of the stomach and rarely cause massive bleeding or perforations. Most ulcers are located in the lesser curvature or prepyloric regions of the stomach or in the duodenal bulb. Although the causes of gastritis and peptic disease in children are variable (see Table 14.2-4), the most common causes of gastritis and ulcers in children and adults with developmental disabilities include *H. pylori* infection, medications, or mechanical trauma from G tubes. The clinical presentation is also highly variable, with common symptoms being abdominal pain, vomiting, melena, bleeding out of a G tube, and occult iron deficiency anemia.

Worldwide, the most common cause of gastritis and duodenal ulcers is *H. pylori.* This gram negative spiral bacterium preferentially colonizes the gastric epithelium within the gastric glands and mucus layer. It

Table 14.2-4. Selected causes of gastritis and peptic ulcer disease

Infectious causes
Helicobacter pylori
Helicobacter heilmannii (Gastrospirillum hominis)
Medications
Nonsteroidal anti-inflammatory drugs
Corticosteroids
Antibiotics
Ethanol
Anticonvulsants
Mechanical
Gastrostomy tubes
Inflammatory
Crohn's disease
Celiac disease
Menetrier disease
Autoimmune (atrophic) gastritis
Eosinophilic (allergic) gastritis
Miscellaneous
Bile reflux gastritis
Stress (e.g., following surgery)

Source: Rowland, Bourke, and Drumm (2000).

also colonizes the duodenum in areas of gastric metaplasia. The bacterium produces cytotoxic proteins and also stimulates the secretion of chemotactic cytokines (e.g., interleukin-8) by the gastric mucosa. The end result is a mucosal inflammatory cellular infiltrate consisting of lymphocytes and neutrophils (gastritis) (McColl, El-Omar, & Gillen, 2000). Approximately 15% of individuals colonized with *H. pylori* go on to develop ulcers, and a much smaller number of adults will develop a low-grade gastric lymphoma (MALToma) from chronic *H. pylori* infection.

H. pylori infection is usually contracted in childhood and persists into adulthood. The overall prevalence worldwide ranges from 20%–80%, with risk factors for infection being poverty, poor hygiene, family history, large number of brothers and sisters, and bed sharing. In developed countries, the prevalence of *H. pylori* is much lower in children (5%–10%) than in adults (50%), presumably because of improved living standards in today's children. Although the exact mode of transmission of *H. pylori* is unknown, it is strongly suspected that person-to-person contact through oral or fecal secretions is the mode of spread (Everhart, 2000; Go, 2002; McColl et al., 2000).

A wide variety of medications may cause gastric inflammation or ulceration. Different medications have different mechanisms of injury. Nonsteroidal anti-inflammatory medicines, including aspirin and ibuprofen, induce peptic injury by causing a local depletion of prostaglandin and possibly vascular injury. Ethanol intake causes a subepithelial hemorrhage with a paucity of inflammatory cells. Chemotherapeutic agents, such as methotrexate, cause ulcers by interfering with cellular replication. It is unclear whether anticonvulsants cause gastritis, though some individuals do complain of epigastric discomfort when taking these medications.

Children and adults with developmental disabilities are frequently fed via G tube. These individuals sometimes experience a small amount of gastric bleeding, which usually is identified when gastric contents are aspirated from the G tube. The most common cause of this problem is mechanical gastritis caused by the inside portion of the tube rubbing against the gastric mucosa. When the internal portion of the tube has a pointed tip, the tip may rub against the opposite gastric wall, causing ulceration and bleeding.

Clinical Symptoms and Diagnosis

Individuals may complain of abdominal discomfort if they can verbalize but may present with more dramatic symptoms, including vomiting blood or passing black stool. The diagnostic test of choice is upper endoscopy, which will establish the severity of the gastric inflammation, identify any bleeding ulcers, and allow biopsy of the affected mucosa to look for infectious organisms. For actively bleeding lesions, endoscopic techniques to control bleeding (e.g., electrocautery) are available. If an individual is too ill or unstable to undergo endoscopy, empiric therapy with proton pump antagonists is appropriate until the procedure is possible (Eisen et al., 2001; Huang & Lichtenstein, 2003).

A variety of noninvasive tests are available to diagnose *H. pylori*, including blood serology, urea breath testing, and fecal antigen testing. Although these tests are relatively specific, their sensitivity in young children is only fair. In addition, these tests may establish if an individual is colonized with *H. pylori*; however, they do not determine whether the *H. pylori* is the cause of the individual's symptoms. Therefore, endoscopy with biopsies should still be considered the gold standard of diagnosis.

Treatment

If an individual has large volume bleeding from a peptic ulcer, he or she should be closely monitored and given hemodynamic support (packed red blood cells and other blood products if necessary). Acutely, intestinal bleeding should be treated with an acid blocking agent. Available agents include proton pump antagonists (e.g. lansoprazole, omeprazole, pantoprazole), and H2 receptor blockers (ranitidine, famotidine). Use of intragastric antacid therapy (e.g., Mylanta, Maalox) may provide additional benefit but should not be instituted if urgent endoscopy is planned because the antacid may coat the stomach and obscure the view of the endoscopist. If significant bleeding persists despite acid blockade, consideration should be given to adding octreotide, a somatostatin analogue that reduces splanchnic blood flow (Rowland, Bourke, & Drumm, 2000).

Once the acute issue has resolved, the underlying cause of the gastritis should be addressed. An individual with *H. pylori* gastritis and peptic ulcer disease should have the *H. pylori* eradicated. Treatment for *H. pylori* typically involves an acid blocking agent and two antibiotics (e.g., lansoprazole, amoxicillin, clarithromycin) given for 14 days. Bismuth subsalicylate may be added for additional efficacy. Given the increasing prevalence of antibiotic-resistant strains, a "test of cure" for *H. pylori* should be performed. A repeat endoscopy is the gold standard for test of cure, but an *H. pylori* breath test is a reasonable noninvasive alternative (Gold et al., 2000). If an individual is on a medication that has caused gastritis, that medication should ideally be discontinued. An individual with a mechanical problem from a specific type of gastrostomy may benefit from having a change in the type of gastrostomy device (e.g., changing from a balloon type gastrostomy to a "button" or a recessed tip device).

CONSTIPATION

Brian is a 30-year-old nonverbal man who lives in a residential nursing home. He eats with assistance by mouth, and his GER is well controlled on medication. The G tube that he needs for supplemental feeds has not required much attention. Despite softening agents, Brian may go 10–12 days without a bowel movement. When he has not defecated, his appetite drops, and he pushes away food. He seems to experience increased regurgitation and will vomit as well. He may then have a "blow-out" stool where he is covered in feces. His caregivers have become very upset as this situation is happening more frequently.

Thyroid testing was done, as Brian had recent weight gain and low energy. There was also a family history of thyroid disease. Brian had normal thyroid functions. An abdominal radiograph done right after a blow out demonstrated a large amount of stool present throughout the colon. Thus, the large amount of stool seen by the caregivers was simply overflow.

Brian was given large doses of bisacodyl laxative to evacuate the accumulated stool and started on a regimen of softeners (polyethylene glycol without electrolytes) and stimulant laxatives (senna) initially. He then began stooling 2–3 times per week. The stimulant laxatives were slowly tapered over 10 months, and the stooling pattern remained stable on softeners alone. He is given a "rescue" dose of a stimulant if no stool has emerged in 3 days. This situation, however, does not occur often now.

Constipation is very common among children and adults with cerebral palsy and neurodevelopmental delays. Prevalence estimates range from 62% to 74% (Bohmer et al., 2001; Del Giudice et al., 1999; Staiano & Del Giudice, 1994). The reason for this high prevalence is not known, but there are many potential causes for constipation in these individuals. Poor fluid intake, poor fiber intake, immobility, and lack of conscious urge to defecate in some individuals are contributing factors.

An increasing amount of literature evaluates colonic motility itself, with the suggestion that disruption in neural modulation or abnormal development of neuromuscular control may be implicated as an underlying cause. One investigator found that colonic transit in children with severe brain damage was slow in the left colon only (18%) or in left colon and rectum (56%) while in neurologically intact children with functional constipation the slow transit was in the left colon in 20% and rectum only in 80% (Staiano & Del Giudice, 1994). Cisapride, which increases colonic contraction amplitude but does not affect contraction propagation, did not change colonic transit time in a heterogeneous population of children with neurological impairment (Staiano et al., 1996). Anorectal manometry results in these children were comparable to asymptomatic controls whereas functional constipation had increased rectal compliance. Therefore, the mechanisms involved seem to be different.

The prevalence of constipation seems to be the same in children and adults with intellectual disabilities, which would suggest that it does not develop over time but is present from early in life. This finding would be consistent with the theory that constipation is an intrinsic motility problem rather than the result of overstretching the rectum, often seen in functional retention.

Signs, Symptoms, and Complications

Constipation can cause early satiety, poor feeding, gassiness, abdominal pain, and vomiting but is rarely associated with soiling. It often causes significant distress, as illustrated by Brian's situation. It can also be associated with behavioral difficulties. In one study, behavioral problems were present in 40% of those with constipation but only 25% of those with normal bowels. Also, one investigator looking at the cessation of laxatives had to stop the study early as almost 80% of the children developed severe behavioral difficulties within a few days (Bohmer et al., 2001). Medicines such as benzodiazepines may be prescribed for behavioral issues, which have the potential of worsening the constipation.

Chronic constipation can cause dilation of the rectum and even megacolon. The sigmoid can become enlarged and elongated, and it may rotate on itself (cecal or sigmoid volvulus). This condition requires immediate intervention, either decompression with colonoscopy or surgical resection. Although this condition is thought to occur mainly in older adults, it has been reported in children as young as 10 years if other factors such as intellectual disabilities or myopathy are present (Al-Kouder et al., 2002).

Differential Diagnosis and Evaluation

History and physical examination alone usually provide adequate diagnostic information. Attention should be paid to delayed meconium passage, early onset of constipation, change of bowel habit with introduction of new foods, trauma with toilet training, and withholding behaviors. Passage of consistent pencil-like stools raises concern about Hirschsprung disease or anal stenosis. Weight loss, new onset of cold intolerance, and lethargy would signal concerns about an organic etiology. A comprehensive list of these organic causes can be found in Table 14.2-5. Dietary history may demonstrate inadequate fluid intake or lack of fiber. Medications should be reviewed to ensure they are not contributing factors. Family history of celiac disease, hypothyroidism, cystic fibrosis, or chronic constipation may heighten concern for organic etiologies.

Physical signs can include a distended or tympanitic abdomen and palpable masses in the abdomen or rectum. On examination, careful attention should be paid to the lower spine, as tethered cord, meningomyocele, or acquired spinal lesions can cause bowel and bladder dysfunction. An absent anal wink, a patulous anal opening, or increased deep tendon reflexes in the lower extremities have been associated with neurological disorders that can cause constipation. A sacral dimple or tuft of hair in the region would be important to observe. The location of the anus should be examined, as anterior placement of the anus has been associated with constipation (Hendren, 1978). For individuals who are difficult to examine, a radiograph of the abdomen will allow a sense of the degree of retained stool in the rectum and colon.

In most cases, further investigation is not necessary. Children with red flags in their history or abnormal physical examination may require further testing. For children and adults with developmental disabilities, the indications for further testing are less clear. In general, investigation is undertaken when a child fails to respond to appropriate treatment for an extended time. In some children, an abdominal radiograph may be useful to evaluate the amount and location of the retained stool and to screen for sacral abnormalities. When Hirschsprung disease is a consideration, rectal suction biopsy or anorectal manometry can be performed. Anorectal manometry, if available, has the additional aspect of determining other abnormalities such as anismus or patterns consistent with spinal pathology; however, rectal suction or full thickness biopsy is the gold standard for the diagnosis of Hirschsprung disease.

To detect spinal abnormalities such as tethered cord or diastematomyelia, magnetic resonance imaging of the lower spine is the test of choice. An ultrasound of the lower spine may be an alternative test in very young (less than 3 months of age) infants. A barium enema is rarely indicated unless a specific anatomic abnormality is suspected. Thyroid function studies should be considered on an individual basis. Lead screening can be done if pica or environmental exposure has occurred. Celiac testing can be done in the appropriate circumstances.

Table 14.2-5. Organic causes of constipation

Structural abnormalities of the rectum or colon
Anterior or ectopic anus
Anal stenosis
Hirschsprung disease
Neuromuscular
Meningomyocele
Tethered cord
Other spinal cord lesions or abnormalities
Hypotonia (i.e., associated with Down syndrome)
Musculodystrophies
Metabolic/toxic/allergic
Hypothyroidism
Celiac disease
Milk protein intolerance
Lead intoxication
Cystic fibrosis
Medications
Analgesics
Anticholinergics
Anticonvulsants
Antidepressants
Bismuth
Iron
Psychotropics

Treatment

Treatment for constipation is the same as for children without neurologic difficulties. The basic approach is to evacuate the accumulated stool and maintain regular soft bowel movements. Table 14.2-6 outlines the medications and doses for both steps. (*Note:* Because doses change over time, verify doses before administering medication.) Evacuation of retained stool is a crucial first step in treatment of constipation.

If the impaction is mainly in the rectum, the use of enemas or suppositories is useful and usually well tolerated in this population. Normal saline or mineral oil enemas can be used repeatedly. Phosphate enemas can be used but should not be repeated frequently as hyperphosphatemia has resulted from retained enemas (Sotos et al., 1977). Tap water or soapsud enemas can be dangerous and should be avoided. On rare occasions, manual disimpaction is required under general anesthesia.

If the accumulated stool is located higher than the rectum or if rectal administration is not advisable for a particular child, evacuation can be accomplished orally with strong laxatives such as bisacodyl, milk of magnesia, or magnesium citrate. Large-dose polyethylene glycol with electrolytes can be given to a child with a G tube, or, less comfortably, via an NG tube. Polyethylene glycol without electrolytes has been given safely to children at doses of 1–1.5 g/kg/day for 3 days (Youssef et al., 2002); however, diarrhea and bloating are significant side effects.

A wide variety of agents are available for maintenance therapy. Generally, bulking and softening or lubricating agents are preferred, although in severe constipation stimulant laxatives may be required on a chronic basis. For mild constipation, the addition of fiber to gastrostomy feeds may be helpful. Few studies have evaluated this action, but one report noted limited success with glucomannan fiber (Staiano et al., 2000). Prune juice and lactulose arc vcry useful and can be titrated easily but at higher doses may cause gassiness. Mineral oil can cause a severe chemical pneumonitis if regurgitated and aspirated, so it should be used with caution in individuals with abnormal swallowing (Bandla, Davis, & Hopkins, 1999). For moderate to severe constipation, the use of polyethylene glycol (PEG) solution, with or without electrolytes, has been increasingly used (Erickson et al., 2003; Loening-Baucke, 2002; Pashankar, Loening-Baucke, & Bishop, 2003). Milk of magnesia is useful, and compliance is less an issue if it can be administered through a G tube.

In individuals with severe chronic constipation that is not expected to improve over time, such as a congenital spinal lesion, the placement of a conduit for antegrade enemas has been beneficial. In an individual with an appendicostomy, the conduit is the appendix, which is tunneled through the cecal wall and brought to the skin. An alternative to appendicostomy is a cecostomy, which allows a catheter to be placed directly into the cecum. The ACE (antegrade colonic enemas) allows instillation of polyethylene glycol or saline through an appendicostomy or cecostomy into the colon. A bowel movement is predictably produced in a relatively short time frame, and often the individual will sit on the toilet during this time. The ACE allows greater independence for many older teens and adults and obviates the need for assistance with invasive toileting regimens (Marshall et al., 2001; Yerkes et al., 2003). In selected individuals, the ACE has improved quality of life.

HEPATOBILIARY DISORDERS

Ben is an 18-year-old man with severe spastic quadreparesis. At age 10, he presented with an episode of pain and mildly elevated transaminases, which resolved after 6 days. As part of his evaluation, he underwent an abdominal ultrasound, which demonstrated multiple gallstones. One gastroenterologist recommended removal of the gallbladder, and a second recommended observation. The family opted for observation, and Ben remained asymptomatic for several years. Eight years later, however, he again developed abdominal pain, lethargy, and fever. Ultrasound followed by exploratory laparotomy demonstrated cholecystitis with a gallbladder perforation and hepatic abscesses. Ben was treated with surgical drainage and intravenous antibiotics for several weeks and subsequently improved.

Biliary tract disease such as cholecystitis, although rare, is potentially life threatening, as in Ben's case. Many individuals with neurodevelopmental disabilities are intermittently placed on parenteral nutrition during times of illness and surgery, and parenteral nutrition is one of the major risk factors for gallstones. Other risk factors for stones include family history, hemolysis, pregnancy, obesity, diabetes, or rapid weight loss. Approximately 1%–3% of individuals with gallstones will develop a complication annually, including cholecystitis (inflammation of the gallbladder), choledocholithiasis (passage of a gallstone into the common bile duct with hepatobiliary obstruction), cholangitis (infection of the bile duct from chronic obstruction), and pancreatitis.

Although "watchful waiting" is advocated for asymptomatic older adults with gallstones, Ben's situation suggests that more aggressive intervention may be warranted in children and adults with disabilities. These

Table 14.2-6. Treatment for constipation

Laxative	Disimpaction dose	Maintenance dose	Considerations
Mineral oil	15–30 mL per year of age up to 240 mL	1–3 mL/kg/d in one or two doses	Lipoid pneumonitis is possible, so avoid use in children younger than 1 year of age or anyone with a swallowing disorder and/or severe reflux.
Polyethylene glycol with electrolytes (Colyte, Golytely, Nulytely)	25 mL/kg/hr (maximum of 1 L/hr) orally or by nasogastric tube until clear or 20 mL/kg/hr for 4 hr/d	Not applicable	Nausea, bloating, abdominal cramps, and vomiting are side effects. Medication is difficult to administer and may require hospital admission.
Polyethylene glycol without electrolytes (Miralax, Glycolax)	1–1.5 g/kg/d for 3 days (maximum of 34 g)	.8 g/kg/d titrated up to 8.5–17 g per day	Abdominal pain, bloating, and cramps are side effects. Electrolyte disturbance can occur if medication is overused
Milk of magnesia	1–3 cc/kg/d (400 mg/5 mL) divided into two doses	1–3 mL/kg/d of (400 mg/5 mL) divided into two doses	Use with caution in infants and individuals with renal impairment. Overdose can lead to hypermagnesemia, hypophosphatemia, and secondary hypocalcemia.
Magnesium citrate	1–3 cc/kg/d (individuals younger than 6 years); 100–150 mL/d (6- to 12-year-olds); 150–300 mL/d (individuals older than 12 years); divide into two doses	Not applicable	Considerations are the same as milk of magnesia. Can mix with soda if taking orally to increase palatability.
Lactulose (Enulose, Duphalac)	1–3 mL/kg/d divided into two doses	1–3 mL/kg/d divided into two doses	Medication can cause flatulence or abdominal cramping and occasionally diarrhea.
Sorbitol	1–3 mL/kg/d divided into two doses	1–3 mL/kg/d divided into two doses	Medication can cause flatulence or abdominal cramping and occasionally diarrhea.
Senna (Senokot, Perdiem)	2.5–7.5 cc/d (2- to 6-year-olds); 5–15 mL/d (6- to 12-year-olds); use a single dose	2.5–7.5 cc/d (2- to 6-year-olds); 5–15 mL/d (6- to 12-year-olds); use a single dose	Long-term melanosis coli is possible. Idiosyncratic hepatitis, osteoarthopathy, and nephropathy (all rare) are also side effects.
Bisacodyl	1–3 tablets per dose	1–3 tablets per dose	Abdominal pain, diarrhea, and hypokalemia are possible.
Phosphate enema	6 cc/kg max of 135 mL	Not applicable	Avoid in children younger than age 2.
Saline enema	5–10 cc/kg	Not applicable	Do not use tap water alone.
Mineral oil enema	15–30 cc per year of age (maximum 240 cc)	Not applicable	Avoid in children younger than age 2.
Bisacodyl suppository	0.5–1 suppository for individuals older than 2 years		Abdominal pain and abnormal rectal mucosa are side effects.

Note: Because doses change over time, verify doses before administering medication.
Source: Baker et al. (1999).

individuals may not be able to communicate symptoms of gallstone disease and, thus, may be at risk for only presenting when hepatobiliary disease is advanced. The predominant treatment of gallstones is cholecystectomy; such a procedure usually cures the problem but carries a 1:200 risk of bile duct injury (Strasberg, 1999). Medical options to treat stones include oral bile acid (ursodeoxycholic acid) treatment of cholesterol stones and lithotripsy; however, the role of medical management of gallstones is limited (Howard & Fromm, 1999).

Although serious chronic liver disease is uncommon in people with developmental disabilities, abnormal liver chemistries are quite common. The biochemical "liver profile" or "liver function tests" consists of the following assays: aspartate aminotranferase (AST), alanine aminotransferase (ALT), alkaline phosphatase, total and direct bilirubin, and gamma glutamyl transpeptidase (GGTP). The AST and ALT usually reflect hepatocellular injury and lysis, with the ALT being more specific for liver injury. In viral hepatitis, both AST and ALT are elevated, with the ALT usually being higher than the AST. Other conditions such as myopathies, rhabdomyolysis, and hemolysis may also cause transaminase elevation, but, in these conditions, the AST will exceed the ALT.

Cholestasis or biliary obstruction (e.g., seen with gallstones in the common bile duct) will usually cause elevations in the direct bilirubin, alkaline phosphatase, and GGTP, with the GGTP being the most specific enzyme for cholestasis. Some anticonvulsant and attention-deficit disorder medications, however, may elevate the GGTP without cholestasis. Elevations of alkaline phosphatase can also be seen in vitamin D–deficient rickets or bone fractures. True synthetic function of the liver can be assayed by measuring albumin, prothrombin time (PT), and partial thromboplastin time (PTT). Evidence of a coagulopathy with no evidence of hemophilia, disseminated intravascular coagulation, or vitamin K deficiency suggests severe liver disease with impairment of synthetic function.

Often, abnormal liver tests are identified during routine screening or monitoring. Drug therapy is the most common cause of such abnormal testing. Therapy with valproic acid carries a small but real risk of fulminant liver failure. A characteristic sign of valproic acid toxicity is evidence of impaired synthetic function, with coagulopathy, hyperammonemia, and hypoalbuminemia. It is thought that valproate is a mitochondrial toxin; therefore, individuals with Rett syndrome, Alpers disease, and other mitochondrial disease may be at increased risk for valproate toxicity. Phenobarbital and phenytoin commonly cause mild elevations (up to 3 times normal) of AST and ALT. More rarely, phenytoin can cause a severe systemic reaction with lymphadenopathy, eosinophilia, and severe hepatitis. Other medications associated with elevation of transaminases or cholestasis are given in Table 14.2-7 (Zimmerman & Ishak, 1995). If abnormal liver function tests are identified in an individual with developmental disabilities, the clinician should thoroughly examine the person's medication list to determine if any of the medications are associated with drug-associated liver disease.

Table 14.2-7. Partial list of drugs associated with liver disease in children with developmental disabilities

Analgesics/muscle relaxants
Acetaminophen
Dantrolene
Diazepam
Ibuprofen
Anticonvulsants
Phenytoin
Valproic acid
Phenobarbital
Carbamazepine
Antimicrobials
Griseofulvin
Isoniazid
Ketoconazole
Sulfonamides
Tetracyclines
Antineoplastics
6-mercaptopurine
Azathioprine
Thioguanine
Cyclophosphamide
Cardiac
Quinidine
Thiazides
Verapamil
Enalapril
Psychotropics
Methylphenidate
Phenothiazines
Tricyclics
Miscellaneous
Sulfasalazine
Vitamin A

Source: Zimmerman and Ishak (1995).

Viral hepatitis is another potential cause of liver injury in individuals with developmental disabilities. Acute viral hepatitis may occur as the result of a number of varied infections, including hepatitis A, hepatitis B, Epstein-Barr virus, cytomegalovirus, and enteroviral infections. Usually, these cases will run a course that is benign and self-limited. In contrast, chronic viral hepatitis is usually caused by hepatitis B or hepatitis C, and the incidence has decreased with improved hygiene and screening of blood products. Both hepatitis B and C are primarily transmitted thorough contaminated bodily fluids or intimate contact. Known risk factors include intravenous drug use, receipt of contaminated blood products, sexual intercourse with an infected individual, or vertical transmission from mother to child. If transaminases are persistently elevated in an individual with disabilities, serologic testing for hepatitis B (including HBsAg, HBcAb, and HepBsAb), and hepatitis C (Hep C Antibody) should be obtained. Medical therapy of chronic viral hepatitis is now available and may include medications such as interferon, lamivudine, and ribavarin. Antiviral treatment should be administered by a physician with experience in these therapies (Jonas, 2000).

Other causes of liver and hepatobiliary injury (including autoimmune hepatitis, hemochromatosis, and Wilson disease) are quite rare; however, if an individual has ongoing abnormalities in liver function testing without a good explanation, referral to a hepatologist is strongly encouraged.

GASTROINTESTINAL CONSIDERATIONS OF SPECIFIC CONDITIONS

A variety of gastrointestinal conditions are associated with Down syndrome and autism. Congenital anomalies associated with Down syndrome include duodenal atresia and Hirschsprung disease. Duodenal atresia typically presents immediately after birth with bilious vomiting. The incidence of duodenal atresia is rare (approximately 1:10,000 live births), but 25% of infants with duodenal atresia have Down syndrome. Abdominal radiographs reveal evidence of high-grade duodenal obstruction (the double-bubble sign); many cases are now diagnosed prenatally with ultrasound. Treatment involves surgical repair of the megaduodenum; children will sometimes have ongoing issues even after surgery secondary to dysmotility and bacterial overgrowth. Duodenal stenosis, a less severe variant, may present later in life with symptoms of partial obstruction and is also associated with Down syndrome (Haddock & Wesson, 2000).

Hirschsprung disease is caused by partial or total aganglionosis of the colon with impaired peristalsis. The prevalence of Hirschsprung disease in infants and children with Down syndrome is approximately 5%, and between 2% and 10% of children with Hirschsprung disease have Down syndrome (Moore & Johnson, 1998). More than 90% of individuals with Hirschsprung disease fail to pass meconium in the first 24 hours of life.

Affected individuals usually present in the first month of life with abdominal distension, inability to defecate, and sometimes bilious vomiting. Diagnosis is established by a combination of barium enema, anorectal manometry, and deep biopsy of the rectum. The treatment of Hirschsprung disease is surgical and involves resection of the aganglionic segment and reanastomosis of the intact segment to the anal verge. Hirschsprung enterocolitis, a life-threatening infection of the bowel secondary to the functional obstruction, may occur either before or after surgical treatment and requires broad spectrum intravenous antibiotics.

As children with Down syndrome grow older, they may develop other acquired disorders. Both GER and constipation are common and most likely are a function of hypotonia. These problems usually improve with time, once children begin ambulating. Celiac disease (gluten-sensitive enteropathy) is present in approximately 5% of older children and adults with Down syndrome (Bonamico et al., 2001). The presentation is highly variable. Infants develop a severe illness with distension, diarrhea, weight loss, and lethargy. In contrast, older children and adults may have less specific signs, including anemia, abdominal pain, and arthralgias.

The screening test of choice is the tissue transglutaminase (TTG) or antiendomysial antibody, but a serum IgA should be concurrently obtained because individuals with IgA deficiency may have false negative tests. Some authors have advocated for genetic screening by identifying individuals whose HLA types put them at risk (Csizmadia et al., 2000). The definitive test is the small bowel biopsy, which demonstrates the flattening of the villi and lymphocytic infiltrate. Clotting studies may be indicated prior to the biopsy as some individuals with celiac disease may have a vitamin K deficiency and resultant coagulopathy. Treatment of celiac disease is a lifelong gluten-free diet.

Children with autism spectrum disorders frequently have gastrointestinal complaints, including vomiting, diarrhea, and constipation (see Chapter 23.1). The prevalence of gastrointestinal evaluations in such children has dramatically increased because of the popular misconception that administration of the gastrointestinal hormone secretin promotes neurologic improvement in children with autism. Unfortunately, controlled clinical studies have failed to show any neurologic benefit of intravenous secretin administration (Lightdale et al., 2001; Sandler et al., 1999).

Children with autism frequently gag and vomit and seem to have exquisite individual sensitivity to different food textures. Solid textured foods are more likely to cause vomiting than pureed foods or liquids. If a child continues to vomit, an empiric trial of antireflux therapy or an attempt to identify the cause with endoscopy may be helpful. In one series of individuals with autism undergoing upper endoscopy, the majority had histologic evidence of esophagitis or gastritis (Horvath et al., 1999).

Chronic diarrhea is also common, particularly in toddlers. In some cases, the "diarrhea" may actually be chronic constipation with fecal overflow. Generally, evaluation for causes of diarrhea fails to identify evidence of infection, malabsorption, or intestinal inflammation.

Some authors have proposed that lactose intolerance and microscopic colonic inflammation may contribute to the diarrhea in these children. There is no proven treatment for this diarrhea; anecdotally, some of the authors' patients have described improvement after a milk- and/or wheat-free diet.

Many parents of children with pervasive developmental disorder, even without diarrhea, are putting children on a gluten-free, casein-free diet (GFCF). No controlled studies have looked at cognitive function of individuals on this diet, but many parents feel very strongly about using the diet. There may be a subset of individuals who in fact have undiagnosed celiac disease or milk protein intolerance who improve on this diet. Alternatively, the high fruit and vegetable content may provide other vitamins or nutrients that are helpful. These very restricted diets, however, often produce growth failure or weight loss, and, thus, individuals on these diets should be monitored carefully. It may be reasonable to screen people before starting the diet, as celiac markers go to normal when on a gluten-free diet. Children with autism do not seem to have increased prevalence of celiac or allergy, yet this relationship has not been carefully evaluated.

CONCLUSION

Gastrointestinal issues in individuals with disabilities are common and can have wide-ranging effects. Many of the problems threaten the health of the individual or his or her quality of life in a significant way. The most common gastrointestinal difficulties in individuals with disabilities are oropharyngeal dysphagia, GER, and constipation. Caregivers and individuals with disabilities should be questioned about these three issues during routine health supervision visits. Providers who recognize these conditions are better prepared to minimize discomfort, recognize potentially dangerous problems, and refer the individual to a specialist if necessary. The gastroenterologist is an essential ally who can aid the primary care physician to improve the health and welfare of their patient.

REFERENCES

Aksglaede, K., Funch-Jensen, P., & Thommesen, P. (1999). Radiological demonstration of gastroesophageal reflux: Diagnostic value of barium and bread studies compared with 24-hour pH monitoring. *Acta Radiologica, 40*(6), 652–655.

Al-Khawari, H.A., Sinan, T.S., & Seymour, H. (2002). Diagnosis of gastro-esophageal reflux in children: Comparison between esophageal pH and barium examinations. *Pediatric Radiology, 32*(11), 765–770.

Al-Kouder, G., et al. (2002). Volvulus of the sigmoid colon in a child. *Saudi Medical Journal, 23*(5), 594–596.

Baker, S.S., et al. (1999). Constipation in infants and children: Evaluation and treatment. A medical position statement of the North American Society for Pediatric Gastroenterology and Nutrition. *Journal of Pediatric and Gastroenterol Nutrition, 29*(5), 612–626.

Bandla, H.P., Davis, S.H., & Hopkins, N.E. (1999). Lipoid pneumonia: A silent complication of mineral oil aspiration. *Pediatrics, 103*(2), E19.

Berezin, S., et al. (1986). Gastroesophageal reflux secondary to gastrostomy tube placement. *American Journal of Diseases of Children, 140*(7), 699–701.

Bohmer, C.J., et al. (2001). The prevalence of constipation in institutionalized people with intellectual disability. *Journal of Intellectual Disability Research, 45*(3), 212–218.

Bonamico, M., et al. (2001). Prevalence and clinical picture of celiac disease in Italian down syndrome patients: A multicenter study. *Journal of Pediatric Gastroenterology and Nutrition, 33*, 139–143.

Csizmadia, C., et al. (2000). Accuracy and cost-effectiveness of a new strategy to screen for celiac disease in children with Down syndrome. *Journal of Pediatrics, 137*, 756–761.

Dahl, M., et al., (1996). Feeding and nutritional characteristics in children with moderate or severe cerebral palsy. *Acta Paediatrica, 85*(6), 697–701.

Del Giudice, E., et al. (1999). Gastrointestinal manifestations in children with cerebral palsy. *Brain Development, 21*(5), 307–311.

Eisen, G., et al. (2001). An annotated algorithmic approach to upper gastrointestinal bleeding. *Gastrointestinal Endoscopy, 53*, 853–858.

Erickson, B.A., et al. (2003). Polyethylene glycol 3350 for constipation in children with dysfunctional elimination. *Journal of Urology, 170*(4 Pt. 2), 1518–1520.

Everhart, J. (2000). Recent developments in the epidemiology of *H. pylori*. *Gastroenterology Clinics of North America, 29*, 559–578.

Galmiche, J.P., & Bruley des Varannes, S. (2003). Endoluminal therapies for gastro-esophageal reflux disease. *Lancet, 361*(9363), 1119–1121.

Gisel, E.G., & Patrick, J. (1988). Identification of children with cerebral palsy unable to maintain a normal nutritional state. *Lancet, 1*(8580), 283–286.

Go, M. (2002). Review article: Natural history and epidemiology of *Helicobacter pylori* infection. *Alimentary Pharmacology and Therapeutics, 16*(Suppl. 1), 3–15.

Gold, B., et al. (2000). North American Society for Pediatric Gastroenterology and Nutrition. *Helicobacter pylori* infection in children: Recommendations for diagnosis and treatment. *Journal of Pediatric Gastroenterology & Nutrition, 31*, 490–497.

Guidice, E.S., Capano, A., et al. (1999). Gastrointestinal manifestations in children with cerebral palsy. *Brain and Development, 21*(307), 307–311.

Hackam, D., et al. (2003). The influence of Down's syndrome on the management and outcome of children with

Hirschsprung's disease. *Journal of Pediatric Surgery, 38*, 946–949.

Haddock, G., & Wesson, D. (2000). The stomach and duodenum: Congenital anomalies. In W. Walker et al. (Eds.), *Pediatric gastrointestinal disease* (pp. 378–382). Hamilton, Ontario: BC Decker.

Hament, J.M., et al. (2001). Complications of percutaneous endoscopic gastrostomy with or without concomitant antireflux surgery in 96 children. *Journal of Pediatric Surgery, 36*(9), 1412–1415.

Hassall, E. (1997). Co-morbidities in childhood Barrett's esophagus. *Journal of Pediatric Gastroenterology and Nutrition, 25*(3), 255–260.

Hendren, W. (1978). Constipation caused by anterior location of the anus and its surgical correction. *Journal of Pediatric Surgery, 13*, 505–512.

Horvath, K., et al. (1999). Gastrointestinal abnormalities in children with autistic spectrum disorder. *Journal of Pediatrics, 135*, 559–563.

Howard, D., & Fromm, H. (1999). Nonsurgical management of gallstone disease. *Gastroenterology Clinics of North America, 28*, 133–144.

Huang, C., & Lichtenstein, D. (2003). Nonvariceal upper gastrointestinal bleeding. *Gastroenterology Clinics of North America, 32*, 1053–1078.

Jonas, M. (2000). Viral hepatitis: From prevention to antivirals. *Clinics in Liver Disease, 4*, 849–877.

Larnert, G., & Ekberg, O. (1995). Positioning improves the oral and pharyngeal swallowing function in children with cerebral palsy. *Acta Paediatrica, 84*(6), 689–692.

Launay, V., et al. (1996). Percutaneous endoscopic gastrostomy in children: Influence on gastroesophageal reflux. *Pediatrics, 97*(5), 726–728.

Lightdale, J., et al. (2001). Effects of intravenous secretin on language and behavior of children with autism and gastrointestinal symptoms: a single-blinded, open-label pilot study. *Pediatrics, 108*, e90.

Loening-Baucke, V. (2002). Polyethylene glycol without electrolytes for children with constipation and encopresis. *Journal of Pediatric Gastroenterology and Nutrition, 34*(4), 372–377.

Mamel, J.J. (1989) Percutaneous endoscopic gastrostomy. *American Journal of Gastroenterology, 84*(7), 703–710.

Marshall, J., et al. (2001). Antegrade continence enemas in the treatment of slow-transit constipation. *Journal of Pediatric Surgery, 36*(8), 1227–1230.

McColl, K., El-Omar, E., & Gillen, D. (2000). *Helicobacter pylori* gastritis and gastric physiology. *Gastroenterology Clinics of North America, 29*, 687–703.

Moore, S., & Johnson, A. (1998). Hirschsprung's disease: Genetic and functional associations of Down's and Waardenburg syndromes. *Seminars in Pediatric Surgery, 7*, 156–161.

Pan, J.J., et al. (2003). Gastroesophageal reflux: Comparison of barium studies with 24-h pH monitoring. *European Journal of Radiology, 47*(2), 149–153.

Pashankar, D.S., Loening-Baucke, V., & Bishop, W.P. (2003). Safety of polyethylene glycol 3350 for the treatment of chronic constipation in children. *Archives of Pediatrics & Adolescent Medicine, 157*(7), 661–664.

Ravelli, A.M., & Milla, P.J. (1998). Vomiting and gastroesophageal motor activity in children with disorders of the central nervous system. *Journal of Pediatric Gastroenterology and Nutrition, 26*(1), 56–63.

Razeghi, S., Lang, T., & Behrens, R. (2002). Influence of percutaneous endoscopic gastrostomy on gastroesophageal reflux: A prospective study in 68 children. *Journal of Pediatric Gastroenterology and Nutrition, 35*(1), 27–30.

Reilly, S., & Skuse, D. (1992). Characteristics and management of feeding problems of young children with cerebral palsy. *Developmental Medicine and Child Neurology, 34*(5), 379–388.

Rowland, M., Bourke, B., & Drumm, B. (2000). Gastritis and peptic ulcer disease. In W. Walker et al. (Eds.), *Pediatric gastrointestinal disease* (pp. 383–404). Hamilton, Ontario: BC Decker.

Samuel, M., & Holmes, K. (2002). Quantitative and qualitative analysis of gastroesophageal reflux after percutaneous endoscopic gastrostomy. *Journal of Pediatric Surgery, 37*(2), 256–261.

Sandler, A., et al. (1999). Lack of benefit of a single dose of secretin in the treatment of autism and pervasive developmental disorder. *New England Journal of Medicine, 341*, 1801–1806.

Shay, S.S., Bomeli, S., & Richter, J. (2002). Multichannel intraluminal impedance accurately detects fasting, recumbent reflux events and their clearing. *American Journal of Physiology. Gastrointestinal and Liver Physiology, 283*(2), G376–G383.

Snyder, J.D., & Goldman, H. (1990). Barrett's esophagus in children and young adults. Frequent association with mental retardation. *Digestive Diseases and Sciences, 35*(10), 1185–1189.

Sotos, J.F., et al. (1977). Hypocalcemic coma following two pediatric phosphate enemas. *Pediatrics, 60*(3), 305–307.

Staiano, A., & Del Giudice, E. (1994). Colonic transit and anorectal manometry in children with severe brain damage. *Pediatrics, 94*(2 Pt. 1), 169–173.

Staiano, A., et al. (1996). Cisapride in neurologically impaired children with chronic constipation. *Digestive Diseases and Sciences, 41*(5), 870–874.

Staiano, A., et al. (2000). Effect of the dietary fiber glucomannan on chronic constipation in neurologically impaired children. *Journal of Pediatrics, 136*(1), 41–45.

Strasberg, S. (1999). Laparoscopic biliary surgery. *Gastroenterology Clinics of North America, 28*, 117–132.

Sulaeman, E., et al. (1998). Gastroesophageal reflux and Nissen fundoplication following percutaneous endoscopic gastrostomy in children. *Journal of Pediatric Gastroenterology and Nutrition, 26*(3), 269–273.

Sullivan, P.B. (1999). Gastrostomy feeding in the disabled child: When is an antireflux procedure required? *Archives of Disease in Childhood, 81*(6), 463–464.

Tutuian, R., et al. (2003). Multichannel intraluminal impedance in esophageal function testing and gastroesophageal reflux monitoring. *Journal of Clinical Gastroenterology, 37*(3), 206–215.

Wheatley, M.J., et al. (1991). Long-term follow-up of brain-damaged children requiring feeding gastrostomy: Should an antireflux procedure always be performed? *Journal of Pediatric Surgery, 26*(3), 301–305.

Yerkes, E.B., et al. (2003). The Malone antegrade continence enema procedure: Quality of life and family perspective. *Journal of Urology, 169*(1), 320–323.

Youssef, N.N., et al. (2002). Dose response of PEG 3350 for the treatment of childhood fecal impaction. *Journal of Pediatrics, 141*(3), 410–414.

Zimmerman, H., & Ishak, K. (1995). General aspects of drug-induced liver disease. *Gastroenterology Clinics of North America, 24*, 739–757.

CHAPTER 15

PULMONOLOGY

David A. Waltz and Eliot S. Katz

Children with developmental disabilities are challenged with a diverse spectrum of impairments that may adversely affect their pulmonary function. Dysfunctional swallowing and gastroesophageal reflux (GER) may produce wheezing and chronic aspiration, resulting in recurrent infection, parenchymal lung disease, and gas exchange abnormalities. Recurrent aspiration may also predispose to airway hyperreactivity, inflammation, or asthma. Muscle weakness and skeletal deformities can give rise to an ineffective cough and hypoventilation, similarly resulting in lung injury and infection. Craniofacial abnormalities and airway hypotonia predispose to obstructive sleep apnea syndrome (OSAS), associated with cardiovascular and neurocognitive impairments.

In addition, many children with disabilities are born prematurely, have a history of mechanical ventilation or prolonged supplemental oxygen requirement, and develop bronchopulmonary dysplasia (BPD). Many of these conditions worsen as individuals with developmental disabilities grow into adulthood. As a result, chronic lung disease and/or recurrent respiratory infections are leading causes of morbidity and mortality in individuals with developmental disabilities. The treatment of respiratory disease in children with developmental delays requires a multidisciplinary approach, including pulmonologists, gastroenterologists, surgeons, physical therapists, and feeding specialists. This chapter describes the pathophysiology of respiratory disease commonly encountered in individuals with developmental disabilities, followed by the pulmonary considerations of specific conditions.

ASPIRATION

Aspiration is a common but frequently unrecognized contributor to lung disease in individuals with developmental disabilities. Central nervous system impairments are often associated with gastrointestinal dysfunction, including dysphagia and GER, which may adversely affect breathing. Wheezing, coughing, and respiratory distress may accompany the introduction of food, upper airway secretions, and stomach contents into the lower respiratory tract. Alternatively, over time, the protective airway reflexes may become tolerant to the acute effects of aspiration, resulting in "silent aspiration."

Severe episodes of aspiration may result in pneumonia, whereas repeated microaspiration may result in irreversible bronchiectasis, fibrosis, and ventilation-perfusion mismatching, characteristics of chronic lung disease. Indeed, the development of chronic lung disease and its sequelae represent a major source of morbidity and mortality in individuals with disabilities (Reddihough, Baikie, & Walstab, 2001). Identification and proper management of these episodes in individuals with developmental disabilities is imperative in promoting long-term health.

DYSFUNCTIONAL SWALLOWING

Swallowing is a complex process involving the sequential activation of cranial nerves V and IX, as well as laryngeal nerves. Under normal conditions, laryngeal reflexes induce vocal cord closure, swallowing, and apnea to prevent aspiration of food and upper airway secretions. Aspiration stimulates coughing and bronchoconstriction to protect the lung parenchyma from damage.

Recurrent aspiration of thin liquids is most common, inducing inflammation and fibrosis in the lung parenchyma. The clinical manifestations include wheezing, coughing, respiratory distress, and recurrent pneumonia. In the presence of these symptoms, recurrent aspiration may be misdiagnosed as asthma. The cumulative effect of chronic aspiration is recurrent pneumonia, irreversible bronchiectasis, fibrosis, and ventilation-perfusion mismatching.

The dysphagia evaluation begins with a physical examination during feeding, including the pace of chewing and swallowing, airway noise, and associated coughing, gagging, or emesis. Swallowing dysfunction may not be readily apparent due to a blunting of the cough observed in "silent" aspirators. Radiological evaluation serves to assess oromotor function, esophageal motility, and anatomical structure. A video-fluoroscopic swallowing study (VFSS) documents the physiology of the oral and pharyngeal phases of swallowing. It may detect aspiration; however, the study requires ingestion of a large volume of fluid with an unpleasant taste, and only a limited number of swallows are evaluated.

A radionucleotide salivagram evaluates whether a sublingual drop of technetium-99m sulfur colloid enters the tracheobronchial tree. The radionucleotide scan utilizes less radiation than VFSS and requires minimal cooperation. It evaluates the handling of oral secretions unrelated to the volitional swallowing of food. Thus, these techniques provide complementary information on swallowing function.

Bronchoscopy permits visualization of mucosal swelling, friability and collapsibility, as well as analysis of bronchoalveolar lavage fluid for lipid-laden macrophages. Insofar as dysphagia may be a manifestation of intracranial pathology, brain and brainstem imaging should also be considered with a compatible clinical history.

Treatment of dysphagia is predicated on the underlying cause but usually entails altering the texture of feedings, positioning, and pace of feeding. Thickening liquids with rice cereal may facilitate oral feeding. Reclined positioning during feedings at 30 degrees with the neck flexed may decrease aspiration in children with cerebral palsy.

If aspiration results in recurrent pneumonia or chronic lung disease, alternative feeding options should be considered. Nasogastric tube feeding is a reasonable alternative for several months in some individuals in whom oral-motor function is likely to improve. In many individuals with dysphagia, a more permanent feeding route, such as a gastrostomy, may be indicated. In some instances of severe oral-motor dysfunction, even nasal and mouth secretions may be difficult to handle.

Pharmacologic therapy with anticholinergics is effective at reducing salivary volume but may be limited by side effects. Injection of botulinum-A toxin into the parotid and submandibular glands reduced sialorrhea for up to 6 months in individuals with cerebral palsy (Suskind & Tilton, 2002) and may be beneficial in reducing salivary aspiration as well. The combination of submandibular gland resection and bilateral duct ligation has been reported to be effective in controlling drooling and possibly decreasing aspiration in some individuals (Gerber, Gaugler, Myer, & Cotton, 1996). Untoward effects of these surgical approaches include injury to the mandibular nerve, xerostomia, and dental caries.

Tracheotomy facilitates suctioning of aspirated secretions but may further weaken swallowing by impairing laryngeal function, thus interfering with supraglottic closure. In addition, individuals with a tracheotomy can continue to aspirate upper airway secretions. In that case, the application of continuous positive airway pressure (CPAP) has been reported to decrease the incidence of pulmonary complications (Finder, Yellon, & Charron, 2001). In severe cases, laryngotracheal separation is an effective surgery for aspiration. The trachea is transected and sutured closed, and a tracheotomy is placed. Speech is lost after surgery, however, and a permanent tracheostomy is necessary.

GASTROESOPHAGEAL REFLUX

GER is a frequent cause of wheezing, coughing, and parenchymal lung disease in children with neurological impairments (Gusafason & Tibbling, 1994; see Chapter 14.2). The presence of gastric acid in the esophagus may produce reflex activation of vagal afferents inducing laryngospasm, bronchospasm, bradycardia, and central apnea. GER is exacerbated by poor esophageal motility, delayed gastric emptying, and elevated intra-abdominal pressure. If frank aspiration occurs, bronchial and lung parenchymal inflammation ensues, which may produce recurrent infections, eventually leading to chronic lung disease.

Many children with developmental disabilities who have aspiration will also have an ineffectual cough and dysphagia, thus contributing to the aspiration. The differential diagnosis of GER in children with neurological impairments includes gastric outlet obstruction, intracranial pathology, superior mesenteric artery syndrome, delayed gastric emptying, and hypotonia. An intraesophageal pH probe is the standard test of the presence and severity of GER; however, the pH probe does not measure nonacidic reflux or the volume of material refluxed.

In some individuals, both vomiting and coughing has been observed without changes in esophageal pH (Gustafsson & Tibbling, 1994). Esophageal probe impedance has recently been introduced to detect nonacidic reflux. A radionucleotide milk scan may provide evidence of aspiration of gastric contents. If a gastrostomy tube is present, Methylene blue may be introduced into the enteral formula. The subsequent observation of a bluish discoloration to oral and/or tracheal secretions is evidence of gastric reflux. Finally, an upper gastrointestinal series under pressure assesses gastroesophageal anatomy and function.

Pharmacological therapy can reduce gastric acid production or increase bowel motility. A percutaneous gastrostomy tube placement may exacerbate GER, particularly in children with neurological impairment. A transgastric-jejunal feeding tube may further lessen GER in some children, but intussusception and bowel obstruction are recognized complications (Wales et al., 2002). Continuous drip feeding regimens seem to produce less GER than bolus feedings. Fundoplication is frequently necessary in children with cerebral palsy, although they have high complication and failure rates.

ASTHMA

Recurrent episodes of coughing, wheezing, and/or respiratory distress are commonly observed in certain individuals with developmental disabilities. In some of these individuals, these episodes represent true asthma, which is relatively common in the general population (5%–10%). In others, these episodes may result from recurrent insults to the lung such as aspiration or respiratory infection. Regardless of the cause, the underlying pathophysiology of these episodes is likely to be similar to that of asthma, which consists of airway obstruction as the results of two main elements: bronchoconstriction and inflammation.

Airway obstruction in asthma results from the release of soluble mediators such as histamine, leukotrienes, and cytokines from airway cells in response to a wide variety of stimuli, including cold air, respiratory viruses, aspiration, and allergenic particles. The release of mediators in response to these stimuli induces airway smooth muscle contraction, increases mucus production, causes submucosal edema, and creates an inflammatory cell infiltrate. As a result, there is narrowing of the airway lumen, increased resistance to airflow, turbulence, and air trapping in lung segments distal to the narrowed airways. The resultant lung hyperinflation places respiratory muscles at a mechanical disadvantage and contributes to the increased work of breathing. Reduced ventilation of selected lung segments relative to their perfusion results in ventilation-perfusion mismatch and hypoxemia.

Treatment of asthma involves a combination of bronchodilators and anti-inflammatory agents. Bronchodilators act to relax airway smooth muscle and thus reverse bronchoconstriction. Commonly used bronchodilators include the short acting beta-2 adrenergic receptor agonist albuterol and its L-isomer, levalbuterol. The latter may have a lower incidence of adrenergic side effects, but it is more costly. Salmeterol is a long-acting beta-2 adrenergic that provides more sustained bronchodilation, but it should not be used as a rescue medication for acute bronchospasm due to a relatively slow onset of action.

Another useful bronchodilator in individuals with developmental disabilities is ipratroprium bromide, an anticholinergic agent, which may also reduce excess oral and airway secretions and is effective when used together with albuterol. These agents are usually administered via nebulizer or metered dose inhaler, as oral formulations are often accompanied by increased systemic adrenergic side effects. If a metered dose inhaler is used, a spacer device is imperative to maximize pulmonary and minimize oropharyngeal deposition.

Treating airway inflammation is of primary importance in the treatment of asthma. Abundant data has accumulated over the last several years that airway inflammation is a major factor in the pathophysiology of asthma and that an element of chronic inflammation may be present even when bronchoconstriction is quiescent. Consideration should be given to anti-inflammatory therapy in any individual with asthma, depending on the frequency of symptoms. National consensus guidelines are available to guide therapeutic decisions. In most cases, anti-inflammatory therapy should take the form of inhaled corticosteroids, although oral leukotriene antagonists are also helpful in selected individuals.

The primary risks of chronic inhaled corticosteroids in children are growth suppression and oral candidiasis. Little data exists regarding the utility of chronic inhaled corticosteroids in preventing recurrent wheezing related to aspiration or recurrent respiratory infections, and, thus, the use of this therapy in individuals without a clear diagnosis of asthma needs to be guided by clinical judgment.

KYPHOSCOLIOSIS

Scoliosis is a lateral curvature of the spine that is often associated with an increased or decreased angulation in the sagittal plane, termed *kyphosis* or *lordosis* (see Chapter 13). Scoliosis may be congenital or acquired and may progress from infancy beyond adolescence. The majority of cases are considered idiopathic, although it is frequently associated with neuromuscular disorders.

Scoliosis results in a chest wall deformity that decreases compliance and impairs the efficiency of respiratory muscles. Individuals with scoliosis are at risk for developing cardiopulmonary insufficiency, although there is a poor correlation between the Cobb angle and lung function (Kearon, Viviani, Kirkley, & Killian, 1993).

Other factors, such as the degree of thoracic lordosis and kyphosis, also contribute to the pulmonary function abnormalities. General guidelines are that a curvature of 50 degrees produces measurable impairments of pulmonary function, and curves beyond 90 degrees may produce respiratory failure. Many individuals with scoliosis have coexistent pulmonary disease that complicates the respiratory function abnormalities observed. Severe kyphoscoliosis may also produce bronchial torsion resulting in airway obstruction.

Simone is a 19 year-old woman with a T-5 myelomeningocele. She had scoliosis repair 5 years ago and has not experienced any respiratory symptomatology. Simone is a sophomore in college and had a part time job at a department store.

During the last semester, Simone noticed that she was falling asleep in class and missing her train stop. She also began having difficulty awakening for work on the weekends. It was not until headaches began occurring in the morning that she sought medical attention. She occasionally snores and reports that her sleep is nonrestorative. She had experienced progression of her lordosis and a 20-lb weight gain over the last 2 years.

An overnight polysomnogram was performed that revealed a few hypopneic events, many arousals, and profound hypoventilation during REM sleep (see Figure 15.1). The combination of restrictive lung disease on the basis of her obesity, scoliosis, and respiratory muscle weakness had combined to produce REM-related hypoventilation. This resulted in poor quality sleep and early morning hypercapnea causing headache.

Simone was placed on nocturnal bi-level ventilation through a nasal mask. A follow-up polysomnogram was performed to titrate the pressure to achieve normal end tidal CO_2 levels. Simone reported that the headache and sleepiness immediately resolved. Referrals were made to a dietician to facilitate weight loss and her orthopedic surgeon to reevaluate the progression in her spinal curvature.

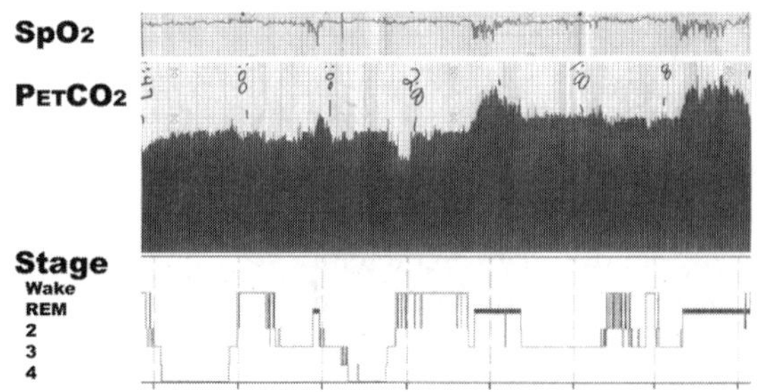

Figure 15.1. An overnight polysomnogram on a 19-year-old woman with a myelomeningocele, sleepiness, and morning headache. The tracing demonstrates a normal baseline oxygen saturation and end tidal CO_2 at sleep onset. The sleep histogram in the third channel reports the sleep state distribution over the night. A marked increase in the end tidal CO_2 and decrease in oxygen saturation occurred during REM sleep, which indicates hypoventilation.

In scoliosis, the respiratory muscles operate at a mechanical disadvantage. Thus, respiratory muscle strength, maximum voluntary ventilation, and exercise tolerance are reduced. Pulmonary function testing indicates a *restrictive* pattern with a decrease in vital capacity (VC), total lung capacity (TLC), and functional residual capacity (FRC) and an increase in the RV/TLC ratio. Individuals with scoliosis rely on a greater contribution of the diaphragm to the tidal volume than normal individuals. In severe scoliosis, individuals develop a compensatory rapid, shallow breathing pattern with an increase in the neuromuscular drive. Autopsy studies in some individuals with scoliosis demonstrate an irregular distribution of alveolar airspaces and vascularity (Davies & Reid, 1971). Scoliosis occurring during the period of lung development in the first 8 years of life may limit alveoli growth.

The most common blood gas abnormality observed with severe scoliosis is normocapnic hypoxemia, suggesting a ventilation-perfusion mismatch. This mismatch is particularly evident during REM sleep. Young children with scoliosis are capable of respiratory compensation by increasing their respiratory rate; however, in older individuals with scoliosis the $PaCO_2$ may increase with age, suggesting alveolar hypoventilation (Kafer, 1976).

A variety of rigid and soft braces have been used in the treatment of scoliosis. No consensus exists on the utility of spinal braces for altering the natural history of scoliosis, but some individuals may benefit. In some children, body braces may be effective in facilitating positioning and head control but can result in decreased lung volumes and increased respiratory effort. This problem especially affects children with neuromuscular weakness (Tangsrud, Carlsen, Lund-Petersen, & Carlsen, 2001).

Surgical intervention to straighten and stabilize the spine can facilitate positioning, thereby improving quality of life. Indications for surgical intervention in scoliosis include progression of the curvature, ease in positioning, nursing care, pain control, and alleviation of pressure sores; however, in Duchenne muscular dystrophy, scoliosis repair does not alter the progressive decline in pulmonary function. Studies evaluating the outcomes of surgical stabilization of idiopathic scoliosis have been disparate. Long-term outcome of pulmonary function has been reported to be improved, unchanged or diminished (Chen, Huang, Lee, & Hsu, 2002; Graham et al., 2000).

The preponderance of evidence supports the view that surgical procedures minimally affect pulmonary function over the long term; however, pulmonary function can be expected to decline during the 3 postoperative months, particularly with anterior spinal instrumentation and fusion (Graham et al., 2000). Surgical outcomes in some special populations, such as children with myelomeningocele, appear to be more favorable (explored in more detail later in this chapter).

OBESITY

Obesity affects 10% of children, with an increased incidence in sedentary individuals and those with endocrine or hypothalamic dysfunction. Excessive adipose tissue poses both a resistive load to the upper airway, and an elastic load to the entire pulmonary system. As the result, OSAS, restrictive lung disease, and dyspnea may be observed.

The decreased compliance of the chest wall and increased airway resistance produce an increased work of breathing and hypoventilation. At rest, individuals who are obese consume more oxygen and produce more carbon dioxide than individuals who are not obese. In response, a rapid, shallow breathing pattern is adopted in obesity, which may result in increased dead space ventilation, and thus, may increase the ventilatory requirement (VE/VO_2). Individuals who are obese have a relative increase in ventilation to the superior lung segments and an increase in perfusion to the lung base, particularly when supine. The resultant ventilation-perfusion mismatching may result in hypoxemia.

Pulmonary function testing in children with isolated obesity, including spirometry and maximal static pressures, are often normal below 200% of ideal body weight (Marcus, Curtis, Koerner, Joffe, Serwint, & Loughlin, 1996); however, in more severe instances, both restrictive and obstructive patterns have been reported. The earliest abnormalities are observed in the static lung volumes, with a decrease in the expiratory reserve volume (ERV) and FRC, due to upward displacement of the diaphragm. Thus, the oxygen reserve is diminished in the setting of increased oxygen utilization, resulting in more rapid hypoxemia during interruptions in ventilation.

In extreme cases, there is a decrease in the VC, forced expiratory volume in 1 second (FEV1), TLC, and an increase in residual volume (RV) due to air trapping. The diffusion coefficient of carbon monoxide (DLCO), a measure of the surface area available for gas exchange, is generally normal in older obese subjects; however, one pediatric study documented a diminished DLCO, corrected for lung volume, in children who were obese (Inselma, Milanese, & Deurloo, 1993). This finding suggests that obesity occurring at an early age may adversely affect alveolar development.

In general, however, the authors believe that a decreased DLCO suggests a mechanism other than obesity. Respiratory muscle strength testing is generally normal in obesity, although the maximal voluntary ventilation is reduced. This finding may reflect the mechanical disadvantage of the respiratory muscles in obesity, as well as changes in airway resistance and pulmonary compliance.

Between 37%–94% of severely obese children with symptoms of sleep-disordered breathing have abnormal polysomnograms (Mallory, Fiser, & Jackson, 1989; Silvestri, Weese-Mayer, Bass, Kenny, Hauptman, & Pearsall, 1993). In addition to the cardiovascular consequences of OSAS, neurocognitive impairment has been reported in obese children with OSAS (Rhodes et al., 1989). The severity of sleep-disordered breathing is related to the degree of obesity. Some obese subjects have hypercapnea, cor pulmonale, and somnolence, termed the *obesity-hypoventilation syndrome.* These individuals have a blunted hypercapnic ventilatory drive that may be congenital or acquired as the result of chronic obesity-induced hypoventilation. Nocturnal ventilation is often effective at correcting gas exchange abnormalities and relieving symptoms. Weight loss has been shown to increase the ERV, FRC, and PaO_2, as well as to relieve upper airway obstruction.

PREMATURITY AND BRONCHOPULMONARY DYSPLASIA

Premature birth is associated with a number of physiological and neurodevelopmental sequelae (see Chapter 10). Among them are chronic lung disease of prematurity, or BPD. The clinical definition of BPD varies but is generally accepted as a need for supplemental oxygen at 36 weeks postmenstrual age (Jobe & Bancalari, 2001). Affected infants may have chronic respiratory distress and a need for supplemental oxygen and frequently have abnormal chest radiographs.

The incidence of BPD has declined as surfactant therapy, improved ventilation strategies, and antenatal glucocorticoid therapy have become more widely adopted. BPD is now relatively uncommon in infants with a birth weight of more than 1,200 grams or a gestational age greater than 30 weeks at birth (Bancalari & Gonzalez, 2000); however, it remains a significant source of mortality and morbidity in younger, smaller premature infants and can also be seen in larger, more mature neonates.

Along with this change in the epidemiology of BPD has come a change in the pathologic appearance of the lungs in infants dying of BPD. Early reports of BPD noted marked airway changes including squamous metaplasia of large and small airways, increased peribronchial smooth muscle with fibrosis, chronic inflammation, and submucosal edema with hypertrophied submucosal glands. These findings are less prominent today, with the most notable findings now being fewer and larger alveoli, suggesting interference with septation and decreased pulmonary microvascular development (Jobe & Bancalari, 2001). Despite the change in the epidemiology and pathology, the etiology of BPD continues to be attributed to the effects of hyperoxia, barotrauma, inflammation, and infection on the immature lung.

Strategies to treat and prevent BPD continue to evolve (Jobe & Ikegami, 2001). As noted previously, the use of antenatal corticosteroids, surfactant therapy, and gentler ventilation strategies in caring for premature newborns has led to a change in the incidence and epidemiology of BPD. For affected infants, supplemental oxygen, bronchodilators, and diuretics remain a mainstay of therapy. Supplemental oxygen therapy should be monitored to ensure pulse oximetry measurements of 92% or greater during sleep to ensure proper growth (Moyer-Mileur, Nielson, Pfeffer, Witte, & Chapman, 1996). Bronchodilators are often used, although their efficacy in individuals should be demonstrated clinically. Diuretic therapy with chlorothiazide and/or spironolactone may be beneficial in selected infants. Furosemide should be used with caution due to its potential nephro- and ototoxic effects.

The use of postnatal steroids has become controversial as concerns over potential adverse effects of glucocorticosteroids on postnatal brain and alveolar development have arisen (Jobe & Ikegami, 2001; Murphy et al., 2001; Wohl & Majzoub, 2000). Indeed, antenatal steroid use may also impair alveolar development (Okajimi, Matasuda, Cho, Matsumoto, Kobayashi, & Fujimoto, 2001). Based on these reports, inhaled corticosteroids should be used cautiously in children with BPD.

RECURRENT RESPIRATORY INFECTIONS

Individuals with developmental disabilities may be prone to recurrent respiratory infections for a number of reasons. Any individual aspiration episode may directly result in infection. Recurrent aspiration, as discussed previously, may contribute to chronic inflammation and impairment of local airway defense mechanisms such as mucociliary clearance. The presence of a poor gag reflex or a weak cough due to neuromuscular disease may lead to stasis of respiratory secretions, increasing the risk of infection. Prematurity and BPD increase the risk of serious sequelae from respiratory viral infections such as respiratory syncytial virus. If the individual is in a group residential setting, then he or she may have increased exposure to viral respiratory infections.

Following appropriate treatment, evaluation for underlying conditions predisposing to recurrent infection should be undertaken. A careful history and physical examination should guide this evaluation. The location and persistence of radiographic abnormalities should be determined. Subsequent investigations may be directed at detecting aspiration due to dysfunctional swallow and/or GER, salivary aspiration, the presence of a foreign body or other localized airway obstruction, an underlying immunodeficiency, or systemic disease.

The airways are normally sterile. Recurrent aspiration or recurrent pneumonia may lead to bronchiectasis, characterized by airway scarring and impairment of mucociliary escalator-driven clearance of bacteria. In the presence of bronchiectasis, it may be difficult or impossible to sterilize the airways, even with prolonged courses of intravenous antibiotics. Typical organisms in this situation include *Staphylococcus aureus*, including Methicillin resistant organisms (MRSA), *Hemophilus influenzae*, and *Pseudomonas aeruginosa*. Routine surveillance cultures in individuals should be performed every few months in order to allow empiric therapy of acute bacterial infections while awaiting culture results during an acute episode.

Strategies for prevention of recurrent pneumonia are predicated by the underlying condition(s). Premature infants and those with BPD should receive palivizumab, a preparation of monoclonal antibodies against respiratory syncytial virus. Consideration should be given to pneumococcal and influenza immunization in individuals with recurrent respiratory infections or, indeed, chronic lung disease from any cause. A therapeutic strategy to reduce chronic recurrent aspiration, as discussed in the section on aspiration, is essential to minimize the effects of these repeated insults to the lung, and to prevent the development of chronic lung disease.

In addition to therapies directed at aspiration, prophylactic antibiotics and airway clearance techniques may be helpful. Although prophylactic oral antibiotics may be effective at reducing the incidence of acute bacterial infections, there is a danger of selecting resistant organisms. In addition, oral antibiotics are unlikely to be helpful in the presence of MRSA or *Pseudomonas aeruginosa*. Chronic inhaled antibiotics, such as tobramycin solution for inhalation (TOBI), may be helpful in individuals chronically infected with *Pseudomonas aeruginosa*. This antibiotic is often administered in 28-day on–off cycles to minimize the development of antibiotic resistance, although the development of resistance remains a concern with chronic use.

Traditional airway clearance techniques, such as chest physiotherapy and postural drainage, may be helpful for individuals with difficulty clearing secretions. In individuals with a weak or dysfunctional cough, the in-exsufflator, a device that alternately delivers positive and negative airway pressure by means of a mask, may be helpful. An effective strategy for the prevention of recurrent pneumonia may well employ many or all of the approaches described.

RESPIRATORY MUSCLE WEAKNESS

Muscle weakness, often involving the respiratory system, is commonly observed in children with developmental disabilities. The etiology includes lesions in the central nervous system, motor neuropathies, transmission defects at the neuromuscular junction, and primary myopathies. Respiratory muscle impairment may be congenital or acquired, and the clinical manifestations are predicated on the severity and distribution of the weakness. Involvement of the upper airway musculature predisposes to obstruction, whereas weakness in the diaphragm and intercostal muscles gives rise to an ineffectual cough and hypoventilation. The clinical pulmonary consequences of muscle weakness include aspiration, obstructive sleep apnea, recurrent infection, atelectasis, hypoxemia, and respiratory failure.

Children with respiratory muscle weakness are at risk for comorbid conditions, obesity, and scoliosis (see Figure 15.2), that may further impair their pulmonary function. These children frequently adopt a breathing pattern that is rapid and shallow. The tidal volume may be supplemented in the upright position using the *abdominal squeeze*. This pattern consists of end-expiratory activity of the abdominal muscles that lowers the end-expiratory lung volume below the relaxation volume of the respiratory system, giving rise to passive descent of the diaphragm during early inspiration. The chest x-ray may reveal low lung volumes with a bell-shaped chest.

Respiratory muscle strength may be evaluated clinically, radiographically, and physiologically. Specific diaphragmatic weakness may be manifested by paradoxical inward motion of the diaphragm during inspiration or dyspnea that develops in the prone position; however, clinical symptomatology may initially be absent in individuals with significant respiratory muscle weakness. Pulmonary function testing in the setting of muscle weakness may reveal a *restrictive* pattern characterized by a reduction in the total lung capacity and vital capacity, with a normal or increased residual volume (depending on the extent of expiratory muscle weakness).

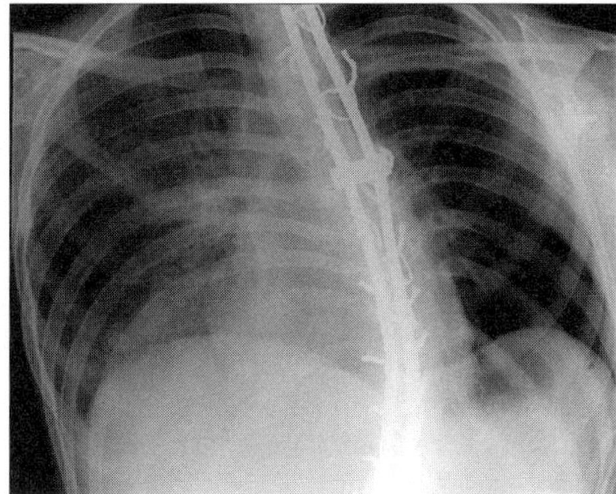

Figure 15.2. Chest x-ray of an 18-year-old with Duchenne muscular dystrophy demonstrating scoliosis with spinal rod placement and right lower lobe atelectasis.

On average, a 50% reduction in muscle strength will result in a decline in vital capacity by only 20% (De Troyer, Borenstein, & Cordier, 1980). The maximum inspiratory pressure (at residual volume) and maximal expiratory pressure (at total lung capacity) are good markers of respiratory muscle strength. The DLCO is reduced in individuals with neuromuscular weakness, but it is normal when corrected for lung volume. The early recognition of respiratory muscle weakness is important to provide supportive care including assisted-cough techniques, secretion clearance, and improved oxygenation and ventilation.

Stephon is a 26-year-old man with a static encephalopathy following a motor vehicle accident at 4 years of age. As the result of the injury, he developed dysphagia and spastic quadriplegia. During the ensuing 6 years, Stephon experienced recurrent episodes of aspiration pneumonia, requiring hospitalization. Though there was no family history of asthma, Stephon frequently developed wheezing during these exacerbations that was responsive to beta-agonists. He was diagnosed with GER and treated pharmacologically, but eventually required a Nissan fundoplication. At 10 years of age, Stephon developed pneumonia and was intubated. After multiple attempts at extubation were unsuccessful, he had a tracheostomy placed.

In the years following the tracheostomy, Stephon required only nocturnal supplemental oxygen. He was generally well, notwithstanding occasional bouts of tracheitis that were treated with inhaled antibiotics. By 20 years of age, Stephon again experienced lobar pneumonia. Stephon now required supplemental oxygen during both the day and night. At 25 years of age, an arterial blood gas obtained while breathing room air revealed a partial pressure of oxygen of 61 mmHg and carbon dioxide of 55 mmHg. A polysomnogram demonstrated worsening hypoventilation, with the end-tidal carbon dioxide reaching 75 mmHg in REM sleep. Bilevel ventilation was started at night.

Stephon's course illustrates how incremental impairments in pulmonary function arise from the combination of progressive kyphoscoliosis, respiratory muscle weakness, and recurrent pneumonia. Thus, individuals are vulnerable to intercurrent viral illnesses and microaspiration. The necessity for a tracheotomy, supplemental oxygen and, ultimately, ventilatory support is common in this setting.

SLEEP-DISORDERED BREATHING PATTERNS

Children with developmental disabilities experience a variety of sleep-disordered breathing patterns, including 1) desaturation, 2) central sleep apnea, 3) OSAS, and 4) hypoventilation. The pathophysiology is often multifactorial, involving the central respiratory pattern generator, airway obstruction, parenchymal lung disease, and unfavorable pulmonary mechanics. Craniofacial dysmorphology, neuromuscular weakness, and an array of genetic conditions may predispose children to have sleep-disordered breathing patterns (see Table 15.1).

The hallmark of pediatric OSAS is loud snoring on most nights that may be associated with witnessed apneic pauses, hyperextension of the neck, and restlessness. Other symptoms include choking noises, increased work of breathing, paradoxical breathing, enuresis, frequent awakenings, and dry mouth. Daytime signs and symptoms are often subtle, involving neurocognitive and behavioral impairments, such as poor school performance, aggressive behavior, hyperactivity, attention-deficit disorder, and morning headaches. These findings may be difficult to observe in children with other developmental disabilities. Excessive daytime sleepiness is common in adults with OSAS but is present in less than 10% of affected children (Gozal, Wang, & Pope, 2001). The physical examination in OSAS is frequently normal, but may reveal anatomical abnormalities (see Table 15.2). The classification of abnormal respiratory events during sleep is summarized in Table 15.3.

Table 15.1. Conditions predisposing to sleep-disordered breathing

Condition	
Craniofacial	
Midface hypoplasia	Apert syndrome
	Marfan syndrome
	Pfeiffer syndrome
	Treacher Collins syndrome
	Achondroplasia
Micrognathia	Pierre-Robin sequence
Macroglossia	Beckwith-Wiederman syndrome
	Down syndrome
Neuromuscular	Cerebral palsy
	Duchenne muscular dystrophy
	Myelomeningocele
	Prader-Willi syndrome
Genetic	Mucopolysaccharidosis
	Sickle cell anemia
	Cohen syndrome
	Prader-Willi syndrome
	Bardet-Biedl syndrome
Miscellaneous	Obesity
	Pharyngeal flap surgery

Table 15.2. Physical examination in obstructive sleep apnea syndrome

General
Sleepiness
Obesity
Failure to thrive

Head
Swollen mucous membranes
Deviated septum
Adenoidal facies
  Infraorbital darkening
  Elongated face
  Mouth-breathing
Tonsillar hypertrophy
High arched palate
Overbite
Crowded oropharynx
Macroglossia
Glossoptosis
Midfacial hypoplasia
Micrognathia/retrognathia

Cardiovascular
Hypertension
Loud second (pulmonary) heart sound (P2)

Extremities
Edema
Clubbing

Adapted from *Principles and practice of pediatric sleep medicine*, S.H. Sheldon, R. Ferber, & M.H. Kryger, Diagnosis of obstructive sleep apnea in infants and children, p. 199, Copyright 2005, with permission from Elsevier.

Table 15.3. Respiratory event classification

Obstructive	
Apnea	Absence of oronasal airflow for any duration with persistent respiratory effort
Hypopnea	Discernable reduction of oronasal flow for two or more breaths with persistent respiratory effort often accompanied by oxygen desaturation or arousal
Respiratory effort-related arousal	Evidence of increased respiratory effort or flow limitation leading to an arousal, followed by normalization of effort and flow
Flow limitation	Flattening of the inspiratory limb of nasal pressure channel
Snoring	Coarse, low-pitched inspiratory sound
Hypoventilation	$P_{ET}CO_2$ greater than 50 mmHg for more than 10% of total sleep time or $P_{ET}CO_2$ greater than 53 mmHg and accompanied by paradoxical breathing or obstructive events
Central	
Apnea	Absence of oronasal airflow for 20 seconds or more without respiratory effort; shorter events are counted if associated with arousal, desaturation, or bradycardia
Hypoventilation	$P_{ET}CO_2$ greater than 50 mmHg for more than 10% of total sleep time or $P_{ET}CO_2$ peak greater than 53 mmHg and accompanied by decreased respiratory effort
Periodic breathing	Succession of 3 central apneas or more of 3 or more seconds in duration separated by less than 20 seconds of normal breathing
Miscellaneous	
Mixed apneas	Cessation of flow with a central and obstructive component
Prolonged expiratory apnea with cyanosis	Prolongation of expiration below the functional residual capacity resulting in ventilation/perfusion mismatching
Apneustic breathing	Marked prolongation of inspiration

Adapted from *Principles and practice of pediatric sleep medicine*, S.H. Sheldon, R. Ferber, & M.H. Kryger, Diagnosis of obstructive sleep apnea in infants and children, p. 206, Copyright 2005, with permission from Elsevier.

The spectrum of obstructive breathing during sleep ranges from the frank, intermittent occlusion seen in OSAS, to persistent, primary snoring. OSAS is characterized by recurrent episodes of partial or complete airway obstruction resulting in hypoxemia, hypercapnea, and/or respiratory arousal. The sleep fragmentation and gas exchange abnormalities observed with OSAS may produce serious cardiovascular and neurobehavioral impairment.

The *upper airway resistance syndrome* (UARS) is characterized by brief, repetitive respiratory effort-related arousals (RERA) during sleep in the absence of overt apnea, hypopnea, or gas exchange abnormalities (Guilleminault, Stoohs, Clerk, Cetel, & Maistros, 1993). It has been linked to significant cognitive and behavioral sequelae in children, including learning disabilities, attention-deficit disorder, hyperactivity, and aggressive behavior (Guilleminault, Korobkin, & Winkle, 1981). *Obstructive hypoventilation* (OH) features prolonged increased upper airway resistance accompanied by gas exchange abnormalities, but not frank apnea or hypopnea (Rosen, D'Andrea, & Haddad, 1992). Primary snoring has been traditionally defined as a benign condition, without polysomnographic abnormalities, although recent neurocognitive data in snoring children may challenge this notion.

At sleep onset, pharyngeal dilator tone decreases, and airway resistance increases, resulting in a reduction in minute ventilation by 20%–30%. In normal individuals, this results in a decrease in PaO_2 by 3–9 torr and an increase in $PaCO_2$ by 5–7 torr. Individuals with normal pulmonary function operate on the plateau of the oxygen dissociation curve and have little change in their arterial oxygen saturation during sleep; however, individuals with restrictive or parenchymal lung disease may have relatively low baseline arterial oxygen saturation, and, therefore, reside near the steep portion of the oxygen dissociation curve.

These individuals may experience profound desaturation during sleep, particularly during rapid eye movement (REM). REM sleep is characterized by intercostal muscle inhibition and irregular breathing, resulting in marked fluctuations in minute ventilation. During nadirs in minute ventilation, hypoxemia and hypercapnea may arise in individuals with respiratory muscle weakness, restrictive lung disease, and parenchymal lung disease. Infants spend approximately 50% of their sleep time in REM sleep. REM sleep time declines to

Table 15.4. Diagnostic classification and severity of sleep-disordered breathing (one or more of the following)

Diagnosis	Apnea index	Arterial oxygen saturation nadir	End tidal Pco_2 peak	End tidal Pco_2 > 50 torr. (percent of total sleep time)	Arousals (events per hour)
Primary snoring	≤ 1 event per hour	> 92%	≤ 53 torr.	< 10%	EEG < 11
Upper airway resistance syndrome	≤ 1 events per hour	> 92%	≤ 53 torr.	< 10%	RERA > 1; EEG > 11
Mild obstructive sleep apnea syndrome (OSAS)	1–4 events per hour	86%–91%	> 53 torr.	10%–24%	EEG > 11
Moderate OSAS	5–10 events per hour	76%–85%	> 53 torr.	25%–49%	EEG > 11
Severe OSAS	> 10 events per hour	< 75%	> 53 torr.	≥ 50%	EEG > 11

Key: EEG = electrocortical findings; RERA = respiratory effort related arousal findings

Adapted from *Principles and practice of pediatric sleep medicine*, S.H. Sheldon, R. Ferber, & M.H. Kryger, Diagnosis of obstructive sleep apnea in infants and children, p. 207, Copyright 2005, with permission from Elsevier.

25% of total sleep time by 2 years old and remains at this level throughout adolescence.

Both intermittent hypoxemia and sleep fragmentation pose a risk to the vulnerable developing brain. The diagnosis and management of pediatric OSAS continues to evolve as more precise measures of flow limitation and sleep fragmentation are introduced. Polysomnography represents the gold standard for establishing the presence and severity of sleep-disordered breathing patterns in children. Guidelines for performing laboratory-based polysomnography in children have been established (American Thoracic Society, 1996).

To the extent possible, sleep studies should conform to the child's usual sleep period. Infants may reasonably be studied during the day, whereas the adolescent studies should generally start later at night. The optimal definition for respiratory events and clinical classification has not been established in children. No clinical studies evaluate the relative merit of specific event definitions in relation to clinical outcomes. The increased recognition of subtle neurocognitive impairments in children with sleep-disordered breathing patterns has forced clinicians to rethink the threshold of disease requiring intervention. The polysomnographic criteria for event scoring and clinical diagnosis, based on the authors' experience, are summarized in Tables 15.3 and 15.4.

The treatment options for OSAS depend on the underlying etiology of airway obstruction and its severity (see Table 15.5). In the general population, adenotonsillar hypertrophy is the major risk factor for OSAS, and adenotonsillectomy successfully alleviates OSAS in 85% of cases. In individuals with airways prone to collapse, such as individuals with neuromuscular disease or obesity, even normal adenotonsillar size may contribute to airway obstruction.

Although an adenotonsillectomy may improve the degree of OSAS, significant residual obstruction often remains. Children with developmental delays and OSAS undergoing an adenotonsillectomy are at risk postoperatively for worsening obstruction due to swelling of the upper airway and postobstructive pulmonary edema. Select individuals may be candidates for additional airway surgery, (see later) and the remainder are given a trial of CPAP.

Although CPAP is efficacious, children with developmental delay often poorly tolerate it. Behavioral therapy training sessions to desensitize the child to the equipment and short-term admission to a developmentally appropriate rehabilitation unit is frequently successful. Despite these efforts, though, many people will not tolerate CPAP. In addition, some individuals will have obstruction during both wakefulness and sleep, making CPAP therapy untenable. In these children, the authors opt for alternative surgical techniques or tracheotomy.

Table 15.5. Management of obstructive sleep apnea syndrome in children

Medical management
Nasopharyngeal airway
Nasal steroids
Weight loss
Nasal corticosteroids
Positive airway pressure
Surgical management
Adenotonsillectomy
Uvulopalatoplasty
Tongue reduction or displacement
Mandibular distraction
Midfacial advancement
Tracheotomy
Things to avoid
Supine positioning
Respiratory depressants
Supplemental oxygen

Some children with cerebral palsy or Down syndrome (Strome, 1986) may benefit from an uvulopalatopharyngoplasty (UPPP); however, the UPPP may be complicated by velopharyngeal incompetence. Individuals with specific craniofacial conditions may benefit from mid-facial reconstruction or mandibular advancement (Cohen, Ross, Burnstein, Lefaivre, Riski, & Simms, 1998). A mandibular advancement device has been used in children with OSAS and malocclusion, but its utility in individuals with developmental delays is uncertain. Tracheotomy is a very effective treatment for OSAS, but it is prone toward infection and may interfere with speech and feeding.

CHRONIC LUNG DISEASE

Chronic lung disease is a major cause of morbidity and mortality in individuals with developmental disabilities. The etiology of chronic lung disease is often multifactorial. The most important contributors are aspiration, leading to recurrent inflammation and pulmonary infections, and poor cough, muscle weakness, and/or scoliosis, leading to atelectasis. The final common pathway of these multiple pulmonary insults often involves bronchiectasis, parenchymal scarring, and, ultimately, respiratory insufficiency.

Treatment of chronic lung disease in individuals with developmental disabilities is predicated on understanding the etiologic factors operative in the individual. As discussed previously, close attention should be paid to methods to minimize aspiration, facilitate airway clearance, treat bronchospasm, and provide assisted ventilation in the presence of sleep-disordered breathing or respiratory insufficiency. Judicious use of antibiotics, either oral or parenteral, is often indicated in the presence of an acute worsening of the underlying clinical state, especially when accompanied by fever or increased respiratory secretions. Antibiotic choices should be directed by the findings on culture of respiratory secretions.

Frank, open, and ongoing discussions with the individual and/or family regarding the overall clinical course and available treatment options are important. These discussions should take place in a culturally sensitive context. At times, the management plan may not be completely optimal from the standpoint of preserving lung function. For instance, a decision to continue oral feeding may be made in an individual with ongoing aspiration for whom a major source of social interaction and enjoyment is mealtimes. In this case, attempts should be made to minimize the potential insult to the lungs while optimizing the benefits to the individual and caregivers.

Finally, these discussions should include advanced care directives and end-of-life decisions (see Chapter 30). The fact that a major cause of death in individuals with developmental disabilities is pneumonia and/or respiratory failure should be discussed with the individual and/or family, and appropriate anticipatory guidance should be given.

ACUTE RESPIRATORY DISTRESS

People with developmental disabilities may develop acute respiratory distress. In general, the approach to these individuals is similar to any patient with respiratory distress; however, clinicians should put the situation in context. Does the individual have a history of recurrent aspiration, asthma, or previous similar episodes? Does the individual have a history of chronic lung disease? What has been done in the past, and was it successful?

The differential diagnosis of acute respiratory distress in an individual with developmental disabilities should include asthma, aspiration (of a foreign body or related to GER or dysfunctional swallowing), an acute respiratory infection (viral, bacterial, or "atypical"), or acute on chronic respiratory failure. General questions about the health of the individual in the past few hours and days, the presence of symptoms of a viral upper respiratory tract illness, and what the individual was doing when respiratory distress was noted are important. The possibility of aspiration should be entertained if the individual was eating or being fed (by mouth or enterally) or has a history of pica. If the individual has chronic lung disease, the clinician should determine if there were precipitating factors that could have led to an "acute-on-chronic" situation? If the individual has a tracheostomy, the clinician should ask if there been a recent change in the amount and/or color of the tracheal secretions.

The physical examination should start with careful observation of the individual to determine the degree of respiratory distress. The presence or absence of nasal flaring, accessory muscle use, and chest wall retractions should be noted. An altered level of consciousness with chronic lung disease may suggest the presence of hypercapnea and impending respiratory failure. A careful set of vital signs should be obtained and reviewed.

In addition to a general systems examination, particular attention should be paid to auscultation and percussion of the chest. Are the breath sounds equal? Can wheezing or crackles be appreciated, and if so, are they focal? Is there dullness to percussion? The answers to these questions may help detect the presence of a respiratory infection, asthma, or foreign body. In an individual with chronic lung disease, the second heart sound should be evaluated for the presence of pulmonary hypertension, and the presence or absence of clubbing should be noted.

Diagnostic testing will be directed by findings on history and examination. Common tests that should be obtained in all cases include a chest radiograph and analysis of gas exchange. The latter could be assessed by pulse oximetry and/or arterial blood gas analysis. Arterial blood gas analysis is extremely important in an individual with a history of chronic lung disease to rule out hypercapnea. Further diagnostic testing will depend on the clinical situation. For individuals with a tracheostomy, an aspirate of tracheal secretions should be sent for gram stain and culture. The presence of abundant neutrophils and bacteria in the gram stain is suggestive of an acute bacterial infection.

The management of an individual with acute respiratory distress should follow the general rule of ABCs: airway, breathing, and circulation. Supplemental oxygen should be given if hypoxia is present, although it should be given with care to individuals with a history of chronic lung disease. In the presence of chronic hypercapnea, correction of hypoxia to an oxygen saturation of greater than 95% may result in blunting of a hypoxic ventilatory drive, which may then result in an increase in hypoventilation, progressively worsening hypercapnea, and the possibly respiratory arrest. In this case, oxygen saturations in the range of 90%–95% should be the goal.

Bronchodilators may be given if wheezing is noted or if the individual has a history of asthma. Ipratroprium bromide is a bronchodilator with anticholinergic properties, which anecdotally can help reduce the volume of oral secretions. Antibiotics should be considered if there is evidence of an acute bacterial process. In individuals with a tracheostomy or chronic aspiration, the results of prior tracheal aspirate or sputum cultures can be used to guide the choice of antibiotics while awaiting contemporaneous culture results. Airway clearance techniques may also be helpful.

Finally, assisted ventilation may be required for those individuals with respiratory failure. Ventilation can take the form of CPAP or bi-level positive airway pressure (BiPAP) and can be delivered by different methods, including via nasal cannula, a tight-fitting nasal or facial mask, or a tracheostomy or endotracheal tube. As with the history and physical examination, the approach to management should take place in the context of the individual's history and should include consideration of prior discussions regarding advanced directives of care such as a Do Not Resuscitate order.

PULMONARY CONSIDERATIONS OF SPECIFIC CONDITIONS

Cerebral palsy is frequently characterized by muscle weakness, decreased compliance of the lung and chest wall, dysfunctional swallowing, GER, scoliosis, and impairments of motor control (see Chapter 11). The bellows action of the lung is diminished, and the resulting restrictive lung disease may produce hypoxemia and hypercapnea, which are particularly pronounced during exercise, feeding, and REM sleep. In addition, aspiration is thought to be the principal cause of the progressive deterioration in pulmonary function characteristic of children with severe cerebral palsy.

Children with cerebral palsy present with infections, ineffective cough, reactive airway disease, central sleep apnea (drooling), and gas exchange abnormalities. They also have an increased incidence of OSAS. Adenotonsillectomy is frequently only partially effective in reducing the severity of OSAS. UPPP has been reported to be successful in some children with cerebral palsy and OSAS. Treating other sites of airway obstruction, including an enlarged and retropositioned tongue, nasal septal deviation, enlarged inferior turbinates, retrognathia, or maxillary hypoplasia, may be more successful.

Craniofacial Abnormalities

Craniofacial anomalies may predispose to upper airway obstruction on the basis of abnormal airway size, collapsibility, or neuromuscular control (see Chapter 8.2). In addition, craniofacial anomalies frequently occur in syndromes that may otherwise adversely affect pulmonary function, including laryngotracheal abnormalities and restrictive lung disease. A retrospective series of 50 micrognathic infants revealed that 72% required an intervention for airway obstruction. Sleep-disordered breathing patterns observed in micrognathic infants often improve during the first year of life. In addition, CPAP, adenotonsillectomy, nasopharyngeal stenting, mandibular distraction, and prone positioning have also been successfully used to treat OSAS (Bull, Givan, Sadove, Bixler, & Hearn, 1990).

Children with craniofacial synostosis syndromes (Apert, Crouzon, Pfeiffer) have a 24%–88% prevalence of OSAS (Kakitsuba et al., 1994; Moore, 1993). In one large series, 48% of individuals with craniofacial synostosis required tracheotomy for airway obstruction (Sculerati, Gottlieb, Zimbler, Chibbaro, & McCarthy, 1998). CPAP has been reported to successfully treat OSAS in young children with Crouzon syndrome (Hui, Wing, Kew, Chan, Abdullah, & Fok, 1998); however, the external maxillary pressure posed by nasal CPAP may retard the growth of the mid-facial bones (Li, Riley, & Guilleminault, 2000) Mid-facial advancement with a Lefort osteotomy or distraction has been reported to improve OSAS in some individuals (McCarthy et al., 1995).

Down Syndrome

The development of subpleural cysts in Down syndrome is associated with impaired lung mechanics and pulmonary hypertension. Upper airway obstruction may result from micrognathia, maxillary hypoplasia, macroglossia, nasopharyngeal narrowing, and hypotonia. In addition, children with Down syndrome with significant left-to-right shunts may develop pulmonary hyper tension and decreased lung compliance. Individuals with Down syndrome may also be at risk for high-altitude pulmonary edema, obesity hypoventilation, congenital chylothorax, tracheal stenosis and pulmonary vascular disease. Respiratory tract pathology, including pneumo nia, croup, OSAS, bronchiolitis, and asthma are common indications for hospitalization (Hilton, Fitzgerald, & Cooper, 1999).

The prevalence of OSAS in Down syndrome is 31%–60% (Marcus, Keens, Bautista, von Pechmann, & Ward, 1991; Stebbins, Dennis, Samuels, Croft, & Southall, 1991). Although an adenotonsillectomy is usually effective in individuals with mild OSAS, it is often insufficient to reverse the upper airway obstruction in severe OSAS (Jacobs, Gray, & Todd, 1996). Removal of the uvula and/or parts of the palate has resulted in favorable outcomes. Following an adenotonsillectomy, children with Down syndrome have a high incidence of postoperative respiratory distress including upper airway obstruction, oxygen desaturation, and hypoventilation (Goldstein, Armfield, Kingsley, Borland, Allen, & Post, 1998). Also, postintubation stridor and subglottic stenosis are commonly reported.

Duchenne Muscular Dystrophy

Most children with Duchenne muscular dystrophy develop sleep-disordered breathing between 15–17 years old, progress to daytime hypercapnea between 16–18 years old, and die between 20–22 years old. Respiratory failure is the cause of death in 80%–90% of cases. During the individual's first 8–10 years, VC increases and remains within the low normal range. During the next 2–3 years, the absolute VC either remains constant or declines minimally, although the percent predicted VC decreases. After this time, the absolute VC declines 150–250 mL/year. After the VC declines below 1 L, only 50% of individuals will survive 3 years, and only 8% will survive 5 years (Phillips, Quinlivan Edwards, & Calverley, 2001).

Respiratory failure in Duchenne muscular dystrophy results from respiratory muscle weakness, decreased compliance of the chest wall and lung, and parenchymal lung disease due to an ineffective cough and recurrent aspiration. The hypercapnic ventilatory response is normal in Duchenne muscular dystrophy, although individuals tend to increase their respiratory rate more than tidal volume. Nocturnal gas exchange abnormalities are frequently observed during adolescence when the VC is less than 1.1–1.2 L. The signs and symptoms of respiratory insufficiency at night are dyspnea, apnea, orthopnea, cyanosis, restlessness, and insomnia. Daytime symptoms include somnolence, morning headache, drowsiness, anxiety, confusion, and polycythemia. Respiratory muscle training may provide some benefit to individuals before VC declines below 25%, although little data has been presented in this regard.

Individuals with Duchenne muscular dystrophy rely on a higher respiratory rate during wakefulness to maintain their tidal volume. During sleep, individuals with Duchenne muscular dystrophy have a greater reduction in their respiratory rate than normal subjects, resulting in a proportionately larger decline in minute ventilation, particularly during REM sleep. REM sleep is particularly problematic due to a reduction in the activity of intercostal muscles and pharyngeal airway dilator muscles, resulting in a decrease in alveolar ventilation and an increase in airway resistance.

The earliest sign of respiratory insufficiency in Duchenne muscular dystrophy is REM-related hypoxemia (Smith, Calverley, & Edwards, 1988). Treatment of nocturnal hypoxemia with oxygen is effective at reversing the desaturation but may worsen the OSAS (Smith, Edwards, & Caverley, 1989). In view of the progressive nature of the disease, early institution of nocturnal ventilatory support should be considered when nocturnal hypoxemia develops.

The use of oral corticosteroids has been shown to increase muscle strength, prolong ambulation, and delay decline in pulmonary function. Although results of treatment with corticosteroids are encouraging, significant steroid-related side effects are common. The use of mechanical insufflation–exsufflation and manually assisted coughing using expiratory abdominal thrusts has been reported to facilitate secretion removal (Bach, 1993).

Mucopolysaccharidosis

For individuals with mucopolysaccharidosis, hypertrophy of structures including the tongue, tonsils, adenoids, and mucus membranes may result in upper airway narrowing that leads to tracheostomy or obligate mouth breathing (see Chapter 7.2). Surgical removal of the adenoids and/or tonsils may help relieve this upper airway obstruction in some individuals, although many individuals have evidence of residual obstruction (Semenza & Pyeritz, 1988). Some individuals may have associated sleep-disordered breathing requiring supplemental oxygen and/or assisted ventilation.

Glycosaminoglycan deposition in tracheobronchial mucosa lining the lower airways may lead to lower airway narrowing. A reduction in tracheal surface area has been documented by computed tomography examination of the airway (Shih, Lee, Lin, Sheu, & Blickman, 2002). This combination of upper and lower airway obstruction may result in acute or subacute respiratory compromise characterized by respiratory distress and hypoxemia as well as difficulties with intubation and even respiratory arrest during surgical procedures (Semenza & Pyeritz, 1988). Persistent or recurrent focal atelectasis and recurrent pneumonia have also been reported as a result of this lower airway obstruction. Positive pressure ventilation may help to maintain airway patency, while the use of intraluminal stents has also been reported (Davitt et al., 2002).

Finally, skeletal dysplasia and abdominal organomegaly may compromise pulmonary function. Kyphoscoliosis and chest wall abnormalities may reduce lung volumes, resulting in restrictive lung disease. Hepatosplenomegaly may be significant, and the resulting upward displacement of the diaphragm further contributes to restrictive lung disease. Functional consequences of this restriction may include focal or "micro" atelectasis, hypoxemia, and recurrent pneumonia (Semenza & Pyeritz, 1988).

Diagnostic evaluation should include arterial blood gas analysis, pulse oximetry, chest radiography, airway computed tomography, and pulmonary function testing. Consideration should be given to polysomnography to evaluate for the presence of sleep-disordered breathing. Careful evaluation should be undertaken prior to any procedures involving sedation or anesthesia. The patency of the airway should be assessed by noninvasive methods, such as airway computed tomography and the analysis of flow-volume loops to detect the presence of upper and/or lower airway obstruction. Direct visualization of the airway via bronchoscopy may be undertaken, but care should be taken to prevent further airway compromise.

Myelomeningocele

Brainstem dysfunction due to anatomic disruption in myelomeningocele may result in vocal cord paralysis, dysphagia, abnormal ventilatory control, and respiratory dysrhythmias (see Chapter 8.1). Symptoms in older children include sleep apnea, headache, dysphonia, and dysphagia. Other respiratory complications include respiratory weakness and ineffective cough. The early recognition and treatment of symptoms of brainstem compression is critical in preserving function.

Exercise capacity may be reduced due to skeletal muscle weakness and pulmonary limitation (Sherman, Kaplan, Effgen, Campbell, & Dold, 1997). A short trachea resulting from a reduced number of tracheal rings has been reported in 36% of children with myelomeningocele, increasing the risk of bronchial intubation (Wells, Jacobs, Senac, & Landing, 1990). Sleep-disordered breathing patterns observed in myelomeningocele include central apnea, obstructive apnea, central hypoventilation, and prolonged expiratory apnea with cyanosis (Ward, Jacobs, Gates, Hart, & Keens, 1986; Waters et al., 1998). Individuals at the highest risk for sleep-disordered breathing include those with a thoracic or thoracolumbar defect, a history of posterior fossa decompression, and pulmonary function abnormalities.

Central apnea may respond to respiratory stimulants such as theophylline. Some individuals are stable on oxygen, and others require positive pressure ventilation either nasally or via a tracheotomy. Prolonged expiratory apnea with cyanosis does not resolve with surgical decompression and may be fatal even after tracheotomy and mechanical ventilation (Cochrane, Adderley, White, Norman, & Steinbok, 1990).

Prader-Willi Syndrome

Children with Prader-Willi syndrome often experience excessive daytime sleepiness, sleep apnea, and hypoventilation deriving from obesity, craniofacial dysmorphism, respiratory muscle weakness, chemoreceptor dysfunction, and/or diencephalic dysfunction (see Chapter 9.4). Significant respiratory muscle weakness may also occur. Spirometry in Prader-Willi syndrome reveals a reduction in FVC and FEV1, while the FEV1/FVC ratio is normal. Lung volume assessment demonstrates an increased RV, with the TLC in the low normal range (Hakonarson, Mokovitz, Daigle, Cassidy, & Cloutier, 1995). Individuals have impaired exercise tolerance and airway clearance, thus predisposing to airway obstruction and pulmonary infections.

Children with Prader-Willi syndrome may have excessive daytime sleepiness even without sleep-disordered breathing (Manni et al., 2001) and after weight loss (Harris & Allen, 1996). Thus, the excessive daytime sleepiness observed in Prader-Willi syndrome suggests a primary hypothalamic dysfunction. Individuals have been successfully treated with nocturnal bi-level ventilation, resulting in normalization of daytime gas exchange (Smith, King, Siklos, & Shneerson, 1998). In addition, growth hormone has been shown to increase respiratory muscle strength, (Carrel, Myers, Whitman, & Allen, 1999) hypercapnic ventilatory response, and basal ventilation (Lindgren, Hellstrom, Ritzen, & Milerad, 1999).

Diego is a 14-year-old with Prader-Willi syndrome who lives at home with his parents, two sisters, and a golden retriever. He is fully bilingual, is interested in gardening, and is a dedicated Red Sox fan. He also enjoys helping his mother with chores around the house.

During the last year, Diego has been hospitalized three times with cardiorespiratory failure. His chest x-ray at the time of an admission revealed an enlarged heart, pulmonary edema, and low lung volumes. He now weighs nearly 300 lb, which has resulted in sleep apnea and nocturnal hypoventilation resulting in heart failure.

Even between admissions, Diego has become dyspniec at rest and is now unable to attend school. He has been prescribed bi-level ventilation during sleep, supplemental oxygen while awake, and a strict dietary regimen. After the third admission, Diego lost 70 lb during a stay in a rehabilitation center and was able to discontinue both daytime oxygen and nighttime ventilation. At that time, it was recommended that he be permanently placed in a residential facility to maintain his strict dietary regimen. Diego's parents were distraught at the prospect of him leaving their household and decided to have him return home with plans to strictly adhere to his caloric restriction.

Over the next several months, Diego regained his weight, and his respiratory failure recurred. Diego had acute respiratory distress with a chest radiograph consistent with atelectasis of the left lung. A computed tomography scan of the chest (see Figure 15.3) revealed that Diego had a foreign body in his left mainstem bronchus. A chicken bone was removed with rigid bronchoscopy.

Diego's parents realized that his school environment was unable to supervise his eating habits effectively. Diego would eat the other students' food and rummage through the garbage for more. Even at home, restricting his intake proved to be difficult. His food-seeking behavior was so intense that he would become violent when he was denied food. His parents now realized that he needed an environment crafted to his special needs, and enrolled him in a residential facility specializing in Prader-Willi syndrome. Diego has lost weight again and returned to his normal level of activity. He is thriving in his new environment and spends the weekends at home with his family.

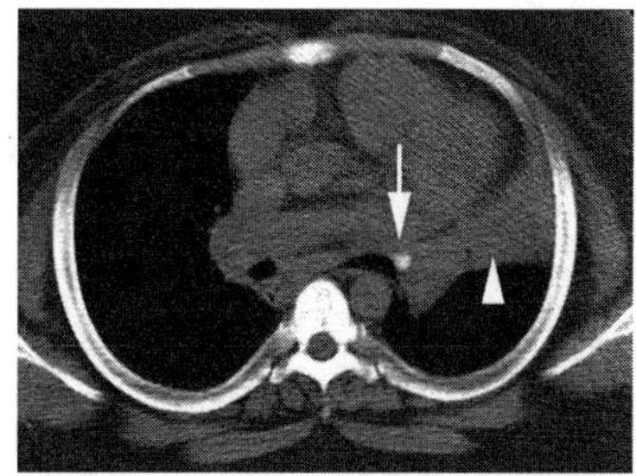

Figure 15.3. Computed tomography scan of Diego's chest. A foreign body can be seen in the left mainstem bronchi (arrow) with atelectasis of the left lower lobe (arrowhead).

Rett Syndrome

Breathing abnormalities in Rett syndrome usually begin after 2 years of age and are largely confined to wakefulness (Julu et al., 2001; see Chapter 9.1). Apneustic and forced breathing patterns predominate in the first 10 years of life. Older individuals demonstrate valsalva breathing, central apnea, and shallow breathing. Brief, nonepileptic staring episodes, dystonic posturing, and repetitive movements may be associated with respiratory dysrhythmias. Breath-holding spells are often interspersed with hyperventilation.

Aerophagia has been reported to occur during hyperventilation and breath-holding episodes resulting in gastric distension that may interfere with respiratory gas exchange. Successful treatment of the gastric distension may require gastrostomy tube placement (Anzai & Ohya, 2001). The termination of inspiration is serotonin-dependent, and agonists to serotonin 1A receptors have been used to treat apneustic breathing in Rett syndrome (Kerr, Julu, Hansen, & Apartopoulos, 1998).

CONCLUSION

Individuals with developmental disabilities commonly experience aspiration, dysfunctional swallowing, GER, and asthma. In addition, kyphoscoliosis, obesity, and prematurity can lead to respiratory problems. Individuals with disabilities also are at risk for recurrent respiratory infections, respiratory muscle weakness, sleep-disordered breathing, chronic lung disease, and acute respiratory distress. This chapter discusses the diverse pulmonary impairments that may affect individuals with developmental disabilities. It also addresses pulmonary conditions associated with specific disorders. Respiratory issues greatly affect quality of life. By addressing these issues, clinicians can ensure that individuals with developmental disabilities live life to its fullest with dignity even in the presence of significant respiratory problems.

REFERENCES

American Thoracic Society. (1996). Standards and indications for cardiopulmonary sleep studies in children. *American Journal of Respiratory and Critical Care Medicine, 153*, 866–878.

Anzai, Y., & Ohya, T. (2001). A case of effective gastrostomy for severe abdominal distention due to breathing dysfunction of Rett's syndrome: A treatment of autonomic disorder. *Brain & Development, 23*(Suppl. 1), S240–S241.

Bach, J.R. (1993). Mechanical insufflation-exsufflation. Comparison of peak expiratory flows with manually assisted and unassisted coughing techniques. *Chest, 104*, 1553–1562.

Bancalari, E., & Gonzalez, A. (2000). Clinical course and lung function abnormalities during development of neonatal chronic lung disease. In R.D. Bland & J.J. Coalson (Eds.), *Chronic lung disease of early infancy* (pp. 41–64). New York: Marcel Dekker.

Bull, M.J., Givan, D.C., Sadove, A.M., Bixler, D., & Hearn, D. (1990). Improved outcome in Pierre Robin sequence: Effect of multidisciplinary evaluation and management. *Pediatrics, 86*, 294–301.

Canny, G.J., Szeinberg, A., Koreska, J., & Levison, H. (1989). Hypercapnia in relation to pulmonary function in Duchenne muscular dystrophy. *Pediatric Pulmonology, 6*, 169–171.

Carrel, A.L., Myers, S.E., Whitman, B.Y., & Allen, D.B. (1999). Growth hormone improves body composition, fat utilization, physical strength and agility, and growth in Prader-Willi syndrome: A controlled study. *Journal of Pediatrics, 134*, 215–221.

Chen, S.H., Huang, T.J., Lee, Y.Y., & Hsu, R.W. (2002). Pulmonary function after thoracoplasty in adolescent idiopathic scoliosis. *Clinical Orthopaedics and Related Research, 399*, 152–161.

Cochrane, D.D., Adderley, R., White, C.P., Norman, M., & Steinbok, P. (1990). Apnea in patients with myelomeningocele. *Pediatric Neurosurgery, 16*, 232–239.

Cohen, S.R., Ross, D.A., Burstein, F.D., Lefaivre, J.F., Riski, J.E., & Simms, C. (1998). Skeletal expansion combined with soft-tissue reduction in the treatment of obstructive sleep apnea in children: Physiologic results. *Otolaryngology—Head and Neck Surgery, 119*, 476–485.

Davies, G., & Reid, L. (1971). Effect of scoliosis on growth of alveoli and pulmonary arteries and on right ventricle. *Archives of Disease in Childhood, 46*, 623–632.

Davitt, S.M., Hatrick, A., Sabharwal, T., Pearce, A., Gleeson, M., & Adam, A. (2002). Tracheobronchial stent insertions in the management of major airway obstruction in a patient with Hunter syndrome (type-II mucopolysaccharidosis). *European Radiology, 12*, 458–462.

De Troyer, A., Borenstein, S., & Cordier, R. (1980). Analysis of lung volume restriction in patients with respiratory muscle weakness. *Thorax, 35*, 603–610.

Finder, J.D., Yellon, R., & Charron, M. (2001). Successful management of tracheotomized patients with chronic saliva aspiration by use of constant positive airway pressure. *Pediatrics, 107*, 1343–1345.

Gerber, M.E., Gaugler, M.D., Myer, C.M., III, & Cotton, R.T. (1996). Chronic aspiration in children: When are bilateral submandibular gland excision and parotid duct ligation indicated? *Archives of Otolaryngology—Head & Neck Surgery, 122*, 1368–1371.

Goldstein, N.A., Armfield, D.R., Kingsley, L.A., Borland, L.M., Allen, G.C., & Post, J.C. (1998). Postoperative complications after tonsillectomy and adenoidectomy in children with Down syndrome. *Archives of Otolaryngology—Head & Neck Surgery, 124*, 171–176.

Gozal, D., Wang, M., & Pope, D.W., Jr. (2001). Objective sleepiness measures in pediatric obstructive sleep apnea. *Pediatrics, 108*, 693–697.

Graham, E.J., Lenke, L.G., Lowe, T.G., et al. (2000). Prospective pulmonary function evaluation following open thoracotomy for anterior spinal fusion in adolescent idiopathic scoliosis. *Spine, 25*, 2319–2325.

Guilleminault, C., Korobkin, R., & Winkle, R. (1981). A review of 50 children with obstructive sleep apnea syndrome. *Lung, 159*, 275–287.

Guilleminault, C., Stoohs, R., Clerk, A., Cetel, M., & Maistros, P. (1993). A cause of excessive daytime sleepiness. The upper airway resistance syndrome. *Chest, 104*, 781–787.

Gustafsson, P.M., & Tibbling, L. (1994). Gastro-oesophageal reflux and oesophageal dysfunction in children and adolescents with brain damage. *Acta Paediatrica, 83*, 1081–1085.

Hakonarson, H., Moskovitz, J., Daigle, K.L., Cassidy, S.B., & Cloutier, M.M. (1995). Pulmonary function abnormalities in Prader-Willi syndrome. *Journal of Pediatrics, 126*, 565–570.

Harris, J.C., & Allen, R.P. (1996). Is excessive daytime sleepiness characteristic of Prader-Willi syndrome? The effects of weight change. *Archives of Pediatrics and Adolescent Medicine, 150*, 1288–1293.

Hilton, J.M., Fitzgerald, D.A., & Cooper, D.M. (1999). Respiratory morbidity of hospitalized children with Trisomy 21. *Journal of Paediatrics and Child Health, 35*, 383–386.

Hui, S., Wing, Y.K., Kew, J., Chan, Y.L., Abdullah, V., & Fok, T.F. (1998). Obstructive sleep apnea syndrome in a family with Crouzon's syndrome. *Sleep, 21*, 298–303.

Inselma, L.S., Milanese, A., & Deurloo, A. (1993). Effect of obesity on pulmonary function in children. *Pediatric Pulmonology, 16*, 130–137.

Jacobs, I.N., Gray, R.F., & Todd, N.W. (1996). Upper airway obstruction in children with Down syndrome. *Archives of Otolaryngology—Head & Neck Surgery, 122*, 945–950.

Jobe, A.H., & Bancalari, E. (2001). Bronchopulmonary dysplasia. *American Journal of Respiratory and Critical Care Medicine, 163*, 1723–1729.

Jobe, A.H., & Ikegami, M. (2001). Prevention of bronchopulmonary dysplasia. *Current Opinion in Pediatrics, 13*, 124–129.

Julu, P.O., Kerr, A.M., Apartopoulos, F., et al. (2001). Characterisation of breathing and associated central autonomic dysfunction in the Rett disorder. *Archives of Disease in Childhood, 85*, 29–37.

Kafer, E.R. (1976). Idiopathic scoliosis. Gas exchange and the age dependence of arterial blood gases. *Journal of Clinical Investigation, 58*, 825–833.

Kakitsuba, N., Sadaoka, T., Motoyama, S., et al. (1994). Sleep apnea and sleep-related breathing disorders in patients with craniofacial synostosis. *Acta Oto-laryngologica. Supplementum, 517*, 6–10.

Katz, E.S. (2005). Diagnosis of obstructive sleep apnea in infants and children. In S.H. Sheldon, R. Ferber, & M.H. Kryger (Eds.), *Principles and practice of pediatric sleep medicine.* New York: Elsevier.

Kearon, C., Viviani, G.R., Kirkley, A., & Killian, K.J. (1993). Factors determining pulmonary function in adolescent idiopathic thoracic scoliosis. *American Review of Respiratory Distress, 148*, 288–294.

Kerr, A.M., Julu, P.O., Hansen, S., & Apartopoulos, F. (1998). Serotonin and breathing dysrhythmia in Rett syndrome. In M.V. Perat (Ed.), *New developments in child neurology* (pp. 191–195). Bologna, Italy: Monduzzi Editore.

Li, K.K., Riley, R.W., & Guilleminault, C. (2000). An unreported risk in the use of home nasal continuous positive airway pressure and home nasal ventilation in children: Mid-face hypoplasia. *Chest, 117*, 916–918.

Lindgren, A.C., Hellstrom, L.G., Ritzen, E.M., & Milerad, J. (1999). Growth hormone treatment increases CO_2 response, ventilation and central inspiratory drive in children with Prader-Willi syndrome. *European Journal of Pediatrics, 158*, 936–940.

Mallory, G.B., Jr., Fiser, D.H., & Jackson, R. (1989). Sleep-associated breathing disorders in morbidly obese children and adolescents. *Journal of Pediatrics, 115*, 892–897.

Manni, R., Politini, L., Nobili, L., et al. (2001). Hypersomnia in the Prader Willi syndrome: Clinical-electrophysiological features and underlying factors. *Clinical Neurophysiologist, 112*, 800–805.

Marcus, C.L., Curtis, S., Koerner, C.B., Joffe, A., Serwint, J.R., & Loughlin, G.M. (1996). Evaluation of pulmonary function and polysomnography in obese children and adolescents. *Pediatric Pulmonology, 21*, 176–183.

Marcus, C.L., Keens, T.G., Bautista, D.B., von Pechmann, W.S., & Ward, S.L. (1991). Obstructive sleep apnea in children with Down syndrome. *Pediatrics, 88*, 132–139.

McCarthy, J.G., Glasberg, S.B., Cutting, C.B., et al. (1995). Twenty-year experience with early surgery for craniosynostosis: II. The craniofacial synostosis syndromes and pansynostosis—results and unsolved problems. *Plastic and Reconstructive Surgery, 96*, 284–298.

Moore, M.H. (1993). Upper airway obstruction in the syndromal craniosynostoses. *British Journal of Plastic Surgery, 46*, 355–362.

Moyer-Mileur, L.J., Nielson, D.W., Pfeffer, K.D., Witte, M.K., & Chapman, D.L. (1996). Eliminating sleep-associated hypoxemia improves growth in infants with bronchopulmonary dysplasia. *Pediatrics, 98*, 779–783.

Murphy, B.P., Inder, T.E., Huppi, P.S., et al. (2001). Impaired cerebral cortical gray matter growth after treatment with dexamethasone for neonatal chronic lung disease. *Pediatrics, 107*, 217–221.

Okajima, S., Matsuda, T., Cho, K., Matsumoto, Y., Kobayashi, Y., & Fujimoto, S. (2001). Antenatal dexamethasone administration impairs normal postnatal lung growth in rats. *Pediatric Research, 49*, 777–781.

Phillips, M.F., Quinlivan, R.C., Edwards, R.H., & Calverley, P.M. (2001). Changes in spirometry over time as a prognostic marker in patients with Duchenne muscular dystrophy. *American Journal of Respiratory and Critical Care Medicine, 164*, 2191–2194.

Reddihough, D.S., Baikie, G., & Walstab, J.E. (2001). Cerebral palsy in Victoria, Australia: Mortality and causes of death. *Journal of Paediatrics and Child Health, 37*, 183–186.

Rhodes, S.K., Shimoda, K.C., Waid, L.R., et al. (1995). Neurocognitive deficits in morbidly obese children with obstructive sleep apnea. *Journal of Pediatrics, 127*, 741–744.

Rosen, C.L., D'Andrea, L., & Haddad, G.G. (1992). Adult criteria for obstructive sleep apnea do not identify children with serious obstruction. *American Review of Respiratory Distress, 146*, 1231–1234.

Sculerati, N., Gottlieb, M.D., Zimbler, M.S., Chibbaro, P.D., & McCarthy, J.G. (1998). Airway management in children with major craniofacial anomalies. *Laryngoscope, 108*, 1806–1812.

Semenza, G.L., & Pyeritz, R.E. (1988). Respiratory complications of mucopolysaccharide storage disorders. *Medicine (Baltimore), 67*, 209–219.

Sherman, M.S., Kaplan, J.M., Effgen, S., Campbell, D., & Dold, F. (1997). Pulmonary dysfunction and reduced exercise capacity in patients with myelomeningocele. *Journal of Pediatrics, 131*, 413–418.

Shih, S.L., Lee, Y.J., Lin, S.P., Sheu, C.Y., & Blickman, J.G. (2002). Airway changes in children with mucopolysaccharidoses. *Acta Radiologica, 43*, 40–43.

Silvestri, J.M., Weese-Mayer, D.E., Bass, M.T., Kenny, A.S., Hauptman, S.A., & Pearsall, S.M. (1993). Polysomnography in obese children with a history of sleep-associated breathing disorders. *Pediatric Pulmonology, 16*, 124–129.

Smith, I.E., King, M.A., Siklos, P.W., & Shneerson, J.M. (1998). Treatment of ventilatory failure in the Prader-Willi syndrome. *European Respiratory Journal, 11*, 1150–1152.

Smith, P.E., Calverley, P.M., & Edwards, R.H. (1988). Hypoxemia during sleep in Duchenne muscular dystrophy. *American Review of Respiratory Distress, 137*, 884–888.

Smith, P.E., Edwards, R.H., & Calverley, P.M. (1989). Oxygen treatment of sleep hypoxaemia in Duchenne muscular dystrophy. *Thorax, 44*, 997–1001.

Stebbens, V.A., Dennis, J., Samuels, M.P., Croft, C.B., & Southall, D.P. (1991). Sleep related upper airway obstruction in a cohort with Down's syndrome. *Archives of Disease in Childhood, 66*, 1333–1338.

Strome, M. (1986). Obstructive sleep apnea in Down syndrome children: A surgical approach. *Laryngoscope, 96*, 1340–1342.

Suskind, D.L., & Tilton, A. (2002). Clinical study of botulinum-A toxin in the treatment of sialorrhea in children with cerebral palsy. *Laryngoscope, 112*, 73–81.

Tangsrud, S.E., Carlsen, K.C., Lund-Petersen, I., & Carlsen, K.H. (2001). Lung function measurements in young children with spinal muscle atrophy: A cross sectional survey on the effect of position and bracing. *Archives of Disease in Childhood, 84*, 521–524.

Vedantam, R., Lenke, L.G., Bridwell, K.H., Haas, J., & Linville, D.A. (2000, September). A prospective evaluation of pulmonary function in patients with adolescent idiopathic scoliosis relative to the surgical approach used for spinal arthrodesis. *Spine, 25*, 82–90.

Wales, P.W., Diamond, I.R., Dutta, S., et al. (2002). Fundoplication and gastrostomy versus image-guided gastrojejunal tube for enteral feeding in neurologically impaired children with gastroesophageal reflux. *Journal of Pediatric Surgery, 37*, 407–412.

Ward, S.L., Jacobs, R.A., Gates, E.P., Hart, L.D., & Keens, T.G. (1986). Abnormal ventilatory patterns during sleep in infants with myelomeningocele. *Journal of Pediatrics, 109*, 631–634.

Waters, K.A., Forbes, P., Morielli, A., et al. (1998). Sleep-disordered breathing in children with myelomeningocele. *Journal of Pediatrics, 132*, 672–681.

Wells, T.R., Jacobs, R.A., Senac, M.O., & Landing, B.H. (1990). Incidence of short trachea in patients with myelomeningocele. *Pediatric Neurology, 6*, 109–111.

Wohl, M.E., & Majzoub, J.A. (2000). Asthma, steroids, and growth. *New England Journal of Medicine, 343*, 1113–1114.

CHAPTER 16

EYE AND VISION CARE

Anne B. Fulton, Luisa Mayer, Kathryn B. Miller, and Ronald M. Hansen

Children and adults with developmental disabilities have special eye and vision care needs because their underlying medical conditions often cause diseases of the visual system (Warburg, 2001). Furthermore, eye and vision assessments are shaped by the physical and cognitive abilities of the individual, and management of eye and vision care must be done in the context of the individual's general condition. Experience indicates that the impact of vision on activities of daily living cannot be overestimated, even though formal study of the relationship of vision and quality of life in individuals with developmental disabilities has yet to be conducted (Mangione, Gutierrez, Lowe, Orav, & Seddon, 1999; Mangione et al., 1994).

This chapter enunciates some of the basic principles for assessment and management of the eye and vision needs of children and adults with developmental disabilities. For those seeking information about eye and vision disorders, the Internet is a strong ally. Families, physicians, and other providers are increasingly consulting web sites, such as http://www.e-Advisor.us, for details about the many ophthalmic disorders that are found in children and adults with development disabilities. These web sites offer current information; link readers to relevant ancillary sources; and facilitate exchange of information among families, physicians, and other therapists.

Table 16.1 lists some ophthalmic features, with definitions of the features, associations, or diagnoses in which the feature is common, and provides web sites with a wealth of additional information on the features. No attempt is made to catalog all eye and vision disorders affecting those with developmental disabilities. Diagrams of the eye and visual pathways (see Figures 16.1 and 16.2) support the definitions in Table 16.1. In Table 16.2, a few systemic conditions that are associated with developmental delays and that have characteristic ocular features are listed. In many of these conditions, the ocular feature leads physicians to the systemic diagnosis. Because the frequency of strabismus (a nonspecific ocular feature, see Table 16.1) and history of preterm birth (see Table 16.2) are quite high in individuals with developmental delays, separate sections on strabismus and the ocular and visual sequelae of prematurity are provided later in this chapter. Further information about ophthalmic disorders and visual impairment in those with special needs may be found in the literature under specific diagnoses and in dedicated journals such as the *Journal of Visual Impairment and Blindness.*

VISION ASSESSMENT AND EYE EXAMINATION

The elements of any eye examination, no matter the diagnosis, include acquisition of information by history taking, sensory testing, and physical examination. The objective is to obtain high-quality data that give information about the structure and function of the eyes (see Figure 16.1) and the visual system (see Figure 16.2). To meet this objective, an approach that has evolved from pediatric ophthalmology practice is used. The results of the examination are the basis for the best possible plan of management for the individual.

Several categories of eye care professionals are involved in the assessment and management of disorders of the eyes and vision (see Table 16.3). Other specialists initiate the process of eye care by referring to an ophthalmologist or optometrist. Based on the details of the examination, a determination is made as to whether the individual should be referred to other eye care professionals.

Logistics are important to the conduct of a successful examination. Prior medical and ophthalmic records should be given to the eye doctor. Consider scheduling the eye examination early in the day or on a day when other examinations and tests are not to be done. After all, the sensory testing part of any eye examination requires a high level of patient participation. Once the eye doctor has been informed of the ophthalmic issues and the medical and developmental condition of the individual, he or she should indicate the expected dura

Table 16.1. Ophthalmic features

Feature	Definition	Common association	Web sites
Cataracts	Opacity of the eye lens	Down syndrome	http://www.geocities.com/catseyeswebsite/gtormondstreet hosp.htm http://www.tc.umn.edu/~chris196/cataracts.htm http://www.heatoneye.com/edu_ped_cataract.html
Coloboma	Failure of closure of fetal fissure leaves a gap in uveal and/or retinal tissue. Coloboma of iris looks like a "keyhole" pupil.	CHARGE association Cat eye syndrome	http://www.eyecare-information-service.org.uk/item_view.php?item_id=68&content_id=4 http://www.emedicine.com/oph/topic673.htm
Glaucoma	High pressure in the eye	Rieger syndrome Neurofibromatosis Fetal alcohol syndrome Sturge-Weber syndrome Peter's anomaly Cockayne syndrome Aniridia	http://www.emedicine.com/oph/topic138.htm http://www.emedicine.com/oph/topic141.htm
Keratoconus	Irregular shape of cornea	Marfan syndrome Down syndrome Aniridia	http://www.nkcf.org/ http://www.kcenter.org/ http://www.uic.edu/com/eye/PatientCare/EyeConditions/Keratoconus.shtml http://www.visionweb.com/content/consumers/dev_consumerarticles.jsp?RID=22# http://www.emedicine.com/oph/topic104.htm
Microphthalmia/ microphthalmos	Very small eye	Congenital cataracts	http://www.nei.nih.gov/health/anoph/index.htm http://www.emedicine.com/oph/topic572.htm
Nystagmus	Involuntary rhythmic eye movements	Albinism Optic nerve atrophy	http://www.lowvision.org/nystagmus.htm http://www.emedicine.com/oph/topic688.htm http://www.emedicine.com/oph/topic339.htm
Optic nerve hypoplasia	Small optic nerves	Septo-optic dysplasia and other midline abnormalities of the brain Rieger syndrome	http://www.blindbabies.org/factsheet_onh.htm http://www.onesmallvoicefoundation.org/images/ONH%20 pamphlet_sm.pdf http://www.tsbvi.edu/Outreach/seehear/spring99/optic nerve.htm http://www.e-advisor.us
Ptosis	Drooping of the upper eyelid	Nerve palsy (III) Kearns-Sayre syndrome Smith-Lemli-Opitz syndrome	http://www.emedicine.com/oph/topic345.htm http://www.iopinc.com/patient_link/ptosis.asp http://www.emedicine.com/OPH/topic201.htm
Retinitis pigmentosa	Retinal degeneration	Usher syndrome Bassen-Kornzweig syndrome Bardet-Biedl syndrome Refsum syndrome Alstrom syndrome	http://www.eyeassociates.com/images/understanding_the_visual_problem1.htm http://www.retina-international.org/rp.htm http://www.visionchannel.net/retinitis/ http://www.rpsa.org.za/retinitis.htm http://www.emedicine.com/oph/topic704.htm http://www.nlm.nih.gov/medlineplus/ency/article/001029.htm
Strabismus	Misaligned eyes	Please see text.	http://www.strabismus.org/all_about_strabismus.html http://www.eyemdlink.com/Condition.asp?ConditionID=421 http://www.bgseyecenter.com/strabismus.html http://www.intelihealth.com/IH/ihtIH/WSIHW000/9339/10805.html http://www.hawaii.edu/medicine/pediatrics/pedtext/s17c03.html

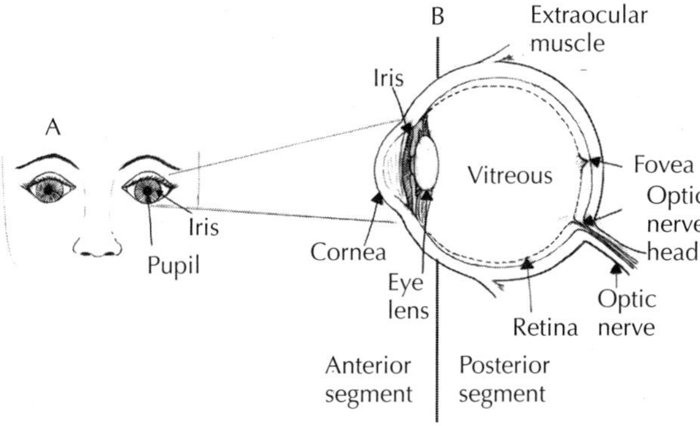

Figure 16.1. The eye. The anterior segment is visible by simple inspection (A). The structures of the anterior segment include the cornea, iris, and eye lens (B). The posterior segment includes the vitreous chamber that is lined by the neurosensory retina (dashed line). The optic nerve head is visible in the eye.

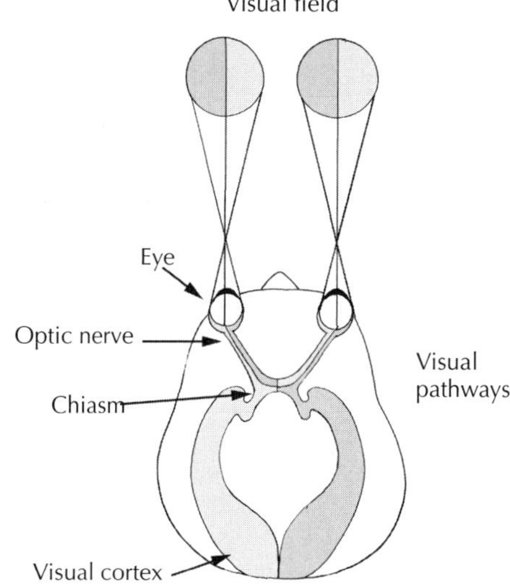

Figure 16.2. Diagram of the visual fields and corresponding pathways.

tion of the visit and the type of participation sought. Some doctors do this through written materials mailed in advance of the visit or through their web sites.

Caregivers can be an enormous help in preparing the individual with developmental disabilities for the visit by practicing how to name or match symbols used for vision tests and discussing the use of eye drops. These simple activities can make the difference between a frustrating visit and one at which reliable, high-quality information is obtained. For optimal performance, the individual must be physically comfortable and calm. Individuals with braces and other appliances must be positioned carefully, and the visit may take extra time. At times, examination under anesthesia may be required.

Acquisition of Information by History Taking

Some history will be obtained from medical and ophthalmic records. The examiner must be apprised of the individual's unifying diagnosis, current medical status, and medications. Some medications may have untoward

Table 16.2. Conditions with characteristic ophthalmic features

Condition	Ophthalmic feature	Web sites
Ataxia telangiectasia	Tortuous and dilated conjunctival and retinal blood vessels	http://www.medhelp.org/lib/ataxia.htm http://www.atcp.org/Clinical/Chap1.pdf
Cytomegalovirus (CMV), systemic	Chorioretinitis; brain injury (encephalopathy)	http://www.cdc.gov/ncidod/diseases/cmv.htm http://home.coqui.net/myrna/cmv.htm http://www.bcm.tmc.edu/pedi/infect/cmv/cmv-updt.htm
Herpes simplex virus (HSV-1), systemic	Retinitis; brain injury (encephalopathy)	http://www.healthandage.com/html/well_connected/pdf/doc52.pdf http://www.ihmf.org/guidelines/summary12.asp http://www.ihmf.org/general/resources04.asp
Neurofibromatosis	Lisch nodules on iris; optic glioma	http://www.nf.org
Prematurity	Retinopathy of prematurity (ROP)	http://www.ropard.org/what_is.shtml http://www.visionchannel.net/retinopathy/index.shtml http://www.nlm.nih.gov/medlineplus/print/ency/article/001618.htm http://www.emedicine.com/ped/topic1998.htm http://www.charles-retina.com/rop-faq.htm http://www.lowvision.org/retinopathy_of_prematurityxx.htm http://www.blindbabies.org/factsheet_rop.htm http://www.e-advisor.us
Tuberous sclerosis	Retinal hamartomas	http://www.nlm.nih.gov/medlineplus/ency/article/000787.htm http://www.ninds.nih.gov/disorders/tuberous_sclerosis/detail_tuberous_sclerosis.htm

Table 16.3. Eye care professionals

Ophthalmologist (M.D.)—Physician and surgeon who evaluates and treats medical and surgical disorders of the eyes and vision

Optometrist (O.D.)—Individual who evaluates and treats refractive and visual disorders

Orthoptist (M.S.)—Individual who evaluates motility and alignment, treats amblyopia, and works with ophthalmologists to evaluate visual function

Optician—Individual who fits eyeglasses and fills prescriptions for eyeglasses

Ocularist—Individual who designs and fits artificial eyes (prostheses) and scleral shells

Psychologist (Ph.D.)—Professional who evaluates visual processes

Teacher of individuals with visual impairments—educational specialist who works with individuals with low vision or blindness

Orientation and mobility instructor—professional who instructs individuals with visual impairments in procedures to navigate independently

effects on visual function. For instance, as many as one quarter to one third of individuals using Vigabatrin for seizures have visual field loss (Johnson, Krauss, Miller, Medura, & Paul, 2000; Krauss, Johnson, Sheth, & Miller, 2003). Brain lesions demonstrated on magnetic resonance imaging (MRI) scans may lead the examiner to anticipate visual field defects.

Potentially of equal importance is the history obtained from the patient, or the patient's proxy, parent, or other provider. Are there complaints about the eyes or vision? There is often a wealth of critical information in the patient's or family's telling of the vision or eye problem from their own perspective. Also, it is important to find out: Has something changed? When did it change? What activities have been affected?

Sensory Testing

Sensory tests are used to evaluate the function of the eye and the visual system. Acuity, the straight-ahead vision mediated by the fovea (see Figure 16.1), and visual field tests are the most frequently performed assessments of visual function.

Acuity Whether the individual has 20/20 vision or less is determined by measurement of acuity. *20/20* is a convention used to indicate that a symbol of a specific size and stroke can be seen 20 ft away. The specific size is one that subtends 5 min. arc visual angle and stroke width of 1 min. arc visual angle. If seven or eight block letters were written equally spaced across a thumbnail, and the thumb were held at arm's length, each letter would subtend approximately 5 min. arc. 20/200 symbols are 10 times larger. 20/200 on a letter test is a criterion for legal blindness, and eligibility for vision support services is often based on this criterion.

Letters are the most common symbols used in charts for acuity tests, and the most common procedure is for the individual to name the letters. However, not all individuals with developmental disabilities can perform such tests. Alternative test materials use letters or other symbols that the individual matches to a sample (Hyvarinen, Nasanen, & Laurinen, 1980; Sheridan & Gardiner, 1970). Such tests have wide application in pediatric ophthalmology and are also very useful in adults with developmental disabilities. Other tests, which originated as procedures for assessment of acuity in infants, have found application in assessment of those who cannot name letters and cannot be instructed in a matching task.

Johanna was a 23-year-old woman with retinal degeneration who had a rapid decline in vision. Examination indicated she had developed cataracts in both eyes. The cataracts were removed surgically, and intraocular lenses were implanted. Her visual acuity needed to be measured in order to monitor her response to treatment, but Johanna could not be tested using symbols or letters. Instead, her acuity was measured using preferential looking procedures such as the black and white stripes of the Teller Acuity Cards (TAC) procedure. The examiner, unaware of the right or left position of the stripes, observed Johanna's responses. Johanna indicated detection of the stripes by pointing, as shown in Figure 16.3, or simply by gazing to the right or left. The smallest stripe detected was taken as her acuity.

Preferential looking procedures (Teller, 1979) depend on the examiner's observation of the individual's looking behavior. The visual targets are stripes, technically called *gratings*. Preferential looking tests have been used to obtain acuities in individuals who could not otherwise have their acuity measured (Friedman, Munoz, Massof, Bandeen-Roche, & West, 2002; Haegerstrom-

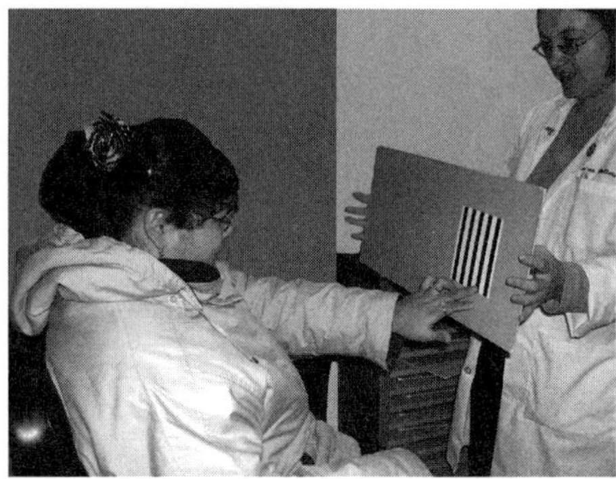

Figure 16.3. Johanna's acuity is tested using Teller Acuity Cards. She appoints to the black and white stripes as the examiner observes her response. The smallest stripe detected determines her visual acuity.

Portnoy, 1993; Mayer, Fulton, & Sossen, 1983). The TAC procedure (Teller, McDonald, Preston, Sebris, & Dobson, 1986) has been normed for clinical use (Mayer et al., 1995; Salomao & Ventura, 1995) and has had wide application in assessment of vision in those with developmental disabilities. A study of the TAC procedure in adults with cognitive impairments showed that a high percentage of these individuals were testable. For individuals who could also perform letter or symbol tests, TAC results correlated well with the letter and symbol acuities (Friedman et al., 2002).

The visual evoked potential (VEP), which has been described as a test of the brain waves from the visual areas of the brain, can also measure acuity (Norcia, 1994). Although not used as widely as preferential looking, eye doctors find VEP tests useful in some individuals with developmental disabilities who cannot have visual acuity measured with conventional tests.

Visual Field Procedures for mapping peripheral vision, known formally as *perimetry*, give information about visual performance in addition to that obtained by tests of acuity. Visual field defects are caused by disorders of the retina, optic nerve, or the brain (see Figure 16.2). They may impair behavior and affect mobility. For instance, in contrast to previously appropriate social behavior, one individual with developmental disabilities stopped shaking hands; an inferior visual field defect caused by retinal degeneration was measured. When this was discovered, a strategy was put into place so that a proffered hand was not ignored, and the individual was no longer considered antisocial. Inferior visual field loss may contribute to difficulties going down stairs and reading and writing. Field cuts to the right or left have predictable effects on navigating through doorways, on scanning the visual scene, and on reading performance.

In all perimetry on individuals with developmental disabilities, the examiner must be able to monitor the individual's fixation directly. Automated perimeters are not, generally speaking, suitable. Ideally, perimetry for individuals with developmental disabilities is performed using the Goldmann perimeter, and each eye is tested separately. For some individuals, the binocular visual field provides important functional information.

Eight-year-old Xander's disorder put him at risk of retinal degeneration. Therefore, he had his visual fields monitored as part of his ophthalmic care. As retinal degeneration progresses, visual field is lost. Xander was positioned in his standing wheelchair at the Goldmann perimeter (see Figure 16.4). His right eye was patched in preparation for testing his left eye, and he was positioned by the chin and brow rest. In his left hand, he held a buzzer used to indicate detection of the test spots. The examiner monitored his fixation through a telescope while controlling the presentation of small test spots on the inner white surface of the perimeter.

Point by point, the examiner mapped Xander's seeing and nonseeing areas to create visual field maps for each eye (see Figure 16.5). Larger, brighter test spots produced bigger fields than smaller, dimmer spots. The small crosshatched area in each map represents the normal blind spot that corresponds to the optic nerve head. Xander was found to have mild constriction of his visual fields.

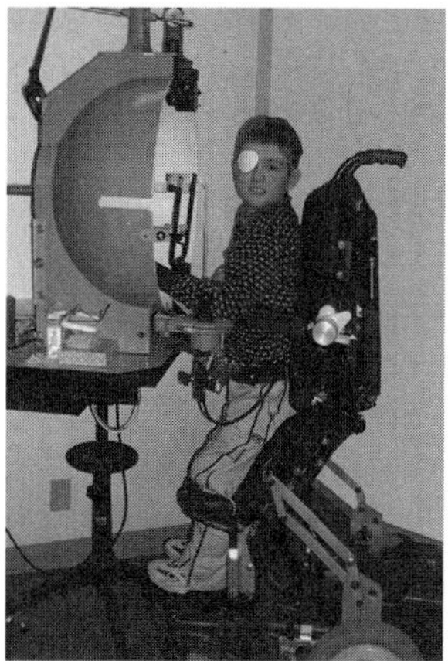
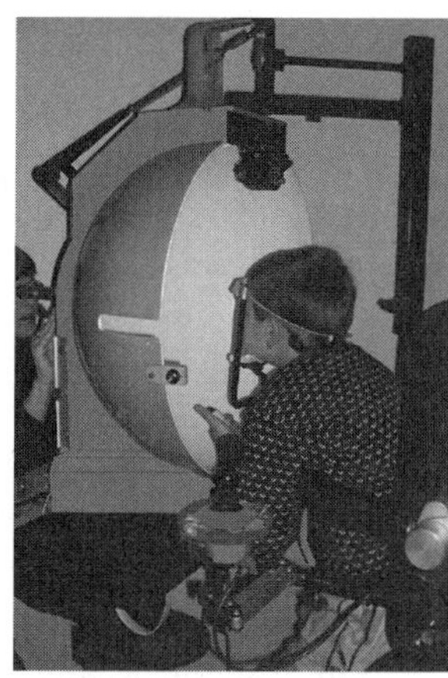

Figure 16.4. Xander positioned in a standing wheelchair at a Goldmann perimeter. His right eye is patched in preparation for the test (left photo). He uses a chin and brow rest to remain in position (right photo).

An example of progressive loss of visual fields in a woman with Bardet-Biedl syndrome and retinal degeneration is shown in Figure 16.6. When the woman was age 17 years, the peripheral islands of vision and the small central field supported her independent navigation. As time went by, the peripheral islands were lost, and progressive constriction of the central field occurred over a 5-year-period. Now, the woman's mobility is aided by cane travel and assistance of sighted individuals.

Gary was a 22-year-old man with a neurodegenerative disorder. He had progressive loss of visual acuity and visual field due to atrophy of the optic nerve. For visual field testing, his mother helped him maintain his position in the perimeter. He was unable to press the buzzer but indicated detection of the test spot verbally. His binocular field (see Figure 16.7) for the largest, brightest test spot in the Goldmann instrument (V-4e, 1.7 degrees) was markedly constricted (solid outline) compared with normal (dashed outline). Besides marked constriction of visual field, he had low acuity, only 20/125 in his better eye, and marked impairments in contrast sensitivity.

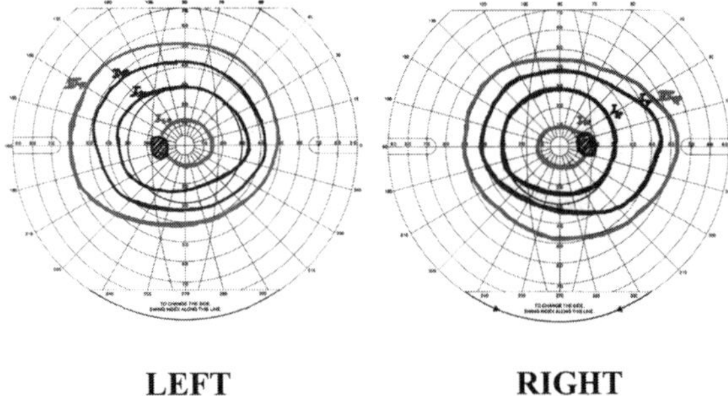

Figure 16.5. Visual field map for Xander's eyes. Heavy lines outline the seeing area at the visual field.

For individuals who cannot perform on the Goldmann instrument, other simpler perimeters, originally designed for infants and young children, have been developed (Cummings, van Hof-van Duin, Mayer, Hansen, & Fulton, 1988; Dobson, Brown, Harvey, & Narter, 1998; Mayer & Fulton, 1993; Mayer, Fulton, & Cummings, 1988; Quinn, Fea, & Minguini, 1991; van Hof-van Duin & Mohn, 1986). In these instruments, a small number of larger test targets are used. Data from typically developing individuals have been obtained, and individuals with ophthalmic and brain disorders have been studied (Mayer & Fulton, 1993; Mohn & van Hof-van Duin, 1983; Quinn et al., 1996; van Hof-van Duin & Mohn, 1986). In short, major visual field defects can be assessed, but refined maps, such as Goldmann maps, are not obtained with the simpler instruments.

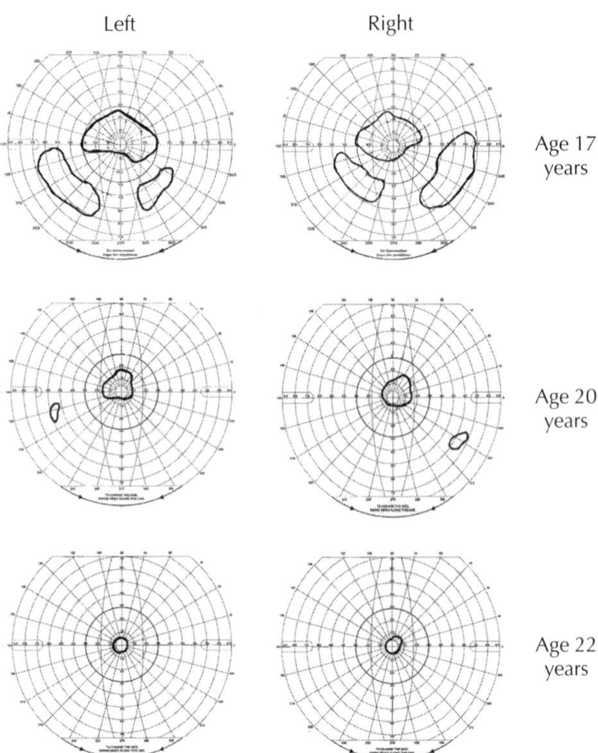

Figure 16.6. Goldmann visual field of both eyes of a woman with Bardet-Biedl syndrome and retinal degeneration. These maps were made using the largest, brightest target (V-e, 1.7 degrees) in the perimeter. Heavy black lines outline the islands of her seeing visual field.

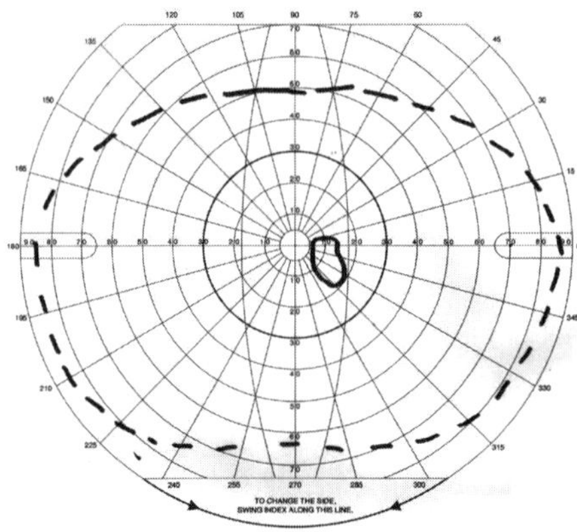

Figure 16.7. Gary's binocular field measured using the Goldmann perimeter. Heavy lines outline the seeing area at the visual field whereas dashed lines show the normal visual field.

The normal visual field, if measured with a 6 mm. white target, subtends nearly 200 degrees visual angle. Visual field constricted to 20 degrees is a definition of legal blindness (see Figure 16.7), just as a letter acuity of 20/200 is another definition of legal blindness. The width of two hands, thumbs abutted, held at arm's length subtends approximately 20 degrees visual angle. Such a limited visual field impairs mobility and orientation and, thus, activities of daily living.

Physical Examination

Assessment of the alignment and motility of the eyes, pupillary responses, and structures in the anterior and posterior segments of the eyes (see Figure 16.1) is performed during an eye examination. The eye doctor uses instruments such as the slitlamp biomicroscope and the indirect ophthalmoscope to obtain magnified, stereoscopic, and panoramic views of the ocular structures. If possible, the intraocular pressure is measured to check for glaucoma (high pressure in the eye). Drops that dilate the pupil are used to facilitate a complete view of the structures in the interior of the eye. Also, measurement of the eyes for glasses, called *refraction*, is often best done after the dilating drops.

Management

A logical plan for management rests on the results of the history and examination with due consideration of the unifying diagnosis, including referral to other eye care specialists if needed (see Table 16.3). A reasonable plan for follow-up must be outlined that ensures sound and appropriate ophthalmic care without making the individual and his or her family feel abandoned.

COMMON EYE AND VISION ISSUES

Some common eye issues are presented next in alphabetical order.

Blepharitis

Blephantis, or chronic crusts and redness along the lid margins, require persistent hygiene and ophthalmic attention. Blepharitis is common in Down syndrome. Regular habits of care are best established early on, even in childhood, and maintained throughout adolescence and adulthood.

Cataracts

Cataracts mean opacification of the eye lens (see Figure 16.1). If the opacity is very tiny, it has no impact on vision. On the other hand, the opacity may be so extensive and dense, or positioned in the lens, as to cause significant defects in vision. Significant defects are those that hinder activities of daily living. Cataracts may be anticipated within the pediatric age range in Smith-Lemli-Opitz (Elias, Hansen, Irons, Quinn, & Fulton, 2003) and Cockayne syndromes and occasionally in retinal degenerations of early onset. In other syndromes, such as Down syndrome, visually significant cataracts become more frequent with increasing age.

Greta, a teenager with Down syndrome, had progressive decline in visual abilities when a cataract developed. Figure 16.8 shows the cataract as seen using a slitlamp biomicroscope. Greta's vision was improved by surgical removal of the cataracts followed by prescription of cataract glasses. To compensate for the optical power previously provided by the eye lens, glasses were prescribed. Cataract glasses are magnifying lenses, so they make the eyes look large.

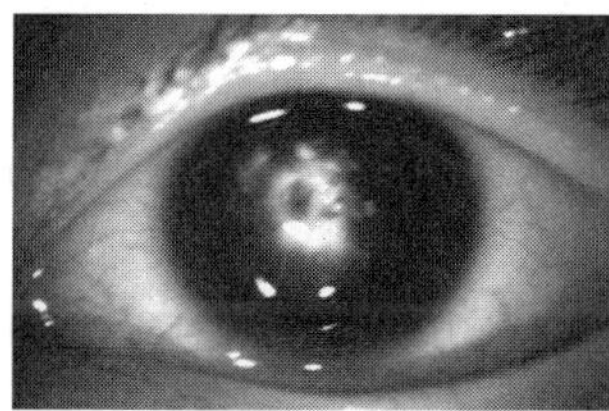

Figure 16.8. A cataract as seen through a slitlamp biomicroscope.

Glasses and Refractive Errors

If the eye's natural optics do not focus a clear image on the retina, glasses may be indicated. In myopia (nearsightedness), the natural optics of the eye focus images in front of the retina. In hyperopia (farsightedness), the image is optically "behind the retina." In astigmatism, the whole image is not in the same focal plane. Eye doctors are trained to measure (refract) the eyes to determine the ophthalmic lenses that put a clear image on the retina. Glasses prescriptions are based on the results of these measurements.

High refractive errors are quite common among individuals with developmental disabilities. Some are associated with a history of retinopathy of prematurity (Quinn et al., 1998) and cerebral palsy. High refractive errors are associated with syndromes that have retinal degeneration as a feature. These include Alstrom, Bardet-Biedl, and Cohen syndromes.

Association of serious eye problems with high refractive errors are recognized. Usually, eye examinations are required to diagnose eye problems. Thus, regular eye care is very important in individuals with high refractive errors, particularly in those with developmental disabilities and limited communication skills. In general, high myopia is associated with a larger, longer eye; stretched retina; and increased risk of retinal detachment, either spontaneous or posttraumatic. Retinal detachment means separation of the retina from the wall of the eye (see Figure 16.1). Eyes with high hyperopia tend to be smaller, with "crowded" anterior segment structures and a relatively higher risk of glaucoma (high pressure in the eyes).

Overall, compliance with eyeglass wear can be achieved in those with developmental disabilities, with the following considerations. If the frame is comfortable and the wearer recognizes improved vision, the glasses are usually accepted. The cooperation of a skilled and knowledgeable optician (see Table 16.3) is needed for successful eyeglass fitting in those with special needs, such as wheelchairs with wrap-around head support. There are cases in which high refractive errors are identified, but the individual's optic nerve, or retina, is diseased, and thus, the individual cannot take advantage of the clear image on the retina. Even in the face of disease, however, some retinal or optic nerve function may persist, and a trial of glasses may be advised, especially if tests indicate acuity is improved by glasses.

Some restless individuals intermittently pull the glasses off. An elastic strap is a gentle deterrent. A more rugged sports frame with a strap has been helpful in securing needed glasses in some active individuals. For individuals with tactile defensiveness, constant reinforcement and, at times, vigorous behavior modification programs have been needed to achieve acceptance of eyeglasses. Some parents have reported success if the eyeglasses are placed on the sleeping individual just before awakening.

Besides refractive errors, glasses are indicated for protection. In functionally monocular individuals, safety glasses are mandatory. Protective eye wear is also recommended for individuals with development delays and low vision who regularly encounter high risks for eye injury. Such individuals do not see and avoid the dangers of eye injury effectively.

Low Vision

Low vision is defined as acuity less than 20/70 with best possible ordinary glasses (Corn & Koenig, 1996). In an individual with visual impairment and developmental disabilities, an evaluation by an eye care specialist with expertise in low vision should be considered. Experience with individuals with developmental disabilities is essential.

Magnification systems and individualized strategies for using residual vision are the mainstays of low vision interventions. In general, the individual must have measurable acuity, albeit low, to benefit from a magnification system. The low vision expert selects these systems based on the visual needs and physical and cognitive abilities of the individual. Among the most effective devices are magnifiers that require little manipulation, such as a spectacle-mounted magnifier. This device takes the form of a high-power bifocal and is highly successful in individuals with cerebral palsy because no hand manipulation is required.

Handheld magnifiers are available in a range of powers. These devices are ideal for short-term use such as finding something on a map, inspecting coins, and reading a limited amount of text. The individual must be able to manipulate the device to find the appropriate focusing distance. Stand magnifiers that are used for reading, require a significant amount of manipulation to move across the reading material. Closed circuit television is an option for some individuals with low acuity. Sharing the joy of an individual with low vision who can now see pictures, books, and other near work with the aid of a closed circuit television is truly heartening.

For distance viewing, monoculars or telescopic devices may be considered. Successful use comes after training to spot street signs, the blackboard, or other distant objects.

Besides magnifying devices, strategies to use residual vision are developed under the guidance of the low vision specialist. Home, classroom, and working environments must be modified to create safe, organized, and visually appropriate settings. Specially marked edges of stairs and boldly marked routes in school and worksites have been helpful for some individuals. Braille (Corn & Koenig, 1996) and other markings with tactile cues are appropriate for others if visual reading is impossible or insufficient to support fluent reading. Large print materials are an alternative or adjunct to magnification. Light sensitivity (photophobia) is addressed by placement to avoid facing light sources; tinted lenses as well as hats and visors may be indicated.

Prematurity and Retinopathy of Prematurity

Visual impairment in individuals with a history of preterm birth may be due to disorders of the eye, the brain, or both. In general, the earlier the preterm birth and the lower the birth weight, the greater the risk of visual impairment. Retinopathy of prematurity (ROP) has its onset at preterm ages when both the retinal vasculature and neural retina are immature (see Chapter 10). The abnormal retinal vasculature, which is the clinical hallmark of ROP, appears to be a response to retinal hypoxia as the oxygen-greedy photoreceptors develop. Approximately 80% of infants with birth weight less than 1,000 g. develop ROP.

Fortunately, the vascular changes of ROP are more likely to resolve than to progress and lead to retinal detachment. The recommendations for treatment of preterm infants with ROP have been revised as the characteristics of high-risk ROP have been defined (Hardy et al., 2003). Laser treatment of earlier stages of ROP has been demonstrated to improve functional outcome, as measured by preferential looking acuity, and structural outcome, as defined by ophthalmoscopic criteria (Early Treatment of Retinopathy of Prematurity Cooperative Group, 2003). Nonetheless, even if an infant has a good response to laser therapy in early infancy or has ROP so mild that it resolves spontaneously, he or she may have future visual impairments and ocular problems. Some develop high myopia in early childhood and have a lifelong risk of retinal detachment. In some, acuity is low, apparently due to retinal changes more subtle than retinal detachment.

Preterm birth is also associated with brain injuries including hypoxic ischemic encephalopathy, hydrocephalus secondary to intraventricular hemorrhage, and periventricular leukomalacia. These children with brain injuries are at risk for cerebral visual impairment and visual field loss, especially from periventricular leukomalacia. The majority of these children have strabismus, and many have nystagmus. The brain injuries of prematurity are the basis for cerebral palsy in some children.

Progressive Visual Loss

Retinal degenerations ("retinitis pigmentosa") are one set of conditions that cause progressive visual loss. The diagnosis of any condition that forecasts progressive visual loss weighs heavily on the individual and his or her family and is particularly tragic if progressive sensorineural hearing loss also occurs. Alström syndrome is an example of a condition in which developmental disabilities and diabetes accompany visual and hearing loss. Vigorous educational and emotional supports must shore up the family's struggle to accept visual loss and prepare them to dream new dreams.

Strabismus

Strabismus (misalignment of the eyes; crossing in or turning out of the eyes) is a common and nonspecific feature among individuals with developmental disabilities. Strabismus does not necessarily mean that vision is poor. However, poor vision in one eye (amblyopia, "lazy eye") is in some cases associated with strabismus. Treatment of amblyopia by patching is important in early childhood. In infancy and the early childhood years, development of the visual system is in progress. In these years, the visual system is plastic and responsive to external influences such as patching ("occlusion therapy"). With increasing age of the child, plasticity gradually diminishes. After age 10 years, patching is much less effective than in early childhood. Strabismus, especially in children, is an indication for prompt referral to an ophthalmologist.

Some types of strabismus, such as accommodative esotropia, are improved with glasses. For strabismus that is not improved with glasses, surgery warrants consideration. As a rule of thumb, strabismus surgery is considered if the angle (the amount) of strabismus is large and stable. Thus, if the strabismus is conspicuous, referral to an ophthalmologist is recommended so that appropriate management may be determined. In fact, many details determine if strabismus surgery is advisable and what procedures are appropriate. The indications for surgery are well known to experts in the management of strabismus, and thorough review of all of the history and current details is needed to make an appropriate plan. Variability in the angle of strabismus is common in individuals with neurological impairments, and, in general, is a reason for a cautious approach to strabismus surgery. On the other hand, changes in the characteristics of strabismus, or sudden onset of strabismus in an older child or adult, warrants prompt investigation by a physician. For instance, sixth nerve palsies and loss of ability to turn an eye outward (abduct) may accompany increases in intracranial pressure.

CONCLUSION

Multiple medical problems are not rare among those with developmental disabilities. Even in the face of serious medical problems, over and over again families tell us that visual impairment ranks as a significant disability. We believe in early, aggressive evaluation to define visual *abilities* because the evaluation is the basis for a plan to ameliorate the visual impairment. The earlier the individual can take advantage of residual vision, the better the long-term outcome. A team consisting of individuals with expertise in low vision, skills in evaluation of eyes and visual pathways using a battery of tests originally developed for infants and young children, and knowledge about vision-impairing ocular and systemic conditions performs these evaluations. Ongoing clinical collaborations with superb colleagues in medical and surgical specialties are critical to good eye and vision care of the individual with multiple medical problems. Links to dedicated vocational, educational, and service professionals make eye and vision care all worthwhile.

REFERENCES

Corn, A.L., & Koenig, A.J. (1996). *Foundations of low vision: Clinical and functional perspectives.* New York: AFB Press.

Cummings, M.F., van Hof-van Duin, J., Mayer, D.L., Hansen, R.M., & Fulton, A.B. (1988). Visual fields of young children. *Behavioural Brain Research, 29*(1–2), 7–16.

Dobson, V., Brown, A.M., Harvey, E.M., & Narter, D.B. (1998). Visual field extent in children 3.5–30 months of age tested with a double-arc LED perimeter. *Vision Research, 38*(18), 2743–2760.

Early Treatment of Retinopathy of Prematurity Cooperative Group. (2003). Revised indications for the treatment of retinopathy of prematurity. *Archives of Ophthalmology, 121,* 1684–1696.

Elias, E.R., Hansen, R.M., Irons, M., Quinn, N., & Fulton, A.B. (2003). Rod photoreceptor responses in children with Smith-Lemli-Opitz syndrome. *Archives of Ophthalmology, 121*(12), 1738–1743.

Friedman, D.S., Munoz, B., Massof, R.W., Bandeen-Roche, K., & West, S.K. (2002). Grating visual acuity using the preferential-looking method in elderly nursing home residents. *Investigative Ophthalmology & Visual Science, 43*(8), 2572–2578.

Haegerstrom-Portnoy, G. (1993). New procedures for evaluating vision functions of special populations. *Optometry and Vision Science, 70*(4), 306–314.

Hardy, R.J., Palmer, E.A., Dobson, V., Summers, C.G., Phelps, D.L., Quinn, G.E., et al. (2003). Risk analysis of prethreshold retinopathy of prematurity. *Archives of Ophthalmology, 121*, 1696–1701.

Hyvarinen, L., Nasanen, R., & Laurinen, P. (1980). New visual acuity test for pre-school children. *Acta Ophthalmologica, 58*(4), 507–511.

Johnson, M.A., Krauss, G.L., Miller, N.R., Medura, M., & Paul, S.R. (2000). Visual function loss from vigabatrin: Effect of stopping the drug. *Neurology, 55*(1), 40–45.

Krauss, G.L., Johnson, M.A., Sheth, S., & Miller, N.R. (2003). A controlled study comparing visual function in patients treated with vigabatrin and tiagabine. *Journal of Neurology, Neurosurgery, and Psychiatry, 74*(3), 339–343.

Mangione, C.M., Gutierrez, P.R., Lowe, G., Orav, E.J., & Seddon, J.M. (1999). Influence of age-related maculopathy on visual functioning and health-related quality of life. *American Journal of Ophthalmology, 128*(1), 45–53.

Mangione, C.M., Phillips, R.S., Lawrence, M.G., Seddon, J.M., Orav, E.J., & Goldman, L. (1994). Improved visual function and attenuation of declines in health-related quality of life after cataract extraction. *Archives of Ophthalmology, 112*(11), 1419–1425.

Mayer, D.L., Beiser, A.S., Warner, A.F., Pratt, E.M., Raye, K.N., & Lang, J.M. (1995). Monocular acuity norms for the Teller Acuity Cards between ages one month and four years. *Investigative Ophthalmology & Visual Science, 36*(3), 671–685.

Mayer, D.L., & Fulton, A.B. (1993). Development of the human visual field. In K. Simons (Ed.), *Early visual development: Normal and abnormal* (pp. 117–129). New York: Oxford University Press.

Mayer, D.L., Fulton, A.B., & Cummings, M.F. (1988). Visual fields of infants assessed with a new perimetric technique. *Investigative Ophthalmology & Visual Science, 29*(3), 452–459.

Mayer, D.L., Fulton, A.B., & Sossen, P.L. (1983). Preferential looking acuity of pediatric patients with developmental disabilities. *Behavioural Brain Research, 10*(1), 189–197.

Mohn, G., & van Hof-van Duin, J. (1983). Behavioural and electrophysiological measures of visual function in children with neurological disorders. *Behavioral Brain Research, 10*, 177–187.

Norcia, A.M. (1994). Vision testing by visual evoked potential techniques. In S.J. Isenberg (Ed.), *The eye in infancy* (2nd ed., pp. 157–173). St. Louis: Mosby-Year Book.

Quinn, G.E., Dobson, V., Hardy, R.J., Tung, B., Phelps, D., & Palmer, E.A. (1996). Visual fields measured with double-arc perimetry in eyes with threshold retinopathy of prematurity from the cryotherapy for retinopathy of prematurity trial. *Ophthalmology, 103*, 1432–1437.

Quinn, G.E., Dobson, V., Kivlin, J., Kaufman, L.M., Repka, M.X., Reynolds, J.D., et al. (1998). Prevalence of myopia between 3 months and 5 ½ years in preterm infants with and without retinopathy of prematurity: Cryotherapy for Retinopathy of Prematurity Cooperative Group. *Ophthalmology, 105*(7), 1292–1300.

Quinn, G. E., Fea, A. M., & Minguini, N. (1991). Visual fields in 4- to 10-year-old children using Goldmann and double-arc perimeters. *Journal of Pediatric Ophthalmology and Strabismus, 28*(6), 314–319.

Salomao, S.R., & Ventura, D.F. (1995). Large sample population age norms for visual acuities obtained with Vistech-Teller Acuity Cards. *Investigative Ophthalmology & Visual Science, 36*(3), 657–670.

Sheridan, M.D., & Gardiner, P.A. (1970). Sheridan-Gardiner test for visual acuity. *British Medical Journal, 2*(701), 108–109.

Teller, D.Y. (1979). The forced choice preferential looking method: A psychophysical technique for use with human infants. *Infant Behavior and Development, 2*, 135–153.

Teller, D.Y., McDonald, M.A., Preston, K., Sebris, S.L., & Dobson, V. (1986). Assessment of visual acuity in infants and children: The acuity card procedure. *Developmental Medicine and Child Neurology, 28*(6), 779–789.

van Hof-van Duin, J., & Mohn, G. (1986). Visual field measurements, optokinetic nystagmus and the visual threatening response: Normal and abnormal development. *Documenta Ophthalmologica, 45*, 305–316.

Warburg, M. (2001). Visual impairment in adult people with intellectual disability: Literature review. *Journal of Intellectual Disability Research, 45*(5), 424–438.

CHAPTER 17

OTOLARYNGOLOGY

17.1 HEARING IMPAIRMENT

Marilyn W. Neault

Hearing loss may be the least visible and most often missed condition affecting individuals with multiple disabilities. Even when hearing loss has been diagnosed properly, remediation rarely optimizes access to spoken language. Hearing aids may not be well tolerated, well maintained, or properly adjusted. In addition, the acoustics of the classroom or workspace of the individual using the hearing aid may be noisy and reverberant, with multiple talkers preventing good reception of a single voice.

The advent of newborn hearing screening has drastically lowered the age of identification of hearing loss in children. Prior to newborn screening, permanent hearing loss in children was diagnosed on average after the second birthday (Harrison, Roush, & Wallace, 2003). A child with a complex medical history or developmental disabilities might have been referred for audiological evaluation as part of a "review of systems" so that the hearing loss was diagnosed after other conditions were unmasked. Now, a hearing loss may be confirmed within the first month of life.

Diagnosis of the hearing loss first in a child with other challenges has advantages for the child but often some wrinkles for the parents, who may have identified themselves with parents of typical deaf and hard of hearing children only to discover that hearing loss is the least of their child's problems (Roush, Holcomb, Roush, & Escolar, 2004). The Annual Survey of Deaf and Hard of Hearing Children and Youth establishes the number of individuals with permanent hearing loss in addition to other conditions (Gallaudet Research Institute, 2003). Table 17.1-1 lists the prevalence of developmental disabilities in more than 40,000 children with hearing loss in the United States.

Jackson spent the first 1½ years of his life in the hospital. Because he was critically ill and underwent many surgeries, his newborn hearing screening test did not take place until he was 13 months old. He did not pass the newborn hearing screening test in either ear. A diagnostic auditory brainstem response (ABR) evaluation at age 14 months showed profound bilateral hearing loss. Although Jackson had not yet been discharged from the hospital, he was fitted with hearing aids, and a teacher of the deaf visited him frequently to introduce sign language to him and his family.

THRESHOLD SENSITIVITY FOR TONES

When an individual is capable of showing awareness of soft sounds, hearing acuity can be tested for tones with the individual's cooperation. Results are displayed on an *audiogram*, a chart of the weakest intensities at which the person can detect each of various frequencies in each ear. Although the human ear is sensitive to frequencies from 20Hz (low frequency, giving a perception of a low pitched or "bass" sound) to 20,000Hz (high frequency, giving a perception of a high pitched or "treble" sound), only the frequencies 250Hz to 8,000Hz typically are tested because nearly all of the acoustic energy in speech falls in that range. The ranges of normal hearing and hearing loss are shown in Figure 17.1-1.

An individual may have normal hearing for sounds in one frequency range but a significant hearing loss for other frequencies. The degree of hearing loss often is described by averaging the thresholds (weakest detected intensity) for the frequencies 500Hz, 1,000Hz, and 2,000Hz in each ear, expressing the degree of hearing loss as the "three frequency pure tone average" hearing level. Table 17.1-2 states rough guidelines for the effect of hearing loss of varying degrees on the ability to hear speech and on educational and vocational needs.

If a hearing loss is unilateral, the listener hears speech at a normal loudness and clarity with the good ear but has difficulty 1) hearing a weak voice on the side of the poorer hearing ear; 2) focusing on one voice in background noise; and 3) localizing the direction from which a sound is coming. Children with unilateral hearing loss, even when diagnosed early, are more likely to need academic support services in elementary school than typically hearing children (Lieu, 2004), presumably because of difficulty hearing the teacher in noise. Teachers and caregivers of a person with unilateral

Table 17.1-1. Percentage of children known to be deaf or hard of hearing who also have other conditions

Condition (more than one may occur in the same child)	Percent of children
None	60.1
Learning disability	10.7
Intellectual disability	9.8
Attention deficit disorder	6.6
Visual impairment	3.9
Cerebral palsy	3.4
Emotional disturbance	1.7
Other conditions	12.1
Not reported	11.9

Note: The total number of children surveyed was 42,361.
Source: Gallaudet Research Institute (2003).

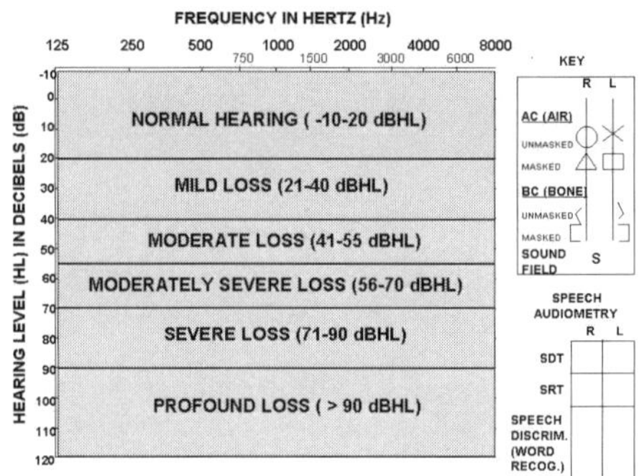

Figure 17.1-1. Ranges of hearing loss in decibels, on an audiogram.

hearing loss and additional disabilities need to have a high level of awareness of presenting sound to the better ear and reducing background noise competition.

Figure 17.1-2 is an audiogram showing normal hearing bilaterally (measured in each ear separately). Thresholds of detection for pure tones presented through earphones (by *air conduction*) are depicted by “O” symbols for the right ear and “X” symbols for the left ear. The person’s speech reception threshold (SRT), which is the weakest intensity at which one can present familiar two-syllable “spondee” words (e.g., airplane, baseball, hotdog) and have the person repeat at least 50% of them correctly, is within 5 decibels of the three frequency pure tone average hearing level, as expected. The person’s speech discrimination (word recognition) score, or the percentage of words repeated (or pictures pointed to) correctly when the words are presented at a comfortably audible intensity, is very good in each ear.

Figure 17.1-3 shows a mild conductive hearing loss for the right ear and a severe sensorineural hearing loss for the left ear. The three frequency pure tone average hearing level by air conduction for the right ear (for which the thresholds are marked with “O” symbols) is 25dBHL, which is in the mild hearing loss range. When the sounds are presented through a *bone conduction oscillator*, which bypasses mechanical attenuation of the sound by outer or middle ear problems, the person has hearing thresholds well within the normal hearing range, marked by “<” symbols.

Because hearing thresholds are normal by bone conduction but reduced by air conduction, the mild hearing loss in the right ear is *conductive*. The amount of the hearing loss between air and bone conduction thresholds is called the *air-bone gap*. This amount helps to predict how much the hearing loss could be improved if the reason for the conductive loss, such as cerumen impaction, middle ear effusion, or tympanic membrane perforation, could be ameliorated. When the bone conduction thresholds agree with the air conduction thresholds in a case of hearing loss, the hearing loss is *sensorineural* (inner ear or, less commonly, auditory nerve in origin). The left ear in Figure 17.1-3 shows a severe hearing loss. The difference between the air conduction thresholds on the left and the bone conduction thresholds on the right (normal hearing range) warranted “masking” while testing the left ear thresholds, which means that a noise was introduced into the right (better ear) earphone while test sounds were being presented to the left ear, to keep the right ear from helping out by detecting sounds that crossed the head.

Figure 17.1-4 shows a profound bilateral sensorineural hearing loss. The three frequency pure tone hearing levels for each ear are greater than 90dBHL by air conduction. Although this person can detect some low frequency bone conducted sounds (as indicated by the “<” and “>” symbols), the bone conduction thresholds fall in an intensity range at which the stimuli can be felt as vibrations on the skin and do not signal a conductive component to the hearing loss.

When the person undergoing the audiological evaluation cannot tolerate wearing earphones for separate-ear threshold measurements, sounds can be presented through calibrated loudspeakers in the audiologist’s sound-treated booth. The resulting thresholds are called *sound field thresholds*. If the person being tested has better thresholds in one ear than the other, the sound field thresholds will reflect the better-ear hearing sensitivity. Without separate-ear measures, one cannot guess which ear is better from the test results alone. One can be assured, however, that at least one ear hears as well as the sound field thresholds indicate.

The audiogram in Figure 17.1-5 is a sound field audiogram showing that either both ears or the better-hearing ear has a mild hearing loss, assuming that the person being tested was able to respond to the weakest

Table 17.1-2. Impact of various degrees of hearing loss

Degree of loss in better ear	Effect on hearing speech	Impact on language, education, and vocation
Mild (21–40dBHL)	The individual can understand speech one-to-one at 3 feet if language development is already established. He or she hears parts of utterance at greater distance. The person misses or mishears word endings. He or she benefits from hearing aids.	The condition causes mild delay in language development. The individual benefits from acoustical treatment of the classroom. He or she attends inclusive educational placement if hearing loss is the only issue.
Moderate (41–55dBHL)	The person can understand speech one-to-one at 2–3 feet only with clear delivery and with lipreading. He or she may not hear 75% of speech sounds without hearing aids. The person benefits from hearing aids.	The condition causes delayed language development and speech articulation errors if present in early childhood. The individual needs educational supports to learn in inclusive classrooms. On the job with hearing aids, the individual needs to look at the talker's face when listening. He or she may use an amplified telephone.
Moderately severe (56–70dBHL)	The individual understands only loud speech close to the ear and catches occasional loud words in an utterance. He or she benefits from hearing aids.	Significant language delay is expected if the condition is present in childhood and not remediated beginning in early infancy. Educational placement depends on spoken language skills. An FM educational amplification system is needed to hear the teacher. On the job, the individual needs readback/feedback of instructions and modified communication strategies to hear in a group.
Severe (71–90dBHL)	The individual may hear a loud voice close to the ear. Without hearing aids, he or she does not detect conversational speech. The person needs early detection, hearing aids, and aggressive therapy to avoid significant language delay. He or she has difficulty monitoring the loudness and clarity of his or her own voice. Cochlear implantation is an option if speech recognition with hearing aids is poor despite training.	Delay in spoken language development is expected if the condition is not remediated beginning in early infancy. The individual needs small specialized class placement unless his or her language skills are robustly normal. Many individuals develop both spoken language and sign language. They should have friends and mentors with hearing loss. On the job, the supervisor and co-workers should be taught how to communicate successfully. The person may be able to use an amplified telephone with a telephone switch on the hearing aid.
Profound (> 90dBHL)	The person is aware of a few loud environmental sounds. He or she does not develop speech without early use of hearing aids and intensive therapy. The individual may rely on sign language to communicate and is unlikely to understand words through hearing aids without visual cues. Cochlear implantation is an option if it is psychoeducationally appropriate for the person.	The individual typically needs a small self-contained class for deaf children unless a cochlear implant in infancy resulted in rapid spoken language development, in which case an inclusive placement with support services may succeed. The individual needs deaf friends and mentors. With hearing aids, the person is unlikely to be able to use the telephone; he or she needs a TTY (teletypewriter) for phone use. E-mail is preferred to telephone use.

intensities he or she could detect. If bone conduction thresholds are obtained through a bone conduction oscillator for this individual and are normal, then the hearing loss is conductive (outer or middle ear in origin) in at least one ear. This degree of hearing loss is the same amount one would expect from an asymptomatic middle ear effusion (Fria, Cantekin, & Eichler, 1985) and in fact is approximately the amount of conductive

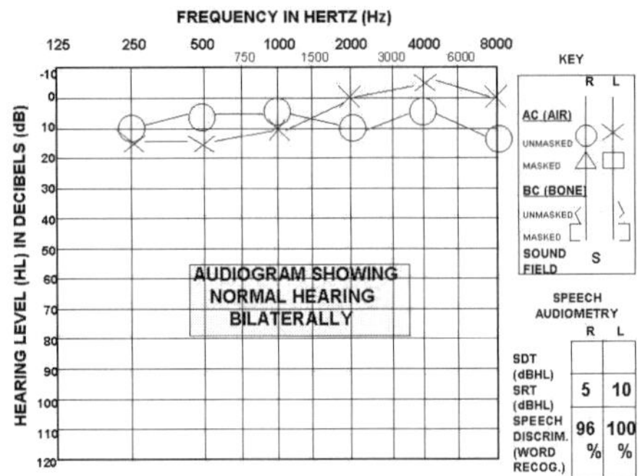

Figure 17.1-2. Audiogram showing normal hearing bilaterally.

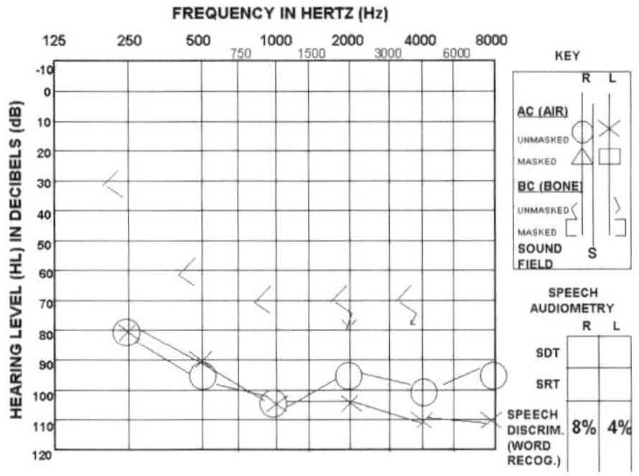

Figure 17.1-4. Profound bilateral sensorineural hearing loss.

hearing loss one has while wearing earplugs for ear protection or while placing one's fingers tightly in one's ears.

The examples of audiograms apply to individuals who can participate in a *behavioral audiological evaluation*, meaning one in which the person is awake and indicates awareness of the presence of the sound. The manner in which the person responds varies with developmental age and motor abilities. Working downward in age, an individual with a developmental age of 6 years and older (sometimes as young as 4 or 5 years) can perform *conventional audiometry* by raising his or her hand or pushing a button every time he or she hears a tone. Individuals with a developmental age of 2½–5 years are best tested using *conditioned play audiometry*, in which they place a block in a bucket, a penny in a bank, or a peg in a pegboard every time they hear a tone. The results of conditioned play audiometry are as reliable as conventional audiometry.

If the developmental level or motor coordination is not high enough for conditioned play audiometry, *visual reinforcement audiometry (VRA)* is used. In VRA, eye-shift or head-turn responses to the sound are rewarded by activation of a lighted mechanical toy. The test can be performed with the sounds coming either from the speakers (sound field testing) or through earphones for separate-ear audiograms. Infants younger than 6 months and older people who do not overtly orient or reliably alert to sounds cannot be tested successfully with VRA. In such cases, behavioral observation audiometry (BOA), or the observation of any behavioral change to sound such as a change in breathing or cessation of sucking on a pacifier, can give some information about hearing but rarely serves as a reliable means of threshold estimation. When hearing cannot reliably be tested by behavioral audiometric methods, the audiologist turns to physiological measures such as the ABR test, which is discussed later.

SPEECH AUDIOMETRY

The speech detection threshold (SDT), also called the speech awareness threshold, can be measured by observing the weakest level at which the individual responds to calibrated speech using the audiometer. The SDT typically agrees with the best of the pure tone thresholds in the lower and middle frequencies on the audiogram. If the individual being tested can repeat words or

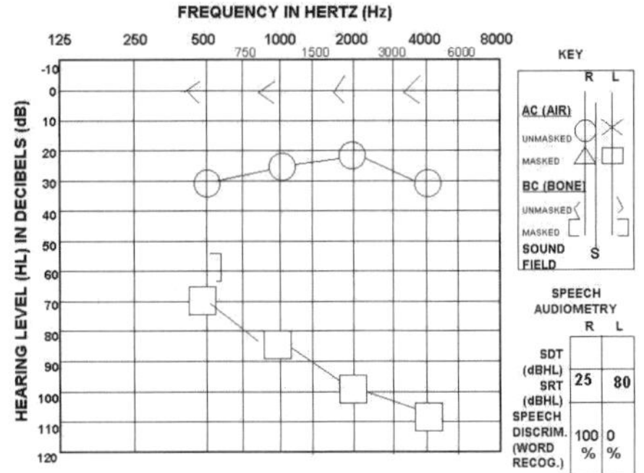

Figure 17.1-3. Mild conductive hearing loss in the right ear, and severe sensorineural hearing loss in the left ear.

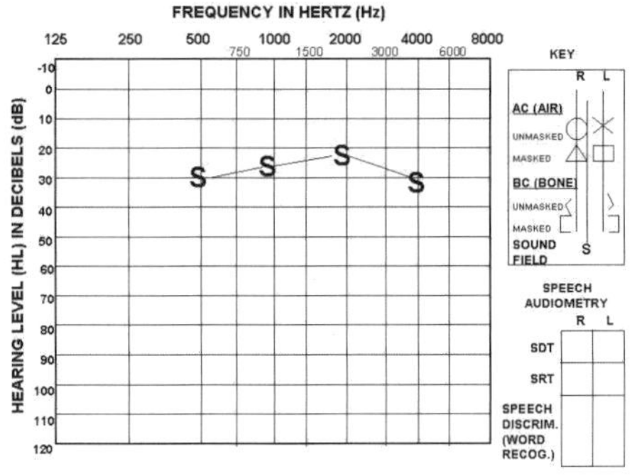

Figure 17.1-5. Mild hearing loss by sound field audiometry.

point to pictures or objects representing words, then the speech reception threshold (SRT), or the weakest intensity at which familiar spondee words are recognized, can be measured. The SRT should be within 5 decibels of the three-frequency pure tone average hearing level.

Word recognition ability for comfortably audible speech is measured either by asking the person to repeat words from standardized lists presented through earphones or loudspeakers or by asking the person to point to pictures corresponding to the words if the person does not have clear speech. Word recognition ability is particularly important to test when the person has sensorineural hearing loss because it gives an estimate of the clarity of hearing, which does not always correlate with the degree of sensorineural hearing loss. The better the word recognition ability, the better the outlook for good benefit from hearing aid use. Word recognition ability usually is very good in conductive hearing loss, which often can be improved medically or surgically rather than through hearing aids.

MODIFYING AUDIOMETRIC TESTS

Behavioral audiological evaluations for individuals with developmental disabilities should be performed by an audiologist who has experience in this area. The audiologist should talk to the individual and the parent or caregiver who brings the person to the test to determine the best way for the person to respond every time a tone is heard. If the person is fearful of wearing earphones, the audiologist can either begin the test through the loudspeakers or begin by playing age-appropriate music through the earphones to entice the person to put them on. When testing older children and adults, the audiologist should be open to the use of a nontraditional response such as making a high five or yelling "yes" each time a sound is heard.

If a conditioned play audiometry task is chosen, the toy should be one within the motor abilities of the person being tested. The audiologist will need to change the play audiometry toy frequently if attention lags. A child with visual impairments will be at a great disadvantage during VRA because the reward for turning to the sound will not be seen, and an alternative reward such as touching a toy after localizing to the side of the sound can be chosen. For any test method used for threshold estimation, the audiologist must remember to leave more time than usual between the stimulus presentation and the expected response before moving on to the next stimulus, as response latency often is increased when developmental disabilities are present.

Speech audiometry can be a rewarding and useful test if words are chosen that are meaningful to the person being tested. For example, a woman with intellectual disabilities might be asked to dump out the contents of her pocketbook on a table and name the items in order to see what she calls them. Then, rather than using potentially unfamiliar vocabulary from a standardized test, the names of the pocketbook's contents can be used as test stimuli, and the woman can be asked to point to items as they are named through the earphones. The caregiver accompanying the person to the test can be most helpful in explaining which words might be most likely to be recognized. Creative modification of behavioral audiometric tests can go a long way toward eliminating the need to sedate or anesthetize older children or adults with developmental disabilities for an ABR test.

NEWBORN HEARING SCREENING

The advent of universal newborn hearing screening, now implemented in nearly all states, changes the landscape for identification of hearing loss in individuals with other disabilities. Most babies now receive a newborn hearing screening test prior to being discharged from the hospital to home. The screening tests, which consist of automated versions of the ABR test or otoacoustic emissions (OAE), are designed to pick up a speech-frequency hearing loss of approximately 30dB or greater in one or both ears.

A "refer" result on a newborn hearing screening test leads to a diagnostic audiological evaluation, which should consist of a frequency-specific ABR test, and other tests that are available to delineate the type of hearing loss if hearing results prove to be abnormal (Joint Committee on Infant Hearing, 2000). Three out of every 1,000 newborns has permanent hearing loss in one or both ears (Finitzo, Albright, & O'Neal, 1998; Van Naarden, Decoufle, & Caldwell, 1999) and of these newborns, at least one will have another condition contributing to developmental disabilities (see Table 17.1-1). The fact that most children born in 2000 or later will have had a newborn hearing screening test helps to plan the monitoring of their hearing levels.

When the newborn hearing screening test is performed using automated ABR, the response being observed is an evoked potential, which, in this case, is a change in the electroencephalogram (EEG) at the brainstem level, evoked by the onset of a rapidly repeated click sound and averaged over trials to extract the response from the background EEG. When a response is present, one may infer not only that the stimulus traversed the outer and middle ear successfully at adequate volume, but also that the inner ear succeeded in stimulating the auditory nerve to fire in a synchronized fashion, causing a cascade of synchronized discharges up the brainstem auditory neural pathway. When the newborn hearing screening test is performed using automated OAE, the response being observed is a preneural activation of outer hair cells in the cochlea, which send a sound back into the ear canal as a result of their mechanical dance in response to the stimulus. Although the OAE requires a clear outer and middle ear for a response to be present, it does NOT require successful activation of the auditory nerve. Therefore, an infant with auditory neuropathy (also known as *auditory dyssynchrony*), a condition in which there is hair cell activity in the cochlea but no synchronized discharge of the auditory nerve and no ABR waveform, will pass the OAE.

As many as 12%–14% of infants with absent ABR waveforms and a significant auditory disorder may have the subtype of hearing loss known as *auditory neuropathy* (Kraus, 2001) and may pass an OAE screen but not pass an ABR screen. Children with auditory neuropathy may detect sounds but hear in a distorted and inconsistent fashion and do not receive the expected benefit from hearing aids. They may benefit from cochlear implantation if the hearing disorder is severe enough to warrant it. Therefore, if a "passed" newborn hearing screening test was performed using OAE but any concern remains regarding the child's auditory responsiveness, the child should have a diagnostic audiological evaluation. This caveat is particularly salient for infants who were born very prematurely and/or had elevated bilirubin levels, as these groups have a higher incidence of auditory neuropathy than the general population of babies.

Infants who pass the newborn screening test but have risk factors for progressive hearing loss also need to have their hearing monitored by diagnostic audiological evaluations. Infants at risk for progressive hearing loss include those with a familial history of early progressive hearing loss, congenital cytomegalovirus, repeated courses of aminoglycosides and diuretics, congenital diaphragmatic hernia, persistent pulmonary hypertension of the newborn, or a history of extracorporeal membrane oxygenation therapy. Children with these conditions should be referred for ABR evaluation in the first few months of life even if they have passed a newborn hearing screening test.

One normal hearing test does not immunize a child against future hearing loss. Careful questioning of the parent at each well-child visit helps to unmask concerns about hearing, based on inattentiveness to sound or lack of expected development of receptive language. Any concern on the part of a parent regarding a child's hearing should be followed by an evaluation by an audiologist, after cerumen impaction and acute otitis media have been ruled out. Tympanometry is advised in the pediatrician's office for frequent monitoring of middle ear status, particularly in conditions that have a high incidence of middle ear disease, such as Down syndrome.

Hearing screening is feasible in the primary care provider's office for children and adults with a developmental age of 4 years and older, using an audiometer in a quiet room. The individual is shown how to raise his or her hand or place a ring on a stick (or peg in a pegboard, or some similar toy) each time a tone is heard. Tones of 20dBHL are presented at 1,000Hz, 2,000Hz and 4,000Hz in each ear. If the room is quiet enough for staff members with normal hearing to detect 500Hz at 20dBHL easily, then this frequency can be tested also. Failure to hear any one of the tones in either ear should result in referral for an audiogram, after cerumen impaction and transient middle ear problems are ruled out.

TYMPANOMETRY

Tympanometry is a middle ear immittance measure, performed with a middle ear analyzer, that tests the function of the tympanic membrane and middle ear system. Although tympanometry does not test hearing, it is a powerful tool in the primary care office for monitoring middle ear status in individuals at high risk for recurrent middle ear disease. After ruling out cerumen impaction or drainage in the outer ear canal by otoscopic exam, a metal probe surrounded by a soft plastic doughnut-shaped tip is placed in the ear canal, achieving an air-tight seal. A steady tone is presented in the ear canal and the intensity of the tone in the canal, consisting of the presented tone and its reflection, is monitored while the air pressure in the canal is varied. The result is a measure of middle ear compliance.

A normal tympanogram shows that the tympanic membrane is most compliant when there is atmospheric pressure in the ear canal. Tympanometric compliance may peak at a positive pressure in a child who is crying vigorously or one who has just awakened from sleep. The tympanogram peaks at a negative pressure when there is negative pressure behind the tympanic membrane as well, as in a case of Eustachian tube dysfunction. When the tympanogram has no peak, the tympanic membrane is not mobile, and the result is highly correlated with the presence of middle ear effusion and conductive hearing loss. An ear with a patent pressure equalization tube or tympanic membrane perforation will show a flat tympanogram as well, but with a high volume measure indicating that the tympanic membrane is not intact. The tympanogram is an excellent way to check for middle ear fluid or patency of pressure equalization tubes, particularly in individuals whose tympanic membranes are not easily seen by otoscopic exam or when the result of the exam is equivocal.

AUDITORY BRAINSTEM RESPONSE

The diagnostic ABR test, which is performed by an audiologist, is the most commonly used tool for hearing threshold estimation in infants younger 6 months of age, toddlers for whom hearing loss cannot be ruled out by VRA, and children or adults who are not developmentally able to give accurate thresholds during behavioral audiological evaluations. Although the ABR test can be given to a quietly resting adult for the purpose of measuring nerve conduction times in response to high-intensity clicks, the use of ABR to measure thresholds requires a sleep state (unsedated, sedated, or anesthetized). Infants younger than 6 months of age can be tested in an unsedated sleep after a feeding if the parent is instructed to bring the child tired but awake and hungry.

To perform the ABR test, three electrodes are placed on the scalp. Repetitive clicks and tone bursts are presented by earphones to each ear separately while a computer uses an averaging program to extract the change in EEG activity time-locked to the onset of the sound from the background EEG. The test should include the presentation of tone bursts at different frequencies to estimate the audiometric threshold contour. The test can be performed through a bone conduction oscillator as well to determine whether a partial hearing loss is conductive or sensorineural. ABR thresholds agree closely with behavioral audiometric thresholds (Stapells & Oates, 1997).

Another evoked potential test, auditory steady state response (ASSR), may also be performed by the audiologist and gives particularly good correlation estimation of audiograms in the severe and profound hearing loss range. Concurrent assessment of middle ear status by tympanometry, and by a physician as well if results are abnormal, is essential on the day of an ABR or ASSR test. If the outer and middle ears are clear and the ABR thresholds are elevated, OAE should be recorded to determine whether there is outer hair cell activity in the cochlea, to distinguish between typical sensorineural hearing loss and auditory neuropathy.

Increasing concern for patient safety has resulted in improved monitoring of the individual during sedation for tests such as the ABR. A limited number of institutions in each state offer the combination of audiology staff, ABR equipment, on-site physician presence, and monitoring of the individual's status by a nurse, necessary for safe sedation using agents such as chloral hydrate. In addition, a child may not be deemed safe to sedate using chloral hydrate if there is a history of gastroesophageal reflux, hypotonia, liver or kidney disease, or cardiac or pulmonary problems.

In such cases, and in cases in which the individual is too large to sedate with chloral hydrate, the ABR exam may best be performed under general anesthesia, along with an exam under anesthesia of the ears by an otolaryngologist. Therefore, if a child older than 6 months of age with medical complications or an adult with developmental disabilities needs an ABR test, the test may need to be accomplished under general anesthesia. The primary care provider may be aware that the individual has a need to be anesthetized for another procedure in the near future and may be able to facilitate combining the tests or procedures under the same anesthesia.

HEARING LOSS IN SPECIFIC DEVELOPMENTAL DISABILITIES

An exhaustive description of the type and incidence of hearing loss with each of the conditions that individuals with developmental disabilities might have is beyond the scope of this chapter. Because of the vast number of genetic syndromes that include hearing loss, the reader is encouraged to refer to a compendium such as Toriello, Reardon, and Gorlin (2004) when caring for an individual with an identified syndrome because knowledge of the degree and time course of hearing loss in a particular syndrome is invaluable in planning care. In this chapter, hearing loss in Down syndrome, CHARGE association, and congenital cytomegalovirus will be considered as examples of conditions in which hearing loss is well enough understood to develop a reasonable plan of care for the ears and hearing.

Hearing Loss in Down Syndrome

Children with Down syndrome have a high incidence of hearing loss (see Chapter 9.2). As infants and toddlers, they are prone to have recurrent and persistent otitis media, sometimes without acute infections. Therefore, they are prone to have conductive hearing loss during the early language-learning years. In a group of 102 children with Down syndrome who received audiometric testing, 57 had hearing loss, of which 50 (88%) were conductive, 4 (7%) mixed conductive and sensorineural, and 3 (5%) sensorineural (Hildmann, Hildmann, & Kessler, 2002). The researchers recommended temporary use of hearing aids in very young children with Down syndrome and conductive hearing loss.

Another group of children with Down syndrome underwent ABR evaluation of hearing levels (Roizen, Wolters, Nicol, & Blondin, 1993). In 47 infants and preschool age children with Down syndrome, 34% had normal hearing, 28% had bilateral hearing loss, and 28% had unilateral loss. These investigators found a higher incidence of sensorineural hearing loss than other studies, showing conductive hearing loss in 19 ears, mixed in 14 ears, and sensorineural in 16 ears. Degree of hearing loss was mild in 33 ears, moderate in 13, and profound in 3 ears.

Early and aggressive identification and follow-up for middle ear effusion may result in improved hearing levels. Shott and Heithaus (2001) reported 5 years of aggressive medical and surgical treatment for otitis media in a group of 48 children with Down syndrome, enrolled during infancy. All but two of the children showed normal hearing levels after treatment intervention, and those two had mild hearing loss. Thus, a variety of studies show a high incidence of conductive hearing loss and otitis media in infants and young children with Down syndrome, with variable findings in regard to the incidence of sensorineural hearing loss.

The high incidence of hearing loss seen in children with Down syndrome appears to have an anatomical basis. Brown, Lewis, Parker, and Maw (1989) showed a significantly smaller nasopharynx and less acute skull base angle in 28 children with Down syndrome as compared with 33 age-matched controls. Examination of 16 temporal bones from 8 individuals with Down syndrome showed both cochlear and middle ear anomalies (Bilgin, Kasemsuwan, Schachern, Paparella, & Le, 1996). Six bones showed cochlear abnormalities, four of which had Mondini deformity of the cochlea. Cochlear length and spiral ganglion cell population were smaller in the study group than in the controls. Middle ear findings included residual mesenchyme and abnormal stapes. In addition, children with Down syndrome may have very narrow ear canals, contributing to occlusion of the canal by ordinary amounts of cerumen or debris, causing conductive hearing loss until the canal is cleaned out by a physician.

The anatomical propensity of children with Down syndrome to have both conductive and sensorineural hearing loss warrants close attention beginning in the early years of life. Children who participate in the Down Syndrome Program at Children's Hospital Boston typically undergo newborn hearing screening, ABR before age 6 months unless the newborn screening was passed bilaterally and the middle ears are clear, and behavioral audiograms and tympanograms every 6 months until their third birthday, with otolaryngology referral and further care as needed. Because the parents are counseled about the likelihood of hearing loss and the possibility of limiting its impact, they are generally eager to obtain and understand measures of their child's hearing and middle ear status.

Fluctuating conductive hearing loss may continue into the school years, affecting classroom performance. Amplification of the teacher's voice using a sound field system, which consists of a wireless microphone/transmitter worn by the teacher and receivers connected to loudspeakers closer to the children, may serve as a way to ensure adequate volume of the teacher's voice without constantly having to assess whether a hearing aid should be used for a mild fluctuating loss. Bennetts and Flynn (2002) measured speech perception in the classroom for four children with Down syndrome with and without a sound field system and found significantly improved speech perception for all four children in all conditions, including high background noise conditions.

Adults with Down syndrome also have a high incidence of hearing loss. Evenhuis, van Splunder, Brocaar, and Roerdinkholder (1992) studied the hearing of 35 adults with Down syndrome who lived in institutions. Using ABR, hearing loss was found in 56 of 59 ears for which accurate data could be obtained. Buchanan (1990) reported audiometric data as a function of age for 152 individuals with Down syndrome age 5 years to 59 years and showed an earlier onset of presbycusis (sensorineural hearing loss related to aging) in the Down syndrome group as compared with a group of nonsyndromic subjects with intellectual disabilities. Thus, hearing screening cannot be discontinued in individuals with Down syndrome after any conductive hearing loss related to middle ear effusion or cerumen impaction has been treated and resolved.

Hearing Loss in CHARGE Association

At Children's Hospital Boston, we have studied the hearing of children with CHARGE association (Shah et al., 1998; see also Chapter 8.2). Ear anomalies are a required characteristic of the condition, and hearing loss is well known to be common in individuals with this constellation of abnormalities. The audiological status of 37 children was examined, 22 being diagnosed with CHARGE and 15 being "CHARGE-like" in that they had most but not all of the required manifestations. Bilateral hearing loss was found in 86% of the children and unilateral hearing loss in 14% of the children when children were tested at a time when their outer and middle ears were confirmed to be clear. No difference was found in incidence or severity of hearing loss between children with CHARGE and CHARGE-like conditions. Therefore, children with CHARGE association or CHARGE-like constellations of abnormalities may be considered to be at or near 100% risk of have hearing loss and should be referred early for audiological management.

From the standpoint of audiological management, CHARGE association poses extreme challenges. The pinnas of the children often are too malformed to obtain a good earmold fit for hearing aid use. Middle ear problems are common, but the ears may drain when pressure equalization tubes are in place, precluding hearing aid use until the ears are dry. The children have so many medical appointments that audiological visits may be cancelled or postponed while other problems are addressed. Delaying audiological management for children with CHARGE, however, can result in unnecessary exacerbation of delayed language development. When the hearing loss is bilaterally profound, the child with CHARGE may be considered to be a candidate for a cochlear implant, pending radiological confirmation of adequate cochlear anatomy for implantation, understanding of the risk of facial nerve damage in a child who already may have facial nerve weakness, and sufficient health to undergo the surgery.

Hearing Loss in Congenital Cytomegalovirus

Congenital cytomegalovirus rates as a major cause of congenital and early progressive hearing loss. Congenital cytomegalovirus infection may be symptomatic or asymptomatic at birth. When symptomatic, the finding of congenital cytomegalovirus typically prompts a referral to audiology, even if the newborn hearing screen is passed. If the congenital cytomegalovirus is asymptomatic and the newborn hearing screen is passed, the child may develop a progressive hearing loss that may go undetected for some time. Stored samples of neonatal dried blood in children later identified with hearing loss reveals a higher than expected incidence of asymptomatic congenital cytomegalovirus as a cause of sensorineural hearing loss in children (Barbi et al., 2003). Because antiviral treatment may prevent deterioration of hearing when ganciclovir is administered during early infancy (Kimberlin et al., 2003), prompt identification of congenital cytomegalovirus as the cause of hearing loss in a young child has implications for treatment.

If a newborn with congenital cytomegalovirus does not pass the newborn hearing screen or is not screened, ABR evaluation is recommended as soon as possible. If the newborn screen was passed, an ABR evaluation should take place at 3 months of age. Hearing levels should be monitored again at age 6 months and then every 6 months during early childhood. Children with identified hearing loss should receive hearing aids, sign language given the possibility of worsening of hearing levels, and early intervention. Cochlear implantation is an option for many deaf children with congenital cytomegalovirus if their associated developmental delay is not so severe that it would preclude the development of symbolic language.

HEARING AIDS AND COCHLEAR IMPLANTS

Once a hearing loss has been confirmed and determined by an otolaryngologist not to be medically or surgically remediable, the individual should be considered as a candidate for a hearing aid fitting by an audiologist. Unilateral hearing loss is managed more often with awareness, preferential seating, and communication strategies rather than hearing aid fitting, although hearing aids can be fitted to unilateral hearing loss in selected cases. If the hearing loss is bilateral, hearing aids typically are fitted on each ear unless there is a reason to fit only one ear. Such reasons may include chronic aural drainage in one ear, head banging on the side of the head not to be fitted with an aid, or a hearing loss too profound to benefit from amplification in one of the ears.

After cerumen removal, an impression is taken of the ear canal. In the case of a behind-the-ear hearing aid fitting, the impression is made into an earmold that holds the hearing aid in place and carries the amplified sound down into the ear canal. In the case of an in-the-ear or canal fitting, the hearing aid is built into a case based on the impression that is taken. Body-level hearing aids rarely are needed but can be helpful when the user has poor manual dexterity and needs large controls on the instrument.

The hearing aid amplifies sounds but does not correct hearing loss. Even the new generation of hearing aids with digital sound processing and noise cancellation circuitry do not enable the individual using the hearing aid to hear easily in background noise and group settings. Accordingly, these individuals continue to need accommodations such as facing the person directly when speaking, having one person speak at a time, using a natural inflection and a slowed rate of presentation, and rephrasing (rather than repeating) sentences that were not heard well the first time.

Background noise in a classroom should not exceed 35 decibels when the classroom is unoccupied but the heating/ventilating/air conditioning system is on. Reverberation time (the amount of time it takes for a sound to subside) should not exceed 0.6 milliseconds for general education but ideally should be even shorter for individuals who use hearing aids (American National Standards Institute, 2002). To achieve reduced background noise and reverberation, carpet, drapes, acoustical ceiling tile, and acoustical wall panels can be used.

The care of the hearing aid for a person with developmental disabilities usually requires the help of a parent or caregiver, who should receive a demonstration by the audiologist regarding how to care for and troubleshoot the hearing aid. The "kit" needed to care for a hearing aid includes a listening tube (hearing aid stethoset) if the user is not a good reporter of malfunctions; a squeeze bulb similar to a baby's nasal syringe to clean the earmold; a hearing aid battery tester; and a dehumidifying jar. Hands should be clean and dry to handle the instrument. The hearing aid should not be dropped on a hard surface. In addition, it should be removed for swimming and showering and should be covered or removed in the rain or snow. The hearing aid should not be left on a counter in a damp bathroom when showering. At night, the hearing aid should be placed in a closed container with a silica gel packet; these dehumidifying containers for hearing aids are available at any business that sells hearing aids. Any hairspray should be applied before the hearing aid is put on.

The earmold must be checked to make certain it is not blocked with cerumen or moisture droplets and may be removed from the aid, washed in warm water, dried, and cleaned with the squeeze bulb before placing back on the hearing aid. If the user has two hearing aids, only one earmold should be removed and cleaned at a time and then replaced, to avoid mixing up the right and left aids. In addition, the earmold must be placed on the hearing aid in the correct orientation (see Figure 17.1-6). When testing hearing aid batteries before putting them in the aid, remember that dead batteries "recover" overnight and work for a minute or two before dying again, so the best time to test hearing aid batteries is at night.

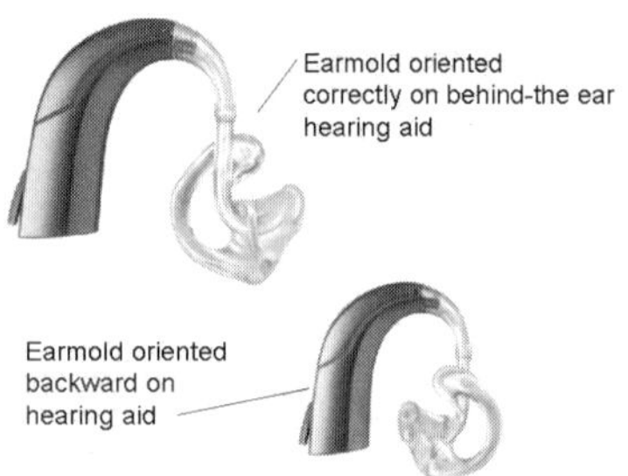

Figure 17.1-6. Behind-the-ear hearing aid and earmold. (Courtesy of Phonak, Inc.)

Older children and adults with developmental disabilities may have difficulty accepting hearing aid use if they were not fitted with hearing aids in infancy. Establishing good hearing aid use may require building the insertion of the aid into the daily routine and using behavior modification strategies such as stickers on a calendar or planned rewards for increasing periods of hearing aid use.

If the individual using the hearing aid has usable ability to understand speech in a quiet environment with the hearing aid but has difficulty hearing a teacher, co-worker, or supervisor, an FM system is recommended for use. The teacher or supervisor wears a wireless microphone/transmitter through which his or her voice is transmitted to a receiver that is coupled to the hearing aid. The FM system can make a difference between success and failure in a school or work situation that involves understanding a voice at varying distances and in typical noisy conditions.

If hearing loss is severe to profound in both ears and the person is unable to recognize words through hearing aids despite training to do so, a cochlear implant may provide better access to sound than hearing aids. Candidates for cochlear implants include very young children, even those with no hearing or spoken language, and older children and adults who have some spoken language but whose hearing is insufficient to support its use. Individuals who use cochlear implants require the same acoustical and communication "helpers" as individuals who use hearing aids and individuals with unilateral hearing loss.

A cochlear implant consists of a surgically implanted receiver/stimulator connected to an electrode array in the cochlea and an externally worn speech processor that is larger than a hearing aid. A hearing aid may continue to be used on the nonimplanted ear if benefit is achieved. Bilateral implantation is performed for selected cases but is not the norm.

For the first several years after cochlear implants were introduced, only candidates without developmental disabilities received the implant. Now, many individuals with developmental disabilities have received cochlear implants after careful screening and consideration and benefit from the use of cochlear implants (Waltzman, Scalchunes, & Cohen, 2000). If a person does not have intellectual disabilities, progress in acquisition of spoken language comprehension is similar to that of typical deaf children. If, however, intellectual disabilities are present, progress through the various stages of learning to listen with the implant is slower and may stop at the level of single word or familiar phrase recognition without understanding of grammatical strings. Children with developmental disabilities who have cochlear implants are more likely to continue to need sign language as a primary rather than supplementary means of communication than typical deaf children who receive implants at a young age.

Cochlear implant teams must consider candidates with developmental disabilities carefully, making an estimation of what the individual would have been able to accomplish in the way of language development if normal hearing had been present. Because a surgical procedure is involved and many children with developmental problems also are medically fragile, the caveat "first do no harm" is foremost in these decisions.

At 2 years of age, Jackson began to acquire sign language but made little progress in the understanding of spoken language using his hearing aids because of the profound degree of his hearing loss. He exhibited global developmental delays. His social interaction was fleeting and poorly focused. His parents were interested in cochlear implantation for him. After careful determination that he was strong enough to undergo an elective surgery, and after careful counseling with his parents that the cochlear implant should improve his access to sound but could not make up for developmental delays, Jackson received a cochlear implant in his left ear shortly before his third birthday. He tolerated his externally worn speech processor well (see Figure 17.1-7). His breathing through his tracheostomy was quite loud, and efforts were made to minimize stimulation on those electrodes corresponding to the frequency of the acoustic energy in his breathing.

Jackson began to develop understanding of spoken words using the cochlear implant, at times showing understanding of the words even when he was not looking at the signs. By age 5 years, his understanding of spoken language became equal to his understanding of sign language, though both remained delayed. During one hospitalization, the value of the cochlear implant became obvious; he was agitated and not getting better until his nurses realized that he wanted to wear his cochlear implant speech processor and hear what was going on, whereupon his condition improved.

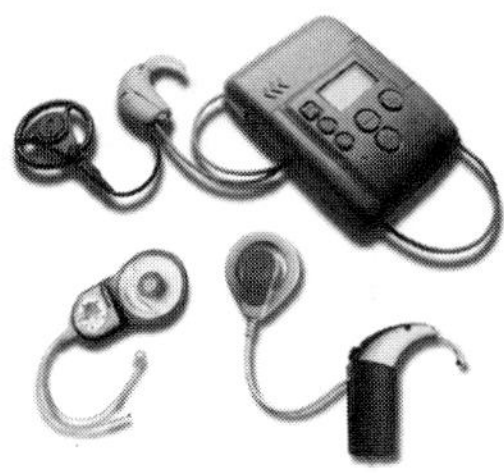

Figure 17.1-7. Cochlear implant (lower left), body-level speech processor (top), and behind-the-ear speech processor. (Photo provided courtesy of Cochlear Ltd.)

At age 6 years, Jackson began to be able to use a speaking valve on his tracheostomy, so that he could vocalize. At last, he was able to begin to speak the words he had learned to understand but thus far had only been able to express in sign language. Early and thoughtful management of Jackson's deafness, with careful planning of medical priorities on the part of his parents and medical team, has resulted in successful communication behavior.

FOCUS ON THE WHOLE PERSON AND FAMILY

Learning that a child with developmental disabilities also has a hearing loss can be unsettling for parents. At times, the diagnosis of the hearing loss may not seem like an additional diagnosis but rather a new package of diagnoses, as the hearing loss changes parents' expectations for communication development and educational methods. Hearing aids may be the first "apparatus" worn by the child that externalizes the impairment and makes it visible.

When hearing loss is found in a newborn before other problems manifest themselves, however, the audiologist must take care to remind the parent that each child is an individual and that this infant's pattern of development has yet to unfold. The diagnosis of hearing loss now can occur so early that it seems to be happening to the parents rather than resulting from the parents' search for an answer to their suspicion of hearing loss. Whenever possible, the audiologist, physicians, and early intervention providers must put the parent in the driver's seat in making informed decisions regarding a plan of care. Explanation of the hearing loss should be expressed in terms related to what it means to the child (e.g., how far away he or she can hear, how it might affect his or her speech) rather than in graphs and wiggly lines on computer screens. Coordination of care through the primary care provider's office as the medical home helps to prioritize the order of appointments and treatment plans.

CONCLUSION

When hearing loss is properly diagnosed and creatively managed in an individual with developmental disabilities at any age, the result can be extremely rewarding for all concerned, as it becomes more and more evident that the person is able to communicate when sounds are made accessible. Treatment not only involves changing the person's auditory access through medical intervention for outer and middle ear problems and through hearing aids for permanent hearing loss, but it also involves changing the communication behaviors of the surrounding caregivers, family members, and friends. Speaking to a person with a developmental disability and hearing loss in a manner in which he or she can understand and using close proximity, natural inflection, slowed rate of speaking, visual focusing, and reduction of background distractions stacks the deck in the person's favor. Teaching a person with a hearing loss how to recognize when he or she has not understood, how to advocate for him- or herself by asking for clarification, and how to use amplification devices properly enables the person's true potential for cognitive development and social prowess to emerge.

REFERENCES

American National Standards Institute. (2002). *American National Standard Acoustical Performance Criteria, Design Requirements, and Guidelines for Schools.* (ANSI S12.60–2002). Melville, NY: Acoustical Society of America.

Barbi, M., Binda, S., Caroppo, S., Ambrosetti, U., Corbetta, C., & Sergi, P. (2003). A wider role for congenital cytomegalovirus infection in sensorineural hearing loss. *Pediatric Infectious Disease Journal, 22*(1), 39–42.

Bennetts, L.K., & Flynn, M.C. (2002). Improving the classroom listening skills of children with Down syndrome by using sound-field amplification. *Down's Syndrome, Research and Practice, 8*(1), 19–24.

Bilgin, H., Kasemsuwan, L., Schachern, P.E., Paparella, M.M., & Le, C.T. (1996). Temporal bone study of Down's syndrome. *Archives of Otolaryngology Head and Neck Surgery, 122*(3), 271–275.

Brown, P.M., Lewis, T., Parker, A.J., & Maw, A.R. (1989). The skull base and nasopharynx in Down's syndrome in relation to hearing impairment. *Clinical Otolaryngology, 14*(3), 241–246.

Buchanan, L. (1990). Early onset of presbycusis in Down syndrome. *Scandinavian Audiology, 19*(2), 103–110.

Evenhuis, H., van Splunder, J., Brocaar, M.P., & Roerdinkholder, W.H. (1992). Hearing loss in middle-age persons with Down syndrome. *American Journal of Mental Retardation, 97*(1), 47–56.

Finitzo, T., Albright, K., & O'Neal, J. (1998). The newborn with hearing loss: Detection in the nursery. *Pediatrics, 102*, 1452–1459.

Fria, T.J., Cantekin, E.I., & Eichler, J.A. (1985). Hearing acuity of children with otitis media with effusion. *Archives of Otolaryngology, 111*(1), 10–16.

Gallaudet Research Institute. (2003). *Regional and national summary report of data from the 2001–2002 Annual Survey of Deaf and Hard of Hearing Children and Youth.* Washington, DC: Gallaudet University.

Harrison, M., Roush, J., & Wallace, J. (2003). Trends in age of identification and intervention in infants with hearing loss. *Ear and Hearing, 24*(1), 89–95.

Hildmann, A., Hildmann, H., & Kessler, A. (2002). Hearing disorders in children with Down's syndrome (German). *Laryngorhinootologie, 81*(1), 3–7.

Joint Committee on Infant Hearing. (2000). Year 2000 position statement: Principles and guidelines for early hearing detection and intervention programs. *Pediatrics, 1006*, 798–817.

Kimberlin, D.W., Lin, C.Y., Sanchez, P.J., Demmler, G.J., Dankner, W., Shelton Jacobs, R.F., et al. (2003). Effect of ganciclovir therapy on hearing in symptomatic congenital cytomegalovirus disease involving the central nervous system: A randomized, controlled trial. *Journal of Pediatrics, 143*(1), 16–25.

Kraus, N. (2001). Auditory neuropathy: An historical and current perspective. In Y. Sininger & A. Starr (Eds.), *Auditory neuropathy: A new perspective on hearing disorders* (pp. 1–14). San Diego: Singular.

Lieu, J.E. (2004). Speech-language and educational consequences of unilateral hearing loss in children. *Archives of Otolaryngology Head and Neck Surgery, 130*(5), 524–530.

Roizen, N.J., Wolters, C., Nicol, T., & Blondin, T.A. (1993). Hearing loss in children with Down syndrome. *Journal of Pediatrics, 123*(1), S9–S12.

Roush, J., Holcomb, M.A., Roush, P.A., & Escolar, M.L. (2004). When hearing loss occurs with multiple disabilities. *Seminars in Hearing, 25*(4), 333–345.

Shah, U.K., Ohlms, L.A., Neault, M.W., Willson, K.D., McGuirt, W.F. Jr., Hobbs, N., et al. (1998). Otologic management in children with the CHARGE association. *International Journal of Pediatric Otorhinolaryngology, 44*(2), 139–147.

Shott, S.R., & Heithaus, D. (2001). Hearing loss in children with Down syndrome. *International Journal of Pediatric Otolaryngology, 61*(3), 199–205.

Stapells, D.R., & Oates, P. (1997). Estimation of the puretone audiogram by the auditory brainstem response: A review. *Audiology and Neuro-Otology, 2*(5), 257–280.

Toriello, H.V., Reardon, W., & Gorlin, R.J. (2004). Hereditary hearing loss and its syndromes *Oxford Monographs on Medical Genetics* (2nd ed.). Oxford, England: Oxford University Press.

Van Naarden, K., Decoufle, P., & Caldwell, K. (1999). Prevalence and characteristics of children with serious hearing impairment in metropolitan Atlanta, 1991–1993. *Pediatrics, 103*, 570–575.

Waltzman, S., Scalchunes, V., & Cohen, N. (2000). Performance of multiply handicapped children using cochlear implants. *American Journal of Otology, 21*, 329–335.

17.2 Ear, Nose, and Throat Care

Margaret A. Kenna

Ear, nose, and throat care in individuals with developmental disabilities has come a long way since the first edition of this book. Diagnostic techniques, especially, have changed dramatically. Airways are routinely evaluated using thin, flexible fiberoptic instruments in the office and rigid fiberoptic rod lens systems in the operating room. Similar endoscopes are also used in the diagnosis and surgical and office management of sinus disease, which especially benefits individuals with cystic fibrosis (Tandon & Derkay, 2003). In addition, digital and programmable hearing aids, bone-anchored hearing aids, and cochlear implants have vastly improved access to sound for many people with permanent hearing loss, with resultant improvement in their communication, social, and academic skills (Copeland & Pillsbury, 2004; Priwin, Stenfelt, Granstrom, Tjellstrom, & Hakansson, 2004). Vascular and lymphatic malformations can now be managed using a combination of surgery and interventional radiologic techniques, and advances in skull base surgery now allow for safer and more effective resection of large head and neck tumors (Giguere, Bauman, & Smith, 2002; Van Aalst, Bhuller, & Sadove, 2003).

Children with developmental disabilities may require otolaryngologic services beginning in the nursery and neonatal intensive care unit and lasting well into adulthood. Many of the most common ear, nose, and throat problems are more frequent, more persistent, and more challenging in children and adults with developmental disabilities. This chapter discusses head and neck examinations, otologic conditions, airway complications, sinus and nasal diseases, and tonsil and adenoid management in individuals with developmental disabilities.

HEAD AND NECK EXAMINATION

Examining any child can be a challenge, but examining children and adults with developmental disabilities can be even more difficult. The individual may have a limited ability to communicate and understand, and physical limitations may make the exam more uncomfortable or difficult for the individual (e.g., individual cannot lie flat, turn his or her head, or open his or her mouth normally). To provide the best care to these individuals and their families, ear, nose, and throat professionals must be able to provide extra help during a visit. Ancillary personnel, including nurses, nurse practitioners, nursing assistants, and physician assistants, make individuals with developmental disabilities and their families feel more comfortable by gathering medical and family information and help parents hold the individual so that the exam can be accomplished efficiently and with the least amount of trauma. Appropriate interpreters (e.g., sign language, Spanish) should be present throughout the visit so that physicians and other care providers can gather important history information, explain the examination process before it takes place, and explain findings and recommendations at the end of the visit.

Although individuals with developmental disabilities may be brought in primarily for an "ear" or "throat" examination, another problem may be present that has been overlooked or underappreciated. For example, an individual may be at the physician's office for evaluation of his or her "large tonsils," but the physician may find that the person's dentition is in poor repair. Or an individual may be at the physician's office to have cerumen removed from his or her ears, but the physician may realize that no recent or thorough evaluation of the person's hearing has taken place. Swallowing, eating, and comfortable breathing should not be taken for granted and should be reevaluated during each visit (Shevell et al., 2003).

In addition, as complete a head and neck exam as possible should be accomplished. The general condition of the individual's skin and hair should be evaluated, as some individuals may have self-abusive behavior or be bedridden and develop pressure-related changes in their head and neck area. Drooling can cause skin changes in the oral cavity and neck areas and may even lead to external otitis or otitis media if the individual lies with his or her head turned in a certain direction so that saliva enters the ear canal or middle ear through a nonintact tympanic membrane (perforation or tympanostomy tube).

In a teaching setting, many individuals have their ears or throats looked at more than once during a visit, as the medical student or resident learns from a more senior physician. Because individuals with disabilities often are difficult to examine, only one examination may be possible. The physician should explain the situation to any trainees present and enlist their assistance in the examination and history-taking process.

If an essential part of the exam cannot be accomplished in the office, general anesthesia may be needed. In this case, the physician should try to coordinate with other providers in order to combine other evaluations and procedures (e.g., making of ear molds for hearing aids, auditory evaluation, cast changes, radiographic procedures, dental examinations and procedures) that need to be performed under anesthesia. This practice saves the individual an extra general anesthetic and the trauma of a trip to the operating room.

OTOLOGIC CONDITIONS

Otologic problems, especially middle ear infections, are the most common of all otolaryngologic concerns for individuals with developmental disabilities. After their airway and other otolaryngologic issues have been long resolved, adults with developmental disabilities may continue to have trouble with hearing, external or middle ear infections, recurrent cerumen impactions, poorly defined ear pain, or trouble wearing their hearing aids (see Table 17.2-1). Middle ear infections are common in all children, but especially children younger than the age of 6 years. The presence of middle ear fluid is often associated with the presence of a conductive hearing loss, which, although temporary, may last weeks to years. This hearing loss can have deleterious effects in children with other medical problems, such as sensorineural hearing loss, cognitive impairments, or severe language delays.

Conditions Related to Craniofacial Anomalies

Children with craniofacial anomalies that predispose them to eustachian tube dysfunction (e.g., cleft palate, Apert or Down syndromes, CHARGE association) are more likely not only to develop otitis media with effusion in the first place, but also to have persistent middle ear problems well into their teen or adult years (Sheahan, Blayney, Sheahan, & Earley, 2002; Shott, Joseph, & Heithaus, 2001). The management of this otitis may involve frequent clinic visits for pneumatic otoscopy, cerumen removal, otomicroscopy, and hearing evaluations. These children often require multiple sets of tympanostomy tubes to manage middle ear fluid and associated conductive hearing loss. Because eustachian tube function in these children is often very abnormal, the children have a high incidence of otitis media and its complications (e.g., tympanic membrane perforation, chronic suppurative otitis media [CSOM] with otorrhea, atelectasis of the tympanic membrane).

Individuals with cleft palate have a higher incidence of cholesteatoma that decreases markedly with the judicious use of frequent ear exams and ventilation tubes when indicated (Sheahan et al., 2002). In children with chronic and more-difficult-to-manage otitis, longer-lasting ventilation tubes may be used. Although these tubes are very effective at providing long-term ventilation of the middle ear, they are more likely than "shorter-term" tubes to result in a persistent tympanic membrane perforation when they extrude. Tympanic membrane perforations are often associated with conductive hearing losses, recurrent otorrhea, and the need for water precautions when swimming and bathing. Closing them requires a surgical procedure.

Table 17.2-1. Potential causes of ear pain in children and adults

Otitis media
Eustachian tube dysfunction
Otitis externa
Cholesteatoma of middle ear/mastoid
Cerumen impaction of the external auditory canal
Foreign body of the ear canal or middle ear
Neoplasm
Temporomandibular joint dysfunction
Referred pain from dental pathology
Referred pain from other head and neck structures

Chronic Suppurative Otitis Media

CSOM can be defined as chronic otorrhea through a nonintact tympanic membrane that is refractory to medical therapy. In children with craniofacial anomalies or underlying immunodeficiency, CSOM can be very difficult to manage effectively due to the severe nature of eustachian tube dysfunction that can be exacerbated by ongoing gastroesophageal reflux, nasopharyngeal reflux, or ciliary dysmotility. Adequately protecting the external ear canal from water may be difficult, and in some children who wear hearing aids with closed ear molds, moisture and built-up cerumen in the ear canal may predispose the child to external otitis as well. Frequent removal of cerumen can help lower the incidence of otitis externa secondary to impaction and facilitate more comfortable and successful hearing aid use.

Even with close and careful management of otitis media, many individuals will have otitis well into adulthood, and many develop chronic, although relatively stable, middle ear disease. Knowledge of an individual's ear status over years or even decades can help formulate an approach that works for the individual and his or her family, hearing, and other developmental needs.

Alex is a 45-year-old man with Down syndrome. During childhood, he had significant problems with otitis media, which improved with age. During that time, he had three sets of tympanostomy tubes placed and underwent a tonsillectomy and adenoidectomy for upper airway obstruction. In his 30s, Alex developed pain and ear drainage in the right ear. He was very difficult to examine in the outpatient department and subsequently underwent examination of his ears in the operating room under general anesthesia. Bilateral cerumen impactions and a right-sided ear canal cholesteatoma were found and removed.

Several years later, Alex's parents and the attendants in his group home noted that he no longer listened to his music box, and hearing loss was suspected. Behavioral audiometric evaluation in the outpatient setting was not successful, and Alex again underwent examination of his ears and auditory brainstem response testing under general anesthesia. A very significant bilateral sensorineural hearing loss was documented, but there was no recurrence of the cholesteatoma. Alex also underwent a dental exam and drawing of blood for thyroid function studies and an electrocardiogram. He continues to be followed as an outpatient.

Sensorineural Hearing Loss

Sensorineural hearing loss is one of the most common birth defects, with a communicatively significant permanent hearing loss present in 1–2/1,000 live births. This number increases to approximately 13/1,000 by the age of 19 years if mild and unilateral hearing losses are included. Hearing loss may occur alone or in association with other syndromes and medical conditions. Diagnostic imaging, including computed tomography and magnetic resonance imaging of the temporal bones, and genetic testing have vastly improved the ability to provide individuals and their families with the cause of the hearing loss (Ohlms, Chen, Stewart, & Franklin, 1999). Some of the more common causes of sensorineural hearing loss include anatomic abnormalities of the inner ear structures, recessively inherited genetic hearing loss, and congenital cytomegalovirus (Kimberlin et al., 2003). Because sensorineural hearing loss is generally a permanent condition, individuals and their families need to know from the beginning that the loss will not improve and may worsen over time.

Conductive Hearing Loss

Some conductive hearing losses (e.g., those associated with external auditory canal stenosis or atresia, those that are the result of severe chronic ear disease) may not be amenable to surgical intervention, or surgical intervention may improve but not completely resolve the hearing loss. In these instances, the hearing loss is also relatively permanent and should be treated with the same degree of seriousness as a permanent sensorineural hearing loss. Bone conduction hearing aids, worn on a headband or bone anchored, provide significant benefit and should always be considered if a conventional hearing aid is not feasible, and the same speech and language services provided to children with sensorineural hearing loss should be considered for children with significant conductive hearing losses (Priwin et al., 2004).

Ongoing Care

Examining the ears of children with anatomic abnormalities of the ear canals and pinnas and children who cannot cooperate adequately for the exam may be next to impossible. General anesthesia in the operating room is sometimes needed to completely examine the ears, remove cerumen, and make ear molds for hearing aids. In addition, if it has not been possible to get an accurate hearing evaluation in the office, auditory brainstem testing and otoacoustic emissions under general anesthesia can also be accomplished. As mentioned previously, combining the ear or hearing exam with another procedure in the operating room is preferable. Imaging studies of the temporal bones can also often be accomplished in this fashion.

AIRWAY COMPLICATIONS

Airway problems are common in all children, although children with developmental disabilities may be more at risk (Boston & Rutter, 2003; Contencin, Guilleminault, & Manach, 2003; Toder, 2000). The most frequently seen conditions are related to adenotonsillar hypertrophy, but other conditions include choanal atresia and other types of congenital nasal obstruction, including encephaloceles, nasolacrimal duct cysts, and nasal aperture stenosis; micrognathia; retrognathia; glossoptosis; cleft palate; laryngomalacia; vocal cord paralysis; subglottic stenosis; tracheomalacia; and tracheal stenosis.

Benign and malignant neoplasms can involve any part of the airway. Benign conditions include dermoids, gliomas, encephaloceles, lymphatic malformations, hemangiomas and other vascular malformations, neurofibromas, thyroglossal duct cysts, and branchial arch anomalies. Malignant neoplasms include rhabdomyosarcoma and lymphoma. In addition, children and adults with neuromuscular or musculoskeletal abnormalities may have severe airway issues that directly or indirectly involve the airway (e.g., severe kyphoscoliosis; see Table 17.2-2).

Nasal obstruction in babies can be life threatening, as infants can only breathe through their noses at birth.

Table 17.2-2. Potential causes of airway obstruction in children

Oral cavity
Adenotonsillar hypertrophy
Palate abnormalities
Neoplasm
Vascular or lymphatic malformation of tongue or other structures
Hypopharynx
Abnormalities of the tongue and tongue base (e.g., macroglossia, lingual tonsillar enlargement, neoplasm)
Micrognathia/retrognathia causing obstruction at the tongue base
Neoplasm or congenital anomaly involving the tongue, tongue base, retropharyngeal, or lateral pharyngeal structures
Nasal cavity
Pyriform aperture stenosis
Nasolacrimal duct obstruction
Nasal septal deviation
Choanal atresia/stenosis
Turbinate enlargement
Encephalocele
Dermoid
Glioma
Nasal polyps
Neoplasm
Foreign body
Deformity or absence of nasal structures
Nasopharynx
Adenoid hypertrophy
Encephalocele
Dermoid
Glioma
Foreign body
Neoplasm
Supraglottis and glottis
Vocal cord paralysis
Subglottic stenosis
Aryepiglottic fold cysts
Vallecular cysts
Respiratory papillomas
Foreign body
Neoplasm
Subglottic hemangioma
Trachea
Congenital or acquired stenosis
Respiratory papillomas
Tracheoesophageal fistula
Vascular anomalies
Foreign body
Neoplasm

Although nasal edema and septal deviation secondary to birth trauma are not uncommon, other causes of congenital nasal obstruction must always be considered. Choanal atresia, seen in more than half of the individuals with CHARGE association, may need to be recognized and bypassed in the newborn period. Although techniques for choanal atresia repair have improved, the child may still have lifelong symptoms of nasal obstruction that may become more apparent with viral upper respiratory tract or sinus infections.

Anterior nasal aperture stenosis may be isolated or associated with other congenital anomalies and also needs to be recognized and addressed early in life. Other less common but important causes of nasal obstruction that may be isolated but also seen in association with other craniofacial anomalies include encephaloceles, gliomas, dermoids, and nasolacrimal duct cysts. Although surgical removal can usually deal with these conditions in a definitive fashion, the residual nasal anatomy may still not be normal, and the child may have long-standing nasal obstruction symptoms or nasal deformity.

Adenotonsillar Hypertrophy

Adenotonsillar hypertrophy is common in all children but may be a more difficult management issue in children and young adults with developmental issues. Although surgery for adenotonsillar hypertrophy in an otherwise normal child usually involves an uneventful general anesthesia, postoperative course, and resolution of the symptoms of airway obstruction, children with developmental disabilities may not have an easy experience. Anesthesia may be complicated by other airway abnormalities and cardiac or pulmonary compromise (Blum & McGowan, 2004). The child may have a prolonged stay in the hospital postoperatively due to feeding issues and the need for oxygen during sleep.

Even after the child has left the hospital and the symptoms that had been associated with adenotonsillar hypertrophy have improved, ongoing airway symptoms from other anatomic abnormalites not related to the tonsils and adenoids (e.g., craniofacial anomalies, musculoskeletal conditions, pulmonary problems) may persist. These other airway issues may even make it more difficult for the child to have the tonsillectomy in the first place. For example, intubation for general anesthesia in a child with severe micrognathia or retrognathia having a tonsillectomy may be much more challenging than the tonsillectomy itself, requiring fiberoptic intubation or even intubation over a bronchoscope. In such a child, tonsillectomy and adenoidectomy may not resolve all of the airway issues, which may be at least in part to the size, shape, or location of the mandible and tongue. Many of these airway issues will follow the child into adulthood, requiring an increased level of vigilance with every anesthetic experience.

Other indications for tonsillectomy and/or adenoidectomy include recurrent/chronic adenotonsillitis, dysphasia, chronic sinusitis, otitis media (usually only the adenoids are an issue), or suspected neoplasm. If a child with developmental disabilities meets the criteria for adenotonsillar removal for one of these diagnoses, the same caution discussed previously for surgery and general anesthesia needs to be observed, but most children do well, and their disability alone should not prevent them from obtaining appropriate medical care.

Craniofacial Surgery

Although craniofacial surgery for mandibular and midface anomalies has advanced significantly, children may continue to have airway compromise into adulthood. For example, early mandibular distraction in infants with both syndromic and nonsyndromic Pierre Robin syndrome may prevent the need for a tracheotomy or allow earlier decannulation (Sidman, Sampson, & Templeton, 2001), but these infants' airways are not necessarily normal, and ongoing vigilance, especially at the time of sedation or general anesthesia, is required. Individuals with severe sleep apnea due to midface anomalies may have improvement in their symptoms and can even be successfully decannulated if they were tracheotomy dependent prior to the surgery, but they may still have some degree of obstruction during sleep or upper respiratory tract illnesses and require continuous positive airway pressure (Van Allen, Fung, & Jurenka, 1999). This situation may also be the case in some individuals who have undergone tonsillectomy and adenoidectomy, whose symptoms are improved but clinically significant obstruction is still detected on polysomnogram. The need for continuous positive airway pressure in these individuals may be lifelong but often allows the individuals to avoid tracheotomy.

Tracheotomy

Although techniques for management of children's airways have significantly improved, some children and adults with developmental disabilities will have airway problems requiring tracheotomy (Kremer, Botos-Kremer, Eckel, & Schlondorff, 2002). Some reasons for tracheotomy include the need for prolonged ventilation for respiratory failure, the need for bypass of a congenital or acquired airway lesion (e.g., subglottic stenosis, vocal cord paralysis, micrognathia, retrognathia), and the need for management of pulmonary toilet due to recurrent aspiration and the inability of individuals to manage their secretions. Depending on the initial reason for the tracheotomy, many individuals can be decannulated during early or middle childhood; however, others are unable to be decannulated, despite surgical intervention to repair the underlying anatomic problem, aggressive management of their lung disease, or management of secretions and aspiration.

Long-term complications of tracheotomy include airway compromise due to the tracheotomy tube coming out, becoming plugged, or becoming obstructed by intrinsic tracheal disease or external compression. The presence of a tracheotomy tube requires family education, home-based nursing support, and nursing support in school. Insurance companies often pay for, and home care companies often provide, suction equipment, extra tracheotomy tubes, oxygen, and other supplies. Simple everyday events like bus or subway travel, vacations, and school attendance can be markedly affected, or even made impossible, by the presence of a tracheotomy tube. Therefore, although a tracheotomy can be life saving and absolutely necessary for the health and safety of the individual, it can also compromise the quality of life of the individual who has it and the family who has to care for it.

Adolescents and adults who have a tracheotomy tube are often very aware of the necessity for the tube, but still have social issues due to secretions and the cosmetic presence of the tube. Although individuals with very severe cognitive impairments may not be aware of the tube's presence, physicians and other care providers still need to recognize the need for ongoing care of the tube and its impact on families or other individuals involved with the individual's care (Kremer et al., 2002).

William is a 15-year-old youth with cerebral palsy and severe kyphoscoliosis. He has recurrent pneumonia due to dysphagia and recurrent aspiration, but he has never required prolonged hospital stays or ventilation for pulmonary insufficiency. After a long and complex spine surgery, which went well, he could not be extubated and required prolonged ventilatory support in the intensive care unit. Multiple attempts at extubation failed due to problems with pulmonary toilet and ongoing need for oxygen, and he subsequently underwent tracheotomy. After several more weeks, William was weaned from the ventilator but was discharged with a 24-hour oxygen requirement.

Ongoing Care

Although the airways of many individuals with disabilities can be managed without an ongoing need for a tracheotomy tube, they often are not normal. Many individuals have neuromuscular problems making airway issues more likely. They may, therefore, have intermittent problems requiring medical attention with upper or lower respiratory tract infections, exercise, or surgery requiring general anesthesia and associated airway management.

As the individual grows and ages, some airway issues may become more apparent. For example, a subglottic or tracheal narrowing that was tolerated when the child was small may now require surgical intervention. Individuals who receive radiation therapy for a head and neck neoplasm may be cured of their underlying disease but develop fibrotic tissue changes making it difficult or impossible to open their mouths, move their necks well, or evaluate their airways. Individuals with cerebral palsy or other neuromuscular diseases may have worsening of their airways with increasing age due to kyphoscoliosis, restrictive lung disease, or decreased neuromuscular control. For example, individuals with mucopolysaccharidoses often develop tracheal narrowing and life-threatening airway problems that did not exist when they were younger (Shinhar, Zablocki, & Madgy, 2004; see Chapter 7.2). Therefore, individuals, their families, and their primary care providers must recognize an ongoing need for vigilance, and physicians who have had little experience with these issues may need to become more aware of the possibility of airway issues in adults with developmental disabilities.

SINUS AND NASAL DISEASES

Sinus disease, already well described in adults, has been increasingly recognized in the pediatric population. Although common in otherwise healthy children, sinus disease is more prevalent and more chronic in certain subpopulations, including those with cystic fibrosis, immunodeficiency, ciliary dyskinesia, and anatomic abnormalities of the paranasal sinus anatomy (Ahmad & Drake-Lee, 2003; Tandon & Derkay, 2003). Advances in both anesthesia and sinus surgical techniques have made the management of chronic sinus disease more effective, but sinusitis remains a disease that often follows children into adulthood. For example, individuals with cystic fibrosis develop chronic sinusitis and nasal and sinus polyps that require frequent removal in the operating room and very frequent outpatient otolaryngology visits. In addition, many individuals with developmental disabilities have other medical problems that may exacerbate their sinus disease, including gastroesophageal and nasopharyngeal reflux.

Not unlike ear disease, the management of sinus disease involves being able to carefully inspect the nose and sinus openings in the office. This procedure may be accomplished with an otoscope, a headlight, and a nasal speculum or, more recently, with rigid and flexible endoscopic instruments. Computed tomographic scans of the paranasal sinuses are now an integral part of both the medical and surgical management of paranasal sinus disease.

If adequate physical examination or computed tomographic scanning cannot be obtained in an outpatient setting due to lack of cooperation, or if more information about the extent or location of the sinus disease is needed, then the individual may need general anesthesia to accomplish the physical examination and needed radiographic studies. The introduction and wide-spread use of functional endoscopic sinus surgery has made the surgery itself more feasible in most individuals and has greatly facilitated complete evaluation of all paranasal sinus cavities, as well as removal of intrasinus disease for both treatment and diagnosis.

Jill is a 27-year-old woman with cystic fibrosis. During adolescence, she developed significant paranasal sinus disease and nasal polyps requiring two surgeries for polyp removal and ventilation of the sinuses. She now comes on a regular schedule to the otolaryngology department for examination and irrigation of her sinus cavities, and she has achieved improved control of both her sinus and her pulmonary diseases.

As in all individuals, underlying causes of sinus disease should be sought and treated, either to avoid surgery or to make surgery more likely to be successful. Immune deficiencies and nasal allergy should be looked for and treated. Ciliary dyskinesia may occur in association with Kartagener syndrome (along with situs inversus and dextrocardia) or as an isolated finding. Diagnosis is made by evaluating nasal ciliary biopsies with electron microscopy (for the anatomy) and microscopic motion studies (for function). Although most ciliary abnormalities are genetic (and therefore permanent) in origin, the identification of the abnormality can greatly facilitate medical management, as well as giving individuals a realistic expectation of the probable lifelong nature of the sinus problem. Individuals with ciliary dyskinesia also frequently have chronic otitis media, something else that should be watched for.

Finally, gastroesophageal reflux is increasingly recognized in all individuals, but is more common in children and adults with developmental disabilities and musculoskeletal problems (see Chapter 14.2). Even in individuals who otherwise do not have significant swallowing issues, gastric contents may reflux onto the larynx and into the nasopharynx, causing or exacerbating sinus disease, otitis media, or other airway problems. In individuals who have other swallowing issues, both gastric and pharyngeal contents may reflux into the nasopharynx causing similar problems. Recognition and management of gastroesophageal reflux and laryngopharyngeal reflux can make these individuals more comfortable and greatly facilitate the management of their underlying sinusitis, otitis, or laryngeal issues.

Although sinus disease is probably the most common nasal disease in children and adults requiring treatment, other problems include epistaxis, foreign bodies, nasal polyps in individuals with cystic fibrosis, allergic rhinitis, and anatomic abnormalities. Epistaxis is usually related to bleeding from the anterior nasal septal area, or Kiesselbach's plexus. It may occur spontaneously but is exacerbated by dry air, nose picking or other nasal traumas, the presence of a foreign body, sinusitis, upper respiratory tract infections, and allergic rhinitis. Much less commonly, epistaxis may be an initial manifestation of an underlying bleeding disorder, such as Von Willebrand's disease, or of a neoplasm, such as an angiofibroma or rhabdomyosarcoma. Persistent and/or severe epistaxis should be investigated with nasal endoscopy, appropriate imaging studies, and laboratory investigations.

Nasal foreign bodies are often present with foul smelling unilateral nasal drainage and/or epistaxis. Although nasal foreign bodies are common in children, recurrent nasal foreign bodies may be more common in individuals with developmental disabilities. Vigilance and a high index of suspicion are needed to diagnose and subsequently prevent further episodes.

TONSIL AND ADENOID MANAGEMENT

Main reasons for removal of the tonsils and/or adenoids are adenotonsillar hypertrophy, recurrent adenotonsillitis, or both conditions. Additional indications for adenoidectomy include chronic and/or recurrent otitis media, especially with chronic effusion, and chronic sinusitis. Less common reasons for removal of tonsils include dysphagia, significant tonsillar asymmetry with a suspicion of malignancy, and halitosis. In individuals who have undergone solid organ transplant, removal or at least biopsy of the tonsil and adenoids may be needed to establish a diagnosis of posttransplant lymphoproliferative disorder.

Adenotonsillar hypertrophy of any etiology may lead to obstructive sleep symptoms and frank sleep apnea. If medical therapy cannot adequately reduce the size of the tonsils and adenoids, removal may be indicated. In addition, recurrent or chronic adenotonsillitis unresponsive to medical therapy may necessitate surgical removal.

In individuals with developmental disabilities who may have concurrent difficulties with swallowing, cognition, or airway anomalies, removal of the tonsils and adenoids can be very challenging. Fiberoptic intubation may be necessary in individuals with micrognathia, glossoptosis, a thick or webbed neck, or other airway anomalies. Many of these individuals require a stay in the intensive care unit postoperatively because their return to baseline pulmonary function may be delayed. They may require oxygen when awake and asleep and close monitoring of end tidal carbon dioxide and oxygen saturations. Although many of these individuals will have dramatic improvement in their breathing, a small percentage will continue to need oxygen during sleep and may even need continuous positive airway pressure to completely alleviate their sleep apnea.

The diagnosis of sleep apnea preoperatively may require a full polysomnogram, especially if the diagnosis is unclear and the risk of surgical intervention more than baseline. In many of these situations, postoperative polysomnography should be performed to determine improvement in symptoms as well as any residual need for nighttime oxygen or even bilevel or continuous positive airway pressure. As mentioned previously, in a small number of individuals, tracheotomy may be indicated if significant sleep apnea remains after tonsillectomy and adenoidectomy is performed.

If the tonsils and adenoids were removed for dysphagia, pre- and postoperative modified barium swallow studies (with both a radiologist and speech pathologist in attendance) may be indicated both for documentation of the preoperative need for intervention as well as to document postoperative improvement and plan any further treatment course.

CONCLUSION

Individuals with developmental disabilities frequently live at home or in small group settings and receive much of their care in outpatient facilities. Coordination of their medical services can be very challenging, and many of these individuals do not outgrow their need for pediatric-based services. Although most children's hospitals routinely only see children until the age of 21, most will continue to take care of adults with a "pediatric" problem. Many individuals with developmental disabilities have a lifelong need for care of their airway issues, hearing and middle ear problems, and sinus disease. For primary care providers who mainly see adults, recognition of the ongoing need for vigilance and management of these problems will allow better patient care and quality of life.

REFERENCES

Ahmad, I., & Drake-Lee, A. (2003, June). Nasal ciliary studies in children with chronic respiratory tract symptoms. *Rhinology, 41*(2), 69–71.

Blum, R.H., & McGowan, F.X., Jr. (2004, January). Chronic upper airway obstruction and cardiac dysfunction: Anatomy, pathophysiology and anesthetic implications. *Paediatric Anaesthesia, 14*(1), 75–83.

Boston, M., & Rutter, M.J. (2003, December). Current airway management in craniofacial anomalies. *Current Opinion in Otolaryngology & Head and Neck Surgery, 11*(6), 428–432.

Contencin, P., Guilleminault, C., & Manach, Y. (2003, December). Long-term follow-up and mechanisms of obstructive sleep apnea (OSA) and related syndromes through infancy and childhood. *International Journal of Pediatric Otorhinolaryngology, 67*(Suppl. 1), S119–S123.

Copeland, B.J., & Pillsbury, H.C., III. (2004). Cochlear implantation for the treatment of deafness. *Annual Review of Medicine, 55*, 157–167.

Giguere, C.M., Bauman, N.M., & Smith, R.J. (2002). New treatment options for lymphangioma in infants and children. *Annals of Otology, Rhinology and Laryngology, 111*, 1066–1075.

Kenna, M.A. (2003, April). Neonatal hearing screening. *Pediatric Clinics of North America, 50*(2), 301–313.

Kimberlin, D.W., Lin, C.Y., Sanchez, P.J., Demmler, G.J., Dankner, W., Shelton, M., et al. (2003, July). National Institute of Allergy and Infectious Diseases Collaborative Antiviral Study Group. Effect of ganciclovir therapy on hearing in symptomatic congenital cytomegalovirus disease involving the central nervous system: A randomized, controlled trial. *Journal of Pediatrics, 143*(1), 16–25.

Kremer, B., Botos-Kremer, A.I., Eckel, H.E., & Schlondorff, G. (2002, November). Indications, complications, and surgical techniques for pediatric tracheostomies—An update. *Journal of Pediatric Surgery, 37*(11), 1556–1562.

Ohlms, L.A., Chen, A.Y., Stewart, M.G., & Franklin, D.J. (1999, February). Establishing the etiology of childhood hearing loss. *Otolaryngology—Head and Neck Surgery, 120* (2), 159–163.

Priwin, C., Stenfelt, S., Granstrom, G., Tjellstrom, A., & Hakansson, B. (2004). Bilateral bone-anchored hearing aids (BAHAs): An audiometric evaluation. *Laryngoscope, 114*, 77–84.

Sheahan, P., Blayney, A.W., Sheahan, J.N., & Earley, M.J. (2002, December). Sequelae of otitis media with effusion among children with cleft lip and/or cleft palate. *Clinical Otolaryngology and Related Research, 27*(6), 494–500.

Shevell, M., Ashwal, S., Donley, D., Flint, J., Gingold, M., Hirtz, D., Majnemer, A., Noetzel, M., & Sheth, R.D. (2003). Quality Standards Subcommittee of the American Academy of Neurology. *Neurology, 60*, 367–380.

Shinhar, S.Y., Zablocki, H., & Madgy, D.N. (2004, February). Airway management in mucopolysaccharide storage disorders. *Archives of Otolaryngology—Head and Neck Surgery, 130*(2), 233–237.

Shott, S.R., Joseph, A., & Heithaus, D. (2001, December 1). Hearing loss in children with Down syndrome. *International Journal of Pediatric Otorhinolaryngology, 61*(3), 199–205.

Sidman, J.D., Sampson, D., & Templeton, B. (2001). Distraction osteogenesis of the mandible for airway obstruction in children. *Laryngoscope, 111* 1137–1146.

Tandon, R., & Derkay, C. (2003, February). Contemporary management of rhinosinusitis and cystic fibrosis. *Current Opinion in Otolaryngology & Head and Neck Surgery, 11*(1), 41–44.

Toder, D.S. (2000, October). Respiratory problems in the adolescent with developmental delay. *Adolescent Medicine, 11*(3), 617–631.

Van Aalst, J.A., Bhuller, A., & Sadove, A.M. (2003, July). Pediatric vascular lesions. *Journal of Craniofacial Surgery, 14*(4), 566–583.

Van Allen, M.I., Fung, J., & Jurenka, S.B. (1999, June 25). Health care concerns and guidelines for adults with Down syndrome. *American Journal of Medical Genetics, 89*(2), 100–110.

Chapter 18

Cardiology

18.1 History of Management of Congenital Heart Disease

Kenneth J. Dooley

Changes in the management of congenital heart disease have occurred over the years. Depending on the approaches used at any one time, different outcomes were expected for children with congenital heart disease. This chapter explores the evolution of the management of congenital heart disease in children with Down syndrome (trisomy 21), the most common developmental disability associated with congenital heart disease (see also Chapter 9.2).

Children with Down syndrome have a 40%–60% chance of having congenital heart disease, the most common form of which is the atrio-ventricular canal defect (AVCD; see Figures 18.1-1 and 18.1-2). This condition may be complicated by having unequal size development of the ventricles or associated pulmonic stenosis, creating a picture similar to tetralogy of Fallot. Children may also have a patent ductus arteriosus in combination with the previously mentioned conditions, which may complicate their presentation. The AVCD can be made up of any combination of ventricular or atrial defects, as well as mitral and/or tricuspid malformation, and the complete form of AVCD will usually have all of these defects. Children with Down syndrome may also have other isolated heart problems such as a membranous/muscular ventricular septal defect, atrial septal defect, coarctation, or patent ductus arteriosus. In addition, they may have cyanotic types of heart disease.

The natural history associated with large ventricular defects involves exposure of the lungs to elevated blood flow and pressure as blood is transmitted from the left ventricle through the defect to the right ventricle and thus the lungs. This condition leads to the lungs attempting to protect themselves by modulating the high flow and pressure, which is done by thickening the muscular wall of the medium and small size vessels, to increase the resistance to flow and thus decrease flow. This is an uncontrolled process that can lead to significant narrowing of the vessels, sometimes to the point of total occlusion.

In the final stages of the process, the vessels try to revascularize with new vessel development, which may erode into a bronchus and may result in hemoptysis. Once the lungs have reached the stage of vascular obstruction, the changes become irreversible (sometimes called Eisenmenger syndrome), and closure of the defect cannot be accomplished successfully. In children with Down syndrome, these irreversible changes may occur as early as 1 year of age.

PAST MANAGEMENT OF CONGENITAL HEART DISEASE

Although doctors can now repair defects in children with congenital heart disease by reducing the child's risk associated with heart failure, these outcomes were not always possible. Consider Antonio's situation in the mid 1950s.

Antonio was born in 1956 with the clinical features of Down syndrome. His family was devastated. The doctor explained to them what the condition meant for Antonio's future so that they would know what to expect. They hoped a heart problem was not present, but several days later, the doctor heard a heart murmur and told them that Antonio might have congenital heart disease. Antonio's family was further devastated when Antonio developed progressive respiratory distress and tachycardia and was not able to eat very well. His nutritional status deteriorated, and he experienced muscle wasting. After several months of struggling, Antonio developed pneumonia, and his doctor discussed the possibility of withholding treatment.

In the 1950s, the decisions placed on parents of children with congenital heart disease were tremendous. In Antonio's situation, if treatment were withheld, then he might be overwhelmed by the infection and die, or respiratory issues might become an ongoing problem

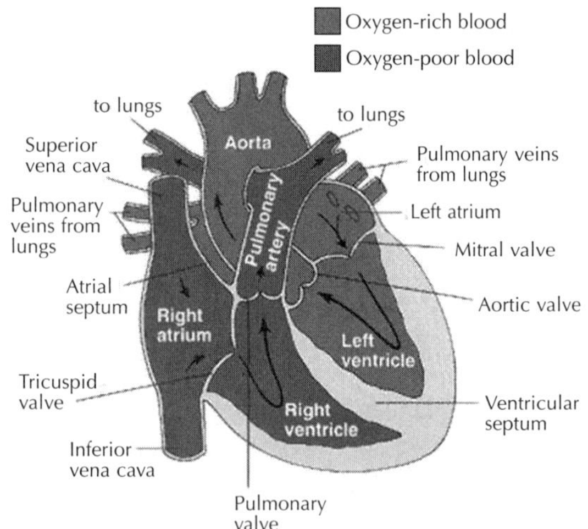

Figure 18.1-1. Normal heart. (Greystone.Net © 2004)

that could take his life. If Antonio survived the respiratory issues and the heart failure, eventually his pulmonary resistance would become elevated and thus his heart failure would improve. At this point, he would stabilize until the pulmonary resistance was higher than the systemic resistance; then he would begin to have a right to left shunt and begin to show evidence of cyanosis. Because of these difficult issues, doctors often suggested that children be institutionalized because there was minimal supportive care available to help families take care their children at home.

By the 1970s, treatment for children with congenital heart disease had advanced. Surgery to attach a pulmonary artery band improved the outcome of many children, and children were often able to be cared for at home. Consider Letitia's situation.

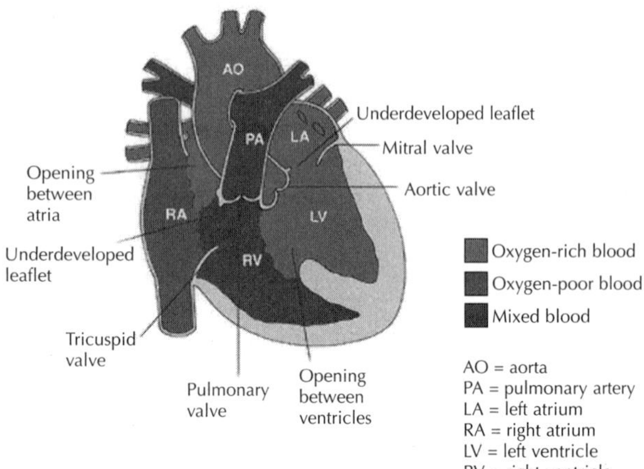

Figure 18.1-2. Heart with an atrio-ventricular canal defect. (Greystone.Net © 2004)

Letitia was born in 1971 with features of Down syndrome. Her family was informed and educated about her outlook and the need for evaluation of multiple systems that might create care issues for them. Letitia had a heart murmur and was referred for evaluation by a pediatric cardiologist. The doctor found a soft heart murmur associated with tachycardia as well as tachypnea and marginal weight gain. An electrocardiogram showed a leftward axis associated with right ventricular hypertrophy and tachycardia, and a chest X-ray showed cardiac enlargement and increased pulmonary vascular markings. An echocardiogram was subsequently performed. The echocardiogram was in its early stages of development, and the doctors thought that Letitia had significant disease—namely, an AVCD. Letitia was started on digoxin and diuretics and sent home with plans for follow-up care during the next several months. She continued to have poor weight gain and developed pneumonia, which required hospitalization.

This scenario repeated itself, and Letitia was scheduled for cardiac catheterization, at which time the defect was defined and demonstrated to be a large left to right shunt with elevated end-diastolic pressures as well as elevated pulmonary artery pressures. Often at this point, the pulmonary resistance was calculated to be low because of the large left to right shunt. Letitia was presented to the cardiac surgeons for consideration of surgical intervention. The surgeons were not enthusiastic about doing anything but decided that they could palliate Letitia with a pulmonary artery band. They hoped that this procedure would help control the heart failure and allow Letitia to grow and not have as many issues requiring hospitalization.

In the 1970s, children such as Letitia with congenital heart disease did remarkably well with pulmonary artery band therapy and were able to grow. Their heart failure often improved to the point where they could be taken off their medications. Decreasing their heart rate and respiratory rate and thus their metabolic demand reduced their nutritional requirements, resulting in improved utilization of calories taken in and better weight gain and growth. Most children responded to this therapy; however, children with significant atrio-ventricular valve regurgitation did not improve with the band as the increased resistance only made the regurgitation worse. Over the following months and years, those benefiting from the surgery grew, and as they grew, their bands became more restrictive and created a right to left shunt and the associated issues of cyanosis, which markedly limited the children's activity.

The advantage at this point was that the children had much larger hearts and their pulmonary resistance was normal because the band had protected their lungs from the high transmitted pressure of the ventricular defect. Surgical repair of the complex cardiac defect was usually attempted. The surgery entailed the closure of the atrial and ventricular defects as well as the creation of two atrio-ventricular valves from the common valve that is often associated with this defect.

Cardiopulmonary bypass was being successfully accomplished, and it allowed about 1 hour to perform the intricate repair under direct vision. Closing the atrial and ventricular defects could be accomplished with good results; however, the separation of the common valve into two competent valves was quite a challenge. Children could be left with regurgitation of the mitral valve, which often caused persistent heart failure, and replacing this valve was not possible because the technology had not been developed to produce valves small enough for children. Sometimes, however, the valves were made too small, and the child was left with mitral stenosis, which often resulted in pulmonary hypertension and right-sided heart failure as the child grew.

In the late 1970s to the 1980s, the scenario for children with congenial health disease remained the same; however, technology and surgical skill had improved, and surgical correction was being performed at more and more centers with increasingly better results. The attitude of the medical community also had changed. The survival of children with congenital heart disease led to the recognition that the children's developmental outlook would improve.

The age at which repair was contemplated was progressively younger, and some institutions attempted neonatal and infant repair once the initial physiologic changes of the newborn had taken place. Echocardiographic evaluation matured, and most children with congenital heart disease no longer required cardiac catheterization to define their anatomy and could be followed in a noninvasive manner. Postoperative management skills also improved, which was one of the major contributors to the improved survival of children with congenital heart disease.

CURRENT MANAGEMENT OF CONGENITAL HEART DISEASE

The Edwards family learned that they were expecting a child. As the baby grew, the obstetrician performed a fetal ultrasound, part of which included an evaluation of the baby's heart. Because Mrs. Edwards was in her late 30s, genetic screening was performed to evaluate for congenital problems. The combined results of these studies allowed for early identification of problems and thus complete fetal cardiac evaluation and an appropriate care plan for their child at birth. The Edwards had their baby, and they were prepared for the cardiac evaluation that took place the day of birth. A congenital heart problem was confirmed.

Children with developmental disabilities are no longer refused surgical interventions for congenital heart disease. Survival of children with complete repair has reached the 95% range in the major cardiac centers. The advancement of echocardiography has lead to the recognition of subsets of the AVCD, and this recognition has also improved survival as the operative approaches have changed and other operations such as the Glenn shunt and Fontan procedure are being used to repair children with the unbalanced form of the disease (Campbell et al., 1998).

Chromosomal analysis has matured and is being used more frequently. In association with this, fetal echocardiography has come of age, and the identification of congenital heart defects can now be established as early as 16–18 weeks. This type of information allows the physician to educate the family about what to expect from their baby when he or she is born and also to be prepared to support the infant if there is hemodynamic instability.

Once the diagnosis and the decision to have surgery have been made, efforts are taken to get the child to gain weight while the pulmonary resistance is allowed to fall as it normally does after birth. Because of the high caloric expenditure associated with congestive heart failure, the child will require a greater intake of calories, and the child is often placed on 30 cal/oz formula (see Chapter 14.1). If the child is tachypneic and cannot suck well, tube feeding is instituted, and, at times, continuous feeds may be necessary. Once the child has reached about 5 kg, he or she is usually large enough to undergo repair with reasonable risk.

In utero, fetal ultrasound in the first trimester can reveal evidence of increased nuchal translucency. Children with nuchal translucency greater than the 95th percentile have an adjusted odds ratio for a cardiac echogenic focus of 2.92 (95% CI 1.83, 4.66; Perfumo, Presti, Thilaganathan, & Carvalho, 2003). Once there is identification of cardiac focus, plans should be made for delivery and management of the child at birth. Referral to a perinatal center will assist in management of any potential issues that may arise. Upon delivery, a complete cardiac exam must be performed, which should include a clinical examination as well as an electrocardiogram, chest x-ray, and echocardiogram.

Echocardiography is the most valuable tool in making the appropriate diagnosis. It should define the presence of any lesions, the direction of blood flow through any defects, and any evidence of atrio-ventricular valve insufficiency. It also has the capability of estimating gradients and intracardiac pressures. The cardiac function should also be measured and used for future comparisons.

The lesions that may be present dictate medical management. An isolated atrial communication will often be well tolerated although weight gain may be slow. Children with this lesion do not usually have overt heart failure, but on occasion, volume management from the left to right shunt may be necessary. Usually, repair is accomplished at 2–4 years of age; however, the presence of recurring pneumonia is an indication to proceed to early correction.

The complete form of AVCD may be made up of an atrial communication, a ventricular communication, as well as insufficiency of the mitral or tricuspid valves (see Figure 18.1-2). Individuals with complete AVCD often present early in life with management problems. In the presence of a large ventricular communication, congestive heart failure will develop from 1 to 4 months after birth, and management of the failure is accomplished with the use of Digoxin, diuretics (Lasix, Diuril, Aldactone), and afterload reduction (Captopril/Enalapril; see Table 18.1-1). (*Note:* Because doses may change over time, verify doses before adminitering any medication.) Monitoring the child's hemoglobin is important, as anemia creates a high output demand and will worsen the heart failure. Most individuals will have elevated pulmonary vascular resistance, and their murmur may not be very loud. The murmur intensity is not a good indication of the significance of heart disease.

Caution must be used in administering oxygen to children with heart failure. Oxygen can decrease pulmonary resistance, which will increase pulmonary flow and actually worsen the heart failure. If a child has heart failure and is somewhat hypoxic, clinicians should be certain there is no evidence of pneumonia and only use oxygen in association with vigorous diuresis and close observation for worsening respiratory status. Respira-

Table 18.1-1. Drugs used for management of congestive heart failure

Drug and concentration	Loading dose	Maintenance dose	Frequency
Digoxin 0.05 mg/cc Oral solution	*Premature* 0.021 mg/kg 50% first dose, 25% next two doses Given every 6–12 hours	*Premature* 12.5% of loading dose, or 0.0035 mg/kg	*Premature* Every 12 hours
	Term and infant 0.04 mg/kg 50% first dose, 25% next two doses Given every 6–12 hours	*Term and infant* 12.5% of loading dose, or 0.005 mg/kg	*Term and infant* Every 12 hours
Diuretics			
Lasix 10 mg/cc Oral solution	None	1 mg/kg	1–4 times per day depending on clinical condition
Diuril 50 mg/cc Oral solution	None	10–20 mg/kg	Divided every 12–24 hours
Aldactone 25 mg Tablet	None	1–3 mg/kg	With other diuretic
Afterload reduction			
Captopril 1 mg/cc Oral solution	0.1–0.3 mg/kg Test dose—monitor for hypotension	*Neonate* 0.1–0.4 mg/kg	*Neonate* Divided every 6–12 hours
		Infant/child 2.5–6 mg/kg	*Infant/child* Divided every 6–12 hours
Enalapril 2.5 mg or 5 mg Tablet	0.08 mg/kg Test dose—monitor for hypotension	0.1–0.5 mg/kg	Divided every 12–24 hours

Note: Because doses change over time, verify doses before administering any medication.

tory failure can occur and sometimes requires management with intubation and positive end expiratory airway pressure.

A vital component in the management of children with heart failure is nutrition. The children's increased heart and respiratory rate requires increased caloric intake. Advancing formula strength to 30 cal/oz (see Table 18.1-2) will often be necessary, and one may also have to make use of nasogastric feeds as the respiratory rate of more than 70 per minute makes sucking very tiring. In order for the child to maintain a good suck, feeds may be started with the nipple and then changed to the tube once the child begins to fatigue.

Clinicians may also use continuous night feeds to further supplement bottle feeds. If they can't get the child to gain a minimum of 0.5 kg per month, surgical correction is indicated. If weight gain is accomplished, repair should be entertained once the child has attained a weight of 5 kg.

Surgical intervention should be entertained once the full diagnosis is known, when management of the heart failure is accomplished well enough to allow some growth, or is preventing growth, and when the pulmonary vascular resistance decrease has occurred. Repair should be performed, if possible, before the child is 6 months of age; when the child has achieved a weight of about 5 kg; or when medical management has not been successful. The mortality rate has been quoted to be as low as 2.5% (Cope, Fraser, Kouretas, & Kron, 2002; Murphy, 1999).

Surgical intervention requires accurate anatomical diagnosis, which can usually be accomplished using echocardiography. Defining the chamber sizes is critical, as it may influence the risk involved with the repair. The use of corrective formulae applied to echocardiography, angiography, or magnetic resonance imaging may be necessary to choose the appropriate surgical approach to these lesions (Drinkwater & Laks, 1997; van Son, 1998). Repairs often require an individualized approach based on the anatomy. The benefits of operating at this age include reduction of the hemodynamic effects of overcirculation on the lungs, reduction in the annular dilatation resulting from long-term shunting and valvar regurgitation, and achievement of a state of nutritional balance to allow growth and physical development.

Cardiac defects that have been surgically repaired, although markedly improved, may have some residual problems. Postoperatively, the atrial and ventricular defects are usually closed; however, children may have some residual mitral insufficiency or tricuspid insuffi-

Table 18.1-2. Nutritional supplementation using polycose and moducal

Infant formula	Starting volume	Amount of supplement to be added	Calories/ounce
Breast milk	3 ounces (90 cc)	1 teaspoon powered formula	24 cal/oz
	3 ounces (90 cc)	1 teaspoon powered formula 1 teaspoon polycose	26 cal/oz
	3 ounces (90 cc)	1 teaspoon powered formula 1.5 teaspoons polycose	28 cal/oz
	3 ounces (90 cc)	1 teaspoon powered formula 2 teaspoons polycose	30 cal/oz
Powered formula	4 ounces of water	2.5 tablespoons of powder	24 cal/oz
	4 ounces of water	2.5 tablespoons of powder 1.5 teaspoons of polycose	27 cal/oz
	4 ounces of water	2.5 tablespoons of powder 3 teaspoons of polycose	30 cal/oz
Liquid concentrate	13 ounces formula 8 ounces water		24 cal/oz
	13 ounces formula 8 ounces water	2 tablespoons of polycose	27 cal/oz
	13 ounces formula 8 ounces water	5 tablespoons of polycose	30 cal/oz
Formula (20 cal/oz) or breast milk	4 ounces formula	0.5 teaspoon of moducal	24 cal/oz
	4 ounces formula	2.5 teaspoons of moducal	26 cal/oz
	4 ounces formula	1 tablespoon of moducal	28 cal/oz
	4 ounces formula	1 tablespoon + 1 teaspoon of moducal	30 cal/oz

ciency. This condition can usually be managed medically using afterload reduction and diuretics; however, on occasion, reoperation is required to again repair the cleft in the valve, and, if that is not possible, then valve replacement may be necessary (Lamberti et al., 1989). In repairing the defect, there may be obstruction to the left ventricular outflow, and, thus, subaortic stenosis becomes an issue to be followed. This condition must be followed closely as it may progress and require resection or valve reorientation to relieve the obstruction.

The use of echocardiography has made quantitative monitoring of any of these residual defects easily done in a noninvasive manner as an outpatient. The evaluation of ventricular function can be compared in sequential visits to be sure that there is no functional deterioration, and gradients can easily be measured and tracked over time. Rhythm disturbances, although rare, may include atrial arrhythmias, particularly in individuals with residual valvar insufficiency. Syncope may be an indication of the presence of heart block. Ventricular ectopy may also be seen in individuals with less-than-normal ventricular function.

Multiple programs have been developed for the improvement of muscle tone and motor coordination, and children after surgery will usually tolerate these programs with little difficulty if they have had a reasonable repair. The presence of any valvar insufficiency or residual shunting warrants that the children receive endocarditis prophylaxis coverage as prescribed by the American Heart Association (Dajani et al., 1997). Other areas that require monitoring that may have cardiovascular consequences include thyroid function and obstructive sleep apnea.

The presence of hypothyroidism may present itself as bradycardia, fatigue, progressive weight gain, and the development of course skin. Children may develop pericardial effusions and present with shortness of breath and some grunting respirations. Echocardiography is helpful in making the diagnosis of effusion and in evaluating myocardial function.

Obstructive sleep apnea also has cardiovascular consequences. The hypoxia associated with the apnea leads to vasoconstriction of both the systemic and pulmonary bed. This condition may present as systemic hypertension (Marcus, Greene, & Carroll, 1998) or pulmonary hypertension (Tal, Leiberman, Margulis, & Sofer, 1988), which may be associated with right-sided heart failure.

The presence of enlarged tonsils and adenoids in association with the small nasopharyngeal airway in children with Down syndrome can often create obstructive airway problems. The children can be diagnosed if they have a history of snoring with sleep, and a sleep study (polysomnograph) is often positive for apnea and hypoxia. Sleep apnea has also been associated with fatigue during the day as the irregular sleep pattern prevents restorative sleep. In normal children, developmental delay patterns will often be seen as well as poor school performance (Brouillette, Fernbach, & Hunt, 1982; Chopo & Lazaro, 2001; Gozal, 1998). Guidelines for the diagnosis and management of childhood obstructive sleep apnea have been developed by the American Academy of Pediatrics (2002).

MANAGEMENT OF CONGENITAL HEART DISEASE IN ADULTS

As children with congenital heart disease enter the adult phase of their lives, they are susceptible to developing aortic and mitral insufficiency. Pueschel and Werner (1994) reviewed echocardiograms on a group of 36 individuals between the ages of 20 and 32. Twenty individuals had abnormal echocardiograms. Thirteen had mitral valve prolapse, three had mitral prolapse and aortic insufficiency, and two had aortic insufficiency only. Of the 16 individuals with mitral valve prolapse, 14 had evidence of a click.

Geggel, O'Brien, and Feingold (1993) evaluated 35 individuals by echocardiogram and had similar findings; however, they discovered that valvar insufficiency was not present in individuals younger than 18 years of age. The etiology of these lesions is uncertain, but there have been suggestions that they may be associated with premature aging because, at times, the aortic valve may show signs of calcification. The presence of these lesions becomes very important to identify, as these individuals require endocarditis prophylaxis for dental and other nonsterile surgical procedures.

Coronary artery disease is thought to be increased in individuals with Down syndrome. Studies have shown that a series of individuals in whom profiles were evaluated had elevated triglyceride levels and decreased levels of HDL cholesterol, apo AI, and HDL cholesterol to total cholesterol ratio—all of which would lead one to suspect a higher incidence of coronary artery disease (Pueschel, Craig, & Haddow, 1992). Monitoring and treatment of abnormal levels may be warranted using diet and/or statin therapy.

Obesity is an all too common finding in young adults. It has been shown to have a high association with obstructive sleep apnea, which in turn creates issues involving hypertension, learning problems, and unusual irritability. Regardless of whether there is the presence of heart disease, weight management is vitally important. Appropriate dietary management and regular exercise are highly recommended. Even the simplest forms of exercise such as walking are beneficial. Walking for 15–20 minutes at a pace to raise the heart rate to 110–120 per minute done 3–4 times a week will definitely improve cardiac fitness and help burn off excessive calories.

Endocarditis prophylaxis is the use of antibiotics to prevent the occurrence of bacterial infection of the cardiac structures. It is commonly used in association with nonsterile procedures such as dental restorations and extractions and ear, nose, and throat procedures such as ear tube insertion (tympanostomy tubes). As children reach the adolescent and adult age range and their clinical exams and echocardiography suggest aortic or mitral insufficiency, prescribing prophylaxis becomes important. The presence of these lesions necessitates using prophylaxis. The types of antibiotics are based on the type of procedure, and dosages may be obtained from the American Heart Association's web site (http://www.americanheart.org). A full description of when prophylaxis is necessary is also found on the web site or in published recommendations in *Circulation* (Dajani et al., 1997).

CONCLUSION

The history of the management of congenital heart disease in children with developmental delays has changed dramatically. No longer are these children treated in isolation, and this progress in care has opened new horizons. Clinicians are now learning about the differences in these children as they mature. They must remain vigilant as the children may present them with challenges they have not anticipated. Careful examination and systematic evaluation will continue to improve the long-term outlook of children with congenital heart disease.

REFERENCES

American Academy of Pediatrics. (2002, April). Clinical practice guidelines: Diagnosis and management of childhood obstructive sleep apnea syndrome. *Pediatrics, 109*(4), 704–712.

Brouillette, R.T., Fernbach, S.K., & Hunt, C.E. (1982). Obstructive sleep apnea in infants and children. *Journal of Pediatrics, 100,* 31–40.

Campbell, R.M., Adatia, I., Gow, R.M., Webb, G.D., Williams, W.G., & Freedom, R.M. (1998, August). Total cavopulmonary anastomosis (Fontan) in children with Down's syndrome. *Annals of Thoracic Surgery, 66*(2), 523–526.

Chopo, G.R., & Lazaro, M.A. (2001, January 1–15). [Obstructive sleep apnea syndrome in childhood]. [article in Spanish]. *Revista de Neurologia, 32*(1), 86–91.

Cope, J.T., Fraser, G.D., Kouretas, P.C., & Kron, I.L. (2002, October). Complete versus partial atrioventricular canal: Equal risks of repair in the modern era. *Annals of Surgery, 236*(4), 514–521.

Dajani, A.S., Taubert, K.A., Wilson, W., et al. (1997). Prevention of bacterial endocarditis: Recommendations by the American Medical Association. *Journal of the American Medical Association, 277,* 1794–1801.

Drinkwater, D.C., Jr., & Laks, H. (1997). Unbalanced atrioventricular septal defects. *Seminars in Thoracic and Cardiovascular Surgery, 9*(1), 21–25.

Geggel, R.L., O'Brien, J.E., & Feingold, M. (1993, May). Development of valve dysfunction in adolescents and young adults with Down syndrome and no known congenital disease. *Journal of Pediatrics, 122*(5 Pt. 1), 821–823.

Gozal, D. (1998). Sleep-disordered breathing and school performance in children. *Pediatrics, 102,* 616–620.

Lamberti, J.J., Jensen, T.S., Grehl, T.M., Oury, J.H., Waldman, J.D., Kirkpatrick, S.E., et al. (1989, April). Late re-operation for systemic atrioventricular valve regurgitation after repair of congenital heart defect. *Annals of Thoracic Surgery, 47*(4), 517–522.

Marcus, C.L., Greene, M.G., & Carroll, J.L. (1998). Blood pressure in children with obstructive sleep apnea. *American Journal of Respiratory and Critical Care Medicine, 157,* 1098–1103.

Murphy, D.J., Jr. (1999, December). Atrioventricular canal defects. *Current Treatment Options in Cardiovascular Medicine, 1*(4), 323–334.

Perfumo, F., Presti, F., Thilaganathan, B., & Cavalho, J.S. (2003, May). Association between increased nuchal translucency and second trimester cardiac echogenic foci. *Obstetrics and Gynecology, 101*(5 Pt. 1), 899–904.

Pueschel, S.M., Craig, W.Y., & Haddow, J.E. (1992, August). Lipids and lipoproteins in persons with Down's syndrome. *Journal of Intellectual Disability Research, 36*(4), 365–369.

Pueschel, S.M., & Werner, J.C. (1994, March–April). Multivalve prolapse in persons with Down syndrome. *Research in Developmental Disabilities, 15*(2), 91–97.

Tal, A., Leiberman, A., Margulis, G., & Sofer, S. (1988). Ventricular dysfunction in children with obstructive sleep apnea. *Pediatric Pulmonology, 4,* 139–143.

van Son, J.A. (1998, July). Correspondence. *Annals of Thoracic Surgery, 66*(1), 310.

18.2 SPECTRUM OF HEART DISEASE

William Mahle

This chapter explores the relationship between congenital heart disease and neurodevelopmental outcome. Newborns with congenital heart disease have a substantially higher incidence of brain abnormalities such as overt cerebral dysgenesis than the general population, as demonstrated by pathologic and neuroimaging studies. Microcephaly has been reported as an associated finding in as many as 36% of neonates with congenital heart disease (Limperopoulus et al., 2000). Glauser, Rorke, Weinberg, and Clancy (1990) reported postmortem examinations in 39 infants with congenital heart disease and found increased operculum in 8 (20%) and absent corpus callosum in 3 (8%). Neuroimaging studies have also demonstrated callosal agenesis, abnormal neuronal migration, temporal lobar hypoplasia, and Chiari I malformations.

An understanding of the expected long-term neurocognitive outcome of children with congenital heart disease is essential to management and appropriate counseling. The potential interactions of underlying central nervous system abnormalities, the hemodynamic effects of complex congenital heart disease, and the sequelae of cardiac surgery are incompletely understood. This chapter explores the neurodevelopment of individuals with congenital heart disease in relation to genetic syndromes and cardiac surgery.

CONGENITAL HEART DISEASE AND GENETIC SYNDROMES

Chromosomal and nonchromosomal syndromes occur in more than 20% of children with significant congenital heart disease. Some of the more common genetic syndromes and associations found in individuals with congenital heart disease are shown in Table 18.2–1. Two genetic syndromes, DiGeorge syndrome and Williams syndrome (see Chapter 9.5), are presented next.

Dana is a 7-year-old girl with tetralogy of Fallot who underwent complete repair of her cardiac defect at 4 months of age. She is followed annually by a cardiologist, and consideration is being given to replacement of her pulmonary valve. Her mother states that Dana is an active girl who has been receiving speech therapy and is due to be evaluated by the school psychologist for learning disabilities. Dana's cardiologist is concerned that she may have 22q11 deletion and arranges for further evaluation.

DiGeorge syndrome (22q11.2) has been found in more than 50% of individuals with interrupted aortic arch (type B) and at least 15% of individuals with tetralogy of Fallot. In most cases, the identification of the congenital heart disease precedes the genetic diagnosis of microdeletion of 22q11.2. The presence of microdeletion of 22q11.2 puts individuals at higher risk following open heart surgery. The risk appears to be more related to the severity of heart disease than to other factors such as predisposition to infection.

Screening individuals with certain high risk lesions such as interrupted aortic arch, tetralogy of Fallot, and truncus arteriosus with *flouresent in situ hybridization* techniques has now become routine. Some lesions, however, such as abnormalities of the aortic arch, may not

Table 18.2-1. Genetic syndromes associated with congenital heart disease and neurodevelopmental risks

Syndromes and associations	Percent of individuals with congential heart disease	Most common lesions	Neurocognitive impairments
Down syndrome (trisomy 21)	40%	Endocardial cushion, VSD, TOF, PDA	Intellectual disabilities (median IQ score 25–50) (Brugge et al., 1994; Byrne, Macdonald, & Buckley, 2002)
DiGeorge syndrome (microdeletion of 22q11)	60%	IAA, TOF, truncus arteriosus	Mean IQ score 70–80, ADHD (Moss et al., 1999)
Turner syndrome (monosomy of chromosome 23)	30%	Bicuspid aortic valve, coarctation of the aorta	Mean IQ score 90 (Swillen et al. 1993; Temple & Carny, 1993)
Williams syndrome (chromosome 7q11 mutation)	60%	Supravalvar AS, PPS	Mean IQ score 56, mild spasticity
Alagille syndrome (chromosome 20p12 mutation)	85%	PPS	Majority with normal intelligence
VACTERL association	53%	VSD, ASD	Majority with normal brain function
CHARGE association	More than 50%	TOF, PDA, VSD, ASD	Intellectual disabilities in almost all cases

Key: ADHD = attention-deficit/hyperactivity disorder; ASD = atrial septal defect; DORV = double outlet right ventricle; IAA = interrupted aortic arch; PDA = patent ductus arteriosus; PPS = peripheral pulmonary stenosis; TOF = tetralogy of Fallot; VSD = ventricular septal defect.

be clinically evident. Although the presence of a perimembranous ventricular septal defect is also associated with microdeletion of 22q11.2, the association is not as strong, and routine screening is not always undertaken. Unlike atrio-ventricular canal defect, for which the majority of individuals will require only one operation in their lifetime, individuals with microdeletion of 22q11.2 often require close follow-up. Further surgery on the right ventricular outflow tract is frequently required by the second decade of life.

The most common congenital heart defect associated with Williams syndrome is supravalvar aortic stenosis. At times, this condition can extend to include a diffuse arteriopathy in which the proximal and distal aorta as well as renal arteries may be stenotic. In advanced forms of supravalvar aortic stenosis, surgery is often indicated. When the distal aorta is involved, surgical options may be limited. Peripheral pulmonary artery stenosis may also occur in Williams syndrome. Interventional catheterization and surgery have had limited success in this lesion. Long-term care of these individuals often focuses on complications of the cardiac and vascular defects such as systemic and pulmonary hypertension.

PREOPERATIVE NEUROLOGIC FINDINGS

In addition to named genetic disorders, individuals with unrepaired congenital heart disease have a higher incidence of neurologic impairments compared with the normal population. Several studies have identified neurologic abnormalities in individuals with congenital heart disease prior to any surgical intervention. A study of newborns with a variety of congenital heart defects demonstrated that more than 50% had at least one abnormal finding on preoperative neurologic examination (Limperopoulos et al., 2000).

Some of the more common abnormalities noted in neonates with congenital heart disease were abnormalities in tone, jitteriness, and poor oromotor coordination. Feeding difficulties were noted in more than one third of newborns. Similarly, Brunberg and associates found abnormalities on neurologic examination in 15 of 21 individuals with congenital heart disease prior to surgical intervention (Brunberg, Reilly, & Doty, 1974).

In addition to congenital neurologic abnormalities, infants with complex congenital heart disease are at risk for preoperative neurologic insult. Factors that can affect preoperative neurologic status include hypoxemia, poor feeding, and congestive heart failure. In particular, newborns with ductal-dependent systemic blood may present with profound acidosis, hypoxic-ischemic injury, and/or shock upon closure of the ductus arteriosus. Preoperative seizures, intraventricluar hemorrhage, and periventricular leukomalacia are known consequences of hypoperfusion in these ductal-dependent lesions (Mahle et al., 2000). Postnatal brain injury primarily involves the white matter and is more likely due to ischemic rather than hypoxic insult (Mahle et al., 2002).

Intraventricular hemorrhage has also been documented in neonates with congenital heart disease. The risk of intraventricular hemorrhage increases when hemodynamic instability is superimposed on the delicate microvasculature of the immature brain. Van Houten and colleagues found intraventricular hemorrhage in 24% of term infants with congenital heart disease (Van Houten, Rothman, & Bejar, 1996). The incidence of intraventricular hemorrhage in premature infants with congenital heart disease is not well described, though presumably the risk would be even higher.

Congestive heart failure also contributes to a poor neurodevelopmental outcome. The association between congestive heart failure and developmental outcome may be related to physical inactivity and failure to thrive. Children with congenital heart disease may not receive sufficient nutrient and caloric intake because of fatigue, recurrent infection, or cardiac decompensation. Because 50% of the normal postnatal brain growth occurs during the first year of life, poor growth and nutrition during this critical period can put the infant at risk.

In addition, studies in adults have shown that heart failure results in impaired cerebral blood flow. Gruhn and colleagues showed that cerebral blood flow is substantially, but reversibly, reduced in individuals with NYHA class III/IV heart failure (Gruhn et al., 2001). This phenomenon suggests that redistribution of cardiac output inadequately secures brain perfusion in individuals with severe congestive heart failure.

Thus, even before the newborn or infant undergoes cardiac surgery, a number of factors—individually or in combination—place the child at increased risk for compromised neurologic and cognitive development. The interactions between genetic predisposition, acquired or congenital structural abnormalities, hypoxemia, low cardiac output, and nutrition must be considered in the overall risk assessment of the infant.

Cardiopulmonary bypass is utilized in many neonatal and infant cardiac surgical procedures. It allows for perfusion of vital organs by providing oxygenated blood via a mechanical pump. During procedures using cardiopulmonary bypass, especially at low-flow rates, neuroprotection may be achieved with concomitant use of hypothermia. Hypothermia protects the brain by decreasing cerebral metabolism. In some procedures, it is necessary to stop blood flow altogether through a process known as deep hypothermic circulatory arrest. Procedures that require deep hypothermia are thought to pose a great risk to the infant brain.

POSTOPERATIVE NEUROLOGIC FINDINGS

Neurologic examinations performed in the postoperative period have identified a variety of abnormalities including hypotonia, pyramidal findings, and asymmetry of tone. Miller and colleagues performed neurologic examinations on 91 young infants undergoing congenital heart surgery (Miller, Mamourian, Tesman, Baylen, & Myers, 1994). In addition to clinical seizures in 15% of infants, the authors found hypotonia in 34% of infants at hospital discharge. Hypertonia was noted in 7% of infants, and asymmetry of tone, in 5%. A decreased level of alertness was noted in 19% of infants at hospital discharge. In the Boston randomized study of low-flow cardiopulmonary bypass and deep hypothermic circulatory arrest, diffuse motor abnormalities were noted in 45%, and cranial nerve abnormalities were noted in 4% of infants at hospital discharge (Newburger et al., 1993).

Neuroimaging studies performed in the early postoperative period have demonstrated a high incidence of abnormalities, though the clinical significance of these findings is unclear. These cystic lesions usually regress after several months. The cysts are often replaced by an astroglial scar resulting in periventricular leukomalacia, which is characterized by a marked deficiency of cerebral white matter. The factors that lead to the development of periventricular leukomalacia after complex congenital heart disease surgery in the neonates have not been well characterized. The white matter is particularly susceptible to injury when cerebral autoregulation is compromised, such as after a period of deep hypothermic circulatory arrest. The subsequent neurologic features of periventricular leukomalacia relate to the topography of this lesion.

Several investigations have addressed the neurocognitive outcome for survivors of complex heart surgery; some are parts of prospective clinical trials, whereas others are retrospective or cross-sectional reviews. The results of some of these studies are summarized in Table 18.2-2. Results of these studies are influenced by many factors, including the era in which individuals underwent surgery, the outcome measures used, and the age at testing. Most standardized tests, such as the Bayley Scales of Infant Development, Second Edition (Bayley, 1993) and the Wechsler Intelligence Scale for Children, Third Edition (Wechsler, 1992) are scored according to the population norms with a mean of 100 and a standard deviation of 15.

Table 18.2-2. Reported outcomes after complex infant heart surgery

Lesion	Full-scale IQ score	Comments
Transposition of the great arteries	92–101 ± 17.4	
Tetralogy of Fallot	100	Significant limitations for individuals with 22q11.2
Single ventricle	95	
Hypoplastic left heart syndrome	86–88	Attention problems common
Heart transplantation	91	

Findings in Transposition of the Great Arteries

The most extensively studied subgroup of individuals is individuals with transposition of the great arteries, most likely due to the high prevalence of transposition of the great arteries (1/5,000), the low mortality of surgical intervention, the long duration of follow-up (early repair was possible in the 1960s), and the low incidence of associated genetic syndromes. At presentation, many of these individuals are profoundly hypoxemic until mixing of oxygenated and deoxygenated blood can be increased by procedures such as balloon atrial septostomy or the institution of prostaglandin E_1. The current approach to tranposition of the great arteries is early reparative surgery with the arterial switch procedure. This operation may require the use of deep hypothermic circulatory arrest with occasional prolonged (> 45 min) periods.

Hesz and Clark studied 10 individuals with transposition of the great arteries after arterial switch and found significantly lower developmental scores when compared with bothers and sisters (Hesz & Clark, 1988). In the Boston prospective randomized trial, the mean full scale IQ score at 4 years of age of individuals with transposition of the great arteries was 92.6 ± 14.7, which was mildly but significantly lower than the normal population (Bellinger et al., 1999). Impairments were most commonly noted in visual-spatial and visual-motor integration. Definite neurologic abnormalities were noted in 30% of individuals. The incidence of speech abnormalities was also higher than the general population. Risk factors for lower, full-scale IQ scores included perioperative seizures and the presence of a coexisting ventricular septal defect.

Findings in Tetralogy of Fallot

Individuals with tetralogy of Fallot have previously been noted to have lower scores on standardized cognitive testing and poorer overall psychological functioning than the normal population. In a study of individuals with tetralogy of Fallot, the majority of whom had undergone complete repair, DeMaso, Beardslee, Silbert, and Fyler (1990) found that 22% scored 80% or less on IQ score testing versus 2.8% of the control population without congenital heart disease. Oates, Simpson, Turnbull, and Cartmill (1995), however, found IQ scores within the normal range for 51 individuals with tetralogy of Fallot (100 ± 13). Potential risk factors in these individuals include prolonged hypoxemia, congestive heart failure, and thrombo-embolic events. An additional risk factor is the association of tetralogy of Fallot and microdeletion of 22q11.2, which is found in more than 15% of individuals with tetralogy of Fallot.

Individuals with tetralogy of Fallot usually undergo complete repair within the first year of life. This strategy reduces the risk of right to left shunting, hypercyanotic spells, and central nervous system damage. Data regarding neurocognitive outcome for individuals with tetralogy of Fallot undergoing early repair and the effects of associated genetic abnormalities is currently under analysis.

Tina is a 32-year-old woman with tetralogy of Fallot who has undergone three cardiac surgeries in her lifetime: a modified Blalock-Taussig shunt at 3 months, surgical repair at 2 years, and replacement of her pulmonary valve at 22 years. She has completed college and works as a systems analyst. Tina is now 16 weeks pregnant and anxious about the outcome for her unborn child. She reports loss of energy and poor appetite.

Adults with tetralogy of Fallot generally have normal cognitive function, and many complete higher education. Most adults with repaired tetralogy of Fallot have mild exercise intolerance. Pregnancy may exacerbate heart failure, so high-risk obstetrics is warranted.

Findings in Single Ventricle Lesions

Individuals with single ventricle lesions who are palliated with the Fontan operation are at considerable risk for neurocognitive impairment. Risk factors include multiple operations requiring cardiopulmonary bypass with or without deep hypothermic circulatory arrest, prolonged hypoxemia, and failure to thrive. Individuals palliated with the Fontan procedure appear to be at particular risk for a cerebrovascular accident. The risk of cerebrovascular accident after Fontan procedure has been reported to be 2.7%–8.8% (Rosti, Colli, & Frigiola, 1997).

Studies have investigated the long-term neurocognitive outcome of individuals palliated with the Fontan operation. Wernovsky and colleagues (2000) evaluated 133 individuals palliated with Fontan surgery at a median age of 11.1 years. The mean full-scale IQ score in this cohort (95.7 ± 17.4) was lower than that in the general population. Intellectual disabilities, defined as full-scale IQ score less than 70, were noted in 7.8% of these individuals.

Additional risk factors for lower scores on cognitive testing included lower socioeconomic status, the use circulatory arrest prior to the Fontan procedure, and anatomic diagnosis. In particular, individuals with hypoplastic left heart syndrome scored significantly lower on standardized testing. Similarly, Uzark and colleagues (1998) reported a mean IQ score of 97.5 ± 12.1 for 32 children with single ventricle palliated with the Fontan procedure. The diagnosis of hypoplastic left heart syndrome was associated with lower scores.

Findings in Hypoplastic Left Heart Syndrome

There are several reasons why individuals with hypoplastic left heart syndrome may be at higher risk for neurodevelopmental impairments than individuals with other forms of single ventricle. Previous investigations have demonstrated a relatively high incidence of congenital brain abnormalities in neonates with hypoplastic left heart syndrome. In addition, these infants have ductal-dependent systemic blood flow; severe acidosis and end-organ injury at the time of presentation are not uncommon. Circulatory arrest is used for surgery. In addition, maintaining adequate systemic blood flow and cerebral perfusion in the postoperative period can be unpredictable. The risk of postoperative seizures is significant, as much as 18% after stage I reconstruction (Clancy et al., 2001).

In 1995, Rogers and colleagues reported the neurodevelopmental outcome of 11 preschool survivors of reconstructive surgery for hypoplastic left heart syndrome at various stages of palliation. The study documented an alarmingly high incidence of neurodevelopmental impairments. Of the 11 children studied, 7 (64%) were found to have intellectual disabilities. Substantial functional disabilities were present in 8 children (73%), and gross motor abnormalities were noted in 5 children (45%).

The author and his colleagues studied the outcome of 115 school-age children with hypoplastic left heart syndrome who had undergone staged palliation before

1992 (Mahle et al., 2000). A questionnaire sent to the study participants and their families revealed that more than 30% of the participants were receiving some form of special education. Standardized neurocognitive testing was performed in 28 local participants. Although the majority of these participants scored within the normal range, the median full scale IQ score was 86—significantly lower than the general population. In addition, 18% of subjects had IQ scores in the mentally retarded range. We also detected minor neurologic abnormalities in 55% of participants. These abnormalities included microcephaly in 13%, fine motor abnormalities in 48%, and gross motor abnormalities in 39%. Cerebral palsy was present in 17%. More than 60% of participants were thought to have problems with attention, and 9% had mood disturbances.

Harith is an 8-year-old boy who was found to have hypoplastic left heart syndrome prenatally. He underwent three palliative surgical procedures at 1 week, 6 months, and 2 years of age. He is currently in second grade and attends special education classes.

Harith participates in sports but tires more easily than his peers. His height and weight are at the 5th and 3rd percentile. He takes three chronic cardiovascular medications (furosemide, aspirin, and enalapril).

Long-term issues for individuals with hypoplastic left heart syndrome include learning disabilities and attention problems. Almost half of individuals receive special education services, and many are underdiagnosed for attention-deficit/hyperactivity disorder because their behaviors are attributed to cardiac problems. Fine motor abnormalities are present in many individuals, but severe motor problems such as cerebral palsy are rare.

Height and weight are significantly less than brothers and sisters, with median height in the 10th percentile and median weight in the 15th percentile. Marked limitation of exercise ability (maximal oxygen consumption 28 l/min./m^2 vs. normal of 40 l/min./m^2) is also a problem. A dynamic exercise regimen is allowed, and exercise rehabilitation programs have been shown to improve exercise ability over time.

Findings in Heart Transplantation

Infant heart transplantation has been undertaken in many centers as an alternative management approach to complex congenital heart disease in which reconstructive surgery is associated with a high mortality. Postoperatively, individuals are at risk for low cardiac output and have an increased risk of seizures, possibly related to immunosuppressive medications or deep hypothermic circulatory arrest. One study of neurologic outcomes in individuals who had undergone infant heart transplantation evaluated 38 infants at 12–30 months of age. The mean scores of both the mental developmental index and psychomotor developmental index, 91 and 88 respectively, were lower than the scores for the normal population (Baum, Freier, Freeman, & Chinnock, 2000).

Neuropsychiatric Issues

Although much has been written about the cognitive outcome after complex congenital heart disease surgery, less is known about neurobehavioral sequelae in these individuals. Several investigators have identified neurobehavioral issues that may contribute significantly to long-term morbidity in individuals with congestive heart failure. Attention deficit disorder has been described in several evaluations of school-age children who underwent surgical repair after congenital heart disease (Clarkson, MacArthur, Barratt-Boyes, Whitlock, & Neutze, 1980; Haka-Ikse, Blackwood, & Steward, 1978). In the evaluation of school-age survivors of staged palliation for hypoplastic left heart syndrome, the author and his colleagues detected a high prevalence of attention problems (Mahle et al., 2000). Both neurologic evaluation and use of standardized behavior batteries suggested a high degree of attention and hyperactivity problems. Why attention-deficit/hyperactivity disorder may be more common in individuals with congenital heart disease is not known. Further analysis will be needed to determine what perioperative factors may be associated with attention problems.

In addition to attention-deficit/hyperactivity disorder, other behavior problems have been identified. In retrospective analysis by the author and his colleagues, 18% of individuals with hypoplastic left heart syndrome had clinically significant anxiety problems (versus 2% in the normal population) as measured by the Achenbach Child Behavior Checklist (Mahle et al., 2000). DeMaso and colleagues also used a standardized instrument to characterize psychological function in individuals who had undergone repair of tetralogy of Fallot and transposition of the great arteries (DeMaso, Beardslee, Silbert, & Fryler, 1990). They demonstrated marked pyschological impairment such as obsessive-compulsive traits and disabling anxiety in more than 15% of individuals. An increased incidence of aggressive behavior was noted among patients with transposition of the great arteries who had undergone the arterial switch under deep hypothermic circulatory arrest (Hesz & Clark, 1988). Others have found an increased incidence of mood disturbances in toddlers with congenital heart disease when compared with control groups.

Brandhagen, Feldt, and Williams (1991) used standardized psychological instruments in the follow-up evaluation of 168 adults with congenital heart disease. They found that adults with congenital heart disease have significantly higher anxiety, hostility, and symptom distress than the normal population. Interestingly, the degree of psychological distress was not correlated to the clinical severity of the cardiac lesions and did not seem to be related to all areas of social function, such as job stability, education attainment, and other factors.

CONCLUSION

Each year, there are more adult survivors of congenital heart disease, a significant number of whom have neurocognitive sequelae. Whether neurocognitive impairments are related to underlying genetic syndromes, to cardiac surgery, or to other factors is not known. An understanding of individuals who are at greater risk and their unique profile of cognitive and behavioral impairments can help clinicians to adequately address these individuals' long-term care and provide appropriate family counseling.

REFERENCES

Baum, M., Freier, M., Freeman, K., & Chinnock, R. (2000). Developmental outcomes and cognitive functioning in infant and child heart transplant recipients. *Progress in Pediatric Cardiology, 11,* 159–163.

Bellinger, D., Wypij, D., Kuban, K., Rappaport, L., Hickey, P., Wernovsky, G. et al. (1999). Developmental and neurological status of children at 4 years of age after heart surgery with hypothermic circulatory arrest or low-flow cardiopulmonary bypass. *Circulation, 100,* 526–532.

Brandhagen, D., Feldt, R., & Williams, D. (1991). Long-term psychologic implications of congenital heart disease: A 25-year follow-up. *Mayo Clinic Proceedings,* 66, 474–479.

Brugge, K.L., Nichols, S.I., Salmon, D.P., Hill, L.R., Delis, D.C., Aaron, L., et al. (1994). Cognitive impairment in adults with Down's syndome: Similarities to early cognitive changes in Alzheimer's disease. *Neurology, 44,* 232–238.

Brunberg, J., Reilly, E., & Doty, D. (1974). Central nervous system consequences in infants of cardiac surgery using deep hypothermia and circulatory arrest. *Circulation,* 50, 1160–1168.

Byrne, A., Macdonald, J., & Buckley, S. (2002). Reading, language, and memory skills: A comparative longitudinal study of children with Down syndrome and their mainstream peers. *British Journal of Educational Psychology, 72,* 513–529.

Clancy, R., Mcgaurn, S., Goin, J., Hirtz, D., Norwood, W., Gaynor, J., et al. (2001). Allopurinol neurocardiac protection trial in infants undergoing heart surgery using deep hypothermic circulatory arrest. *Pediatrics, 108,* 61–70.

Clarkson, P., Macarthur, B., Barratt-Boyes, B., Whitlock, R., & Neutze, J. (1980). Developmental progress after cardiac surgery in infancy using hypothermia and circulatory arrest. *Circulation, 62,* 855–861.

DeMaso, D., Beardslee, W., Silbert, A., & Fyler, D. (1990). Psychological functioning in children with cyanotic heart defects. *Journal of Developmental and Behavioral Pediatrics, 11,* 289–294.

Glauser, T., Rorke, L., Weinberg, P., & Clancy, R. (1990). Congenital brain anomalies associated with the hypoplastic left heart syndrome. *Pediatrics, 85,* 984–990.

Gruhn, N., Larsen, F., Boesgaard, S., Knudsen, G., Mortensen, S., Thomsen, G., et al. (2001). Cerebral blood flow in patients with chronic heart failure before and after heart transplantation. *Stroke, 32,* 2530–2533.

Haka-Ikse, K., Blackwood, M., & Steward, D. (1978). Psychomotor development of infants and children after profound hypothermia during surgery for congenital heart disease. *Developmental Medicine and Child Neurology, 20,* 62–70.

Hesz, N., & Clark, E. (1988). Cognitive development in transposition of the great vessels. *Archives of Disease in Childhood, 63,* 198–200.

Limperopoulos, C., Majnemer, A., Shevell, M., Rosenblatt, B., Rohlicek, C., & Tchervenkov, C. (2000). Neurodevelopmental status of newborns and infants with congenital heart defects before and after open heart surgery. *Journal of Pediatrics, 137,* 638–645.

Mahle, W., Clancy, R., Moss, E., Gerdes, M., Jobes, D., & Wernovsky, G. (2000). Neurodevelopmental outcome and lifestyle assessment in school-aged and adolescent children with hypoplastic left heart syndrome. *Pediatrics, 105,* 1082–1089.

Mahle, W., Tavani, F., Zimmerman, R., Nicolson, S., Galli, K., Gaynor, J., et al. (2002). An MRI study of neurological injury before and after congenital heart surgery. *Circulation, 106,* 1109–1114.

Miller, G., Mamourian, A., Tesman, J., Baylen, B., & Myers, J. (1994). Long-term MRI changes in brain after pediatric open heart surgery. *Journal of Child Neurology, 9,* 390–397.

Moss, E.M., Batshaw, M.L., Solot, C.B., Gerdes, M., McDonald-McGinn, D.M., Driscoll, D.A., et al. (1999). Psychoeducational profile of the 22q11.2 microdeletion: A complex pattern. *Journal of Pediatrics, 134,* 193–198.

Newburger, J., Jonas, R., Wernovsky, G., Wypij, D., Hickey, P., Kuban, K., et al. (1993). A comparison of the perioperative neurologic effects of hypothermic circulatory arrest versus low-flow cardiopulmonary bypass in infant heart surgery. *New England Journal of Medicine, 329,* 1057–1064.

Oates, R., Simpson, J., Turnbull, J., & Cartmill, T. (1995). The relationship between intelligence and duration of circulatory arrest with deep hypothermia. *Journal of Thoracic and Cardiovascular Surgery, 110,* 786–792.

Rogers, B., Msall, M., Buck, G., Lyon, N., Norris, M., Roland, J., et al. (1995). Neurodevelopmental outcome of infants with hypoplastic left heart syndrome. *Journal of Pediatrics, 126,* 496–498.

Rosti, L., Colli, A., & Frigiola, A. (1997). Stroke and the Fontan procedure. *Pediatric Cardiology, 18*, 159.

Swillen, A., Fryns, J.P., Kleczkowska, A., Massa, G., Vanderschueren-Lodeweyckx, M., & Van den Berghe, H. (1993). Intelligence, behaviour and psychosocial development in Turner syndrome: A cross-sectional study of 50 preadolescent girls. (4–20 years). *Genetic Counseling, 4*, 7–18.

Temple, C.M., Carney, R.A. (1993). Intellectional functioning of children with Turner syndrome: A comparison of behavioral phenotypes. *Developmental Medicine and Child Neurology, 35*, 691–698.

Uzark, K., Lincoln, A., Lamberti, J., Mainwaring, R., Spicer, R., & Moore, J. (1998). Neurodevelopmental outcomes in children with Fontan repair of functional single ventricle. *Pediatrics, 101*, 630–633.

Van Houten, J., Rothman, A., & Bejar, R. (1996). High incidence of cranial ultrasound abnormalities in full-term infants with congenital heart disease. *American Journal of Perinatology, 13*, 47–53.

Wernovsky, G., Stiles, K., Gauvreau, K., Gentles, T., Duplessis, A., Bellinger, D., et al. (2000). Cognitive development after the Fontan operation. *Circulation, 102*, 883–889.

CHAPTER 19

ENDOCRINOLOGY

Diego Botero and Amy Fleischman

Individuals with developmental disabilities often have associated endocrine abnormalities. They may have disabilities caused by endocrinopathies (e.g., hypothyroidism, hypoglycemia), endocrine conditions associated with chromosomal and nonchromosomal syndromes that have diverse physical and neurodevelopmental characteristics (e.g., Down syndrome, Turner syndrome), or secondary symptoms to underlying disorders of the central nervous system (e.g., those that trigger the onset of pubertal development at an early age). In addition, medications utilized in the treatment of children and adults with developmental disabilities can cause or confound endocrine disorders. Individuals with developmental disabilities require a comprehensive evaluation of endocrine function, including growth and pubertal development.

ENDOCRINE DISORDERS THAT CAUSE DEVELOPMENTAL DISABILITIES

Congenital Hypothyroidism

Harry was discharged from the hospital 3 days after birth. His mother had had a normal pregnancy, labor, and delivery. On Harry's eighth day of life, his pediatrician was contacted by the regional neonatal screening program due to an abnormally elevated thyroid-stimulating hormone. A complete thyroid profile confirmed the diagnosis of congenital hypothyroidism. Harry underwent a thyroid scan that revealed the presence of a hypoplastic thyroid gland. With diagnosis of sporadic congenital hypothyroidism, Harry was started on thyroid hormone replacement at 10 days. He is now 2 years old and has a normal neurological development.

Congenital hypothyroidism is a common preventable cause of intellectual disabilities with an overall incidence of approximately 1:4,000. At birth, the clinical picture may not be obvious because typical signs appear only after several weeks, but a delayed diagnosis could have severe consequences in neurological development. Less than 5% of affected infants are diagnosed on clinical grounds before the screening report. Maternal supply of thyroid hormones explains why most of the athyreotic newborns usually do not show any signs of hypothyroidism at birth. Affected infants may present with poor feeding, lethargy, constipation, prolonged jaundice, large fontanelles, prolonged hyperbilirubinemia, macroglossia, hoarse cry, distended abdomen, umbilical hernia, and hypotonia (see also Figure 19.1).

Most regional screening programs employ measurements of thyroxine in blood collected on filter paper before the newborn is discharged from the hospital (see Chapter 7.1). Before the implementation of neonatal screening programs, the mean IQ score of children with congenital hypothyroidism was 76, and 40% required special education. The prognosis has improved, and the neurological gap between infants with congenital hypothyroidism and children without the disorder has been closed due to early, high-dose treatment. Frequent monitoring of thyroid function is recommended every 1–3 months.

Hypoglycemia

Seraphine's birth weight was normal, but she had severe hypoglycemia in the first 24 hours of life. Despite being fed every 2 hours, her glucose readings were below 50 mg/dL. She was placed on intravenous 10% Dextrose solution providing 6 mg/kg/min of glucose. A critical sample obtained at the time of a hypoglycemic episode revealed a serum insulin level of 30 uU/mL concomitant with a blood glucose of 25 mg/dL. Seraphine did not have ketonemia, and the levels of growth hormone and cortisol were appropriately elevated.

Considering her elevated insulin in the setting of a low blood sugar, Seraphine was diagnosed with hyperinsulinism and was placed on diazoxide. It was necessary to increase the 10% Dextrose infusion to provide 15 mg/kg/min in order to control her low blood sugars. In the second week of life, she was still having episodes of hypoglycemia despite receiving the maximal dose of diazoxide and a Dextrose infusion rate to 20 mg/kg/min. The decision was made to perform a near-total pancreatectomy.

Seraphine tolerated the procedure. One day after the surgery, she experienced persisting hyperglycemia. Serum levels of insulin and C-peptide were undetectable. With di-

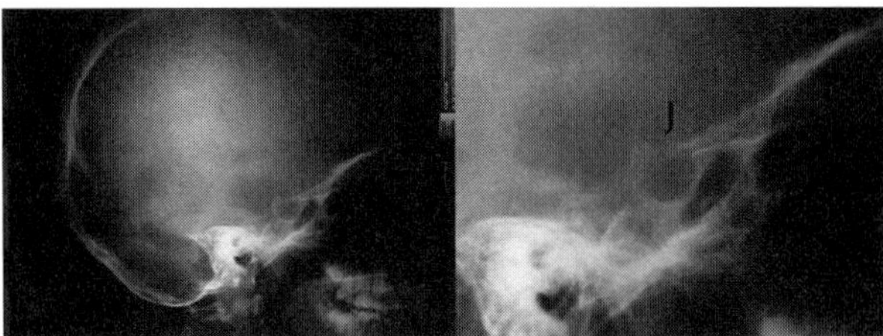

Figure 19.1. A 4-year-old child with untreated congenital hypothyroidism. Significant sclerosis of the base of the skull and enlargement of the Sella turcica (J) are noted.

agnosis of diabetes mellitus secondary to pancreatectomy, she was placed on subcutaneous insulin. Seraphine also received pancreatic enzymes to treat her exocrine pancreatic dysfunction. Histological analysis of her pancreas revealed the presence of a mutation in the sulfonylurea receptor.

Early recognition and treatment of hypoglycemia can prevent the large majority of sequelae including cognitive and motor impairments and seizure disorders. Hypoglycemia is more common in premature infants, small for gestational age infants, infants of diabetic mothers, and infants who had significant stressors at the time of delivery. More permanent and serious causes of neonatal hypoglycemia include hyperinsulinemia, metabolic deficiencies, and endocrinopathies (e.g., panhypopituitarism).

A thorough physical exam may also provide clues to the etiology of hypoglycemia. Poor growth, microphallus, or midline facial impairments are suggestive of a pituitary abnormality such as growth hormone deficiency or hypopituitarism. A large liver found on examination should suggest an evaluation for disorders of glycogen storage, gluconeogenesis, fatty acid oxidation, or carnitine metabolism. Hyperventilation or respiratory distress without obvious pulmonary pathology should suggest a state of metabolic acidosis or hyperammonemia. Global cardiac abnormalities can be associated with impairments in fatty acid oxidation or carnitine metabolism. The steps in Table 19.1 may be used as a guideline in the diagnosis of hypoglycemia in children.

Table 19.1. Guidelines for the diagnosis of hypoglycemia in children

Confirm hypoglycemia with serum blood sample processed in timely manner.

Conduct a physical examination.

- Small child, midline defects—suggestive of endocrine etiology (hypopituitarism)
- Large liver size—suggestive of glycogen storage diseases or disorder of gluconeogenesis

Assess the timing of the event.

- Less than 4 hours—hyperinsulinemia or defect in glycogenolysis
- 10–12 hours—defect in gluconeogenesis or fatty acid oxidation

Conduct a laboratory evaluation of first urine for ketones.

- Negative/small ketones—suggestive of hyperinsulinism or a fatty acid oxidation defect
- Moderate to large (appropriate)—further evaluation needed for abnormalities in urine organic acid patterns suggestive of specific metabolic defect

Source: Wolfsdorf and Weinstein (2003).

Hyperinsulinism often manifests in the neonatal period but can reveal itself later in childhood. Children with hyperinsulinism also have decreased utilization of fatty acids and ketones, increasing their risk for neurologic damage due to lack of alternate fuel sources. Therapy for hyperinsulinism is focused on the prevention of neurologic sequelae by preventing severe hypoglycemia. Initial therapy involves adequate intravenous or parenteral glucose to prevent hypoglycemia. Surgical interventions are utilized in those children who fail medical management.

CHROMOSOMAL AND NONCHROMOSOMAL SYNDROMES ASSOCIATED WITH ENDOCRINOPATHIES

Septo-Optic Dysplasia (DeMorsier Syndrome)

Gregory is a 12-year-old boy with septo-optic dysplasia. He was noted to have microphallus and prolonged jaundice at birth, and wandering nystagmus was noticed at 4 months of age. Ophthalmologic evaluation revealed the presence of hypoplastic optic nerves. Brain magnetic resonance imaging (MRI) showed hypoplasia of the hypothalamic-pituitary area, bilateral optic nerve hypoplasia, and a normal septum pellucidum.

At 5 years of age, Gregory's growth rate was 3.5 cm/year (greater than 4.5 cm/year is normal for a prepubertal child). He underwent a growth hormone stimulation test with a subnormal response. His levels of cortisol and thyroid hormones were normal. With the diagnosis of partial growth hormone deficiency, Gregory was placed on biosynthetic growth hormone. Gregory is legally blind but has had normal neurological development. He is still prepubertal.

Septo-optic dysplasia, also known as DeMorsier syndrome, is characterized by varying degrees of hypoplasia of the optic nerves, chiasm, and infudibular region of the hypothalamus. The septum pellucidum may be absent. The syndrome has an incidence of 1:16,000 live newborns.

The etiology of septo-optic dysplasia is still unknown. Different hypotheses including sagital midline dysplasia, vascular disruptive sequence, or abnormal midline neuronal migration have been proposed. As many as 50% of cases are diagnosed or suspected in the newborn period. Neonates may present with hypoglycemia, apnea, cyanosis, bradychardia, jaundice, hypotonia, hypothermia, seizures, polyuria, nystagmus, microgenitalia, and craniofacial abnormalities. Visual impairment, the most frequent finding of the syndrome, is reported in 62%–80% of individuals.

Other clinical features include growth failure, epilepsy, intellectual disabilities, hemiplegia, spasticity, athetosis, autism, learning disabilities, and attention-deficit disorder (Williams et al., 1993). The most common endocrinologic abnormality is growth hormone deficiency reported in 50%–80% of individuals. Combined pituitary growth hormone deficiency (CPHD), including growth hormone, thyroid-stimulating hormone, and prolactin deficiencies, has been reported in 50% of individuals, and complete panhypopituitarism has been reported in 11% of individuals. Diabetes insipidus may also be found in 8%–38% of individuals. Cases of central precocious puberty have also been published (Siatkowski et al., 1997).

Individuals with septo-optic dysplasia need a careful assessment by a multidisciplinary team including neurologist, endocrinologist, and ophthalmologist. Treatment with human growth hormone will be implemented frequently as growth hormone deficiency is the most frequent endocrine abnormality found. If thyroid-stimulating hormone and adrenocorticotropic hormone deficiencies are also present, replacement therapy with thyroid hormones and corticosteroids should be started. For those individuals with diabetes insipidous, desmopressin acetate (an arginine-vasopressin synthetic analogue) is the drug of choice.

Down Syndrome (Trisomy 21)

Rhonda is a 9-year-old girl who was diagnosed at birth with Down syndrome. Newborn screening for thyroid function was normal. Her height has been consistently at the 75th percentile on the Down syndrome growth chart. She is obese with a body mass index higher than the 95th percentile.

Rhonda does not have symptoms of diabetes mellitus. Her thyroid-stimulating hormone and thyroid antibodies are measured annually. At age 6 years, her levels of thyroid peroxidase antibodies became positive. Free thyroxine and thyroid-stimulating hormone were normal. Rhonda was diagnosed with chronic lymphocytic thyroiditis (Hashimoto thyroiditis). Four months later, her thyroid-stimulating hormone was elevated, and her free thyroxine count was slightly low.

With diagnosis of primary hypothyroidism secondary to chronic lymphocytic thyroiditis, Rhonda was placed on thyroid hormone replacement. Her thyroid function is monitored every 4 months. Rhonda is on a low glycemic index diet, and her nutritional plan also provides an adequate supply of calcium and vitamin D. A program for regular physical activity has been also implemented.

Down syndrome is associated with several endocrine autoimmune disorders, including type I diabetes mellitus, chronic lymphocytic thyroiditis, acquired hypothyroidism, and Graves disease (Ivarsson et al., 1997). Short stature, obesity, gonadal dysfunction, and osteoporosis also occur with a higher prevalence in individuals with Down syndrome. Diabetes mellitus develops in at least 1% of children and adolescents with Down syndrome. A higher prevalence of alopecia, celiac disease, and pernicious anemia has also been reported in children with the disorder. Individuals with Down syndrome experience an increased frequency of acquired and congenital thyroid disorders, and newborns with Down syndrome have a higher prevalence of compensated and decompensated primary congenital hypothyroidism.

Down syndrome is also associated with autoimmune thyroid disease. Thyroid autoantibodies are found in 13%–34% of individuals. Chronic lymphocytic thyroiditis and subclinical hypothyroidism (defined as an elevated thyroid-stimulating hormone level in the setting of a normal free thyroxine level), occur with a higher prevalence in Down syndrome. The presence of thyroid antibodies constitutes a risk factor for developing clinically overt thyroid disease (Rubello et al., 1995). Levels of free thyroxine and thyroid-stimulating hormone should be determined at birth and at 6 months of age. Thereafter, annual screening is appropriate. The frequency of autoimmune hyperthyroidism (Graves disease) is also higher in children with Down syndrome compared with the general population.

As in children, the prevalence of thyroid disease and other autoimmune disorders is higher in adults with Down syndrome. Acquired hypothyroidism and chronic lymphocytic thyroiditis occur frequently in adults with Down syndrome, and annual determinations of thyroid-stimulating hormone are recommended. Untreated hypothyroidism in individuals with Down syndrome can contribute to dementia.

Down syndrome is the most common chromosomal abnormality associated with short stature. On average, newborns with Down syndrome are 2–3 cm shorter and have birth weights 400–600 g less than normal full-term infants. Shortness of stature continues throughout life and is typically associated with a delay in skeletal maturation and in the pubertal growth spurt. Growth and weight gain may also be affected by an associated hypothyroidism and/or congenital heart disease (present in 50% of newborns with Down syndrome).

The ranges of adult heights vary from 135 cm to 170 cm in men and 127 cm to 158 cm in women (Anneren et al., 1990). The administration of biosynthetic growth hormone to individuals with Down syndrome and short stature may accelerate growth velocity, but long-term follow-up data are not available. The appropriateness of growth hormone therapy in children with Down syndrome has also raised ethical concerns.

Children with Down syndrome have a higher prevalence of obesity than other individuals. Thus, by 2–3 years of age, more than 30% of children with Down syndrome will be overweight (Chumlea & Cronk, 1981). Obstructive sleep apnea is common and is likely due to obesity as well as the presence of midfacial hypoplasia and hypotonia. Total caloric intake should be less than the recommended daily allowance to manage obesity. A program of physical activity through adulthood is also important for control of weight and for good bone density.

Different factors contribute to the higher prevalence of osteoporosis reported in adults and children with Down syndrome (Angelopoulou et al., 2000). Thyroid disease, disorders of sexual development, administration of anticonvulsant medications, low daily dairy intake, hypotonia, low muscle strength, delay of development of gross motor skills, and sedentary lifestyle are risk factors that may compromise the bone mineral density. Early implementation of an active lifestyle in childhood and puberty, increased physical activity to improve muscular strength, and adequate calcium and vitamin D intake are essential to prevent or postpone the development of osteoporosis (Roizen & Patterson, 2003).

Limited information is available on gonadal function and sexual development in Down syndrome. Although the age of onset of puberty is similar to that of typically developing adolescents, an increased frequency of primary gonadal dysfunction has been reported. Women are able to have children, but men have diminished fertility (Hsiang et al., 1987). The onset of menopause for women with Down syndrome occurs earlier compared with typically developing women.

Turner Syndrome

Twelve-year-old Jewel was taken to the Endocrinology Clinic for an evaluation of her short stature. On physical exam, Jewel was noted to have short stature, a low hairline, and a wide chest with a widened carrying angle with extended arms. She had no evidence of pubertal progression and appeared younger than her chronological age. Initial laboratory evaluation revealed a marked elevation in her follicle-stimulating hormone level, a delayed bone age of 10 years, and a karyotype of 45XO, consistent with Turner syndrome. A thyroid screen was normal, but a bone age evaluation showed a delay at 10 years old. The physician discussed growth hormone and estrogen therapy with Jewel and her family.

Turner syndrome is a common chromosomal disorder, occurring in approximately 1 girl per 2,000 live births. The disorder should be considered in an evaluation of a girl with short stature or delayed puberty, particularly if any additional suggestive clinical features are present (Bertelloni et al., 2003). Short stature and gonadal dysgenesis with delayed pubertal development are the most common presenting complaints.

Primary amenorrhea is a common presentation for young adolescent girls with Turner syndrome. In children diagnosed with Turner syndrome prenatally by amniocentesis or in early childhood due to clinical characteristics, anticipatory guidance is important to ease the psychological stress of delayed pubertal progression. Estrogen therapy is necessary for the induction and maintenance of pubertal development in the large majority of girls with Turner syndrome; however, estrogen also promotes rapid bone maturation and subsequent cessation of growth. Therefore, the coordination of growth hormone and estrogen therapy is essential to maximize final adult height and maintain a normal pubertal progression. Estrogen should be initiated in a slow, step-wise progression with progestin therapy added only after evidence of adequate estrogenization has occurred (Bertelloni et al., 2003).

Short stature is a major clinical factor in individuals with Turner syndrome. Slow growth begins in utero and persists throughout adolescence with the lack of the pubertal growth spurt. The average final adult height for women with Turner syndrome is 143 cm (56.5 in) with two standard deviations yielding the range of 132–155 cm or 52–61 in. Growth hormone causes acceleration in height and an increase in final adult height (Bertelloni et al., 2003; Rosenfeld et al., 1998; Sas et al., 1999). Therefore, early recognition of Turner syndrome and treatment with growth hormone can result in near normalization of adult height in many women.

Hypothyroidism occurs in 10%–30% of females with Turner syndrome, often associated with thyroid autoantibodies (Radetti et al., 1995). Obesity may be more common in women with Turner syndrome, which may lead to the possible increase of insulin resistance. Adults with Turner syndrome are also at increased risk for multiple elements of the metabolic syndrome including insulin resistance and progression to type 2 diabetes, obesity, hypertension, and dyslipidemia.

Osteoporosis and fractures are increased in adults with Turner syndrome (Landin-Wilhelmsen et al., 1999).

Baseline screening and adequate calcium and vitamin D intake should be emphasized in all adults with this syndrome. Adults continue to require hormonal supplementation and further assessment of fertility options and gynecologic care. They also continue to need general medical, cardiac, renal, otologic, gynecologic, and endocrinologic evaluations. Standard screening should continue as required based on childhood diagnoses. In addition, emphasis on physical activity and dietary discretion is important.

Klinefelter Syndrome

Jerzy met with an endocrinologist at the age of 16 years. During his annual physical exam, his pediatrician had noted small, firm testicles that were out of proportion to his clinically advanced pubertal development. After discussion with Jerzy's family, the endocrinologist learned that Jerzy had been struggling in school and with his social interactions for several years. Jerzy's family had had no physical health concerns but did note that Jerzy was taller and leaner than other members of his family. They had sought educational and psychological consultation for his school difficulties and anxiety but had not been presented with a formal diagnosis. A karyotype was sent, revealing 47XXY, Klinefelter syndrome. A discussion of fertility issues was initiated, and the possibility of testosterone therapy was addressed with Jerzy and his family.

Klinefelter syndrome, an aneuploidy of 47XXY, is found in 1 in 500–1,000 boys. Approximately 10% of infants with Klinefelter syndrome are diagnosed by amniocentesis, approximately 25% are diagnosed by clinical findings, and the remaining 65% are undiagnosed at least into adulthood. Klinefelter syndrome is characterized by tall stature; increased limb length, particularly of the lower extremities; small, firm gonads; and variability in the degree of virilization, gynecomastia, and fertility in adults (see Figure 19.2). Infants may be normal or slightly below normal in weight and length and may have an increase in minor congenital anomalies. The timing and extent of puberty is variable,

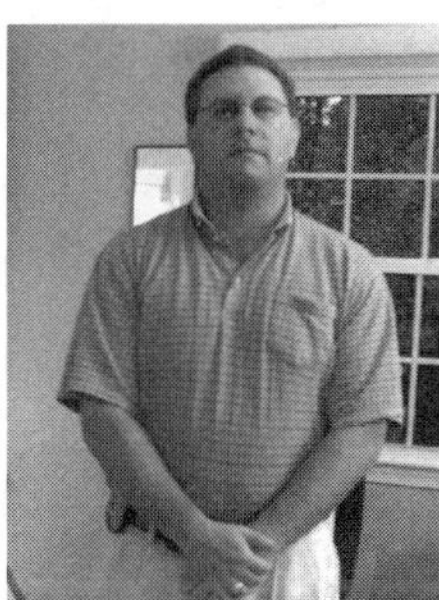

Figure 19.2. It is difficult at times to identify an individual who has a particular condition, such as this man with Klinefelter syndrome, who was diagnosed at age 25. For this reason, doctors must be clinically vigilant.

with some individuals experiencing normal pubertal development and others presenting with absence of secondary sexual development. Gynecomastia is present in boys with Klinefelter syndrome at puberty at an increased incidence from the general population of boys (Ratcliffe, 1999).

Boys with Klinefelter syndrome have normal pituitary response to pubertal initiation and many subsequently develop hypergonadotrophic hypogonadism by the age of 14 years. Some boys will require testosterone therapy to progress through a normally timed puberty. Adolescents and adults with Klinefelter syndrome are at increased risk for decreased bone density and subsequent osteoporosis in those individuals with early diminution of testosterone levels without adequate replacement. Adequate calcium and vitamin D intake is also important.

Limited data is available as to whether learning and behavioral abnormalities are improved by testosterone treatment. Adult studies have indicated improvement in mood, energy, strength, concentration, and behavior in the large majority of men surveyed (Nielsen, Pelsen, & Sorensen, 1988). In Nielsen et al. (1988) and other descriptive, noncontrolled studies, men were found to have improved success in social and professional interactions when treated with testosterone therapy; however, controlled clinical trials have not been performed. Insulin resistance is associated with this syndrome and may be improved by dietary changes, testosterone, and insulin sensitizing agents (Ota et al., 2002). Some instances of autoimmune disorders, including diabetes, associated with Klinefelter syndrome have been reported.

Prader-Willi Syndrome

Prader-Willi syndrome is one of the most frequent microdeletion syndromes and the most commonly recognized genetic form of obesity (see Chapter 9.4). Individuals with Prader-Willi syndrome have a higher prevalence of diabetes mellitus, which may not be only the result of the insulin resistance associated to obesity, but also may be due to a primary impairment in insulin secretion. Individuals with Prader-Willi syndrome have short stature of unknown etiology. The average height for men is 155 cm and 148 cm for women. Although Prader-Willi syndrome may be associated with intrauterine growth retardation, the growth arrest usually occurs postnatally.

Growth hormone therapy for individuals with Prader-Willi syndrome, short stature, and growth failure has been approved by the Food and Drug Administration. Therapy with growth hormone in for these individuals has shown benefits in growth velocity, body composition, physical strength, agility, fat distribution, and bone mineral content (Burman, Ritzen, & Lindgren, 2001). Seven deaths of individuals with Prader-Willi syndrome treated with biosynthetic growth hormone have been reported by the Pharmacia International Growth Study (Eiholzer, Nordmann, & L'Allemans, 2002). All of these individuals were morbidly obese, and five had preexisting respiratory difficulties prior to starting growth hormone therapy. The company recommends not administering growth hormone to individuals with Prader-Willi syndrome who are severely obese, have severe respiratory impairment, or experience sleep apnea.

Individuals with Prader-Willi syndrome have hypogonadotropic hypogonadism (central hypogonadism) as a result of a congenital hypothalamic dysfunction. Infant boys may experience genital hypoplasia including microphallus, cryptorchidia, and scrotal hypoplasia. Infants girls may have absence or severe hypoplasia of labia minora and/or clitoris. Later manifestations of central hypogonadism include primary amenorrhea and pubertal insufficiency. Genitalia remain hypoplastic, sexual activity is rare, and infertility is the rule. Hypogonadism may persist into adult life, which may lead to osteoporosis and lifelong hypotonia. Replacement therapy with sex hormones (testosterone gel in men and oral contraceptives in women) should be initiated in adolescence.

Obesity is the major cause of morbidity and mortality in Prader-Willi syndrome and is caused by an impaired mechanism of satiety due to hypothalamic dysfunction. The lack of satiety and hyperphagia result in morbid obesity, which may begin in the first 2 years of life. A study in individuals with Prader-Willi syndrome reported increased levels of a novel peptide, Ghrelin, which is an acylated peptide hormone recently purified from rat stomach (Haqq et al., 2003). Acting as an endogenous ligand of the growth hormone secretagogue receptor, Ghrelin contributes to the regulation of growth hormone secretion. In children with Prader-Willi syndrome, fasting Ghrelin concentrations were higher (3- to 4-fold elevation) compared with all obese groups, which may explain its a role as an orexigenic factor driving the insatiable appetite and obesity found in this syndrome.

The treatment of obesity in individuals with Prader-Willi syndrome is complicated. Appetite suppressants have not been useful. The total caloric intake needs to be restricted. A low glycemic index diet has the potential benefit of decreasing the appetite and will also improve the insulin sensitivity that is compromised in obese individuals. An early implementation of an active lifestyle in childhood and puberty and a program of physical activity through adulthood are also essential for control of weight

Glycemic index refers to the relative rise in blood glucose occurring after consumption of a food containing a standard amount of carbohydrate. Most refined grain products and potatoes have a high glycemic index, whereas nonstarchy vegetables, legumes, and fruits generally have a low glycemic index. Recently, a low glycemic index diet has been proposed as a novel treatment for obesity (Ludwig, 2000). In this diet, most carbohydrates come from nonstarchy vegetables, fruits, legumes, nuts, and dairy.

A low glycemic index diet will prevent abnormal postprandial excursions of blood sugar as well as postprandial hyperinsulinism (Ludwig et al., 1999). Insulin secretion has been shown to be greater after consuming a high glycemic index meal compared with a low glycemic index meal. Similarly, higher elevations of counter-regulatory hormones epinephrine and growth hormone occur after consuming a high glycemic index meal compared with a low glycemic index meal. Several studies relating glycemic index to hunger, satiety, or voluntary food intake have demonstrated beneficial effects of low glycemic index means compared with high glycemic index meals (Ludwig et al., 1999). Although the low glycemic index diet appears to be promising in weight reduction, long-term studies are not available yet.

Noonan Syndrome

Ming is a 14-year-old boy who was diagnosed at birth with valvular pulmonic stenosis and bilateral cryptorchidism. His testicles were surgically descended in the first year of life. Ming has short stature, mild developmental delays, obesity, and a syndromic facies. He is advancing into puberty normally and has a normal karyotype 46XY. Genetic analysis revealed a mutation on chromosome 12q22-qter, confirming the diagnosis of Noonan syndrome.

Noonan syndrome is an autosomal dominant disorder with a candidate gene mapped to chromosome 12 (12q42 24.1). This mutation has now been found to be present in approximately 50% of individuals with a clinical diagnosis of Noonan syndrome (Tartaglia et al., 2001), which includes features of distinct facies, heart disease (valvular pulmonic stenosis and hypertrophic cardiomyopathy), short stature, webbed neck, square chest, cryptorchidism, and mild intellectual disabilities. The incidence of the syndrome is 1 in 1,000–2,500 live births.

Hypothyroidism is a less-common component of this syndrome, but physicians should screen for it. Theintz and Savage (1982) reported delayed puberty and gonadal failure in men with Noonan syndrome, and they also found that bilateral testicular maldescent occurred in 6 of 11 adults with Noonan syndrome. In three men, puberty was delayed. Four of the men had fathered children. Although the luteinizing hormone and testosterone levels were normal in all men, the follicle-stimulating hormone levels were elevated in the group with testicular maldescent. Four of five men from whom semen samples were obtained showed azoospermia or oligozoospermia. Bilateral testicular maldescent may compromise the fertility in men with Noonan syndrome and should be evaluated.

Williams Syndrome

The earliest endocrinologic manifestation of Williams syndrome is that of idiopathic hypercalcemia (see Chapter 9.5). Infants often present with symptomatic hypercalcemia, including evidence of poor feeding, muscle cramps, and irritability. The presence of hypercalcemia in infants with Williams syndrome is variable, and serum calcium may be normal, but the presence of nephrocalcinosis and soft tissue calcifications suggests that hypercalcemia may have occurred previously. The etiology of the hypercalcemia remains unclear. Low-calcium vitamin D–free formula should be provided for those infants with hypercalcemia. Occasionally, short-term therapy with glucocorticoid may be necessary.

Both prenatal growth deficiency and short stature are features of this syndrome. Early pubertal progression with diminished growth acceleration may also contribute to a decreased final adult height (Partsch et al., 2002). Standardized Williams syndrome growth charts are available and should be utilized to follow the growth of these individuals (see Table 19.2). As many as 15% of individuals will develop diabetes mellitus related to obesity and insulin resistance (Morris & Mervis, 2000). Hypothyroidism is a less-common component of this syndrome, occurring in approximately 2% of individuals. Hypertension is also a common finding in this syndrome. Adults with Williams syndrome continue to require screening for hypercalcemia, hypothyroidism, hypertension, renal dysfunction, cardiac complications, diabetes, and other complications of obesity.

OTHER ABNORMALITIES OF GROWTH AND DEVELOPMENT

Central Precocious Puberty

Zara is a 9-year-old girl with a history of congenital obstructive hydrocephalus, cerebral palsy, developmental delay, and seizures. At age 4 years, she exhibited bilateral breast enlargement and a growth velocity of 9 cm/year (normal for a prepubertal child is 5 cm/year). She had no history of expo-

Table 19.2. Growth charts, support groups, and other resources

Down syndrome growth chart	Cronk, C., Crocker, A.C., Pueschel, S.M., Shea, A.M., Zackai, E., Pickens, G., et al. (1985, January). Growth charts for children with Down syndrome: 1 month to 18 years of age. *Pediatrics, 81,* 102–110.
Down syndrome support group	http://www.nas.com/downsyn/
Klinefelter Syndrome and Associates	http://www.genetic.org/ks/
Noonan syndrome growth chart	Witt, D.R., Keena, B.A., Hall, J.G., & Allanson, J.E. (1986, September). Growth curves for height in Noonan syndrome. *Clinical Genetics, 30,* 150–153.
Noonan Syndrome Support Group	http://www.noonansyndrome.org/
Pediatric Endocrinology Nursing Society (patient information sheets)	http://www.pens.org
Septo-optic Dysplasia (DeMorsier syndrome) support group	http://www.focusfamilies.org/focus/
Turner syndrome growth chart	Lyon, A.J., Preece, M.A., & Grant, D.B. (1985, October). Growth curve for girls with Turner syndrome. *Archives of Disease in Childhood, 60,* 932–935.
Turner Syndrome Society	http://www.turner-syndrome-us.org/
Williams syndrome growth chart	Greenwood Genetic Center. (1998). Third trimester to adulthood: Growth curve for Williams syndrome. Greenwood, SC: Author.
The Williams Syndrome Association	http://www.williams-syndrome.org/

sure to exogenous estrogens. Family history was negative for precocious puberty.

On physical examination, Zara had a Tanner stage II for breast development (pubertal). She did not have pubic hair, vaginal discharge, hyperpigmentation, or café-au-lait spots. Zara underwent a gonodotropin-releasing hormone stimulation test, which showed a pubertal response (elevated luteinizing hormone and follicle-stimulating hormone). Her bone age was advanced more than three standard deviations for her chronological age. A brain MRI did not reveal the presence of intracranial masses.

Following a diagnosis of central precocious puberty, Zara was started on suppressive therapy with a long-acting gonodotropin-releasing hormone analogue (Leuprolide, intramuscular, monthly dose). A repeat gonodotropin-releasing hormone stimulation test obtained 2 months after onset of therapy showed a prepubertal response with complete suppression of gonadotropins. Her breast development regressed. Similarly, her growth velocity decreased to 5 cm/year (prepubertal). Her more recent bone age was 11 years for a chronological age of 10 years. Zara's predicted final height based on her current bone age reached her mid parental target height. Gonadotropin-releasing hormone therapy will be discontinued when Zara is 12 years old.

Traditionally, precocious puberty has been defined as the development of secondary sexual characteristics before the age of 8 years in girls and 9 years in boys. Although the Lawson Wilkins Pediatric Endocrine Society has recently proposed not to evaluate Caucasian girls with onset of puberty after the age of 7 years or African American girls with onset of puberty after the age of 6 years (Kaplowitz & Oberfield, 1999), careful evaluation of girls with onset of puberty before 8 years of age is still advisable.

Precocious puberty is classified as central, or gonadotropin dependent, and peripheral, or gonadotropin independent (often called *pseudoprecocious puberty*). Central precocious puberty can result from a variety of intracranial disturbances (see Table 19.3). These disorders may cause sexual precocity by affecting neurologic tracts carrying inhibitory signals to the hypothalamus.

Evaluation of precocious puberty includes a careful clinical and family history and physical examination. Height, weight, growth curves, and bone age determinations need to be obtained. On physical examination, the growth of pubic hair, penis, and testes is usually evident in males and that of breast enlargement and/or pubic hair in females. The skeletal maturation is advanced, which may compromise the final height.

Endocrine analysis includes determinations of serum concentrations of gonadotropins and sex hormones. The measurement of gonadotropin levels following a gonadotropin-releasing hormone stimulation test is the gold standard for the diagnosis of central precocious puberty. Central nervous system lesions can be assessed by computed tomography or MRI scanning (Robben et al., 1995). A pelvic ultrasound will be useful to determine the uterine length and the ovarian volume. The use of a functional vaginal cytology will help to determine the duration and degree of estrogenization.

Untreated precocious puberty has significant effects on growth, skeletal maturation, and psychological development. Psychological counseling should be offered not only for the affected child but also for the parents. The libido of these children is usually not increased. Some children may be at increased risk for sexual abuse considering their advanced sexual maturity. Untreated precocious puberty may also lead to an early rapid pubertal growth spurt and premature epiphysial fusion, compromising the child's final adult height. Effective suppression of gonadotropin release with gonodotropin-releasing hormone long-acting analogues (Leuprolide) will result in cessation or regression of physical pubertal development and attenuation of the increased growth rate and skeletal maturation (Klein et al., 2000).

Table 19.3. Central nervous system abnormalities associated with central (true) precocious puberty

Brain tumors
Hypothalamic hamartomas
Astrocytomas
Craniopharyingiomas
Dysgerminomas
Ependymomas
Pinealomas
Ganglioneuromas
Neuroblastoma
Congenital anomalies
Myelomeningocele
Hydrocephalus (congenital and acquired)
Midbrain developmental defects
Septo-optic dysplasia (SOD)
Solitary maxillar incisor
Cysts
Neurocutaneous syndromes
Tuberous sclerosis
Neurofibromatosis type 1
Inflammatory/infectious/granulomatous
Meningitis
Encephalitis
Brain abscess
Histiocitosis
Tuberculosis
Vasculitis
Miscellaneous
Cranial irradiation
Brain surgery
Brain trauma

Intrauterine Growth Retardation

Intrauterine growth retardation is defined as a birth weight of under the 10th percentile for gestational age (Goldberg et al., 1989). Intrauterine growth retardation is associated with potential long-term complications in adulthood, including neurological and developmental disabilities, and an increased risk of reduced rate of postnatal growth with ultimate short stature. About 10%–15% of babies with intrauterine growth retardation do not show catch-up growth and remain short through life.

Fetal growth failure may be caused by extrinsic factors such as placental disorders or maternal disease, including chronic undernutrition, which is prevalent in underdeveloped countries. Intrinsic factors are usually responsible for early onset intrauterine growth retardation and have more significant consequences. They include infectious agents associated with TORCH syndrome (toxoplasmosis, other infections, rubella, cytomegalovirus, and herpes simplex), and chromosomal and nonchromosomal syndromes.

Although the U.S. Food and Drug Administration (FDA) approved the use of biosynthetic growth hormone in individuals with intrauterine growth retardation, short stature, and lack of catch-up growth by 2 years of age, the treatment of this group of individuals should be very thoughtfully considered and should take into account several factors, including psychosocial, ethical, and safety issues. Although treatment with growth hormone may stimulate growth rate during the first 2 years of treatment, data on final height are not yet available (De Zegher et al., 2000).

The association of intrauterine growth retardation with several adult-onset disorders has been described and is the aim of broad research (Lucas, 1991). An increased prevalence of essential hypertension, impaired glucose tolerance, type 2 diabetes mellitus, polycystic ovary syndrome (PCOS), ischemic heart disease, hypertriglyceridemia, and low–high density lipoprotein (HDL) (all components of the dysmetabolic syndrome or syndrome X) have been reported in adults with a clinical history of low birth weight (Rich-Edwards et al., 1999).

MEDICATIONS ASSOCIATED WITH ENDOCRINE EFFECTS

Thyroid-stimulating hormone can be suppressed by dopamine or dopamine agonists, corticosteroids, or severe intercurrent illness (see Table 19.4). Drugs containing iodides can have a significant suppressive effect on the thyroid, including amiodarone, an antiarrythmic.

Table 19.4. Commonly used medications affecting endocrine function and testing

Drug	Hormonal effect
Dopamine Dopamine agonists Corticosteroids (Iodine)	Thyroid-stimulating hormone suppression
Iodide-containing drugs Lithium* Amiodarone**	Thyroid suppression
Estrogens Phenytoin Phenobarbital	Effects on thyroid binding proteins
Phenobarbital Phenytoin Primidone Carbamazepine	Inactivation of vitamin D
Corticosteroids	Osteoporosis
Atypical antipsychotics Clozapine Quetiapine	Diabetes/obesity
H2-receptor antagonists Cimetidine Ranitidine Metoclopramide	Galactorrhea
Amphetamines (Adderall) Methylphenidate (Ritalin) Corticosteroids	Growth retardation

*Nephrogenic diabetes insipidus (NDI) may be associated with lithium therapy.

**Administration of amiodarone has been also associated with hyperthyroidism.

Of note, amiodarone has also been shown to produce hyperthyroidism with chronic use. In addition, lithium, a medication used for mood stabilization can suppress thyroid hormone release, leading to a hypothyroid state. All individuals taking amiodarone or lithium should be screened for thyroid dysfunction prior to medication initiation, as hypothyroidism is more likely to occur in individuals with baseline thyroid abnormalities. Ongoing screening during the course of therapy is also essential.

Several medications can alter the thyroid binding proteins and therefore alter measured total levels of thyroxine without altering the active thyroid hormone or the clinical thyroid status. Estrogen therapy and pregnancy can increase binding proteins. Phenytoin also alters the ability of thyroid binding proteins to bind thyroid hormone, altering the thyroid studies without affecting clinical status. A measure of thyroid-stimulating hormone is an appropriate screen in these individuals (Surks & Defesi, 1996); however, phenytoin may also alter the metabolism of thyroid hormone. Therefore, individuals who require thyroid hormone replacement in addition to phenytoin may require larger doses to remain in the therapeutic range. Phenobarbital may have similar effects on thyroid hormone metabolism.

Antiepileptic medications have also been shown to have effects on bone metabolism, and chronic use may lead to osteoporosis and rickets. Other factors pertinent to individuals with disabilities also contribute to bone health, such as an individual's ability to ambulate and level of physical activity, sunlight exposure, and vitamin D intake. Several of the antiepileptic medications, including phenobarbital, phenytoin, primidone, and carbamazepine, have been shown to accelerate the inactivation of vitamin D, increasing the daily needs of individuals on chronic therapy. In addition, phenytoin and carbamazepine may have direct effects on bone cells (Feldkamp et al., 2000). Other direct and indirect mechanisms have also been postulated for the observed effect of decreased bone density and increased fracture risk. Therefore, maintaining adequate calcium and vitamin D intake in individuals receiving anticonvulsant therapy or individuals who are otherwise at risk for deficient states is essential to their bone formation and prevention of osteoporosis.

Diabetes or impaired glucose metabolism may be exacerbated by many commonly used medications. Because many syndromes predispose individuals to progression to impaired glucose tolerance or diabetes, clinicians should be cautious in utilizing these medications in susceptible individuals, particularly those with obesity. Atypical antipsychotic medications have been shown to both induce weight gain and to increase the risk of progression to diabetes mellitus. The mechanism for the induction of hyperglycemia remains unclear; however, increasing numbers of cases indicate that diabetes can present very early after the introduction of medications such as clozapine or quetiapine, implicating a diabetogenic effect of the medication not directly related to weight gain. Children or adults on atypical antipsychotic therapy should be monitored for early signs of hyperglycemia and/or excessive weight gain (Clark & Burge, 2003).

Stimulant medications used for attention disorders or other behavioral concerns may cause poor weight gain and poor linear growth. Stimulant medication is associated with a decrease in height and weight during the first 6–30 months of administration (Poulton & Cowell, 2003). More recent studies describe the effects on the final height of children with ADHD who are treated with methylphenidate (MPH) as only slight. Only a handful of reports have attributed severe growth impairments to MPH, which were associated with gastrointestinal side effects. Evidence shows that growth suppression accompanies weight loss, and possibly some suppression of stature, but these effects are not long-lasting and, from existing evidence, seem to have little effect on adult height or weight. Some evidence exists of catch-up growth and normal final adult height in individuals who completed stimulant therapy during childhood. Although, for most children, extended treatments with MPH do not have negative effects on growth, children who are prescribed stimulant medications should have meticulously measured growth parameters on a frequent basis in order to detect any nutritional deficits or suppression of growth (Clark & Burge, 2003).

In addition, some controversy surrounds the growth effects of inhaled corticosteroids utilized for respiratory ailments. Inhaled corticosteroids at size-appropriate dosages have a better safety profile than recurrent oral corticosteroids; however, a level of systemic absorption exists, particularly with high doses of inhaled corticosteroids that can have at least transient effects on growth velocity, bone density, and adrenal function (Allen et al., 2003). Clinicians should be aware of these possible effects of inhaled steroids and attempt to wean or discontinue these medications as respiratory symptoms allow. In addition, the possibility of adrenal suppression should be considered and screened for with morning cortisol levels and subsequent stimulation testing as required.

Finally, galactorrhea may result from common medications that effect the dopamine and prolactin pathways, such as or H2-receptor antagonists or metoclopramide. Medication effects should be considered when a child or adult has unexplained galactorrhea.

CONCLUSION

Endocrine abnormalities are common in individuals with developmental disabilities. Providers should be knowledgeable about the common endocrinopathies and introduce lifetime screening for alterations in hormonal functioning. In addition, the promotion of a healthy lifestyle that includes healthy food choices with weight control, physical activity (as appropriate), and adequate vitamin and mineral intake will improve or prevent some of the common endocrinopathies in people with developmental disabilities.

REFERENCES

Allen, D.B., Bielory, L., Derendorf, H., et al. (2003). Inhaled corticosteroids: Past lessons and future issues. *Journal of Allergy and Clinical Immunology, 112*, S1–S40.

Angelopoulou, N., Matziari, C., Tsimaras, V., et al. (2000). Bone mineral density and muscle strength in young men with mental retardations (with and without Down syndrome). *Calcified Tissue International, 66,* 176.

Anneren, G., Gustavson, K.H., Sara, V.R., et al. (1990). Growth retardation in Down syndrome in relation to insulin-like growth factors and growth hormone. *American Journal of Medical Genetics (Suppl), 7,* 59.

Bertelloni, S., Baroncelli, G.I., Fruzzetti, F., Spinelli, C., Simi, P., & Saggese, G. (2003). Growth and puberty in Turner's syndrome. *Journal of Pediatric Endocrinology & Metabolism, 16,* 307–315.

Burman, P., Ritzen, E.M., & Lindgren, A.C. (2001). Endocrine dysfunction in Prader-Willi syndrome: A review with special reference to GH. *Endocrine Review, 22,* 787.

Chumlea, W.C., & Cronk, C.E. (1981). Overweight among children with trisomy 21. *Journal of Mental Deficiency Research, 25,* 275.

Clark, C., & Burge, M.R. (2003). Diabetes mellitus associated with atypical anti-psychotic medications. *Diabetes Technology Therapy, 5,* 669.

De Zegher, F., Albertsson-Wikland, K., Wollmann, H.A., et al. (2000). Growth hormone treatment of short children born small for gestational age: Growth responses with continuous and discontinuous regimens over 6 years. *Journal of Clinical Endocrinology and Metabolism, 85,* 2816.

Eiholzer, E., Nordmann, Y., & L'Allemand, D. (2002). Fatal outcome of sleep apenoea in PWS during the initial phase of growth hormone treatment. *Hormone Research, 58,* (Suppl. 3), 24–26.

Feldkamp, J., Becker, A., Witte, O.W., et al. (2000). Long-term anticonvulsant therapy leads to low bone mineral density–evidence for direct drug effects of phenytoin and carbamazepine on human osteoblast-like cells. *Experimental and Clinical Endocrinology and Diabetes, 108,* 37.

Goldberg, R.L., Cutter, G.R., Hoffman, H.J., et al. (1989). Intrauterine growth retardation: Standards for diagnosis. *American Journal of Obstetrics and Gynecology, 161,* 271.

Haqq, A.M., Farooqi, S., O'Rahilly, S., et al. (2003). Serum ghrelin levels are inversely correlated with body mass index, age, and insulin concentrations in normal children and are markedly increased in Prader-Willi syndrome. *Journal of Clinical Endocrinology and Metabolism, 88,* 174.

Hsiang, Y.-H.H., Bercovitz, G.D., Bland, G.L., et al. (1987). Gonadal function in patients with Down syndrome. *American Journal of Medical Genetics, 27,* 449.

Ivarsson, S.A., Ericsson, V.B., Gustafsson, J., et al. (1997). The impact of thyroid autoimmunity in children and adolescents with Down syndrome. *Acta Paediatrica, 86,* 105.

Kaplowitz, P.B., & Oberfield, S.E. (1999). Reexamination of the age limit for defining when puberty is precocious in girls in the United States: Implications for evaluation and treatment. Drug and Therapeutics and Executive Committees of the Lawson Wilkins. *Pediatric Endocrine Society Pediatrics, 104*(4 Pt. 1), 936–941.

Klein, K.O., et al. (2001). Increased final height in precocious puberty after long-term treatment with LHRH agonists: The National Institutes of Health experience. *Journal of Clinical Endocrinology and Metabolism, 86,* 4711–4716.

Landin-Wilhelmsen, K., Bryman, I., Windh, M., et al. (1999). Osteoporosis and fractures in Turner syndrome–importance of growth promoting and oestrogen therapy. *Clinical Endocrinology, 51,* 497.

Lucas, A. (1991). Programming by early nutrition in man. In D.P.J. Barker (Ed.), *The childhood environment and adult disease: CIBA Symposium 156* (p. 38). Chichester, UK: John Wiley & Sons.

Ludwig, D.S. (2000). Dietary glycemic index and obesity. *Journal of Nutrition, 130*(Suppl.), 280S–283S

Ludwig, D.S., Majzoub, J.A., Al-Zaharani, A., et al. (1999). High glycemic index foods, overeating, and obesity. *Pediatrics, 103,* E26.

Morris, C.A., & Mervis, C.B. (2000). Williams syndrome and related disorders. *Annual Review of Genomics and Human Genetics, 1,* 461.

Nielsen, J., Pelsen, B., & Sorensen, K. (1988). Follow up of 30 Klinefelter males treated with testosterone. *Clinical Genetics, 33, 262.*

Ota, K., Suehiro, T., Ikeda, Y., et al. (2002). Diabetes mellitus associated with Klinefelter's syndrome: A case report and review in Japan. *Internal Medicine, 41,* 842–847.

Partsch, C.J., Japing, I., Siebert, R., Gosh, A., et al. (2002, Sept.). Central precocious puberty in girls with Williams syndrome. *Journal of Pediatrics, 141*(3), 441–444.

Poulton, A., & Cowell, C.T. (2003). Slowing of growth in height and weight on stimulants: A characteristic pattern. *Journal of Pediatrics and Child Health, 39,* 180–185.

Radetti, G., Mazzanti, L., Paganini, C., et al. (1995). Frequency, clinical and laboratory features of thyroiditis in girls with Turner's syndrome: The Italian Study Group for Turner's syndrome. *Acta Paediatrica, 84,* 909.

Ratcliffe, S. (1999). Long term outcome in children of sex chromosome abnormalities. *Archives of Disease in Childhood, 80,* 192.

Rich-Edwards, J.W., Coldtiz, G.A., Stamfer, M.J., et al. (1999). Birthweight and the risk for type 2 diabetes mellitus in adult women. *Annals of Internal Medicine, 130,* 278.

Robben, S.G., et al. (1995). Idiophatic central precocious puberty: Magnetic resonance findings in 30 patients. *British Journal of Radiology, 68,* 34–38.

Roizen, N., & Patterson, D. (2003). Down's syndrome. *The Lancet, 361,* 1281.

Rosenfeld, R.G., Attie, K.M., Frane, J., et al. (1998). Growth hormone therapy of Turner's syndrome: Beneficial effect on adult height. *Journal of Pediatrics, 132,* 319.

Rubello, D., Pozzan, G.B., Casara, D., et al. (1995). Natural course of subclinical hypothyroidism in Down's syndrome: Prospective study results and therapeutic considerations. *Journal of Endocrinological Investigation, 18,* 35.

Saenger, P., et al. (2001). Endocrinc care of special interset to the practice of endocrinology: Recommendations for the diagnosis and management of turner syndrome. *Journal of Clinical Endocrinology and Metabolism, 86,* 3061.

Sas, T.C., de Muinck Keizer-Schrama, S.M., Stijnen, T., et al. (1999). Normalization of height in girls with Turner syndrome after long-term growth hormone treatment: Results of a randomized dose response trial. *Journal of Clinical Endocrinology and Metabolism, 84,* 4607.

Siatkowski, R.M., Sanchez, J.C., Andrade, R., et al. (1997). The clinical, neuroradiographic, and endocrinologic profile of patients with bilateral optic nerve hypoplasia. *Ophthalmology, 104,* 493.

Surks, M.I., & Defesi, C.R. (1996). Normal serum free thyroid hormone concentrations in patients treated with phenytoin or carbamazepine: A paradox resolved. *Journal of the American Medication Association, 275,* 1495.

Tartaglia, M., Mehler, E.L., Goldberg, R., et al. (2001). Mutations in PTPN11, encoding the protein tyrosine phosphatase SHP-2, cause Noonan syndrome. *Nature and Genetics, 29*, 465.

Theintz, G., & Savage, M.O. (1982). Growth and pubertal development in five boys with Noonan's syndrome. *Archives of Diseases in Children, 57*, 13.

Williams, J., Brodky, M.C., Griebel, M., et al. (1993). Septo-optic dysplasia: The clinical insignificance of an absent septum pellucidum. *Developmental Medicine and Child Neurology, 35*, 490.

Wolfsdorf, J., & Weinstein, D.A. (2003). Hypoglycemia in infants and children. *Pediatric Endocrinology*, 575.

CHAPTER 20

DERMATOLOGY

Brian P. Pollack, Jason C. Hadley, and Jack L. Arbiser

This chapter addresses dermatological conditions that are commonly experienced by children and adults with developmental disabilities. Some of the conditions are etiologically associated with developmental disabilities because the embryonic origin of the skin and nervous system are both ectodermal. The most commonly recognized of these conditions are neurofibromatosis and tuberous sclerosis (see Chapter 9.7). This chapter describes other, less common neurocutaneous syndromes (e.g., LEOPARD syndrome). Common skin disorders and drug eruptions are explored. The chapter concludes with a look at skin disorders associated with Down syndrome.

Melanocytes are derived from the neural crest and represent the pigment producing cells of the body. During embryogenesis, they migrate to multiple sites, including the eye (uveal tract), ear (cochlea), mucous membrane epithelium, and the skin. In the skin, these cells reside in the basal layer of the epidermis, and each melanocyte usually contacts and can transfer pigment to 30–40 keratinocytes (Bolognia et al., 2003; Odom & Berger, 2000). In both benign and malignant neoplasms, these cells can grow in cohesive groups known as nests. Collections of benign nested melanocytes form a *nevus* (pleural, *nevi*), or common mole.

The cells of a nevus are known as *nevus cells* (or nevomelanocytes). Unlike melanocytes, they do not possess dendrites. Based on the histologic location of these nevus cells, the nevus is described as junctional (cells are located at the dermal:epidermal junction), dermal (cells are located in the dermis only), or compound (having both a dermal and junctional component). Junctional nevi are macular, whereas compound nevi have a macular and papular component. Dermal nevi are typically skin-colored papules. Hairs may emanate from compound or dermal nevi. Nevi typically appear during the first years of life (they can be present at birth) and peak in incidence during the second and third decades. They then decline in number.

Readers are referred to http://dermis.multimedica/de/ to view photographs of the conditions discussed in this chapter.

A *lentigo* (plural, *lentigines*) represents a pigmented macule typically 1–5 mm in size that can appear on any surface or mucous membrane. They have little or no relation to sun exposure. They can range from light brown to dark-brown/black in color and are well demarcated. They can be present at birth or acquired (as can occur with ultraviolet light therapy). Multiple lentigines can occur as an isolated finding or be associated with LEOPARD syndrome, Peutz-Jeghers syndrome, or Carney complex.

Ephelides, commonly known as freckles, appear in sun-exposed areas and are more common in individuals with fair skin. Unlike other pigmented macules, ephelides become less apparent and may disappear in the absence of sun exposure. Histologically, they represent increased melanin with no increase in the number of basilar melanocytes. In addition, the overlying epidermis is normal.

Café au lait macules (and the darker café noir macules) are well-demarcated macules or patches that are several shades darker than the surrounding skin. They are typically present at birth and can range in size from 1.5 cm to 15 cm in diameter (Odom & Berger, 2000). The majority of individuals with café au lait macules have no associated abnormalities; however, these lesions can be a marker of several systemic diseases, including neurofibromatosis, Watson syndrome, Noonan syndrome, McCune-Albright syndrome, tuberous sclerosis, piebaldism, Mukamel syndrome, Bannayan-Riley-Ruvalcaba syndrome, Cowden's disease, gastrocutaneous syndrome, Fanconi's anemia, and partial unilateral lengtiginosis (Bolognia et al., 2003).

SPECIFIC NEUROCUTANEOUS SYNDROMES

Many inherited and acquired disorders have both dermatologic and neurologic manifestations (Bolognia et al., 2003; Odom & Berger, 2000; Schepis & Romano, 1996; Spitz, 1996). This section focuses on diseases and syndromes not covered elsewhere in this book, including disorders with cutaneous findings, particularly pigmented lesions that have been associated with developmental disabilities. Special emphasis on the cutaneous features of these syndromes is provided to help the reader approach individuals with developmental disabilities and skin findings. Some of these syndromes are covered in the following section, whereas others are included in Table 20.1.

LEOPARD Syndrome

LEOPARD syndrome is a complex autosomal dominant disorder affecting multiple organs. Additional names for this syndrome include cardiocutaneous lentiginosis syndrome, multiple lentigines syndrome, and Moynahan syndrome. The acronym LEOPARD represents the key features of the disorder that include lentigines, electrocardiographic conduction anomalies, ocular hypertelorism, pulmonary stenosis, abnormalities of genitalia, retardation of growth, and deafness (Sarkozy et al., 2004). LEOPARD syndrome has variable expressivity. Not all features are present in any one individual, and members of the same family may have different features. Cases of LEOPARD syndrome have been found to be allelic to Noonan syndrome. Indeed, the majority of cases of LEOPARD syndrome represent mutations in the *PTPN11* gene that encodes the protein tyrosine phosphatase SHP2.

Lentigines are mostly on the face, neck, and upper trunk but can be widely distributed (generalized) and may involve the sclera. The mucous membranes are spared. Additional cutaneous findings include café au lait macules, café noir spots, axillary freckling, localized hypopigmentation, hyperelastic skin, onychodystrophy, and other pigmented lesions. Absence of lentigines does not exclude the diagnosis of LEOPARD syndrome, and some features of LEOPARD syndrome develop with age. Other features of LEOPARD syndrome that may be present include triangular facies or other facial dysmorphism, broad nasal root, ocular hypertelorism, ptosis, low set ears, growth retardation, pectus excavatum, or pectus carinatum.

The most life-threatening feature of LEOPARD syndrome is cardiac involvement. Hypertrophic cardiomyopathy has been reported to be the most prevalent cardiac impairment in individuals with mutations in the *PTPN11* gene (Sarkozy et al., 2004). Because the cutaneous features may be variable, hypertrophic cardiomyopathy should be searched for in otherwise asymptomatic individuals from affected families. Other cardiovascular features that may be present include pulmonic stenosis, aortic stenosis, and arrhythmia and conduction defects. Other features of LEOPARD syndrome include genital abnormalities such as hypospadias and cryptorchidism. Intellectual disabilities, present in 20%–30% of individuals, are usually mild.

Basal Cell Nevus Syndrome

Basal cell nevus syndrome (BCNS), also called Gorlin syndrome or nevoid basal cell carcinoma syndrome, is an autosomal dominant disorder linked to mutations in the *PTCH* tumor-suppressor gene that can affect many organ systems (Gorlin, 1995). BCNS is characterized by an increased risk of malignancy (internal and cutaneous), sensitivity to ionizing and ultraviolet radiation, neurologic abnormalities (which may include intellectual disabilities, congenital communicating hydrocephalus, medulloblastoma, and seizures), genitourinary system abnormalities, dental and skeletal abnormalities, and congenital malformations. Major criteria include greater than two basal cell carcinomas (or one in someone younger than 20 years) and odontogenic keratocysts of the jaw. Minor criteria include congenital malformations such as cleft lip and medulloblastoma. Congenital blindness, strabismus, and skeletal abnormalities may also be found. The features of BCNS can present at different times, making an early diagnosis challenging. In addition, due to the potentially serious aspects of BCNS, long-term surveillance of individuals with this disorder is warranted.

In addition to multiple and early basal cell carcinomas, palmar and plantar pits are another important cutaneous sign of BCNS. The pits are small (a few millimeters at most), shallow depressions of the palmar or plantar skin. They are visible to the naked eye but may be more easily seen with a magnifying lens. Pits may be found in children younger than 10 years.

Piebaldism

Piebaldism is an autosomal dominant disorder characterized by areas (patches) of skin and hair without pigmentation. The condition is caused by mutation in the gene encoding the tyrosine kinase receptor, c-Kit, or mutation in the gene encoding the transcription factor SLUG. The hair and skin findings are present at birth and are static throughout life.

The characteristic area of poliosis is the central frontal part of the scalp. Areas of the eyebrows may also be affected. The depigmented patches may be present on the face, trunk, or extremities and may have a hyperpigmented border as well as islands of hyperpigmentation within them.

Although piebaldism is not classically associated with systemic disease, similar cutaneous features of de-

Table 20.1. Syndromes featuring developmental disabilities with prominent cutaneous features

Disorder	Genetics/mutations	Cutaneous features	Systemic features
Sjögren-Larsson syndrome	Autosomal recessive (AR), fatty aldehyde dehydrogenase (FALDH)	Generalized ichthyosis in infancy with erythroderma, scaling, areas of lamellar scaling, hyperkeratosis, and pruritus; darker scale without erythroderma after infancy, most pronounced in flexures and lower abdomen; spares the central face	Intellectual disabilities, spastic diplegia or tetraplegia, seizures, atypical retinitis pigmentosa, dental dysplasia, scissor gate
Conradi-Hunerman syndrome (X-linked dominant chondrodysplasia punctata)	X-linked dominant, emopamil binding protein (EBP; also known as the sterol-$\Delta^8\Delta^7$-isomerase gene)	Ichthyosiform erythroderma in Blashko's lines in infancy, resolves with follicular atrophoderma with or without hyperpigmentation, course hair with patchy alopecia	Facial asymmetry, frontal bossing, macrocephaly, short stature, flat nasal root, asymmetric limb shortening, stippled epiphyses (radiographic), scoliosis, cataracts
Richner-Hanhart syndrome (tyrosinemia type II)	AR, tyrosine aminotransferase	Palmoplantar keratoderma focal or diffuse, can occur on weight-bearing areas and result in pain with ambulation, hyperkeratotic plaques on the elbows and knees	Intellectual disabilities; pseudoherpetic keratitis with photophobia, corneal ulceration, neovascularization, and blindness
Darier disease	Autosomal dominant (AD), ATP2A2 encoding the sarcoplasmic/endoplasmic reticulum Ca^{2+} ATPase (SERCA)2	Hyperkeratotic yellow-brown papules that coalesce to plaques in a seborrheic distribution, verrucous papules on the dorsum of the hands, palmoplantar punctate keratoses and pits, nail changes including red/white longitudinal bands and V-shaped nicking at the distal edge, subungual hyperkeratosis, cobblestone papules on the oral and anogenital mucosa	Intellectual disabilities and schizophrenia reported in some families
Epidermal nevus syndrome	Sporadic	Epidermal nevi present as skin colored to hyperpigmented verrucous plaques that can involve large portions of the body surface; plaques can follow Blashko's lines; epidermal nevi including nevus Unius Lateralis, inflammatory linear verrucous epidermal nevi (ILVEN) and nevus sebaceous (an orange-tan waxy plaque on the scalp that can extend to the face); localized pigmented papillomas; hemangiomas, capillary malformations, hypopigmentation, and café au lait macules possible	Intellectual disabilities; seizures; spastic hemiparesis/paralysis; sensorineural deafness; cerebral hemangiomas; vascular malformations; hemihypertrophy; kyphoscoliosis; ankle/foot deformities; vitamin D–resistant rickets; extension of the epidermal nevi to the eyelid and bulbar conjunctiva; colobomas; corneal opacity; nystagmus; cortical blindness; multiple tumors reported including Wilm's tumor, rhabdomyosarcoma, salivary gland adenocarcinoma, and syringocystadenoma papilliferum
Sturge-Weber syndrome	Sporadic	Facial capillary malformation in a trigeminal nerve distribution, unilateral more common than bilateral, progressive soft tissue and skeletal hypertrophy beneath the malformation is possible	Seizures, intellectual disabilities, and hemiparesis possible; cerebral atrophy; arteriorvenous malformations involving the central nervous system ipsilateral to the skin involvement; choroid malformation of the eyes; ipsilateral glaucoma and visual loss
Ataxia-telangiectasia	AR, ATM gene	Telangiectasias first in the bulbar conjunctiva then ear, eyelid, cheeks, upper chest, and flexor forearms; granulomas; café au lait macules	Ataxia (typically presents before telangiectases), nystagmus, slurred speech, recurrent (especially sinopulmonary) infections, lymphoma, ovarian dysgenesis, radiation sensitive, heterozygotes (parents) at risk for breast cancer
Cutis marmorata telangiectasia congenita	Sporadic	Atrophic reticulated vascular patches occurring on the extremities, trunk, or face; extremities most common site of involvement	Ipsilateral hemihypertrophy or hemiatrophy of extremity, intellectual disabilities, glaucoma

(continued)

Table 20.1. *(continued)*

Disorder	Genetics/mutations	Cutaneous features	Systemic features
Focal dermal hypoplasia (Goltz syndrome)	X-linked dominant	Asymmetric atrophic dyspigmented telangiectatic linear streaks in Blashko's lines on the trunk and extremities; soft red-yellow nodules due to fat herniation in Blashko's lines; ulcers at sites of congenital absence of skin that heal with atrophy; papillomas on the lips, perineum, axilla, and periumbilical area; sparse, brittle hair; patchy alopecia of the scalp or pubic areas; absent or dystrophic nails	Short stature; intellectual disabilities; small, rounded facies; notched alae; mandibular prognathism; hypo- or oligodontia; small teeth with dysplastic enamel; syndactlyly; polydactyly; oligodactyly with "lobster claw" deformity; asymmetric trunk and limbs; osteoopathia striata (radiographic); coloboma; strabismus; microphthalmia
Aplasia cutis congenita	AD, AR, or sporadic; many subtypes	Solitary or multiple erosions, deep ulcerations with thin membrane or atrophic scars with alopecia on the scalp (80%) or other areas, areas heal with scarring weeks after birth, larger lesions possible with extension into the dura	Increased risk of meningitis, venous thrombosis, and sagittal sinus hemorrhage due to communication between area of tissue defect and deeper structures; many possible anomalies depending on subtype involving limbs, central nervous system, and gastrointestinal tract
Xeroderma pigmentosum	AR, XPA–XPG (complementation groups A–G) mutation results in deoxyribonucleic acid repair defects	Acute sun sensitivity in infancy with sunburnlike reaction; erythema, inflammation, and bullae; pigmented macules and telangiectasias (photodistributed) in childhood or adolescence can give rise to areas of atrophy with scaling; greatly increased risk for skin cancer, both melanoma and nonmelanoma	Progressive neurologic degeneration in some complementation groups with intellectual disabilities; sensorineural deafness; microcephaly; hyporeflexia; spasticity and ataxia; progressive symptomatology of eyes with photophobia, conjunctivitis, telangiectasia, and pigmention of the lid and conjunctiva; ectropion; corneal vascularization; opacification; benign lid papillomas; basal cell carcinoma; melanoma
Dyskeratosis congenita	X-linked and autosomal dominant, Dyskerin (DKC1) and hTR (RNA component of telomerase)	Reticulate gray-brown hyper- and hypopigmentation with telangiectasia and atrophy (poikoliderma) on the face, neck, trunk, and upper thighs; palmoplantar keratoderma; hyperhidrosis; friction bullae; acrocyanosis; thinning alopecia on scalp eyelashes and eyebrows; absent, atrophic, or dystrophic nails; longitudinal ridges; pterygium; premalignant leukoplakia of any mucosal surface; dental caries with early loss of teeth	Mild to moderate intellectual disabilities, Fanconi's type pancytopenia with secondary infection and hemorrhage, blepharitis, conjunctivitis, lacrimal duct obstruction with overflow of tears (epiphora), ectropion
Rothmund-Thompson syndrome	AR, RECQ4	Photosensitivity with or without bullae; initial erythema/edema on face rapidly replaced by red-brown patches of poikiloderma; telangiectasia on the face, buttocks, and extensor extremities; acral verrucous keratoses after puberty that may precede squamous cell carcinoma; alopecia of the scalp, eyebrows, and lashes; dystrophic nails	Short stature; small hands and feet; hypoplastic or absent thumbs; various skeletal abnormalities; juvenile cataracts beginning at 3–7 years of age; hypogonadism; dental dysplasia; reports of neoplasia including osteosarcoma, fibrosarcoma, and squamous cell carcinoma

Table 20.1. *(continued)*

Disorder	Genetics/mutations	Cutaneous features	Systemic features
Cockayne syndrome	AR, CSA/CKN1, CSB	Photosenitivity, erythema and scaling in a butterfly distribution on the face that may resolve with hyperpigmentation and atrophy, subcutaneous fat loss on the face with sunken eyes and aged appearance, alopecia	Short stature, microcephaly, thin nose, large ears, disproportionately long limbs with joint contractures, large feet and hands, progressive neurologic deterioration with intellectual disabilities, intracranial calcifications, diffuse demyelination of the central nervous system and peripheral nerves, sensorineural deafness, salt and pepper retinal pigment, miotic pupils, cataracts, optic atrophy, dental carries
Hartnup disease	AR, SLC6A19 encoding a neutral amino acid transporter	Photodistributed erythema and scale with or without bullae on forehead, cheeks, extensor arms, and dorsum of the hands	Cerebellar ataxia, mild intellectual disabilities, psychiatric disturbances
Menkes kinky hair syndrome	X-linked recessive, ATP7A	Hypopigmented, "doughy" skin with laxity; pudgy cheeks; Cupid's bow upper lip; hypopigmented, sparse, short, brittle hair with "steel wool" quality; sparse broken horizontal eyebrows; sparse eyelashes; pili torti most common hair finding	Progressive deterioration with lethargy, seizures, mental and motor retardation, hypertonia, and hypothermia; failure to thrive; wormian bones in sagittal and lambdoid sutures; metaphyseal widening with spurs in long bones; tortuous arteries; multiple genitourinary anomalies
Monilethrix	AD, hHb1 and hHb6 (hair keratins 1 and 6)	Keratosis pilaris on the upper back, nape of neck, and arms; structural defect results in dry, brittle, lusterless, and short hair; brittle nails	Intellectual disabilities (rare), cataracts (rare), teeth abnormalities
Trichothiodystrophy	AR, XPB, XPD (xeroderma pigmentosa complementation groups B and D)	Ichthyosis of variable morphology and severity; short, brittle, and sparse hair on scalp, eyebrows, and eyelashes; polarizing microscopy reveals alternating light and dark bands; dystrophic nails	Short stature, intellectual impairments, ataxia, protruding ears, micrognathia, decrease fertility with hypogonadism, photosensitivity, cataracts
Niemann-Pick disease	AR, sphingomyelinase deficiency	Xanthomas, yellow/brown induration on exposed surfaces	Progessive psychomotor retardation, hypotonicity, and muscle weakness; hepatosplenomegaly; failure to thrive; vomiting; generalized lymphadenopathy; blindness; cherry red spots; deafness; bronchopneumonia
Phenylketonuria	AR, phenylalanine hydroxylase	Blond/light hair (increased phenylalanine inhibits melanogenesis), sclerodermoid changes, generalized hypopigmentation, eczematous dermatitis	Intellectual disabilities, seizures, hyperreflexia, psychomotor delay, blue eyes
Mucopolysaccharidoses	AR; MPS I—(Hurler) α-L-iduronidase; MPS II (Hunter)—iduronate sulfatase; MPS IIIA (Sanfilippo A)—heparan N-sulfatase; MPS IIIB (Sanfilippo B) — α-N-acetyl-glucosaminidase; MPS IIIC (Sanfilippo C)—acetyl CoA: α-glucosaminide acetyltransferase; MPS IIID (Sanfilippo D)—N-acetylglucosamine 6-sulfatase; MPS IVA (Morquio A)—galactose-6-sulfatase;	Thick and course skin, firm ivory-colored papules between angles of the scapulae and posterior axillary line (Hunter), generalized hirsutism	Unusual facies with thick nose and depressed nasal bridge, thick lips and tongue, short neck, macrocephaly, intellectual disabilities, progressive neurologic impairment, deafness, behavioral disturbances, hydrocephalus, short stature, broad hands and short fingers, multiple skeletal/joint problems, corneal clouding, cardiovascular disease (valvular and coronary), hepatosplenomegaly, bronchopneumonia

(continued)

Table 20.1. *(continued)*

Disorder	Genetics/mutations	Cutaneous features	Systemic features
	MPS IVB (Morquio B)—β-galactosidease; MPS VI (Maroteaux-Lamy)—arylsulfatase B; MPS VII (Sly)—β-glucuronidase; MPS IX—hyaluronidase		
Wilson disease	AR, ATP7b	Pretibial hyperpigmentation, blue lunulae	Dementia, decreased motor coordination, ataxia, dysarthria, Kayser-Fleischer ring
Multiple carboxylase deficiency	AR, biotinidase or holocarboxylase deficiency	Periorificial/generalized dermatitis, sparse hair to total alopecia	Hypotonia, seizures, ataxia, coma, vomiting (holocarboxylase deficiency), optic atrophy (biotinidase deficiency), high-frequency hearing loss (biotinidase deficiency)
Homocystinuria	AR, cystathionine β-synthetase deficiency	Malar flush; livedo reticularis; leg ulcers; fine, sparse hair	Intellectual disabilities, seizures, psychiatric disturbances, Marfanoid body habitus, osteoporosis, kyphoscoliosis, pectus excavatum, thromboses/emboli of the arterial and venous systems, downward lens displacement
Cornelia de Lange syndrome	Sporadic	Cutis marmorata, hirsutism, hypoplastic nipples and umbilicus, low hairline, synophrys, long eyelashes	Microcephaly, small nose, anteverted nostrils, long philtrum, downturned thin lips, late-erupting widely-spaced teeth, micrognathia, low-set ears, short neck
Rubinstein-Taybi syndrome	Sporadic, creb binding protein (CREBBP)	Keloid formation in surgical scars, café au lait macules, hirsutism, capillary malformation	Short stature, large-beaked nose, nasal septum below alae, broad nasal bridge, downslanting palpebral fissures, high-arched palate, epicanthal folds, mild micrognathia, microcephaly, severe intellectual disabilities with speech delay and motor retardation, strabismus, cryptochordism, congenital heart defects

Source: Bolognia et al. (2003).

pigmentation can be seen in association with immunodeficiency (Griscelli syndrome), intellectual disabilities, Waardenburg syndrome, deafness, cerebellar ataxia, and Hirschprung disease. Treatment of piebaldism includes use of the erbium:YAG laser and autologous cultured epidermis (Guerra et al., 2004). Areas without pigment are at increased risk for ultraviolet-induced damage and skin cancer and thus should be protected from sun exposure.

Waardenburg syndrome

Ty, a recently adopted 5-year-old boy, was brought in for an evaluation of delayed speech and communication skills. On examination, he was noted to have a white forelock, heterochromatic irides, and several hypopigmented patches on his trunk. The physician also observed a high, broad nasal root, laterally displaced medial canthi (dystopia canthorum), and synophrys. During Ty's evaluation, the physician also detected sensorineural hearing loss and mild developemental delays. The findings suggested a diagnosis of Waardenburg syndrome.

Waardenburg syndrome is characterized by abnormalities in pigment of the skin, hair, and eyes; congenital deaf-mutism; facial features; and other impairments that are attributed in part to abnormal migration of cells derived from the neural crest (Dourmishev, Dourmeshev, Schwartz, & Janniger, 1999; Spitz, 1996). Individuals may have depigmented patches on the body with islands of hyperpigmentation within them. Hyperpigmented macules on normally pigmented background skin can also be present.

A white forelock is present less than half of the time, and confluent eyebrows (synophrys) can be seen in 70%. Premature graying of the scalp hair, eyebrows, or body hair is another possible finding. Ocular findings include dystopia canthorum, partial or complete heterochromatic (different colored) irides, bilateral isohypo-

Table 20.2. Types of Waardenburg syndrome

Waardenburg syndrome subtype	Key features	Gene mutation
I	Presence of dystopia canthorum	*PAX3*
II	Absence of dystopia canthorum	*MITF*
III	Limb/musculoskeletal abnormalities	*PAX3*
IV	Aganglionic megacolon	*EDNRB, EDN3, SOX10*

From Dourmishev, A.L., Dourmishev, L.A. Schwartz, R.A., & Janniger, C.K. (1999). Waardenburg syndrome. *International Journal of Dermatology, 38,* 657; adapted by permission.

chromatia irides (pale blue eyes), strabismus, and alterations in the pigmentation of the fundus. Facial findings may include facial asymmetry, dystopia canthorum, broad nasal root, narrow nose, short philtrum, and retropositioned maxilla.

Individuals with Waardenburg syndrome may not have all of the key features, and members of the same family may not share the same features. These "forme fruste" cases can be a diagnostic challenge because the characteristic features may be absent. Based on clinical features, Waardenburg syndrome has been divided into four types, and mutations in different genes have been associated with different phenotypes (see Table 20.2). The inheritance of Waardenburg syndrome is autosomal dominant for Types I–III. Type IV is autosomal recessive.

One of the most important features of Waardenburg syndrome is congenital deaf-mutism. Hearing loss can be unilateral or bilateral, can range from total to partial, and can be moderate or severe. Due to the possibility of deafness, any child suspected of having Waardenburg syndrome should have a thorough hearing evaluation. Hirschsprung disease is associated with Type IV Waardenburg syndrome, and musculoskeletal abnormalities associated with Type III include arm abnormalities involving the muscle and bone, aplasia of the first two ribs, underdeveloped carpal bones, cystic formation of the sacrum, and bilateral syndactyly. Microcephaly, macrocephaly, intellectual disabilities, and other central nervous system abnormalities have been reported.

Hypomelanosis of Ito

Swirled hypopigmented patches that can be unilateral or bilateral characterize Hypomelanosis of Ito (Bolognia et al., 2003; Odom & Berger, 2000). These hypopigmented areas follow the lines of Blaschko. In addition, other patterns of hypopigmentation have been described, including a checkerboard pattern, dermatomal pattern, and a plaque-like arrangement (Kuster & Konig, 1999). The ability to recognize these patterned skin signs as hypopigmentation can vary depending on the individual's underlying skin pigmentation.

This disorder represents a cutaneous marker of genetic mosaicism. Internal involvement varies greatly and has been reported to range from 33% to 75% (Nehal, PeBenito, & Orlow, 1996; Zvulunov & Esterly, 1995). When present, anomalies can involve the central nervous system (e.g., intellectual disabilities, motor disabilities, microcephaly, seizures, deafness), the eyes (e.g., microphthalmia, retinal degeneration, ptosis, nonclosure of upper eyelid, strabismus), the teeth (e.g., enamel changes, hamartomatous cusps, anodontia), and the skeletal system (e.g., short stature, facial and limb asymmetry, pectus carinatum or excavatum). These varied findings are due to differences in the underlying genetic defect(s).

Incontinentia Pigmenti

Incontinentia pigmenti is an X-linked dominant multisystem disorder caused by mutation in the *NEMO* (NF-kB essential modulator) gene (Shah, Gibbs, Upton, Pickworth, & Garioch, 2003; Smahi et al., 2000). Characteristic of many X-linked dominant disorders, incontinentia pigmenti is lethal to boys in utero. Rare case reports of boys with incontinentia pigmenti have been reported but are usually associated with Klinefelter syndrome or other chromosomal anomalies. Individuals with incontinentia pigmenti are, therefore, nearly always girls and characteristically have neurologic, ophthalmologic, and dental manifestations of the disorder as well as typical cutaneous findings. Ninety percent of individuals with incontinentia pigmenti develop the characteristic skin lesions of the disease within the first year of life, which may help in the diagnosis. The skin lesions of incontinentia pigmenti are separated into four stages (see Table 20.3).

In addition to the cutaneous manifestations of the disease, involvement of other neuroectodermal structures has been described. Common organs affected include hair (vertex alopecia, agenesis of eyebrows and eyelashes), nails (intermittent ridging, pitting, or nail disruption; subungual or periungual keratotic tumors), teeth (partial anodontia, pegged and conned teeth, supernumeracy), and eyes (vascular occlusive events, strabismus). Incontinentia pigmenti can also involve the central nervous system and cause seizures before the age of 1. Also, intellectual disabilities, ataxia, spastic anomalies, microcephaly, cerebral atrophy, hypoplasia of the corpus callosum, and periventricular edema are associated with

Table 20.3. Clinical characteristics of cutaneous stages of incontinentia pigmenti

Stage	Frequency	Typical age of onset	Typical age of resolution	Clinical findings
1. Vesicular	90%	Birth to 2 weeks	4 months	Erythema, vesicles in linear distribution on torso and/or extremities
2. Verrucous	70%	2–6 weeks	6 months	Verrucous hyperkeratotic papules and plaques on extremities
3. Pigmented	98%	12–36 weeks	Puberty	Whorls and streaks of brown pigmentation following lines of Blaschko on torso
4. Depigmented	42%	Early teens to adulthood	None	Pale, hairless, atrophic patches and/or hypopigmentation

the disease. Typically, the prognosis of incontinentia pigmenti is variable but depends most heavily on the degree to which the central nervous system is involved.

McCune-Albright Syndrome

McCune-Albright syndrome (MAS) is characterized by the triad of polyostotic fibrous dysplasia, café-au-lait macules, and endocrine hyperfunction (Ringel, Schwindinger, & Levine, 1996). This syndrome is due to activating mutations in the *GNAS1* gene, which is involved in the regulation of adenylate cyclase ($G\alpha_s$). Mutation in the *GNAS1* gene does not occur in all of the cells in those affected with MAS, even within the same organ. Indeed, mutations in the *GNAS1* gene have been shown to occur as a postzygotic somatic mutation, which supports early clinical reports of individuals with MAS characterized by variable involvement of the endocrine and skeletal systems as well as skin lesions in arrangements corresponding to lines of embryonic development. The absence of inherited cases of MAS suggests that germline mutation would be lethal. The clinical manifestations of MAS from 158 reported cases are shown in Table 20.4.

The main cutaneous feature of MAS is the café au lait macule. Affected individuals have pigmented patches with irregular borders that have been likened to the "coast of Maine." These patches are in contrast to other syndromes characterized by café au lait macules, such as neurofibromatosis, where the café au lait macules have a smooth border. The distribution of café au lait macules in MAS is characteristic as well. These patches rarely extend beyond the midline and tend to be on the same side of the body affected by skeletal abnormalities. The most common regions involved are the buttock and lumbosacral areas and the lesions follow the lines of Blashko. These lines represent clonal expansions from embryonic precursor cells during skin development. Because of their clonal nature, cells in these areas have the same pattern of X chromosome inactivation (i.e., all have the same X chromosome inactivated) and thus phenotypic expression of mutated alleles on the X chromosome.

Polyostotic fibrous dysplasia (i.e., skeletal lesions) typically develops during the first decade and can cause serious neurologic and/or skeletal problems, including nerve entrapment, deformity, and fractures. These lesions are very common in MAS and are present in nearly all individuals with MAS. The most commonly involved sites are the femur and pelvis. These growths appear as lytic lesions with a scalloped border and "ground glass pattern" on radiographs (Ringel et al., 1996). Most individuals with MAS develop multiple areas of involvement, but single lesions can occur. Fatal osteosarcomas have occurred in individuals with MAS, and thus individuals with MAS should be carefully monitored for the development of osteosarcomas.

Endocrinopathies are common in individuals with MAS and are due to autonomous and excessive function of hormone-producing tissues. As such, levels of tropic or stimulating hormones are normal or decreased. The most common endocrinopathy is gonadal hyperfunction. Precocious puberty is more common in girls (Ringel et al., 1996). In addition, growth hormone excess (with or without hyperprolactinemia) is common in individuals with MAS and, as such, acromegaly, gigantism, and galactorrhea have been described. Not all individuals with growth hormone excess have radiographic evidence of a pituitary tumor. Thyroid nodules and hyperthyroidism occur in individuals with MAS. Although the thyroid gland will often be normal on physical exam, nodules are nearly always detectable by sonography.

Table 20.4. Features of McCune-Albright Syndrome

Clinical feature	Age at diagnosis	Comments
Fibrous dysplasia	7.7 (0–52)	Polyostic is more common than monostotic.
Café au lait macules	7.7 (0–52)	Macules are variable in size and number with irregular border.
Precocious puberty	4.9 (0.3–9)	This symptom is a common initial manifestation.
Acromegaly/gigantism	14.8 (0.2–42)	17/26 of individuals have adenoma on magnetic resonance imaging/computed tomography.
Hyperprolactinemia	16 (0.2–42)	23/42 of individuals are acromegalics with elevated prolactin.
Hyperthyroidism	14.4 (0.5–37)	Euthyroid goiter is common.
Hypercortisolism	4.4 (0.2–17)	All cases are primary adrenal.
Myxomas	34 (17–50)	Extremity myxomas are the most common.
Osteosarcoma	36 (34–37)	This condition is found at sites of fibrous dysplasia and is not related to prior radiation therapy.
Rickets/osteomalacia	27.3 (8–52)	This condition is responsive to phosphorus plus calcitriol.
Cardiac abnormalities	33.1 (0.1–66)	Arrhythmias and congestive heart failure have been reported.
Hepatic abnormalities	1.9 (0.3–4)	Neonatal icterus is most common.

From Ringel, M.D., Schwindinger, W.F., & Levine, M.A. (1996). Clinical implications of genetic defects in G proteins: The molecular basis of McCune-Albright syndrome and Albright hereditary osteodystrophy. *Medicine (Baltimore), 75,* 175; adapted by permission.

Primary hypercortisolism occurs occasionally in individuals with MAS and can occur at a young age. Abnormal phosphate metabolism can occur with or without the MAS phenotype and can lead to hypophosphatemic rickets and osteomalacia in those with fibrous polyostotic dysplasia. Although most individuals with MAS have some form of endocrinopathy, nonendocrine organs can be involved as well. Activating mutations of the *GNAS1* gene have been found in peripheral blood leukocytes, the liver, the heart, the thymus, and the gastrointestinal tract with associated hepatitis, arrhythmias, and polyps (Ringel et al., 1996). A more severe form of MAS has been reported with jaundice, hepatitis, extramedullary hematopoiesis, gastrointestinal polyps, thymic hyperplasia, acute pancreatitis, neurodevelopmental disorders, and sudden cardiac death.

Carney Complex

Carney complex is an autosomal dominant disorder characterized by cardiac, endocrine, neural, and cutaneous tumors as well as pigmented lesions of the skin and mucous membranes. Due to the multiple endocrine tumors (two or more are often present) that can occur in Carney complex, it has been described as a type of multiple endocrine neoplasia (Stratakis et al., 1996). Individuals with some components of Carney complex have been described as having syndromes using the acronyms NAME (Nevi, Atrial Myxomas, and Ephelides) and LAMB (Lentigines, Atrial Myxomas, and Blue nevi).

Mutation in the *PRKAR1A* gene encoding the type 1α regulatory subunit of protein kinase A (PKA) has been linked to several families with Carney complex (Sandrini & Stratakis, 2003). Like other neurocutaneous syndromes, the clinical manifestations can vary significantly, even within the same family. Such variability has been responsible for the apparent "skipping" of a generation. With this in mind, it is doubtful that individual cases are sporadic unless detailed analysis (clinical, radiological, and biochemical) of all first-degree relatives is performed.

"Spotty skin pigmentation" is the most common clinical finding in individuals with Carney complex. These skin findings can include different dermatologic entities including pigmented lesions and tumors. The pigmented lesions can include lentigines, blue nevi, combined nevi, café au lait macules, and areas of depigmentation. In addition, cutaneous myxomas are classically found on the eyelid, external ear canal, and nipple. The lentigines typically appear in the peripubertal period, although individuals may be born with these or other pigmented lesions. The café au lait macules and other pigmented lesions can sometimes be found at birth, although they typically appear in early childhood. Both the lentigines and café au lait macules tend to fade with time, although they may be detected as late as the eighth decade.

The systemic features of Carney complex include a variety of tumors, as well as endocrine dysfunction. Heart myxomas can occur at a young age and may recur. Myxomas can occur at other sites including skin, breast, tongue, hard palate, pharynx, genital tract (for girls), and pelvis (for girls). Endocrine tumors can include primary pigmented nodular adrenocortical disease, growth hormone and prolactin secreting pituitary adenomas, testicular neoplasms (primarily large-cell calcifying Sertoli cell tumor), thyroid adenoma or carcinoma, and ovarian cysts (Stratekis et al., 1996). Additional manifestations include psammomatous melanotic schwannoma, breast ductal adenoma, and osteochondromyxoma. Acromegaly can occur, albeit infrequently. The life expectancy of individuals with Carney complex has been reported to be decreased primarily due to cardiac or cardiac-related causes.

COMMON DERMATOLOGIC CONDITIONS

Common dermatologic conditions seen in individuals with developmental disabilities include acne vulgaris, warts, and tinea infection.

Acne Vulgaris

Acne vulgaris is a common disorder of the pilosebaceous unit that has a peak incidence during adolescence, although all age groups can be affected (Bolognia et al., 2003; Jansen, Burgdorf, & Plewig, 1997; Oberemok & Shalita, 2002; White, 1998). Although an incidence of 85% for individuals between the ages of 12 and 24 has been reported, the disease can affect adults into their 40s. The clinical spectrum of acne vulgaris is great and can range from mild asymptomatic comedones to fulminant acne fulminans with systemic symptoms. In addition to the cosmetic component of acne, acne can have a substantial psychological impact on individuals.

The pathogenesis of acne vulgaris involves four key components, each of which needs to be considered when initiating therapy. In addition, understanding the basic structure of the pilosebaceous unit is extremely helpful. The four components to acne pathogenesis include ductal hypercornification, sebaceous hyperplasia with seborrhea, *Propionibacterium acnes* colonization of the duct, and the inflammatory response (Gollnick et al., 2003). Comedones (and microcomedones), the starting lesions of acne, begin at the opening of the hair follicle. The corneocytes (fully differentiated dead skin keratinocytes) are retained in the follicle instead of being shed and extruded through the follicular ostia, which leads to blockage of the pilosebaceous unit with subsequent accumulation of sebum (the sebaceous glands enter into the follicle below the blockage) and shed corneocytes. This initial lesion presents clinically as a small skin-colored papule or comedone. As the comedone expands, the wall can rupture, releasing the immunogenic contents into the surrounding dermis, thus triggering an immune response. This response can present as a small inflammatory papule or may be more exuberant, leading to deep-seated painful cysts. In addition to keratin, *P. acnes*, which requires the sebaceous lipids, also contributes to the immune response (Bolognia et al., 2003).

The response of the sebaceous glands to hormonal influences, particularly androgens, also plays a key role in the pathogenesis of acne. This explains the typical pubertal onset of acne as well as the clinical picture seen in syndromes with androgen excess (Bolognia et al., 2003; Gollnick et al., 2003). Any girl or woman with unresponsive, severe, or atypical acne should be questioned regarding other clinical features of androgen excess, such as irregular menses, voice changes, and excess hair growth. Laboratory evaluation should be performed on any individual with a suspected androgen excess.

The differential diagnosis of acne is large, as are the number of variants of acne. Diagnosis depends on the type of clinical lesions that predominate. The typical age of onset, distribution, and presence of comedones usually allow for the diagnosis; however, when the clinical picture is more confusing, a broad differential needs to be considered, particularly for individuals who are immunocompromised because many infections can present with skin-colored or inflammatory papules on the face (Bolognia et al., 2003). The differential diagnosis of acne and variants of acne can be seen in Tables 20.5 and 20.6, respectively.

Treatment of acne depends on the severity of the eruption. In addition, education is crucial, as most of the effective therapies require several weeks before improvement can be seen. Topical therapy should be maximized as most individuals can benefit from topical therapy alone. Effective use of topical therapy also helps reduce the individual's exposure to and risk from systemic medication; however, some individuals do not respond sufficiently to topical therapy and require systemic therapy at least for a period of time. Therapy is aimed at clearing lesions and reducing the risk of scarring. Scarring can be severe and can have a long-lasting impact.

Table 20.5. The differential diagnosis of acne vulgaris

Comedonal acne	Inflammatory acne	Infantile acne
Milia	Rosacea	Miliaria rubra
Trichoepitheliomas	Perioral dermatitis	Milia
Nevus comedonicus	Folliculitis: gram negative, *Staphylococcus aureus*	Candida infection
Molluscum contagiosum	Eosinphilic folliculitis	Sebaceous hyperplasia
Deep fungal infection	Pseudofolliculitis barbae	
Eruptive vellus hair cysts		

From Bolognia, J.L., Rapini, R.P., Horn, T.D., Mascaro, J.M., Mancini, A.J., Salasche, S.J., et al. (2003). *Dermatology* (p. 538). St. Louis: Mosby; adapted by permission.

Numerous studies have indicated that the cornerstone of acne treatment is retinoid therapy (Gollnick et al., 2003). Retinoids help decrease ductal hypercornification and sebaceous gland production and have anti-inflammatory properties. Numerous compounds are available, including tretinoin, adapalene, and tazarotene. Newer products, including azaleic acid, also have multiple beneficial properties. Other topical agents include benzoyl peroxide alone or in combination with topical antibiotics, which may be more effective than either product alone.

Systemic therapy for acne includes several classes of medications, including antibiotics, hormonal therapies, and systemic retinoids. Antibiotics reduce *P. acnes*, and some (particularly the tetracycline class) have anti-inflammatory properties. The tetracycline antibiotics (tetracycline, doxycycline, and minocycline) are the most commonly used antibiotics for the treatment of acne. Although they are a useful adjunct, they are not without their risks, and thus therapy needs to be individualized based on disease severity and the individual's comorbidities and other medications.

Systemic therapy should be used for defined periods of time to help minimize risk. Some systemic therapies can have serious effects on a developing fetus, and thus the possibility of pregnancy needs to be addressed. Hormonal therapy can be very effective for girls and women and may be necessary if considering therapy with systemic retinoids. Spironolactone has antiandrogen activity and can also be used effectively to treat acne. Isotretinoin is another useful medication for the treatment of acne unresponsive to other therapies or scarring acne. Its possible association with mood disturbances as well as its known teratogenicity require that individuals be monitored closely. The clinician must be familiar with the side effects of isotretinoin. In addition, regular clinical and laboratory evaluations are required both prior to and during therapy.

Table 20.6 Variants of acne vulgaris

Acne variant	Features
Acne fulminans	This severe suppurative and nodulocystic acne is associated with systemic symptoms of fever, osteolytic bone lesions, arthralgias, myalgias, and prostration.
Acne conglobata	This severe nodulocystic acne does not have systemic symptoms.
Acne mechanica	Comedones form due to repeated mechanical and frictional forces that occlude the pilosebaceous duct.
Excoriated acne	Comedones and inflammatory papules are excoriated, leaving crusted erosions. This variant typically occurs in young women.
Drug-induced acne	Acneiform eruptions can occur due to numerous medications, including steroids (anabolic and corticosteroids), phenytoin, lithium, isoniazid, iodides, bromides, corticotropin, azathioprine, and tetracyclines. An abrupt monomorphic eruption of inflammatory papules is characteristic.
Occupational acne and chloracne	Exposure to substances that occlude the follicles are the culprits. These substances commonly include cutting oils and petrolatum-based products. Comedones predominate particularly on exposed areas. Chloracne occurs after several weeks of exposure to chlorinated aromatic hydrocarbons that may be found in insecticides, fungicides, electrical insulators/conductors, and herbicides.
Neonatal acne (neonatal cephalic pustulosis)	This condition occurs in more than 20% of healthy newborns. Lesions appear at 2 weeks and resolve by 3 months. The acne typically presents as small, inflamed papules on the cheeks and nose and is due (at least in part) to Malassezia species.
Infantile acne	This variant presents at 3–6 months with more comedonal formation than seen in infantile acne. It is due to hormonal imbalances intrinsic to this age and typically resolves by 1–2 years of age.

Source: Bolognia et al. (2003).

Warts

Warts, or verruca, are caused by any one of a number of deoxyribonucleic acid (DNA) viruses known as human papilloma viruses (HPV). These viruses can infect the skin or mucosa and cause a wide range of growths ranging from common warts to large disfiguring condyloma. In addition, some of the HPV subtypes have been shown to be the major cause of cervical cancers as well as other types of cancer, including cancers of the vagina, vulva, anus, and penis (Munger, 2002; Stratakis et al., 1996; Tyring, 2000; zur Hausen, 2000).

Infection with HPV may be clinical, subclinical, or latent. Clinical disease is seen on inspection whereas subclinical disease requires an aid for examination (e.g., acetic acid soaking). Latent disease refers to the presence of HPV particles or DNA in normal skin and may account for the refractive nature of some HPV infections. Based on their clinical appearance, several types of warts have been described along with their HPV etiologies.

In addition to affecting the cutaneous and gential areas, verrucae can also occur on the oral mucosa. Oral warts appear as whitish to pink to red papules or larger plaques that occur on the buccal, gingival, labial, or lingual surfaces as well as on the hard palate. They are associated with HPV types 6 and 11. Other types of intraoral verrucae include Heck's disease (focal epithelial hyperplasia) that presents with multiple flat or condylomatous papules on the intraoral mucosa.

Four types of verrucous carcinoma are worth mentioning because of their bland histologic picture: Buschke-Lowenstein tumor (giant condylomata acuminata), oral florid papillomatosis, epithelioma cuniculatum of the sole, and papillomatosis cutis carcinoides of the skin. These growths can invade and cause local destruction. They can also occassionally metastasize to regional lymph nodes. Because of their benign histologic picture, they can be confused with benign verrucae both clinically and histologically.

Treatment of HPV infection depends on several factors. Common warts frequently resolve spontaneously within 1–2 years (Bolognia et al., 2003). Most therapies are aimed at the destruction of visible lesions or induction of cytotoxicity against infected cells. Many options are available including over-the-counter preparations. Vaccine development is promising for some HPV infections that have been linked to cervical cancer (Brentjens, Yeung-Yue, Lee, & Tyring, 2003). New agents, such as imiquimod cream, have been approved for use in the treatment of genital warts, and its use in the treatment of other warts has been reported (Hengge & Cusini, 2003). In addition, the use of skin test antigens for the treatment of warts is a promising new area under investigation (Johnson, Roberson, & Horn, 2001).

Tinea Infection

Tinea infection, or dermatophytosis, represents superficial infection of the skin, hair, or nails by a group of fungi known as dermatophytes, which include members of three genera: *Microsporum*, *Trichophyton*, and *Epidermophyton*. The infection is given a different name depending on the site of involvement. Entities include tinea capitis (scalp), tinea barbae (beard), tinea faciei (face), tinea corporis (trunk and proximal extremities), tinea manuum (hand), tinea pedis (feet), and tinea cruris (groin). Infection of the nail is known as onychomycosis (or tinea unguium). Tinea incognito is the name given to tinea infections whose clinical picture is modified by the application of topical steroids or other topical immunomodulators.

The clinical picture of tinea infections depends on several factors, including host response to the organism (immune status of the individual), organism involved (some species are more likely to cause a brisk inflammatory response), location, and prior therapy. Although the classic tinea infection (especially tinea corporis) presents as an erythematous annular plaque with scale (so-called "ring worm"), the differential diagnosis can be large depending on the clinical picture. Examination of scrapings with potassium hydroxide solution should be done on any individual considered to have a tinea infection. Other options includes culture, clippings of nail for microscopic examination (for onychomycosis), or skin biopsy if the diagnosis is in question. A list of types of tinea infections and their differential diagnosis is seen in Table 20.7.

Tinea capitis typically occurs in school-age children; however, it can occur in infants and adults (in-

Table 20.7. Differential diagnoses of dermatophyte infections

Tinea capitis	Tinea faciei	Tinea corporis	Tinea cruris	Tinea pedis
Seborrheic dermatitis	Seborrheic dermatitis	Nummular eczema	Inverse psoriasis	Contact dermatitis
Alopecia areata	Perioral dermatitis	Atopic dermatitis	Erythrasma	Dyshidrotic eczema
Psoriasis	Contact dermatitis	Pityriasis rosea	Intertrigo	Psoriasis
Trichotillomania	Lupus erythematosus	Pityriasis versicolor		Secondary syphilis
Lichen planus		Psoriasis		
Discoid lupus		Subacute lupus erythematosus		
Folliculitis		Secondary syphilis		
Secondary syphilis				

From Bolognia, J.L., Rapini, R.P., Horn, T.D., Mascaro, J.M., Mancini, A.J., Salasche, S.J., et al. (2003). *Dermatology* (p. 1176). St. Louis: Mosby; reprinted by permission.

cluding the elderly) sometimes without many of the typical features seen in children. It is divided into inflammatory and noninflammatory types. The noninflammatory types can be an area of alopecia that is dry and scaly, so called "gray patch" tinea capitis, or as "black dot" tinea capitis with multiple areas of alopecia studded with black dots representing hairs broken off at or below the surface. The inflammatory type of tinea capitis can start as a scaly, erythematous, papular eruption with alopecia and can progress to a large, boggy purulent, indurated area known as a kerion. If extensive, pain can occur, as can systemic symptoms of fever and adenopathy. A widespread dermatophytid, or "id," reaction can also occur on other areas of the body. Kerion formation can lead to permanent scarring and alopecia.

Diagnosis can be made by microscopic examination and culture. Treatment requires systemic therapy with antifungal medication because the infecting organism penetrates deeply into the hair follicle. Systemic medications include griseofulvin, itraconazole, terbinafine, and fluconazole (Chan & Friedlander, 2004). Adjuvant therapy with an antifungal shampoo (e.g., ketoconazole) may be helpful.

Tinea coporis represents tinea infection on any part of the body other than those where tinea infection is given an alternative name (scalp, groin, feet, hands, beard, and face). It typically presents as an erythematous annular plaque with scale. The raised border and central clearing produces the so-called "ring worm." Hypopigmentation may be present. In the elderly or individuals who are immunosuppressed, the plaques can become large and cover large body surface areas. Diagnosis like other tinea infections depends on demonstrating the organism in skin scrapings with the use of potassium hydroxide. Culture or biopsy may be helpful if no organisms are demonstrable using potassium hydroxide preparations. Treatment is usually with topical antifungal preparations unless the infection is extensive. A low-potency topical steroid may be used in conjunction with the antifungal medication to help reduce the inflammation if it is symptomatic.

Variants of tinea corporis include tinea profunda, Majocchi's granuloma, and tinea imbricata. Tinea profunda results from an extensive inflammatory response to the dermatophyte. It can appear verrucous or infiltrative. Majocchi's granuloma represents a deeper follicular infection and may occur in the setting of topical steroids or on the legs of women after shaving. Tinea imbricata is an infection with a specific type of dermatophyte (*T. concentricum*) that causes a unique pattern of concentric annular rings.

Tinea manuum represents infection of the hand, and palmar involvement has a different clinical picture than infection of the dorsal hand. Tinea pedis frequently coexists ("two feet and one hand syndrome"). The palm(s) are most commonly hyperkeratotic. Vesicular and papular variants can occur. Tinea barbae usually presents as an inflammatory eruption in the beard area, frequently with multiple pustules. Sinus tracts, abscesses, and bacterial superinfection may also occur. Tinea faciei may present as other classic tinea infections, although others can be more atypical, and a high index of suspicion is necessary.

Tinea pedis ("athlete's foot") is an extremely common tinea infection occurring more often in adults. There are four major types: mocassin, interdigital, inflammatory, and ulcerative. Bacterial superinfection can occur including a gram-negative toe web infection. Other complications include a dermatophytid reaction (a distant eczematous eruption), cellulitis, and even osteomyelitis. Treatment is usually with topical antifungals although oral antifungals may be warranted in diabetics and individuals who are immunosuppressed. Hyperhidrosis is a predisposing factor, and the feet should be kept as dry as possible. Tinea unguum or onychomycosis is discussed in the section on Down syndrome.

DRUG ERUPTIONS

Individuals with developmental disorders often take medications that cause skin eruptions. Among these medications are corticosteroids (e.g., prednisone, prednisolone), anticonvulsants (e.g., phenytoin, phenobarbital, valproic acid, carbamazepine), and psychotropic medicines (e.g., lithium). Prednisone is commonly used to decrease intracranial pressure and is used as an anti-inflammatory. Administration of prednisone can cause steroid acne during treatment, and rebound eruptions of other types may occur after prednisone is tapered. If an individual has a drug eruption masked by prednisone, it becomes evident after the prednisone is removed. Similarly, prednisone can mask mild psoriasis, that upon steroid withdrawal, may flare and even result in pustular psoriasis.

Anticonvulsants are frequent causes of drug eruptions ranging from macular and urticarial eruptions, which are self-limited, to life-threatening eruptions (e.g., toxic epidermal necrolysis, anticonvulsant hypersensitivity syndrome). Toxic epidermal necrolysis frequently occurs with the administration of anticonvulsants in the setting of cranial irradiation. Anticonvulsant hypersensitivity syndrome is thought to occur as a result of metabolic intermediates binding to the liver, followed by an immune response directed against the liver-metabolite adduct. This hypersensitivity syndrome is characterized by eosinophilia, macular eruption, and increased liver function tests and can be due to any of the aromatic anticonvulsants (phenytoin, carbamazepine, and Phenobarbital), but is not associated with the non-aromatic valproic acid (Arbiser, Goldstein, & Gordon, 1993).

Other skin eruptions are thought to be associated with reactivation of herpes virus 6. Of note, valproic acid causes reactivation of HHV8/KSHV, and reactivation of HHV6 may occur in a similar fashion (Zeller, Schuab, Steffen, Battegay, Hirsh, & Bircher, 2003). Lithium is commonly used for bipolar disorder. It is a potent inducer of psoriasis, and caution should be utilized in the treatment of individuals with preexisting psoriasis, even if mild. Lithium inhibits glycogen synthase kinase 3, thus potentiating growth factor mediated signal transduction, and this may underlie its ability to cause and potentiate psoriasis (Chalecka-Franaszek & Chuang, 1999).

DERMATOSES ASSOCIATED WITH DOWN SYNDROME

Individuals with Down syndrome (see Chapter 9.2) have an increased incidence of several cutaneous conditions that may or may not be clinically problematic for the individual (Barankin & Guenther, 2001; Dourmishev, Miteva, Mitev, Pramatarov, & Schwartz, 2000; Ercis, Balci, & Atakan, 1996; Schepis, Barone, Siragusa, Pettinato, & Romano, 2002). They have been reported to experience cutaneous signs of accelerated aging (Brugge, Grove, Clopton, Grove, & Piacquadio, 1993). Features such as premature graying of the hair, alopecia, and wrinkling have been reported. The mechanisms underlying these processes are not well understood but may be linked to damage by free radicals.

Alopecia Areata

Alopecia areata is felt to represent an autoimmune-mediated loss of hair that can vary from discrete nummular patches on the scalp to complete loss of scalp hair (alopecia totalis) or total body hair loss (alopecia universalis) (Bolognia et al., 2003; Odom & Berger, 2000). Alopecia may also occur in a bandlike pattern on the periphery of the scalp (ophiasis) or in a diffuse pattern. The scalp is otherwise normal in alopecia areata. "Exclamation point" hairs represent short, broken hairs, often at the periphery of areas of alopecia, whose distal ends are broader than their proximal ends. Biopsy reveals an infiltrate of T-lymphocytes and macrophages consistent with an immunologically mediated process.

Anetoderma

Anetoderma presents as localized areas of flaccid or saclike skin often with herniation of underlying adipose (Bolognia et al., 2003). The condition is due to a focal loss of dermal elastic tissue. It can occur secondary to an inflammatory process (folliculitis or cutaneous vasculitis) or penicillamine use, or it may be idiopathic.

Atopic Dermatitis

Atopic dermatitis represents a chronic pruritic dermatosis that typically starts in early infancy (95% by the age of 5 years). Reports of both increased and decreased prevalence in individuals with Down syndrome exist in the literature. It is clinically characterized by eczematous patches and plaques. In infants, the areas of involvement are typically the scalp, face, cheeks, and extensor surfaces of the extremities. In those older than 2 years, the involved areas are typically the flexural regions of the extremities, especially the antecubital and popliteal fossae.

Over time, areas of involvement are frequently lichenified due to chronic scratching and/or rubbing. Young infants may lose hair on the posterior scalp due to the chronic rubbing done in response to the pruritus. Xerosis and colonization with *Staphylococcus aureus* are other important features of atopic dermatitis. Individuals with atopic dermatitis are also at risk of disseminated herpes infection (eczema herpeticum), erythroderma, and vaccinia (after vaccination) (Odom & Berger, 2000). Atopic dermatitis is associated with a personal or family history of other atopic diseases such as allergic rhinitis or asthma. Treatment is aimed at hydration of the skin with regular application of emollients, topical anti-inflammatory medications (steroids and calcineurin inhibitors such as tacrolimus and pimecrolimus), and systemic medications to control infection, if present, and pruritus (typically with antihistamines).

Cheilitis

Cheilitis, or inflammation of the lips, is more common in those with Down syndrome compared with the general population. Although the cause is unknown, chronic exposure to saliva (due to macroglossia) may play a role. The lips frequently develop vertical fissures and crusting. Infection with candida is a possibility in any warm, moist environment. Bacterial superinfection is also a risk in any area that is chronically inflamed. Lip licking, mouth breathing, and a decrease in the separation between the mandible and maxilla are all potential contributors.

Treatment should be aimed at protecting the lips with petrolatum ointment (Vaseline) as well as anticandidal medications such as nystatin cream. Low-potency topical steroids can be used alone or in combination with anticandidal topical medications to help decrease inflammation. Actinic cheilitis, due to chronic sun exposure, typically presents as a hyperkeratotic papule or scaly macule or patch on the lower lip. Palpation for induration and lesion depth is always indicated as these lesions can give rise to squamous cell cancer on the lip.

Cutis Marmorata

Cutis marmorata presents as a transient reticulate and or mottled erythematous/vascular patch typically on the extremities (Bolognia et al., 2003). It is made worse by exposure to cold and is decreased with warming. This condition can be physiologic and may be seen in normal infants. A similarly patterned finding is livedo reticularis that may be present in those with underlying disease (i.e., infection, collagen vascular disease, vasculitis).

Elastosis Perforans Serpiginosa

Dwayne, a 25-year-old man with Down syndrome, was noted on physical examination to have a group of pink-red papules as well as an annular plaque on his lateral and posterior neck. He had no history of pruritus or trauma. Microscopic examination of the annular plaque revealed no evidence of dermatophyte. Biopsy revealed evidence of a perforating disorder consistent with the diagnosis of elastosis perforans serpiginosa.

Elastosis perforans serpiginosa (EPS) represents one type of perforating disorder in which there is transepidermal elimination of dermal connective tissue. Although the elimination of collagen characterizes some types of perforating disorders, EPS is characterized by the elimination of elastic tissue. Typically, EPS manifests itself in childhood or early adulthood with hyperkeratotic pink-red papules that may coalesce to form annular or arcuate plaques. The typical area of involvement is the lateral or posterolateral neck; however, other areas that can be involved include the arms, face, or other flexural areas. Involvement of the penis has been reported. EPS can be idiopathic, although 40% of cases occur in association with genetic disorders including Down syndrome. Other disorders associated with EPS include acrogeria, Ehlers-Danlos syndrome, Marfan syndrome, osteogenesis imperfecta, pseudoxanthoma elasticum, and Rothmund-Thomson syndrome. Treatment of EPS is difficult, but individual lesions may respond to liquid nitrogen therapy. In addition, tazarotene and various lasers have been reported to be of benefit in treating EPS.

Fissured Tongue

Numerous furrows and grooves on the dorsal aspect of the tongue characterize fissured tongue (Barankin & Guenther, 2001; Dourmishev et al., 2000; Ercis et al., 1996; Schepis et al., 2002). It is a benign condition and has been reported with a prevalence of 2%–5% of individuals with Down syndrome.

Folliculitis

Folliculitis represents inflammation of the hair follicle. This inflammation may be secondary to infection (bacterial, fungal, or viral), mechanical causes (e.g., persistent trauma, tight clothing), or idiopathic inflammation (e.g., eosinophilic folliculitis). Eosinophilic folliculitis may be associated with human immunodeficiency virus (HIV) infection. Bacterial folliculitis is most commonly caused by *S. aureus.*

Infection may be superficial or may involve deeper portions of the follicular unit. On examination, pink-to-red papules and/or pustules are seen around the hair follicle. Any area of the body may be involved. Deep folliculitis is characterized by larger papules or nodules (with or without an obvious pustule) that are more likely to be painful or tender. Sycosis barbae is an example of such a deep folliculitis that occurs in the beard area.

Treatment with topical antimicrobial therapy such as mupirocin ointment, clindamycin, or erythromycin solution along with use of an antibacterial soap is usually sufficient to treat superficial bacterial folliculitis. More extensive or deep infections frequently require antistaphylococcal oral antibiotics. Culture is indicated if there are systemic symptoms, no response to treatment, or risk factors for acquiring resistant strains of bacteria, such as incarceration, hospitalization, or exposure to someone harboring a resistant strain.

Folliculitis caused by dermatophyte is termed *Majocchi's granuloma* or *tinea profunda* and can occur when superficial dermatophyte infection is treated with topical steroids. It may also occur in individuals that are immunosuppressed such as transplant recipients or those infected with HIV. There are no reports of Majocchi's granuloma occurring in individuals with Down syndrome. Clinically, there are inflammatory papules, pustules, and or plaques, typically with some scaling. Potassium hydroxide examination is usually positive, although a negative KOH does not exclude the diagnosis. Diagnosis may require a skin biopsy to reveal fungal organisms. Treatment frequently requires systemic antifungal therapy because penetration deep into the hair follicle may not occur with topical therapy.

Furunculosis

Furuncle is the medical term for boil—a deep follicular-based skin infection that is painful, firm, or fluctuant. The process represents a collection of pus that has been walled off by the individual's immune response. A carbuncle represents an interconnecting collection of furuncles. Most individuals are immunocompetent, although certain conditions may predispose the development of furuncles, such as Chediak-Higashi syndrome, diabetes, hyperimmunoglobulin E syndrome, immunosuppression, malnutrition, or obesity. Any hair-bearing area may be affected. Areas of increased friction and/or sweating are most commonly affected, such as the buttocks, anterior thighs, axillae, and groin. There may be increased risk in areas recently shaven.

Depending on the extent of the process, there may be systemic symptoms of fever, malaise, and chills. The pain may be excruciating. Treatment involves warm compresses, drainage of flucuant lesions (with or without packing with iodoform gauze), and appropriate systemic antibiotics if there are systemic symptoms or in an immunocompromised individual. Recurrent disease may warrant attempts aimed at eradication of nasal carriage of *S. aureus* with topical mupirocin ointment (Raz, Miron, Colodner, Staler, Samara, & Keness, 1996), although this may benefit only selected individuals and a recent analysis found no evidence for its routine use as prophylactic therapy (Laupland & Conly, 2003). Of note is the increasing prevalence of community acquired methicillin resistant *S. aureus* (CA-MRSA) (Eady & Cove, 2003; Said-Salim, Mathema, & Kreiswirth, 2003).

Geographic Tongue

Geographic tongue can be a manifestation of atopy or psoriasis, although it is usually an isolated finding. The incidence in Down syndrome has been reported to be 11% (Ercis et al., 1996). The clinical and histopathologic findings of geographic tongue are identical to the tongue lesions seen in pustular psoriasis and Reiter syndrome. Geographic tongue has also been reported in an individual with AIDS and as a result of lithium therapy. It can also coexist with fissured tongue.

Clinically, geographic tongue usually affects the dorsal surface with well-demarcated red patches surrounded by a thin white-yellow border. The initial appearance may be a smooth red patch on the tip or lateral surface of the tongue. The appearance can remain stagnant or can change daily, with some patches disappearing and new ones developing. Periods of exacerbation or quiescence are often experienced. Geographic tongue is usually asymptomatic, although glossodynia may occur occasionally. Although no therapy is usually needed, topical treatment with 0.1% tretinoin solution has produced clearing, and topical antihistamine solution mouth rinses may be helpful during exacerbations (Assimakopoulos, Patrikakos, Fotika, & Elisaf, 2002).

Keratosis Pilaris

Keratosis pilaris is an autosomal dominantly inherited condition that is due to a keratotic plug occurring within the hair follicles of the affected area. Mild cases are usually confined to the posterior proximal upper extremities although other areas can be involved including the upper thighs, face, forearms, and legs. The small follicular papules may be erythematous or have a grayish appearance. Keratosis pilaris usually appears by age 2 or 3 and subsides after early adulthood. Treatment can be difficult for moderate or severe cases. Therapies include 12% lactic acid, topical tretinoin, and topical tazarotene.

Milia-Like Calcinosis Cutis

Milia-like idiopathic calcinosis cutis presents as small, smooth, whitish, firm papules resembling milia. Central crusting may result from transepidermal elimination of calcium or surrounding erythema. Milia-like idiopathic calcinosis cutis has been reported primarily in those with Down syndrome, although healthy children have been reported to have milia-like idiopathic calcinosis cutis as well (Becuwe, Roth, Villedieu, Chouvet, Kanitakis, & Claudy, 2004). The papules occur primarily on the hands. Other locations include the feet, elbows, knees, thighs, and even face. The lesions may heal with or without scarring and usually disappear before adulthood.

Norwegian (Crusted) Scabies

Seventy-year-old Phyllis, who had moved in with her family 3 weeks ago, was brought in for evaluation of a scaly eruption of several months duration. She presented with mild pruritus, although several members of her family complained of severe pruritus over the last few days. The pruritis had little to no response with the use of topical steroids and topical antifungal medications. On examination, Phyllis was noted to have several red plaques with thick hyperkeratotic scale. Examination with potassium hydroxide revealed no evidence of hyphae; however, numerous ovoid forms were noticed, as were several moving insectlike creatures. Based on this evidence, Norwegian scabies was diagnosed, and Phyllis was treated with oral ivermectin. All contacts were treated with topical permethrin. The eruption slowly resolved in Phyllis and her family members.

Norwegian scabies is a term used to describe a severe type of infestation by the mite *Sarcoptes scabiei.* The condition occurs in individuals who are immunocompromised, institutionalized, or malnourished or who have neurologic disorders including Down syndrome. Cutaneous immunosuppression with potent topical steroids has also been associated with the development of Norwegian scabies.

Rather than the typical scabies infection presenting with pruritic papules, burrows, and nodules and caused by a small number of mites, Norwegian scabies are crusted or scaly (can be psoriasiform) plaques teeming with mites. The distribution is also more widespread and can involve atypical areas of the body including the scalp and face. In addition, the nails can be involved along with the fingertips. There can be fissuring of the trunk, buttocks, or genitals as well as subungual and palmar hyperkeratosis. Pressure-bearing areas may have hyperkeratotic lesions as well. Lesions can become secondarily infected and eczematous. Pruritus may be mild.

Treatment is aimed at preventing the spread of the mite and treating all close contacts. Therapies include permethrin cream and systemic treatment with oral ivermectin. Although both treatments are usually well tolerated, infants, pregnant or nursing women, and older adults may be at risk for adverse effects with commonly used therapies topical and systemic. Therapy must, therefore, be tailored to the individual (Chouela, Abeldano, Pellerano, & Hernandez, 2002; Scheinfeld, 2004; Wendel & Rompalo, 2002).

Onychomycosis

Onychomyosis is any fungal infection of the nail plate. Most commonly, the disease is due to dermatophyte species. It can be divided into several clinical types, including distal subungual, white superficial, proximal subungual (which may be a cutaneous indication of HIV infection), and candidal onychomycosis. Treatment is usually not necessary if there are no symptoms; however, the nails may be a reservoir for fungus, causing superficial skin infections (e.g., tinea pedis), and quality-of-life issues must be considered in individuals with onychomycosis (Elewski, 1998a, 1998b, 2000).

Fungal elements should be documented prior to antifungal therapy because other nail diseases can cause a similar clinical picture. Evidence of fungus can be obtained by KOH examination, culture, or microscopic examination of nail plate clippings. If treatment is desired, topical therapy with ciclopirox or systemic therapy with terbinafine, itraconazole, or fluconazole may be tried. Recurrence is common, and more than one course of therapy may be required (Seebacher, 2003).

Palmoplantar Hyperkeratosis

Palmoplantar hyperkeratosis represents a thickened keratotic stratum corneum on the palms or soles. It typically is observed after 5 months of age in those with Down syndrome and was reported in 40.8% of children with Down syndrome admitted to a clinical genetics unit (Ercis et al., 1996). A similar picture can occur in a group of diseases (the keratodermas) characterized by a thickened hyperkeratotic stratum corneum of the palms and soles. Diffuse or focal thickening may occur, and palmoplantar hyperkeratosis may or may not be associated with internal features. Many inherited forms of palmoplantar keratoderma exist for which a genetic mutation has been identified (Kelsell & Stevens, 1999). Acquired forms of keratoderma may be associated with internal malignancies.

Pityriasis Alba

Pityriasis alba is hypopigmented to light pink round to oval patches most commonly on the face but also occurring on the upper arms, shoulders, and neck. There is commonly fine adherent scale. Mild pruritus may occur, but it is usually asymptomatic. Two uncommon variants are pigmenting pityriasis alba and extensive pityriasis alba. The etiology is unknown, although it is considered to be a manifestation of atopic dermatitis. It does, however, occur in the absence of atopic dermatitis. Treatment with emollients and low-potency topical steroids is usually helpful. Lesions usually clear with time.

Pityriasis Rubra Pilaris

Pityriasis rubra pilaris is a chronic papulosquamous skin disease characterized by keratoderma (classically smooth and yellow), small follicular papules frequently with a central keratotic plug and yellowish-pink scaling patches. Islands of sparing are classic and represent patches of normal skin within an involved patch or plaque. Scalp erythema and scaling can be an early feature. Over time, large symmetric areas of involvement can occur. The nails may be brittle, thickened, and fragile. Generalized erythroderma and koebnerization may occur. Associated malignancies have included leukemia, Kaposi's sarcoma, lung cancer, unknown primary cancer, and hepatocellular carcinoma. Pityriasis rubra pilaris has also been reported in individuals with HIV who responded to antiretroviral therapy. Whether these are chance findings is unknown. Familial forms and several subtypes have been reported as well (Alpert & Mackool, 1999). Treatments include systemic retinoids and immunosuppressive agents as well as emollients.

Psoriasis

Psoriasis is a chronic papulosquamous skin disease characterized by well-demarcated erythematous plaques with overlying typically "silvery" scale (Gottlieb, 2001; Myers, Opeola, & Gottlieb, 2004). Areas of involvement are classically the elbows, knees, trunk, and gluteal cleft. The genitals may be involved as well. There are several variants including guttate, inverse, and pustular psoriasis. The incidence in Down syndrome has been reported to be 0.5%–8%. The prevalence of psoriasis in the general population is between 1% and 2%. Associated psoriatic arthritis can lead to marked joint destruction.

Therapy depends on the extent of the disease and the impact on the quality of life of the individual. Therapies are categorized as topical therapy, phototherapy, and systemic therapy. Newer agents have recently been developed that include a broad class of agents termed *biologic* that target cytokines, cytokine receptors, and other specific immunologic targets.

Seborrheic Dermatitis

Seborrheic dermatitis is a chronic skin condition characterized by erythema and yellow-brownish scaling (typically described as somewhat greasy) localized in a "seborrheic distribution" (Bolognia et al., 2003; Odom & Berger, 2000). The typical distribution includes the scalp, brows, nasolabial creases, nasal alae, and sternal area. Other regions of involvement may include the postauricular area, axillae, groin, gluteal crease, eyelids, beard area, lips, and umbilicus. Pruritus, if present, is usually mild. Several diseases other than Down syndrome are associated with seborrheic dermatitis including HIV, Parkinson disease, diabetes, sprue, and malabsorption syndromes.

Treatments can control the disease but are usually required chronically (although a few times per week may be enough). Mild topical steroids (e.g., over-the-counter preparations) are a mainstay of therapy, as is topical antifungal therapy (e.g., ketoconazole cream). Steroids should not be used around the eyes, and usage should be tapered to the minimal amount needed to control the disease to avoid adverse effects of the medications. Other options include selenium sulfide lotions or shampoos, tar preparations, and zinc pyrithionate. Newer medications such as topical tacrolimus and pimecrolimus may also be effective (Braza, DiCarlo, Soon, & McCall, 2003).

Syringoma

Syringomas are benign tumors typically seen as skin-colored to yellow-brownish papules around the eyes, especially the lower eyelids and upper cheeks. Eruptive, generalized, and plaque-type variants have been reported. They occur with increased frequency in individuals with Down syndrome (reportedly around 18%) and often appear in adolescence (Barankin & Guenther, 2001; Dourmishev et al., 2000; Ercis et al., 1996; Schepis et al., 2002). Newer lesions can develop during adulthood. Syringomas are thought to be related to eccrine ducts due to their histological appearance. Options for therapy include lasers, cryotherapy, electrodessication, and electrocautery alone or in combination with chemical peeling.

Vitiligo

Vitiligo is caused by the loss of melanocytes characterized clinically by hypo- and depigmented patches. Based on the extent and distribution, different types have been described that include localized/asymmetric (focal or segmental) and generalized (disseminated, universal and acrofacial). The most common type is generalized, and the pattern of involvement is symmetrical. The distribution most commonly involves the face, upper chest, dorsal hands, axillae, and groin. Periorificial sites such as the eyes, nose, mouth, ears, nipples, umbilicus, and genitals are also affected preferentially. The hairs in an affected area can also lose their color. The psychological impact of this disorder can be severe. Treatments include topical steroids, topical calcineurin inhibitors (e.g., tacrolimus), laser therapy, various grafts, and the use of cultured cells.

Xerosis

Xerosis refers to dryness of the skin. It can manifest as patches of fine scale overlying normal skin. When severe, xerosis can lead to nummular eczema in some individuals. Treatment involves the use of emollients that are best applied within 3 minutes of bathing. Creams and ointments are preferred to lotions. Ammonium lactate 12% is a prescription emollient that can be helpful. Humidification of a very dry environment may also help.

CONCLUSION

This chapter explores various dermatological conditions that may affect individuals with developmental disabilities. Because all aspects of these conditions could not be covered, the chapter provides guidance on how to examine dermatological conditions and make diagnoses or, if necessary, seek an experienced opinion. Neurocutaneous lesions, neurocutaneous syndromes, skin lesions, and drug eruptions are discussed as well as specific conditions associated with Down syndrome.

REFERENCES

Albert, M.R., & Mackool, B.T. (1999). Pityriasis rubra pilaris. *International Journal Dermatology, 38*, 1.

Arbiser, J.L., Goldstein, A.M., & Gordon, D. (1993). Thrombocytopenia following administration of phenytoin, dexamethasone and cimetidine: A case report and a potential mechanism. *Journal of Internal Medicine, 234*, 91.

Assimakopoulos, D., Patrikakos, G., Fotika, C., & Elisaf, M. (2002). Benign migratory glossitis or geographic tongue: An enigmatic oral lesion. *American Journal of Medicine, 113*, 751.

Barankin, B., & Guenther, L. (2001). Dermatological manifestations of Down's syndrome. *Journal of Cutaneous Medicine and Surgery, 5*, 289.

Becuwe, C., Roth, B., Villedieu, M.H., Chouvet, B., Kanitakis, J., & Claudy, A. (2004). Milia-like idiopathic calcinosis cutis. *Pediatric Dermatology, 21*, 483.

Bolognia, J.L., Rapini, R.P., Horn, T.D., Mascaro, J.M., Mancini, A.J., Salasche, S.J., et al. (2003). *Dermatology*. St. Louis: Mosby.

Braza, T.J., DiCarlo, J.B., Soon, S.L., & McCall, C.O. (2003). Tacrolimus 0.1% ointment for seborrhoeic dermatitis: An open-label pilot study. *British Journal Dermatology, 148*, 1242.

Brentjens, M.H., Yeung-Yue, K.A., Lee, P.C., & Tyring, S.K. (2003). Vaccines for viral diseases with dermatologic manifestations. *Dermatologic Clinics, 21*, 349.

Brugge, K.L., Grove, G.L., Clopton, P., Grove, M.J., & Piacquadio, D.J. (1993). Evidence for accelerated skin wrinkling among developmentally delayed individuals with Down's syndrome. *Mechanisms of Ageing and Development, 70*, 213.

Chalecka-Franaszek, E., & Chuang, D.M. (1999). Lithium activates the serine/threonine kinase Akt-1 and suppresses glutamate-induced inhibition of Akt-1 activity in neurons. *Proceedings of the National Academy of Sciences of the United States of American, 96*, 8745.

Chan, Y.C., & Friedlander, S.F. (2004). New treatments for tinea capitis. *Current Opinion in Infectious Disease, 17*, 97.

Chouela, E., Abeldano, A., Pellerano, G., & Hernandez, M.I. (2002). Diagnosis and treatment of scabies: A practical guide. *American Journal of Clinical Dermatology, 3*, 9.

Dourmishev, A.L., Dourmishev, L.A. Schwartz, R.A., & Janniger, C.K. (1999). Waardenburg syndrome. *International Journal of Dermatology, 38*, 656.

Dourmishev, A., Miteva, L., Mitev, V., Pramatarov, K., & Schwartz, R.A. (2000). Cutaneous aspects of Down syndrome. *Cutis, 66*, 420.

Eady, E.A., & Cove, J.H. (2003). Staphylococcal resistance revisited: Community-acquired methicillin resistant Staphylococcus aureus—an emerging problem for the management of skin and soft tissue infections. *Current Opinion in Infectious Disease, 16*, 103.

Elewski, B.E. (1998a). Once-weekly fluconazole in the treatment of onychomycosis: Introduction. *Journal of the American Academy of Dermatology, 38*, S73.

Elewski, B.E. (1998b). Onychomycosis: Pathogenesis, diagnosis, and management. *Clinical Microbiology Review, 11*, 415.

Elewski, B.E. (2000). Onychomycosis: Treatment, quality of life, and economic issues. *American Journal of Clinical Dermatology, 1*, 19.

Ercis, M., Balci, S., & Atakan, N. (1996). Dermatological manifestations of 71 Down syndrome children admitted to a clinical genetics unit. *Clinical Genetics, 50*, 317.

Gollnick, H., Cunliffe, W., Berson, D., Dreno, B., Finlay, A., Leyden, J.J., et al. (2003). Management of acne: A report from a Global Alliance to Improve Outcomes in Acne. *Journal of the American Academy of Dermatology, 49*, S1.

Gorlin, R.J. (1995). Nevoid basal cell carcinoma syndrome. *Dermatology Clinics, 13*, 113.

Gottlieb, A.B. (2001). Psoriasis: Immunopathology and immunomodulation. *Dermatologic Clinics, 19*, 649.

Guerra, L., Primavera, G., Raskovic, D., Pellegrini, G., Golisano, O., Bondanza, S., et al. (2004). Permanent repigmentation of piebaldism by erbium: YAG laser and autologous cultured epidermis. *British Journal of Dermatology, 150*, 715.

Hengge, U.R., & Cusini, M. (2003). Topical immunomodulators for the treatment of external genital warts, cutaneous warts and molluscum contagiosum. *British Journal of Dermatology, 149*(Suppl. 66), 15.

Jansen, T., Burgdorf, W.H., & Plewig, G. (1997). Pathogenesis and treatment of acne in childhood. *Pediatric Dermatology, 14*, 17.

Johnson, S.M., Roberson, P.K., & Horn, T.D. (2001). Intralesional injection of mumps or Candida skin test antigens: A novel immunotherapy for warts. *Archives of Dermatology, 137*, 451.

Kelsell, D.P., & Stevens, H.P. (1999). The palmoplantar keratodermas: Much more than palms and soles. *Molecular Medicine Today, 5*, 107.

Kuster, W., & Konig, A. (1999). Hypomelanosis of Ito: No entity, but a cutaneous sign of mosaicism. *American Journal of Medical Genetics, 85*, 346.

Laupland, K.B., & Conly, J.M. (2003). Treatment of *Staphylococcus aureus* colonization and prophylaxis for infection with topical intranasal mupirocin: An evidence-based review. *Clinical Infectious Diseases, 37,* 933.

Munger, K. (2002). The role of human papillomaviruses in human cancers. *Frontiers in Bioscience, 7,* d641.

Myers, W., Opeola, M., & Gottlieb, A.B. (2004). Common clinical features and disease mechanisms of psoriasis and psoriatic arthritis. *Current Rheumatology Reports, 6,* 306.

Nehal, K.S., PeBenito, R., & Orlow, S.J. (1996). Analysis of 54 cases of hypopigmentation and hyperpigmentation along the lines of Blaschko. *Archives of Dermatology, 132,* 1167.

Oberemok, S.S., & Shalita, A.R. (2002). Acne vulgaris: I. Pathogenesis and diagnosis. *Cutis, 70,* 101.

Odom, R.B., & Berger, T.G. (2000). *Andrews' diseases of the skin.* Philadelphia: W.B. Saunders.

Raz, R., Miron, D., Colodner, R., Staler, Z., Samara, Z., & Keness, Y. (1996). A 1-year trial of nasal mupirocin in the prevention of recurrent staphylococcal nasal colonization and skin infection. *Archives of Internal Medicine, 156,* 1109.

Ringel, M.D., Schwindinger, W.F., & Levine, M.A. (1996). Clinical implications of genetic defects in G proteins: The molecular basis of McCune-Albright syndrome and Albright hereditary osteodystrophy. *Medicine (Baltimore), 75,* 171.

Said-Salim, B., Mathema, B., & Kreiswirth, B.N. (2003). Community-acquired methicillin-resistant *Staphylococcus aureus*: An emerging pathogen. *Infection Control and Hospital Epidemiology, 24,* 451.

Sandrini, F., & Stratakis, C. (2003). Clinical and molecular genetics of Carney complex. *Molecular Genetics and Metabolism, 78,* 83.

Sarkozy, A., Conti, E., Digilio, M.C., Marino, B., Morini, E., Pacileo, G., et al. (2004). Clinical and molecular analysis of 30 patients with multiple lentigines LEOPARD syndrome. *Journal of Medical Genetics, 41,* 68.

Scheinfeld, N. (2004). Controlling scabies in institutional settings: A review of medications, treatment models, and implementation. *American Journal of Clinical Dermatology, 5,* 31.

Schepis, C., Barone, C., Siragusa, M., Pettinato, R., & Romano, C. (2002). An updated survey on skin conditions in Down syndrome. *Dermatology, 205,* 234.

Schepis, C., & Romano, C. (1996). Cutaneous findings in the mentally retarded. *International Journal of Dermatology, 35,* 317.

Seebacher, C. (2003). Action mechanisms of modern antifungal agents and resulting problems in the management of onychomycosis. *Mycoses, 46,* 506.

Shah, S.N., Gibbs, S., Upton, C.J., Pickworth, F.E., & Garioch, J.J. (2003). Incontinentia pigmenti associated with cerebral palsy and cerebral leukomalacia: A case report and literature review. *Pediatric Dermatology, 20,* 491.

Smahi, A., Courtois, G., Vabres, P., Yamaoka, S., Heuertz, S., Munnich, A., et al. (2000). Genomic rearrangement in *NEMO* impairs NF-kappaB activation and is a cause of incontinentia pigmenti. The International Incontinentia Pigmenti (IP) Consortium. *Nature, 405,* 466.

Spitz, J.L. (1996). *Genodermatoses.* Philadelphia: Lippincott, Williams and Wilkin.

Stratakis, C.A., Carney, J.A. Lin, J.P., Papanicolaou, D.A., Karl, M., Kastner, D.L., et al. (1996). Carney complex, a familial multiple neoplasia and lentiginosis syndrome: Analysis of 11 kindreds and linkage to the short arm of chromosome 2. *Journal of Clinical Investigation, 97,* 699.

Tyring, S.K. (2000). Human papillomavirus infections: Epidemiology, pathogenesis, and host immune response. *Journal of the American Academy of Dermatology, 43,* S18.

Wendel, K., & Rompalo, A. (2002). Scabies and pediculosis pubis: An update of treatment regimens and general review. *Clinical Infectious Diseases, 35,* S146.

White, G.M. (1998). Recent findings in the epidemiologic evidence, classification, and subtypes of acne vulgaris. *Journal of the American Academy of Dermatology, 39,* S34.

Zeller, A., Schaub, N., Steffen, I., Battegay, E., Hirsch, H.H., & Bircher, A.J. (2003). Drug hypersensitivity syndrome to carbamazepine and human herpes virus 6 infection: Case report and literature review. *Infection, 31,* 254.

zur Hausen, H. (2000). Papillomaviruses causing cancer: Evasion from host–cell control in early events in carcinogenesis. *Journal of the National Cancer Institute, 92,* 690.

Zvulunov, A., & Esterly, N.B. (1995). Neurocutaneous syndromes associated with pigmentary skin lesions. *Journal of the American Academy of Dermatology, 32,* 915.

CHAPTER 21

UROLOGY

Bartley G. Cilento, Jr., and Stuart B. Bauer

This chapter focuses on urologic issues in children with developmental disabilities. Most genitourinary (GU) abnormalities are congenital disorders such as the spinal cord abnormalities (myelodysplasia, sacral agenesis, and spinal dysraphisms). Others are acquired (spinal cord trauma), but the diagnosis, evaluation, and management are similar to congenital disorders. Less serious but more common GU disorders seen in individuals with developmental disabilities, such as enuresis, incontinence, toilet training, and urinary tract infections (UTI), are also discussed. The chapter concludes with a discussion of issues faced in adulthood, such as sexuality, benign prostatic hypertrophy, and renal failure.

CONGENITAL GENITOURINARY AND RENAL ANOMALIES

Although 10% of all newborns have a malformation of the urinary system, only 1% of malformations are significant—remarkably low given the complex nature of the embryologic development of the GU system. GU development involves three embryonic structures: the pronephros, the mesonephros, and the metanephros. The pronephros and mesonephros become vestigial. The metanephros becomes the definitive kidney at 5 weeks of gestation. The collecting system is derived from the ureteral bud of the Wolffian duct that branches as it enters the metanephric tissue, inducing nephron formation.

Teratogenic influences on renal development also affect other organ systems that are developing concurrently. Therefore, many nonrenal malformations are associated with GU tract anomalies. The anomalies listed in Table 21.1 are commonly associated with GU tract abnormalities. Identification of these nonrenal malformations should prompt the clinician to search for associated urologic abnormalities.

The association between otic and renal anomalies is well documented but poorly understood. Individuals with abnormally shaped pinnae have an increased incidence of nonspecific renal abnormalities. Abnormalities in ocular structure are also associated with renal anomalies. A number of syndromes with particular facies, unusual head shape, or palatal clefts have known associated renal anomalies (e.g., Potter syndrome, Fraser syndrome, Meckel syndrome).

Vertebral anomalies are commonly associated with abnormal renal development. The most common example is myelodysplasia, and other anomalies include Goldenhar syndrome, Klippel-Feil syndrome, and Smith-Lemli-Opitz syndrome. One quarter of the individuals with horseshoe kidneys also have vertebral anomalies, and approximately 14% of individuals with unilateral renal agenesis have abnormalities of their vertebrae. Limb abnormalities and abnormally shaped digits, particularly polydactyly or syndactyly, are seen in association with renal anomalies in a number of syndromes, including Rubinstein-Taybi, Robert, and Apert syndromes.

Embryologic development of the heart and kidney occurs simultaneously. Many syndromes involve both congenital heart disease and renal anomalies (e.g., Down syndrome, velo-cardiofacial syndrome, neurofibromatosis). The VATER association (vertebral anomalies, anal atresia, tracheoesophageal fistula, and radial dysplasia) is a good example of the complexity of extra renal involvement that may be found in association with renal anomalies. Another example, the prune belly syndrome, is a triad of inadequately formed abdominal musculature, cryptorchidism, and renal anomalies. Certain female genital anomalies (bifid or septate vagina, didelphia, uni- or bicornate uterus) are frequently associated with unilateral renal agenesis or upper urinary tract abnormalities. Polycystic kidney may be found in association with hepatic or pancreatic cysts.

Some syndromes of chromosomal aberrations also contain known urologic pathology. Examples include Turner syndrome (XO), which is associated with various renal anomalies in 60% of cases; Down syndrome (trisomy 21), in which 7% of individuals have cystic and other renal abnormalities; cat-eye syndrome (extra material from chromosome 22), which is associated with renal agenesis and other anomalies in 60%–100% of individuals; and cri-du-chat syndrome (deletion of short

Table 21-1. Nonrenal anomalies associated with urologic defects

Craniofacial anomalies
Retinal dysplasia
Cataracts
Cryptorchidism
Retinitis pigmentosa
Craniosynostosis
Abnormal pinnae
Middle ear anomalies
Cleft lip/palate
Macroglossia
Dysmorphic facies
Skeletal anomalies
Syndactyly
Polydactyly
Phocomelia
Hemihypertrophy
Spina bifida
Sacral agenesis
Vertebral anomalies
Visceral anomalies
Congenital heart disease
Liver cysts
Pancreatic cysts
Imperforate anus
Female reproductive tract anomalies
Ambiguous genitalia
Tuberous sclerosis
Visceromegaly
Single umbilical artery
Tracheoesophageal fistula
Hirshsprung disease
Absent abdominal musculature with cryptorchidism
Neurofibromatosis
CHARGE association
Small genitalia
Coloboma
Heart defects
Ear anomalies

arm of chromosome 5), which is also associated with various anomalies. Inborn errors of metabolism are not usually associated with anatomic abnormalities; however, they are often associated with intrinsic renal dysfunction (vice structural renal abnormalities). The renal problems associated with these disorders include renal tubular dysfunction, calculi, enlarged kidneys, and aminoaciduria.

Clinical Presentation

With the advent of prenatal ultrasonography, most renal anomalies are now detected prenatally or in early infancy. Findings on a prenatal sonogram that may suggest a urologic problem include oligohydramnios; hydronephrosis; and abnormal size or configuration of the kidney, ureter, or bladder. In infancy, clinical clues include failure to thrive, acidosis, anemia, unexplained dehydration, or an abdominal mass. In childhood, common presentations include episodic abdominal pain, hematuria, UTIs, persistent day and night incontinence, and an abnormal urinary stream. Nevertheless, many renal anomalies are often asymptomatic and may go undiagnosed for long periods of time, sometimes into adolescence or adulthood. Clinical suspicion or any of these common signs should prompt a further evaluation.

Screening and Diagnosis

Laboratory screening of individuals suspected of renal or urinary tract anomalies should include a routine urinalysis, serum electolytes, including urea nitrogen and creatinine, and a urine culture. If chronic renal disease is suspected, the measurement of serum calcium, phosphorous, alkaline phosphatase, hemoglobin, and hematocrit is helpful because hypocalcemia, hyperphosphatemia, hyperphosphatasia, and anemia are common findings in chronic renal disease. These studies indicate the degree of functional renal impairment but not the type of structural anomaly that may be present.

The three most common methods to evaluate anatomic abnormalities are 1) ultrasonography, 2) renal scintigraphy, and 3) voiding cystourethrogram (VCUG). Ultrasonography is noninvasive, is easily available, and provides information about size and location of the kidneys. It can also assess the presence or absence of hydronephrosis or hydroureteronephrosis. Bladder characteristics such as size, shape, and bladder wall thickness can also be assessed. For example, a distended but thick-walled bladder may be an indication of an abnormality of the urethra (i.e., posterior urethral valves or urethral stricture).

The renal scan is a radioisotope imaging technique. The two most common types of renal scintigraphy are the MAG3 (mercaptoacetyltriglycine) Lasix renal scan and the DMSA (dimercaptosuccinic acid) renal scan. The MAG3 Lasix renal scan provides information about renal function from which creatinine clearance can be calculated and the ability of the kidney to drain when stressed. The DMSA scan gives an indication of tubular function but no information regarding drainage. In clinical terms, the DMSA is a cortical imaging agent that detects renal scars and determines percent function of each kidney. The MAG3 Lasix renal scan provides differential percentage function but also is excreted by the kidney and helps to determine the presence or absence of obstruction to urine flow. The renal scan has supplanted the intravenous pyelogram (IVP) as the means of assessing renal function and drainage. Advantages of the renal scan include reduced exposure to radiation and avoidance of a potential allergic reaction to the iodinated contrast material.

The VCUG is used to determine the presence or absence of vesicoureteral reflux (VUR), bladder diverticulae, posterior urethral valves, and possibly voiding dysfunction (spinning top urethra). A simple radiologic procedure, the abdominal flat plate, or KUB, may be helpful in selected instances. For example, medial deviation of the splenic flexure gas pattern is a sign of an absent or malpositioned left kidney. Its most important function may be the appearance of the vertebrae (e.g., spina bifida occulta, sacral agenesis, absent rib). Table 21.2 lists the recommended laboratory and radiologic studies to aid in the diagnosis of suspected renal or urinary tract anomalies.

Management

In many instances, the medical (nonsurgical) management of renal and GU tract anomalies is the first line of treatment. The goal of medical treatment is preservation of renal function and prevention of infection. In some cases, surgery is required to meet these objectives (i.e., correction of VUR). In general, early diagnosis and management provides a greater chance of controlling infection, which will preserve renal function and prevent further complications. Some of the common but less serious urologic problems such as cryptorchidism, hernia, hydrocele, and hypospadias are described in Table 21.3, along with a recommended timetable for surgical repair. Circumcision is described in Table 21.4. Table 21.5 describes the evaluation and management of obstructive uropathies.

Table 21-2. Recommended studies for the evaluation of urologic defects

Urine tests
Routine urinalysis
Urine culture
24-hour collection for creatinine clearance and protein excretion (if earlier studies are abnormal)
Blood tests
Serum electrolytes—sodium, potassium, bicarbonate, chloride
Blood urea nitrogen, creatinine
Calcium, phosphorus, alkaline phosphatase
Hematocrit
Anatomic tests
Renal and bladder ultrasound
Renal scan—MAG3 and/or DMSA
Intravenous pyelogram (if renal scan not readily available)
Roentgenogram of kidney, ureter, and bladder (KUB)
Voiding cystourethrogram (VCUG)

Advances in perinatology and neonatology have made it possible for more newborns with multiple congenital anomalies to survive into infancy, early childhood, and even adulthood with excellent renal function. The goals of long-term management of individuals with urologic anomalies remain unchanged and include preservation of renal function, prevention of infection, and attainment of a socially acceptable lifestyle.

VESICOURETERAL REFLUX

VUR is a common condition that occurs in healthy children and children with developmental anomalies. It is secondary to an abnormally positioned ureter within bladder (detrusor) muscle that results in an incompetent ureterovesical junction, allowing urine to freely reflux from the bladder into the ureter during filling and emptying of the bladder. In fact, 15%–35% of girls with infection have VUR. Although UTI is less common in boys, VUR is found in as many as 50% of boys who are investigated for infection (Belman, 1976). Infants have an almost equal incidence of VUR in boys and girls.

VUR should never be considered a normal phenomenon considering that reflux with infection could have a devastating effect on renal function. Before the availability of diagnostic studies, reflux was the cause of chronic renal failure in one third of individuals undergoing renal transplantation. Today, prompt evaluation in children with any signs of hydronephrosis, UTIs, and known syndromes associated with VUR has dramatically reduced the incidence to chronic renal failure secondary to VUR. Consequently, VUR is being discovered sooner and the sequelae of chronic infection are being prevented.

Grading of Vesicoureteral Reflux

VUR is graded according to its severity. An international classification has been devised with reflux being graded on a scale of I to V, with V being the most severe, and I the least. The grading of VUR allows clinicians to estimate the probability of spontaneous resolution. For example, Grades I and II reflux have an 80%–90% chance of spontaneous resolution during a 3- to 5-year observation period. Grade III has approximately a 50% spontaneous resolution rate during the same period of time. Grade IV has a relatively low

Table 21.3. Urologic problems

Problem	Frequency	Complications	Management
Cryptorchidism	3% in full-term infants 0.7% in 6-month-olds 0.7% in adults 60% of cases are in inguinal canal 22% of cases are prescrotal 8% of cases are intra-abdominal 10% of cases are ectopic	If found in association with hypospadias, 50% chance of abnormal sex chromation Infertility in as many as 70% (histologic changes develop after age 1, increases with age) Commonly associated with hernias Increased incidence of testicular torsion	Orchiopexy between 6–12 months If hypospadias present, do karotype Laparoscopy useful to locate abdominal testes Ultrasounds not helpful in evaluation of nonpalpable testis Voiding cystourethrogram if associated with hypospadias
Hypospadias	0.82% in live male births Less severe forms more common 12% when another family member has hypospadias 26% if brother or father has hypospadias Increased incidence if mother took progestational agents Increased incidence if fetus has abnormality of testosterone, chromosomal abnormalities, or Beckwith-Wiedemann syndrome	Usually associated with chordee If found in association with cryptorchidism, 50% chance of abnormal sex chromation Seen in association with Wilms tumor, aniridia, and hemihypertrophy Ambiquous genitalia	Correct between 5 and 18 months of age If associated with cryptorchidism, do karotype If associated with aniridia and hemihypertrophy, evaluate for Wilms tumor and continue surveillance for Wilms tumor every 6 months until age 10 with renal ultrasonography Voiding cystourethrogram if associated with hypospadias
Hernia and hydrocele	Hernia eight times more frequent in boys than in girls Peak incidence birth to 1 year old	Incarceration of intestines more common in younger children In girls, herniation of ovary or fallopian tube more common than bowel herniation	Consider bilateral exploration in boys to 2 years old and in girls to age 6 Small hydroceles may resolve spontaneously—consider waiting until 6 months of age for repair Weigh risks of incarceration versus risk of anesthesia in deciding appropriate time for surgical repair of hernia

Table 21.4. Circumcision

Incidence and evaluation	Complications	Management
1.5 million operations are performed per year. Medical indications (phimosis, paraphimosis, balanitis) are rare. Adhesions of prepuce occur in 10% of boys 6 years old and less than 1% of postpubertal men. For children with neurogenic bladders who require intermittent catheterization, the family must make a private decision.	The frequency of the following complications is 1%–35%: • Bleeding • Separation of wound • Cyanosis of penis • Injury to glans • Iatrogenic hypospadias or epispadias • Urethral fistula • Lymphedema • Penile loss • Meatal stenosis (8%–30%) • Phimosis (if insufficient skin is removed) • Concealed penis (if too much shaft skin is excised or a child has a very prominent pubic fat pad) • Psychological trauma (if performed in older children)	General anesthesia is required if circumcision is performed on a child older than 2 weeks.

Table 21.5. Obstructive uropathy

Location	Presentation	Diagnosis	Treatment
Ureteropelvic junction	Prenatal—sonogram Newborns—abdominal mass, urinary tract infection Older children—abdominal mass, gastrointestinal symptoms, urinary tract infection, hematuria following mild abdominal trauma, intermittent flank pain with or without vomiting	Excretory urogram Renal sonogram Renal scan (mercaptoacetyltriglycine, or MAG3) to determine renal function and degree of obstruction	Surgically correction of obstruction if 10% renal function is preserved
Ureterovesical junction	Prenatal—hydroureteronephrosis Any age—urinary tract infection May be found in association with distal bladder obstruction or neurogenic bladder	Renal ultrasound and/or excretory urogram, MAG3 renal scan Voiding cystourethrogram/radionucleotide cystogram to rule out vesicoureteral reflux as a cause	Removal of abnormal portion of ureter along with reimplantation Nephroureterectomy rarely necessary (only if function < 10%)
Posterior urethral valves	Prenatal—ultrasound reveals hydronephrosis or thick-walled bladder Newborns—renal failure, electrolyte imbalance, abnormal urinary stream Infants and young children—failure to thrive Older children—incontinence Any age—urinary tract infection	Voiding cystourethrogram Cystoscopy	Transurethral fulguration of valves Urinary diversion in small infants (rarely necessary)
Meatus	Does not usually produce obstructive uropathy Usually see irritative symptoms (frequency, dysuria, dribbling) Found in 10% of circumcised boys	Urinary stream fine, forceful, or deflected Urinary frequency Blood-stained underwear	Meatotomy Possibly urethral dilation

spontaneous resolution rate in the range of 10%–20%. Most children have mild to moderate grades of reflux (I–III) and can be managed with long-term low-dose antibiotic therapy while awaiting spontaneous resolution. It should be noted that the spontaneous resolution rates have not been well studied in children with congenital or developmental abnormalities.

Pathologic Consequences of Vesicoureteral Reflux

Reflux with infection can produce renal parenchymal damage. Inoculation of the kidney papillae with bacteria from the refluxed urine results in colonization. The inflammatory response to this bacterial growth leads to pyelonephritic scarring, papillary damage, and cortical loss. Prophylactic antibiotics should be used to prevent infection while reflux is present. Many parents express concern with long-term antibiotic use, but low-dose prophylactic use has proven to be safe and effective. A prophylactic antibiotic for prevention of infection in reflux is defined as 20%–25% of the normal antibiotic dosing. Higher doses can lead to higher serum levels and potentially induce bacterial resistance of the intestinal bacteria that colonize the perineum. Lower dosing reduces serum concentration of antibiotics, reducing the pressure for the development of bacterial resistance. Because these antibiotics are excreted in the urine, the antibiotic concentrations are sufficient to prevent bacterial colonization of the urinary tract.

Diagnosis

VUR is diagnosed with a voiding cystourethrogram (VCUG) that uses fluoroscopic imaging and should include a voiding phase. Often, reflux will not occur during filling of the bladder but may be seen only during the voiding, illustrating the importance of the voiding phase of the cystogram. It is preferable that all boys and infant girls undergo a VCUG as their initial study whereas older girls with their first UTI may have a radionucleotide cystogram (RNC). The VCUG provides more anatomic detail than the RNC. RNC is being used with increasing frequency for screening for reflux in children with suspected infection, brothers and sisters of children with reflux, and as follow-up for children with a past history of reflux. It is not good, however, for delineating other anatomic conditions associated with reflux, such as bladder diverticulae or posterior urethral valves. Ultrasound and IVP are poor screening tests for reflux because 50% or more individuals with reflux will have a normal study.

Management

All children with one febrile UTI, symptoms of pyelonephritis, or difficulty in clearing their first infection should undergo a radiologic evaluation (renal/bladder ultrasound and VCUG). Once the diagnosis of Grade I, II, or III reflux is established, antibiotic therapy is begun. Children with Grades IV and V are usually surgical candidates. Children with nonfebrile UTIs (cystitis) may be screened with a renal and bladder ultrasound alone. In voiding individuals, infrequent voiding behaviors are the most likely reason for recurrent cystitis, and a careful voiding history is essential. In individuals performing clean intermittent catheterization (CIC), recurrent cystitis is likely secondary to infrequent CIC or incomplete emptying.

Some clinicians advocate that urine cultures be obtained every 3 months; however, others recommend only obtaining urine cultures when there are signs or symptoms of a UTI. Either method is acceptable and should be individualized according to the individual's circumstances and the health care providers' philosophy. Bag specimens are notoriously inaccurate, particularly in girls and non–toilet-trained children. A catheterized urine specimen in babies and pre–toilet-trained infants is the only way to accurately detect an infection. In addition, individuals performing CIC are almost universally colonized with bacteria that exist symbiotically with the individual. Follow-up radionuclide studies are obtained on a yearly basis with renal ultrasound performed periodically to assess renal growth. Indications for antireflux surgery include breakthrough infections despite prophylactic antibiotics, reflux with an anatomic abnormality at the ureterovesical junction (i.e., diverticulum), development or progression of renal parenchymal scarring, poor compliance in taking antibiotics, and persistent reflux.

Surgery

Ureteroneocystostomy (antireflux surgery) involves repositioning of the affected ureter within the bladder in such a way as to create a longer tunnel through the bladder wall to prevent reflux. Various operations have been devised to achieve this result. The ureter can be repositioned somewhat higher in the bladder and advance toward the trigone (Politano-Leadbetter), or the same ureteral hiatus can be maintained with the ureter advanced either across the trigone toward the opposite side (Cohen), or downward toward the bladder neck (Glen-Anderson). In recent years, some surgeons have advocated cystoscopic injection therapy to the ureteral orifice in order to "bulk up" the intramural tunnel and prevent reflux. The cystoscopic injection therapy is a brief outpatient procedure. Polytef paste (Teflon) was first recommended, but its ability to migrate to the lungs and brain has limited its use in children. Other agents such as collagen, chrondrocytes, and fat are reabsorbed and are not good long-term solutions. Hyaluronic acid (Deflux) is now approved by the Food and Drug Administration (FDA) for the treatment of VUR. It has a 70%–80% success rate, but its long-term efficacy remains to be determined.

Postoperatively, all children are maintained on antibiotics for approximately 3–4 months. A renal and bladder ultrasound is obtained 4 weeks following surgery to assess for hydronephrosis. A radionuclide cystogram is performed 4 months after surgery to document resolution of the reflux. Antibiotics are discontinued at this point if the operation has been successful and the individual is reminded to void regularly (every 3 hours). Some children do develop postoperative UTIs (approximately 15% of girls and 1% of boys), but pyelonephritis is unusual (Pope & Rink, 1999). In most instances, postsurgical nonfebrile UTIs are the result of infrequent daytime voiding and/or voiding dysfunction. Postoperatively, continuing to assess the child's voiding habits is important in order to identify this condition and suggest corrective behavioral management.

MYELODYSPLASIA

Historically, renal failure secondary to recurrent pyelonephritis was the leading cause of early death in children with myelodysplasia. With appropriate therapy, much of this deterioration of renal function can be prevented. This section outlines the recommended urologic management of children with myelodysplasia and other spinal defects such as sacral agenesis and spinal dysraphisms (see also Chapter 8.1).

Management

The vast majority of infants born with myelodysplasia undergo surgical repair within 24 and 48 hours of life. Most of these children have normal functioning kidneys. Individuals with a high spinal lesion have a greater incidence of upper urinary tract abnormalities.

The initial workup should include a serum creatinine, urinalysis, urine culture, urodynamic evaluation, renal ultrasonography, and VCUG (Shurtleff, 1980). The VCUG is always done, even with a normal renal ultrasonogram, because significant reflux may be present even with normal renal ultrasound. Prophylactic antibiotics to prevent infection should be started at birth until the VCUG is performed. Prophylaxis can be stopped if there is not evidence of reflux or obstruction. If functional renal assessment is necessary, a renal scan can be performed.

After the neurosurgical repair, trauma to the spinal cord may induce cord shock resulting in urinary retention. This symptom is often temporary (2–6 weeks), and treatment includes CIC. The Crede maneuver to help empty the bladder is controversial when reflux is present because the increased intra-abdominal pressure that results from external palpation of the bladder exacerbates the VUR and may cause renal damage (Shurtleff, 1980). Therefore, CIC is the preferred method of managing urinary retention. After 4–6 weeks, the CIC should be stopped, and the baby should be retested for urine residuals because the spinal cord shock may have resolved.

Bladder management has three main objectives: 1) minimize urine residuals, 2) prevent UTI, and 3) keep the perineal area free of rashes. Urine residuals are minimized by CIC. This method is safe and effective and can be used in either sex at any age (Perez-Marrero, Dimmock, Churchill, & Hardy, 1982). The success of this procedure depends on frequent and regular catheterization to completely empty the bladder. Residuals should be checked every 6 months. A renal ultrasound is recommended every 6 months to monitor renal growth and to detect hydronephrosis.

Repeat urodynamic testing is individualized and depends primarily on the presence or absence of hydronephrosis and recurrent UTIs. In infants, reflux is suspected if hydronephrosis is seen on the renal ultrasound or with recurrent febrile UTIs. The most common presenting sign of reflux in a slightly older child is a febrile UTI. In infants, symptoms include nonspecific fever, vomiting, diarrhea, and failure to thrive. The kidney is most sensitive to injury early in life; therefore, good urologic management beginning at birth is critical to the prevention of renal parenchymal loss.

Amelia is a 27-year-old ambulatory woman with a lumbar 3 level myelodysplasia. She had her back closed in the neonatal period and a ventriculo-peritoneal shunt placed. In infancy, she was found to have left-sided reflux into a duplex collecting system but was followed expectantly at the time with just antibiotics. Because of recurrent UTI, however, she had a left duplicate ureteral reimplantation at age 4, and postoperatively she was started on CIC.

Amelia's reflux was cured, but as she aged, she remained incontinent between catheterizations despite adjunctive therapy with anticholinergic medication. Urodynamic studies at age 11 revealed a good capacity bladder with excellent compliance on oxybutynin. Her urethral sphincter electromyogram revealed complete denervation, and her incontinence was thought to be secondary to low urethral resistance. An artificial urinary sphincter was inserted around her bladder neck at age 13, and, for the first time, she was continent day and night.

Within 2 years following the placement of the sphincter, she developed left hydroureteronephrosis. A repeat cystometrogram exhibited detrusor hypertonicity, which proved to be responsible for the left upper urinary tract dilation. She was started on oxybutynin, which controlled her hypertonicity and improved her hydoureteronephrosis. She remained stable for the next 10 years but has had very close surveillance with frequent urine cultures, periodic renal ultrasounds, and yearly cystometrograms to ensure that her kidneys stay normal and her bladder filling pressures remain low.

Amelia did not let the numerous visits to the Myelodysplasia Program deter her goals. She was a dedicated student and did very well in high school. She attended college and lived away from home. Amelia found college studies stimulating and the social activities rewarding. She is now married and is planning on having a family of her own in the near future.

Vesicoureteral Reflux and Myelodysplasia

Management of reflux in individuals with myelodysplasia is identical to management in individuals with reflux from other causes and has been detailed previously. Intermittent catheterization may be successful in treating reflux in children with myelodysplasia (Bauer, Colodny, & Retik, 1982). When antibiotics and CIC prove ineffective in preventing recurrent UTIs, surgical intervention is necessary. Rarely, a cutaneous vesicostomy (often a temporary measure) is necessary in young babies, in whom it is impractical to perform CIC on a routine basis. Parents usually can perform CIC on their child, especially with appropriate teaching and support. Indications for surgery in older children include recurrent infection, progression of renal scarring, persistent hydronephrosis, a documented anatomic abnormality of the ureterovesical junction, and failure of spontaneous resolution.

Historically, ileal conduit diversion was the therapy of choice for VUR; however, many complications have occurred from this procedure, including recurrent pyelonephritis, nephrolithiasis, renal insufficiency, loop strictures, and stomal stenosis (Crooks & Enrile, 1983; Shurtleff, 1980). These complications occur in as many as 80% of individuals with ileal conduits. Since 1972, when Lapides introduced the concept of CIC, ileal conduits are no longer the recommended therapy for individuals with myelodysplasia. In fact, many individuals whose urinary tracts had been diverted are now considered candidates for undiversion procedures.

Neurogenic Bladder and Myelodysplasia

Neurogenic bladder dysfunction in children with myelodysplasia is varied and complex. The abnormality may involve the nerves to the bladder, the internal and external sphincters, and the spinal cord above the sacral nerve roots. The degree or type of bladder dysfunction cannot be accurately predicted based on the location of the anatomic lesion, which illustrates the need for urodynamic evaluation. Clinically, the two problems are failure to retain urine (caused by hypertonic or uninhibited detrusor contractions, excessive parasympathetic activity, or inadequate sphincter function) and excess urine retention (caused by an adynamic detrusor and/or a spastic or dyssynergic sphincter). Many individuals have an indeterminate picture with mixed degrees of incontinence and retention. Less than 10% of individuals with neurogenic bladder have the ability to voluntarily control bladder or sphincter function and become completely toilet trained.

In most cases, medical management is the first line of therapy, which includes CIC and anticholinergic medicines, such as oxybutynin hydrochloride (Ditropan), tolterodine tartrate (Detrol), and propantheline bromide (Pro-Banthine). These medications increase the bladder capacity and, in conjunction with CIC, can be very effective in achieving continence and reducing UTIs. Children with a neurogenic bladder can do well with CIC alone as long as there is sufficient resistance in the sphincter to allow storage of the urine between each bladder emptying. Sometimes alpha-sympathomimetic drugs (i.e., phenylpropanolamine [Ornade] and ephedrine) are used for increasing resistance to the bladder neck or internal sphincter mechanism, thereby achieving continence.

Failure of medical management usually results in surgical intervention. Ureteral reimplantation, performed to correct the VUR and bladder augmentation, is often necessary to increase bladder storage capacity. As long as the bladder outlet resistance is adequate, increases in bladder capacity result in reduced storage pressures and urinary continence. Various intestinal segments used to augment the bladder include the stomach, small intestine, and colon. In certain circumstances, dilated ureters that service poorly functioning or nonfunctioning renal units can be used to augment the bladder. The ureter is lined with normal nonabsorptive urothelium, whereas intestinal segments are absorptive, resulting in electrolyte disturbances that must be carefully managed. Some bladder augmentations can be performed by way of minimally invasive surgical techniques involving laparoscopic surgery (Cilento et al., 2003). More recently, tissue engineered autologous bladder augmentation techniques have been developed and hold promise for the future.

Another huge advancement in the care of these individuals involves the creation of a catheterizable continent stoma. Many individuals with disabilities are unable to perform CIC via the native urethra due to positional restrictions, manual dexterity, or social issues. In addition, urethral incontinence may be persistent despite CIC and anticholinergic therapy. In these situations, the appendix or a tapered segment of intestine can be used to create a catheterizable channel from the bladder to the anterior abdominal wall. The preferred site on the abdominal wall is the umbilicus, which provides an excellent cosmetic appearance. If urethral resistance is very low, a fascial sling around the bladder neck, an artificial urinary sphincter, or closure of the bladder neck may be necessary.

Incontinence and Myelodysplasia

Starting at preschool age, bowel and bladder continence becomes increasingly important from a social perspective. Urodynamic evaluation is important to help individualize management. Most children use a combination of CIC and medications. Five- to seven-year-old children can master CIC as long as they have free use of their hands, can maintain an appropriate position, and have mature adaptive skills. The Crede or Valsalva maneuvers have been used if the child can empty the bladder in this manner (Barrett & Furlow, 1982; Shurtleff, 1980). Failure of these techniques usually results in surgical intervention.

If there is some reactivity in the external sphincter, the bladder neck can be reconstructed to improve urethral resistance and prevent leakage of urine. If the external sphincter is completely denervated and the urethral resistance is low, an artificial urinary sphincter or fascial sling can used to achieve continence. Bulking agents to increase bladder outlet resistance have been used, but no good sustainable agent has been identified.

If CIC and medication fail and bladder capacity is inadequate, bladder augmentation with a segment of bowel may be necessary. These operations are usually combined with medications and CIC to achieve continence and complete bladder emptying. Panty-liner inserts are available for children with constant dribbling (seen with low outlet resistance, a hypertonic detrusor muscle, or uninhibited detrusor contractions). As children become teenagers, they may prefer a continent catheterizable abdominal wall stoma for bladder emptying rather than urethral catheterization. The convenience and ease of the abdominal stoma may also lead to increased compliance with routine CIC. In individuals who are wheelchair bound, ease of emptying makes this procedure an attractive option.

Fecal continence is also important but difficult to manage. The continent fecal stoma (MACE or Malone Antegrade Continent Enema) has come into vogue. A catheterizable conduit from the abdominal wall to the cecum can be fashioned from the appendix or a small segment of intestine. It can then be used to instill an enema solution (saline, tap water, Golytely) every other day into the cecum to initiate complete colonic emptying within half an hour and fecal continence for up to 48 hours.

SACRAL AGENESIS AND SPINAL DYSRAPHISM

The urologic problems in sacral agenesis are similar to myelodysplasia—namely, neurogenic bladder. A neurogenic bladder is usually present if sacral nerves 2–4 are involved. Fortunately, sacral agenesis is rare. It occurs in 1% of infants of insulin-dependent diabetic mothers. Other anomalies are associated with sacral agenesis, such as orthopedic deformities, imperforate anus, renal ectopia, and renal agenesis.

Physical findings suggestive of sacral agenesis include a shortened gluteal cleft and flattened buttocks. The diagnosis is commonly missed because innervation of the lower extremities and sacral area is not affected and the gait is normal. Delay of diagnosis until the age of 3, when the child comes to medical attention because of delays in toilet training, is not uncommon.

The recommended diagnostic workup for suspected sacral agenesis is listed in Table 21.6. In addition to the roentgenograms of the spine, a workup for associated renal anomalies, a urodynamic assessment of the bladder function, a complete neurologic examination, and evaluation of the gait are advised. An MRI of the spine will demonstrate a sharp, abrupt cutoff to the spinal cord at T-12 with individual nerve roots streaking distally. The neurologic level has little correlation with the vertebral bony defect, particularly if the lesion was below S2 (Bauer et al., 1980). Motor roots are affected more often than sensory afferents (70% of individuals with normal sensation). The VCUG is always abnormal, ranging from the absence of the sacral spine to failure of emptying. Management of individuals with sacral agenesis is similar to that for the child with myelodysplasia, including CIC, pharmacologic (anticholinergic) agents, an artificial urinary sphincter, or bladder augmentation as dictated by the urodynamic findings or the initial response to therapy.

Table 21-6. Recommended diagnostic workup for sacral agenesis

Lateral and anteroposterior spine films
Intravenous pyelogram or renal/bladder ultrasound
Voiding cystourethrogram
Urodynamic studies (cystometrogram, urethral pressure profile, electromyogram of external urethral sphincter)
Neurologic examination
Spinal ultrasonography if child is younger than 3 months
Magnetic resonance imaging of spine for children diagnosed at an older age

Spinal dysraphism refers to a group of abnormalities of the caudal end of the spinal cord, including diastematomyelia (sagittal splitting of the spinal cord from an intervertebral bony spur or fibrous band), lipoma, dermoid cyst or sinus, aberrant spinal roots, and fibrous tethering of the conus medullaris or filum terminale. These lesions are grouped together because they produce a similar urologic and neurologic picture.

Children with spinal dysraphism may present with gait disturbances (usually broad-based), abnormalities of the lower extremities, a skin lesion overlying the midline lumbosacral area, and urinary or fecal incontinence. The individual may experience pain and/or numbness radiating down the lower extremities, particularly after awakening. Deformities of the lower extremities include high-arched feet, clawing of the toes, and leg length or muscle mass discrepancies. Cutaneous lesions overlying the spinal cord abnormality are seen in 75% of individuals with spinal dysraphism. The two most common lesions are hypertrichosis (hairy patch) and hyperpigmentation (Gusman et al., 1983), or vascular malformation. Lipomas, or skin dimples, are also presenting signs.

Twenty to forty percent of children with spinal dysraphism develop neurogenic bladder dysfunction. Lower urinary tract dysfunction caused by spinal dysraphism commonly presents with continuous dribbling during infancy, day and night incontinence in the older child, and/or UTI. Signs and symptoms are sometimes not evident until puberty, when a growth spurt accentuates tethering of the spinal cord. The type of neurologic picture that develops clinically is variable and depends on which nerve roots and/or segments of the spinal cord are involved. Therefore, each child should have a complete urodynamic evaluation so that the therapeutic intervention can be individualized.

ENURESIS

Nocturnal enuresis is defined as an episode of voiding that occurs during sleep. Children between the ages of 3 and 10 years who have no other overt neurologic or structural urologic abnormality have *primary nocturnal enuresis.* Urinary incontinence, in contrast, occurs in the setting of urinary tract or neurologic pathology.

In infants, the bladder functions automatically. When it is filled to capacity (usually about 2 ounces), the stretch reflex activates a detrusor contraction, forcing a stream of urine that fully empties the bladder. An infant does not appreciate bladder fullness and can neither voluntarily stop nor start voiding. With maturation of the central nervous system, a toddler gradually becomes aware of the active voiding and the sensation of bladder fullness. A child of 2–2½ also develops the ability to hold urine for brief periods of time and acquires the verbal ability to communicate the need to void. A 2-year-old still may not be able to voluntarily initiate voiding or to void if the bladder is not full. By age 2½–3, a normal child has the motor skills to independently get to the lavatory and remove clothing in order to urinate.

By age 3, most children have control over the levator ani and other pelvic muscles to allow postponement of voiding and to limit the number of voids to 6–8 per 24 hours. Bladder capacity also increases during this time. By age of 3, most children can achieve daytime dryness. Nocturnal dryness occurs later, usually by 3–4 years. Some time between ages 3–6, children learn to contract the diaphragm and abdominal muscles while simultaneously relaxing those of the pelvic floor, to voluntarily initiate voiding at varying degrees of bladder filling. Children at 4–5 years also learn that they can voluntarily stop the urinary stream by contracting the levator ani muscles.

Classification and Etiology

The first distinction of enuresis is between primary enuresis, when a child has never achieved bladder control, and secondary enuresis, when a child has been dry for a prolonged period of time and then resumes wetting. Another distinction refers to what time the enuresis occurs: diurnal involves daytime wetting, and nocturnal involves nighttime wetting. The vast majority of children with enuresis (about 85%), have primary nocturnal enuresis. Encopresis is an associated problem in about 10%–25% of children with enuresis. The majority of children with enuresis are boys (ratio of 3:2).

Many hypotheses attempt to explain the etiology of enuresis. Some consider that environmental factors play a major role because there is an increased incidence of enuresis in children from broken homes and lower socioeconomic status groups. A genetic component, most likely autosomal dominant with a fairly high penetrance, exists because 1) there is an increased incidence of enuresis in monozygotic versus fraternal twins and 2) children have a much higher likelihood of being enuretics if either one or both parents were enuretic. Recent investigation has attempted to locate the genetic locus, and there appears to be three candidate genes. Some investigators think that enuresis occurs as a result of a disorder of arousal in the normal sleep cycle (Stage IV). Others think that psychologic factors play a major role, particularly in children with known emotional disturbances. In addition, a small number of children develop a decreased bladder capacity after eating certain foods (i.e., caffeine), and their enuresis improves when these foods are withheld from the diet.

The most accepted hypothesis to explain enuresis suggests that it is caused by delay in the maturation of the central nervous system. Evidence to support this hypothesis includes the persistence of an infantile pattern on the cystogram (uninhibited bladder contractions or reduced functional capacity) in about half of individuals with enuresis. Other authors cite an increased incidence of delays in other developmental processes such as walking, cognitive function, and fine motor coordination. A small functional bladder capacity results in an increased diurnal frequency and urgency commonly seen in children with nocturnal enuresis. Finally, there is an increased incidence of minor abnormalities in the electroencephalograms of children with enuresis, which is thought to be another manifestation of the immaturity of the central nervous system.

Another hypothesis involves the decreased nocturnal secretion of the naturally occurring vasopressin from the posterior pituitary, with the result being an inappropriate polyuria during sleep. In this fashion, synthetic vasopressin (DDAVP) was developed in order to supplement this decreased nocturnal secretion. A certain subset of children with enuresis will respond to this medication therapy. In all likelihood, the etiology is multifactorial. Fortunately, primary nocturnal enuresis is a self-limited condition.

Clinical Evaluation

The clinical evaluation of enuresis is not standard and is controversial. In otherwise healthy children with normal daytime voiding patterns and primary nocturnal enuresis, evidence can be found to support no further evaluation beyond a history and physical examination. Others feel that, in addition to history and physical examination, several laboratory studies are necessary. The history helps to differentiate primary from secondary, and diurnal from nocturnal enuresis. In the history, clinicians should elicit prenatal factors, developmental issues, symptoms of UTI, disorders of sleep, relationships to certain foods, or history of recent emotional stress. The family history is significant because the likelihood of enuresis increases from 15% if neither parent was enuretic to 44% if one parent was enuretic and to 77% if both parents were enuretic.

The physical examination includes an abdominal palpation to rule out a mass (i.e., hydronephrosis, hydroureter, large bladder), a genital examination to rule out genital anomalies (i.e. meatal stenosis, subsymphyseal epispadias), and possibly a rectal examination to rule out a pelvic mass, assess rectal tone and sensation, and check for evidence of chronic constipation. A neurologic examination, including examination and palpation of the lower spine, is important to rule out occult vertebral anomalies or sacral agenesis. Neurologic examination should also include assessment of perineal sensation, high-arched feet, hyperactive lower-extremity deep tendon reflexes, and discrepancy in the muscle mass and leg length.

Laboratory Evaluation

The initial laboratory examination includes a urine culture as well as a urinalysis. No further workup is necessary if the physical examination is normal, the urinary stream and urinalysis are normal, the urine culture is negative, and particularly if the family history is positive. Further evaluation is indicated for a history of abnormal urinary stream, diurnal incontinence, an abnormal physical examination, or a diagnosis of UTI. Organic causes of nocturnal enuresis are rare. Urinary tract lesions are found in 2%–10% of individuals with nocturnal enuresis. Bladder outlet obstruction is also rare. If a further evaluation is indicated, the workup should include an IVP or a renal and bladder ultrasound and a VCUG.

Management

Many remedies for enuresis have been tried, with varying rates of success. Some methods, such as psychotherapy for children with known emotional problems and dietary therapy (eliminating foods such as eggs, chocolate, and colas or other caffeinated beverages) are only useful in certain children. More generalized treatments include conditioning techniques, medication, behavioral modification, and urodynamic biofeedback approaches. These techniques are all based on the presumption that the person with enuresis has normal anatomy, physiology, and cognitive and motor abilities.

"Conditioning therapy" and "nonbiofeedback biobehavioral management" are the terms used for the approach in which behavioral modification techniques are used in conjunction with an alarm system. The alarm is a sensing apparatus or pad that is placed either in the bed or inside the child's underpants. It is activated by moisture voiding, to set off a bell, light, buzzer, music, or a combination. Ideally, the alarm wakes the child, who turns it off, finishes voiding in the bathroom, and then returns to bed. This method can be somewhat cumbersome and requires cooperation and motivation on the part of the child and his or her family. The average duration of the treatment is long, 8–10 weeks, as reported by some clinicians, and 16–17 weeks by others. The cure rate is 75%–80%; almost twice as good as imipramine, and the relapse rate of 25%–30% is much lower than imipramine.

Drug therapy is useful in some instances. Imipramine, a tricyclic antidepressant, is a drug that was once commonly used but not any longer. Its mechanism of action is poorly understood, although it has anticholinergic activity, antihistamine activity, and antiserotonin and central nervous system effects. The dosage is 0.9–1.5 mg/kg/day, which usually works out to be 25 mg. for 5- to 8-year-olds and 50 mg for older children given once a day at bedtime. About one half of children with enuresis are cured with Imipramine, and another 10%–20% experience improvement. The relapse rate is very high, with about two thirds resuming wetting once the medicine is stopped. There are also many known side effects, including sleep disorders, personality changes, dry mouth, and gastrointestinal symptoms.

In addition, high-dose tricyclic antidepressants can produce cardiac conduction delay abnormalities.

Other tricyclic antidepressants have an effect similar to Imipramine and can be tried if Imipramine fails. Currently, the only FDA-approved medication for the use of nighttime wetting is DDAVP. DDAVP is now the most common medicine used for enuresis. It comes in a tablet form of 0.2 mg. per tablet. The usual dose is titrated from one to three tablets depending on the effect. A few side effects occur with DDAVP, such as headache or dizziness. In very rare instances, hyponatremia may be a side effect in children who are allowed unrestricted and free access to water. There is no consensus as to appropriate duration in therapy, but a trial of 6–8 weeks is usually initiated. Other drugs, such as oxybutynin hydrochloride (Ditropan), tolterodine tartrate (Detrol), and flavoxate hydrochloride (Urispas), alone or in combination with imipramine, have been used with reasonable rates of success when single drug therapy fails.

Behavioral modification techniques include *responsibility reinforcement* (rewarding dryness with prizes or working toward a desired goal) and *bladder training* (keeping a daily log of voided volumes, forcing fluids, and gradually increasing the time interval between voids). These techniques are the treatments of choice for enuresis because they can be implemented by the pediatrician and are effective about 80% of the time. The relapse rate is about 20%.

An individual with disabilities may have cognitive, neurologic, physical, or emotional limitations that preclude development of bladder control. For example, a person with intellectual disabilities or a language disorder may not have the verbal ability to communicate his or her needs, may lack the neurologic maturity to appreciate or control his or her body signals, or may have a neurological impairment (e.g., myelodysplasia) that prevents normal bladder function. A person with cerebral palsy may not have the mobility to get to the lavatory or to remove his or her clothing independently. Because enuresis and encopresis are both common manifestations of emotional disturbance in children, clinicians should consider not only the common causes of enuresis but also each person's limitations when evaluating abnormal maturation in an individual with disabilities.

INCONTINENCE

Individuals with physical disabilities that preclude toilet training present a special challenge. These individuals have incontinence rather than enuresis. Incontinence may be associated with obstruction (posterior urethral valves, urethral stricture, sphincter dysfunction, or prostatic enlargement), retention (secondary to a neuromuscular disease such as meningomyelocele, transverse myelitis, or spinal cord trauma), or both. The incontinence may be congenital or acquired, total or partial, continuous or intermittent.

Evaluation of incontinence includes the same history, physical examination, and laboratory studies as for enuresis. In addition to the IVP or VCUG, further surgical evaluation may include a cystourethroscopy. In nearly all cases, urodynamic studies are indicated. Parameters that current urodynamic studies can evaluate include uroflowmetry (measures urine flow rate and voided volume), cystometry, urethral pressure profilometry, and external urethral sphincter electromyography. These studies may be needed to precisely define the neuromuscular abnormality.

Achieving continence is possible in some individuals with an organic lesion, especially with the advent of new urodynamic biofeedback techniques. These techniques consist of monitoring detrusor pressure or external urethra sphincter activity using a visual or auditory feedback mechanism in conjunction with behavioral modification. Biofeedback techniques were first used primarily in individuals with "nonneurogenic bladder," or bladder–sphincter dysfunction, despite normal neurologic function. Biofeedback techniques have been successful in individuals with normal anatomy and physiology whose enuresis was refractory to the usual behavioral approaches and pharmacologic agents. A new hope for the future is the recent use of urodynamic biofeedback techniques in individuals with spinal cord trauma, sacral agenesis, and meningomyelocele. Some of these children have actually achieved continence despite neurologic pathology. A few investigators have employed botulin toxin (Botox) to paralyze the sphincter and improve emptying, but long-term results are not available.

Kwan is an 18-year-old boy with a sacral 1 level myelodysplasia whose back was closed and a ventriculo-peritoneal shunt placed within his first day of life. A urodynamic study in the neonatal period revealed a hypertonic and hyperreflexic bladder with normal sphincter electromyogram activity and normal sacral reflexes but bladder sphincter dyssynergy when his bladder contracted at capacity. Kwan was started on prophylactic CIC and oxybutynin to prevent VUR and upper urinary tract deterioration.

Kwan's bladder responded only partially, eventually leading to left VUR and hydronephrosis. Kwan required frequent catheterizations, about every 2 hours, to stay reasonably dry during the day. He was incontinent at night and had recurrent UTIs that lead to a successful left ureteral reimplantation performed when he was 8 years of age. Kwan's bladder-filling pressure continued to stay elevated despite increasing doses of anticholinergic medication, and he could not maintain his continence. His serum creatinine gradually increased to 1.5 mg/dl.

At age 12, Kwan underwent bladder augmentation with a segment of stomach to increase his bladder capacity, reduce his hydronephrosis, and achieve continence. This surgery was technically successful and achieved all of its objectives. Throughout high school, however, Kwan had occasional episodes of gross hematuria and lower abdominal pain, which are known complications of gastric augmentation. He was admitted to the hospital three times with hyponatriemic acidosis secondary to his gastroenteritis.

Kwan understands his suspectiblity to sensitive electrolyte balance during episodes of vomiting or diarrhea and is quick to seek appropriate care. He has a dry sense of humor and is accepting of his medical condition. After graduating from high school, he applied and was accepted to a local community college, where he continues to excel. He has found college life rewarding and enjoys most of the social activities associated with it.

URINARY TRACT INFECTIONS

UTIs are a common urologic problem, especially in individuals with developmental disabilities. One recent study has shown that residents of a state institution for individuals with intellectual disabilities had a 14% incidence of UTI, which is almost three times greater than the 5% incidence sited in the general adult population. Several anatomic and nonanatomic explanations exist for this observation. Anatomic abnormalities that lead to incomplete emptying or bacterial colonization include neurogenic bladder, VUR, urethral stricture, benign prostatic hypertrophy, and an indwelling urethral catheter. Nonanatomic conditions include voiding dysfunction, hormonal influences, chronic constipation, intellectual disabilities with poor perineal hygiene, and chronic vaginitis.

A UTI is defined by a positive urine culture with equal to or greater than 100,000 colonies per milliliter of a single organism. The most accurate method of obtaining a culture specimen is urethral catheterization. The alternate method is a clean catch midstream urine specimen, but this method may not be possible in many individuals with developmental disabilities. As mentioned previously, bagged urine specimens are notoriously unreliable.

A number of symptoms related to UTI vary with the age of the individual. Small infants and young children may have a fever, vomiting, diarrhea, and/or failure to thrive. Preschoolers often have fever, enuresis, and abdominal pain. A period of increased frequency, increased urgency, urinary incontinence (especially at night), and dysuria is often only seen in older children and adults who develop a UTI.

The most common organism is *Escherichia coli*, a common fecal resident that ascends into the urinary tract via the urethra. Hematogenous spread of bacteria causing UTI is usually seen only in neonates. Other urinary tract pathogens include *Klebsiella*, *Enterococcus*, *Salmonella*, *Proteus mirabilis*, *Staphylococcus* (especially in boys), *Haemophilus influenza*, and *Pseudomonas*.

Associated Factors

Factors thought to contribute to the development of UTI include anatomic abnormalities, abnormal voiding patterns (i.e., overt or occult neurogenic bladder dysfunction), hormonal influences (i.e., pregnancy, birth control pills), VUR, urinary tract obstruction, and trauma (i.e., foreign body, sexual intercourse, or sexual abuse). Many of these factors exist in the individuals with disabilities and contribute to the higher incidence of UTIs than the general population. Examples include inadequate perineal and perianal hygiene, chronic constipation (thought to cause a functional obstruction to the urine flow as well as increasing the potential for swelling and feeding the lower urinary tract with fecal bacteria), abnormal voiding patterns, and the increasing predisposition to infectious diseases inherent in a residential setting.

Individuals with cerebral palsy severe enough to have developed joint contractures of the hip are at particular risk for poor perineal hygiene, chronic vaginitis, and recurrent UTIs. Individuals who require an indwelling catheter are also at extremely high risk because bacterial colonization of the catheter is inevitable. Other predisposing factors include benign prostatic hypertrophy in older men and postsurgical instrumentation.

Prostatitis has been shown to be a cause of recurrent UTI in men and boys. It may not respond to a customary 10-day course of antibiotics and can cause chronic feeding of the bladder with bacteria if not treated for a prolonged period (3–4 months) with antibiotics (Bactrim or ciprofloxacin). Antibiotics alone may not be effective in controlling infection. Other measures are also important, including vigorous measures to control constipation, improvement of perineal hygiene, and local treatment of chronic vaginitis. Decreasing urinary retention by increasing voiding frequency, improving toilet practices, or increasing the frequency of CIC is an important strategy. Physical therapy is important in individuals with cerebral palsy because tight hip adductors reduce good perineal hygiene technique. Some orthopedists have even recommended surgical procedures to release contracted hips in order to improve perineal care and help prevent UTI.

Diagnosis

In individuals with disabilities, a UTI must be suspected because the symptoms may be subtle. Nonspecific symptoms are common, particularly in young children, or insidious in adults who are nonverbal, nonambulatory, and incontinent—fever, anorexia, or a change in urine odor or color. The urine culture will provide the diagnosis. In older individuals who are able to provide a "clean catch" midstream specimen, this sample may be appropriate. In young children, bladder catheterization is recommended. Suprapubic aspiration is rarely necessary. Urine from a bagged collection is easily and rapidly contaminated and is the less-desirable method. If a urine culture from a bagged specimen is negative, however, it is usually significant, indicating the absence of infection. In older individuals who cannot provide a clean catch urine, catheterization using sterile technique is the method of choice.

A urinalysis is important because the presence of leukocytes, nitrites, red blood cells, and bacteruria suggest that an infection is present. Several assays have been developed to detect bacteruria and to localize the infection to the upper or lower urinary tract. These methods include Uricult slides, nitrite indicator strips, antibody-coded bacteria, sedimentation rate, C-reactive protein, LDH isoenzyme, and antibodies against Tamm-Horsfall protein. The Uricult slides are particularly useful in following a child with an anatomic abnormality because the parents can screen the urine at home with this inexpensive test, and any growth can be sent for analysis. The other tests are not completely reliable, and some are not easily obtainable. The urine culture remains the one absolute indicator for UTI.

Management

Antibiotic treatment depends on the sensitivity of the infecting organism. A complete and comprehensive review of all antibiotics available to treat uncomplicated and complicated UTIs is beyond the scope of this chapter. Traditionally, ampicillin (Omnipen), sulfamethoxazole (Gantrisin), trimethoprim sulfamethoxazole (Bactrim), and nitrofurantin (Macrodantin) are the usual drugs of choice for the uncomplicated infection. More current choices include amoxicillin (Amoxil) and other cephalosporins. In the case of recurrent infections, organisms resistant to ampicillin are often the pathogens. Medications such as Bactrim, nitrofurantoin, carbenicillin (Geopen), and tetracycline are used. In addition, ciprofloxacin (Cipro) has also been used with increasing frequency.

Ciprofloxacin is commonly used in adults and is now commonly administered to children with good safety and efficacy. The pediatric dosing of ciprofloxacin is 10–15 mg/kg/day. The new aminoglycosides are very effective against gram-negative organisms, but they must be used parentally, and doses must be modified in individuals with renal insufficiency.

Single-day dosing of aminoglycosides provides better bacterial kill and less renal toxicity due to lower trough levels. When nephrotoxicity is a concern, antibiotics such as piperacillin/tazobactam (Zosyn) and aztreonam (Azactam) can be used. The usual course of therapy is 7–10 days, although a single dose has been shown to be effective in some adult studies. In individuals with disabilities, however, the incidence of anomalies and other predisposing factors is so high (45% in one recent study) that a full 10-day course is recommended (Kunin, 1981). A repeat urine culture after 72 hours of treatment is recommended to establish the efficacy of therapy. Follow-up cultures are also recommended, and they should be obtained 3–4 days after completing therapy.

Any neonate who develops a UTI should be treated with parenteral ampicillin and gentamicin pending culture results. Neonates with UTIs should have a full urologic evaluation including a VCUG and renal/bladder ultrasound. Men and boys with one UTI or women and girls with recurrent infections deserve a workup.

ISSUES IN ADULTHOOD

Sexuality

Sexuality is an important and often an overlooked issue for individuals with developmental disabilities. It is important to address issues of sexuality with growing children as well as with parents, who are sure to be concerned but often not willing to address the issues without prompting. In girls with myelodysplasia, menarche often occurs early (8–10 years of age), and fertility is possible. Girls can be normal sexual partners, but there are some risks during pregnancy, including UTI, hydronephrosis, worsening urinary tract pathology, back pain, disk herniation, premature delivery, and even loss of neuromuscular function. The risk of having an infant with myelodysplasia is 5% and is the same for men and women (Bauer, 1984; Shurtleff, 1980). Serum alpha-fetoprotein (AFP) determination between the sixteenth and nineteenth weeks of gestation has a high rate of detection of myelodysplasia. Individuals must decide for themselves if they would like to have AFP determination.

Men have more complex issues (Bauer, 1984; Shurtleff, 1980). Fertility rates among men and boys with myelodysplasia is decreased secondary to neurologic injury affecting potency and ejaculation, chronic UTIs, mechanical trauma to the urethra, and testicular hypoplasia (in conjunction with cryptorchidism). Some boys can achieve erections, but sometimes not until puberty. About 30% can ejaculate, but usually in a retrograde fashion into the bladder due to bladder neck dysfunction. If the sperm can be recovered from the bladder, the wife of an individual with meningomyelocele can be artificially inseminated. The psychological issues for boys are more problematic, because of an altered body image and low self-esteem. Physicians should be supportive during these difficult teenage years or even arrange for psychological or psychiatric support.

Benign Prostatic Hypertrophy

Enlargement of the prostate is a common problem in men older than 50 years of age. It is rarely present in men younger than 50, but its prevalence increases steadily with age. By the time they are 80, most men have some signs of obstruction. Its inception is insidious, with minimal symptoms that progress slowly until one day an individual realizes his voiding characteristics have changed. In individuals with disabilities, this condition may not become apparent until an obvious sign occurs, such as urinary incontinence, urinary infection, hematuria, or retention.

Symptoms include frequency, urgency, nocturia, hesitancy, decrease in stream size, force, straining to void, postvoid dribbling, hematuria, and urinary infection. Acute urinary retention is a rather late manifestation of the disease. On physical exam, the size of prostate on rectal examination is a poor predictor of the degree of obstruction. A large intravesical component of the gland can never be appreciated by rectal palpation and is only evidenced by ultrasonography or cystoscopic visualization of the bladder and posterior urethra. Measurement of urinary flow rate and postvoid residual urine are important objective tests to assess the degree of obstruction. An excretory urogram or renal ultrasound should be obtained in every individual suspected of having BPH to assess its effect, if any, on the upper urinary tract.

Medical management is usually the first line of therapy, and surgery is usually indicated with failure of medical management. Today, most operations are performed transurethrally to remove the hyperplastic elements of the prostate gland. The open (suprapubic or retropubic) approach is reserved for men with excessively large prostates (Fitzpatrick & Mebust, 2002).

Renal Failure

Renal failure may be the endpoint of many of the conditions mentioned previously in this chapter, including congenital anomalies, VUR, and recurrent UTI. Renal failure can be acute or chronic. Acute renal failure is caused by 1) decreased glomerular filtration (e.g., dehydration, hypertension), 2) injury to renal parenchyma (e.g., nephrotoxic drugs, acute tubular necrosis), and 3) obstructive uropathy (much more common in adults than children). Depending on the etiology, acute renal failure may be reversible, particularly in children. Chronic renal failure, in contrast, is usually progressive and leads to end-stage renal disease.

A helpful mnemonic for remembering the causes of renal failure is *VITAMIN C*. The *V* is for vascular causes, *I* for infection (e.g., chronic pyelonephritis), *T* for traumatic, *A* for allergic, *M* for metabolic, *I* for iatrogenic, *N* for neoplastic, and *C* for congenital etiologies (Urizer, Largent, & Gilboa, 1983). The five most common causes of chronic renal failure (CRF) in children include glomerular disease, obstructive uropathy occurring prenatally, renal hypoplasia, hereditary nephropathies, and vascular nephropathies (Gauthier, Edelmann, & Barnett, 1982). The prevalence of an obstructive uropathy (e.g., secondary to myelodysplasia or a congenital anomaly and renal hyperplasia) is greater in individuals with disabilities than in the general population; thus, these conditions are likely to be a cause of renal failure in individuals with disabilities (Shurtleff, 1980).

Renal failure presents with two main features: oliguria and azotemia. Other important signs include seizures, hyperkalemia, acidosis, hypertension, hyponatremia, hyperuricemia, hypokalemia, and altered mental status. Some of the clinical features of renal failure deserve special mention in reference to children with physical and cognitive disabilities. The first of these is growth failure. Growth deficiency is thought to be secondary to deficient caloric intake, acidosis, vitamin D deficiency, and low levels of somatomedin. Children with developmental disabilities often have feeding difficulties that contribute to caloric deficiency, and they may have little exposure to sunlight, which contributes to vitamin D deficiency. Second, children with renal insufficiency tend to have delayed sexual development. This symptom is also commonly seen in individuals with disabilities who are malnourished.

The psychosocial impact of renal failure on individuals is significant. Individuals may have problems coping with the chronic nature of their disease, the painful medical procedures, frequent hospitalizations, dietary restrictions, and dependency on dialysis. Individuals with anatomic urologic abnormalities may find that the frequent surgical and medical focus on the genital area may be upsetting and invasive. The medical management of renal failure is the same for any individual regardless of the presence of a disability. It involves correcting the chemical abnormalities, normalizing fluid status, controlling neurologic complications, and treating hypertension.

Because chronic renal failure is a progressive disease, the final outcome is end-stage renal disease. Once end-stage renal disease is present, there are two options available to support life—dialysis and transplantation. Dialysis can be hemodialysis or peritoneal. Hemodialysis may be difficult to perform in small children because it requires vascular access, which is created surgically via a subcutaneous arteriovenous fistula (A-V), a synthetic A-V graft, or an external A-V shunt. Peritoneal dialysis is another alternative that is useful in small infants because no vascular access is necessary. The major advantage of peritoneal dialysis is the potential for performing continuous ambulatory peritoneal dialysis (CAPD) through permanent peritoneal catheters. Parents and patients can be taught to perform daily CAPD at home. Recurrent peritonitis is the major risk of indwelling peritoneal catheters.

Renal transplantation is the other alternative. Organs are obtained either from living related donors or from deceased organ donors. Transplantation can be performed relatively safely and is favored over dialysis in the pediatric age group because it leads to improve somatic growth and offers a greater chance for a normal lifestyle. Transplantation is also less expensive than a chronic dialysis program. The morbidity and mortality associated with the surgical procedure and the necessity of taking immunosuppressive drugs indefinitely are its major disadvantages.

CONCLUSION

Urologic anomalies are common, but only a small percentage are severe and clinically significant. These urologic anomalies are frequently found in association with other congenital anomalies. The diagnosis and evaluation of these urologic anomalies in children with congenital disabilities is the same as in children without congenital disabilities; however, the management and treatment may vary depending on the impact of the associated anomalies on the natural history of the urologic condition. Clinical outcomes continue to improve as a result of advancement in urologic management and routine follow-up.

REFERENCES

Barrett, D.M., & Furlow, W.L. (1982). The management of severe urinary incontinence in patients with myelodysplasia by implantation of the AS 791/792 urinary sphincter device. *Journal of Urology, 128*, 484.

Bauer, S.B. (1984). Genitourinary problems in adolescence. *Journal of Reproductive Medicine, 29*, 385.

Bauer, S.B., Colodny, A.H., & Retik, A.B. (1982). The management of vesicoureteral reflux in children with myelodysplasia. *Journal of Urology, 128*, 102.

Bauer, S.B., Retik, A.B., Colodny, E.H., et al. (1980). The unstable bladder of childhood. *Urologic Clinics of North America, 7*, 321.

Belman, A.B. (1976). The clinical significance of vesicoureteral reflux. *Pediatric Clinics of North America, 23*, 707.

Cilento, B.G., Jr., Diamond, D.A., Yeung, C.K., Manzoni, G., Poppas, D.P., & Hensle, T.W. (2003). Laparoscopically assisted ureterocystoplasty. *British Journal of Urology, 91*, 525–527.

Crooks, K.K., & Enrile, B.G. (1983). Comparison of the ileal conduit and clean intermittent catheterization for myelomingocele. *Pediatrics, 72*, 203.

Fitzpatrick, J.M., & Mebust, W.K. (2002). Minimally invasive and endoscopic management of benign prostatic hypertrophy. In P.C. Walsh, A.B. Retik, E. Darracott Vaughan, & A.J. Wein (Eds.), *Campbell's urology* (8th ed., pp. 1379–1416). Philadelphia: W.B. Saunders.

Gauthier, B., Edelmann, C.M., Jr., & Barnett, H.L. (1982). *Nephrology and urology for the pediatrician.* Boston: Little, Brown & Co.

Gusman, L., et al. (1983). Evaluation and management of children with sacral agenesis. *Urology, 22*, 506.

Kunin, C.M. (1981). Duration of treatment of urinary tract infections. *American Journal of Medicine, 71*, 849.

Perez-Marrero, R., Dimmock, W., Churchhill, B.M., & Hardy, B.E. (1982). Clean intermittent catheterization in myelomeningocele children less that three years old. *Journal of Urology, 128*, 779.

Pope, J.C., & Rink, R.C. (1999). Surgical options in the management of the neurogenic bladder. In E.T. Gonzales & S.B. Bauer (Eds.), *Pediatric urology practice* (pp. 401–419). Philadelphia: Lippincott, Williams & Wilkins.

Shurtleff, D.B. (1980). Myelodysplasia management and treatment. In L. Gluck (Ed.), *Current problems in pediatrics* (Vol. 10, pp. 53–64). Chicago: Year Book Publishers.

Urizar, R.E., Largent, J.A., & Gilboa, N. (1983). *Pediatric nephrology: New directions in therapy.* New Hyde Park, NY: Medical Examination Publishing.

CHAPTER 22

DENTISTRY

Joel Pearlman and Edward Sterling

In the past, many thought that dental disease was an inevitable problem for people with developmental disabilities and, as a result, many individuals have suffered from dental disease and its resultant discomfort, disfigurement, dysfunction, and social and psychological isolation. Much of their suffering was needless. Dental disease is preventable and therefore avoidable (Kay et al., 1982; Plotnick, 1975; Tesini, 1980). Individuals with developmental disabilities can and deserve to have good oral health. The cornerstone supporting this right is a commitment to a program of prevention that combines early intervention with consistent effective daily oral hygiene and thorough, comprehensive professional care (Nowak, 1984).

EXPERIENCED DENTISTS

No dental specialty deals particularly with developmental disabilities—only pediatric dentistry includes individuals with special health care needs in its definition. Thus, resources for children are more readily available than for adults. Pediatric dentistry, unlike any other recognized specialty in dentistry, does not limit the range of services provided but rather limits *for whom* the services will be provided. In many instances, young children with developmental disabilities begin dental care with a pediatric dentist and never leave the practice due to the limited availability of resources for adults (Grant, Carlson, & Cullen-Reikson, 2004; Reichard, Turnbull, & Turnbull, 2001; U.S. Department of Health and Human Services, 2000; Waldman & Perlman, 2002).

Very few dental schools provide much more than a few lectures on disabilities to their students (Haden et al., 2003; Wolff et al., 2004). Students leave school with little understanding and even less experience in providing services to people with developmental disabilities, so it is no wonder that studies conducted in various states invariably conclude that dental care is one of the top three issues facing people with developmental disabilities, along with employment and housing.

ACCESS TO APPROPRIATE DENTAL CARE

Access to care has been an ongoing problem for people with developmental disabilities. For many years, this concern has been raised, discussed, and given some token support by various dental organizations, including the American Dental Association and the Council on Dental Education, but dentistry only began to truly work to solve the problem after the Surgeon General's report of 2000 (Honig, 2004; U.S. Department of Health and Human Services, National Institute on Dental and Craniofacial Research, & National Institutes of Health, 2000). In reality, the Surgeon General's report merely reiterated what had been known from previous studies and what dental health professionals working in this area had known.

In 1993, in "Access to Health Care: Key Indicators for Policy," prepared by the Center for Health Economics Research and supported by The Robert Wood Johnson Foundation, dentistry was described as a sentinel indicator of inadequate access to care because "dental problems are largely preventable through routine, periodic dental care" (pp. 109–112). The report went on to recommend that the first visit to a dentist should occur during early childhood. The American Academy of Pediatric Dentistry recommends that a child's first visit to the dentist be at 1 year of age or 6 months after the first tooth erupts, whichever comes first. The intents are to provide anticipatory guidance, promote health, establish a dental home (i.e., someplace and someone to turn to when the individual has questions, concerns, or an injury), and provide treatment, if necessary. The data suggests that children who are not impoverished are more likely to be seen by a dentist and at an earlier age (Casamassimo, 2003; Honig, 2004).

Parents or caregivers of children with developmental disabilities share some responsibility in this problem, as well. Often, dental care is not a high priority until there is a problem or suspected problem. In such a situation, the dentist is faced with providing secondary or tertiary level care and not primary prevention, which is less invasive, less time consuming, and less expensive.

The vast majority of children and adults with disabilities can and should be able to receive dental care in a normalized environment—a dental office in their community—and do not require a specialized setting or special equipment. They should be able to gain access to almost any office and receive the care they need to maintain oral health. What is lacking mostly in the system is confidence and not competence to meet these needs. It is hoped that in the near future, all dental schools will be required to include significant clinical experiences with people with disabilities for their students as part of accreditation (Fenton, 2003; Haden, 2003).

Harvey did not receive proper dental care for the majority of his adult life. His caregiver, Iris, would schedule appointments, but he would refuse to go. This situation perplexed Iris because Harvey had loved going to the dentist as a child and had received excellent care from a pediatric dentist for several years. In fact, Harvey used to stop by the dentist's office for a quick hello when he was in the neighborhood. Unfortunately, the pediatric dentist retired, and Harvey was unable to tolerate treatment from a new dentist.

Iris decided that a personal relationship was the missing element with the new dentists. She spoke to several dentists before she found one who was interested in fostering a relationship with Harvey. She invited the dentist over for dinner so that he could get to know Harvey. Her effort worked. Now, Harvey keeps his visits only when the dentist promises to take him out for lunch after the visit.

THE FIRST VISIT

Dental care begins with the initial visit, which includes the following:

1. A thorough history
2. An assessment of caries risk
3. A review of dental development
4. An oral examination
5. Guidance with home care
6. Anticipatory guidance
7. Establishment of a Dental Home

The history will include a review of the prenatal, perinatal, and postnatal periods and any problems the mother or child may have had during that time. Primary teeth begin to form during about the fifth month of pregnancy, so impairments in the structure, hypoplasias, and hypocalcifications in the primary dentition reflect disruptions in tooth formation during the pregnancy. The impairments provide an indication that something happened, and their location and extent of involvement give an indication of time and duration of the insult. Likewise, insults early in the child's life may be reflected in the structure, shape, or color of the teeth, both primary and permanent teeth. These impairments are not pathognomonic but open the door for further discussion with the parent. The history should also review current diet habits. The kinds of foods the infant is eating are significant and have implications for caries risk along with the bottle- or breast-feeding habits. Along with these are the obvious considerations of heart problems, seizure disorder, allergies, medications, and/or supplements the infant is receiving.

Caries risk assesses the likelihood that dental decay is or will be a problem for this infant. In 2002, the American Academy of Pediatric Dentistry developed, published, and adopted the Caries Risk Assessment Tool (CAT), which categorizes a child with developmental disabilities or special health care needs in the high-risk group (American Academy of Pediatric Dentistry, 1998, 2001). The CAT enables dental and nondental health care providers to establish a framework for classifying caries risk based on a set of clinical conditions, environmental characteristics, and general health factors. This risk assessment needs to be reviewed periodically to assess changes in an individual's caries risk status.

Reviewing normal dental development provides the parents with an overview of what to expect, especially regarding eruption of primary teeth. In Down syndrome, for example, dental eruption is commonly delayed. In addition, the eruption pattern and sequence is often quite different from the usual. Parents may be concerned whether their child has any teeth at all; dental health professionals need to alleviate and respond to these concerns.

The oral examination of a very young child is most likely to occur with the parent and dental professional sitting knee to knee with the child resting in the dental professional's lap, and a parent assisting to stabilize the child. The child's lips are parted, and the dental professional will carefully examine 1) the oral structures for symmetry, size, shape, and color; 2) the child's dental development as reflected in tooth eruption; 3) health of the gingival tissues; and 4) oral hygiene status. The dental professional will also assess motor control by running a finger around the outer surface of the gingival tissue to determine whether the tongue follows. The dental professional may then demonstrate how to provide oral hygiene for the child and how to stabilize the child to make the procedure safe for the parent and the child.

Many parents are quite timid and uncertain as to how to accomplish oral hygiene. Many use a washcloth because they lack the confidence to use a toothbrush. Unfortunately, in too many instances, the parent still uses a washcloth many years later and has not graduated to a toothbrush, whether manual or powered. A washcloth or small sponge is totally inadequate to provide thorough cleansing once the child has more than a couple of teeth, and parents would probably be wise to avoid the washcloth or sponge entirely and use a small toothbrush from the beginning. Whether toothpaste is incorporated into the procedure is a judgment decision. If the child likes the toothpaste and it allows the parent to brush longer and better, then it is fine. Otherwise, toothpaste is not required. If it is used, a small, pea-sized amount of toothpaste is all that is necessary. Ingestion of this small an amount will not cause any problems such as fluorosis or an upset stomach. Using an electric toothbrush is a matter of personal preference. The choice of inexpensive battery powered brushes sold at retail stores may offer the advantage of a low-cost trial run and possible segue to a more advanced product such as Sonicare or Braun Oral-B.

Anticipatory guidance is intended to provide the parent with information as to what is likely to occur within the next year or less. During this time, the dental professional can explain which teeth are likely to erupt next and the steps the parents should be making in diet, hygiene, or bedtime bottle/nursing. Based on the findings of the dental professional, an individualized follow-up regimen will be recommended, which may be anywhere from 2 or 3 months to a year depending on the findings. The aim is to establish a regimen that meets the child's needs and not some arbitrary average of once every 6 months. This regimen is periodically reviewed to determine whether it is continuing to meet the child's needs, and it is modified accordingly. The first visit procedures lead to the establishment of a dental home for the child and family, and this relationship may last well into adulthood.

CONTRIBUTING FACTORS FOR DENTAL PROBLEMS

Individuals with developmental disabilities are at a higher risk for developing dental problems for a variety of environmental factors and reasons.

Feeding Difficulty and Diet

The abnormal function of the tongue, lips, and cheek and the abnormal patterns of swallowing adversely affect mastication and deglutition. These problems lead to diet selections that are soft, easy to eat, and rich in carbohydrates, with resulting overretention of food debris in the oral cavity. Retention of food debris, combined with the individual's general coordination problems, makes oral hygiene a difficult task. As might be expected, caries and periodontal disease are more prevalent and more severe. Trouble swallowing can also mean difficulty drinking, which leads to a decreased fluid intake, less cleansing and rinsing action of liquids, and less than optimal intake of fluorides (if the water is fluoridated).

Meal Patterns

As infants, children with metabolic disorders may use a bottle longer before developing regular meal patterns and are at greater risk of developing "nursing bottle syndrome" if allowed to fall asleep with a bottle of juice or formula. When these children are not nursing, they must have carbohydrate-rich diets at frequent intervals, but the consistency and texture of these foods and the frequency of intake can affect decay rates by exposing teeth to more acid attacks (Bibby, 1975). Diet imbalances and inadequate nutritional intake can also contribute to the development of periodontal disease or a decreased resistance to it and can even lead to a diminished response to its treatment.

Children with disabilities may be indulged by parents and other adults who give them candy and sweets. Sometimes this indulgence is done intentionally in conjunction with a behavior program through rewards; at other times, it is a result of babying the child. Alternatives to these rewards should be encouraged that are less harmful to oral health. For all individuals with developmental disabilities, early intervention is necessary, with specific preventive treatment plans including fluoride supplements, affirmative dental health dietary practices, and effective plaque control (Ripa, 1981). In conjunction with these home measures, clinical preventive procedures such as oral prophylaxis, topical fluoride treatments, and pit and fissure sealants should be used to maintain good oral health (Pinkham, 1999; Plotnick, 1975).

Medications

The sugar contained in syrup-based medications can promote decay, especially if medications are taken often or for a long period of time. Two prescribed anticonvulsants, phenytoin (Dilantin) and valproic acid (Depakene) in liquid form, contain 1 g and 3 g of sucrose per teaspoon, respectively. Two commonly prescribed agents, chloral hydrate and hydroxyzine hydrochloride (Atarax), contain 3.5 g and 5.9 g of sucrose per teaspoon, respectively.

In addition, drug therapies or prescribed medications taken on a regular basis increase the risk for dental problems. The most obvious association is that between phenytoin therapy and gingival hyperplasia. Gingival hyperplasia is the overgrowth of the tissue surrounding the teeth seen in individuals with seizure disorders treated with phenytoin therapy. With effective oral hygiene, the thickened fibrotic tissues can remain pink and firm, thus avoiding the secondary inflammation and hyperemic condition that can grossly exaggerate this condition (Baer & Benjamin, 1974; Jenson, 1980).

Advanced gingival hyperplasia in individuals with intellectual disabilities, however, presents an especially difficult treatment and management problem. The grossly enlarged gingiva can obscure the clinical crowns, causing teeth to drift and rotate and interfere with normal function. When surgical treatment cannot be followed by controlled oral hygiene and other anticonvulsant therapies cannot be substituted for phenytoin, then the generally accepted treatment modalities do not apply (O'Donnell & Cohen, 1984; Pinkham, 1999). If surgery is undertaken, excessive bleeding, difficulty in tissue contouring, difficulty with periodontal pack placement and retention, and postoperative tooth mobility and sensitivity are all complications that can be anticipated.

Antianxiety medications (Valium, Tranxene, Xanax) and the common preparations for coughs and colds (Dimetapp, Robitussin, Actifed, and Triaminic) can cause motor restlessness and irritability. This condition can adversely affect behavior and interfere with the delivery of dental care. Barbiturates can cause dizziness, drowsiness, and lethargy. Neuroleptics and antidepressants both have been known to result in orthostatic hypotension. Constipation, the chronic side effect of all these medications, cannot be overlooked as contributing to irritability and motor restlessness as well.

Saliva Flow

Xerostomia (reduced saliva flow) induced by drugs can make teeth more vulnerable to decay. Anticholinergics reduce secretions, and widely used antidepressants such as amitriptyline (Elavil), imipramine (Tofranil), and trazodone (Desyrel) have this as a major side effect. Neuroleptic medications including phenothiazines (e.g., Thorazine, Mellaril, Stelazine, Trilafon) all may cause xerostomia. Saliva also acts as a lubricating medium, and in individuals who are edentulous geriatric or chronically ill, a dry mouth increases the potential for trauma. Wearing dentures can be difficult and uncomfortable for a person with a dry mouth, and the oral mucosa may exhibit a lowered resistance to irritation.

Physical Limitations

Individuals with a convulsive disorder are more prone to trauma during a seizure, and often anterior teeth are fractured, avulsed, or devitalized as a result (see Table 22.1). The same is true of people with cerebral palsy, muscular dystrophy, physical disabilities, and motor function impairments. These physical limitations can also mean a higher risk of developing dental disease because of the person's inability to care for his or her oral hygiene needs (Miller & Taylor, 1970).

Muscle function impairments can also result in poor oral hygiene. If the individual's physical disability prevents adequate performance of daily care, even with adaptive aids, the individual becomes totally or partially dependent on caregivers. This dependency can also add to the risk of dental disease if care is erratic and irregular. The longer the plaque is in contact with the teeth and gums, the greater the risk of dental disease. Toothbrushing and other proven oral hygiene techniques should be totally familiar to the parent, surrogate, or institutional staff in order to provide the necessary care.

Whenever possible, independent activity is preferable. Individuals with disabilities should be encouraged to clean their own teeth, and their effectiveness should be assessed. Goals that are practical and realistic can be set to develop self-care skills. If the individual is hindered by a mental or physical limitation, then the oral health maintenance plan should always strive for maximum effectiveness in any combination of self-care and assisted direct care.

Risk of Infection

As part of routine dental care, practitioners treating individuals with disabilities should be familiar with a number of commonly encountered problems. Specifically, the higher frequency of infection in individuals with valvular heart disease, congenital heart disease, mitral valve prolapse, idiopathic hypertrophic subaortic stenosis, and prosthetic heart valves requires an antibiotic (infective endocarditis) prophylaxis regimen. For individuals with scoliosis, respiratory function impairments due to postural limitations or depressed function secondary to premedication deserve attention. The

Table 22.1. Dental management for individuals with epilepsy/seizure disorder

Symptoms	Major oral conditions	Prevention and dental treatment	Medications
Seizures may be triggered by external stimuli: • Stress • Anxiety • Pain • Sensory overload Individual may also experience • Strange sensations, emotions, and behavior • Convulsions • Muscle spasms • Loss of consciousness	Gingival hyperplasia associated with phenytoin (Dilantin) Uncontrolled clenching Trauma from falls during seizures	Start a strict daily oral hygiene regimen at an early age. Adapt toothbrushing skills to the individual's abilities and strengths. Repair fractured teeth and gaps in between teeth to prevent injury to oral tissues during a seizure. Provide routine exams and prophylaxis. Use mouth props in the event of a seizure during treatment. Perform surgery to remove excessive gingival tissue if indicated. Alter anticonvulsant medications to reduce the incidence of gingival hyperplasia. Use mechanical toothbrushes. Use oral antimicrobial agents (chlorhexidine eluconate). Use fluoride therapy/varnish. Apply sealant. Offer nutrition counseling.	Seizure medication such as phenytoin (Dilantin) may cause gingival hyperplasia. Valproic acid (Depakene) and carbamezapine (Tegretol) may cause excessive bleeding. Sucrose-based medications may increase susceptibility to dental caries. Do not give erythromycin to individuals taking Tegretol.

Sources: http://www.ninds.nih.gov/disorders/epilepsy/epilepsy.htm and http://specialcaredentistry.com/sneeds/epilepsy.htm.

chronic nature of periodontal disease means that it cannot be overlooked in any differential diagnosis of head and neck problems (Butts, 1967; Goyings & Riekse, 1968; Gullikson, 1959).

Oral Problems and Habits

A number of commonly encountered oral habits can be challenging to caregivers. Individually or in combination, they can make it difficult to achieve and maintain good dental hygiene. The spastic, clonic jaw movements of an individual with cerebral palsy can result in biting on the toothbrush or gagging as a result of it. Tight perioral musculature can almost certainly frustrate anyone unaware of techniques for retracting the lips. Some individuals with disabilities are hypersensitive about having their mouths and lips touched and become resistive when any attempt is made to do so. Individuals who breathe through their mouths or thrust their tongues may have chronic mouth irritation that can result in less-than-optimal oral hygiene.

DENTAL PROBLEMS ASSOCIATED WITH DISORDERS

At an early stage, most individuals are dentally comparable. With age, a number of factors related to different disabilities make prevention more difficult (American Dental Association, 1982). Tables 22.2–22.4 present dental concerns related to sensory impairment, muscular dystrophy, and spina bifida. Dental disease for the most part falls into two general categories: caries and periodontal disease. Both are chronic conditions that can involve acute episodes and can afflict individuals throughout their life spans. When dealing in generalities, keep in mind that each person is an individual and therefore unique. Actual dental findings vary from person to person.

Down Syndrome

Experience has shown the dental profile of an individual with Down syndrome would take the following form: a low caries index or incidence of decay, a predisposition for periodontal disease with early onset and greater severity, malocclusion with delayed eruption of the primary and permanent dentition, spacing or diastemas between teeth or significant crowding, and malformed or congenitally missing permanent teeth (Cohen & Winer, 1965; Dicks, 1978; Sindoor & Desai, 1997; Sterling, 1992; Pilcher, 1998; see Table 22.5). The tongues of many individuals with Down syndrome assume a forward position caused by underdevelopment of the maxilla, and chronic mouth breathing is often secondary to persistent rhinitis. This tongue position manifests as pseudomacroglossia (O'Donnell & Cohen, 1984). The lower incidence of decay can be attributed to the spac-

Table 22.2. Dental issues related to sensory impairment

Symptoms	Major oral conditions	Prevention and dental treatment	Medications
Causes of sensory impairment may include • Rh incompatibility • Maternal diabetes • Prematurity • Rubella	Bruxism and tooth grinding during waking hours are common in deaf-blind individuals. This habit appears frequently during periods of inactivity and may serve to fill the sensory void left by the disability. Increased prevalence of enamel dysplasia may exist.	Start a strict daily oral hygiene regimen at an early age. Adapt toothbrushing skills to the individual's abilities and strengths. Provide routine exams and prophylaxis. Communicate using the method(s) that is familiar to the individual. Speak clearly and slowly and avoid background noise when communicating with an individual with acquired hearing loss. Maintain eye contact with a person with a hearing impairment. If applicable, develop an oral desensitization program. Use mechanical toothbrushes. Use oral antimicrobial agents. Use fluoride therapy/varnish. Apply sealants. Offer nutrition counseling.	Sucrose-based medications may increase susceptibility to dental caries.

Sources: http://www.sense.org.uk/deafblindness/causes.htm; Kanar (1976); Wolf and Anderson (1969).

Table 22.3. Dental issues related to muscular dystrophy

Symptoms	Major oral conditions	Prevention and dental treatment	Medications
Progressive weakness and degeneration of skeletal or voluntary muscles that control movement are present. Depending on form of muscular dystrophy, age of onset can vary from infancy to middle age. There is a high incidence of heart disease.	Greater prevalence of gingival and periodontal disease due to lack of muscle control Malocclusion	Start a strict daily oral hygiene regimen at an early age. Adapt toothbrushing skills to the individual's abilities and strengths. Provide routine exams and prophylaxis. Use mechanical toothbrushes. Use oral antimicrobial agents. Use fluoride therapy. Apply sealants. Offer nutrition counseling.	Due to the high percentage of cardiovascular conditions, individuals should be screened for subacute bacterial endocarditis and infective endocarditis premedication. Individuals taking phenytoin (Dilantin) for myotonic dystrophy (a delayed relaxation of a muscle after a strong contraction) should be monitored for gingival hyperplasia.

Source: http://www.ninds.nih.gov/disorders/md/md.htm.

Table 22.4. Dental issues related to spina bifida

Symptoms	Major oral conditions	Prevention and dental treatment	Medications
Failure of the fetus's spine to close properly during the first month of pregnancy causes neural tube disorder. Individual may need braces, crutches, or a wheelchair to be ambulatory. Individual may also experience • Learning disabilities • Lack of bowel and bladder control • Hydrocephalus • Latex allergy	Increased risk of dental disease when learning disability is present	Start a strict daily oral hygiene regimen at an early age. Adapt toothbrushing skills to the individual's abilities and strengths. Use positive reinforcement to develop good oral hygiene practice. Provide routine exams and prophylaxis. Use mechanical toothbrushes. Use antimicrobial agents. Use fluoride therapy/varnish. Apply sealants. Offer nutrition counseling. Use latex-free products.	Sucrose-based medications may increase susceptibility to dental caries.

Source: http://www.ninds.nih.gov/disorders/spina_bifida/spina_bifida.htm.

Table 22.5. Dental issues related to Down syndrome

Symptoms	Major oral conditions	Prevention and dental treatment	Medications
Growth deficiency and intellectual disabilities are present. Approximately 33% of babies born with Down syndrome have congenital heart impairments, especially ventricular septal defect. Individuals have increased risk of Alzheimer dementia at an early age.	High valued palate Small oral cavity Large, fissured and/or scalloped protruding tongue Mouth breathing Shorter crowns and roots Enamel hypoplasia Congenitally missing teeth Slightly reduced risk of dental caries Greatly increased risk of periodontal disease Malocclusion—usually Class III due to underdeveloped maxilla and midface Bruxism Marked gag reflex Angular cheilitis Xerostomia Delayed eruption of first and second teeth	Start a strict daily oral hygiene regimen at an early age. Adapt toothbrushing skills to the individual's abilities and strengths. Provide frequent exams and prophylaxis to avoid periodontal disease and maintain periodontal health. Tell, show, and do when teaching oral hygiene. Use mechanical toothbrushes. Use oral antimicrobial agents. Use fluoride therapy. Apply sealants. Offer nutrition counseling.	Due to high percentage of cardiovascular conditions, screen for subacute bacterial endocarditis premedication. Sucrose-based medications may increase susceptibility to dental caries.

Sources: http://www.altonweb.com/cs/downsyndrome/desai.html; http://www.kidsource.com/NICHCY/downs.html; http://content.health.msn.com/content/asset/adam_disease_mongolism.

ing between teeth, the excessive wear of occlusal surfaces, and the increased buffering capacity of saliva.

Periodontal disease tends to have an earlier onset in most individuals with disabilities than in the general population. In individuals with Down syndrome, periodontal disease is caused in part by the physical characteristics of the syndrome and in part by a decreased immunologic response. In most other individuals with disabilities, the main contributing factor is poor oral hygiene. Several factors predispose a person with Down syndrome to develop early periodontitis: 1) poor occlusal relationships place inordinate stress on the developing periodontium; 2) high labial frenum attachments lead to mucogingival impairments, resulting in early detachment of the gingiva from the mandibular incisors; and 3) the anterior position of the tongue creates abnormal forces on the teeth. For these reasons, treatment considerations should include frenectomy and interceptive orthodontics when possible (Pilcher, 1998). See Chapter 9.2 for more information on Down syndrome.

Cerebral Palsy

Individuals with cerebral palsy encounter a higher incidence of dental problems (see Table 22.6). Enamel hypoplasia in primary teeth, higher rates of decay, gingivitis, malocclusion, bruxism, and temporomandibular joint (TMJ) dysfunction are some common findings. The hypoplastic enamel corresponds to the dentochronology or time of insult in odontogenesis. Individuals with both athetoid and spastic cerebral palsy tend to brux and abrade their teeth (Massler, 1957; Miller & Taylor, 1970), and the result is a decreased vertical dimension or overclosure of the bite, which can ultimately contribute to a TMJ problem. For more information on cerebral palsy, see Chapter 11.

Congenital Anomalies

Most disturbances of growth and development have a genetic basis and are sometimes traceable to a specific prenatal problem in embryogenesis, including cleft lip, cleft palate, median rhomboid glossitis, bifid tongue, amelogenesis, and dentinogenesis imperfecta. In conditions such as amelogenesis and dentinogenesis imperfecta, teeth have defective structures and are, therefore, more prone to decay. Cleft lip and palate can be accompanied by an increased frequency of congenitally missing teeth, supernumerary teeth, and teeth that are fused, malformed, or malposed. Dental texts cover in detail the characteristics of medical problems and syndromes that can have dental implications (Little & Falace, 2002; Magalini et al., 1997; Pinkham, 1999).

Table 22.6. Dental issues related to cerebral palsy

Symptoms	Major oral conditions	Prevention and dental treatment	Medications
Nonprogressive disorder caused by damage to the immature brain. Motor dysfunction Individual may also experience • Learning disabilities • Psychological problems • Sensory impairments • Seizure disorders	Greater prevalence of gingival and periodontal disease due to lack of control of oral muscles and inability to perform daily oral hygiene regimen Malocclusion—especially Class II Division I Grinding/attrition Drooling Enamel hypoplasia of primary teeth Hyperactive gag reflex Difficulty with clearing food from mouth when eating Limited volitional tongue control Primitive bite reflex	Start a strict daily oral hygiene regimen at an early age. Adapt toothbrushing skills to the individual's abilities and strengths. Provide routine exams and prophylaxis. Modify toothbrush handles if needed. Use mechanical toothbrushes. Use oral antimicrobial agents. Use fluoride therapy/varnish. Apply sealants. Offer nutrition counseling. Consider a drooling device. Use mouth prop to maintain oral access.	Seizure medication such as phenytoin (Dilantin) may cause gingival hyperplasia. Anticholinergic drugs used to control drooling may cause increased susceptibility to dental caries. Sucrose-based medications may cause increased susceptibility to dental caries due to the inability of the individual to self-cleanse. Psychotropic drugs should be monitored for xerostomia, which may increase susceptibility to dental caries.

Sources: http://www.ninds.nih.gov/health_and_medical/disorders/cerebral_palsy.htm; http://www.ninds.nih.gov/health_and_medical/pubs/cerebral_palsyhtr.htm; http://www.geocities.com/HotSprings/Sauna/4441/dental.htm.

TREATMENT APPROACHES AND RATIONALE

In many cases, the treatment and management of individuals with developmental disabilities are similar to treatment and management of typically developing individuals. This scenario is especially true for individuals with mild intellectual disabilities, and some individuals with profound intellectual disabilities also respond well in a dental treatment situation. Treatment planning is designed to respond immediately to the elimination of pain, to restore and maintain existing dentition, to achieve an acceptable level of oral hygiene, and to restore and maintain function and aesthetics. Frequent recall, staff in-service training, and dental health education complete the picture of total patient care (Center for Development and Learning Disorders, 1967; Nicolai & Tesini, 1982).

Initially, all treatment is attempted on an outpatient basis. Various management adjuncts, such as behavior modification, nitrous oxide, premedication, protective restraints (e.g., Pedi-Wrap, papoose board), and mild physical restraint are commonplace. Mouth props and headrests are used routinely to maximize access. In a clinical situation, the presence of direct care staff who accompany and often know an individual, extra dental assistants, and other dental personnel can offer a staff-to-patient ratio that generally does not exist in private practice. In addition, the lack of time constraints and costs to the individual are positive factors that help to establish a successful treatment program for individuals with disabilities.

Another important consideration in treating individuals with special needs is weighing the risks, benefits, and costs of mild physical and chemical restraints versus general anesthesia. The ability to provide routine prophylaxis on an outpatient basis is important if it can prolong the intervals between reliance on general anesthesia. Frequent recalls may, over time, reduce resistance and lead to gradual acceptance or tolerance of routine care. In any event, frequent visits (2- or 3-month intervals) can ensure that acute or potentially acute problems are carefully monitored and kept to a minimum.

Some individuals require general anesthesia and hospital admission for any definitive treatment. Also included in this group are individuals who are physically hyperactive; individuals who exhibit impulsive behavior that can be harmful to themselves and others; and individuals who clench their jaws, purse their lips, or otherwise aggressively avoid treatment. Individuals with concomitant behavioral problems can present real challenges in dental management, thus requiring alternative modes of service delivery (Capute, 1974).

Familiarization/Conditioning

The long-term goals of dental compliance and tolerance can be attained through the technique of familiarization (desensitization and successive approximation), a form of behavior modification, positive reinforcement, and operant conditioning. Over time, individuals with disabilities can learn to accept the dental setting and dental treatment. Serious consideration should be given to this method of gaining cooperation when evaluating other options such as premedication and intravenous sedation (O'Donnell, 1975). Enlisting the cooperation of parents or staff to participate in practice sessions between visits with individuals who are capable of learning simple tasks may make the use of other behavior modifiers unnecessary.

Doctor–patient rapport is not always easily established. The dental professional can conduct a safe, nonthreatening examination while brushing the individual's teeth. The toothbrush is a familiar object, and its introduction is not likely to cause apprehension when used, resulting in more compliant behavior. It can provide a baseline response and can even be used in conjunction with other instruments to maintain the level of familiarity. Swabbing with gauze impregnated with fluoridated mouth rinse serves the same purpose.

The success of a visit often depends on criteria that have been predetermined. If an individual's limited attention span precludes extensive treatment, the treatments can be broken down into units. Cleaning one quadrant and rescheduling the individual for additional treatment may be a more "successful" approach than attempting to clean all four quadrants during the same visit.

Determining an Individual's Preferences

Some individuals will accept conventional treatment in an unconventional manner. For example, an individual may be quite cooperative if allowed to stand up or sit on the floor or on a chair other than the dental chair. Individuals with idiosyncratic behaviors should be identified; it is useful to know that a specific person can be pacified by merely holding a doll, toy, or other familiar object or by being accompanied by a specific individual. Although the delivery of clinical care may be easiest for the dentist and assistant in a conventional sit-down, four-handed approach, the comfort of the individual with disabilities should come first.

Individuals with gastrostomies and those with kyphosis, scoliosis, osteoporosis, quadriplegia, or joint contractures all require special consideration when positioning. They may need to be treated on stretchers or in wheelchairs. In addition, many individuals, including those who are blind (Lebowitz, 1974), are easily startled and are especially aware of postural changes, so even seating and positioning an individual in the dental chair require care and understanding. For explaining procedures and describing what will happen next, variations of tell, show, and do can be very helpful and appropriate.

Idealism must be balanced with reality, and the ability to improvise is essential to successfully treat individuals who are not always totally cooperative. Flexibility, perseverence, patience, humor, and dedication, combined with a practical yet casual informality that mixes care and concern with a modicum of firmness, usually constitutes "management." In most forms of treatment, management is the variable, and the dental procedure is the constant. Treatment plans may have to be altered according to the physical or other aspects of the person's condition, but the principles of good dental care do not.

A thorough individual assessment based on the medical, physical, emotional, and social history helps shape the management aspects of the treatment plan. What may be more helpful in the long run is documentation of the individual's tolerances: responses, both positive and negative, to sounds, instruments, and touching; responses to premedication dosages and combinations; and time tolerances for treatment. One should approach the person with an open mind, always willing to review individual needs and treatment options.

Modifying Treatment

Modifications in the delivery of treatment usually must be made due to difficulties regarding mobility, stability, communication, and medical problems (see Table 22.7). Most disabilities have no direct dental manifestations, and, therefore, treatment is usual and customary. Modifications in treatment, however, must be made in the following clinical situations: congenital or hereditary disabilities that have dental manifestations, disabilities that limit jaw mobility, psychomotor imbalances with predisposition for facial trauma, conditions that cause attrition and abrasion of the dentition, congenital or acquired physical disabilities limiting maintenance of oral hygiene, and congenital or acquired intellectual disabilities that render individuals dependent (Ettinger & Pinkham, 1976; Pinkham, 1999).

Treatment limitations relate directly to the individual's ability to cooperate with or without special delivery modifications. Lack of cooperation can mean a paucity of intraoral radiographs and can impede other diagnostic procedures as well as necessitate restraint or positive support. When it is necessary to control body movements, the use of physical restraints should be explained so that their purpose is not misinterpreted as punishment or undue force. When a dental professional uses chemical restraint in the form of premedication or sedation, he or she must be aware of possible drug interactions because many individuals with developmental disabilities take daily medications. Phenothiazines and their derivatives can potentiate sedatives

Table 22.7. Modifications in dental treatment per disability

Disabilities with no direct dental manifestations	Disabilities that make individuals trauma-prone (*continued*)
Hemiplegia	Chronic vertigo
Blindness	Lesch-Nyhan syndrome
Deafness	Disabilities accompanied by abrasion
Poliomyelitis	Cerebral palsy
Autism spectrum disorders	Epilepsy
Juvenile diabetes	Psychogenic disturbances
Klinefelter syndrome	Chorea
Mild muscular dystrophy	**Physical disabilities that limit maintenance of oral hygiene**
Congenital heart disease	Cerebral vascular accident
Turner syndrome	Amputation
Cystic fibrosis	Paralysis
Hemophilia	Cerebral palsy
Hereditary or congenital disabilities with dental manifestations	Muscular dystrophy
Amelogenesis imperfecta	Parkinson disease
Dentinogenesis imperfecta	Multiple sclerosis
Dentinal dysplasia	Rheumatoid arthritis
Severe enamel hypoplasia	**Intellectual disabilities that limit maintenance of oral hygiene**
Disabilities that limit oral opening	Severe intellectual disabilities
Juvenile rheumatoid arthritis	Hydrocephaly
Temporomandibular joint ankylosis	Down syndrome
Facial burn contractures	Meningitis
Discoid lupus erythematosus	Cranial trauma
Scleroderma	Anoxia
Trismus	Encephalitis
Myositis ossificans	Brain tumor
Cicatricial trismus	Senility
Disabilities that make individuals trauma-prone	Alzheimer disease
Epilepsy	Cerebral vascular accident
Cerebral palsy	

Source: Ettinger and Pinkham (1976).

and narcotic analgesics. Antidepressants can enhance the effects of barbiturates and other central nervous system depressants. Anesthetics containing epinephrine should be used cautiously because tricyclic antidepressants can potentiate the effect of catecholamines (O'Donnell & Cohen, 1984).

In cases in which lack of cooperation ultimately leads to performing dental procedures under general anesthesia, the preoperative workup and hospital admission may be the first comprehensive medical evaluation an individual has ever received. Often, previously unknown medical problems are revealed. When possible, day surgery is preferable as the least disruptive procedure for individuals who react adversely to unfamiliar settings and situations. In addition, it represents an attempt at cost containment and reduces the demands on hospital staff, who are less familiar with handling behavioral problems.

Replacing Missing Teeth

Usually the lack of cooperation and limited comprehension, understanding, and desire of the individual are the determining factors for the replacement of missing teeth. Other considerations are existing aesthetics, the individual's ability to function as is, and the potential ability of the individual to adapt to a prosthesis. Predicting long-term response to either fixed or removable prostheses is the most difficult consideration.

Twenty-eight-year-old Roselani has autism, psychosis, and intellectual disabilities. She was taken by her mother to the dentist because of loose teeth. Acute situational anxiety necessitated general anesthesia. Roselani received the necessary medical care, and a partial denture was fabricated at that time for some teeth that Roselani was missing. Roselani's mother noticed significant behavioral changes when Roselani wore the prosthesis. She attributed the positive changes to Roselani's improved appearance and comfort.

An individual's definite desire to have missing teeth replaced is a fairly good indication that the prosthesis will be worn. Many times, however, the request for tooth replacement is generated by parents or other caregivers. In any event, the dentist must ultimately decide whether to undertake the steps involved in fabrication of a removable prosthesis. Usually at least one appointment is necessary before the expenditure of a laboratory fee. These visits enable the dentist to become more familiar with the individual, and vice versa. The dentist is then in a better position to assess the individual's tolerances and gag reflex control with and without premedication and to predict whether the individual will tolerate a prosthetic device.

The real challenge begins when the denture is made and delivered, when the etched-metalresin retained bridge is inserted, and when the temporary crowns or ceramic bridges are cemented. One-to-one coverage for the first 24–48 hours has worked with some success. Phased-in delivery of prostheses, when possible, has also made transition and adjustment easier. There are still many cases, however, of complete dentures and partial dentures that are not worn. Partial dentures are probably the most complicated prosthesis to adjust to.

Bent or broken clasps and frameworks are not uncommon, and they represent forced or incorrect insertion or removal or damage from dropping. High-impact or impact-resistant acrylics reduce breakage and should be part of a lab prescription. In addition, the individual's name should be placed in each removable prosthesis by the lab before final insertion.

Prosthetic replacement of missing teeth can be the most rewarding dental service for individuals with developmental disabilities, but it can also be frustrating. When prostheses are worn regularly, sudden behavior changes often result in removable prostheses being thrown, discarded, or flushed down the toilet and so-called "fixed" prostheses actually being removed. Some individuals inadvertently lose their dentures after many weeks or months of successful wear and care. This scenario is particularly common in an institutional setting. A duplicate denture or jump case can be made by the dental laboratory at the time of remaking the denture and can reduce the number of appointments needed in the future if a remake again becomes necessary.

Considerable care must be taken by the dentist and laboratory in the fabrication of a removable dental prosthesis for a person with developmental disabilities. The chances of success are enhanced if the device initially fits properly with minimal adjustment and is aesthetically pleasing. Both are motivating factors that encourage wear.

For the questionable full-denture candidate, the dentist may decide to fabricate only the upper denture, and if this is successful, then make a lower one at a later time. The upper denture generally tends to be more easily retained and more stable. As a result, it is easier to adjust to. The motivational responses and postinsertion tolerances to dental prostheses are probably similar to an individual's tolerance for eyeglasses and hearing aids. In fact, tolerance of such devices can help serve in the determination of whether a prosthesis should be undertaken at all.

The development of the etched-metalresin retained bridge was of considerable benefit to individuals with developmental disabilities. In some cases, the etched-metalresin retained bridge can be an alternative to either a removable partial denture or a fixed bridge. It is essentially a reversible procedure when compared with a conventional bridge. The remaining teeth are not significantly altered and need no further treatment if the bonded bridge cannot be tolerated. Fabrication of a resin-bonded bridge requires less appointment time, can he done on minimally cooperative individuals, and does not require the administration of local anesthetics.

For individuals who require extensive maxillofacial reconstruction or orthognathic surgery, a team workup representing various disciplines is indicated. Again, the results can be profound and dramatic, but serious questions must be asked, answered, and reviewed before treatment is attempted.

Improving Access to Care

Access to care in the community remains problematic. Experienced and knowledgeable providers are few and far between. A survey of dental school curricula found that in 53% of schools, the number of lecture hours devoted to special care dentistry dropped from an average of 10 hours to fewer than 5 (Fenton & Horbelt, 2002; Ostrove, 2003; Ozar & Sokol, 2002). In addition, many states do not have differential Medicaid rates that recognize the added demands of providing care for individuals with disabilities. Dental care for adults is not even covered under Medicaid in many states. In other states, reimbursement rates have been poor, and the relationship between the state agency and dental providers has been acrimonious (American Academy of Pediatric Dentistry, 2001; Farsai & Calabrese, 2002; Reichard, Turnbull, & Turnbull, 2001).

In Ohio, for example, besides an overall reimbursement rate of 35% of usual and customary fees, the state agency has taken 35 years to adopt the American Dental Association standard insurance form, codes, and format for billing purposes. Prior to 2004, Medicaid in Ohio had its own unique billing form and many unique codes for dental procedures. Those dentists wishing to participate in the Medicaid program needed to use different forms, formats, and codes. Unfortunately, many providers and potential providers still believe this system is in place.

Dental care under Medicaid represents approximately 1% or less of the budget for many states, so it is frequently on the chopping block when agencies need to reduce budget deficits. In Ohio during fiscal year 2004, adult dental services under Medicaid were "up for review" three times. So far, thanks to the organized efforts of the Ohio Dental Association and other concerned stakeholders, adult dental services have avoided being cut or significantly reduced. Community safety net programs that help individuals with disabilities often have no safety net themselves and are frequently understaffed and underfunded. As a result, many safety net programs around the country have open positions for dentists.

Advances in aesthetic dentistry have widened a service gap for most individuals with developmental disabilities. The number and types of aesthetic materials have increased dramatically. More posterior composites than amalgams are now placed daily in the United States. Exciting technological advances include dentin bonding, tooth whitening, veneers, electronic tooth shading, CAD/CAM (computer aided design/manufacture) techniques, light emitted diode curing lights, digital photography, along with integrated dental software, and intraoral cameras. Much of these advances, however, are not necessarily available or accessible to individuals with developmental disabilities.

Individuals with developmental disabilities should also have access to preventive products. Fluoride varnishes (i.e., duraphat) may be an effective tool because they are easy to apply and can be used at each prophylaxis appointment for caries-active patients. Prescription items such as Prevident 5000+ Booster toothpaste and Prevident gel or rinse are also beneficial. Many of these products require manual application by a caregiver using a toothbrush because most individuals with moderate or severe developmental disabilities cannot reliably rinse for the designated 30–60 seconds and then expectorate. The use of chlorhexidine rinses (Peridex, Periogard) and Xylitol gum may reduce inflammation and bleeding and even inhibit caries, but the efficacy for long-term use or level of benefit in the presence of poor oral hygiene is questionable (Glassman, 2003).

Pain management, an essential criterion in dental care delivery with the general population, is just as important for individuals with disabilities. The advent of Septocaine (articaine HCL 4% with epinephrine 1:100,000) means more options for infiltration versus nerve blocks. Of course, lasting local anesthetics can present a postoperative problem as individuals may be more inclined to "test" or bite their lips, tongue, or cheeks if not supervised.

THE TUFTS DENTAL PROGRAM

The experiences of Tufts Dental Program, a university-affiliated dental service program for individuals with developmental disabilities, can serve as a model for service provision. This program is a statewide network of dental facilities funded on a contractual basis through an agreement with the Massachusetts Department of Public Health. It offers and provides comprehensive clinical care in all specialty areas and in preventive education.

More than 16,000 individuals with developmental disabilities who either live in institutions or in community residences, supervised apartments, halfway houses, group homes, homes with parents or relatives, or homes with a foster family or surrogate are served by the Tufts Dental Program. As an American Dental Association–accredited program, it operates much like a large multispecialty group practice. The program is characterized by providers with an advanced level of training, qualified personnel, adequate staff, state-of-the-art equipment, and supplies and clinical facilities that are adapted to meet special needs (Kay et al., 1982).

Until the 1990s Tufts Dental Program maintained an open-door policy and eliminated fee and predetermination barriers. It still serves as a referral center to supplement community care. An individual can be referred for a specific procedure or for multiple scalings, which Medicaid does not cover. A treatment fund has been established to bridge the gap and cover a wider range of services, but there is still a substantial difference from usual and customary fees.

Record Keeping

Treatment and documentation follow a prescribed format (Kay et al., 1982). A treatment plan is developed after a medical history review, including the results of a complete head and neck examination and radiographs whenever possible. Reports of consultations and regular treatment provided are sequentially recorded in abbreviated fashion on a record-of-treatment sheet and in considerably more detail as a continuing-progress note. The signed and dated continuing-progress note serves to identify behavioral responses, including reactions to premedication, treatment provided, prevention measures needed or provided, and recommendations for future visits. A separate medication log identifies the premedication ordered, dosage and form given, the individual's response to it, and recommendations for successive visits. Review of the medication log helps the prescribing dentist decide whether to increase, decrease, modify, or discontinue premedications. Precaution stickers placed inside the record covers alert providers to drug allergies, idiosyncracies, and special care considerations.

Scheduling

Individuals' complex health needs, their care programs, and their involvement in school, sheltered workshop activities, and jobs all require scheduling consideration. An attempt is made to coordinate services in the most sensitive and least disruptive manner. Those holding jobs may be the last hired and first fired, so scheduling becomes a delicate compromise. Frequent recall is an important adjunct to the prevention program. The optimal interval is that which a dentist or hygienist considers to be the most likely to be successful for any individual's oral health maintenance program.

Standard of Care

Constant peer reviews take place because of 1) the staffing patterns of the clinic, which are similar to that of a large multispecialty group practice; 2) the advanced level of training of the providers; and 3) the educational nature of this accredited program. To supplement this internal review process, the quality of care is periodically reviewed by an external review committee of unbiased dental service providers. The quality and quantity of services provided, appropriateness of treatment plans, and accuracy of records are assessed (Weintraub, 1983). In addition to current competence in cardiopulmonary resuscitation (annual recertification), continuing education is encouraged, required, and supported.

All of these steps help to establish and ensure a certain standard of care. At the community level, the quality and nature of dental care is not checked. Usually, the only control is the conscience of the provider. This lack of review represents a potential weakness in the process of normalization and mainstreaming. A review mechanism should exist to protect individuals unable to make competent decisions concerning their own health needs.

Changing Dental Needs

Initially, when the dental program began, the individuals served had a backlog of unmet oral health needs. As their basic needs were addressed, fewer restorations and extractions were necessary. Greater emphasis was placed on prevention. Frequency of maintenance therapies and the demand for prosthetic services increased. If adequate treatment cannot be provided in the dental clinic on an outpatient basis either with or without premedication, relative analgesia, or intravenous sedation, elective dental procedures under general anesthesia must be considered. Therefore, affiliation with a hospital with a well-equipped operating room is a necessary part of the delivery of care.

Complementing the clinical component is a dental health education program designed to be responsive to and responsible for their preventive care. This is accomplished through in-service training programs for individuals with developmental disabilities, parents, and other caregivers (Nicolai & Tesini, 1982). Through ongoing instruction, supervision, motivation, and follow-up—coordinated with periodic clinical assessments—an accountable preventive program is leading to improved oral health.

The implementation and continuity of preventive programming rest almost exclusively on a group of relatively new dental health personnel—dental health educators. These professionals select, design, and present materials and audiovisual aids in conveying the message of proper oral physiotherapy. In addition, they must 1) be an efficient administrator to oversee any structured oral hygiene program and provide detailed, concise, and appropriate records to measure the progress of that program; 2) implement constructive programs that may benefit individuals or groups of individuals; 3) become sensitive and open-minded in the area of public relations as it applies to participation in the administration of the institution and/or the individual residences in the community setting; and 4) become totally familiar with all departments in the institution and work closely with them to expedite complete care, to correct perceived program deficiencies, and to collaborate on policy making. In short, dental health educators must be able to do a little of everything. They mainly concentrate on their expertise but are proficient in all aspects of care provision to individuals with developmental disabilities.

CONCLUSION

Advocacy efforts on behalf of individuals with special needs have to be more diligent than ever before. Medicaid fees require continual examination and upgrading to cover specialized services and procedures. The coverage for preventive and rehabilitative services must be expanded. Grants and funds for clinical research and treatment facilities are necessary. Dental school education should continue to offer sufficient courses and clinical experiences that emphasize the management and treatment of individuals with special needs. Above all, dental professionals must remain aware of the complex and essential needs of individuals with developmental disabilities.

REFERENCES

Albertson, D. (1974). Prevention and the handicapped child. *Dental Clinics of North America, 18*, 595.

American Academy of Pediatric Dentistry. (1998). *Risk assessment: ABC's of infant oral health.* Chicago: Author.

American Academy of Pediatric Dentistry. (2001). *Caries Risk Assessment Tool.* Chicago: Author.

American Dental Association. (1982). *Caring for the disabled child's dental health.* Chicago: Author.

American Dental Association. (1995, June). Caries diagnosis and risk assessment: A review of preventive strategies and management. *Journal of the American Dental Association (Supplement), 126*, 1–S.

American Dental Association. (1998). *The ADA guide to dental therapeutics* (1st ed., pp. 298–319). Chicago: Author.

American Dental Association. (2003). *Dental health policy analysis series: Medicaid and dental care for children: A review of the literature.* Chicago: Author.

Baer, P.N., & Benjamin, S.D. (1974). *Periodontal disease in children and adolescents.* Philadelphia: Lippincott, Williams & Wilkins.

Bhaskar, S.N. (1986). *Synopsis of oral pathology* (7th ed.). St. Louis: Mosby.

Bibby, B.C. (1975). Cariogenicity of snack foods and confections. *Journal of the American Dental Association, 90*, 121.

Butts, J.E. (1967). Dental status of mentally retarded children. *Journal of Public Health Dentistry, 27*(4), 195.

Capute, A.J. (1974). Developmental disabilities. *Dental Clinics of North America, 18*, 557.

Casamassimo, P.S. (1996). *Bright futures in practice: Oral health.* Washington, DC: National Center for Education in Maternal and Child Health.

Casamassimo, P.S. (2003). Dental disease prevalence, prevention and health promotion: The implications on pediatric oral health of a more diverse population. *Pediatric Dentistry, 25*(1), 16–18.

Center for Development and Learning Disorders. (1967). *Dental care for the mentally retarded: A handbook for ward personnel.* Birmingham: University of Alabama in Birmingham.

Center for Health Economics Research. (1993). *Access to health care: Key indicators for policy.* Princeton, NJ: The Robert Wood Johnson Foundation.

Cohen, L.A., Manski, R.J., Magder, L.S., & Mullins, C.D. (2002). Dental visits to hospital emergency departments by adults receiving Medicaid: Assessing their use. *Journal of the American Dental Association, 133*, 715–724.

Cohen, M.M., Sr. (1977). Stomatologic alterations in childhood. *ASDC Journal of Dentistry for Children, 44*, 396.

Cohen, M.M., Sr., & Winer, R.A. (1965). Dental and facial characteristics in Down's Syndrome. *Journal of Dental Research, 44*, 197.

Dicks, J.L. (1978). *Dental implications of Down's syndrome.* Atlanta: Georgia Retarded Center.

Dolinsky, E.H., & Dolinsky, H.B. (1984). Infantilization of elderly patients by health care providers. *Special Care in Dentistry, 4*, 150.

Ettinger, R.L., & Pinkham, J.R. (1976). Modifications in restorative dentistry for the handicapped patient. In A.J. Novak (Ed.), *Dentistry for the handicapped patient* (pp. 276–301). St. Louis: Mosby.

Farsai, P., & Calabrese, J. (2002, September) Oral health for adults with disabilities: Dental treatment for adults. *Exceptional Parent*, 111–115.

Fenton, S.J. (2003, April). Universal access to healthcare: Making a difference. *Exceptional Parent*, 65–68.

Fenton, S.J., & Horbelt, C.V. (2002, October). The keys to ensure access to dental care. *Exceptional Parent*, 109–112.

Garrard, S.D. (1982). Health services for mentally retarded people in community residences: Problems and questions. *American Journal of Public Health*, 72, 1226.

Gellis, S.S., & Feingold, M. (1968). *Atlas of mental retardation syndromes.* Washington, DC: U.S. Department of Health Education and Welfare.

Glassman, P. (2003). Practical protocols for the prevention of dental disease in community settings for people with special needs. *Special Care in Dentistry, 23*(5), 157–188.

Gorlin, R.J., & Pindborg, J.J. (1964). *Syndromes of the head and neck.* New York: McGraw Hill.

Gotowka, T.D., Johnson, ES., & Gotowka, C.J. (1982). Costs of providing dental services to adult mentally retarded: A preliminary report. *American Journal of Public Health*, 72, 1246.

Goyings, E.D., & Riekse, D.M. (1968). Periodontal condition of institutionalized children: Improvement through oral hygiene. *Journal of Public Health Dentistry, 28*, 5.

Grant, E., Carlson, G., & Cullen-Erickson, B. (2004). Oral health for people with intellectual disability and high support needs: Positive outcomes. *Special Care in Dentistry*, 70–79.

Gullikson, J.S. (1959). Oral findings of mentally retarded children. *ASDC Journal of Dentistry for Children, 36*, 59.

Haden, N.K., et al. (2003, March). *Improving the oral health status of all Americans: Roles and responsibilities of academic dental institutions: The report of the ADEA President's commission.* Chicago: American Dental Education Association.

Honig, A. (2004, April 5). *Guest essay: Disparities in access to Pediatric dental care.* Washington, DC: Children's Dental Health Project.

Jenson, L.G. (1980). Clinical management of the epileptic dental patient. In T.M. Hassell et al. (Eds.), *Phenytoin induced teratology and gingival pathology* (pp. 129–132). New York: Raven Press.

Johnson, H., & Alhertson, D. (1972). Plaque control for handicapped children. *Journal of the American Dental Association, 84*, 824.

Kamen, S. (1976). Mental retardation. In A.J. Nowak (Ed.), *Dentistry for the handicapped patient* (pp. 39–53). St. Louis: Mosby.

Kanar, H.L. (1976). The blind and the deaf. In A.J. Nowak (Ed.), *Dentistry for the handicapped patient.* St. Louis: Mosby.

Kay, L., et al. (1982). *Guidelines for dental programs in institutions for developmentally disabled persons.* Denver: National Foundation for Dentistry for the Handicapped.

Kraus, B.S., Clark, C.S., & Oka, S.W. (1968). Mental retardation and abnormalities of dentitions. *American Journal of Mental Deficiency, 72,* 905.

Lebowitz, E.J. (1974). An introduction to dentistry for the blind. *Dental Clinics of North America, 18,* 3.

Leviton, F.J. (1980). The willingness of dentists to treat handicapped patients: A summary of eleven surveys. *Journal of Dentistry for the Handicapped, 5*(1), 13.

Little, J.W., & Falace, D.A. (2002). *Dental management of the medically compromised patient* (6th ed.). St. Louis: Mosby.

Magalini, S., et al. (1997). *Dictionary of medical syndromes* (4th ed.). Philadelphia: Lippincott, Williams & Wilkins.

Massler, N.I. (1957). Review of problems in dealing with the handicapped. *Journal of Dental Education, 21,* 62.

Miller, J.B., & Taylor, P.P. (1970). A survey of the oral health of a group of orthopedically handicapped children. *ASDC Journal of Dentistry for Children, 37,* 31.

National Foundation of Dentistry for the Handicapped. (1976). *Campaign of concern.* Denver, CO: Author.

Nicolaci, A.B., & Tesini, D.A. (1982). Improvement in the oral hygiene of institutionalized mentally retarded individuals through training of direct care staff: A longitudinal study. *Special Care in Dentistry, 2*(5), 217.

Nowak, A.J. (1984). Dental disease in handicapped persons. *Special Care in Dentistry, 4,* 66.

O'Donnell, J.P. (1975). Dental familiarization for the handicapped. *Journal of Dentistry for the Handicapped, 1,* 1.

O'Donnell, J.P. (2004, February). *Dentistry for special needs individuals in Massachusetts: A 30-year perspective.* Unpublished manuscript.

O'Donnell, J.P., & Cohen, N.I.M., Sr. (1984). Dental care for the institutionalized retarded individual. *Journal of Pediatrics, 9,* 3.

Office of the Surgeon General. (2002). *Closing the gap: A national blueprint to improve the health of persons with mental retardation. Report of the U.S. Surgeon General's Conference in Health Disparities and Mental Retardation.* Rockville, MD: U.S. Department of Health and Human Services.

Ostrove, L. (Ed.). (2003). Oral health care for people with special needs: Guidelines for comprehensive care. *Exceptional Parent Monograph.*

Ozar, D.T., & Sokol, D.J. (2002). *Dental ethics at chairside: Professional principles and practical applications* (2nd ed.). Washington, DC: Georgetown University Press.

Pearlman, J. (1975). *Dental treatment needs of the mentally retarded in state schools: Survey, report assessment, and proposal for corrective measures.* Boston: Massachusetts Department of Mental Retardation.

Pilcher, E.S. (1998). Dental care for the patient with Down syndrome. *Down Syndrome Research and Practice, 5*(3), 111–116.

Pinkham, J.R. (Ed.). (1999). *Pediatric dentistry: Infancy through adolescence* (3rd. ed.). Philadelphia: W.B. Saunders.

Plotnick, S. (1975). A survey of preventive dental programs for the handicapped child. *New York Dental Journal, 45*(5), 160.

Pnsnick, W.R., & Posnick, I.H. (1976). Dental care in private practice. In A.J. Nowak (Ed.), *Dentistry for the handicapped patient* (pp. 193–208). St. Louis: Mosby.

Reichard, A., Turnbull, H.R., & Tumbull, A.P. (2001). Perspectives of dentists, families and case managers on dental care for individuals with developmental disabilities in Kansas. *Mental Retardation, 39*(4), 268–285.

Ripa, L. (1981). *A guide to the use of fluoride for the prevention of dental caries, with alternative recommendations for patients with handicaps.* Denver, CO: National Foundation for Dentistry for the Handicapped.

Romer, M., Dougherty, N., & Amores-Lafleur, E. (1999). Predoctoral education in special care dentistry: Paving the way to better access? *ASDC Journal of Dentistry for Children,* 132–135.

Sindoor, S., & Desai, B.D.S. (1997, September). Down syndrome: A review of the literature. *Oral Surgery, Oral Pathology and Endodontics, 84*(3), 279–285.

Sterling, E. (1992). Oral and dental considerations in Down syndrome. In I. Lott & E. McCoy (Eds.), *Down syndrome: Advances in medical care* (pp. 135–145). New York: John Wiley & Sons.

Tesini, D.A. (1980). Age, degree of mental retardation, institutionalization and socioeconomic status as determinants in the oral hygiene status of mentally retarded individuals. *Community Dentistry and Oral Epidemiology, 8,* 355.

Tesini, D.A. (1982). *Developing dental health education programs for the handicapped: A training manual and reference text.* Springfield, MA: Area Health Education Center of Pioneer Valley.

U.S. Department of Health and Human Services. (2000). *Healthy people 2010.* Retrieved from http://www.healthypeople.gov

U.S. Department of Health and Human Services, National Institute of Dental and Craniofacial Research, & National Institutes of Health. (2000, May). *Oral health in America: A report of the surgeon general. Executive summary.* Rockville, MD: Author.

Waidman, H.B., & Penman, S.P. (2000, July). Dental care for people with disabilities: Prospects and problems. *Exceptional Parent,* 26–30.

Waidman, H.B., & Penman, S.P. (2003). Why dentists shun Medicaid: Impact on children, especially children with special needs. *ASDC Journal of Dentistry for Children, 70*(1), 5–9.

Waldman, B., & Perlman, S. (2002). Why is providing dental care to people with mental retardation and other developmental disabilities such a low priority? *Public Health Reports,* 12–14.

Walton, S.M., Byck, G.R., Cooksey, J.A., & Kaste, L.M. (2004, May). Assessing differences in hours worked between male and female dentists. *Journal of the American Dental Association, 135,* 637–645.

Wei, S.H.Y. (Ed.). (1978). *Pediatric dental care: An update for the dentist and for the pediatrician.* New York: Medcom.

Weintraub, J.A. (1983). *Utilization review and quality assessment of Tufts Dental Facilities for the Handicapped.* Boston: Massachusetts Department of Public Health.

Wolf, J.M., & Anderson, R.M. (1969). *The multiply handicapped child.* Springfield, IL: Charles C Thomas.

Wolff, A.J., Waidman, B., Milano, M., et al. (2004). Dental students' experiences with and attitudes toward people with mental retardation. *Journal of the American Dental Association, 135,* 353–357.

CHAPTER 23

MENTAL HEALTH AND BEHAVIOR

23.1 AUTISM SPECTRUM DISORDERS

Raun Melmed, Kerim Munir, and Peter Tanguay

Autism as a diagnostic term has captivated American society if not the world, and the condition can no longer be regarded as rare (Yeargin-Allsopp et al., 2003). The appreciation clinicians have of this condition and its associated medical, genetic, educational, social, recreational, and vocational factors has changed the way they view children and adults who have developmental disabilities. This chapter has been constructed by three authors who represent different perspectives of the clinical and social phenomenology of autism, have experience that spans 4–5 decades, and inhabit different parts of the country and world. In this chapter, the authors use the term *autism spectrum disorders* (ASD) for three reasons: 1) it defines the set of characteristics that are exemplified in the diagnostic criteria of autism; 2) the authors recognize that there is a wide spectrum of presentation that reflects both the degree of severity of autistic features and the intellectual and functional ability of affected individuals; and 3) autism is a "spectrum" of human variation, and to recognize it as such is to appreciate that although individuals may have varying degrees of social and emotional difficulties, many can become functional and successful in life.

Individuals with ASD have been recognized in the literature for more than 100 years (Barr, 1898). The term *autism* itself was first used by the Swiss psychiatrist Bleuler to describe a disturbance in social withdrawal along with disturbances in association, affect, and ambivalence. Kanner (1943), a leader in American child psychiatry, described a series of 11 children, some of whom appeared to have normal intelligence, who failed to establish normal social relationships. Around the same time, Asperger in Vienna, was preparing a doctoral thesis, eventually published as a monograph in German, *Die 'Autischen Psychopathen' in Kindesalter*. It was published during World War II, and although Asperger became a very well-regarded behavioral pediatrician and educator in later years, the monograph was not widely known or appreciated in the English world until Wing called attention to it in 1981. A full translation did not appear until 1991 (Wing, 1991).

Asperger emphasized that the disorder was quite variable in its severity, ranging from a condition of profound disability to milder versions, which were not incompatible with gainful employment and even a degree of success. He noted that even successful individuals with the condition remained socially "odd" and isolated and that their successes were often a result of a single-minded, dogged pursuit of a special personal interest. In contrast to Kanner, Asperger believed that the syndrome was more a personality trait than a developmental disorder. The diagnosis of Asperger disorder in the United States lay dormant until the publication in 1994 of the fourth edition of the *Diagnostic and Statistical Manual* (DSM–IV; American Psychiatric Association, 1994).

EVOLUTION OF THE DSM AND ICD DEFINITIONS

Autism was not included as a diagnosis in the first edition of the DSM (DSM–I), which was published by the American Psychiatric Association (APA) in 1952. The second edition, DSM–II (APA, 1968) also did not include *autism* as a separate diagnostic category. By mid 1960, research had begun to point to sensory and perceptual disturbances in children with an expanded description of Kanner's infantile autism. In 1964, Rimland published a keynote review of existing literature, challenging the lack of evidence for psychogenic factors in the etiology of autism and pointing to biological mechanisms (Rimland, 1964). The turning point for autism in its current form occurred with the publication of the third edition of the DSM (DSM–III; APA, 1980) because prior to that time there was a great deal of confusion about the diagnosis, etiology, and treatment of autism. Many children that would be characterized as

This chapter was supported, in part, by the National Institutes of Health/Fogarty grant D43 TW05807(KM).

having autism were mislabeled as having *childhood psychosis* or *childhood schizophrenia.*

The diagnosis of *infantile autism* consistent with the four *Rutter Criteria* was adopted in the third edition of the DSM–III. The publication of the DSM–III, therefore, marked a breakthrough in American psychiatry in the modern conceptualization of autism. The new criteria included 1) age of onset younger than 30 months; 2) lack of relatedness; 3) communications impairments; and 4) perseverative behaviors. The DSM–III emphasized the core symptoms of autism in young children with less recognition of developmental variation by age.

With the introduction of the DSM–III–R (APA, 1987) the age of onset criterion was dropped, leaving only three domains: 1) social reciprocity, 2) communication, and 3) special interests/repetitive behaviors. The criteria count was increased to 16 with minimum of 8 needed for the diagnosis with at least 2 under social reciprocity, 1 under communication, and 1 under special interests/repetitive behaviors. The intent was to broaden the diagnosis of *autism* compared with the DSM–III definition. The DSM–III–R changes led to increased use of the diagnosis of autism over time.

The DSM–IV (APA, 1994) was an attempt to compromise between the clinical and the research needs inherent in the definitions of *autism.* In the tenth edition of the International Classification of Disease (ICD–10; World Health Organization, 1993), pervasive developmental disorders were grouped under several subcategories; the ICD–10 approach influenced the DSM–IV classification under *pervasive developmental disorders* (see Table 23.1-1), which include 1) autistic disorder; 2) Asperger disorder; 3) Rett syndrome; 4) childhood disintegrative disorder; and 5) pervasive developmental disorder–not otherwise specified (PDD-NOS). The diagnosis of autistic disorder listed in the DSM–IV specifies symptoms to be of sufficient severity to result in a marked degree of impairment of function, under three domains:

1. *Impairments in social interaction*—impairment in eye contact, facial expression, body posture and gesture; failure to develop peer relationships; no seeking to share enjoyments or interests; lack of social and emotional reciprocity; and obliviousness to the needs and interests of others

2. *Impairment in verbal and nonverbal communication*—delay or lack of spoken language; marked impairment in the ability to initiate or sustain a conversation; stereotypical and repetitive use of language; and lack of varied, spontaneous make believe or socially imitative play

3. *Restrictive, repetitive, and stereotyped patterns of behavior*—preoccupation with restricted patterns of interest; inflexible adherence to nonfunctional routine or ritual; stereotypies and repetitive motor mannerisms; and persistent preoccupation with parts of objects

Table 23.1-1. DSM–IV and ICD–10 categories of pervasive developmental disorders

DSM–IV Classification (American Psychiatric Association, 1994)	ICD–10 Classification (World Health Organizaztion, 1993)
299 Pervasive developmental disorders	F84 Pervasive developmental disorders
299.00 Autistic disorder	F84.0 Childhood autism
	F84.1 Atypical autism
299.80 Rett syndrome	F84.2 Rett syndrome
299.10 Childhood disintegrative disorder	F84.3 Other childhood disintegrative disorder
	F84.4 Overactive disorder with mental retardation and stereotyped movements
299.80 Asperger disorder	F84.5 Asperger syndrome
	F84.8 Other pervasive developmental disorders
299.80 Pervasive developmental disorder not otherwise specified	F84.9 Pervasive developmental disorder, unspecified

Reprinted with permission from the *Diagnostic and Statistical Manual of Mental Disorders, Fourth Edition* (Copyright 1994). American Psychiatric Association.

Not all of the previous symptoms need be present for the diagnosis to be made. At a minimum, there must be a total of six symptoms, with at least two from the first category and one from each of the remaining categories.

Much like autism, PDD-NOS is a highly heterogeneous disorder with a great deal of variation based on age, gender, and social and educational environment. The original term used in the DSM–III was *childhood onset PDD*—a subthreshold, *atypical* or *residual* form of infantile autism. When children did not meet the requisite symptom number or severity, the term *childhood onset PDD* was utilized to capture the subthreshold manifestations of autism proper. In addition, the suffix *-NOS,* widely used for many other conditions, has both added to the confusion and diluted the impact of the PDD-NOS diagnosis.

The DSM–IV Text Revision (TR) (APA, 2001) added a minor but fundamentally important change for the definition of PDD-NOS. Prior to the DSM–IV–TR definition, only one symptom criterion was adequate from any of the three major autistic symptom domains: 1) social interaction; 2) communication and imaginative activity; or 3) restricted repetitive and stereotyped behavior, interests, and activities. The DSM–IV–TR stipulates that at least one symptom from the social interaction domain is now *necessary* for a diagnosis of PDD-NOS. Wing (1997) suggested that it may be appropriate to consider autistic disorder, Asperger disorder, and other pervasive developmental disorders as representing an *autism spectrum* of social and language impairment, communication impairment, limited imagination, and narrow and repetitive patterns of behavior. Although the idea may appear clinically persuasive to some, the notion of a spectrum may be no more than a concatenation of symptoms representing a range of genetically influenced impairments.

Given the current state of knowledge and the various preferences in diagnostic thinking, a consensus on diagnostic labels is needed. For these reasons, *ASD* is used in this chapter except for historical, collective, or colloquial contexts in which the term *autism* is used. The following excerpt of personal notes from a 30-year-old man with Asperger disorder describes some of his experiences, which can be extrapolated to reflect the experiences of children and adults with other ASD but who are unable to articulate their experiences. It may be helpful to consider that individuals who have ASD have different experiences and incorporate that thinking into our diagnostic considerations.

I do not view Asperger syndrome as the manifestation of some neurological mishap. I have no shame in being identified as autistic, nor do I feel that my opportunities in life are unusually limited. Rather, I feel uniquely qualified for certain roles in life, and proud of my natural abilities. I appreciate that I am able to use logic and discern details with an unusual acuity. My lack of interest of in social activities only serves to accommodate me, as I'm able to use time others would waste in socializing for more personally rewarding activities, such as writing computer programs, reading or making music.

Rather than attribute the difficulty I have in interacting with the ordinary world as a failing on my part, as some undesirable deviance from the norm, I believe that the gap between the autistic and ordinary worlds is a difference of culture. Every day, I prepare myself for the effort of bridging that gap. The responsibility is mine—after all, how many people in the ordinary world would even know how? I am an alien in a foreign culture, and while my skills at interaction have improved over the years, I am still and will always be an *auslander.*

Take eye contact, for example, maintaining an appropriate level of eye contact is an unconscious effort for most people. In autistic culture, however, eye contact is largely inappropriate, as it causes discomfort. Failure to make and maintain eye contact is expected. In the ordinary every day culture, eye contact is a critical communication point. Failure to maintain eye contact can represent either deceit or guilt; too much eye contact can represent either intimacy or threat. It can be very difficult to find the right balance.

Consider environment factors. Most people with Autism have a much greater sensitivity to sensory stimuli than do people in the outside world. I, myself, prefer working in a quiet, dimly lit room. Occasionally, I'll be happy to listen to loud music, but I try to be considerate of incursions into others' sensory borders. Since I am so distressed by stimuli I cannot control, I try not to impose on others the stimuli I choose for myself. My sense of peace is truly damaged when I'm forced to endure unwanted stimuli, especially sound.

Self-stimulating activities, called "stims," can serve as minor stress release activities. In my case, these are often rocking, bouncing, grinding and clicking my teeth, flicking my fingers, or kicking my legs or feet. And I'd prefer to do those things in quiet isolation, away from unwanted stimuli, until my energy reserves are restored.

Perhaps the most important imperative in communication is this: *listen to my words.* Do not try to understand me by reading into my tone of voice, my facial expressions, my body language, my pheromone levels, my horoscope. . . whatever. Like everybody else, I have body language, emotions, and spoken language. Apparently unlike everyone else, you're not likely to understand me better if you add meaning to my words by "reading between the lines." In fact, you're almost certain to get it wrong.

Furthermore, what I say can truly be taken at face value. I almost never lie. Lying makes me feel physically ill. If I sound upset and don't mention it in relation to our conversation, it's probably not relevant! Maybe there was a loud sound that upset me just before we started talking. Maybe I'm not upset and you've misread me altogether. Maybe I am distressed about something immediately relevant, but choose not to discuss it. In any event, literally *any event,* let it go!

EPIDEMIOLOGY

Since the 1960s, more than 30 epidemiological studies of ASD have shown an increase in prevalence from 4.4 per 10,000 during the period of 1966–1991 to an average of 12.7 per 10,000 during the period of 1992–2001 (Fombonne, 2001; see Figure 23.1-1). Gillberg, Steffenburg, and Schaumann (1991), in a total population study involving children 13 years and younger, suggested that the prevalence of autism and related conditions (excluding Asperger disorder) was 4 per 100,000 in 1980, 7.5 per 10,000 in 1984, and 11.6 per 10,000 in 1988.

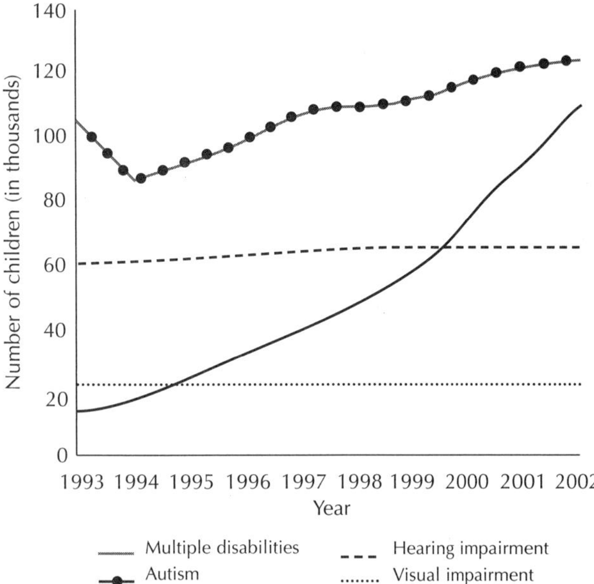

Figure 23.1-1. Trend in the number of children age 6–21 with certain low-incidence disabilities. (Reprinted from the U.S. Government Accountability Office. [2005, January]. *Special education: Children with autism* [p. 17]. Washington, DC: Author.)

Following a pilot prevalence study in Brick Township in New Jersey in 1988, a more recent Centers for Disease Control estimate of 3.4 per 1,000 for the prevalence of autism represents an almost eightfold increase from 1966–1991 and threefold increase from 1992–2001 (Yeargin-Allsopp et al., 2003). The observed increases in prevalence have been attributed to the broader DSM–IV (APA, 1994) definition of the disorder, increased public awareness, earlier diagnosis, change in diagnostic practices, better ascertainment of individuals with varying degrees of severity, and "diagnostic substitution" of autism for what in the past were attributed to mental retardation (Volkmar et al., 2004). Important methodological deficiencies in the data make it difficult to determine whether there has been a true increase in the prevalence of ASD since the case definition has been expanded and the age at diagnosis has decreased, both of which contribute to increased diagnosis (Fombonne, 2001). Nonetheless a true increase cannot as yet be ruled out.

Both the educational and health services have witnessed a dramatic rise in the number of younger children with autism and its broader subcategory of PDD-NOS. Furthermore, this pattern of administrative increase has risen consistently across all the states with three prevalence bands, 0–1.9, 2.0–3.9, and 4–6 per 1,000 children ages 6–17 in public schools in the United States with a total of 130,000 children with autism.

Neurobiology and Causal Factors

Several postmortem studies have highlighted areas of neuroanatomic abnormalities in the brains of individuals with ASD. Consistent findings have been observed in the limbic system, cerebellum, and related inferior olive. In the limbic system, the hippocampus, amygdala, and entorhinal cortex have shown small cell size and increased cell packing density at all ages, suggesting a pattern consistent with development curtailment. Findings in the cerebellum have included significantly reduced numbers of Purkinje cells, primarily in the posterior inferior regions of the hemispheres. A different pattern of change has been noted in the vertical limb of the diagonal band of broca, cerebellar nuclei, and inferior olive, with plentiful and abnormally enlarged neurons in the brains of young people with ASD, and small, pale neurons that are reduced in number in the brains of adults with ASD. These findings, combined with reported age-related changes in brain weight and volume, have raised the possibility that the neuropathology of ASD may represent an ongoing process.

Other anomalies described include larger third ventricles and smaller caudates, abnormal forebrain structures, a smaller right anterior cingulate gyrus, and smaller parietal lobes. A consistent finding has been that 14%–30% of individuals with ASD have a significant increase in head circumference, which has not been correlated with IQ score, verbal ability, seizure disorder, or medical illness. MRI studies have confirmed the increase in brain volume with an increase in the temporal, parietal, and occipital areas but not in the frontal lobes. The cause and specificity of this increase in size remain unexplained (Bauman & Kemper, 2005).

Twin studies have indicated that genetic factors play an important etiological role. A reexamination of the expanded set of individuals seen in the first British twin study found that 60% of monozygotic twins and 0% of dizygotic twins were concordant for the ICD–10 diagnosis of autism (Bailey et al., 1995). The variation was as great within monozygotic twins as between dizygotic twins. Because monozygotic twins share 100% of their genomic architecture, this finding suggested that the varying symptoms seen in autism were not a result of different sets of genes acting to produce different clinical features. It would appear that autism is under a high degree of genetic control but also that what is inherited is a broader spectrum of related cognitive and social abnormalities. Family studies have shown an increased loading for both autism and related disorders in the first-degree relatives of individuals with autism (Piven, Saliba, Bailey, & Arndt, 1997).

Approximately 2%–5% of children diagnosed with ASD have a concomitant fragile-X anomaly (Bailey et al., 1993). This statistic is not particularly high, but it does suggest that children with autism be screened for presence of a CGG triple-repeat abnormality in the Xq27 region. ASD and autism-like syndromes have been reported in approximately 40% of individuals with tuberous sclerosis, often associated with a seizure disorder.

Numerous reports describe putative chromosome abnormalities in individuals or small groups of individuals with ASD, but diagnostic shortcomings and failure to replicate the findings have left many of the findings in doubt. The most important studies have been the large multisite investigations whose initial findings are currently being reported. Investigators from the International Molecular Genetic Study of Autism Consortium (1998) carried out a two-stage genome search for susceptibility loci for ASD on 87 affected sibling pairs and 12 nonsibling affected relatives. The highest lod scores were obtained for regions on chromosome 7q and 16p, with lesser scores of interest on chromosomes 4, 10, 19, and 22. A few specific genes, such as the *RELN* gene on 7q and the *WNT2* gene, both expressed in the central nervous system, have also been linked to ASD in some families (Persico, D'Agruma, & Mairano, 2001; Wassink, Piven, & Vieland, 2001). Maternal transmission of genetic variations in the glutamate receptor 6 gene *(GRIK2)* on chromosome 6q21 has been seen in one sample (Jamain, Beatncur, & Quach, 2002). Another multicenter group has reported that the results of their linkage analysis studies were compatible with a model specifying a large number of loci (greater than 15), and less so with models specifying less than 10 loci.

Based on published studies, several different genes are likely to be implicated, and they may be different in different families (Folstein & Roren-Sheidly, 2001). Individuals with similar physical or behavioral findings might suggest a phenotype with a common underlying genetic cause. These findings might include macrocephaly, the presence of severe gastrointestinal symptoms, a history of developmental skill regression, and the presence of repetitive behaviors more evident than that seen in the typical phenotype.

Gene expression studies will hopefully help elucidate the role of environmental factors, such as neurotoxins, which have been posited to have a role in the etiology of ASD. Although these have not yet been proven, the interaction between these implicated genes and environmental factors are under investigation. For some time, there had been a concern about the etiological role of vaccines and, in particular, of the mercury-containing preservative Thimerosal in the vaccines; however, epidemiological studies have thus far failed to prove this association (Institute of Medicine, 2004; see Figure 23.1-2).

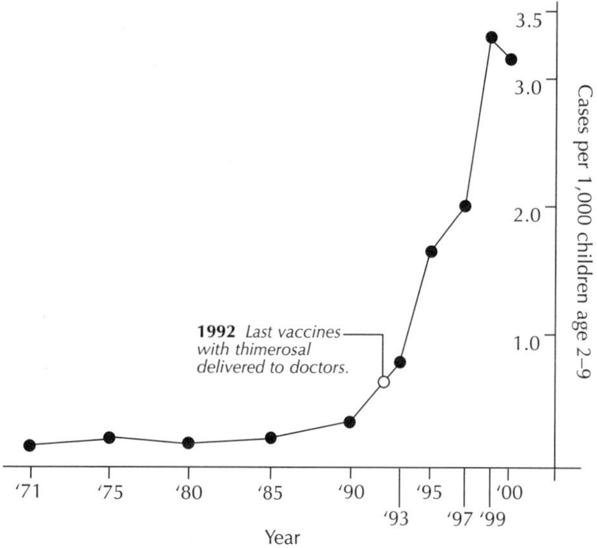

Figure 23.1-2. Autism rates in Denmark. Cases rose sharply even after the banning of Thimerosal, a mercury-containing vaccine preservative thought to cause autism. (From Madsen, K.M., Lauritsen, M.B., Pedersen, C.B., Thorsen, P., Plesner, A.M., Andersen, P.H., et al. [2004, September 13]. [Thirmerosal and the occurrence of autism: Negative ecological evidence from Danish registry data]. *Ugeskrift for Laeger, 166*(38), 3291–3293; reprinted by permission.)

DIAGNOSTIC ASSESSMENT MEASURES

For infants and young children, the diagnosis of ASD should be suspected if there has been a delay or unusual pattern of speech development often first noted in the first year of life, along with unusual patterns of communication, interaction, and socialization and unusual patterns of behavior that tend to be repetitive and/or ritualistic. The definitive diagnosis then can be made by using the DSM or ICD criteria listed previously or the diagnostic tests described below.

Screening

ASD must be diagnosed as early as possible so that appropriate intervention for the child and family can be instituted and an optimal outcome can be facilitated. The Centers for Disease Control have taken an initiative in this area and have developed nationwide strategies to alert the public as well as pediatricians, who are likely to be the first, and at times the only, professionals to see infants and young children during their critical developmental stages. Screening and developmental surveillance are primary functions of the physician in the context of the medical home (AAP, 1993; Johnson & Blasdo, 1997). Several screening programs are available to help facilitate screening within the medical community, including First Signs (www.firstsigns.org) and the Autistic Disorders Screening Kit from the Southwest Autism Research and Resource Center (SARRC) (Melmed, 2003).

Screening programs that incorporate tools such as the M-CHAT, a modified version of the Checklist for Autism in Toddlers (CHAT; Baird et al., 2000), require less than 10 minutes to administer and are early attempt to identify ASD in toddlers. The M-CHAT was developed as a consequence of the low sensitivity of the CHAT in the general population (Robins, Fein, Barton, & Green, 2001). Screening instruments are not used to make a definitive diagnosis of ASD but can and should be used to identify infants and young children who are in need of further diagnostic workup and/or referral for therapeutic services. The Childhood Autism Rating Scale (CARS; Schopler, Reichler, & Renner, 1988) is a more reliable instrument and is used diagnostically; however, reliance on parental information and perspective can reflect a bias in reporting.

Diagnosis

The "gold standard" research diagnostic instruments include the ADI-R, a semistructured parent or key caregiver interview (LeCouteur, Rutter, & Lord, 2003), and the ADOS (Lord et al., 2000), involving standardized judgments of a child's activities based on measures conceptualized on the three autism domains. The Diagnostic Interview for Social and Communication Disorders (DISCO; Wing et al., 2002) is another important semistructured interview that compiles extensive information on a subject's developmental history over a wide range of developmental domains. All three diagnostic instruments take considerable time to administer and require meticulous investment in training of raters to achieve 90% interrater reliability or higher.

Medical Diagnostic Consideration

The medical management of an individual with ASD typically involves the collection and interpretation of information regarding health and behavior. As appropriate, the child should be referred for speech therapy, occupational therapy, or any other necessary therapy. In addition, the family should be provided with information on the condition and referred to parent support groups in the community. Family members have many questions about the future, alternative therapies, and how much can and should be done. Clinicians should schedule a follow-up appointment because, when parents go home and ask questions of relatives or acquaintances and search on the Internet, even more questions will arise.

On general examination, the individual is assessed for nutritional status as a measure of health and growth, especially considering that many individuals with ASD have unusual dietary preferences and habits. Clinicians should look at any unusual physical characteristics that may suggest dysmorphic syndromes, though these represent a recognizable disorder in less than 25% of individuals (Gillberg & Coleman, 1996). A Wood's light examination to detect early hypopigmented lesions consistent with ash leaf macules is appropriate, particularly in children suspected of having seizures. These lesions might be the only sign suggestive of tuberous sclerosis as, in the younger child, facial angiofibromata may not yet be evident. Long facies, large ears, and large testes in postpubertal men are suggestive of fragile X syndrome, often accompanied by severe hyperactivity and gaze aversion (Gillberg & Coleman, 2001). An ataxic gait and broad mouth with persistent smile in a child with ASD might suggest Angelman syndrome.

When an underlying syndrome is suspected, a high-resolution chromosomal analysis and a deoxyribonucleic (DNA) analysis to detect fragile X syndrome is warranted. It is of particular importance to obtain these analyses in situations in which there is a family history of ASD, intellectual disabilities, or related disorders. Autistic behaviors are seen at an increased rate in individuals with several genetic, chromosomal, and metabolic disorders, such as tuberous sclerosis, fragile X syndrome, and a growing number of other conditions (e.g., duplication of 15q 11-13; Cook, Courchesne, & Cox, 1998).

FUNCTIONAL COMORBIDITIES

Communication/Language Disorders

Much of the research on language disorders in general separates the phenomenology into the four domains of phonology (sounds of language), syntax (grammar rules of language organization), semantics (content and vocabulary), and pragmatics (communicative competence). Individuals with impairments in social interaction and communication, or *semantic-pragmatic language deficits*, typically misunderstand implicit or explicit verbal messages and violate rules of conversational exchange. The issue that is present within this similarity of symptomatology is whether the communication impairments are part of ASD or whether they justify a secondary diagnosis of a language disorder.

It may be helpful to consider that the primary impairments observed in strict language disorders are in the area of language/communication. As opposed to the severe social impairments in ASD, social skills in language disorders are relatively preserved, and unusual restricted interests and repetitive movements are not present. The presence of receptive or comprehension language disorders, although highly underdiagnosed, is an important indicator of other phonological and pragmatic concerns and worsening social competence, which calls immediate attention to the need for detection of broad-based language disorders and for referral to speech-language pathologists.

Nonverbal Learning Disorder

Both Asperger disorder and PDD-NOS can co-occur in the presence of nonverbal learning disabilities, as noted by neuropsychological data cited by Klin et al. (1995) with impairments in visual-spatial organization, tactile-perceptual skills, psychomotor coordination, nonverbal problem solving, concept formation, sense of time, and social perception. Nonverbal learning disabilities involve dimensions that are strikingly similar to that of Asperger disorder because a child with nonverbal learning disabilities may have a behavior pattern of psychosocial and adaptive difficulties manifested by a marked failure to appreciate the nonverbal aspects of communication while maintaining well-developed language and verbal skills. Whereas nonverbal learning disability and Asperger disorder tend to share a neurocognitive profile, observable differences exist in terms of their manifestations of social relatedness. Individuals with Asperger disorder typically have a much more severe social disability. Further research will need to be conducted into the differences in social disability and neurological etiology of Asperger disorder and nonverbal learning disabilities in order to better understand their complex interrelationship.

Intellectual Disabilities

About 75% of children diagnosed with ASD meet criteria for intellectual disabilities, and this percentage is higher when the cognitive capacity is assessed by full-scale IQ scores (Volkmar et al., 2004). With increasing degree of cognitive and adaptive delays, the frequency of symptoms of ASD intensifies with an increased potential for diagnostic confusion. In an individual with a severe degree of intellectual disabilities, a comorbid diagnosis of ASD must include a careful evaluation of the social, communicative, sensory, and educational impairments relative to the person's overall developmental and intellectual levels. Once the developmental perspective has been considered as part of a thorough evaluation, a comorbid diagnosis of ASD with intellectual disabilities should not be made unless the individual demonstrates significant impairments in social skills (verbal or nonverbal), which are uncharacteristic of uncomplicated intellectual disabilities.

Although intellectual disabilities can often coexist with autism or related conditions, by definition, Asperger disorder *cannot* be comorbid with intellectual disabilities according to the cognitive nonimpairment criterion as delineated by the DSM-IV. Assessing cognitive and intellectual function on standard tests is difficult when an individual has a limited ability to communicate. Ultimately, however, the IQ score is not as critical as the Social Quotient.

BEHAVIORAL COMORBIDITIES

ASD has a significant association with behavior disorders. Questions arise whether the specific "behavior" or behavioral profile is in fact a "true comorbidity" or an exaggerated or unusual expression of an emotional reaction or an attempt to communicate in an individual who is nonverbal. Regardless of the underlying reason for the behavior, clinicians should try to sort out what the cardinal elements are in the individual and in the environment through a careful and thorough history, review of past medical and behavior treatments, and observations over a period of time.

PSYCHIATRIC COMORBIDITIES

True comorbidity can only adequately be determined in representative population-based studies that compare frequencies in contrasting groups and develop plausible etiological hypotheses. To date, the comorbidity of autism and associated conditions have not been systematically studied. In ASD, nonetheless, comorbidity is the rule rather than the exception. Comorbid conditions can interfere with functioning and can be an impediment to progress in educational or vocational settings. Irrespective of the ASD and Asperger disorder dichotomy, considerable interest in various case reports have focused on the issue of psychiatric comorbidity with conditions such as obsessive-compulsive disorder, psychotic disorder-NOS, schizophrenia, attention-deficit/hyperactivity disorder (ADHD), depression, Tourette syndrome (see Chapter 12.4), and mood or bipolar disorder.

The critical issues surrounding an association between these developmental and behavioral conditions are whether such associations occur at levels greater than would be expected by chance alone and whether the symptoms and behavioral manifestations observed are best viewed as part of ASD, Asperger disorder, or PDD-NOS, or as the manifestation of some other condition. The ability to effectively discriminate between a comorbid diagnosis and varied symptomatology is further hindered when evaluating younger children who are nonverbal or who have significant intellectual disabilities. Sometimes, the true nature of the disorder(s) becomes clear only over the course of development with longitudinal evaluations.

EVALUATING BEHAVIORAL DISORDERS

Antecedents and consequences of any symptom, along with the context and the timing of that symptom, will help distinguish between symptoms that are either situational or pervasive in nature. Whether a symptom occurs in a variety of settings (e.g., at home, on the school bus, in the work place) and throughout the course of the day or manifests only in the evenings might be helpful. Determining the temporal relationship of the symptoms to mealtimes, to toileting events, and to other activities of daily living, especially those demanding attention and effort, might help distinguish various types of gastrointestinal symptomatology. The time of onset of a symptom, its frequency and duration, and the individual's developmental stage are also useful to examine. The identification of psychological stressors, such as a move, a new teacher, and a new roommate is important. Consider Zachary's situation.

Zachary was diagnosed as having ASD at a relatively young age. At 45, he was nonverbal, had limited eye contact and communication, and preferred to be on his own. Although he did know and relate to his family members, he did not care for unfamiliar people. He had very specific likes and dislikes that included a real dislike for noises and bright lights. He also had repetitive mannerisms and patterns of activity. His medical conditions included a seizure disorder, which, was managed on medication, and constipation which was managed by diet.

Zachary lived at home with his parents until they passed away when he was 40 years old. His two devoted sisters arranged for him to live in a group where they could visit often. When his sisters brought him to the residential facility, they reported that he needed 12 hours of sleep and that if he did not have enough sleep, he became agitated. They also reported that he became agitated with constipation or any kind of pain. They described some obsessive elements and some self-injurious behaviors, particularly if he became anxious.

Zachary seemed to do well in the group home for about 4 years but experienced a sudden change in behavior. Whereas in the past he liked to sit in a rocking chair and rock back and forth, he now paced the floor. In fact, his intense and persistent pacing would cause him to sweat. In addition, his sleeping patterns changed. His need for sleep seemed to diminish, and he only needed a few hours sleep. Sometimes, he did not sleep at all and instead paced all night. Because of his insomnia, Zachary was prescribed lorazepam, which worked initially but soon wore off. The dose was steadily increased until it reached a dose of 2 mg in the morning and 4 mg at night.

Zachary was also having behavioral outbursts day and night, which were managed with lorazepam prn, and, if this medication did not work, Zachary was given haloperidol. Zachary was seeing a psychiatrist for his challenging behaviors and was treated on a variety of psychoactive medications. In addition, Zachary's seizures had increased, so his neurologist had modified his anticonvulsants.

A review of Zachary's situation revealed that multiple physicians were prescribing medications. The consultant decided that the first step to understand the causes and therefore the management of Zachary's behavior was to appoint one physician in charge of changing his medication. The lorazepam was clearly not helping Zachary sleep as much as he should and was making him drowsy and weak. For this reason, the physician decided to wean Zachary quite rapidly off the lorazepam and haloperidol.

Second, Zachary's history of constipation led to a review of his bowel charts. An x-ray of his abdomen revealed stool throughout his ascending transverse and descending colon. Aggressive management of his constipation was recommended. In addition, a gastrointestinal workup revealed *Helicobacter pylori,* which was also treated.

A review of a videotape of Zachary's behavior revealed Zachary pacing back and forth in his residence with his left hand cupped over his left ear, his right-hand fingers across his eyes, and his right-hand thumb across the opening of his right ear. In the background, one could hear a lot of noise from a television set and people talking and shouting. On direct questioning the staff recalled that Zachary preferred quiet and dark environments to noisy and bright ones.

Apparently, when Zachary first moved into the residential facility from home, his roommate understood and respected his need for darkness and quiet and would even tiptoe around when he was near. This roommate was moved from the residence around July, and a new roommate took his place. The new roommate liked to play the guitar, listen

Table 23.1-2. Potential side effects of medications in individuals with autism

Medication class	Potential side effects
Decongestants	Agitation
Antihistamines	Sedation, disinhibition
Anticonvulsants	Irritability, activation, drowsiness, dizziness, personality changes, clumsiness, nystagmus, gingival hypertrophy, rash, hirsutism, alopecia, diploplia, confusion, dyspepsia, photophobia, hyperphagia
Stimulants and nonstimulants	Agitation, aggressiveness, stereotypies, tics, isolatory behaviors, loss of appetite, nausea, lethargy
Mood stabilizers, neuroleptics	Tremor, weakness, posturing, dyskinesias, autonomic movements, agitation, weight gain
Serotonin reuptake inhibitors	Agitation, hyperactivity, sleep disruption, constipation, weight gain, constipation

to the radio, and keep the lights on. If Zachary would try and switch off the lights, the roommate would turn them back on. This change coincided exactly with Zachary's change in sleeping patterns, pacing back and forth, increased outbursts of agitation, and change in seizure activity, which resulted in changes to his medication and worsening of his symptoms.

In light of this knowledge, Zachary's living arrangement was changed, his roommate was moved out, the television set was kept off when Zachary was there, and the lights were dimmed. After the treatment of Zachary's constipation, the rearrangement of his environment, and the reduction in his medication, his sleep pattern and behavior began to improve. The physician then proceeded to slowly wean him off all of his psychotropic medication. At the time of writing, Zachary is only an anticonvulsant medication, which is controlling his seizures very well, and his behavior has returned to his previous status.

Table 23.1-3. Common symptoms of distress expressed by individuals with autism

Self-injurious behaviors including head banging
Aggressive behaviors
Agitation
Self-stimulatory behaviors
Sleep disorders (e.g., increased difficulty in going to sleep, more frequent nighttime wakening)
Regression and loss of skills
Regression in toilet training
Behavior regression
Masturbation
Poor attention and increased distractibility and hyperactivity
Rectal digging and fecal smearing
Excessive eating
Weight gain or weight loss
Increase in toe walking

An inquiry into all medications as well as nutritional supplements is very important, as some may be a clue to the etiology of many symptoms. Side effects from medications include sleep disruption and neuromotor symptoms such as tics, dyskinesias, and alterations of temperament (see Table 23.1-2). In addition, medical conditions can cause discomfort or distress and trigger behavioral manifestations. Gastrointestinal symptoms (e.g., abdominal pain associated with gastroesophageal reflux and/or *H. pylori*) and constipation are perhaps the most common conditions associated with unexplained expressions of distress, including what is commonly termed "intermittent explosive behavior." Table 23.1-3 lists possible behavioral manifestations, and Table 23.1-4 lists medical conditions that should be explored in a systematic way.

Table 23.1-4. The range of possible medical conditions that should be explored when an individual with autism presents with one of the symptoms in Table 23.1-3

Head and neck
Head—headache, migraine
Eyes—visual disturbances, eye pain
Ear, nose, and throat—sore throat, ear infections, sinusitis, headache, dental pain
Dental—toothache, abscess, nerve root sensitivity
Jaw—temporomandibular joint dysfunction
Neck—muscle spasm, cervical spine problems
Chest
Lungs—difficulty breathing (e.g., asthma, pain, pleurisy)
Heart—palpitations, ischemic heart disease
Ribs—fracture
Abdomen, gastrointestinal, and genitourinary tracts
Upper gastrointestinal tract—gastroesophageal reflux, gastritis, *Helicobacter pylori*
Lower gastrointestinal tract—constipation, colic, hemorrhoids, appendicitis, obstruction, volvulus
Other gastrointestinal areas—hepatitis, pancreatitis, cholecystitis
Renal—infection, renal colic
Bladder—urinary tract infection, urethritis, bladder spasm
Female genitalia—menstrual discomfort, uterine pain, vaginitis (commonly monilial), other infections (especially if sexually active)
Male genitalia—orchitis, epididymitis, testicular torsion
Musculoskeletal system
Muscles—synovitis, myalgias/fibromyalgia, stiff muscles from excessive exercise, myositis, muscle spasm
Bones and joints—fractures, bursitis, arthritis, osteomyelitis
Vertebral column—backache, nerve root compression
Systemic issues
Medications—side effects, adverse effects, drug interactions
Infections—flu
Autoimmune—juvenile rheumatoid arthritis, discoid lupus erythematosus
Environment—sensory, allergies, toxins, changes in place, objects or people

NEUROLOGICAL AND MEDICAL COMORBIDITIES

As noted previously, as many as 30% of children with isolated ASD have an occipitofrontal circumference greater than the 97th percentile (Lainhart, Piven, & Wzorek, 1997; see Chapter 12.1). Macrocephaly evident at 1 or 2 years of age might not have been apparent at birth. In the absence of focal neurological signs, computed tomography or magnetic resonance imaging is not usually helpful.

Common comorbid neuromotor disorders include muscle hypotonia and coordination disorders that manifest in motor planning problems and can result in fine, gross, oral, and visual motor dysfunction and dyspraxias, which significantly affect the acquisition of functional skills. In addition, sensory integration disorders are common diagnoses that are made particularly by occupational therapists and reflect a set of unusual sensory-driven reactions and behaviors. Hypersensitivities to sound and touch can result in agitation, irritability, and other behaviors. Taste sensitivities can result in severely restricted diets. Insensitivity to pain can even result in delayed identification of fractures. Sensitivities to smell and temperature can also manifest in unusual ways.

Tic-like behaviors appear to occur not infrequently and may be confused with the repetitive stereotypic behaviors common to ASD. They can present in a variety of ways, and exploration of other repetitive behaviors of recent onset, including blurting out, might point to comorbid Tourette syndrome or may be an expression of an underlying anxiety disorder. Tic-like behaviors might even reflect underlying medical conditions (e.g., chronic sniffing and repetitive coughing could indicate environmental allergies) or they can be exacerbated by the use of psychostimulant medications and by any anxiety-provoking situation, including exposure to noxious sensory stimuli and novel social situations.

Seizures

Seizures are present in approximately 20%–35% of children with ASD and have two peaks of onset—during early childhood and during adolescence, at which time they are often accompanied by behavioral regression (Minshew, 1991; see Chapter 12.2). Seizures are more common in those with severe cognitive impairments and are also more likely to occur in girls. Concern exists as to whether seizures might herald the sudden onset of regression sometimes seen in toddlers with ASD (Minshew, Sweeney, & Bauman, 1997). Landau-Kleffner syndrome (acquired epileptic aphasia) is characterized by language regression, presenting often in the second and third year of life. A sleep electroencephalogram (EEG) throughout all four stages of sleep is indicated in those with symptoms of developmental regression along with clinical seizures or in situations in which there is a high suspicion of subclinical seizures (Filipek, Accardo, & Baranek, 1999; Tuchman, Rapin, & Shinnar, 1991). Concomitant medications may alter the seizure threshold or may interact with anticonvulsants to either enhance or to diminish their effectiveness.

Fourteen-year-old Abdul experienced unexplained aggression. He had been diagnosed with ASD at age 2 years and had always had a very easy-going temperamental style. His adjustment to a middle school program for individuals with special needs had been unremarkable. His teachers and parents had reported a recent onset of frequent violent outburst that were both uncharacteristic as well as unexplained by any environmental factors. An EEG was performed, and a pattern consistent with minor motor seizures was seen. Anticonvulsants were initiated, with an almost immediate cessation of any violent behaviors.

Some seizures can be subclinical (see Table 23.1-5); thus, a high index of clinical suspicion is called for. These signs include poor memory for routine events (e.g., getting on the bus, getting undressed), a loss of speech and memory skills, diminished responsiveness in general, and engaging in behaviors outside of the individual's usual repertoire. More commonly seen are staring spells, spacing out, dizzy spells, eye blinking, repetitive mouth movements, and unexplained aggression.

Seizures can be difficult to identify because of the child's atypical, repetitive, and/or ritualistic behaviors. Effective treatment can, however, be achieved with an early and accurate diagnosis, though individuals with ASD are likely to require long-term anticonvulsant therapy. If localizing findings are present in an individual with unexplained neurological symptomatology, such as loss of consciousness or ataxia, magnetic resonance

Table 23.1-5. Subclinical signs of seizures

Poor memory (out of character)
Staring, spacing or dizzy spells
Eye blinking
Repetitive mouth movements
Speech or memory loss
Poor response to name and diminished responsiveness in general
Unexplained aggression
Behaviors outside the individuals usual repertoire

imaging may be helpful. It is not likely, however, to be helpful when neurological symptoms are absent or with isolated macrocephaly (Filipek, Accardo, & Ashwal, 2000; Filipek, 1999).

Sleep Disorders

Anywhere between 56% and 83% of individuals with ASD have sleep-related challenges (Clements, Wing, & Dunn 1986). A variety of symptoms such as daytime irritability, inattention, and lethargy can result as a consequence of inadequate sleep. Types of sleep problems commonly encountered include refusing to go to bed, getting out of bed, tantrums at bedtime, early waking, and requiring a parent to sleep with the child. Richdale and Prior (1995) reported that 50%–80% of individuals with ASD have difficulty falling asleep, 60% have difficulty staying asleep, and 25%–50% have early morning arousal difficulties.

As the severity of developmental challenges increases, so does the prevalence and severity of sleep disorders. Although typically developing infants appear to learn very early on from environmental cues how, when, and for how long to sleep, those with cognitive challenges might not respond as readily to such cues. This underlines the importance of establishing firm and highly regulated sleep hygiene schedules from very early on (Jan & Freeman, 2004; Rivkees, 2003).

It can be helpful to provide families with a template to document the individual's sleep–wake cycle. This provides both the clinicians and parents a more objective measure of the number of hours of sleep as well as the sleep–wake pattern. It is also helpful in observing changes when instituting and monitoring interventions. At times, the graph can indicate either that the number of hours of sleep (although reduced) is adequate for the individual or that a small modification in the ritual of going to sleep (e.g., eliminating sensory distractions before bed, no television in the bedroom) makes a big difference.

Sleep difficulties can also be a consequence of side effects of medications (including psychostimulants), environmental allergies, asthma, gastroesophageal reflux, and other pain syndromes. Pain is a common cause of irritability, particularly of nighttime irritability. For example, a child who wakens in the middle of the night screaming, agitated, and irritable might have an underlying esophagitis secondary to reflux. This condition might explain reports of a subgroup of children with nighttime wakening and irritability being responsive to treatment with Pepcid (Linday, Tsiouris, et al., 2001). Sleep apnea is sometimes accompanied by snoring and bruxism and can be a significant cause of hyperactivity and irritability the next day.

In a review of pharmacological interventions, melatonin has been found to be helpful and safe in inducing and maintaining sleep in some children with ASD and sleep disorders (Niederhofer, Staffen, Mair, & Pittschieler, 2003); however, when considering other medications, caution must be exercised as the side effects of the medications may outweigh the benefits they provide. Clonidine is commonly used at night but should likely be preceded with an electrocardiogram and frequent checks of pulse and blood pressure. It can be started at very low doses and titrated slowly up to efficacy. If untoward side effects occur, clonidine should be discontinued and tapered cautiously.

Medication in general (including antihistamines, antidepressants, and hypnotics) should be used with extreme caution as paradoxical effects and other undesirable side effects are common. Even when medications prove to be effective, periodic attempts at discontinuing them is appropriate to evaluate continuing positive effects and to ensure that those outweigh any possible adverse effects.

Gastrointestinal Disorders

Mining of the database of individuals with ASD at SARRC has lead to several findings including the co-occurrence of significant gastrointestinal symptomatology in individuals with autism. In that unselected population, 25% of the individuals had chronic diarrhea and a further 25% had chronic constipation (see Chapter 14.2). In total, approximately 50% of the individuals had chronic gastrointestinal dysfunction, which was significant when compared to their brothers, sisters, and unrelated controls (Melmed, Schneider, et al., 2000). Others have reported a high prevalence of mild to moderate degrees of inflammation in both the upper and lower intestinal tract along with pathological intestinal permeability, as well as decreased digestive enzyme activity (Horvath & Perman, 2002). Treatment of these gastrointestinal problems appeared to have positive effects on certain presenting problematic behaviors.

Genitourinary Disorders

The most common genitourinary symptoms seen in ASD are enuresis and polyuria (see Chapter 21). Nighttime dryness before age 7 is unusual. For those with nocturnal enuresis at older than 7 years of age who fail to respond to behavioral or nonmedical means, desmopressin (DDAVP) and imipramine may be considered.

In the presence of polyuria, polydypsia should be excluded. Masturbation is a common concern of caregivers. In the case of priapism, a close medication review is warranted and in other situations urethritis needs to be considered.

Caregivers of 19-year-old Jared, a nonverbal man living in a group home, were concerned about his excessive masturbatory behavior. Behavioral treatments to address what was considered to be a self-stimulatory behavior were unsuccessful. A urinanalyis and a urethral swab were performed, and a non-specific urethritis was diagnosed, which was responsive to treatment. The masturbation ceased.

Dental Conditions

Individuals with ASD may resist tooth brushing, which puts them at higher risk for dental caries and periodontal disease (see Chapter 22). Pain caused by dental problems will very likely aggravate any underlying behavioral challenges an individual with ASD might have. Unrecognized dental problems have been reported to result in face slapping in an adolescent with cognitive impairment (Lacamera & Lacamera, 1997). Extra vigilance of dental health is required if gums are swollen or bleeding, if food intake has dropped off, or if oral self-stimulatory behaviors are present.

Nine-year-old Kaili had a history of extreme nighttime irritability and disordered sleep. After weeks of unsuccessful treatment with psychoactive medications, examination of her gum margin revealed a draining dental abscess. Following treatment of the abscess, her sleep patterns returned to normal, and her irritability resolved.

Ear, Nose, and Throat Conditions

In early infancy, hearing impairment is often a concern because of the delay in speech development. One of the common features of ASD is the situation in which the individual does not respond to his or her name being called (even though he or she might hear a softer sound from another source). Hearing testing should be performed regularly. Sensitivity to sound is more common with individuals covering their ears in noisy environments or crowds. In this situation, earplugs can be very helpful. In a group of 199 children and adolescents with ASD, mild to moderate hearing loss was diagnosed in 7.9%, and unilateral hearing loss in 1.6%, of those who could be tested. Severe to profound bilateral hearing loss or deafness was diagnosed in 3.5% of all cases, representing a prevalence considerably more than that seen in the general population and comparable to the prevalence found in individuals with intellectual disabilities.

Otitis media can be a common problem and can either cause pain, which may be expressed in a change in behavior, or go undetected because of insensitivity to pain. Chronic otitis can result in a conductive hearing loss, which in turn can manifest as increased withdrawal, confusion, or even disorientation. Hearing loss can aggravate underlying communication and behavior problems, such as frustration and ease of agitation. Otitis media should thus be considered and ruled out in the face of a prolonged "cold," increased irritability or lethargy, head-banging, and lack of responsiveness to sound. In addition, the rate of serous otitis media (23.5%) and related conductive hearing loss (18.3%) appeared to be increased in ASD. Similar concerns have been seen in adults with ASD (Stoddart, McColl, Lowe, & Temple, 2003).

Overall these issues emphasize the need for close audiological scrutiny of individuals with ASD in order to detect possible deterioration of hearing status, to uncover reasons for unexplained behavioral regression, and to identify comorbid or confounding disorders.

Eye Conditions

Ophthalmological problems are more common in ASD than in the typical population. These problems are often missed but can be misdiagnosed, as was the case with 8-year-old Joseph, as a behavior problem. His story, which is described by his mother, concerned an unrecognized error in prescription lenses.

Nothing is obvious when your child can't communicate. At Joseph's eye check-up, we discovered his lenses had been reversed since being replaced 6 months earlier—his right lens was ten times too powerful, and he had almost no correction for his legally blind left eye. I replayed in my mind all these times I had forced him to wear the glasses. He would have a tantrum and throw them off his face. He couldn't say, "Mommy, I can't see."

Cardiovascular

Palpitations can be a side effect of psychostimulant medications, nonstimulants, as well as antidepressants and antihypertensives. Orthostatic hypotension and fainting can result from the use of clonidine and guanfacine. Again, the expression of the symptoms may be unusual; hence, the critical need to be aware of conditions that might occur and constantly look for medical conditions that may explain unusual behaviors (see Table 23.1-4).

INTERVENTIONS

Psychosocial and Educational Programs

The most important psychosocial and educational interventions for children with ASD and related disorders include the Treatment and Education of Autistic and Related Communication Handicapped CHildren (TEACCH), Applied Behavioral Analysis (ABA), Floor Time, social stories, and Picture Exchange Communication System (PECS). The TEACCH approach, established by Mesibov and Schopler at the University of North Carolina, is one of the oldest strategies with a worldwide following that supports individuals with ASD throughout the life span. It is based on a person's interests and motivation to learn in a structured educational environment. The approach is clearly organized with an emphasis on visual learning modalities; it uses functional concepts and individualized curricula. Strategies in special education, such as speech therapy and occupational therapy, are supported, and additional therapies such as PECS and Floor Time, among others, are accommodated. The TEACCH approach identifies the individual's emerging skill sets and targets them for highest probability of success, rewards, and reduction of stress. For the program to be properly implemented, training and consultation are necessary, in addition to collaborative work with parents as cotherapists.

ABA is also known as the Lovaas (1987), Discrete Trials (DT), or Intensive Behavioral Interventions (IBI) methods. It involves intensive social and language one-on-one sessions through the use of positive reinforcement based on the ABC model (i.e., A = antecedent, B = behavior, and C = consequence). The child develops skills in receptive and expressive language, attending, listening, imitation, and self-help. The ABA approach seems to be most effective for those children with mild to moderate functional impairments. The cost of the more intensive treatment schedules may prohibit equal access to ABA treatment in some communities. It is also important to recognize that a given child's unique set of neurological, sensory, and processing characteristics may modify the interpretation of behavioral outcomes in using this approach.

Floor Time is a developmental, individual-difference and relationship-based (DIR) approach stressing social and personal interactions that are child directed (Greenspan, 1995). The approach targets a child's emotional developmental capacity and is highly dependent on intuitive observations of a child's responses. The Floor Time, or Greenspan approach, incorporates semi-structured, sensory, and motor play components. Floor Time views the child as a functionally integrated unit and does not focus on specific cognitive impairments areas. The program is implemented in 20-minute sessions with alternating 20-minute breaks addressing developmental delays through sensory modulation, motor planning, and perceptual processing elements.

Social Stories, or social scripts, developed by Gray in 1991, help a child with ASD to understand social rules, address theory of mind deficits, and provide a guide for self-management in specific social situations. Social scripts are specific to the child's needs. There are three types of scripts: perspective taking, descriptive, and directive. The strategy addresses social impairments to help alleviate anxiety and improve social behaviors. A balanced mix of sentences is important as is a program that is not excessively directive. The stories should not use overly complex language or writing cues. Modification of this strategy may include classwide group activities, peer-based interactions, videotaped sessions stressing acquisition of social skills in everyday contexts, transitional situations, and play to gain insight into another's social perspectives.

PECS helps young children with ASD who are preverbal to build language skills through the use of pictures, encouraging them to spontaneously initiate communicative interactions and to develop communicative competence. The PECS approach is based on a broader appreciation of communication (i.e., the differentiation between communicating and talking). This program assists the child to progress through eight steps beginning with initially rewarded functional acts. In addressing social-communication impairments in autism, the program appears to augment language development rather than hinder it.

These approaches, among many others, have been based on specific theoretical frameworks rather than founded on empirical research establishing their validity (Volkmar et al., 2004); nonetheless, children with ASD benefit greatly from psychoeducational and behavioral programs when 1) observational data is integrated in evaluating individual outcomes; 2) flexible and creative strategies are used that accommodate other therapies and supports; and 3) learning strategies are

Table 23.1-6. Model educational and vocational programs

Support the individual's unique learning needs
Are fun, predictable, and routine without tedium and television
Encourage family involvement on a regular basis
Teach behavioral skills training for family members
Incorporate a wide range of modalities, including speech therapy, augmentative communication, occupational therapy, social skills training, recreational opportunities, and animal assisted therapy
Foster inclusion and integrating opportunities

introduced that emphasize visual rather than auditory presentations (see Table 23.1-6).

Medical Treatment Approaches

The goal of all interventions, therapies, and medical treatments is to promote optimal growth and development and ensure optimal physical, emotional, and social well-being (World Health Organization definition of *health*). Medical, developmental, behavioral, and educational intervention strategies can reduce the frequency and intensity of behavioral and physical disturbances, such as seizures, sleep disorders, agitation, encopresis, self-injurious behavior, anxiety, hyperactivity, impulsiveness, and aggression (AAP Guidelines, 2001). Treatment of individuals with ASD involves multimodal approaches. Interventions such as parental support and counseling, behavior modification, special education, sensory integration therapy, speech ther-apy, and social skill training will help to assure optimal outcome.

The goals of treatment programs are to minimize core symptoms, prevent harmful behaviors (e.g., aggression, self-injurious behaviors), facilitate access to intervention programs, maximize beneficial effects of non-medical interventions, and improve the quality of life for the child and the family (AAP Guidelines, 2001). Treatment is aimed at helping to facilitate improved functionality in community settings. All concerned parties should understand the indications for, side effects of, and limitations of any therapeutic intervention.

The individual with ASD should be involved in the treatment process as much as possible, despite any developmental limitations. Every effort should be made to help the individual understand the reasons for the treatment, expected results, and possible side effects. This approach will prevent the development of negative attitudes or misperceptions toward the use of the medication in these individuals. When this is done, the individual with ASD becomes an effective partner in the intervention (Tsai, 2001).

MANAGEMENT OF CHALLENGING BEHAVIORS

Where necessary and possible, a functional behavioral analysis should be carried out before the initiation of pharmaceutical intervention. Other factors to be considered, aside from the appropriateness of an individual's educational or vocational program, include deciding whether the targeted symptoms might more likely respond to educational or behavioral interventions. When considering pharmacological intervention, one or two behaviors are targeted at a time.

Once target outcomes are identified, they are assigned a rating of frequency, duration or severity. Baseline ratings of these symptoms are obtained. These target behaviors may change as the child grows older or progresses developmentally or more likely when the goals are either met or missed and a reassessment becomes necessary. If target outcomes are not met, a re-evaluation of the treatment plan is in order to reconsider the scope of treatments and the challenges with compliance or adherence to the plan by all those involved in the individual care. The presence of other disorders that might be compounding or aggravating the underlying problems is considered. Specifying appropriate target outcomes, especially when long-term treatment is envisioned, can help parents who are often overwhelmed and need encouragement. Symptom severity monitoring should in and of itself help to provide positive reinforcement to caregivers, especially when improvements in functioning, however small, can be ascertained.

Pharmacological Interventions

Pharmacological intervention should be carefully considered in association with a clear sense of what is being treated and what the expected outcomes are. Intervention can be grouped into three categories, with the goal of

1. Improvement of interfering symptoms associated with the *core syndrome* (e.g., interfering stereotyped repetitive behaviors, regressive social withdrawal); however, to date, despite much controversy, there is no medication (psychotropic or otherwise) that is specifically effective in treating the social and relationship problems in ASD.

2. Improvement of *secondary symptoms* commonly associated with ASD (e.g., inattention, disruptive behaviors, tantrums, self-injurious, or aggressive behaviors). These symptoms can also occur as a

maladaptive response to transitions, sensory stimulation, poor communication ability, and regulatory skills; thus, it is important to address these concerns with a combined behavioral modification and pharmacological approach.

3. Improvement of *co-occurring disorders and symptoms* comorbid with ASD as outlined previously

There is a paucity of well-designed randomized clinical trials in children and adolescents with ASD. As a first general principle, it is important to start with the lowest recommended dose and titrate it upward slowly, as individuals with ASD, particularly in the presence of intellectual disabilities, may be particularly sensitive to side effects, such as disinhibition, irritability, and reduced sleep. Their interpretation of the physical sensation of the side effect might also vary significantly. Principles of prescribing medication in individuals with ASD are outlined in Table 23.1-7.

Periodic discontinuation of medication can be appropriate. Treatment may not be needed when behavioral and environmental variables are in flux. These variables would include biorhythms, home stressors, paternal or maternal depression, school difficulties, and problems with inclusion. October and February are good times to consider discontinuation as routines are then usually set and no major disruptions in school are expected. Weaning must be performed slowly. Discontinuity syndromes may result from accelerated weaning schedules from stimulants as well as antidepressants.

Clinicians working with individuals with ASD should familiarize themselves with the need for combined psychosocial and educational strategies and should not prescribe medications with inadequate information, aiming, for example, for symptom suppression seemingly without consideration of the potential negative impact of the medication on the demeanor, adaptive functioning, or quality of life of the individual. A child who is acting up secondary to a great deal of sensory stimulation in an inappropriate educational setting is unlikely to respond to short-term pharmacological strategies, especially if this strategy is urgently requested as a means of behavioral control. Pharmacological interventions, therefore, should be integrated as part of a child's individualized educational program.

Obstacles to the success of such an integrated approach might be 1) lack of any defined behavioral interventions; 2) lack of communication between the prescribing physician and the behavior therapist in the presence of a specific behavioral plan; 3) no systematic behavioral data collection; 4) poorly justified use or inappropriate choice of medications; 5) misclassification of symptoms and secondary disorders (e.g., calling all problems with inattention ADHD, labeling transitional difficulties as overanxious disorder and poor frustration tolerance and irritability as mood or bipolar disorder); 6) prescription of medications for extended periods of time with limited consideration of dynamic changes in the child's environment and availability (or lack thereof) of supports; and 7) use of polypharmacy regimens with little or no attempt over time to reduce medication doses, document ongoing overall needs, and achieve the lowest effective dose.

Table 23.1-7. Principles in prescribing medication for behavior

1. Monotherapy is best!
2. Start low, and increase slowly.
3. Taper any medication slowly and cautiously.
4. Monitor side effects at each visit by history, physical, and laboratory testing.
5. See patient frequently, and measure vital signs and growth parameters.
6. Periodic discontinuation is advisable.

Reproduced with permission from *Pediatrics,* Vol. 107(5), Pages 1221–1226, Copyright © 2001 by the AAP.

REVIEW OF MEDICATIONS

The topography of medication for individuals with ASD is changing rapidly. For example, the traditional antidepressants (e.g., tricyclics), antianxiety medications (e.g., benzodiazepines), and antipychotics or neuroleptic agents (e.g., thioridazine, haloperidol) that were once popular are no longer recommended. In the following discussion, only the salient usages of major groups of pharmacological agents are discussed.

Stimulants and Nonstimulant Medications

Individuals with ASD can have comorbid ADHD regardless of their level of functioning (Ehlers & Gilberg, 1993). Clinical manifestations of both disorders have neurodevelopmental and executive functioning impairments in common. A number of long-acting stimulant medications (e.g., Adderall XR, Concerta, Metadate, Ritalin-LA) and new noradrenergic agents (e.g., Strattera [atomoxetine], Focalin-LA) have been successful in targeting individuals with ADHD, which has translated to their use in targeting symptoms of ADHD in children with ASD and related disorders. A concern with the use of stimulants in ASD has been the observation that they can be "activating" and lead to irritability, lability, and agitation. Sleep difficulties, overly selective patterns of food preference, increased social isolation, aggression, agitation, and an increase in stereotypical behaviors may be seen (Aman & Langworthy, 2000).

When using stimulants in young children with ASD, particular caution is advised. The efficacy of the stimulants for improving attention span in children with ASD has not been systematically appraised, with the exception of suggestions that individuals with Asperger disorder with higher cognitive, verbal, and adaptive functioning might be more responsive. Pharmacological studies of the treatment of ADHD in ASD have at best led to mixed results. Nonetheless, as the relative index of safety of these medications is quite high, many clinicians nevertheless initiate an empirical trial of a stimulant or nonstimulant under circumstances that are clinically warranted. Starting at lower than typically recommended dosages and titrating slowly is the rule.

Antidepressants

Although tricyclic antidepressants, such as imipramine and desipramine, were initially popular, potential cardiovascular side effects along with lack of perceived efficacy have led to their being supplanted by newer antidepressants. The selective serotonin reuptake inhibitors (SSRIs) appear to be moderately effective in decreasing interfering symptoms of anxiety associated with transitions and sensory stimulation, as well as in aiding with interfering repetitive thoughts, rituals, and preoccupations akin to obsessive-compulsive behaviors. The SSRIs also may decrease hyperactivity, restlessness, and agitation if they mitigate underlying interfering symptoms (often interpreted as anxiety) that may lead to such secondary behaviors.

No single SSRI has been shown to be superior for this purpose. Controlled trials with fluoxetine and fluvoxamine in adults with ASD showed significant benefits over placebo, although a subsequent controlled trial of fluvoxamine in children and adolescents revealed a lower response (McDougle et al., 2000). A recent open-label study using low-dose fluvoxamine reported a response in only 17% of individuals (Martin et al., 2003). SSRIs are used in practice to treat depression, anxiety, and obsessive, compulsive and ritualistic behaviors (Delong, Teague, & McSwain Kamran, 1998; Steingard, Zimnitzky, DeMaso, Bauman, & Bucci, 1997). Once again, the rule of starting at dosages lower than those used in the typical population and titrating very slowly will help alleviate many adverse effects.

Alpha agonists

The use of clonidine hydrochloride and guanfacine hydrochloride can effect a modest reduction in impulsivity, hyperactivity, and irritability; it is less beneficial in ameliorating social behaviors (McDougle, 1997; Jaselskis, Cook, & Fletcher, 1992). Drowsiness has been reported as a main side effect and often can target sleep difficulties commonly reported in young children with autism and related disorders.

Atypical Neuroleptics

The main target symptoms potentially responsive to atypical neuroleptics include severe tantrums and disruptive behaviors, agitation, aggressive behaviors, comorbid major affective disorders, and, more rarely, psychosis. In those who are unresponsive to behavioral interventions, psychopharmacological treatments are considered. Risperidone is the most studied among the major atypical neuroleptics among children and adolescents with ASD (McDougle et al., 1998). The Research Units in Pediatric Psychopharmacology (RUPP) Autism Network (2002), funded as part of a National Institutes of Health multisite trial, looked at the safety and efficacy of risperidone in 100 children and adolescents with ASD.

The atypical neuroleptics can help address interfering stereotyped repetitive behaviors and social withdrawal and can allow the person with ASD to be more amenable to social interactions and communication. Social relatedness, a core symptom of ASD, will improve when hostility, aggression, irritability, agitation, and hyperactivity are treated, which may, in turn, result from overstimulation or frustration. Often, no clear cause is apparent.

In low-dosage ranges, the atypical neuroleptics are rarely associated with extrapyramidal symptoms or long-term risk of tardive dyskinesia. Self-injurious behaviors seen in ASD and intellectual disabilities are poorly responsive to pharmacological interventions in general as well as to atypical neuroleptics. The major undesirable effects of "atypicals" include significant weight gain and metabolic problems ranging from minor blood sugar elevations to potential difficulties in glucose tolerance and risk of diabetes.

Clinicians prescribing these medications need to obtain baseline and follow-up weights of all individuals. Nutritional intervention is recommended for individuals who demonstrate significant weight gain during treatment or who are overweight at the outset. A full lipid panel with fractionation of cholesterol has been recommended annually, with quarterly fasting total triglycerides and cholesterol during the first year of treatment. Fasting blood sugar levels, liver function tests, and electrocardiograms are also monitored.

Anticonvulsants

As noted previously, individuals with ASD experience clinical or subclinical seizures at a much higher risk than in the general population and, therefore, should have baseline neurological assessments. *Significant* clinical and subclinical seizures, if left untreated, can lead to deleterious effects. As seizures can emerge at any time, they should be ruled out as possible contributory factors for any change in behavior (tantrums, irritability, and agitation), sleep, and regulatory functions. There is also an increased incidence of newly onset seizures in seizure-free individuals with ASD as they progress through puberty and adolescence.

Pharmacological treatment with sodium valproate has been used in particular children with ASD who present with a developmental regression in milestones or seizures, sometimes in the context of Landau-Kleffner syndrome. Sodium valproate has also been used with modest success in the treatment of secondary symptoms of hypomania in association with irritability, silly or elated moods, temper outbursts, and agitation. Clinicians have been apt to translate their experience from sodium valproate to other anticonvulsants; lamotrigine has not been as effective, and the most commonly used anticonvulsants after valproate for targeting behaviors have been carbamazepine and oxycarbamazepine.

Adverse Reactions

This following story, provided by an individual with Asperger disorder, illustrates that when an individual has an adverse reaction to medication there are often associated sensory and emotional experiences. Therefore, medications must be very carefully prescribed and very closely monitored.

I have taken medication before for depression and anxiety—specifically, paroxotine, lorazepam and an SSRI. I felt that I was largely unaffected by paroxotine, though it did make me feel emotionally numb. Not disconnected, but dulled, as if I was still feeling things, but with less intensity. I approached lorazepam with understandable apprehension. I took one to alleviate an approaching panic attack. It produced an effect I can only think to describe as "layered." On the sublayer, I continued to experience generalized fear that, without the medicine, would have become a panic episode. I experienced the episode from a layer on top, this lorazepam layer, where I realized I was panicking, but did not seem to mind at all. If I remember correctly, I remarked detachedly to no one in particular of the duality of my feelings shortly before falling asleep.

On the SSRI, I experienced a severe panic attack. I suddenly felt as if I was suffocating and my heart was beating wildly. After a time, the episode had largely abated, leaving me feeling exhausted and bewildered.

It is worth noting that while I continue to experience anxiety today, it is not unmanageable, nor is it overwhelming. I very rarely suffer true panic attacks, and the episodes I do have are minor, more annoying than controlling.

ALTERNATIVE TREATMENTS

Autism is a lifelong condition that does not have a clear singular etiology nor does it have a singular "cure." For this reason, it has become the focus of many unconventional alternative and experimental therapies, some of which are taxing to families and may cost inordinate amounts of money. The AAP has suggested guidelines to consider when evaluating controversial treatment choices for those with developmental disabilities, outlined in Table 23.1-8.

At the same time, it behooves the clinician to become familiar with alternative and controversial therapies since many families pursue them (Hyman & Levy, 2000). Support of a trial of therapy in select situations is called for by helping to establish clear treatment objectives while remaining actively involved, even if in disagreement with the family's decision. Some examples of commonly adopted alternative treatments include gluten- and casein-free diets (GFCF) and the use of antifungal therapies. Studies funded by the National Institutes of Health are underway to determine the diet's efficacy in blinded situations.

Table 23.1-8. Controversial therapy guidelines

Are based on overly simplified scientific theories
Claim to be effective for more than one condition
Caim that children will respond dramatically and even be cured
Use anecdotal data rather than carefully designed studies to support claims for treatment
Fail to identify specific treatment objectives or target behaviors
Are stated to have unremarkable or no adverse effects; thus, proponents deny the need to conduct controlled studies

Reproduced with permission from *Pediatrics*, Vol. 107(5), Pages 1221–1226, Copyright © 2001 by the AAP.

Individuals on these regimens need to be followed with emphasis on the critical importance of concomitant behavioral and developmental interventions, the avoidance of any undue financial burdens, the monitoring of the nutritional status, and most important with the setting of appropriate expectations regarding the treatment. Accurate delineation of specific target treatment goals helps ascertain the extent to which interventions are beneficial or not. Alternative treatments include the use of nutritional supplements with high-dose pyridoxine and magnesium, ascorbic acid, and dimethylglycine, which have not passed the muster of double-blind scrutiny. Ongoing research is warranted to substantiate anecdotal claims and some has already been done. For example, double-blind, placebo-controlled trials of secretin, including some performed at SARRC, failed to demonstrate significant improvement in ASD behaviors. Comprehensive reviews of alternative approaches differentiate between proven, disproved, and unproven therapeutic modalities. That approach is helpful in the context of family counseling regarding intervention options.

Within the culture of ASD, there are those who have very differing world views and very different perspectives on what is to be done for ASD and why. An integrative approach, which combines the best of what research and experience has to offer, along with a strong respect for the culture of the family, is helpful.

CONCLUSION

A World Health Organization (2003) report on caring for children and adolescents with mental disorders has emphasized the disproportionately high burden of ASD and developmental disabilities. Furthermore, the treatment gap in diagnosis and available interventions for young children remains almost nonexistent even in many developing nations (Erol, Simsek, Oner, & Munir, 2005). The National Research Council (2001) on educational interventions for children with ASD identified seven key areas for needed improvement for care of individuals with ASD. These include better appreciation of:

1. Early diagnostic assessments
2. Effect on and role of families
3. Appropriate goals for educational services
4. Characteristics of effective interventions and educational programs
5. Need for public policy initiatives to ensure access to education
6. Need for improvements in the training of educational personnel
7. Need for future research

Awareness of the condition is critical, and the efforts of the Centers for Disease Control and Prevention and other public and private organizations toward early identification and early intervention are in process and should continue to advance the cause. In addition, there is the need to provide effective interventions toward assuring optimal outcome, and, in this context, training and education of professionals is imperative. Parent-driven and parent-supported organizations are critical to the optimal outcome for children. The partnership that has developed between the families and the community of providers of services, teachers of professionals, and researchers is a model for how societies should operate in improving the well-being of all its citizens.

REFERENCES

Aman, M.G., & Langworthy, K.S. (2000). Pharmacotherapy for hyperactivity in children with autism and other pervasive developmental disorders. *Journal of Autism and Developmental Disorders, 30*(5), 451–459.

American Academy of Pediatrics. (1993, November). The medical home statement addendum: Pediatric primary health care. *AAP News,* 7.

American Academy of Pediatrics. (2001). The pediatrician's role in the diagnosis and management of autistic spectrum disorder in children. *Pediatrics, 107,* 1221–1226.

American Psychiatric Association. (1952). *Diagnostic and statistical manual of mental disorders.* Washington, DC: Author.

American Psychiatric Association. (1968). *Diagnostic and statistical manual of mental disorders* (2nd ed.). Washington, DC: Author.

American Psychiatric Association. (1980). *Diagnostic and statistical manual of mental disorders* (3rd ed.). Washington, DC: Author.

American Psychiatric Association. (1987). *Diagnostic and statistical manual of mental disorders* (3rd ed., revised). Washington, DC: Author.

American Psychiatric Association. (1994). *Diagnostic and statistical manual of mental disorders* (4th ed.). Washington, DC: Author.

American Psychiatric Association. (2001). *Diagnostic and statistical manual of mental disorders* (4th ed., text revision). Washington, DC: Author.

Asperger, H. (1991). "Autistic psychopathology" in childhood. In F. Uta (Ed.), *Autism and Asperger syndrome* (pp. 37–92). Cambridge, England: Cambridge University Press.

Bailey, A., Bolton, P., Butler, L., LeCouteur, A., Murphy, M., Scott, S., et al. (1993). Prevalence of the fragile X anomaly amongst autistic twins and singletons. *Journal of Child Psychology and Psychiatry, 34,* 673–678.

Bailey, A., LeCouteur, A., Gottesman, I., Bolton, P., Simonoff, E., Yuzda, E., et al. (1995). Autism as a strongly genetic disorder: Evidence from a British twin study. *Psychological Medicine, 25,* 63–77.

Baird, G., Charman, T., Baron-Cohen, S., Cox, A., Swettenham, J., Wheelwright, S., Drew, A., & Kemal, L. (2000). A screening instrument for autism at 18 month of age: A six-year follow-up study. *Journal of the American Academy of Child & Adolescent Psychiatry, 39* (6), 694–702.

Barr, M.W. (1898). Some notes on echolalia, with the report of an extraordinary case. *Journal of Nervous and Mental Diseases, 25,* 21–30.

Bauman, M.L., & Kemper, T.L. (2005). Neuroanatomic observations of the brain in autism: A review and future directions. *International Journal of Developmental Neuroscience, 23*(2–3), 183–187.

Clements, J., Wing, L., & Dunn, G. (1986). Sleep problems in handicapped children: A preliminary study. *Journal of Child Psychology and Psychiatry,* 27(3), 399–407.

Cook, E.H., Jr., Courchesne, R.Y., & Cox, N.J. (1998). Linkage-disequilibrium mapping of autistic disorder, with 15q11-13 markers. *American Journal of Human Genetics, 62,* 1077–1083.

DeLong, G.R., Teague, L.A., & McSwain Kamran, M. (1998). Effects of fluoxetine treatment in young children with idiopathic autism. *Developmental Medicine and Child Neurology, 40,* 551–562.

Ehlers, S., & Gilberg, C. (1993). The epidemiology of Asperger syndrome: A total population study. *Journal of Child Psychology and Child Psychiatry, 34,* 1327–1350.

Erol, N., Simsek, Z., Oner, O., & Munir, K. (2005). Behavioral and emotional problems among Turkish children at age 2–3. *Journal of American Academy of Child and Adolescent Psychiatry, 44,* 80–87.

Filipek, P.A. (1999). Neuroimaging in the developmental disorders: The state of the science. *Journal of Child Psychology and Psychiatry, and Allied Disciplines, 40,* 113–128.

Filipek, P.A., Accardo, P.J., & Ashwal, S. (2000). Practice parameter: Screening and diagnosis of autism. Report of the Quality Standards Subcommittee of the American Academy of Neurology and the Child Neurology Society. *Neurology, 55,* 468–479.

Filipek, P.A., Accardo, P.J., & Baranek, G.T. (1999). The screening and diagnosis of autistic spectrum disorders. *Journal of Autism and Developmental Disorders, 29,* 439–484.

Folstein, S., & Roren-Sheidly, B. (2001). Genetics of autism: Complex etiology for a heterogeneous disorder. *Genetics, 2,* 943–955.

Fombonne, E. (2001). Is there an epidemic of autism? *Pediatrics, 107*(2), 411–412.

Gillberg, C., & Coleman, M. (1996). Autism and medical disorders: A review of the literature. *Developmental Medicine and Child Neurology, 38,* 191–202.

Gillberg, C., & Coleman, M. (2001). *The biology of the autistic syndromes* (3rd ed.). London: MacKeith Press.

Gillberg, C., Steffenburg, S., & Schaumann, H. (1991). Autism epidemiology: Is autism more common now than 10 years ago? *British Journal of Psychiatry, 158,* 403–409.

Greenspan, S.I. (1995). *The challenging child: Understanding, raising, and enjoying the five "difficult" types of children.* Reading, MA: Addison Wesley.

Horvath, K., & Perman, J.A. (2002). Autistic disorder and gastrointestinal disease. *Current Opinion in Pediatrics, 14*(5), 583–587.

Hyman, S.L., & Levy, S.E. (2000). Autistic spectrum disorders: When traditional medicine is not enough. *Contemporary Pediatrics, 10,* 101–116.

Institute of Medicine. (2004). *Immunization safety review: Thimerosal-containing vaccines and neurodevelopmental disorders.* Washington, DC: National Academies Press.

International Molecular Genetic Study of Autism Consortium. (1998). A full genome screen for autism with evidence for linkage to a region on chromosome 7q. *Human Molecular Genetics,* 7, 571–578.

Jamain, S., Betancur, C., et al. (2002). Paris Autism Research International Sibpair (PARIS) Study: Linkage and association of the glutamate receptor 6 gene with autism. *Molecular Psychiatry,* 7(3), 302–310.

Jan, J. & Freeman, R. (2004). Melatonin therapy for circadian rhythm sleep disorders with multiple disabilities. *Developmental Medicine and Child Neurology, 46,* 776–782.

Jaselskis, C.A., Cook, E.H., & Fletcher, K.E. (1992). Clonidine treatment of hyperactive and impulsive children with autistic disorder. *Journal of Clinical Psychopharmacology, 12,* 322–327.

Johnson, C.P., & Blasco, P.A. (1997). Infant growth and development. *Pediatric Review, 18,* 224–242.

Kanner, L. (1943). Autistic disturbances of affective contact. *Nervous Child, 2,* 217–250.

Klin, A., Volkmar, F.R., Sparrow, S.S., Cicchetti, D.V., & Rourke, B.P. (1995). Validity and neuropsychological characterization of Asperger syndrome: Convergence with nonverbal learning disabilities syndrome. *Journal of Child Psychology and Psychiatry, and Allied Disciplines, 36,* 1127–1140.

Lacamera, R., & Lacamera, A. (1997). Routine health care. In D.J. Cohen & F.R. Volkmar (Eds.), *Handbook of autism and pervasive developmental disorders* (2nd ed., pp. 730–742). New York: John Wiley and Sons.

Lainhart, J.E., Piven, J., & Wzorek, M. (1997). Macrocephaly in children and adults with autism. *Journal of the American Academy of Child and Adolescent Psychiatry, 36,* 282–290.

LeCouteur, A., Lord, C., & Rutter, M. (2003). *The Autism Diagnostic Interview (ADI-R).* Los Angeles: Western Psychological Services.

Linday, L., Tsiouris, J., Cohen, I., Shindledecker, R., & DeCresce, R. (2001). *Journal of Neural Transmission, 5,* 593–611.

Lord, C., Risi, S., Lambrecht, L., Cook, E.H., Leventhal, B.L., DiLavore, P.C., et al. (2000). The Autism Diagnostic Interview schedule-Generic: A standard measure of social and communication deficits associated with the spectrum of autism. *Journal of Autism and Developmental Disorders, 30,* 205–223.

Lovaas, O.I. (1987). Behavioral treatment and normal educational and intellectual functioning in young autistic children. *Journal of Consulting and Clinical Psychology, 55,* 3–9.

Madsen, K.M., Lauritsen, M.B., Pedersen, C.B., Thorsen, P., Plesner, A.M., Andersen, P.H., et al. (2004, September 13). [Thirmerosal and the occurrence of autism: Negative ecological evidence from Danish registry data]. *Ugeskr Laeger, 166*(38), 3291–3293.

Martin, A., Koenig, K., Anderson, G.M., & Scahill, L. (2003). Low-dose fluvoxamine treatment of children and adolescents with pervasive developmental disorders: A prospective, open-label study. *Journal of Autism and Developmental Disorders, 33*(1), 77–85.
McDougle, C.J. (1997). Psychopharmacology. In D.J. Cohen & F.R. Volkmar (Eds.), *Handbook of autism and pervasive developmental disorders* (2nd ed., pp. 707–729). New York: John Wiley & Sons.
McDougle, C.J., Holmes, J.P., Carlson, D.C., Pelton, G.H., Cohen, D.J., & Price, L.H. (1998). A double-blind, placebo-controlled study of risperidone in adults with autistic disorder and other pervasive developmental disorders. *Archives of General Psychiatry, 55*, 633–641.
McDougle, C.J., Kresch, L.E., & Posey, D.J. (2000). Repetitive thoughts and behavior in pervasive developmental disorders: Treatment with serotonin reuptake inhibitors. *Journal of Autism and Developmental Disorders, 30*(5), 427–435.
Melmed, R. (2003, September). *Physicians' outreach program: Autistic disorders screening program.* Poster presented at the American Academy of Cerebral Palsy Annual Meeting, Montreal, Canada.
Melmed, R.D., Schneider, C., Fabes, R.A., Philips, J., & Reichelt, K. (2000). Metabolic markers and gastrointestinal symptoms in children with autism and related disorders. [Abstract]. *Journal of Pediatric Gastroenterology and Nutrition, 31*(Suppl. 2), S31.
Minshew, N.J. (1991). Indices of neural function in autism: Clinical and bilogical implications. *Pediatrics, 87*, 774–780.
National Research Council. (2001). *Educating young children with autism.* Washington, DC: National Academies Press.
Niederhofer, H., Staffen, W., Mair, A., & Pittschieler, J. (2003). Brief report: Melatonin facilitates sleep in individuals with mental retardation and Insomnia. *Journal of Autism and Developmental Disorders, 33*(4), 469–472.
Persico, A.M., D'Agruma, L., Maiorano, N., et al. (2001). Reelin gene alleles and haplotypes as a factor predisposing to autistic disorder. *Molecular Psychiatry, 6*(2), 150–159.
Piven, J., Saliba, K., Bailey, J., & Arndt, S. (1997). An MRI study of autism: The cerebellum revisited. *Neurology, 49*, 546–551.
Research Units in Pediatric Psychopharmacology (RUPP) Autism Network. (2002). Risperidone in children with autism and serious behavioral problems. *New England Journal of Medicine, 347*, 314–321.
Richdale, A.L., & Prior, M.R. (1995). The sleep/wake rhythm in children with autism. *European Child and Adolescent Psychiatry, 4*(3), 175–186.
Rimland, B. (1964). *Infantile autism: The syndrome and its implications for a neural theory of behavior.* New York: Appleton-Century-Crofts.
Rivkees, S. (2003). Developing circadian rythmicity in infants. *Pediatrics, 112*, 373–381.
Robins, D.L., Fein, D., Barton, M.L., & Green, J.A. (2001). The Modified Checklist for Autism in Toddlers: An initial study inverstigating the early detection of autism and pervasive developmental disorders. *Journal of Autism and Developmental Disabilities, 31*, 131–144.
Schopler, E., Reichler, R., & Renner, B.R. (1988). *The Childhood Autism Rating Scale (CARS).* Los Angeles: Western Psychological Services.
Steingard, R.J., Zimnitzky, B., DeMaso, D.R., Bauman, M.L., & Bucci, J.P. (1997). Sertraline treatment of transition-associated anxiety and agitation in children with autistic disorder. *Journal of Child and Adolescent Psychopharmacology, 7*, 9–15.
Tsai, L. (2001). *Taking the mystery out of medications in autism/Asperger syndromes.* Arlington, TX: Future Horizons.
Tuchman, R.F., Rapin, I., & Shinnar, S. (1991). Autistic and dysphasic children: I. Clinical characteristics. *Pediatrics, 88*, 1211–1218.
U.S. Government Accountability Office. (2005, January). *Special education: Children with autism* (p. 17). Washington, DC: Author.
Volkmar, F.R., Lord, C., Bailey, A., Schultz, R.T., & Klin, A. (2004). Autism and pervasive developmental disorders. *Journal of Child Psychology and Psychiatry, and Allied Disciplines, 45*, 135–170.
Wassink, T.H., Piven, J., Vieland, V.J., et al. (2001). Evidence supporting WNT2 as an autism susceptibility gene. *American Journal of Medical Genetics, 105*(5), 406–413.
Wing, L. (1981). Asperger's syndrome: A clinical account. *Psychological Medicine, 11*, 115–129.
Wing, L. (1997). The autistic spectrum. *Lancet, 350*, 1761–1766.
Wing, L., Leekam, S.R., Libby, S.J., Gould, J., & Larcombe, M. (2002). The Diagnostic Interview for Social and Communication Disorders: Background, inter-rater reliability and clinical use. *Journal of Child Psychology and Psychiatry, and Allied Disciplines, 43*, 307–325.
World Health Organization. (1993). *International classification of diseases* (10th ed.). Geneva: Author.
World Health Organization. (2003). *Caring for children and adolescents with mental disorders: Setting WHO priorities.* Geneva: Author.
Yeargin-Allsopp, M., Rice, C., Karapurkar, T., Doernberg, N., Boyle, C., & Murphy, C. (2003). Prevalence of autism in a U.S. metropolitan area. *Journal of the American Medical Association, 289*, 49–55.

23.2 ATTENTION-DEFICIT/HYPERACTIVITY DISORDER

Mark L. Wolraich

Attention-deficit/hyperactivity disorder (ADHD) is a behavioral disorder characterized by inattention and a combination of impulsivity and hyperactivity. It has the distinction of being both the most extensively studied behavioral disorder and the most controversial. Most of the public controversies surrounding ADHD have focused on the existence of the condition and the extensive use of stimulant medication. Concern was first raised by Maynard (1970), who claimed that 5%–10% of the children in the Omaha, Nebraska, school system were receiving stimulant medications to control their behavior. Although the report was not substantiated, it led to a Congressional investigation and was the impetus for further research about stimulant medications.

In the 1980s, the Church of Scientology, through its Citizen's Commission on Human Rights, questioned the existence of the diagnosis of ADHD and pushed for the banning of stimulant medications, emphasizing and exaggerating the potential side effects. This action led to a decrease in the use of methylphenidate in the late 1980s (Safer & Krager, 1992); however, use of stimulant medications has considerably increased since 1990. During the 5-year period of 1990–1995, a double (Safer, Zito, & Fine, 1996) to a six-fold increase (Drug Enforcement Administration, 1995) in the use of stimulant medications led to further concerns in both the scientific (Diller, 1996) and lay (McGinnis, 1997) literature about the excessive use of and rationale for stimulant treatment.

The controversy has been difficult for individuals and families. The implications of denying the disorder status of ADHD are that parents are drugging their children to be more compliant and that teachers are suggesting the diagnosis so they can be more controlling. In both scenarios, parents and teachers are seen as incompetent. The identification of an efficacious treatment for a condition in most cases would be considered a scientific advance, but the increased use of stimulant medication is looked at with suspicion. The confusing and contradictory messages make it difficult for individuals and their families to seek and obtain appropriate diagnostic and treatment services.

HISTORY

Although ADHD may seem to be a new condition, it actually has a long history. In the mid-19th century, the characteristics of ADHD were described by Heinrich Hoffman, a German physician, and represented in his children's book by two characters, Fidgety Phil and Harry Who Looks in the Air. At a meeting of the Royal College of Physicians in 1902, George Still described a disease he characterized as resulting from an impairment in moral character. He noted that the problem resulted in a child's inability to internalize rules and limits and also manifested itself in patterns of restless, inattentive, and overaroused behaviors. He suggested that the children had likely experienced brain damage but that the behavior could also arise from hereditary and environmental factors.

The connection of ADHD with brain damage became more clear after 1918, following a worldwide epidemic of influenza with encephalitis that in some recovering children resulted in symptoms of restlessness, inattention, impulsivity, easy arousability, and hyperactivity. When many cases were seen with similar behavioral manifestations but no clear evidence of brain damage, the condition of *minimal cerebral/brain dysfunction/damage* (MBD) was defined.

A shift from a primary etiologic focus of brain damage to a focus on behavioral manifestations first began to appear in the 1960s, as reflected in the *Diagnostic and Statistical Manual of Mental Disorders, Second Edition* (DSM–II) definition of *hyperkinetic impulse disorder* (American Psychiatric Association, 1968). In 1980, due to the work of Virginia Douglas (1974) and others, the focus shifted from considering the primary impairment to be hyperactivity to considering inattention to be the primary impairment. This change is reflected in the shift of the diagnostic label to *attention deficit disorder* in the *DSM, Third Edition* (DSM–III; American Psychiatric Association, 1980) and to *attention deficit hyperactivity disorder* in *DSM, Third Edition, Revised* (DSM–III–R; American Psychiatric Association, 1987) and *DSM, Fourth Edition* (DSM–IV; American Psychiatric Association, 1994).

Use of Medication

The first description of a successful intervention with stimulant medication was reported by Bradley in 1937. Children had initially received Benzedrine to relieve their headaches caused by spinal taps performed as part of diagnostic procedures. The added benefit of improved behavior was noted. Little research was conducted subsequent to Bradley's work until the 1950s, when clinicians rediscovered his work, and methylphenidate was released for commercial use in 1957.

The use of stimulants specifically for MBD was provided a boost by reports of positive effects in both the psychiatric and pediatric literature. Early studies set the guidelines for controlled studies to determine efficacy. By 1977, 62 double-blind placebo controlled studies had been reported in the literature (Wolraich, 1977). Since that time, the number of controlled studies has increased so that a review in 1998 utilizing rigorous research criteria and only including studies from 1981 found 123 studies (Miller et al., 1998).

The initial interest was in dextroamphetamine; however, adverse publicity from the use of dextroamphetamine as a treatment for weight reduction and its addictive properties when used in that context diminished its popularity at about the time that methylphenidate became commercially available and known to clinicians. The psychological literature is also quite extensive with research pertaining to psychosocial interventions and behavior modification techniques. Although many early studies were not specific to children diagnosed with MBD or attention-deficit disorder, subsequent studies demonstrated its applicability specifically to children with ADHD (Pelham, Wheeler, & Chronis, 1998).

ETIOLOGY

ADHD is a heterogeneous disorder whereby multiple etiologies can manifest similar behavioral symptoms. Impairments due to genetic effects or brain injuries affecting the same central nervous system areas most likely will cause similar manifestations. By far, the most common cause of ADHD has been genetic transmission, which is manifested in twin studies with a heritability of 0.75 (75% of the variance in phenotype can be attributed to genetic factors). Family studies have also shown that adoptive relatives of children with ADHD are less likely to have the disorder (Alberts-Corush, Firestone, & Goodman, 1986) and first-degree relatives have a greater risk compared with controls (Biederman, Faraone, Keenan, Knee, & Tsuang, 1990). Specific gene associations have been identified in a portion of individuals with ADHD. These associations include the dopamine transporter gene, the D4 receptor gene, and the human thyroid receptor-b gene (Swanson & Castellanos, 1998).

Insults to the brain also can result in the behaviors characteristic of ADHD. Children who are born premature have a higher incidence of ADHD as well as learning disabilities (Klebanov, Brooks-Gunn, & McCormick, 1994). Traumatic injuries to the brain and exposures in utero, particularly to alcohol, cause ADHD symptomatology. Lead or infections such as meningitis in young children can also result in similar behavioral symptoms (Tuthill, 1996). Symptoms of ADHD, particularly hyperactivity, can be seen in children with pervasive developmental disorders (PDD). The current classification system (American Psychiatric Association, 1994) precludes a concurrent diagnosis between PDD and ADHD; however, it is not clear that there is clear empiric evidence why PDD subsumes ADHD and that the conditions are indeed mutually exclusive.

Further progress has been made in identifying some of the preliminary central nervous system mechanisms. Studies of brain anatomy have demonstrated that, on average, individuals with ADHD have smaller prefrontal cortex, basal ganglia, or cerebellar vermix. Functional studies, such as positron emission tomography, single photon emission computed tomography, and functional magnetic resonance imaging, have shown striatal hypoperfusion in individuals with ADHD compared with individuals in a control group. On a neurotransmitter level, functions relate to the dopamine and norepinephrine systems in the same areas of the brain identified by anatomical studies (Castellanos et al., 1996).

Although research has progressed significantly in helping to identify possible underlying mechanisms in individuals with ADHD, the sophisticated assessment techniques now available do not help to facilitate the clinical diagnosis. There is such wide variation in both individuals with and without ADHD in size and activity—with a good deal of overlap between the two groups—that the assessments cannot adequately predict who has ADHD on an individual basis.

PREVALENCE

Determining the true prevalence rate of ADHD has been a challenging task. It is also a main source of controversy in the popular press—namely that too many children are being diagnosed as having ADHD and being treated with stimulant medication. First, the diagnosis is dependent on the presence of specific behaviors that are observed and reported by the child's caregivers. The diagnosis must rely on these subjective judgments because no biological markers (lab tests or image studies) exist. In addition, no clear normative criteria are available for caregivers to judge against when determining the normal frequency of a given behavior at a given age.

Another major challenge is that no clear demarcation exists between appropriate behavior and inappropriate behavior. Although a child can be diagnosed with schizophrenia by the presence of any hallucinations, the behaviors in ADHD follow a more normal distribution. A defined cut-point must be set in establishing diagnostic criteria. This phenomenon especially creates a problem for primary care clinicians because they are likely to see cases that are on or close to the borderline.

In addition, the modifications in criteria over time have further complicated the process of determining the true prevalence of ADHD. The most recent change from only one subtype in DSM–III–R to three subtypes in DSM–IV is likely to increase the prevalence rates (American Psychiatric Association, 1987, 1994). Besides the challenges in making accurate diagnoses, studies of prevalence rates are dependent on the sample studied. The rates are different when one examines a mental health clinic referred sample versus a primary care sample versus a community/school sample.

Given the challenges, the varying rates of ADHD are not surprising. The prevalence has ranged from 4% to 12% (median 5.8%). Rates are higher in community samples (10.3%) compared with school samples (6.9%), and they are higher in boys (9.2%) than girls (3.0%) (Brown et al., 2001).

PROGNOSIS

ADHD is a chronic illness that has no cure. Ongoing management is required to minimize the extent of impairment. Contrary to earlier beliefs, ADHD will not necessarily disappear by puberty. Approximately half of those who have the condition will, with maturity, be able to sufficiently compensate for the impairments created by having ADHD such that they no longer have the disorder. The more intelligent the individual, the better he or she will be able to compensate for the impairments. About half of the individuals diagnosed with ADHD will continue to require treatment even as adults, and because many children with ADHD still go through childhood without being identified, there continue to be individuals who are not diagnosed until they are adults. Adults with ADHD are at greater risk for substance abuse and smoking, in particular, and are at greater risk for automobile accidents.

DIAGNOSIS

As noted previously, the diagnosis of ADHD remains dependent on obtaining information about an individual's behavior from those who most frequently observe the behavior. For children, at a minimum, the sources need to include both parents and teachers (Perrin et al., 2000). Teachers observe children for up to 6 hours a day in comparison with a group of same-age peers and in situations that require the children to pay attention and control their activity level and impulsivity. Where possible, information should be obtained from other observers, such as coaches, scout leaders, and grandparents. Direct observations of a child's behavior in the classroom can provide some of the most objective information if it is available, but it is labor intensive and therefore has to be limited to small samples of time (American Psychiatric Association, 1994; Perrin et al., 2000).

Observations in the physician's office are frequently not useful because they do not correlate well with the child's behavior in the classroom. The physician's office is a different-enough setting that either the anxiety will worsen the child's behavior or the novelty will improve his or her behavior.

Table 23.2-1. DSM–IV definition of attention-deficit/hyperactivity disorder

Inattention dimension

1. Makes careless mistakes
2. Has difficulty sustaining attention
3. Seems not to listen
4. Fails to finish tasks
5. Has difficulty organizing
6. Avoids tasks requiring sustained attention
7. Loses things
8. Is easily distracted
9. Is forgetful

Hyperactivity-impulsivity dimension

Hyperactivity

1. Fidgets
2. Is unable to stay seated
3. Moves excessively (is restless)
4. Has difficulty engaging in leisure activities quietly
5. Is "on the go"
6. Talks excessively

Impulsivity

7. Blurts answers before questions are completed
8. Has difficulty awaiting turn
9. Interrupts/intrudes on others

To be considered as having the symptoms in each dimension, a child must display the "often" occurrence of at least six of the dimension's nine behaviors. The behaviors must

- Be inappropriately often for the developmental level of the child
- Have an onset before 7 years of age
- Be present for at least 6 months
- Be present in two or more settings (e.g., home, school, work)
- Create significant clinical impairment in social, academic, or occupational functioning

The three subtypes consist of:

1. *Predominantly inattentive type*—children who meet the criteria on the inattention dimension
2. *Predominantly hyperactive-impulsive type*—children who meet the criteria on the hyperactivity-impulsivity dimension
3. *Combined type*—children who meet the criteria on both dimensions

Diagnostic Criteria

DSM–IV defines two dimensions of core symptoms for ADHD: inattention and a combination of impulsivity and hyperactivity (American Psychiatric Association, 1994). The two dimensions have been found consistently when studying varied populations of children from different countries. Each dimension consists of nine behaviors presented in Table 23.2-1. The behaviors need to occur inappropriately often for what is expected for the individual's age. For the hyperactive/impulsive dimension, there are six hyperactive behaviors and three impulsive behaviors. Some of the inattentive behaviors reflect activities of executive function, including being able to organize activities, sustain attention, and filter out extraneous stimuli. These functions help individuals organize and execute their activities.

In addition to the presence of the core symptoms, ADHD symptoms 1) need to have been present for at least 6 months; 2) need to have started before the age of 7 years; 3) need to cause significant impairment in more than one setting (e.g., school and home); and 4) should not be the result of another mental disorder. The requirement for at least 6 months duration reflects the chronic nature of the condition, and the requirement of the age of 7 years is included to reflect a biologic basis for the condition starting in childhood. The exact age is not necessarily based on strong evidence, and some debate exists that some children with the inattentive subtype may not experience symptoms until an older age, when they have a greater need to be able to concentrate. The most important aspect of the diagnosis is the concept that the core symptoms impair the individual's ability to function. Some individuals have many of the core symptoms, but their strengths (e.g., above average intelligence) enable them to compensate well enough to prevent the symptoms from causing significant dysfunction (American Psychiatric Association, 1994).

Because the behaviors fall on a spectrum, some children may have some of the problem behaviors, but these behaviors are not severe enough to warrant a diagnosis of ADHD. These children have been referred to as *subsyndromal* and are defined in the *DSM for Primary Care Child and Adolescent Version* (Wolraich, 1996) as being inattentive and having hyperactive/impulsive problems. The diagnoses may be more challenging in primary care settings. Considering the conditions presented in Table 23.2-2 in the differential diagnosis is important.

Table 23.2-2. Differential diagnosis for attention-defecit/hyperactivity disorder

Developmental disorder
Learning disabilities
Intellectual disabilities
Pervasive developmental disorder
Medical
Anemia
Lead intoxication
Medications
Asthma
Antiepileptic
Allergy
Seizure disorder
Sensory impairments
Hearing
Vision
Sleep apnea
Substance abuse
Thyroid disease
Behavioral
Adjustment disorder
Mood disorder
Depression
Manic-depression
Psychotic disorder
Anxiety disorder
Substance abuse disorder

Limitations of the Diagnostic Criteria

The current diagnostic criteria for ADHD are less than perfect. First, the DSM system does not include a developmental perspective. The diagnostic criteria were derived primarily from research in children 6–13 years of age. Second, the behaviors are contextually dependent. The greater the adult-to-child ratio, the stronger the interest the child has in the activity, or the greater the structure in the environment, the easier it is for a child to control his or her behaviors. Third, there are also no specific guidelines for an observer such as a parent or teacher to precisely decide that a behavior is occurring inappropriately often.

Generally, teacher reports have correlated well with direct observations of the children in the classroom (Kazdin, Esveldt-Dawson, & Loar, 1983). The teacher's reports will be more accurate in elementary school, where the teacher is likely to have a child for a good portion of the day. They are less accurate in middle and high school, where teachers may only have a student for 45 minutes each day. Little is known about the accuracy of preschool teachers and child care workers, but it is likely to be similar to that of elementary school teachers. Gathering as much information as possible from multiple sources—at the very least from parents and teachers—is important.

Physicians should obtain enough information to make a diagnosis based on DSM–IV criteria (American Psychiatric Association, 1994). Using rating scales that base a child's behavioral symptoms on DSM–IV can help to shorten the time required to obtain the information. This fact is particularly true in obtaining information from teachers when direct contact may be difficult. Several scales are available, including the Vanderbilt Parent and Teacher ADHD Rating Scales (Wolraich, Hannah, Baumgaertel, Pinnock, & Feurer, 1998), the SNAP (Swanson, Nolan, & Pelham, 1982), the ADHD–IV Parent and School Versions (DuPaul et al., 1997), the Disruptive Behavior Disorder Rating Scale–IV (Bagwell, Molina, Pelham, & Hoza, 2001), and the Revised Conners Teacher and Parent Rating Scales (Conners, Sitarenios, Parker, & Epstein, 1998).

Diagnostic Issues in Adulthood

Going in reverse order from many of the psychiatric disorders, ADHD started as a childhood disorder and is now being considered as a disorder in adults as well. This process makes the diagnosis in adults challenging. As stated previously, the current behavioral criteria are primarily based on the behaviors of elementary school–age children, mostly boys. In addition, the most reliable sources of behavioral information, parents and teachers, are usually not available for adults.

Many of the behaviors of ADHD (e.g., impulsivity) decrease with age, so adolescents and adults with ADHD do not tend to have hyperactive symptoms, although adults may describe a sense of restlessness. Inattention and difficulties with executive function are likely to continue into adulthood. Specific adult criteria will need to be developed to more accurately diagnose those individuals who are not initially identified in childhood.

Other Diagnostic Tests

Other tests have not been found to be useful in making the diagnosis. Although physicians should screen children with ADHD for lead as they would other children who live in a high-risk area, ADHD does not necessitate more extensive evaluation. Thyroid abnormalities are not likely to be present without other thyroid symptoms, and although there is an increased incidence of nonspecific EEG changes, the changes have little diagnostic utility at this time (Brown et al., 2001; Perrin et al., 2000).

COMMON COMORBID CONDITIONS

The majority of individuals with ADHD will also have at least one other comorbid condition. The comorbid conditions are listed in Table 23.2-3. The mental disorders consist of internalizing and externalizing conditions. Cognitive impairments include intellectual and learning disabilities, motoric conditions (e.g., clumsiness, developmental coordination disorder, motor dysfunction), and general medical conditions (e.g., unresponsiveness to thyroid hormone).

STIMULANT MEDICATIONS

Stimulant medications are the most studied psychotropic medications. They consist of dextroamphetamine, methylphenidate, mixed amphetamine salts, and pemoline. More than 300 studies with 6,000 participants demonstrate short-term efficacy of these medications (Swanson, Gupta, et al., 1999). Most researchers have studied the effects of methylphenidate on elementary school–age children. With appropriate titration, approximately 70% will respond to the stimulant medication with which they are treated initially. If those who do not respond are systematically tried on a second stimulant medication in the same manner, a total of approximately 80%–90% will respond.

The stimulant medications reduce the core symptoms of inattention, hyperactivity, and impulsivity. They also improve academic productivity, although they do

Table 23.2-3. Comorbid conditions with attention-deficit/hyperactivity disorder

Mental conditions
Externalizing disorders
- Oppositional defiant disorder
- Conduct disorder

Internalizing disorders
- Mood disorders
    - Major depressive disorder
    - Dysthymic disorder
- Anxiety disorders
    - Posttraumatic stress disorder
    - Obsessive-compulsive disorder
    - Panic disorder
    - General and over anxiety disorder
    - Phobias

Cognitive impairments
Learning disabilities
Language and communication disorders

Motoric conditions
Developmental coordination disorder
Tourette syndrome or chronic tic disorder

Medical conditions
Generalized unresponsiveness to thyroid hormone
Sleep problems

not improve cognitive abilities or academic performance. Furthermore, in some children, they will reduce oppositional and aggressive behaviors. Although the evidence for the short-term efficacy of stimulant medications is quite clear, the evidence for long-term efficacy is not as clear. Evidence from the National Institute of Mental Health Multi-modal Therapy of ADHD supports efficacy for 24 months, but the long-term studies are less well designed and provide equivocal results (Jensen et al., 2001).

When Chad was 2½ years old, his parents were concerned because he was very oppositional and had frequent temper tantrums. He also was overactive and had a short attention span. Chad had difficulty in preschool and child care situations and was removed several times. After starting kindergarten, Chad was referred for evaluation because of his continuing behavior problems. Psychoeducational assessment determined that he had cognitive impairments, and he was initially placed in a resource classroom. Continuing problems resulted in Chad's placement in a self-contained classroom.

By age 8, Chad had been diagnosed by his primary care physician as having ADHD and was placed on mixed amphetamine salts at 10 mg twice a day. Although the medication was initially very effective in reducing his hyperactivity and oppositional behavior, the effects diminished during a 4-month period, and the medication was gradually increased to 20 mg twice a day. Six months later, the medication seemed to have a further diminished effect, and the doctor switched Chad to methylphenidate and increased the dose to 60 mg per day in three divided doses. The methylphenidate demonstrated a similar effect with diminishing benefits occurring over a 6-month period. Chad was then given alternating methylphenidate mixed amphetamine salts when tolerance developed. Most recently, he was started on atomoxetine while maintaining his stimulant regimen with the intent to taper the stimulants if he responds well to the atomoxetine.

Dextroamphetamine, methylphenidate, and mixed amphetamine salts have similar effects, side effects, and safety; however, differences exist in lengths of action dependent on the delivery systems of the medication. In addition, although methylphenidate may lower the seizure threshold and dextroamphetamine does not, both medications have been used to treat children with ADHD and seizure disorders with no recurrence of seizures as long as the children's seizure disorders are adequately treated (Gross-Tsur, Manor, van der Meere, Joseph, & Shalev, 1997; see Chapter 12.2). Even in children with other comorbid conditions, such as anxiety or mood disorders, treating the ADHD first with stimulant medications is preferable because the mood or depressive symptoms may diminish significantly if the stress caused by the ADHD is reduced.

Misconceptions

Several misconceptions remain about stimulant medications. The effects of the medications are not paradoxical; the same effects are seen in children without ADHD and in adults. Response to stimulant medications is idiosyncratic and is not based on the diagnosis. Therefore, a response to medication cannot be used as a diagnostic test. Children do not find stimulant medication pleasurable and do not commonly abuse them. In fact, there is some suggestion that those children with ADHD who are appropriately treated have a lower risk of substance abuse (Biederman et al., 1995).

New delivery systems to administer methylphenidate help to extend the duration of action of the medication to reduce the frequency of doses required for treatment so as to increase adherence with treatment and, particularly, to avoid having to administer the medications at school. The oldest compound is methylphenidate-sustained release. The extension of duration of this delivery system has been less than initially expected. It generally lasts approximately 5 hours. A newly improved system that utilizes microbead technology (methylphenidate-extended release, or Metadate CD) has extended the duration to 8 hours (equivalent to twice a day dosing of regular methylphenidate) (Adesman, 2002), and a system that utilizes an osmotic pump system (OROS methylphenidate, or Concerta) has extended the duration to 12 hours (Wolraich et al., 2001). The actual duration of action will vary from individual to individual. A methylphenidate patch is currently under study as is an isolated d-isomer.

Side Effects

The most common side effects are anorexia, headache, and sleep disturbance. The anorexia will frequently diminish after several months. If the individual's weight is affected, use of calorie-enriched food may be helpful. Determining the individual's current and past history of sleep and headaches is important because sleep problems are frequently present in individuals with ADHD independent of their treatments. When the dose is too high or is taken by individuals who are overly sensitive to the medication, individuals may develop psychotic symptoms or become overfocused. These side effects can sometimes be resolved with lowering the dose. Over-focusing usually manifests by the individual becoming listless or what parents refer to "as appearing like a zombie."

The medications can increase tics, but determining the relationship between stimulant medications and tics is difficult because the usual course of tics is to wax and wane. If children have tics and require treatment with stimulant medication, about one third will have an increase in the tics, about one third will have a decrease in the tics, and about one third will have the same amount of tics. The side effects profile between methylphenidate and amphetamines are essentially the same, with the exception of several minor differences. Dextroamphetamine leads to more appetite suppression. It also does not lower the seizure threshold, whereas methylphenidate does slightly. Although tolerance is not widely reported, occasional cases can occur.

Titration

Because the response of stimulant medication is so variable, doses related to the size of the individual (mg/kg) are not as relevant as they are in treating children with other medications. The most appropriate process is to start at the lowest dose (5 mg/dose for methylphenidate or 2.5 mg/dose in children under 5 years) and gradually increase the dose until the optimal dose is achieved with the least side effects up to the maximum dose of 60 mg per day or 20 mg per dose. The methylphenidate can be given twice or three times a day based on the individual's need for symptomatic relief and the family's preferences. For example, children whose inattentiveness creates school dysfunction may get by with morning and noon dosing or single doses lasting 8 hours, whereas individuals who experience dysfunction at school *and* at home are more likely to require three times a day dosing or single doses lasting 12 hours.

Because the main reason for treating individuals with ADHD is to alleviate their dysfunction, the best method for titrating the dose is by monitoring an individual's function. Although core behaviors are frequently monitored via completion of rating scales by parents and teachers, they are only important to the extent that they affect the individual's function. The domains to follow with regard to functioning are school/work, peers, family (parents, brothers, and sisters), community (organized activities), relationships, and leisure activities.

Although obtaining a complete blood count periodically has been in the original and ongoing instructions for the prescription of methylphenidate, it has not been found to be necessary, and no specific laboratory assessments are required. Because the blood levels do not correlate well with behavioral changes, they are also of little clinical use. Close monitoring to obtain and maintain adequate dosing is essential.

Dextroamphetamine is about twice as potent as methylphenidate because it only contains the dextro isomer. Mixed amphetamine salts (Adderall) is a mixture of 75% dextroamphetamine and 25% levo-amphetamine. It appears to have a longer duration of action than methylphenidate, but it has never been assessed compared with dextroamphetamine. Whether it is any

Table 23.2-4. Pharmacologic interventions for attention-deficit/hyperactivity disorder

Medication	Brand names	Starting dosage recommendations	Dosing intervals	Onset	Duration (hours)	Maximum dose
Mixed salts of amphetamine	Adderall	2.5–5 mg	QD–BID	20–60 minutes	6	40 mg/day
	Adderall XR	5 mg	QD	20–60 minutes	12	
Dextroamphetamine	Dexedrine/Dextrostat	2.5 mg	BID–TID	20–60 minutes	4–6	40 mg/day
	Dexedrine Spansule	5 mg	QD–BID	60 + minutes	6 +	40 mg/day
Methylphenidate	Concerta	18 mg	QD	20–60 minutes	12	54 mg/day
	Methylin	5 mg	BID–TID	20–60 minutes	3–5	60 mg/day
	Methylin ER	20 mg	QD–BID	1–3 hours	2–6	60 mg/day
	Ritalin	5 mg	BID–TID	20–60 minutes	3–5	60 mg/day
	Ritalin-SR	20 mg	QD–BID	1–3 hours	2–6	60 mg/day
	Ritalin-LA	20 mg	QD	8 hours		
	Metadate CD	20 mg	QD	8 hours	6–8	60 mg/day
Dextro-methylphenidate	Focalin	2.5 mg	BID–TID	20–60 minutes	3–5	20 mg/day
	Focalin XR 7	5 mg	QD	20–60 minutes	4.5–7	20 mg/day
Atomoxetine	Strattera	0.5 mg/kg	QD	2–6 weeks	Probably 24	1.4 mg/kg/day

Key: BID = twice a day; TID = three times a day; QD = every day

Note: Because doses may change over time, verify doses before administering medication.

different in its treatment or side effects profile is unknown. A sustained release form of mixed salts of amphetamine (Adderall-XR) was released in 2002 and has a 10–12 hour effect.

Because of the rare but severe side effects of liver toxicity and, in a few cases, liver failure and death, pemoline is no longer recommended as a first line treatment. The Food and Drug Administration recommends monitoring liver function tests every 2 weeks as well as making sure that the individual and parents are aware of the hepatic side effects. Information about the dosing and pharmacokinetic information is provided in Table 23.2-4. (*Note:* Because doses may change over time, verify doses before administering medication.)

Use in Individuals with Intellectual Disabilities

Although most of the studies of efficacy have been performed on children with ADHD and normal intelligence, stimulant medications also are effective for many children with intellectual disabilities (Handen et al., 1992). The reported use of stimulant medication for children with moderate intellectual disabilities is 3.4% (Gadow, 1985) and 15% for children with mild intellectual disabilities (Cullinan, Gadow, & Epstein, 1987). Although individuals with mild intellectual disabilities respond essentially as individuals without intellectual impairments, those with severe intellectual impairments are much less likely to respond to stimulant medications (Aman, Marks, Turbott, Wilsher, & Merry, 1991).

OTHER MEDICATIONS

In addition to stimulant medications, other drugs that physicians may prescribe for ADHD include atomoxetine, tricyclic antidepressants, alpha-adrenergic medications, and buprorion.

Atomoxetine

Atomoxetine is a selective norepinephrine reuptake inhibitor. Its efficacy in treating individuals with ADHD is based on several multisite phase III and IV studies. Atomoxetine appears to have similar effects and side effects to stimulant medications except for the effects on sleep. It also appears to have a more extended duration of action beyond the serum half-life and takes longer initially to manifest effects. Slower titration can reduce the effect of drowsiness, and positive effects emerge more slowly than those seen with stimulant medications.

Tricyclic Antidepressants

The tricyclic antidepressants used to treat individuals with ADHD have generally been imipramine (Tofranil), desipramine (Norpramin), and nortrptyline (Pamelor). Their mechanism of action is to inhibit the reuptake of seratonin and norepinephrine, but they also have anticholinergic effects. Their efficacy in the treatment of ADHD has been supported by approximately 20 randomized control trial studies. The side effects of the tricyclic antidepressant medications include sedation, anticholinergic effects, and anorexia, but the most troublesome side effect is cardiac arrhythmia. Most of the arrhythmia has related to overdoses because of the narrow margin of safety, but for desipramine, there may have been a sudden death at a therapeutic level. Because of the side effects, tricylic antidepressant medications should not be used unless an adequate trial of stimulant medication and behavioral interventions has been tried first (Pliszka et al., 2000).

Alpha-Adrenergic Medications

The alpha-adrenergic medications used to treat individuals with ADHD are clonidine (Catapres) and guanfacine (Tenex). Although they were approved as antihypertensive agents, they are alpha noradrenergic agonists that affect the central nervous system. Their evidence of efficacy in treating individuals with ADHD is limited to a few studies (Weisz & Jensen, 1999). The side effects for the alpha-adrenergic medications include sedation, fatigue, anorexia, dry mouth, and hypotension. Several cases of sudden death in individuals treated with a combination of clonidine and methylphenidate have been reported, but the deaths could not be confirmed as definitely due to the medications, (Swanson, Conner, & Cantwell, 1999; Wilens & Spencer, 1999). Because of potential side effects and the limited evidence for efficacy, alpha-adrenergic medications should only be prescribed if stimulant medications and tricyclic antidepressants/bupropion have failed after adequate trial (Pliszka et al., 2000).

Bupropion

Bupropion (Wellbutrin) is an antidepressive medication whose mechanism of action is mostly unclear. It is a weak dopamine agonist, and it decreases whole body norepinephrine, but neither of these effects would explain its clinical results. Its efficacy in treating individuals with ADHD is based on one multisite study where it was significantly better than placebo, but not as potent as stimulant medications (Conners et al., 1996). The side effects of buproprion include agitation, reduction in the seizure threshold, anorexia, insomnia, and nausea/vomiting. Because buproprion has more sedative effects and less evidence for its efficacy, it should only be prescribed if stimulant medications and behavioral interventions have failed after adequate trials.

PSYCHOSOCIAL INTERVENTIONS

Psychosocial interventions include all of the interventions that employ counseling or behavior management. The one most frequently employed, and the one with the strongest scientific evidence for its efficacy is behavior modification training for the significant caregivers in the child's environment. Social skills therapy tries to address the impairment that many children with ADHD have in social situations, but because of the difficulty that the children have in generalizing what they learn, there is limited evidence for its efficacy unless the training takes place in actual situations with other children. Family therapy may be helpful, particularly on issues such as relationships with brothers and sisters, but the evidence for its efficacy is weaker. Play and cognitive therapy have not been found to be efficacious treatments for children with ADHD (Pelham et al., 1998).

Parent training comes in different forms depending on the severity of the child's behavioral problems. With children whose behavioral problems are mild and with parents adept at behavior management, simple advice from their primary care clinician combined with reading material may suffice, although this scenario has not been studied to determine its efficacy. Most parents are likely to require more intense instruction, which is available in most communities and consists of training groups for parents in behavior modification techniques.

When parents find it difficult to understand or implement the techniques and/or their children demonstrate more severe behavior problems, individualized training tailored to their needs is required such as Parent Child Interaction Therapy (Herschell, Calzada, Eyberg, & McNeil, 2002). The most severe situations, short of removing a child from the home, may require implementing the parent training directly in the home or utilizing a day treatment situation that can help the parent while intensely shaping the child's behavior. Access to parent training services can be challenging, and the time demand may be too much for a one-parent family or a two-parent family with both parents working.

Parent training usually consists of three elements: 1) providing clear commands and rules to the children and keeping children aware of the rules, 2) providing positive attention and reinforcing the children for positive behaviors, and 3) providing punishment and the removal of the positive attention for rule violations and inappropriate behaviors (Hannah, 1999). Parents must provide positive attention and reinforcement to their children. Many times, because of their child's difficult behaviors, parents with children with ADHD get into a cycle where most of their interactions are negative and involve punishment for negative behaviors. Unless they are able to develop a systematic method for providing quality time in the form of positive attention and for reinforcing the children for appropriate behaviors, the punishments will be less effective and the desired goals will not be achieved. Positive attention requires providing undivided attention to the child for activities that are mutually enjoyed by both parties. The parents also need to learn to recognize and reward appropriate behaviors.

One systematic method for providing reinforcement is a token system. A token system consists of identifying the appropriate behaviors parents want to increase in their child. The three or four most appropriate behaviors are targeted, and the child can earn points for performing the appropriate behavior. As an example, if the parents want their child to say *please* when the child requests something, the child can earn points every time he or she uses *please* appropriately. For young children between 3 and 6 or 7 years of age, tangible tokens may work better than points. The parents need to set up a system such as a chart to keep track of the points, and the child needs to know how many points are needed to achieve a reward. The target behaviors and the number of points required to earn rewards can be revised as the child progresses or if the system does not seem to be working. The rewards can be special privileges like increased television time or increased time with a parent, or they can be tangible such as baseball cards. Immediate praise for earning points can help to enhance the effects.

A positive system alone is usually not sufficient to control the behavior of a child with ADHD. Some punishment system is also required for rule violations and inappropriate behaviors. Effective forms of punishment are time-out for younger children and removal of privileges for older children. With a token system, a cost response can also be employed. In that system, points are removed for rule violations and inappropriate behaviors. The child requires clear messages about the rules and what are inappropriate behaviors.

SCHOOL INTERVENTIONS

Children with ADHD can receive services from their schools based on Section 504 the Rehabilitation Act of 1973 (PL 93-112) for milder cases and the Individuals with Disability Education Act (IDEA) of 1990 (PL 101-476) for more severe cases. Section 504 requires the schools to provide accommodations so that the child can function in his or her class. All children with the diagnosis of ADHD are eligible; however, the legislation does not provide any added compensation to the school. Therefore, the adaptations provided can be of a limited nature, and the procedures, not well defined or scrutinized. Adaptations may include preferential class seating, assignment and homework reduction, and consultation for the teacher to help him or her set up a behavioral program.

IDEA is a much more comprehensive program, but it is only available to those children whose ADHD interferes with their ability to learn or who have cognitive comorbidities such as learning disabilities. The school system is required to provide comprehensive assessment that includes intellectual and achievement assessment as well as speech and language and more assessment if appropriate. Assessment provided by an external source such as a private psychologist can be used in place of the school assessment if the school personnel feel it is accurate, but most frequently that assessment has to be obtained at the parents' expense.

Based on the assessment, the school system must develop an individualized education program with clearly measurable goals. Services must be provided in as inclusive a setting as possible (least restrictive environment). Most children with ADHD spend a short portion of the day in a resource room with a teacher trained in special education or in an inclusive classroom with help from an aid. Speech-language and occupational therapy services are also provided as necessary. Social skills training may be helpful if it is provided in social situations such as the classroom or other group activities so that the training can be applied in the real context with the opportunity for practice and feedback.

The daily report card is a useful tool to coordinate behavior management between teachers and parents

Table 23.2-5. Other treatments for attention-deficit/hyperactivity disorder

Intervention	Description	Scientific evidence
Diets		
Feingold	Individuals restrict additives, preservatives, and food dyes from their diet.	About 1% of individuals may respond to this diet.
Oligoantigenic	Individuals eat a restricted diet to prevent presumed sensitivity reactions.	About 5 controlled studies with methodologic weaknesses exist.
Sugar restrictions	Individuals reduce the amount of refined sugars in their diet.	Repeated controlled studies show no effect.
Diet supplements		
Essential fatty acids	Individuals take supplements of linoleic and linolenic acids.	No objective evidence exists of benefits or harm.
Megavitamins	Individuals take at least 10 times the recommended daily amount of vitamins.	No objective evidence exists of benefits. These supplements can elevate hepatic enzymes.
Zinc	Zinc is given to individuals because of presumed deficiency.	No objective evidence exists of benefits or harm.
Antioxidants	Individuals take melatonin, ginko biloba, and/or pycnogenol.	No objective evidence exists of benefits or harm.
Herbal compounds	Individuals take chamomile, kava hops, lemon, valerian root, and/or passion flower.	No objective evidence exists of benefits or harm.
Alternative medicine		
Antifungal agents	Individuals are given antifungal agents in the hopes of reducing fungal toxins.	No objective evidence exists of benefits or harm.
Nootropic agents	Individuals take piracetam and/or dimethylaminoethanol.	No objective evidence of benefits or harm.
Training		
Electroencephalogram (EEG) biofeedback	Individuals use EEG feedback to suppress theta waves and enhance alpha waves.	No randomized control trials demonstrating efficacy exist.
Sensory integration	Individuals practice exercises to improve the integration of their senses.	No randomized control trials demonstrating efficacy exist.

Sources: Arnold (1978); Baumgaertel (1999); Feingold (1975); Goldstein and Goldstein (1998); Haslem, Dalby, and Rademaker (1984); Wender (1986); Wolraich, Wilson, and White (1995).

and to provide the clinician with useful information by which he or she can measure the effects of medication on the performance of the child in the classroom. It provides a good means of communication between parents and teachers, is inexpensive, requires a minimal effort on the teacher's part, and provides documented benefits (Pelham & Gnagy, 1999). The teacher, parent, and child together define 4–5 activities that have been problematic for the child. To be successful, the daily report card needs to target individualized problems, establish procedures for monitoring, give feedback to the child for the problems, provide feedback to the parents for the problems, and provide a reward for positive consequences.

Generally, a 20% improvement over baseline is targeted for each goal, and the child should have a success rate of 66% (Pelham & Gnagy, 1999). If the success rate is lower, it will not provide enough encouragement, and if it is close to 100%, the tasks are too easily accomplished. As the child improves, the requirements for success should be modified to maintain the same level of success. Positive report cards should be rewarded with reinforcements that are of value to the child, such as increased privileges or tangible prizes.

Using behavioral interventions does have some limitations. The behavioral interventions often will not be sufficient alone to bring a child with ADHD to the normal range of function and will not be effective for all children (Jensen et al., 2001). In addition, the interventions are costly compared with medication, and it is difficult to get parents and teachers to maintain the intervention. Hence, there is also no evidence of long-term benefits. The effects of combining both stimulant medications and behavioral interventions can provide additive effects for many children with ADHD and particularly those with significant comorbidity. It also can lower the dose of medication required and possibly allow for a less-intense behavioral intervention.

When students with ADHD make the transition to college, they can seek out colleges that have adaptations and support services on campus. College routines tend to be less structured and more variable than many students have experienced. Classes also place a greater demand on organizational skills and executive function. Students may benefit from a counselor or coach who can help them adjust. Continued close contact with their physician or referral to a clinician near the campus for ongoing management is also advised.

Adaptations in the work environment including clear rules and a reminder system can be helpful for adults with ADHD. There also are a growing number of ADHD coaches to help adults in need; however, only anecdotal impressions are available about the efficacy of these interventions. Other treatments, such as diets, dietary supplements, alternative medications, exercises, and biofeedback, are presented in Table 23.2-5.

CONCLUSION

Most of the controversy surrounding ADHD involves the condition's existence and the extensive use of stimulant medication. This negative attention can prevent many individuals and families from seeking appropriate diagnostic and treatment services. Although no cure exists for ADHD, stimulant medications and psychosocial and school interventions can improve the affected individual's ability to function in home, school, and work environments. Associations such as Children and Adults with Attention-Deficit/Hyperactivity Disorder (http://www.chadd.org) are an excellent source of information and support for individuals with ADHD and their families.

REFERENCES

Adesman, A. (2002). New medications for treatment of children with attention-deficit/hyperactivity disorder: Review and commentary. *Pediatric Annals, 31*, 514–522.

Alberts-Corush, J., Firestone, P., & Goodman, J.T. (1986). Attention and impulsivity characteristics of the biological and adoptive parents of hyperactive and normal control children. *American Journal of Orthopsychiatry, 56*, 413–423.

Aman, M.G., Marks, R.E., Turbott, S.H., Wilsher, C.P., & Merry, S.N. (1991). Clinical effects of methylphenidate and thioridazine in intellectually subaverage children. *Journal of the American Academy of Child and Adolescent Psychiatry, 30*, 246–256.

American Psychiatric Association. (1968). *Diagnostic and statistical manual of mental disorders* (2nd ed.). Washington, DC: Author.

American Psychiatric Association. (1980). *Diagnostic and statistical manual of mental disorders* (3rd ed.). Washington, DC: Author.

American Psychiatric Association. (1987). *Diagnostic and statistical manual of mental disorders* (3rd ed., revised). Washington, DC: Author.

American Psychiatric Association. (1994). *Diagnostic and statistical manual of mental disorders* (4th ed.). Washington, DC: Author.

Arnold, L.E. (1978). Megavitamins for MBD: A placebo-controlled study. *Journal of the American Medical Association, 20*, 24.

Bagwell, C., Molina, B., Pelham, W.J., & Hoza, B. (2001). Attention-deficit hyperactivity disorder and problems in peer relations: Predictions from childhood to adolescence. *Jour-*

nal of the American Academy of Child and Adolescent Psychiatry, 40, 1285–1292.

Baumgaertel, A. (1999). Alternative and controversial treatments for attention-deficit/hyperactivity disorder. *Pediatric Clinics of North America, 46,* 977–992.

Biederman, J., Faraone, S.V., Keenan, K., Knee, D., & Tsuang, M.T. (1990). Family-genetic and psychosocial risk factors in DSM–III attention deficit disorder. *Journal of the American Academy of Child and Adolescent Psychiatry, 29,* 526–533.

Biederman, J., Wilens, T., Mick, E., Milberger, S., Spencer, T.J., & Faraone, S.V. (1995). Psychoactive substance use in adults with attention deficit hyperactivity disorder (ADHD): Effects of ADHD and psychiatric comorbidity. *American Journal of Psychiatry, 52,* 1652–1658.

Bradley, C. (1937). The behavior of children receiving benzedrine. *American Journal of Psychiatry, 94,* 577–585.

Brown, R.T., Freeman, W.S., Perrin, J.M., Stein, M.T., Amler, R.W., Feldman, H.M., et al. (2001). Prevalence and assessment of attention-deficit/hyperactivity disorder in primary care settings. *Pediatrics, 107,* e43.

Castellanos, F.X., Giedd, J.N., Marsh, W.L., Hamburger, S.D., Vaituzis, A.C., Dickstein, D.P., et al. (1996). Quantitative brain magnetic reasonance imaging in attention deficit-hyperactivity disorder. *Archives of General Psychiatry, 53,* 607–616.

Conners, C.K., Casat, C.D., Gualtieri, T.C., Weller, E., Reader, M., Reiss, A., et al. (1996). Buproprion hydrochloride in attention deficit disorder with hyperactivity. *Journal of the American Academy of Child and Adolescent Psychiatry, 35,* 1314–1321.

Conners, C.K., Sitarenios, G., Parker, J.D., & Epstein, J.N. (1998). Revision and restandardization of the Conners Teacher Rating Scale (CTRS-R): Factor structure, reliability, and criterion validity. *Journal of Abnormal Child Psychology, 26,* 279–291.

Cullinan, D., Gadow, K.D., & Epstein, M.H. (1987). Psychotropic drug treatment among learning-disabled, educable mentally retarded, and seriously emotionally disturbed students. *Journal of Abnormal Child Psychology, 15,* 469–477.

Diller, L.H. (1996). The run on Ritalin: Attention deficit disorder and stimulant treatment in the 1990's. *Hastings Center Report, 26,* 12–18.

Douglas, V.I. (1974). Differences between normal and hyperkinetic children. In C. Conners (Ed.), *Clinical use of stimulant drugs in children* (pp. 12–23). Amsterdam: Excerpta Medica.

Drug Enforcement Administration, Office of Public Affairs. (1995). *Yearly aggregate production quotas.* Washington, DC: Author.

DuPaul, G.J., Power, T.J., Anastopoulos, A.D., Reid, R., McGoey, K.E., & Ikeda, M.J. (1997). Teacher ratings of attention deficit hyperactivity disorder symptoms: Factor structure and normative data. *Psychological Assessment, 9,* 436–444.

Feingold, B. (1975). *Why your child is hyperactive.* New York: Random House.

Gadow, K.D. (1985). Prevalence and efficacy of stimulant drug use with mentally retarded children and youth. *Psychopharmacology Bulletin, 21,* 291–303.

Goldstein, S., & Goldstein, M. (1998). *Managing attention deficit hyperactivity disorder in children: A guide for practitioners* (2nd ed.). New York: John Wiley & Sons.

Gross-Tsur, V., Manor, O., van der Meere, J., Joseph, A., & Shalev, R.S. (1997). Epilepsy and attention deficit hyperactivity disorder: Is mehtylphenidate safe and effective? *Journal of Pediatrics, 130,* 670–674.

Handen, B.L., Breaux, A.M., Janosky, J., McAuliffe, S., Feldman, H., & Gosling, A. (1992). Effects and non-effects of methylphenidate in children with mental retardation and ADHD. *Journal of the American Academy of Child and Adolescent Psychiatry, 31,* 455–461.

Hannah, J.N. (1999). *Parenting a child with attention-deficit/hyperactivity disorder.* Austin, TX: PRO-ED.

Haslam, R., Dalby, J., & Rademaker, A. (1984). Effects of megavitamin therapy on children with attention deficit disorders. *Pediatrics, 74,* 103–111.

Herschell, A.D., Calzada, E.J., Eyberg, S.M., & McNeil, C.B. (2002). Parent–child interaction therapy: New directions in research. *Cognitive and Behavioral Practice, 9,* 9–16.

Individuals with Disabilities Education Act (IDEA) of 1990, PL 101–476, 20 U.S.C. §§ 1400 *et seq.*

Jensen, P.S., Hinshaw, S.P., Swanson, J.M., Greenhill, L.L., Conners, C.K., Arnold, L.E., et al. (2001). Findings from the National Institute of Mental Health multimodal treatment study of ADHD (MTA): Implications and applications for primary care providers. *Journal of Developmental and Behavioral Pediatrics, 22,* 60–73.

Kazdin, A.E., Esveldt-Dawson, K., & Loar, L.L. (1983). Correspondence of teacher ratings and direct observations of classroom behavior of psychiatric inpatient children. *Journal of Abnormal Child Psychology, 11,* 549–564.

Klebanov, P., Brooks-Gunn, J., & McCromick, M. (1994). Classroom behavior of very low birth weight elementary school children. *Pediatrics, 94,* 700–708.

Maynard, R. (1970, June 29). Omaha pupils given "behavior" drugs. *Washington Post,* p. A8.

McGinnis, J. (1997, September 18). Attention deficit disaster. *The Wall Street Journal,* pp. A–14.

Miller, A., Lee, S.K., Raina, P., Klassen, A., Zupanic, J., & Olsen, L. (1998). *A review of therapies for attention deficit/hyperactivity disorder.* Vancouver: University of British Columbia, Research Institute for Children's and Women's Health.

Pelham, W.E., & Gnagy, E.M. (1999). Psychosocial and combined treatments for ADHD. *Mental Retardation and Developmental Disabilities Research Reviews, 5,* 225–236.

Pelham, W.E.J., Wheeler, T., & Chronis, A. (1998). Empirically supported psycho-social treatments for attention deficit hyperactivity disorder. *Journal of Clinical Child Psychology, 27,* 190–205.

Perrin, J.M., Stein, M.T., Amler, R.W., Blondis, T.B., Feldman, H.M., Meyer, B.P., et al. (2000). Diagnosis and evaluation of the child with attention-deficit/hyperactivity disorder. *Pediatrics, 105,* 1158–1170.

Pliszka, S.R., Greenhill, L.L., Crimson, M.L., Sedillo, A., Carlson, C., Conners, C.K., et al. (2000). The Texas Children's Medication Algorithm Project: Report of the Texas Consensus Conference Panel on Medication Treatment of Childhood Attention-Deficit/Hyperactivity Disorder. *Journal of the American Academy of Child and Adolescent Psychiatry, 39,* 920–927.

Rehabilitation Act of 1973, PL 93–112, 29 U.S.C. §§ 701 *et seq.*

Safer, D.J., & Krager, J.M. (1992). Effect of a media blitz and a threatened lawsuit on stimulant treatment. *Journal of the American Medical Association, 268,* 1004–1007.

Safer, D.J., Zito, J.M., & Fine, E.M. (1996). Increased methylphenidate usage for attention deficit disorder in the 1990's. *Pediatrics, 98*, 1084–1088.

Swanson, J., & Castellanos, F.X. (1998). *Biological bases of ADHD: Neuroanatomy, genetics, and pathophysiology.* Paper presented at the NIH Consensus Development Conference on Diagnosis and Treatment of Attention Deficit Hyperactivity Disorder, Bethseda, MD.

Swanson, J.M., Conner, D.F., & Cantwell, D. (1999). Ill-advised. *Journal of the American Academy of Child and Adolescent Psychiatry, 35*, 5.

Swanson, J.M., Gupta, S., Guinta, D., Flynn, D., Agler, D., Lerner, M., et al. (1999). Acute tolerance to methylphenidate in the treatment of attention deficit hyperactivity disorder in children. *Clinical Pharmacology and Therapeutics, 66*, 295–305.

Swanson, J.M., Nolan, W., & Pelham, W.E. (1982). *SNAP rating scale for the diagnosis of attention deficit disorder.* Paper presented at the meeting of the American Psychological Association, Los Angeles.

Tuthill, R.W. (1996). Hair lead levels related to children's classroom attention-deficit disorder. *Archives of Environmental Health, 51*, 214–220.

Weisz, J.R., & Jensen, P.S. (1999). Efficacy and effectiveness of child and adolescent psychotherapy and psychopharmacology. *Mental Health Services Research, 1*, 125–157.

Wender, E.H. (1986). The food additive-free diet in the treatment of behavior disorders: A review. *Journal of Developmental and Behavioral Pediatrics*, 7, 35–42.

Wilens, T.E., & Spencer, T.J. (1999). A clinically sound medication option. *Journal of the American Academy of Child and Adolescent Psychiatry, 38*, 5.

Wolraich, M.L. (1977). Stimulant drug therapy in hyperactive children: Research and clinical implications. *Pediatrics, 60*, 512–518.

Wolraich, M.L. (1996). *The classification of child and adolescent mental conditions in primary care: Diagnostic and statistical manual for primary care (DSM–PC) child and adolescent version.* Elk Grove, IL: American Academy of Pediatrics.

Wolraich, M. (2000). *Attention deficit hyperactivity disorder: Current diagnosis and treatment.* Retrieved from http://medscape.com/viewarticle/420198

Wolraich, M., Greenhill, L.L., Pelham, W., Swanson, J., Wilens, T., Palumbo, D., et al. (2001). Randomized controlled trial of OROS methylphenidate once a day in children with attention-deficit/hyperactivity disorder. *Pediatrics, 108*, 883–892.

Wolraich, M.L., Hannah, J.N., Baumgaertel, A., Pinnock, T.Y., & Feurer, I. (1998). Examination of DSM–IV criteria for ADHD in a county-wide sample. *Journal of Developmental and Behavioral Pediatrics, 19*, 162–168.

Wolraich, M.L., Wilson, D.B., & White, J.W. (1995). The effect of sugar on behavior or cognition in children: A meta-analysis. *Journal of the American Medical Association, 274*, 1617–1621.

23.3 ANXIETY

Alya Reeve

Anxiety is a normal physiologic and psychologic response to change in or around an individual. *Signal anxiety* occurs normally to alert the individual that there is something not right with the environment—that a potential danger exists. This response involves a helpful increase in attention, a focusing of mental, physical, sensory, and emotional systems toward analysis of the environment for the seriousness of threat to oneself and to choose the best response to this threat (Gross & Hen, 2004) . This *fight-or-flight* response helps many people make lifesaving decisions.

Pathological anxiety states of a similar magnitude, however, can override daily functions and render an individual dysfunctional because a truly dangerous situation is not present, yet the person is acting as if his or her life were in extreme danger. People with developmental disabilities encounter many situations that challenge their abilities and put them in positions of making decisions for which they feel unprepared. This chapter offers the reader a framework for assessing the appropriateness of an individual's or group's response to such situations and for developing a supportive reaction to achieve the most functional behavior possible.

PATHOPHYSIOLOGY OF ANXIETY RESPONSES

Meaningful emotional events enter a person's memory storage and retrieval systems through activity in the hippocampus. Activating serotonin receptors in the hippocampus may reduce worry, irritability, and distractibility symptoms in generalized anxiety disorder (Rynn & Brawman-Mintzer, 2004); however, numerous clinical studies have found that pharmacological strategies alone do not address the biological tendencies to have dysfunctional anxious responses. Cognitive behavioral therapy and psychotherapy techniques have been used in conjunction with medications to address basic skill deficits, improve anger management, improve coping skills under stressful conditions, decrease automatic worry patterns, and decrease substance abuse (Hammer, Robert, & Frueh, 2004; Rynn & Brawman-Mintzer, 2004).

The basal ganglia and limbic systems of the brain are coupled for goal-setting and goal-attaining functions. Rewarding events and objects are experiences that need to be remembered and differentiated from experiences that are undesirable. Activity can then be directed toward desired goals but must be monitored for effectiveness and feedback information.

In early infancy, these activities are totally focused on the goal of feeling fed and rested. Distress and anxiety rise when these needs are met in an untimely fashion, in insufficient amount, or in overabundance. In adulthood, information about potential dangerousness moves beyond feeding oneself to complex situations that require figuring out which is the best of several possible actions. The amygdala must provide modulating information to the motor control systems so that meaningful actions can be made (Gray, 1995).

Anxiety reflects activity within a behavioral inhibition system in response to threat of punishment, to omission of anticipated reward, and to perceived extreme novelty. Ongoing behavior is inhibited, and increased attention is given to environmental cues. This model includes neuroanatomic structures based on empirical evidence: anxiolytic drugs have primary action on sites in the septohippocampal system; anxiety evoked by fear conditioning involves the amygdala; and fight-or-flight behavior involves the amygdala, medial hypothalamus, and central gray area. Cue–reinforcement associations (fear conditioning) are formed in the amygdala and transferred by way of the entorhinal cortex to the hippocampus. Results of past and current motor actions (programs) are relayed from the prefrontal cortex by way of entorhinal pathways to the hippocampus. Ascending noradrenergic and serotonergic neurons modulate the input and relative gain in this system. Output from the hippocampus through the cingulate cortex, or through nucleus accumbens can interrupt motor behaviors and complex automatic behaviors.

Symptoms of anxiety may be organized into three broad categories: autonomic, behavioral, and cognitive. The neuroanatomic model illustrates connections by which arousal symptoms and avoidant behavior can assume progressively intrusive roles in a person's life. Words can amplify the activity in these circuits, bringing new meaning and impact from frontal and prefrontal areas with stored experiences and becoming as effective as danger at activating these interrelated systems.

Attributing meaning to physiologic symptoms does not indicate abnormal peripheral nervous system activity as shown by objective markers of autonomic arousal in individuals with panic disorder, individuals with obsessive-compulsive disorder, individuals with anxiety disorder, and normal controls (Roy-Byrne et al., 1997). No differences were found between any of the groups on any measure of autonomic arousal, although the individuals with panic disorder, obsessive-compulsive disorder, and anxiety disorder endorsed significant clinical symptoms.

Twenty-eight-year-old Alison, who had been nonverbal since childhood, was brought to a specialist's office by her mother for evaluation of unremitting anxiety. She refused to sleep in her own bed, pulled her hair out (even in her sleep), no longer left the house, and stuck by her mother. The onset of Alison's symptoms had been gradual after she injured her thumb in a van's wheelchair lift at her day habilitation program. After the initial trauma was repaired and healed, Alison started to refuse to ride in the van, then refused to attend the day program, and eventually refused to leave the house. Alison presented on initial evaluation as withdrawn, stiff, and worried. She had little eye contact and meekly followed her mother.

The specialist prescribed tricyclic medication (imipramine) at 25 mg at bedtime for 4 months, but Alison experienced no change in sleep or daytime behavior. Imipramine was titrated gradually to 125 mg nightly. Alison progressively resumed her old patterns of activity and interests: helping prepare meals at home, attending some day programs, traveling with family out of state to go to baseball games, and riding in public transportation without difficulties. The trichotillomania ceased once the dose of imipramine was raised from 100 mg/d to 125 mg/d.

A marked clinical improvement was noted at subsequent visits, with spontaneous smiling in agreement with her mother's statements, nonverbal gestures to enhance her mother's reporting of activities, direct eye contact with the examiner, and relaxed normal physical movements. Once clinical stability was maintained, Alison was referred to her primary care physician for maintenance prescriptions.

Alison's story illustrates one woman's experience with posttraumatic stress disorder (PTSD) and trichotillomania.

DIAGNOSTIC CONSIDERATIONS

Anxiety disorders are the major cause of disability and lost productivity in typically developing individuals (Blazer, George, & Hughes, 1991). They frequently present with other medical and psychiatric illnesses, particularly depression. The National Comorbidity Study reported a lifetime prevalence of any anxiety disorder as 25% in the adult population in the United States (Kessler et al., 1994). Although genetic predispositions exist in the development of anxiety disorders (i.e., anxiety disorders run in families), anxiety disorders also arise spontaneously and as secondary conditions to other medical conditions. Untreated anxiety disorder symptoms are associated with inappropriate under-usage of health care (de Beurs et al., 1999; Iwamasa & Hilliard, 1999).

The prevalence of anxiety disorders among individuals with intellectual disabilities was reported as 60%

(Barrios, Gonzalez-Gordon, & Ruiz, 1999). People with developmental disabilities are at increased lifetime risk for emotional, physical, and/or sexual abuse (Cook et al., 1993), and individuals with severe-profound levels of intellectual disability may not express their experiences of stress directly. Any assessment of these individuals has to focus on overall changes in behavior, rather than on direct expressions of anxiety (Matson et al., 1997).

Generalized anxiety disorder, phobias, panic disorder, and obsessive-compulsive disorder were the most common late-life anxiety problems reported in a review of primary care practices (Banazak, 1997). The rates of these disorders and PTSD are somewhat higher in psychiatric clinics, ranging from 10% to 73%. PTSD, like generalized anxiety disorder, usually lasts for years or decades, waxing and waning in intensity of symptoms and often generalizing to similar situations. One of the diagnostic criteria for PTSD is having an initial triggering event that caused the traumatic, anxiety response (see Table 23.3-1). When exposed to a similar trigger or part of the trigger, an individual may experience all of the extreme hyperarousal symptoms as inspired by the original trigger.

The societal burden of having anxiety disorders is seen in increased medical morbidity and health care cost over the life span. Early recognition of anxiety disorders may lessen the overall health care and financial burden by increasing the likelihood of successful treatment (Ronalds et al., 1997). Nonetheless, the burden of anxiety disorder extends into the indirect costs of impaired social function. Studies of the cost of specific mental illnesses cannot be made in isolation from other values of society.

Individuals with developmental disabilities are an identified vulnerable population and merit special attention and support. Recognition of anxiety disorders is important for the individuals' health and quality of life, as well as for the people who support these individuals within the community. Appropriate treatment with medication and therapy can improve function and communication for people with anxiety disorders and developmental disabilities.

Table 23.3-1. Diagnostic categories of anxiety disorders

Generalized anxiety disorder
- The person experiences uncontrollable, excessive anxiety for more days than not for at least a 6-month period.

Panic disorder
- The individual has intense escalating fear accompanied by at least 4 of 13 somatic and cognitive symptoms.
- The person may feel as if he or she is having a heart attack.
- The individual may or may not have agoraphobia.

Agoraphobia
- The person pervasively avoids certain situations that bring on excessive anxiety or panic.

Specific phobia
- The individual has a persistent fear of exposure to possible scrutiny by others.
- The person's avoidant behavior interferes with his or her functioning at work or in social situations.
- The individual is markedly distressed about the problem.

Obsessive-compulsive disorder
- The person has recurrent, distressful obsessions (thoughts) or compulsions (behaviors) that significantly interfere with his or her social, academic, and daily function.
- Resisting the obsession or compulsion causes anxiety to rapidly escalate to intolerable levels.

Posttraumatic stress disorder
- The onset of symptoms was some time after a traumatic event.
- The experience produced intense fear, helplessness, or horror.
- The individual experiences flashbacks or recurrent and intrusive recollections of the event(s).
- The person has feelings of detachment, guilt, sleep problems, and many anxious and somatic symptoms of arousal.

Acute stress disorder
- This disorder is similar to posttraumatic stress disorder but is limited from 2 days to 4 weeks.

Anxiety disorder due to general medical condition
- The symptoms of anxiety, obsessive-compulsive disorder, or panic are directly linked to a medical condition.
- The symptoms are often atypical for age of onset, course of symptoms, and family history.

Substance-induced anxiety disorder
- The anxiety symptoms, which may not meet full criteria of above disorders, are due to direct exposure to drugs, medications, or toxins.

CLINICAL MANIFESTATIONS OF ANXIETY

People who are worried commonly are irritable and short-tempered. For example, people who have trouble controlling their impulses may express this irritability with increased, rapid-onset violence toward themselves or others. Individuals frequently find an action or actions that reduce the tension caused by underlying anxiety and have a hard time not repeating the action until it becomes habitual. Often, the behavior doesn't express directly what is troublesome or anxiety provoking. The challenge for the clinical provider is to help the individual with developmental disabilities to cope with many different anxiety-inducing experiences and to develop a flexible array of adaptive, effective responses.

A confusing aspect for both the treatment and diagnosis of anxiety in individuals who depend on others is the interaction between the individual and his or her support people (e.g., family, professionals, direct care staff). The parent, relative, or professional must attempt to differentiate normal worries, personality traits, and anxiety disorders within a context of multiple interpersonal interactions. Different experiences pose greater or smaller threats to people based on their prior experience, their life experiences, their personalities, and their overall perception of well-being and safety.

Rose, Jones, and Fletcher (1998) noted the differences in staff reports of anxiety and stress from six residential homes for people with developmental disabilities. The group homes that conducted more outings in the community and were generally more community oriented had higher stress levels reported by the staff. A higher level of interaction was reported between staff and residents in the group homes with a low stress level. These reports show that stress alone does not guarantee severe anxiety. Some family groupings induce more anxiety than others. These findings from non–family living environments mirror general experience.

Before concluding that any person, including someone with developmental disabilities, has an anxiety disorder, a clinician should make every reasonable attempt to rule out medical causes of anxiety, including hyperthyroidism, hypoglycemia, hypoxia, seizure disorders, substance withdrawal states (e.g., alcohol), caffeinism, or rare tumors such as pheochromocytoma. In adolescence and adulthood, substance use may be a hidden factor because individuals are trying to fit in with age-matched peers. Valid diagnostic assessment techniques include gathering historical observations from different people who encounter the individual in different settings; careful history about onset of symptoms and exacerbating or alleviating conditions; subtle, nonverbal communications by the individual when accompanied by staff, guardians, or family; and opportunities for the individual to report his or her concerns independently (without fear of retribution as in the case of ongoing abuse by care providers). In other words, the evaluation may take a number of sessions while the clinician builds a therapeutic alliance with the individual and while clinical hypotheses are assessed for their likely contribution to the entire clinical picture.

AUTISM AND ANXIETY

Anxiety may be expressed through more rigid cognitive or behavioral rituals in people with autism spectrum disorders. Separation anxiety symptoms have been noted in children with autism (Gillot, Furniss, & Walter, 2001), although the symptoms were more varied than increased physical, clinging behavior. Increased symptoms of feeling unsettled, worried, or irritated may be expressed by more physical activity, poor sustained attention, or prolonged intense attention, and even aggression. Obsessive-compulsive disorder is found so frequently among children and adults with autism spectrum disorders, including Asperger syndrome, that some authors suggest that these disorders would be conceptualized more correctly as being on a continuum of clinical expression (Fontenelle et al., 2004; Gross-Isseroff, Hermesh, & Weizman, 2001; Harris, 2003; Hollander et al., 2003; Sturm, Fernell, & Gillberg, 2004; see also Chapter 23.1).

Often, people observing an individual with autism spectrum disorders only note overt behaviors. Increased frequency or severity of dysfunctional behaviors merit active generation of hypotheses about the circumstances contributing to the situation. Even if a normal child or adult would think nothing of an occurrence, circumstances must be analyzed for their impact on a person who is sensitive to specific stimuli (e.g., noises, lights, order). Because obsessive-compulsive disorder has a high prevalence among individuals with autism spectrum disorders, observers need to be aware when interruptions in routine and order are causing increased drive in the individual to control routines as a way to tolerate the increased anxiety.

Paulo was a tall, obese, 45-year-old man with autism. He was referred for evaluation of loud vocalizations (between a roar and a grunt), episodic physical violence toward staff and his immediate environment (e.g., car, kitchen), and concerns over drooling noted since he began taking antipsychotic medications. Over the course of 9–12 months of return visits, the antipsychotic medication was reduced (with permission of Paulo's guardian). Repetitive behaviors were noted (e.g., insistence on certain items of clothing, flicking motions with his hands), and clinical history revealed that Paulo was much attached to routines. He seemed to have less aggression and violence when given ample warning that changes in his routine were being made.

On the hypothesis that Paulo's behaviors might be manifestations of obsessive-compulsive disorder, a trial of Luvox was started and slowly titrated (at 6-week intervals) to 100 mg twice daily. Once the total daily dose reached 150 mg/d, a marked change in tolerance to activities occurred. Paulo started going out into community settings (e.g., sitting on the local university campus while people walked by) and walking off the porch of his house into the yard. He no longer rocked back and forth in the kitchen doorway before entering the kitchen. Most notably, he started speaking single and few-word phrases in response to direct questions and conversations with him.

Paulo is an example of a man with autism and obsessive-compulsive disorder. Just because a behavior is repetitive, though, does not mean that the behavior is obsessive or compulsive. It may be a mannerism, learned affectation, tic, or involuntary movement. Treatment has to be directed to the underlying cause(s) driving the symptoms or behaviors to be properly effective.

TREATMENT APPROACHES

Environmental assessment is needed for every individual who has a new onset of anxiety spectrum disorders for several reasons. First, the clinician should determine if there are any known traumatic events that preceded the anxiety symptoms for a possible diagnosis of PTSD. Second, the clinician should assess for changes in the environment that may be disturbing the individual. Third, the clinician should evaluate the individual's present reality to determine *real* versus *threatened* dangers. Finally, the clinician should determine a baseline of experience against which to measure therapeutic intervention.

Environmental assessments involve a range of settings and include all aspects of immediate sensory experience—from the ambient temperature, to background sounds, to stress level. Indoor and outdoor environments have different effects on individuals. Analyzing an individual's response to his or her environment allows a team (either relatives or paid staff) to determine how the environment can be modified and whether there are characteristic responses of the individual under certain conditions.

Saul, an 8-year-old boy with autism, was very unsettled, restless, and irritable when he got off the bus from school. Looking for factors that typically induced this behavior, his father asked some questions about Saul's school day and bus trip home. He could discover nothing out of the ordinary. Because Saul's shoelace was untied, his father went to retie it. He discovered sand in Saul's sneakers. He checked further and found a small sharp rock in Saul's other shoe. He promptly and gently cleaned out both sneakers and checked Saul's feet, which had no cuts. With the accumulated sand and stone gone from his shoes, Saul turned to getting his usual after-school snack.

Saul's story illustrates a boy with autism who has an environmental irritant.

Behavioral and cognitive therapy techniques are essential tools in long-term improvement of function in people with anxiety disorders. Cognitive rehearsals increase an individual's awareness of anxious states, provide a framework for assessing real and apparent danger, and help the individual to implement behavioral relaxation techniques. Massage therapy has also been demonstrated to have clinical efficacy in reducing anxiety (Chen & Chen, 1998). In a case report, cognitive behavioral therapy treatment for severe obsessive-compulsive behavior produced clinical improvement after 6 months in a 7-year-old girl with Asperger syndrome (Reaven & Hepburn, 2003).

Pharmacotherapy has had the most extensive documentation in the literature (see Table 23.3-2). (*Note:* Because doses change over time, verify doses before

Table 23.3-2. Medications recognized to reduce anxiety

Drug class	Drug name	Dose (mg/d)	Comments
Benzodiazepines	Alprazolam	0.5–6	T ½ = 6–14 hours
	Lorazepam	2–10	T ½ = 12–18 hours
	Diazepam	5–60	T ½ = 20–36 hours
	Clonazepam	1–4	T ½ = 30–40 hours
Antipsychotics	Thioridazine	12.5–125	Has the lowest risk for tardive dyskinesia among typical antipsychotics
	Olanzapine	5–10	Atypical with side effects of weight gain and blood dyscrasias
Selective serotonin reuptake inhibitors	Paroxetine	10–40	Side effects include anxiety and depression
	Fluoxetine	10–40	Has an akathisia risk
	Sertraline	25–200	May cause sedation
	Fluvoxamine	25–200	Most individuals take at night because of sedation
	Venlafaxine	37.5–300	Approved for generalized anxiety disorder
Buspirone	Buspirone	15–80	Has slow onset
ß-blocker	Propranolol	60–240	More than 80 mg/d has decreased risk of further hypotensive side effects

Note: Because doses may change over time, verify doses before administering any medication.

administering any medication.) Medications include benzodiazepines, antidepressants (tricyclics, serotonin reuptake inhibitors, and monoamine oxidase inhibitors), buspirone, beta-blockers, and even antipsychotics. Placebo response rates are reported as high in generalized anxiety conditions and low in obsessional conditions (Piercy, Sramek, & Kurtz, 1996).

Dosages published in the *Physician's Desk Reference* or package inserts must be interpreted cautiously. People with developmental disabilities are often more sensitive to the side effects on visual, gastrointestinal, vascular, or vestibular systems. When individuals have any cerebral atrophy, benzodiazepine, in particular, may cause behavioral disinhibition. In general, clinicians should "start low and go slow," meaning they should start at a dose that does not cause visible side effects and slowly titrate the dosage upwards over weeks, being alert to new onset of disturbing side effects.

Sturmey (1999) reviewed clinical indications for the use of psychotropic medications, even for behaviors that do not have a clear diagnosis in the *Diagnostic and Statistical Diagnostic and Statistical Manual of Mental Disorders, Fourth Edition, Text Revision* (DSM–IV; American Psychiatric Association, 2000):

1. The behavior has a clearly stated diagnostic hypothesis or drug-responsive target symptom or DSM–IV diagnosis.
2. The medication corresponds to this hypothesis or diagnosis.
3. The person benefits substantially from the medication.
4. There are no credible alternatives.
5. There are few or no significant side effects of taking the medication.

Alternative therapies and physical manipulation in addition to massage can enhance sensory integration. Acupuncture is a well-established Eastern medicine therapy. Weighted vests and regularly applied sensory stimulation can assist people with autism spectrum disorder to tolerate more interpersonal and physical motion in their immediate environments.

Careful observation of the effects of the interventions on the individual is critical to all therapeutic approaches. The focus must remain on assisting the individual to become more functional, not just to suppress *inconvenient* mannerisms, actions, or verbalizations.

Louisa, a 49-year-old woman with intellectual disabilities, was referred for outpatient care after she was discharged from the institution where she had lived since the age of 8 years. She had a persistent delusion that her baby had been killed by the University Hospital's medical staff. Louisa's primary care physician, listening to her detailed descriptions of her concerns, insisted on digging up Louisa's old medical records from storage. The records documented that Louisa had in fact given birth to a baby girl at the University Hospital. The baby had died in the pediatric intensive care unit at age 4 months from cardiac complications.

After the physician and other staff learned Louisa's 19-year-old history, Louisa started psychotherapy to help her deal with her unresolved grief issues. The physician also determined that Louisa had borderline personality disorder because she projected her impulses, emotions, and motivations on others. She also had rash decision making and impulsive anger.

Cognitive improvement was noted after Louisa's previous antipsychotic, thioridazine, was completely discontinued, and valproic acid (Depakote), which had been prescribed to reduce Louisa's impulsivity, was also discontinued. Discontinuing these medications assisted Louisa in her psychotherapy and improved her ability to communicate her observations and responses to staff. Louisa's anxiety symptoms in response to changes in expectations were clinically responsive to verbal reassurance and lorazepam (a benzodiazepine) at 1 mg twice daily.

In her third year of treatment, Louisa started a trial of stimulant medication for symptoms of not staying on task long either at home or at her supervised work setting or in community settings (e.g., supermarkets). She continued to take methylphenidate SR 20 mg every morning, with sustained improvement in psychotherapy, work, and community functioning. For the last 4 years, Louisa has participated in the local civic club. She has a job in a pet grooming business and has gone on trips out of state with her staff.

Louisa's story illustrates a woman with intellectual disabilities, borderline personality disorder, posttraumatic stress disorder, generalized anxiety disorder, and attention-deficit disorder.

CONCLUSION

Anxiety is a common human condition. "Signal anxiety" occurs normally to alert the individual that potential danger exists. The efficiency with which humans can activate this sensory and mental system is very great and assists in many life-saving decisions. Individuals with developmental disabilities may have difficulty expressing themselves; therefore, anxiety can manifest in unique ways that may be misdiagnosed as maladaptive behaviors or even as psychiatric illnesses as severe as psychosis.

Anxiety disorders that have an onset in late life are under-recognized in the general population, probably more so in those with intellectual disabilities, autism spectrum disorders, or developmental disabilities. Outcome studies of single mode treatment and combined treatments are urgently needed for these individuals. These studies are needed to document the rationale for treatment and to learn about efficacious therapeutic modalities. As professionals, we have historically erred on the side of making assumptions about the experiences of persons with developmental disabilities. Careful research, with the informed consent of participants, will decrease the need for extrapolation and increase our understanding of what constitutes the most therapeutic modalities in the treatment of psychiatric disorders in people with developmental disabilities.

REFERENCES

American Psychiatric Association. (2000). *Diagnostic and statistical manual of mental disorders* (4th ed., text revision). Washington, DC: Author.

Banazak, D.A. (1997). Anxiety disorder in elderly patients. *Journal of the American Board of Family Practice, 10*, 280–289.

Barrios, J.A., Gonzalez-Gordon, R.G., & Ruiz, J.P.N. (1999). Medical and psychosocial evaluation of a mentally retarded adult population. *Revista Española de Salud Publica, 73*, 383–392.

Blazer, D., George, L.K., & Hughes, A. (1991). The epidemiology of anxiety disorder: An age comparison. In C. Salzman & B.D. Lebowitz (Eds.), *Anxiety in the elderly* (pp. 17–30). New York: Springer.

Chen, Z., & Chen, Z. (1998). Forty-eight cases of anxiety syndrome treated by massage. *Journal of Traditional Chinese Medicine, 18*, 282–284.

Cook, E.H.J., et al. (1993). Autistic disorder and post-traumatic stress disorder. *Journal of the American Academy of Child and Adolescent Psychiatry, 32*(6), 1292–1294.

de Beurs, E., et al. (1999). Consequences of anxiety in older persons: Its effect on disability, well being, and use of health services. *Psychological Medicine, 29*, 583–593.

Fontenelle, L.F., et al. (2004). Asperger syndrome, obsessive-compulsive disorder, and major depression in a patient with 45,X/46,XY mosaicism. *Psychopathology, 37*(3), 105–109.

Gillot, A., Furniss, F., & Walter, A. (2001). Anxiety in high-functioning children with autism. *Autism, 5*(3), 277–286.

Gray, J.A. (1995). A model of the limbic system and basal gangila: Applications to anxiety and schizophrenia. In M.S. Gazzaniga (Ed.), *The cognitive neurosciences* (pp. 1165–1176). Cambridge, MA: MIT Press.

Gross, C., & Hen, R. (2004). The developmental origins of anxiety. *Nature Reviews: Neuroscience, 5*(7), 545–552.

Gross-Isseroff, R., Hermesh, H., & Weizman, A. (2001). Obsessive compulsive behaviour in autism—towards an autistice-obsessive compulsive syndrome? *World Journal of Biological Psychiatry, 2*(4), 193–197.

Hammer, M.B., Robert, S., & Frueh, B.C. (2004). Treatment-resistant posttraumatic stress disorder: Strategies for intervention. *CNS Spectrums, 9*(10), 740–752.

Harris, S.L. (2003). Adolescent with autistic spectrum disorder and some obsessive-compulsive disorder behavior. *Journal of Autism and Developmental Disorders, 33*(6), 709.

Hollander, E., et al. (2003). Obsessive-compulsive behaivors in parents of mulitplex autism families. *Psychiatry Research, 117*(1), 11–16.

Iwamasa, G.Y., & Hilliard, K.M. (1999). Depression and anxiety among Asian American elders: A review of the literature. *Clinical Psychology Reviews, 19*, 343–357.

Kessler, R.C., et al. (1994). Lifetime and 12-month prevalence of DSM–III–R psychiatric disorders in the United States. *Archives of General Psychiatry, 51*, 8–19.

Matson, J.L., et al. (1997). Do anxiety disorders exist in persons with severe and profound mental retardation? *Research in Developmental Disabilities, 18*, 39–44.

Piercy, M.A., Sramek, J.J., & Kurtz, N.M. (1996). Placebo in anxiety disorders. *Annals of Pharmacotherapy, 30*, 1013–1019.

Reaven, J., & Hepburn, S. (2003). Cognitive-behavioral treatment of obsessive-compulsive disorder in a child with Asperger syndrome: A case report. *Autism, 7*(2), 145–164.

Ronalds, C., et al. (1997). Outcome of anxiety and depressive disorders in primary care. *British Journal of Psychiatry, 171*, 427–433

Rose, J., Jones, F., & Fletcher, B. (1998). Investigating the relationship between stress and worker behavior. *Journal of Intellectual Disability Research, 42*, 163–172.

Roy-Byrne, P., et al. (1997). Cardiovascular and catecholamine response to orthostasis in panic and obsessive-compulsive disorder and normal controls: Effects of anxiety and novelty. *Depression & Anxiety, 6*, 159–164.

Rynn, M.A., & Brawman-Mintzer, O. (2004). Generalized anxiety disorder: Acute and chronic treatment. *CNS Spectrums, 9*(10), 716–723.

Sturm, H., Fernell, E., & Gillberg, C. (2004). Autism spectrum disorders in children with normal intellectual levels: Associated impairments and subgroups. *Developmental Medicine & Child Neurology, 46*(7), 444–447.

Sturmey, P. (1999). Integration of pharmacotherpy and functional analysis. *The NADD Bulletin, 2*, 97–99.

23.4 DEPRESSION

Robert J. Pary, Mohamed El-Defrawi, Imran Khan, Matthew Parvin, and Nancy Hatch-Warner

Martha was a "hard-to-place" child with moderate intellectual disabilities who was eventually adopted into a family that already had three biological children. She exhibited challenging behaviors, such as self-injurious behaviors. As a teenager, she was suicidal and depressed, which led to a month stay in a psychiatric hospital. The staff had no experience with individuals with developmental disabilities. Furthermore, no follow-up care could be arranged for Martha. Perhaps most frustrating for the family was that the hospital did not prepare them for what Martha's dual diagnosis of intellectual disabilities and affective disorder would entail.

The dual diagnosis meant numerous struggles. Martha saw 12 psychiatrists before finding the "right one." She endured numerous psychiatric diagnoses; three psychiatric hospitalizations; and negative side effects from medications that she was prescribed. Martha's family also soon realized that resources did not cover the two diagnoses as a whole. Finding staff to deal with vocational and residential skills and long-term psychotherapy was a challenge. The family finally hired an attorney from the Disability Law Center to file a discrimination complaint to the Office of Civil Rights and a plan to develop a Self-Directed Support Corporation.

The struggle of Martha's family is important to keep in mind while reading this chapter's discussion of assessment, differential diagnosis, and treatment. Martha's family gave up hope that the "system" will ever understand how to deal with their daughter. For some, this chapter will be a review of largely known material. For others, the chapter will be an opportunity to familiarize with the dual diagnosis of depression and developmental disabilities. Someday, perhaps families of children like Martha will be not so frustrated in dealing with the "system."

PREVALENCE

In the 1800s, clinicians started to describe depressive symptoms in individuals with intellectual disabilities (Smiley & Cooper, 2003). During the mid 1900s, however, psychoanalytic theorists questioned whether individuals with intellectual disabilities were capable of having depressive symptoms (Earl, 1961). Nevertheless, case reports of individuals with developmental disabilities and depressive disorders continued to appear. Sovner and Hurley (1983) directly addressed affective disorder and intellectual disabilities by reviewing case reports and research literature. Their paper was influential, and acceptance that individuals with developmental disabilities can have significant depression is now universal.

Depression in individuals with developmental disabilities appears at least as common as in the general population. A population-based survey and random sample of 10,438 children age 5–15 years found no difference in the rates of depression in children with intellectual disabilities and those in the general population (Emerson, 2003). A fundamental issue for determining how many individuals with developmental disabilities have depression, however, is whether to use standardized criteria for mood disorders or use modified diagnostic criteria.

Historically, diagnostic systems were intended for individuals who could communicate and were able to reflect on abstract concepts such as hopelessness or worthlessness. Sovner (1986) proposed modified criteria for depression in individuals with developmental disabilities. Unfortunately, no systematic attempt has been made to standardize the modification of criteria. Smiley and Cooper (2003) concluded that the existing literature indicated a point prevalence around 4%. They noted, however, that there is a lack of population-based epidemiological studies using contemporary assessment and diagnoses. This situation may change as the formalized diagnostic criteria for psychiatric disorders for use with adults with learning disabilities and intellectual disabilities is used clinically. A similar project is underway as a companion to the *Diagnostic and Statistical Manual of Mental Disorders, Fourth Edition* (DSM–IV) (American Psychiatric Association [APA], 1994), through the APA and National Association of the Dually Diagnosed (NADD) (R. Fletcher, 2004, personal communication).

Dekker and Koot (2003a) took a different approach and *did not modify* standard criteria. They targeted all 6- to 18-year-olds who attended school (borderline intellectual functioning to moderate intellectual disability) in a province in Zuid, Holland. They did a random selection from each of 115 schools. In their first phase, nearly 70% (968 children and adolescents) of all eligible individuals participated. In a second phase, 58% of a random sample from the first phase were eligible, and 474 home interviews were conducted with children and families. Investigators used the Dutch translation of the Diagnostic Interview Schedule–Parent Version (DISC–IV–P).

Dekker and Koot (2003a) determined that 4.4% of individuals tested had some type of mood disorder. This figure included 1.7% with a major depressive disorder; 2.3% with dysthymia; 0.2% with mania; and 0.4% with hypomania. Of the children and adolescents who met criteria for major depressive disorder, 88% were severely affected by the symptoms. For dysthymic disorder, however, only 17% were judged to be severely affected.

In a companion study, Dekker and Koot (2003b) determined what factor(s), if any, predicted a DSM–IV (APA, 1994) psychiatric disorder, including a mood disorder. A previous study had looked at 10 possible factors—previous psychopathology in the child; chronic physical illness; school/learning problems; stressful life events; gender; maternal psychopathology; paternal sociopathy; family dysfunction; single parenthood/divorce; and low socioeconomic status—to predict behavioral or emotional childhood disorders (Williams, Anderson, McGee, & Silva, 1990). Dekker and Koot (2003b) found that mood disorders were uniquely predicted by 16 negative life events, including 1) parent leaving home in past 2 years; 2) at least a 20% decline in family income; 3) hospitalization of a parent for 2 weeks; and 4) death of a friend (Berden, Althaus, & Verhulst, 1990). As Dekker and Koot (2003b) pointed out, stressful life events seemed to trigger depression in both children and adults.

A related issue is the prevalence of depressive disorders in a specific population, such as Down syndrome. A population-based study of 11,277 individuals with Down syndrome found 2.3% with depressive-like behavior compared with a control group of 7.1% with depressive-like behavior (Pary, Strauss, & White, 1997). Another group, however, diagnosed depression in 42 of 371 persons with Down syndrome (11.3%) (Collacott, Cooper, & McGrother, 1992). At this time, whether depression is increased, decreased, or similar in individuals with Down syndrome compared with other individuals with developmental disabilities is unknown.

DIFFERENTIAL DIAGNOSIS FOR DEPRESSIVE EPISODES

The Diagnostic and Statistical Manual of Mental Disorders, Fourth Edition, Text Revision (DSM–IV–TR; APA, 2000) lists several medical illnesses that can cause mood symptoms, including autoimmune, cardiovascular, endocrine, infective, oncologic, metabolic, and neurologic conditions (see Table 23.4-1). Other conditions include hypothyroidism (Sovner & Pary, 1993) and sleep apnea presenting as depression (Smith, 2001). Both hypothyroidism and sleep apnea are important conditions to rule out in individuals with Down syndrome who present with depressive symptoms. Dinani and Carpenter (1990) reported that 40% of 106 adults with Down syndrome had hypothyroidism. Celiac disease may also present with depressive symptoms. In an English abstract of an article in French, psychotic and depressive symptoms improved after 12 months of a gluten-free diet in a 41-year-old with Down syndrome (Serratrice et al., 2002).

Dementia is part of the differential diagnosis of apathy in older adults, especially those with Down syndrome. Evenhuis (1990) noted that symptoms of dementia presenting in the first year were apathy, withdrawal, daytime sleepiness, and loss of self-help skills. Less frequently seen was memory disturbance. Burt, Loveland, and Lewis (1992) proposed that depression and dementia were associated in Down syndrome but not in other etiologies of intellectual disabilities. Alzheimer dementia is the most common dementia in Down syndrome. Unfortunately, there is no treatment that reverses Alzheimer dementia. Consequently, if a clinician is uncertain whether an individual with Down syndrome has Alzheimer dementia or depression, it may be more prudent to first treat depression because a mood disorder has a greater chance to respond to treatment.

Dementia is in the borderland between medical and psychiatric conditions. Other psychiatric conditions also are part of the differential diagnosis. An important differential is bipolar disorder because antidepressants can worsen manic symptoms. Another important psychiatric differential is substance-induced (e.g., steroids, reserpine, Phenobarbital, alpha methyldopa, alcohol) mood disorder. Diagnosing a substance-induced disorder is important because treatment should focus on removing the offending drug.

Finally, four conditions should be included in the differential. First, almost everyone experiences depressed feelings at some point in one's life. For one to be concerned about depression, the duration should be a minimum of 2 weeks and usually longer. Second, depression may serve as a signal that a person needs help and is overwhelmed. Third, depression may be adaptive at times because dangerous goals are not pursued and unpropitious situations are better tolerated (Nesse, 2000). Fourth, and perhaps the most important differential, depression may be a sign of bereavement.

Table 23.4-1. Differential diagnosis of depressive episodes

Medical causes
Acquired immunodeficiency syndrome (AIDS)
B_{12} deficiency
Cancer
Cushing disease
Diabetes mellitus
Huntington disease
Hypothyroidism
Migraines
Multiple sclerosis
Parkinson disease
Perimenopausal hormonal changes
Sleep apnea
Stroke
Viral illness
Psychiatric causes
Adjustment disorder
Bipolar disorder
Dementia
Substance-induced
Other
Grief
Expected [disappointed]

Reprinted with permission from *American Psychiatric Press Textbook of Neuropsychiatry.* (Copyright 1987). American Psychiatric Press.

BEREAVEMENT

Regardless of the level of functioning, everyone experiences losses. Some grieving individuals react to a loss with symptoms characteristics of a major depressive episode (e.g., feeling sad, eating poorly, having disrupted sleep). Individuals in the general population who are grieving typically regard depressed moods as "normal," although the individuals (or their caregivers) may seek professional help for relief of associated symptoms such as insomnia or anorexia. According to DSM–IV–TR (APA, 2000), the duration and expression of "normal" bereavement vary considerably among different cultural groups.

Hollins and Esterhuyzen (1997) reported that when people with developmental disabilities experience bereavement, they were likely to be irritable, lethargic, or hyperactive. Service providers were likely to attribute these changes in behavior to disability rather than to bereavement, and subsequently, to respond to them in ways other than addressing the person's grief. The phenomena following bereavement include a wide range of behaviors such as withdrawal, tearfulness, weight loss, obsession with death, health problems, fecal incontinence, and regressive behavior.

Although bereavement in individuals with developmental disabilities has received increasing attention from researchers and clinicians, prevalence of complicated bereavement is unknown. Some individuals with developmental disabilities are denied an opportunity to participate in the funeral or sometimes even hear about the death of a family member. Hollins and Esterhuyzen (1997) interviewed staff of 50 individuals with developmental disabilities who lost a parent within the past 2 years. Only two individuals refused to go to the funeral. Eleven (22%) individuals did not attend the funeral because another person (usually a family or staff member) made the decision for them not to go. Only 27 individuals (54%) attended the funeral. For the remaining 10 people, researchers could not determine if the person attended. Even fewer people, 8 (16%), had an opportunity to visit the gravesite or place where the ashes were scattered. Hollins and Esterhuyzen concluded that most of the 50 individuals were not assisted in saying goodbyes to their dying parents and were even excluded from the rituals surrounding dying and death.

Bonnell-Pascual et al. (1999) were able to follow 41 of the original 50 people in the Hollins and Esterhuyzen (1997) study. The follow-up was between 6 and 8 years after the parental death. Only a quarter of the sample had received any grief support such as 1) receiving an explanation of the death, 2) attending the funeral, 3) getting opportunities to talk about the loss, 4) visiting the grave, 5) having individual or art therapy, or 6) attending a bereavement-support group.

Yanok and Beifus (1993) believed that individuals with developmental disabilities benefited from a curriculum on death education and grief counseling. The curriculum included such questions as 1) Can a chair die? 2) If you wish hard enough can you make a dead person return to life? and 3) If you wished someone were dead and that person died the next day, would it be your fault?

COMORBIDITY

Individuals with developmental disabilities may have comorbid conditions that are also a treatment target in addition to a depressive episode. About 80% of children diagnosed with any mood disorder also had a comorbid disorder such as an anxiety disorder or disruptive disorder (Dekker & Koot, 2003a). Aman, Arnold, and Armstrong (1999) noted that serotonin selective-reuptake inhibitors (SSRIs) were given for depressive episodes and 1) compulsive behavior; 2) trichotillomania; 3) self-injurious behavior; and 4) aggression. Both Sovner and Pary (1993) and Di Martino and Tuchman (2001) suggested that autism, epilepsy, and affective disorders co-occur. Individuals with developmental disorders, epilepsy, and affective disorders may be at increased risk for suicidal behavior. Di Martino and Tuchman noted that abnormalities in serotonin are common to both autism and affective disorders, which suggests that individuals with autism may be at increased risk for affective disorders.

DIAGNOSIS IN INDIVIDUALS WITH INTELLECTUAL DISABILITIES

As long as a person with mild intellectual disabilities has adequate receptive and communicative skills, DSM–IV (APA, 1994) unmodified criteria for depression can be used. Clinicians can also use behavioral presentations listed in Table 23.4-2 to guide the diagnosis. Sometimes, individuals with mild intellectual disabilities will excessively talk about deceased people and make frequent negative statements about being stupid or no good. Lowry (1993) emphasized that some individuals will focus on somatic physical complaints that often defy explanation after a thorough workup.

Table 23.4-2. Behavioral equivalents of depressive diagnostic criteria for individuals with intellectual disabilities

Diagnostic criteria	Behavioral equivalent
Depressed mood	The individual experiences episodes of crying/whining and rarely smiles.
Irritable mood	The individual is easily provoked to scream, swear, or spit at others.
Loss of interest in previously enjoyable activities	The individual refuses most work or social activities that were once enjoyed. He or she changes from being social to spending excessive time alone.
Loss of appetite	The individual refuses meals.
Excessive appetite	The individual changes eating habits by gorging food, eating too quickly, or stealing food.
Insomnia	The individual has difficulty falling asleep or staying asleep and wakes up too early.
Excessive sleep	The individual sleeps more than 12 hours and takes excessive naps.
Psychomotor agitation	The individual paces, runs, and rarely sits down.
Psychomotor retardation	The individual has extremely slow body movement and stops talking.
Loss of energy	The individual spends excessive time lying or sitting down.
Diminished ability to concentrate	The individual has reduced work productivity (in absence of external causes) and diminished self-care skills.
Feelings of worthlessness	The individual makes negative self-statements.
Excessive physical illness (an associated feature, though not a diagnostic criteria in DSM–IV)	The individual has repeated focus on and complaints of aches, pains, or physical complaints that have no physical basis following examination.

Sources: American Psychiatric Association (2000) and Lowry (1993).

Diagnosis is more challenging for individuals with severe to profound intellectual disabilities because DSM–IV (APA, 1994) unmodified criteria for depression do not apply. Reid (1983) emphasized that psychiatric disorders are largely language based. In individuals without adequate language skills, Reid (1976) suggested that a decline in previous skills (e.g., onset of urinary incontinence) or a significant increase in physical aggression or self-injurious behavior may signal a depressed mood. Sovner (1986) included positive family history as a criterion that would require one fewer criteria to diagnose depression. Meins (1996) designed a depression scale specifically created for individuals with severe and profound intellectual disabilities. His scale includes items such as inner tension; inability to feel; lassitude; reduced sleep; apparent sadness; hostility; withdrawal; agitation; and muscular tension.

Lowry (1993) provided a useful guide of behavioral presentations of depressive diagnostic criteria, shown in Table 23.4-2. Although this table includes an item (feelings of worthlessness) seen primarily in individuals with higher functioning, most of the behavioral presentations are practical for determining depression in individuals who are either nonverbal or are unable to adequately reflect on their own thoughts and feelings. Children with depression may show irritability, have temper tantrums, and indicate that they have somatic complaints. Di Martino and Tuchman (2001) suggested that in some individuals with autism, affective disorder may manifest as an exacerbation of autistic symptoms.

SUICIDAL BEHAVIOR

Davis, Judd, and Herrman (1997) believed that suicidal behavior in individuals with developmental disabilities has been largely neglected. Individuals with intellectual disabilities attempt suicide, and some case reports exist. Walters (1990) presented one such individual, and Hurley (1998) described two individuals with Down syndrome who attempted suicide. Pary et al. (1997) examined suicidal behavior in a population survey of 154,420 individuals receiving support from the California Department of Developmental Services. Two findings from the study were 1) individuals with Down syndrome had significantly fewer incidences of suicidal behavior compared with the control group, and 2) attempted suicide was significantly more likely if the individual also had epilepsy.

Patja, Iivanainen, Raitasuo, and Lonnqvist (2001) conducted a survey of completed suicides among Finnish individuals with intellectual disabilities. From a population-based cohort of 2,369 with intellectual disabilities, 10 people committed suicide based on the Finnish registry of causes of death. Women had a comparable completed suicide rate to the general population, but men with intellectual disabilities had only one third of the expected rate. The study mentioned that 2 of the 10 individuals had epilepsy and another had childhood seizures; however, the authors did not indicate whether individuals with epilepsy had a higher, lower, or comparable rate of suicide.

The issue of epilepsy and suicidal behavior or completed suicide is complicated by the frequent use of phenobarbital for seizure control in the past. Historically, as many as 40% of individuals with intellectual disabilities and epilepsy were prescribed phenobarbital (Kalachnik & Hanzel, 2001). Phenobarbital is associated with numerous behavior and mood problems. Poindexter and Koltsoe (1992) described improvements in alertness and decreases in aggression and explosiveness when phenobarbital was tapered and discontinued.

PHARMACOLOGIC TREATMENT

Sovner et al. (1998) reviewed antidepressants in individuals with developmental disabilities. They concluded that antidepressant therapy is the first choice of medication if the individual meets criteria for major depression or dysthymic disorder. The suggestion of Sovner et al. to use an antidepressant for someone meeting criteria of major depression may seem too obvious. It *is* obvious, until one realizes that later articles noted the inappropriate use of antipsychotics. Santosh and Baird (1999) reminded readers that often individuals with mild or moderate intellectual disabilities and depression *inappropriately* are given antipsychotics.

The *Expert Consensus Guidelines Series* (2000) is a good resource for antidepressant dosing/trials in individuals with intellectual disabilities. The series provides information for 8 (citalopram, fluoxetine, fluvoxamine, paroxetine, sertraline, nefazodone, venlafazine, and bupropion) of the 10 antidepressants on the market (see also Table 23.4-3). Escitalopram dosing is one half that of citalopram. The series does not give dosing guidelines for mirtazapine, and there is a paucity of information about its use in individuals with intellectual disabilities (Patel, Crismon, Rush, & Frances, 2001). Duloxetine was scheduled for release in the United States in 2004, but as of 2005, there have been no studies in individuals with intellectual disabilities.

Thase (2004) outlined three strategies when an initial antidepressant trial fails. The new drug could 1) replace the previous one and be from the same class; 2) replace the previous one and be from a different class; or 3) be added to the current drug. Thase (2004) emphasized that there is very limited evidence-based support for combining antidepressants. A National Institute of Mental Health (NMH) multicenter study on combining antidepressants is expected to be completed in 2005 (Rush, 2004).

Side Effects

Tricyclic antidepressants (TCAs), such as imipramine, amitriptyline, and desipramine, are less often used because of the increased risk of lethality with overdose. TCAs have anticholinergic side effects such as blurred vision, constipation, urinary hesitancy, tachycardia, or delirium (Israel, Georgiopoulos, & Fava, 2004). They can also cause weight gain, orthostatic hypotension, and sedation. In addition, a weak association exists between the tricyclic antidepressant desipramine and sudden death in children (Santosh & Baird, 1999). Other side effects of TCAs include insomnia, weight change (loss followed by gain or just gain), headache, sedation, jitteriness, rash, dry mouth, excessive sweating, and sexual dysfunction (Israel et al., 2004). Hyponatremia can occur rarely with SSRIs.

Venlafaxine is a serotonin-norepinephrine reuptake inhibitor. Side effects are similar to SSRIs. In addition, sustained increases in diastolic blood pressure can occur. Bupropion, mirtazapine, and nefazodone are considered as atypical antidepressants (Israel et al., 2004). Bupropion increases dopamine and norepinephrine turnover. Bupropion is associated with tremor, agitation, weight loss, dry mouth, headache, constipation, insomnia, and seizures at higher doses (e.g., above 450 mg/d). Main side effects with mirtazapine include weight gain, sedation, constipation, orthostatic hypotension, and dizziness. Nefazodone has been associated with catastrophic liver failure, especially if there was preexistent liver disease. It can lead to prolongation of the QT interval. Other side effects include sedation, dizziness, blurred vision, headache, constipation, gastrointestinal upset, and dry mouth.

SSRIs and newer antidepressants may possibly increase the risk of suicide in depressed children and adolescents (Sood, Weller, & Weller, 2004). A dearth of literature exists about increased suicidality in individuals with developmental disabilities. Consequently, the focus will be on the general population. Sood and colleague's (2004) group noted that in May 2003, the Food and Drug Administration (FDA) received unpublished data from placebo-controlled trials of paroxetine in children and adolescents that suggested an increase of possible suicide-related events. No completed suicides were reported at that time. As of December, 2003, the United

Table 23.4-3. Dosages for antidepressant medications in adults with intellectual disabilities and depression

Medication	Pediatric dose	Adult dose	Older adult dose	Comments
Citalopram	N/A	Starting dose 20 mg; usual daily dose 20–40 mg	Usual daily dose 10–30 mg	Use with caution in individuals with hepatic impairment.
Escitalopram	N/A	Starting dose 5 mg; usual daily dose 10–20 mg	Usual daily dose 10 mg	Use with caution in individuals with severe renal impairment.
Fluoxetine	Starting dose of 10 mg; may increase to 20 mg/d after several weeks	Starting dose 10–20 mg; usual daily dose 20–40 mg	Usual daily dose 5–40 mg	Active metabolite, norfluoxetine, has a half-life of 4–16 days. Use with caution in individuals with hepatic impairment.
Fluvoxamine	Starting dose for ages 8–17 years 25 mg; usual daily dose 50–200 mg	Starting dose 50 mg; usual daily dose 50–300 mg	Usual daily dose 50–150 mg	Medication has approval by the Food and Drug Administration for treatment of obsessive-compulsive disorder. Titrate slowly in individuals with hepatic impairment.
Paroxetine	N/A	Starting dose 10–20 mg; usual daily dose 20–40 mg	Usual daily dose 5–20 mg	Avoid abrupt discontinuation.
Sertraline	Starting dose for 6–12 years 25 mg	Starting dose 50 mg; usual daily dose 50–200 mg	Usual daily dose 12.5–150 mg	Use with caution in individuals with hepatic impairment.
Bupropion-SR	N/A	Starting dose 150–200 mg; usual daily dose 200–450 mg	Usual daily dose 75–225 mg	Medication has increased risk of seizures at higher doses. Use with caution in individuals with hepatic or renal impairment.
Mirtazapine	N/A	Starting dose 15 mg; usual daily dose 15–45 mg	Reduce dose; use caution in older adults	Use with caution in individuals with renal or hepatic impairment.
Nefazodone	N/A	Starting dose 100 mg; usual daily dose 100–600 mg	Usual daily dose 50–200 mg	This medication has a reported case of life-threatening liver disease.
Venlafaxine–XR	N/A	Starting dose 75 mg; usual daily dose 75–225 mg	Usual daily dose 12.5–200 mg	Use with caution in individuals with renal or hepatic impairment. Hypertension may be seen at higher doses.

Key: N/A = not applicable because not approved for pediatric use.
Note: Because doses may change over time, verify doses before administering medication.
Sources: Expert Consensus Guidelines (2000) and Mosby's Drug Consult (2005).

Kingdom's Medicines and Healthcare Products Regulatory Agency (MHRA) mandated that the following medications be labeled as contraindicated for major depression in children under 18 years: paroxetine, venlafaxine, sertraline, citalopram, and es-citalopram.

In March 2004, the FDA issued a warning on the pediatric use for major depression of the five drugs in the MHRA warning and added: bupropion, fluoxetine, fluoxamine, mirtazapine, and nefazodone. The FDA did *not* indicate that these drugs caused increased suicidality, but that the possibility existed and increased vigilance was needed. Also, a study was commissioned to review more than 400 clinical vignettes from placebo as well as medication-treated arms to determine if there was an increase in suicidality.

Sood and colleague's (2004) group noted that the FDA heard testimony from families of two youths who committed suicide while taking SSRIs. The American College of Neuropharmacology (ACNP; 2004), however, reviewed the published clinical studies of more than 2,000 youths on SSRIs as well as unpublished data. The ACNP concluded that no youth completed suicide in any clinical trial, and no statistically significant association existed between SSRIs and suicidal ideation or behavior. Mann, co-chair of the ACNP report, believed that not treating severe depressive illness in youth was a greater risk than side effects of SSRIs.

LIGHT THERAPY

In seasonal affective disorder (SAD), individuals typically become depressed during winter. A leading hypothesis of SAD is that decreased light in winter is responsible for the depressed state, and light therapy can help alleviate the depression. Cooke and Thompson (1998) suggested that if an individual has a pattern of worsening target behaviors in winter, then light therapy may be a consideration. They described two individuals with developmental disabilities in their article who responded to light therapy, but more research is needed on this topic.

ELECTROCONVULSIVE TREATMENT

In severe depression, electroconvulsive treatment (ECT) works when medication trials have failed (Lazarus, Jaffe, & Dubin, 1990; Warren, Holroyd, & Folstein, 1989). Furthermore, ECT has been advocated as a maintenance treatment (Ruedrich & Alamir, 1999). Some clinicians, families, and guardians, however, are very reluctant to even consider it because of fear of further cognitive deterioration (Friedlander & Solomons, 2002). Permanent brain damage from ECT is unproven. Posttreatment confusion and delirium, however, can occur. Individuals with moderate or severe intellectual disabilities are probably at greater risk for developing delirium.

If ECT is contemplated, clinicians should be careful to monitor pretreatment orientation and memory and continue to reassess memory and orientation throughout the course of treatments. If there is evidence of confusion during treatments, the frequency of treatments should be decreased. With the paucity of research, ECT for depression in individuals with intellectual disabilities is a treatment of last resort.

PSYCHOTHERAPY

Ample evidence shows that psychotherapy (individual, group, and family) can benefit an individual with developmental disabilities if it is adapted to the individual's mental age and communication abilities (Hollins, Sinason, & Thompson, 1994; Nezu & Nezu, 1994; Sigman, 1985). Goals of therapy are 1) to relieve symptoms, 2) to help the individual understand the nature of his or her distress/feelings, and 3) to encourage the individual to appreciate his or her strengths (Reber, 2002). Dagnan and Sandhu (1999) studied self-esteem, depression, and social comparison (i.e., evaluating one's self in contrast with others) in 43 individuals with mild or moderate intellectual disabilities. They found that depression correlated with thoughts of being worse than other people or not as good at things as other people. This finding suggested to the authors that individuals with mild or moderate intellectual disabilities may benefit from cognitive therapy.

CONCLUSION

Depression in individuals with intellectual disabilities is at least as common as it is in the general population. The evaluation and treatment processes remain taxing for individuals and their families. Suicidal behavior can occur in individuals with intellectual disabilities and should be considered during assessment and treatment. Treatment with psychotherapy and/or SSRIs is standard.

Compared with mood disorders in the general population, research on depression in individuals with intellectual disabilities is still at a very elementary level. Standardization of modified criteria and testing these criteria against standard criteria for depression in a multicenter study is waiting to be done. Clinicians need to know if and how standard criteria should be modified for individuals with intellectual disabilities and possible depression.

Areas for further investigation include negative life events and future depressive episodes in children with developmental disabilities. The possibility that epilepsy increases the risk of suicidal behavior should also be studied. In addition, studies assessing psychotherapy alone and antidepressants alone versus antidepressants combined with psychotherapy are needed. Light therapy for SAD demands further research as well.

REFERENCES

Aman, M.G., Arnold, L.E., & Armstrong, S.C. (1999). Review of serotonergic agents and perseverative behavior in patients with developmental disabilities. *Mental Retardation and Developmental Disabilities, 5,* 279–289.

American College of Neuropsychopharmacology. (ACNP). (2004). *Preliminary report of the task force on SSRIs and suicidal behavior in youth.* Retrieved from http://www.acnp.org/exec_summary.pdf

American Psychiatric Association. (1994). *Diagnostic and statistical manual of mental disorders* (4th ed.). Washington, DC: Author.

American Psychiatric Association. (2000). *Diagnostic and statistical manual of mental disorders* (4th ed., text revision). Washington, DC: Author.

Berden, G.F.M.G., Althaus, M., & Verhulst, F.C. (1990). Major life events and changes in the behavioural functioning of children. *Journal of Child Psychology and Psychiatry, and Applied Disciplines, 31*(6), 949–959.

Bonell-Pascual, E., Huline-Dickens, S., Hollins, S., Esterhuyzen, A., Sedgewick, P., Abdelnoor, A., et al. (1999). Bereavement and grief in adults with learning disabilities: A follow-up study. *British Journal of Psychiatry, 175*, 348–350.

Burt, D.B., Loveland, K.A., & Lewis, K.R. (1992). Depression and the onset of dementia in adults with mental retardation. *American Journal of Mental Retardation, 96*(5), 502–511.

Collacott, R.A., Cooper, S.-A., & McGrother, C. (1992). Differential rates of psychiatric disorders in adults with Down syndrome compared with other mentally handicapped adults. *British Journal of Psychiatry, 161*, 671–674.

Cooke, L.B., & Thompson, C. (1998). Seasonal affective disorder and response to light in two patients with learning disability. *Journal of Affective Disorders, 48*(2–3), 145–148.

Dagnan, D., & Sandhu, S. (1999). Social comparison, self esteem, and depression in people with intellectual disability. *Journal of Intellectual Disability Research, 43*(5), 372–379.

Davis, J.P., Judd, F.K., & Herrman, H. (1997). Depression in adults with intellectual disability: Part I: A review. *Australian and New Zealand Journal of Psychiatry, 31*(2), 232–242.

Dekker, M.C., & Koot, H.M. (2003a). DSM–IV disorders in children with borderline to moderate intellectual disability: I: Prevalence and impact. *Journal of the American Academy of Child and Adolescent Psychiatry, 42*(8), 915–922.

Dekker, M.C., & Koot, H.M. (2003b). DSM–IV disorders in children with borderline to moderate intellectual disability: II: Child and family predictors. *Journal of the American Academy of Child and Adolescent Psychiatry, 42*(8), 923–931.

Di Martino, A., & Tuchman, R.F. (2001). Antiepileptic drugs: Effective use in autism spectrum disorders. *Pediatric Neurology, 25*, 199–207.

Dinani, S., & Carpenter, S. (1990). Down syndrome and thyroid disorder. *Journal of Mental Deficiency Research, 43*, 187–193.

Earl, C.J.C. (1961). *Subnormal personalities.* London: Balliere, Tindal & Cox.

Emerson, E. (2003). Prevalence of psychiatric disorders in children and adolescents with and without intellectual disability. *Journal of Intellectual Disability Research, 47*(1), 51–58.

Evenhuis, H.M. (1990). The natural history of dementia in Down's syndrome. *Archives of Neurology, 47*, 263–267.

Expert consensus guideline series: Treatment of psychiatric and behavioral problems in mental retardation. (2000). *American Journal of Mental Retardation, 105*(3), 159–226.

Friedlander, R., & Solomons, K. (2002). ECT: Use in individuals with mental retardation. *Journal of ECT, 18*(1), 38–42.

Hales, R.E., & Yudofsky, S.C. (1987). *The American Psychiatric Press textbook of neuropsychiatry.* Washington, DC: American Psychiatric Association.

Hollins, S.A., & Esterhuyzen, A. (1997). Bereavement and grief in adults with learning disabilities. *British Journal of Psychiatry, 170*, 497–501.

Hollins, S., Sinason, V., & Thompson, S. (1994). Individual group and family therapy. In N. Borus (Ed.), *Mental health in mental retardation.* Cambridge, England: Cambridge University Press.

Hurley, A.D. (1998). Two cases of suicide attempt by patients with Down syndrome. *Psychiatric Services, 48*, 1618–1619.

Israel, J., Georgiopoulos, A., & Fava, M. (2004). Antidepressants and somatic therapies. In T.A. Stern & J.B. Herman (Eds.), *Massachusetts General Hospital psychiatry update and board review preparation* (pp. 343–348). New York: McGraw-Hill.

Kalachnik, J.E., & Hanzel, T.E. (2001). Behavioral side effects of barbiturate antiepileptic drugs in individuals with mental retardation and developmental disabilities. *NADD Bulletin, 4*(3), 49–54.

Lazarus, A., Jaffe, R.L., & Dubin, W.R. (1990). Electroconvulsive therapy and major depression in Down's syndrome. *Journal of Clinical Psychiatry, 51*, 422–425.

Lowry, M.A. (1993). Behavioral psychology update—A clear link between problem behaviors and mood disorders. *Habilitative Mental Healthcare Newsletter, 12*(6), 105–110.

Meins, W. (1996). A new depression scale designed for use with adults with mental retardation *Journal of Intellectual Disability Research, 40, 222–226.*

Mosby's Drug Consult [on-line database]. (2005). Available on-line at http://www.mosbysgrugconsult.com

Nesse, R.M. (2000). Is depression an adaptation? *Archives of General Psychiatry, 57*(1), 14–20.

Nezu, C.M., & Nezu, A.M. (1994). Outpatient psychotherapy for adults with mental retardation and concomitant psychopathology: Research and clinical imperatives. *Journal of Consulting and Clinical Psychology, 62*, 34–42.

Pary, R.J., Strauss, D., & White, J.F. (1997). A population survey of suicide attempts with and without Down syndrome. *Down Syndrome Quarterly, 2*, 12–13.

Patel, N.C., Crismon, M.L., Rush, A.J., & Frances, A. (2001). Practitioner versus medication-expert opinion on psychiatric pharmacotherapy of mentally retarded patients with mental disorders. *American Journal of Health-System Pharmacy, 58*(19), 1824–1849.

Patja, K., Iivanainen, M., Raitasuo, S., & Lonnqvist, J. (2001). Suicide mortality in mental retardation: A 35-year follow-up study. *Acta Psychaitrica Scandanavica, 103*(4), 307–311.

Poindexter, A.R., & Kolstoe, P.D. (1992). Effects of barbiturate withdrawal on behavior—Results from a barbiturate discontinuation program. *Habilitative Mental Healthcare Newsletter, 11*(10), 63–66.

Psychiatry. (2004). *Mental Fitness, 3*(2), 12.

Reber, M. (2002). Dual diagnosis: Mental retardation and psychiatric disorders. In M.L. Batshaw (Ed.), *Children with disabilities* (5th ed., pp. 347–363). Baltimore: Paul H. Brookes Publishing Co.

Reid, A.H. (1976). Psychiatric disturbances in the mentally handicapped. *Proceedings of the Royal Soc of Medicine, 69*, 509–512.

Reid, A.H. (1983). Psychiatry of mental handicap: A review. *Journal of the Royal Society of Medicine, 76*, 376–592.

Ruedrich, S.L., & Alamir, A. (1999). Electroconvulsive therapy for persons with developmental disabilities: Review, case report and recommendations. *Mental Health Aspects of Developmental Disabilities, 2*(3), 83–91.

Rush, A.J. (2004). Treatment-resistant depression: Choices that improve response rates. *Current Psychiatry, 3*(3), 10–19.

Santosh, P.J., & Baird, G. (1999). Psychopharmacology in children and adults with intellectual disability. *Lancet, 354*, 233–242.

Serratrice, J., Disdier, P., Kaladjian, A., Granel, B., Azorin, J.M., Laugier, R., et al. (2002). [Psychosis revealing a silent celiac disease in a young women with trisomy 21.] [Article in French.] *Presse Medicale, 31*(33), 1551–1553.

Sigman, M. (1985). Individual and group psychotherapy with mentally retarded adolescents. In M. Sigman (Ed.), *Children with emotional disorders and developmental disabilities* (pp. 259–276). New York: Grune & Stratton.

Smiley, E., & Cooper, S.-A. (2003). Intellectual disabilities, depressive episode, diagnostic criteria and diagnostic criteria for psychiatric disorders for use in adults with learning disabilities/mental retardation (DC/LD). *Journal of Intellectual Disability Research, 47*(s1), 62–71.

Smith, D.S. (2001). Health care management of adults with Down syndrome. *American Family Physician, 64*(6), 1031–1038.

Sood, A.B., Weller, E., & Weller, R. (2004). SSRIs in children and adolescents—Where do we stand? *Current Psychiatry, 3*(3), 83–89.

Sovner, R. (1986). Limiting factors in the use of DSM-III criteria with mentally ill/mentally retarded persons. *Psychopharmacology Bulletin, 22*, 1055–1059.

Sovner, R., & Hurley, A.D. (1983). Do the mentally retarded suffer from affective disorder? *Archives of General Psychiatry, 40*, 61–7.

Sovner, R., & Pary, R.J. (1993). Affective disorders in developmentally disabled persons. In J.L. Matson & R.P. Barrett (Eds.), *Psychopathology in the mentally retarded* (2nd ed., pp. 87–148). Boston: Allyn & Bacon.

Sovner, R., Pary, R.J., Dosen, A., Gedye, A., Barrerra, F.J., Cantwell, D.P., et al. (1998). Antidepressant drugs. In S. Reiss & M.G. Aman (Eds.), *Psychotropic medications and developmental disabilities: The international consensus handbook* (pp. 179–200). Columbus: The Ohio State University, Nisonger Center.

Thase, M.E. (2004). What to do for SSRI nonresponders? *American Psychiatric Association Annual Meeting Syllabus and Proceedings Summary*, 27.

Walters, R.M. (1990). Suicidal behavior in severely mentally retarded patients. *British Journal of Psychiatry, 157*, 444–446.

Warren, A.C., Holroyd, S., & Folstein, M.F. (1989). Major depression in Down's syndrome. *British Journal of Psychiatry, 155*, 202–205.

Williams, S., Anderson, J., McGee, R., & Silva, P.A. (1990). Risk factors for behavioral and emotional disorder in preadolescent children. *Journal of the American Academy of Child and Adolescent Psychiatry, 29*(3), 413–419.

Yanok, J., & Beifus, J.A. (1993). Communicating about loss and mourning: Death education for individuals with mental retardation. *Mental Retardation, 31*(3), 144–147.

23.5 SELF-INJURY, AGGRESSION, AND PICA

Henry Roane, Wayne Fisher, Nathan A. Call, and Michael E. Kelley

Behaviors that place an individual or his or her caregivers at risk for physical harm may be generally classified as *destructive behavior problems*. Common topographies of destructive behaviors include self-injurious behavior (SIB), physical aggression, and property destruction. SIB has been defined as behavior in which an individual produces physical damage to his or her body (Tate & Baroff, 1966). Examples of frequently observed SIB among individuals with developmental disabilities include head banging, self-hitting, self-biting, self-pinching, self-scratching, pica, hand-mouthing, eye poking, and hair pulling (Iwata, Dorsey, Slifer, Bauman, & Richman, 1982/1994; Johnson & Day, 1992). The outcome of chronic SIB ranges from hematomas and severe tissue damage to death. SIB can also affect the social and educational development of individuals who engage in these behaviors in that appropriate social behavior may be sacrificed for aberrant behavior. Furthermore, others may avoid social interaction with these individuals due to the frequency and severity of the behavior.

Physical aggression commonly includes hitting, kicking, or pinching others; tearing or breaking objects; throwing objects; climbing or taking other unnecessary risks; and pushing objects over (Fisher, Lindauer, Alterson, & Thompson, 1998; Iwata, Pace, et al., 1994). In contrast to SIB, aggression generally poses the most significant health risks to others. For example, Piazza et al. (1994) noted that aggressive behavior caused an average of 20 staff injuries, 2 emergency room visits, and 8 sick days monthly on a 6-bed inpatient unit that served individuals with destructive behavior.

Nationwide, destructive behavior problems affect more than 160,000 individuals with developmental disabilities (Thompson & Gray, 1984). In general, the prevalence of severe destructive behaviors (i.e., those requiring intervention) has been estimated to occur among 10%–20% of individuals with developmental disabilities, although these estimates may vary dramatically (Schroeder, 1991). For example, Schroeder, Schroeder, Smith, and Dalldorf (1978) interviewed employees of residential facilities on multiple occasions across a 4-year period. Data were compiled on a sample of 208 individuals, and "chronic" destructive behavior was noted to occur in approximately 10% of the sample. Using interviews of psychologists, psychiatrists, physicians, and other care providers, Oliver, Murphy, and Corbett (1987) collected prevalence data on 596 individuals with developmental disabilities and found that approximately 19% of the sample engaged in repeated occurrences of destructive behavior.

Among individuals with developmental disabilities, the occurrence of destructive behavior seems to be highly correlated with a number of variables. In a review of 34 studies related to the prevalence of SIB, for example, Johnson and Day (1992) concluded the following: 1) boys and men were more likely to engage in SIB than girls and women, 2) SIB did not consistently vary with age, 3) SIB was associated more with the severe to profound range of intellectual disabilities than with the mild to moderate range, and 4) SIB was associated with institutional placement for individuals with profound intellectual disabilities.

PROPOSED ETIOLOGY

Psychoanalytic theory posits that destructive behavior patterns are related to unconscious feelings or improper development of the ego (Spitz & Wolfe, 1949); however, little empirical support exists for a psychodynamic model of SIB (Carr, 1977; Schroeder, 1991). An alternative epidemiological explanation for destructive behaviors is that certain organic variables predispose an individual to engage in severe destructive behavior. This organic hypothesis is supported by the prevalence of destructive behaviors among specific sex-linked and chromosomal disorders. For example, individuals diagnosed with Lesch-Nyhan disorder engage in severe self-biting and often other forms of SIB (Little & Rodemaker, 1998). Likewise, children with Cri-du-chat syndrome are likely to engage in behaviors that are dangerous to themselves and others (Wilkins, Brown, & Wolf, 1980). Finally, pain insensitivity or endogenous opiate release have been discussed as potential factors underlying the emergence of SIB and aggression (Cataldo & Harris, 1982).

Although some evidence suggests that organic variables play a role in the development of destructive behavior, incidences of these problems cannot be attributed entirely to organic aberrations. For example, fragile X syndrome and Down syndrome are sometimes associated with the emergence of self-injurious and aggressive behaviors; however, these behaviors do not occur in all individuals diagnosed with these disorders (Schroeder, 1991). Likewise, biochemical origins of SIB may be applicable to some individuals but not others (see Cataldo & Harris, 1982, for a review).

An alternative to the hypotheses listed previously is that SIB and aggression are learned responses that are maintained by environmental consequences. Carr (1977) theorized that destructive behavior and SIB (and aggression) are maintained by different events that precede or follow their occurrence. Central to this *operant* hypothesis is the idea that destructive behaviors operate on their environment to produce consequences that influence their future probability. Carr presented three mechanisms that may be associated with the occurrence of destructive behavior.

The *positive reinforcement hypothesis* suggests that destructive behavior is maintained by pairing the behavior with a preferred outcome. For example, a child may have a history of receiving social attention (e.g., verbal reprimands, hugs) for engaging in destructive behavior. Although these reactions may be intended to "calm" the child or make the behavior stop, the delivery of attention following SIB may pair the behavior with the consequence, thereby increasing the future likelihood of SIB. When the presentation of some stimulus or event results in an increase in the response it is made contingent upon, the stimulus is referred to as a *positive reinforcer.*

The second operant mechanism described by Carr involves pairing destructive behavior with removal of an aversive stimulus. In this *negative reinforcement hypothesis,* destructive behavior results in the avoidance or cessation of an aversive event (e.g., instructional activities). In much the same way that presentation of a preferred outcome increases the behavior that preceded the presentation, the removal of an aversive event can function to strengthen the future occurrence of the maladaptive response. For example, a child for whom self-help tasks are aversive may act aggressively toward caregivers during these activities. As a result, caregivers may stop presenting such tasks to the child because of the probability of destructive behavior. Thus, the child's behavior is negatively reinforced because aversive activities are avoided by engaging in destructive behavior.

The final operant mechanism described by Carr was the "self-stimulation" hypothesis. This hypothesis purports that *automatic reinforcement* (i.e., reinforcement directly produced by the maladaptive response, independent of the external environment; Vaughn & Michael, 1982) may function in the development and maintenance of SIB. Just as events that are produced by others (e.g., attention, breaks from tasks, access to preferred items), or *social reinforcers,* can be subdivided into positive and negative reinforcers, automatic reinforcers can be positive or negative. For example, children who hand-mouth may be presumed to do so because hand-mouthing is a pleasurable event (i.e., *automatic positive reinforcement*). In contrast, some behaviors may occur because they alleviate an aversive stimulus. For example, an individual may engage in head hitting to attenuate pain caused by an ear infection (i.e., *automatic negative reinforcement*; O'Reilly, 1997).

Carr's (1977) operant account of SIB suggested that in some cases these behaviors are used by the individual as a method of controlling or interacting with surroundings. Numerous research findings support Carr's (1977) hypotheses by empirically demonstrating that an individual's destructive behavior occurred predictably when it resulted in certain consequences and stopped occurring when those consequences were discontinued. Lovaas and Simmons (1969), for example, showed that rates of SIB increased when the behaviors resulted in attention (i.e., positive reinforcement). Carr, Newsome, and Binkoff (1980) showed that, for one participant, aggression occurred at high rates when it resulted in escape from academic demand situations (i.e., negative reinforcement). Also, rates of aggression dropped to low levels when aggression no longer produced escape. Berkson and Mason (1964) showed that when participants were deprived of alternative stimulation (e.g., toys) they engaged in high rates of SIB, supporting the hypothesis that those participants' SIB was maintained by self-stimulation (i.e., automatic reinforcement). Furthermore, low rates of SIB occurred when alternative stimulation was provided continuously. Finally, both De Lissovoy (1963) and O'Reilly (1997) noted that some cases of SIB occurred only in the presence of ear infections, presumably to alleviate painful stimulation (i.e., automatic reinforcement).

STRUCTURAL VERSUS FUNCTIONAL ASSESSMENT

Treatments for behavior problems often are based on the particular behavior (i.e., topography) and the extent to which behavior problems co-occur (Kratochwill & McGivern, 1996). Unfortunately, two individuals who display topographically similar behaviors (e.g., aggression) may require different treatments because their behaviors are maintained by different consequences (Carr & Durand, 1985; Demchak, 1993; Iwata, Pace, Kalsher, Cowdery, & Cataldo, 1990). Behavioral intervention is maximally effective when it matches the consequences that motivate or reinforce the problem behavior (Day, Rea, Schussler, Larsen, & Johnson, 1988; Repp, Felce, & Barton, 1988). Thus, when assessing an individual's destructive behavior, practitioners should consider methods for identifying the underlying reasons that maintain the behavior.

One important step is to examine the *function*, of the behavior. How is the behavior related to events that occur before (antecedents) and after (consequences) the behavior? The following section provides an overview of some common assessments that are used to determine the function of problematic behavior.

IDENTIFYING FUNCTIONAL RELATIONSHIPS

Iwata, Dorsey, et al. (1982/1994) presented a methodology designed to assess potential operant mechanisms responsible for the maintenance of SIB in individuals. Their methodology directly tested the hypotheses put forth by Carr (1977). In three test conditions, relevant antecedent (i.e., presence or absence of social attention, aversive stimulation, or alternative stimulation) and consequent events (i.e., delivery of attention, escape from tasks, or level of stimulation) varied. Each condition was developed to test a particular operant hypothesis.

The *social disapproval condition* was designed to test whether behavior was maintained by positive reinforcement in the form of attention. A therapist who was in the room did not interact with the participant but sat nearby and was engaged in another activity. The participant had continuous access to toys but was ignored otherwise. Contingent on the occurrence of SIB, the therapist immediately ceased his or her activity and provided the participant with attention in the form of disapproving comments (e.g., "Stop that," "Don't do that"). From this arrangement, participants for whom attention was reinforcing and who had a history of receiving attention for SIB were expected to engage in SIB in this condition.

The second test condition was the *academic demand condition*. In this condition, a therapist was present in the room with the participant. Instructional activities were presented to the participant once every 30 seconds. If SIB occurred, instructional items were removed, the therapist turned away from the participant, and the participant was given a 30-second break from instructions. This condition was designed to test the negative reinforcement hypothesis because participants were likely to engage in SIB in this condition if breaks from aversive demands were negatively reinforcing.

In the final test condition (*alone*), the participant was observed alone in a therapy room. No toys were present, and no social consequences were provided for

SIB. The purpose of this condition was to determine if SIB would occur in the absence of social stimulation, which would suggest an automatic reinforcement function. That is, if the participants engaged in SIB when there was no social consequence (e.g, attention, breaks for demands) for doing so, some automatic reinforcer was probably maintaining the behavior.

In addition to these test conditions, a control condition (*unstructured play*) also was conducted in which participants had continuous access to preferred stimuli and received attention every 30 seconds. The analysis continued until 1) stable responding occurred in one of the test conditions, 2) unstable responding persisted for 5 days, or 3) 12 days of sessions were completed. Results indicated that higher levels of SIB were associated with one test condition for 6 of the 9 participants. Furthermore, response patterns differed among these 6 participants, suggesting that the reinforcer maintaining SIB (i.e., the function of SIB) varied across individuals. Thus, the data presented by Iwata, Dorsey, et al. (1982/1994) provided evidence for an operant account of SIB. Furthermore, the authors demonstrated an efficient methodology for studying the relationship between problem behavior and specific environmental events.

Since its development, the functional analysis methodology has been extended to other topographies of destructive behavior, including aggression (Marcus, Vollmer, Swanson, Roane, & Ringdahl, 2001; Thompson, Fisher, Piazza, & Kuhn, 1998), disruption (e.g., Fisher, Adelinis, Thompson, Worsdell, & Zarcone, 1998), screaming (Lalli, Mace, Wohn, & Livezy, 1995), and stereotypy (Vollmer, Marcus, & LeBlanc, 1994; see also Hanley, Iwata, & McCord, 2003, for a comprehensive review). Functional analyses also are effective prescriptive tools because events that maintain problem behavior can be manipulated as part of treatment (Mace, 1994).

For example, Day et al. (1988) used functional analysis–based treatments for three individuals who engaged in SIB. Two participants' behavior was maintained by positive reinforcement in the form of access to leisure items or toys. Treatment consisted of teaching an alternative method of obtaining the same stimuli (i.e., teaching participants to request materials) while no longer providing items for SIB. For a third participant, the functional analysis revealed that SIB was maintained by automatic reinforcement. Treatment consisted of blocking SIB (via restraints) and providing alternative stimulation (i.e., music via headphones).

Steege et al. (1990) demonstrated that two participants' SIB was maintained by escape from tasks (i.e., self-grooming). Treatment consisted of teaching the participants to engage in an alternative response (i.e., pressing a microswitch) to escape tasks. In both the Day et al. (1988) and Steege et al. investigations, functional analyses were used to determine what type of reinforcement to manipulate in treatments. These reinforcers were made available to the participant for emitting an alternative response and withheld when the participant engaged in the inappropriate behavior.

TREATMENT DEVELOPMENT

When behavioral interventions are selected based on the function of the problem behavior, the response–reinforcer relationship that maintains the maladaptive behavior can be disrupted, and the same consequences that maintain the behavior can be differentially delivered for alternative behaviors. Thus, a situation can be arranged in which the probability of receiving reinforcement for problem behavior is 0, and the probability of receiving reinforcement for desirable behavior is 1.0 (Pelios, Morren, Tesch, & Axelrod, 1999). The most basic process consists of discontinuing the delivery of the reinforcer when the individual engages in the target behavior (i.e., *extinction*). For example, if a functional analysis has demonstrated that a child's aggression is maintained by parental attention, no longer delivering attention following acts of aggression could be expected to result in a decrease in aggression.

Extinction is a core component of many behavioral treatments; however, it is sometimes associated with negative side effects, including an initial increase in problem behavior (i.e., *extinction burst*), the occurrence of new forms of problem behavior, or emotional responding (e.g., Cowdery, Iwata, & Pace, 1990). Despite concerns about side effects, extinction bursts occur in approximately one third of individuals (Lerman, Iwata, & Wallace, 1999). Furthermore, the side effects of extinction are generally ameliorated when extinction is accompanied by additional treatment components.

An individual is rarely entirely prevented from gaining access to a reinforcer that was previously available for problem behavior. That is, despite the best intentions of caregivers, not responding to severe destructive behavior is often difficult or dangerous. Therefore, one alternative to extinction consists of delivering the maintaining reinforcer at set time intervals. This procedure, known as *noncontingent reinforcement* (NCR; Mace & Lalli, 1991), involves the delivery of the reinforcer that maintains destructive behavior on a time-based schedule (e.g., once every 60 seconds) rather than contingent on the child's behavior. The rational for this approach is that the child should be less motivated to use destructive behavior to obtain reinforcement if he or she is essentially receiving reinforcement "for free." NCR procedures have been effective in a number of cases (Lalli, Casey, & Kates, 1997; Roane, Fisher, & Sgro, 2001; Vollmer, Iwata, Zarcone, Smith, & Mazaleski, 1993); however, NCR may be limited in its practicality because it does not develop an appropriate form of behavior to replace destructive behavior.

Another treatment procedure, *differential reinforcement,* involves reinforcing a response other than the targeted (maladaptive) response (Vollmer & Iwata, 1992). The term differential reinforcement refers to an arrangement in which some behaviors result in delivery of the reinforcer while others (i.e., destructive behaviors) are placed on extinction. Several variations of differential reinforcement have been demonstrated to be effective, with the difference between them primarily being the behaviors that are reinforced. For example, differential reinforcement of other behavior (DRO; Repp & Deitz, 1974) specifies that any behaviors other than the targeted problem behavior result in reinforcement. Thus, after a certain period of time without engaging in the target behavior, the individual receives reinforcement. In contrast, when reinforcement is contingent on a specific alternative behavior, the procedure is referred to as differential reinforcement of alternative behavior (DRA; e.g., Mazaleski, Iwata, Vollmer, Zarcone, & Smith, 1993; Vollmer & Iwata, 1992). For example, a child whose SIB in the form of hitting his head is maintained by access to a preferred toy might only receive the same toy when he engages in some behavior that is incompatible with head hitting (e.g., doing a puzzle).

A variation of DRA, called functional communication training (FCT), specifies that the alternative behavior be a communicative response. FCT involves the delivery of a previously identified functional reinforcer contingent on the individual emitting an appropriate request (e.g., saying, "Toy, please," or emitting a manual sign; Carr & Durand, 1985). FCT is a beneficial treatment because it allows for the development of a response that may be understood by a variety of caregivers. Furthermore, FCT has been used in combination with a number of consequences for problem behavior, including extinction (Day et al., 1988; Fisher et al., 1993; Lalli et al., 1997), punishment (Fisher, et al., 1993; Wacker et al., 1990), extinction plus redirection (Steege, Wacker, Berg, Cigrand, & Cooper, 1989), and extinction plus response blocking (Carr & Durand, 1985; Durand & Carr, 1991). In a comparison of these procedures, Hagopian, Fisher, Sullivan, Acquisto, and LeBlanc (1998) demonstrated that FCT appeared to be effective at increasing communication and reducing problem behavior regardless of the accompanying consequence for problem behavior. The lone exception to this finding was that FCT did not result in reductions in problem behavior when it was the sole treatment component. In addition, when problem behaviors continued to result in reinforcement, FCT was not effective.

Although research has demonstrated that treatments based on functional analysis outcomes are generally robust given less-than-perfect implementation (Vollmer, Roane, Ringdahl, & Marcus, 1999), poor treatment integrity can influence the effectiveness of treatments. For example, if an extinction procedure is not implemented consistently, an intermittent schedule of reinforcement is established in which some responses are reinforced whereas others are not. This schedule of reinforcement has been associated with higher rates of responding as well as greater resistance to future attempts to implement extinction procedures (Ferster & Skinner, 1957). Thus, if treatment integrity is poor, counter-therapeutic results may occur.

Providing appropriate care for individuals who display severe aggression and self-injury is often difficult. Many placements do not have the training, staff, or other resources that are necessary to provide intervention services for these types of problems. The Severe Behavior Disorders (SBD) Program at the Marcus Institute in Atlanta, Georgia, is based on the treatment programs developed at the Neurobehavioral Unit (NBU) at the Kennedy Krieger Institute in Baltimore. The SBD Program and the NBU have been extremely successful in treating individuals with behavior problems.

Children are typically admitted to the SBD Program for a period of 12–16 weeks in which they receive services for 6 hours per day. Each day, three specially trained therapists, under the supervision of a licensed psychologist, conduct assessment and treatment sessions in which data are collected on all occurrences of targeted maladaptive and adaptive responses. During the initial part of the admission, a functional analysis is conducted to identify the environmental conditions associated with the occurrence of self-injurious or aggressive behavior. Following the functional analysis, treatments are developed to decrease the occurrence of problem behavior in the clinic setting. Finally, all caregivers are trained in treatment implementation in the natural environment, and ongoing outpatient follow-up is provided for a period of 2 years postdischarge. Mitchel's story presents a typical course of assessment and treatment of severe behavior problems.

Mitchel, an 8-year-old boy with Down syndrome and severe intellectual disabilities, had a history of aggressive behavior (hitting, kicking, pinching, scratching, head butting, and throwing objects at others), SIB (face slapping, head banging), and property destruction (breaking glass). Most recently, Mitchel had released his seatbelt in the family car, become aggressive, and grabbed the steering wheel while his mother was driving. Throughout his life, Mitchel's behaviors had led to repeated hospitalizations for medical treatment (e.g., treatment of broken bones, removal of glass from his hands) as well as a variety of environmental manipulations (e.g., placing deadbolt locks on all doors and Plexiglas in all windows in the home) designed to maintain the safety of Mitchel and his family. Mitchel was admitted to the SBD Program at the Marcus Institute due to the severity of his behaviors and the harm they posed to both himself and his caregivers.

Prior to his admission to the SBD Program, Mitchel had been evaluated and treated by a number of medical specialists. Previous medications included methylphenidate, dextroamphetamine, clonidine, fluoxetine, guanfacine, and bupropion. Mitchel had also received speech and occupational therapies in an attempt to decrease his problematic behavior. Despite these therapies, little change occurred in the rate and intensity of his behavior problems. Moreover, Mitchel's behavior had continued to deteriorate significantly during the months that preceded his admission. At the time of his enrollment, Mitchel was receiving citalopram and buspirone to manage his problematic behaviors.

Following a parent interview, a functional analysis was conducted to identify which environmental variables maintained Mitchel's problem behavior. During this assessment, Mitchel's problem behavior was monitored and recorded on laptop computers under different environmental conditions. One therapist was in the room with Mitchel during all sessions, and two observers were seated behind one-way observation windows collecting data on the occurrence of problem behavior. All sessions were conducted in a padded room and were 10 minutes in length. The assessment consisted of social disapproval, academic demand, alone, and unstructured play.

Figure 23.5-1 shows the results of Mitchel's functional analysis. Each data point represents one 10-minute observation of Mitchel's behavior under the various experimental conditions. The rates of Mitchel's problem behavior were highest and most consistent (averaging 6.6 responses per minute) during the social disapproval condition of the functional analysis. By contrast, near-zero rates of aggressive behavior were observed across all other conditions of the functional analysis. Based on these results, clinicians concluded that

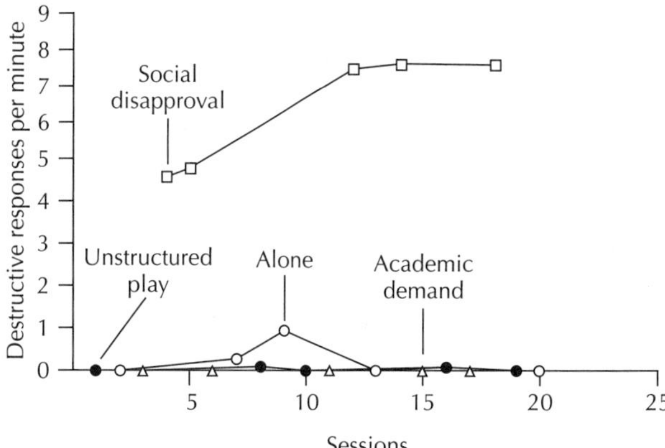

Figure 23.5-1. Destructive responding during the functional analysis for Mitchel. Each data point represents a 10-minute observation of behavior under one of the four test conditions.

Mitchel's problem behavior appeared to be maintained by socially mediated positive reinforcement.

Following the functional analysis, a treatment was developed to reduce the occurrence of Mitchel's problem behavior. The baseline condition was identical to the social disapproval condition of the functional analysis. Mitchel received a brief reprimand and physical interaction contingent on each occurrence of problem behavior. The treatment condition consisted of a type of DRA in which Mitchel could only get adult attention by engaging in a more appropriate form of behavior. Specifically, Mitchel was taught an idiosyncratic manual sign to request attention. In addition, problem behavior no longer resulted in access to adult attention (i.e., extinction).

Results of the treatment analysis are shown in Figure 23.5-2. As in Figure 23.5-1, each data point represents a different 10-minute observation period. During baseline, problem behavior averaged 8.7 responses per minute. Conversely, problem behavior decreased to an average of 1.0 response per minute during the treatment condition. Clinicians then focused on helping Mitchel transfer the treatment effects to more naturalistic settings (e.g., home, school).

PICA

Pica is from the Latin word for magpie, a bird that characteristically finds unusual objects and brings them to its nest. The condition includes three basic criteria: "(a) persistent eating of non-nutritive substances for a period of at least one month. (b) the eating of non-nutritive substances is inappropriate for the individual's developmental level. (c) the eating behavior is not part of a culturally sanctioned practice" (American Psychiatric Association, 2000, p. 103).

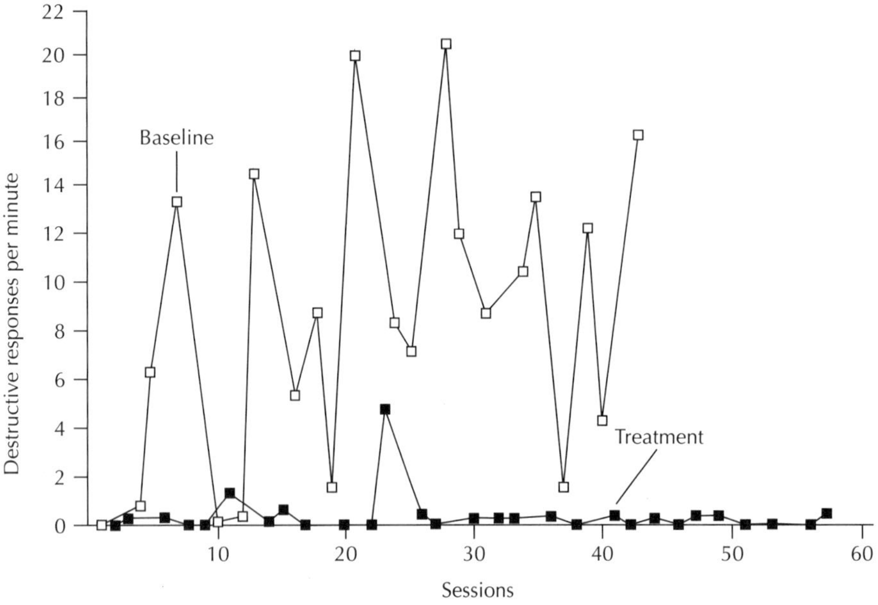

Figure 23.5-2. Destructive responding during the treatment analysis. Each data point represents a 10-minute observation of behavior under either the baseline or treatment condition.

From a clinical perspective, pica has been considered the ingestion of nonnutritive substances (e.g., plastic) or the unsanitary ingestion of edible items (e.g., food from a trashcan; Piazza, Roane, Keeney, Boney, & Abt, 2002). It is a potentially life-threatening behavior depending on the types of substances ingested, and the behavior has been estimated to occur in approximately 25% of individuals with intellectual disabilities (Danford & Huber, 1982). The negative outcomes of pica may range widely from very little harm to intestinal blockage, accidental poisoning, parasitic infection, surgical removal of objects, and death (Fisher et al., 1994; Motta & Basile, 1998).

Proposed Etiology

One explanation for the occurrence of pica views the behavior as a biologically driven, adaptive response to a nutritional deficiency. This theory is unclear about whether ingesting nonnutritive items directly compensates for, or alters the absorption of, the deficient minerals or nutrients in the individual's diet. Such hypotheses are supported by instances in which pica is associated with preexisting medical conditions (e.g., pregnancy; Motta & Basile, 1998).

In some cases, pica may be symptomatic of obsessive-compulsive disorder (OCD; Gundogar, Demis, & Eren, 2003; Zeitlin & Polivy, 1995); however, this research has largely consisted of participants who were typically developing and who also displayed other symptoms of OCD (e.g., handwashing, obsessions of contamination). Although it has been suggested that some individuals with developmental disabilities may display characteristics of comorbid OCD (Luiselli, 1996), little research supports this hypothesis, and future research on this topic is warranted.

Functional analysis can be used to identify variables that maintain pica (Hanley et al., 2003). In the majority of published research, pica has been shown to be maintained by automatic reinforcement. For example, an individual with profound intellectual disabilities may have few appropriate skills for interacting with his or her surroundings. In such cases, the placement of nonnutritive substances into the mouth might be one way of producing stimulation.

When a behavior like pica is maintained by automatic reinforcement, it produces a special dilemma for clinicians for a number of reasons (Vollmer, 1994). First, identification of automatic reinforcement as the maintaining variable describes what the reinforcer is not (i.e., not a social variable), but does not identify what the actual reinforcer is. As a result, prescription of treatment is less clear. Second, automatic reinforcers are not typically within the control of a therapist and cannot be manipulated directly. The clinician cannot simply ignore the behavior and expect it to decrease.

Third, automatic reinforcers are available constantly because the behavior and the reinforcer are inseparably tied. Thus, it is often difficult to teach the individual to engage in some other response that requires him or her to forgo engaging in pica.

Prevention and Treatment

Clinicians should start by considering pica in relation to the individual's culture. In some cultures, the ingestion of nonnutritive substances is an accepted practice and does not involve the consumption of dangerous materials (Motta & Basile, 1998). As such, the behavior may not require direct intervention.

Because the occurrence of pica may be associated with nutritional variables, blood levels can be drawn to identify the specific nutritional deficit. Treatments include supplemental access to the deficient mineral or nutrient (e.g., Pace & Toyer, 2000). The literature describes successful treatment of pica through administration of iron (Moore & Sears, 1994) and zinc (Lofts, Schroeder, & Maier, 1990) supplements, as well as through the use of a supplemental diet (Bugle & Rubin, 1993) and multivitamins (Pace & Toyer, 2000). Despite these findings, most examples of this treatment approach have been with individuals in the normal range of intellectual functioning (see reports by Bugle & Rubin, 1993, and Pace & Toyer, 2000, for notable exceptions). Nevertheless, treatment with nutritional supplements, when successful, would appear to be much less effortful for care providers and far less intrusive for individuals with developmental disabilities than other potential treatments

Efforts have been made to decrease pica with treatments that are commonly used for OCD, including the use of exposure and response prevention techniques (Zeitlin & Polivy, 1995) and pharmacological treatment consisting of selective seratonin reuptake inhibitors (Gundogar et al., 2003). Limited research, however, is available on these approaches to treatment, and additional research examining the use of these treatments is needed.

If the occurrence of pica is not related to cultural factors, nutritional variables, or comorbid OCD, the first order of treatment often includes taking steps to maintain a safe environment. Modifications to the environment primarily consist of the removal of objects that have a high probability of being ingested or that would prove dangerous if swallowed. In many instances, individuals are likely to engage in pica with certain types of items. Thus, limiting the presence of those items within the environments where the individual spends most of their time can significantly reduce the occurrence of pica.

For example, cigarette butt pica is a specific form of pica exhibited by many individuals with developmental disabilities (Piazza, Hanley, & Fisher, 1996). The ingestion of cigarette butts is associated with the additional risks that occur when nicotine is consumed orally such as oral cancer, gingival recession, periodontal disease, and elevation of blood pressure (Larsen, Haag, & Silvette, 1961; McMahon et al., 1986). Also, consuming cigarette butts that have been previously smoked may result in exposure to saliva-borne pathogens. Caregivers can modify the environment by making sure that no one smokes cigarettes in or around the house or making sure that cigarette butts are disposed of.

Not all individuals are as selective about the items they will consume. Furthermore, maintaining control over all of the environments an individual might encounter is not always feasible. Thus, when it is not possible to eliminate items from the environment or to restrict the individual to environments that are under the control of care providers, more intrusive procedures, such as mechanical restraints, may be required.

The literature has examples of reductions in pica and pre-pica behavior (e.g., foraging for pica items) with the use of mechanical restraints such as helmets or face shields (Rojahn, Schroeder, & Mulik, 1980). Another potential benefit of using protective equipment is that it may be possible to decrease the amount of effort expended by care providers in supervising the individual. Evidence shows, however, that this benefit cannot be assumed for every individual that engages in pica. For example, at least one study showed that pica was more likely when protective equipment was applied (Mace & Knight, 1986). Mace and Knight also noted that, when an individual wore a protective helmet, staff were less likely to provide direct supervision or deliver reprimands as a punishing consequence for pica. In other words, protective equipment may not always allow care providers to relax their supervision.

Even in cases in which protective equipment eliminates the possibility of pica, applying and maintaining the equipment may be more effortful than supervision in the absence of restraint devices (LeBlanc, Piazza, & Krug, 1997). The supervision required to remove protective equipment and pica related to the equipment itself may be difficult in itself. Furthermore, use of restraints and other protective equipment can decrease quality of life as measured by limitations of the individual's ability to engage in leisure activities or social interactions.

A number of other variables may affect the efficacy of mechanical restraints for treating pica. For example, the type of items the individual tends to ingest may influence the effectiveness of a helmet or facemask because some items may be more difficult to insert through a mask than others. Such variables should be considered before the decision is made to use protective equipment as a treatment for pica.

Behavioral Interventions

Behavioral interventions are another class of treatment for pica exhibited by individuals with disabilities. Rather than preventing the opportunity to, or restraining the individual from, engaging in pica, these interventions attempt to manipulate the individual's environment in such a way that alters the motivation to engage in pica.

The assessment and treatment of pica may be difficult for clinicians because the response and the reinforcer are inherently linked to one another (unlike social reinforcers described previously). Thus, rather than attempting to disrupt the relationship between pica and its outcome, many investigators have attempted to reduce pica by providing access to alternative (i.e., appropriate) stimulation that can be safely placed in the mouth. Favell, McGimsey, and Shell (1982) found that when toys were provided to participants, individuals stopped engaging in pica. The participants, however, initially placed the toys in their mouths instead. Thus, additional procedures have been developed to decrease the placement of objects into the mouth in general. In the Favell et al. study, for example, providing access to an alternative but more appropriate source of oral stimulation (popcorn), further reduced pica as well as mouthing of the toys. This general procedure has been applied with success in a number of subsequent investigations (LeBlanc, Piazza, & Krug, 1997; Piazza et al., 1998; Piazza et al., 2002; Roane, Kelly, & Fisher, 2003).

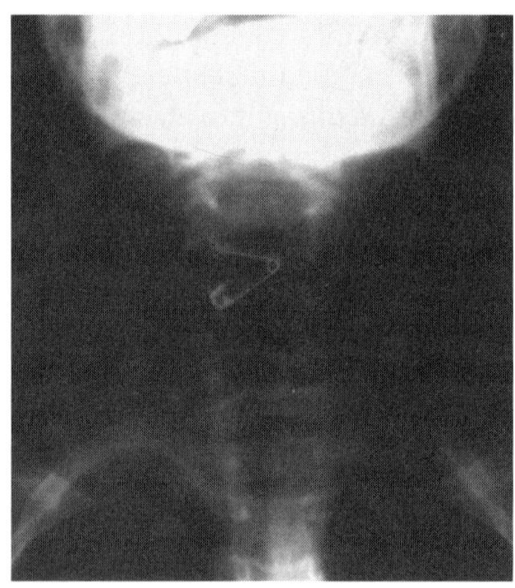

Figure 23.5-3. X-ray showing physical evidence of the severity of Calvin's pica.

Calvin was a 9-year-old boy with autism who had a lifelong history of pica, which primarily consisted of ingesting metal objects (e.g., paperclips) and rocks. Calvin had ingested a variety of objects throughout his life, and, at the time of his referral to the SBD, he had been hospitalized to remove a foreign object that had lodged in his esophagus (see Figure 23.5-3).

Calvin was admitted to the SBD program for 4 weeks of intensive assessment and treatment to reduce his pica. Clinicians conducted a functional analysis in which Calvin was exposed to several experimental conditions. Each condition was an analogue of situations in which his parents reported that Calvin was likely to engage in pica. Alternative items that were similar in texture and size to those that Calvin typically ingested but that were safe for human consumption were identified and used (e.g., uncooked beans instead of rocks).

In one condition (demand), Calvin was given a series of instructions to complete. If he engaged in pica instead of completing his work, the therapist would remove the work and allow Calvin to have a brief break. In the second condition (attention), Calvin was given attention in the form of reprimands and statements of concern if he engaged in pica. In the third condition (alone), Calvin was observed while he was alone in the therapy room. This condition was conducted to assess the rates of his pica in the absence of supervision. Finally, a toy play condition was conducted as a control comparison. In this condition, Calvin had free access to his preferred activities and also had continuous interaction from a therapist.

Throughout this assessment, 16 10-minute sessions were conducted in a randomized order. During all sessions, an observer was seated behind a one-way observation window and collected data using a laptop computer. Data were collected on the frequency of pica across all conditions, and the frequencies were converted to a response rate (pica responses per minute). The data were visually compared across all conditions. Treatment was developed based on the condition associated with the highest level of pica.

Results of the functional assessment are shown in Figure 23.5-4. High rates of pica were observed across the alone, attention, and demand conditions with lower rates occurring in the toy play condition. Based on this pattern of responding, clinicians concluded that Calvin engaged in pica regardless of any social manipulations, unless he had free access to preferred stimuli (e.g., toys in the control condition). That

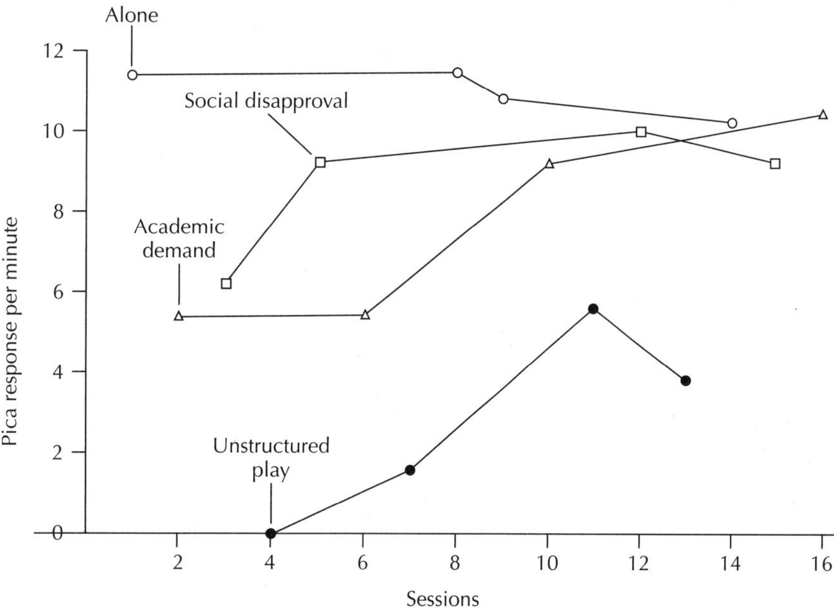

Figure 23.5-4. Pica responding during the functional analysis for Calvin. Each data point represents a 10-minute observation of behavior under one of the four test conditions.

is, his behavior appeared to be maintained by automatic reinforcement.

Treatment for Calvin involved the presentation of two types of items that differed in their properties. One class of items was not similar to those that Calvin typically ingested. Items in this category included a preferred video, a television, a sit and spin, and toy cars. The other class of items was stimuli that shared properties with the items that Calvin typically ingested (e.g., hard breadsticks, celery stalks, hard sugar-free candies). During both conditions, Calvin was in a room by himself and had free access to either the similar or the dissimilar items throughout the session. The similar items and dissimilar items conditions were alternated with a baseline condition, which was identical to the alone condition of the

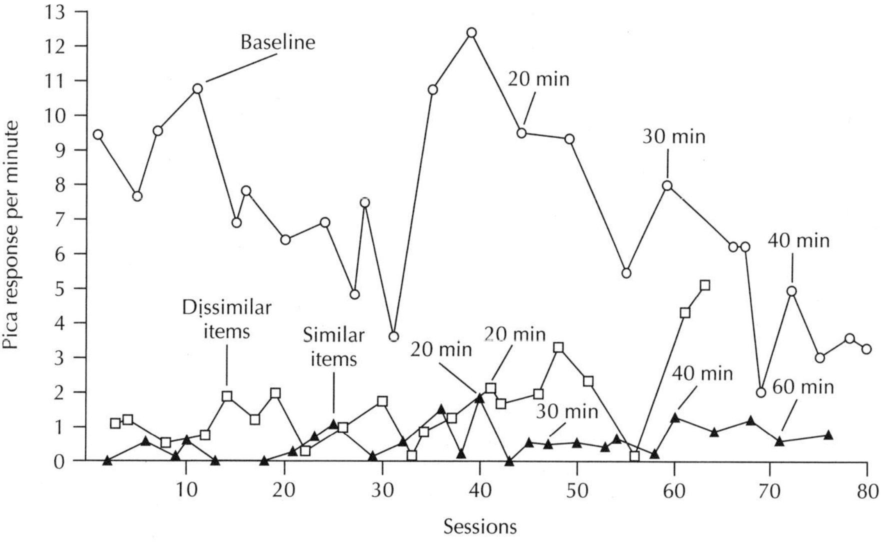

Figure 23.5-5. Pica responding during the treatment analysis for Calvin. The numbers on the graph represent changes in the length of each observation session.

functional assessment. Results of the treatment analysis are shown in Figure 23.5-5. Both conditions produced decreased rates of pica, even as session length was increased from 10 to 20 minutes.

CONCLUSION

SIB, aggression, and pica can threaten the safety of an individual and his or her care providers, place the individual at risk of more restrictive placements, and prevent the individual from engaging in or acquiring more adaptive behaviors. Although several etiological variables may account for the development of these behaviors, the operant hypothesis has been associated with the most substantiating research. Functional analysis has been shown to be highly effective at identifying the variables that maintain an individual's problem behavior within a variety of naturalistic and clinical settings. This methodology has led to the development of new treatment approaches for severe behavior problems, leading to more effective treatment of those behaviors (Hanley et al., 2003).

REFERENCES

American Psychiatric Association. (2000). *Diagnostic and statistical manual of mental disorders* (4th ed., text revision). Washington, DC: Author.

Berkson, G., & Mason, W.A. (1964). Stereotyped movements of mental defectives: IV. The effects of toys and the character of the acts. *American Journal of Mental Deficiency, 68,* 511–524.

Bugle, C., & Rubin, H.B. (1993). Effects of a nutritional supplement on coprophagia: A study of three cases. *Research in Developmental Disabilities, 14,* 445–456.

Carr, E.G. (1977). The origins of self-injurious behavior: A review of some hypotheses. *Psychological Bulletin, 84,* 800–816.

Carr, E.G., & Durand, V.M. (1985). Reducing behavior problems through functional communication training. *Journal of Applied Behavior Analysis, 18,* 111–126.

Carr, E.G., Newsome, C.D., & Binkoff, J.A. (1980). Escape as a factor in the aggressive behavior of two retarded children. *Journal of Applied Behavior Analysis, 13,* 101–117.

Cataldo, M.F., & Harris, J. (1982). The biological basis for self-injury in the mentally retarded. *Analysis and Intervention in Developmental Disabilities, 2,* 21–39.

Cowdery, G.E., Iwata, B.A., & Pace, G.M. (1990). Effects and side effects of DRO as treatment for self-injurious behavior. *Journal of Applied Behavior Analysis, 23,* 497–506.

Danford, D.E., & Huber, A.M. (1982). Pica among mentally retarded adults. *American Journal of Mental Deficiency, 87,* 141–146.

Day, R.M., Rea, J.A., Schussler, N.G., Larsen, S.E., & Johnson, W.L. (1988). A functionally based approach to the treatment of self-injurious behavior. *Behavior Modification, 12,* 565–589.

De Lissovoy, V. (1963). Head banging in early childhood. *Journal of Genetic Psychology, 102,* 109–114.

Demchak, M. (1993). Functional assessment of problem behaviors in applied settings. *Intervention in School and Clinic, 29,* 89–95.

Durand, V.M., & Carr, E.G. (1991). Functional communication training to reduce challenging behavior: Maintenance and application in new settings. *Journal of Applied Behavior Analysis, 24,* 251–264.

Favell, J.E., McGimsey, J.F., & Schell, R.M. (1982). Treatment of self-injury by providing alternative sensory activities. *Analysis and Intervention in Developmental Disabilities, 2,* 83–104.

Ferster, C.B., & Skinner, B.F. (1957). *Schedules of reinforcement.* Acton, MA: Copley.

Fisher, W.W., Adelinis, J.D., Thompson, R.H., Worsdell, A.S., & Zarcone, J.R. (1998). Functional analysis and treatment of destructive behavior maintained by termination of "don't" (and symmetrical "do") requests. *Journal of Applied Behavior Analysis, 31,* 339–356.

Fisher, W.W., Lindauer, S.E., Alterson, C.J., & Thompson, R.H. (1998). Assessment and treatment of destructive behavior maintained by stereotypic manipulation. *Journal of Applied Behavior Analysis, 31,* 513–527.

Fisher, W.W., Piazza, C.C., Bowman, L.G., Kurtz, P.F., Sherer, M.R., & Lachman, S.R. (1994). A preliminary evaluation of empirically derived consequences for the treatment of pica. *Journal of Applied Behavior Analysis, 27,* 447–457.

Fisher, W., Piazza, C., Cataldo, M., Harrell, R., Jefferson, G., & Conner, R. (1993). Functional communication training with and without extinction and punishment. *Journal of Applied Behavior Analysis, 26,* 23–36.

Gundogar, D., Demir, S.B., & Eren, I. (2003). Is pica in the spectrum of obsessive-compulsive disorders? *General Hospital Psychiatry, 25,* 293–294.

Hagopian, L.P., Fisher, W.W., Sullivan, M.T., Acquisto, J., & LeBlanc, L.A. (1998). Effectiveness of functional communication training with and without extinction and punishment: A summary of 21 inpatient cases. *Journal of Applied Behavior Analysis, 31,* 211–235.

Hanley, G.P., Iwata, B.A., & McCord, B.E. (2003). Functional analysis of problem behavior: A review. *Journal of Applied Behavior Analysis, 36,* 147–185.

Iwata, B.A., Dorsey, M.F., Slifer, K.J., Bauman, K.E., & Richman, G.S. (1994). Toward a functional analysis of self-injury. *Journal of Applied Behavior Analysis, 27,* 197–209. (Reprinted from *Analysis and Intervention in Developmental Disabilities, 2,* 3–20, 1982.)

Iwata, B.A., Pace, G.M., Dorsey, M.F., Zarcone, J.R., Vollmer, T.R., Smith, R.G., et al. (1994). The functions of self-injurious behavior: An experimental-epidemiological analysis. *Journal of Applied Behavior Analysis, 27,* 215–240.

Iwata, B.A., Pace, G.M., Kalsher, M.J., Cowdery, G.E., & Cataldo, M.F. (1990). Experimental analysis and extinction of self-injurious escape behavior. *Journal of Applied Behavior Analysis, 23,* 11–27.

Johnson, W.L., & Day, R.M. (1992). The incidence and prevalence of self-injurious behavior. In J.K. Luiselli, J.L. Matson, & N.N. Singh (Eds.), *Self-injurious behavior:*

Analysis, assessment, and treatment (pp. 21–56). New York: Springer-Verlag.

Kratochwill, T.R., & McGivern, J.E. (1996). Clinical diagnosis, behavioral assessment, and functional analysis: Examining the connection between assessment and intervention. *School Psychology Review, 25*, 342–355.

Lalli, J.S., Casey, S.D., & Kates, K. (1997). Noncontingent reinforcement as treatment for severe problem behavior: Some procedural variations. *Journal of Applied Behavior Analysis, 30*, 127–137.

Lalli, J.S., Mace, F.C., Wohn, T., & Livezy, K. (1995). Identification and modification of a response-class hierarchy. *Journal of Applied Behavior Analysis, 28*, 551–559.

Larsen, P.S., Haag, H.B., & Silvette, H. (1961). *Tobacco-experimental and clinical studies.* Baltimore: Williams & Wilkens.

LeBlanc, L.A., Piazza, C.C., & Krug, M.A. (1997). Comparing methods for maintaining the safety of a child with pica. *Research in Developmental Disabilities, 18*(3), 215–220.

Lerman, D.C., Iwata, B.A., & Wallace, M.D. (1999). Side effects of extinction: Prevalence of bursting and aggression during the treatment of self-injurious behavior. *Journal of Applied Behavior Analysis, 32*, 1–8.

Little, S.G., & Rodemaker, J.E. (1998). Lesch-Nyhan disease. In L. Phelps (Ed.), *Health-related disorders in children: A guidebook for understanding and educating.* Washington, DC: American Psychological Association.

Lofts, R.H., Schroeder, S.R., & Maier, R.H. (1990). Effects of serum zinc supplementation of pica behavior of persons with mental retardation. *American Journal on Mental Retardation, 95*, 105–109.

Lovaas, O.I., & Simmons, J.Q. (1969). Manipulation of self-destruction in three retarded children. *Journal of Applied Behavior Analysis, 2*, 143–157.

Luiselli, J.K. (1996). Pica as obsessive-compulsive disorder. *Journal of Behavior Therapy and Experimental Psychiatry, 27*(2), 195–196.

Mace, F.C. (1994). The significance and future of functional analysis methodologies. *Journal of Applied Behavior Analysis, 27*, 385–392.

Mace, F.C., & Knight, D. (1986). Functional analysis and treatment of severe pica. *Journal of Applied Behavior Analysis, 19*, 411–416.

Mace, F.C., & Lalli, J.S. (1991). Linking descriptive and experimental analyses in the treatment of bizarre speech. *Journal of Applied Behavior Analysis, 24*, 553–562.

Marcus, B.A., Vollmer, T.R., Swanson, V.A., Roane, H.S., & Ringdahl, J.E. (2001). An experimental analysis of aggression. *Behavior Modification, 25*, 189–213.

Mazaleski, J.L., Iwata, B.A., Vollmer, T.R., Zarcone, J.R., & Smith, R.G. (1993). Analysis of the reinforcement and extinction components in DRO contingencies with self-injury. *Journal of Applied Behavior Analysis, 26*, 143–156.

McMahon, B., Cataldo, M.F., Collier, M.E., Haggerty, R.J., Holford, T.R., Hulka, B.S., et al. (1986). Health applications of smokeless tobacco use. *Journal of the American Medical Association, 255*, 1045–1048.

Moore, D.F., & Sears, D.A. (1994). Pica, iron deficiency, and medical history. *American Journal of Medicine, 97*, 390–393.

Motta, R.W., & Basile, D.M. (1998). Pica. In L. Phelps (Ed.), *Health-related disorders in children: A guidebook for understanding and educating.* Washington, DC: American Psychological Association.

Oliver, C., Murphy, G.H., & Corbett, J.A. (1987). Self-injurious behavior in people with mental handicap: A total population study. *Journal of Mental Deficiency Research, 31*, 147–162.

O'Reilly, M.F. (1997). Functional analysis of episodic self-injury correlated with recurrent otitis media. *Journal of Applied Behavior Analysis, 30*, 165–167.

Pace, G.M., & Toyer, E.A. (2000). The effects of a vitamin supplement on the pica of a child with severe mental retardation. *Journal of Applied Behavior Analysis, 33*, 619–622.

Pelios, L., Morren, J., Tesch, D., & Axelrod, S. (1999). The impact of functional analysis methodology on treatment choice for self-injurious and aggressive behavior. *Journal of Applied Behavior Analysis, 32*, 185–195.

Piazza, C.C., Fisher, W.W., Hanley, G.P., LeBlanc, L.A., Worsdell, A.S., Lindauer, S.E., et al. (1998). Treatment of pica through multiple analyses of its reinforcing functions. *Journal of Applied Behavior Analysis, 31*, 165–189.

Piazza, C.C., Fisher, W., Hyman, S.L., Fleishell, J., Lou, K.K., & Cataldo, M. (1994). Evaluation of pharmacologic treatment of destructive behaviors: Aggregated results from single-case experimental studies. *Journal of Developmental and Physical Disabilities, 6*, 149–168.

Piazza, C.C., Hanley, G.P., & Fisher, W.W. (1996). Functional analysis and treatment of cigarette pica. *Journal of Applied Behavior Analysis, 29*, 437–449.

Piazza, C.C., Roane, H.S., Keeney, K.M., Boney, B.R., & Abt, K.A. (2002). Varying response effort in the treatment of pica maintained by automatic reinforcement. *Journal of Applied Behavior Analysis, 35*, 233–246.

Repp, A.C., & Deitz, S.M. (1974). Reducing aggressive and self-injurious behavior of institutionalized retarded children through reinforcement of other behaviors. *Journal of Applied Behavior Analysis, 7*, 313–325.

Repp, A.C., Felce, D., & Barton, L.E. (1988). Basing the treatment of stereotypic and self-injurious behaviors on hypotheses of their causes. *Journal of Applied Behavior Analysis, 21*, 281–289.

Roane, H.S., Fisher, W.W., & Sgro, G.M. (2001). Effects of a fixed-time schedule on aberrant and adaptive behavior. *Journal of Applied Behavior Analysis, 34*, 333–336.

Roane, H.S., Kelly, M.L., & Fisher, W.W. (2003). The effects of noncontingent access to food on the rate of object mouthing across three settings. *Journal of Applied Behavior Analysis, 36*, 579–582.

Rojahn, J., Schroeder, S.R., & Mulik, J.A. (1980). Ecological assessment of self-protective devices in three profoundly retarded adults. *Journal of Autism and Developmental Disorders, 10*, 59–66.

Schroeder, S.R. (1991). Self-injury and stereotypy. In J.L. Matson & J.A. Mulick (Eds.), *Handbook of mental retardation* (pp. 382–396). Elmsford, NY: Pergamon.

Schroeder, S.R., Schroeder, C.S., Smith, B., & Dalldorf, J. (1978). Prevalence of self-injurious behaviors in a large state facility for the retarded: A three-year follow-up study. *Journal of Autism and Childhood Schizophrenia, 8*, 261–269.

Spitz, R.A., & Wolfe, K.M. (1949). Autoeroticism. *Psychoanalytic Studies of the Child, 3*, 85–120.

Steege, M.W., Wacker, D.P., Berg, W.K., Cigrand, K.K., & Cooper, L.J. (1989). The use of behavioral assessment to

prescribe and evaluate treatments for severely handicapped children. *Journal of Applied Behavior Analysis, 22*, 23–33.
Steege, M.W., Wacker, D.P., Cigrand, K.C., Berg, W.K., Novak, C.G., Reimers, T.M., et al. (1990). Use of negative reinforcement in the treatment of self-injurious behavior. *Journal of Applied Behavior Analysis, 23*, 459–467.
Tate, B.G., & Baroff, G.S. (1966). Aversive control of self-injurious behavior in a psychotic boy. *Behavior Research and Therapy, 4*, 281–287.
Thompson, R.H., Fisher, W.W., Piazza, C.C., & Kuhn, D.E. (1998). The evaluation and treatment of aggression maintained by attention and automatic reinforcement. *Journal of Applied Behavior Analysis, 31*, 103–116.
Thompson, T., & Gray, D.B. (1984). *Destructive behavior in developmental disabilities.* London: Sage Publications.
Vaughn, M.E., & Micheal, J.L. (1982). Automatic reinforcement: An important but ignored concept. *Behaviorism, 10*, 217–228.
Vollmer, T.R. (1994). The concept of automatic reinforcement: Implications for behavioral research in developmental disabilities. *Research in Developmental Disabilities, 15*, 187–207.
Vollmer, T.R., & Iwata, B.A. (1992). Differential reinforcement as treatment for behavior disorders: Procedural and functional variations. *Research in Developmental Disabilities, 13*, 393–417.
Vollmer, T.R., Iwata, B.A., Zarcone, J.R., Smith, R.G., & Mazaleski, J.L. (1993). The role of attention in the treatment of attention-maintained self-injurious behavior: Noncontingent reinforcement and differential reinforcement of other behavior. *Journal of Applied Behavior Analysis, 26*, 9–21.
Vollmer, T.R., Marcus, B.A., & LeBlanc, L. (1994). Treatment of self-injury and hand mouthing following inconclusive functional analyses. *Journal of Applied Behavior Analysis, 27*, 331–344.
Vollmer, T.R., Roane, H.S., Ringdahl, J.E., & Marcus, B.A. (1999). Evaluating treatment challenges with differential reinforcement of alternative behavior. *Journal of Applied Behavior Analysis, 32*, 9–23.
Wacker, D.P., Steege, M.W., Northup, J., Sasso, G., Berg, W., Reimers, T., et al. (1990). A component analysis of functional communication training across three topographies of severe behavior problems. *Journal of Applied Behavior Analysis, 23*, 417–429.
Wilkens, L.E., Brown, J.A., & Wolf, B. (1980). Psychomotor development in 65 home-reared children with cri-du-chat syndrome. *Journal of Pediatrics, 97*, 401–405.
Zeitlin, S.B., & Polivy, J. (1995). Coprophagia as a manifestation of obsessive-compulsive disorder: A case report. *Journal of Behavior Therapy and Experimental Psychiatry, 26*(1), 57–63.

23.6 CRISIS PREVENTION AND MANAGEMENT

Joan B. Beasley

Perhaps as many as one in four individuals with intellectual disabilities exhibits challenging behavior (Reiss, 1990). In order to meet the needs of these individuals, comprehensive assessment and coordination of services by trained professionals are needed. This chapter provides an overview of diagnostic, treatment, and service considerations in order to effectively support individuals with intellectual disabilities and problem behavior.

PROBLEM BEHAVIOR AND INTELLECTUAL DISABILITIES

Many studies have shown that individuals with intellectual disabilities have a high degree of problem behavior, and many individuals have co-occurring mental disorders (Chapman & Hesketh, 2000; Deb, Thomas, & Bright, 2001; Emerson, 2003; Freidlander, 2004; Gillberg, Persso, Grufman, & Themner, 1986; Hastings, Hatton, Taylor, & Maddison, 2004; Hurley, 1996). In the Isle of Wight study, Rutter, Tizard, Yule, Graham, and Whitmore (1976) found that 50% of children age 9–11 with neurological and developmental disabilities had behavioral disorders. This research project incorporated the examination of a normative population, rating scales completed by parents and teachers, and an individual diagnostic interview.

According to parent interviews, 30% of children with developmental disabilities had behavior disorders, but teacher ratings alleged that 42% of the children had behavior disorders. Psychiatric interviews found that 50% of the children had a behavior disorder versus 7% in the general population. This landmark study concluded that children with neurological impairments and developmental disabilities were at significant risk for behavioral and mental health problems.

In another study, Gillberg and colleagues (1986) followed 149 youngsters in a 4-year birth cohort at ages 13–17 and found a 57% rate of behavior disorder among those with mild intellectual disabilities and 64% among those with severe intellectual disabilities. Gath and Gumley (1986) studied 346 children with Down syndrome in a health care region in England and determined that 38% had behavior disorders; a matched group of children with disabilities who did not have Down syndrome had a rate of 49%. Reiss's (1990) meta-analysis of adult studies found that approximately 25%

of individuals with intellectual disabilities were likely to experience problem behaviors, including those related to mental illness, at one point in their life span.

AGGRESSION

Perhaps the most common concern found in the literature is the management of aggression. In numerous settings, aggression was found to be the most common reason for referral to psychiatric or crisis evaluation for people with intellectual disabilities (Beasley, 2002; Davidson, Morris, & Cain, 1999; Davidson et al., 1994). Aggressive behavior is defined here as physical harm to others and often coincides with other behavior problems such as property destruction and self-injury.

Charlot, Doucette, and Mezzacampa (1993) found that aggression is often a common motivating factor for evaluation, largely due to the fact that the caregiver initiates the referral, and aggression is a problem for the caregiver. The result was similar for Edelstein and Glenwick (1997) in a study of 391 individuals with intellectual disabilities seeking outpatient services at a specialty clinic. They found "externalizing" behaviors (e.g., aggression) to be the most frequent referral problem.

King, DeAntoni, McCracken, Forness, and Ackerland (1994) found aggression and self-injury were among the most common reasons for referral to his psychiatric consultation service at a state facility serving individuals with severe and profound intellectual disabilities. Of 251 individuals referred, 30% were referred due to aggression; 36% due to self-injury; 35% due to medical problems; and 47% due to "behavior." Aggression and self-injury were jointly noted in 23% of all referrals.

Aggression is very rare among typically developing adults and adults with normal intelligence who are referred for mental health care. Hurley, Folstein, and Lam (2003) found aggression to be the most frequent chief complaint for individuals with intellectual disabilities (40%) compared with individuals with normal intelligence (6%) in an outpatient hospital setting. In a study examining aggressive assault, 2,916 outpatients seen by psychiatric residents in clinics of two private psychiatric hospitals found 3% having actually assaulted a person, and these individuals were more likely to have childhood onset disorders, intellectual disabilities, or personality disorders (Tardiff & Koenigsberg, 1985). Because aggression and other related behavioral difficulties are not typically seen as a presenting symptom for adults with normal intelligence, the adult psychiatric community has little practical clinical experience assessing this situation. As a result, people with intellectual disabilities and problem behaviors such as aggression are often misdiagnosed, are incorrectly treated with pharmacotherapy to suppress the symptom, or are believed to have the behavior as a symptom of intellectual disabilities.

The occurrence of aggression may be exacerbated by multiple disabilities. Freeman, Fast, and Burd (2000) conducted a meta-analysis of selected findings for 3,500 individuals in 22 countries with Tourette syndrome. They not only found that comorbidity is common, but that each additional comorbidity progressively increases the rate of behavioral problems, such as aggression. A subsequent study of the subset of individuals with Tourette syndrome and developmental delays showed the same trend (Friedlander, 2004).

HEALTH FACTORS

Health problems are significant contributors to behavioral difficulties and are all too often overlooked. Individuals with intellectual disabilities have a higher incidence of physical problems including epilepsy, hearing loss, visual problems, gastroesophageal reflux, constipation, muscular-skeletal impairments, dental problems, or hypothyroidism, and any or all of these issues can lead to behavioral difficulties (Bradley, 2002). Some individuals with specific syndromes, such as Down syndrome, have an even larger number of potential physical problems (Van Allen, Fund, & Jurenka, 1999). Furthermore, epilepsy is more common in people with intellectual disabilities (Barnhill & Hurley, 2003; Benjamin, 2000).

Seizures may be provoked by acute events including infection, head injury, chemical imbalance, stroke, or brain tumor. Epilepsy occurs in 2% of the general population and more frequently (25%–35%) in people with neurological-based disabilities. It is another manifestation of brain injury or differences in brain development. Active seizures affect the mental status and, therefore, the behavioral presentation of the person. In addition, psychiatric symptoms may be directly or indirectly related to the seizure disorder.

Beange and her colleagues (1995) in Australia found that individuals with intellectual disabilities had an average of 5.4 medical disorders, half of which had not been detected prior to the study's health survey. When health problems are not diagnosed, behavior problems related to undetected health problems are likely to be attributed to the person's intellectual disabilities (Kastner, Walsh, & Fraser, 2001). Undiagnosed or improperly treated physical or medical problems can affect a person's behavior and may lead to overdiagnosing of "behavior" problems; misdiagnosis of personality disorder; or even psychosis resulting in overprescribing of psychotropic medications, especially antipsychotic medications, which in turn can result in increasing behavior problems. Lunsky, Emery, and Benson (2002) found deficiencies in reports of health behaviors, physical complaints, and medication facts.

The presence of aggression and self-injury in many individuals with intellectual disabilities has led to a historical trend for overuse and misuse of antipsychotic medications in these individuals (Branford, 1997; Burd et al., 1997; Robertson et al. 2000). These medicines were often prescribed for behavior without an understanding of what was behind the behavior (Singh, Ells, & Wechsler, 1997). Due to better knowledge about the medications and their usefulness, the trend in recent years has been to reduce the use of the older antipsychotic medications whenever possible; however, weaning off antipsychotic medication must be a slow process (5%–10% every 2 months) in order to minimize serious withdrawal effects (Friedlander, Lazar, & Klancnik, 2001). When medications are discontinued too quickly, individuals may experience increased agitation, insomnia, confusion, or aggression—which in turn can result in an increase in prescription medication. Without the proper information and supports, service providers, family members, and mental health professionals may falsely conclude that the person obviously needs the medication, and it is reinstated for many more years.

With the development of newer medicines, especially the atypical antipsychotics, enthusiasm has renewed for the use of these drugs in people with intellectual disabilities. Although they are widely used, and can be very effective, it is also likely that they are again overused, as the traditional antipsychotics were in the past. Thus, caution and close monitoring are still required (Friedlander et al., 2001). Medical problems that may also lead to an increase in behavior problems associated with the use of the newer medications also require a different approach than was previously thought.

PSYCHOSOCIAL CONTEXT

Multiple psychological and environmental factors may contribute to a significantly high rate of mental health and problem behaviors in individuals with intellectual disabilities. First, due to developmental delays, many of these individuals have relatively poor verbal and communication abilities. Thus, they are not able to use language for coping skills. They often cannot analyze situations; develop coping statements and strategies; or use language as an alternative to better control their behavior or to report accurately on feelings, emotions, or symptoms (Gardner, 2002).

Social rejection is another continual stressor for people with intellectual disabilities. They are aware that rejection they experience in the community has something to do with their disabilities. Attempts to develop relationships with people with normal intelligence are often rudely rejected. Social rejection becomes a major issue at many life-developmental stages (Levitas & Gilson, 2001). Evidence directly links life stresses with psychiatric illnesses such as depression and anxiety disorders in individuals with developmental disabilities (Hastings et al., 2004). Furthermore, two studies conducted by Lunsky and her colleagues linked the level of social support to stress and psychiatric problems (Lunsky & Benson, 2001; Lunsky & Havercamp, 1999).

Higher rates of physical, emotional, and even sexual abuse may also be responsible for a higher rate of mental illness. Sobsey, Sharmaine, Well, Pyper, and Reimer-Heck (1992) developed an annotated bibliography documenting research on the extent of abuse for people with disabilities. The authors noted that post-traumatic stress disorder, depression, and anxiety disorders are often unrecognized and undertreated in these individuals.

Analysis of problem behaviors must also include applied behavior analysis to better understand whether some of the behavior was learned in a partcular environment. For many individuals, problem behavior may be encouraged by environmental conditions that can be understood by looking at the context in which that behavior is more (or less) likely to occur (O'Neill et al., 1997). Psychosocial factors that result in behavior problems are rarely, if ever, easily defined by one predominant contributor; therefore, remedies must go beyond basic behavioral learning programs in order to be effective. Optimally, approaches to assessment and management must be multifactorial and interdisciplinary.

DIAGNOSIS OF A MENTAL DISORDER

Although individuals with intellectual disabilities and co-occurring disorders are likely to have problem behaviors, not all individuals with intellectual disabilities and problem behaviors have co-occurring disorders. Therefore, accurate diagnosis and treatment of mental disorders is often key to understanding and managing problem behaviors. The overriding effects of intellectual disabilities on the individual's presentation often require that clinicians have special clinical skills in the diagnosis and treatment of mental illness as well as other medical conditions (Borthwick, 1988; Bouras, Kon, & Drummond, 1993; Bregman, 1991; Campbell & Malone, 1991; Criscione, Kastner, Walsh, & Nathanson, 1993; Dosen, 1988; Evangelista, 1988; Jacobson, 1990; Menolascino, Gilson & Levitas, 1986; Sovner, 1986).

In 1986, Sovner described four major factors that influence the diagnosis of mental illness in individuals with intellectual disabilities (Sovner, 1986), which he called intellectual distortion, psychosocial masking, cognitive disintegration, and baseline exaggeration. *Intellectual distortion* refers to the inability of an individual with developmental and intellectual disabilities to think abstractly and communicate verbally. It undermines the results of a diagnostic interview because the person with intellectual disabilities may be unable to respond to questions accurately. The use of general mental health diagnostic instruments that rely heavily on the individual's ability to self-report is often compromised by the person's inability to articulate internal abstract experiences as well as the experience of concrete thinking, aphasia, limited vocabulary, and hearing impairments. This situation greatly hampers the clinician's ability to use these tools effectively in diagnosing a specific disorder, especially because so much is weighted on the clinical interview (Carlson, 1981; McCracken & Diamond, 1988).

During the clinical interview, people with intellectual disabilities may acquiescence to the interviewer (Matikka & Vesala, 1997). The individual will typically want to please the examiner and may think of the exchange as a test in school. He or she may be anxious to produce the "right answer" to gain approval. Lack of contextual understanding of the psychiatric process usually results in less than adequate and reliable answers to most of the typical questions of the psychiatric interview. As a result, the language of the interview must be significantly altered. The physician/clinician may be required to simplify or slow down the presentation so that the person has time to digest the information (Levitas, Hurley & Pary, 2001).

Psychosocial masking describes the effects of intellectual disabilities on the content of psychiatric symptoms. The individual's limited knowledge of the world along with his or her limited life experience may restrict the detail, range, and richness of delusions and hallucinations that the individual experiences. The clinician has a harder time determining whether the individual with developmental disabilities is experiencing a "fear" or a "delusion" (Carlson, 1981).

Cognitive disintegration describes the tendency for some individuals with intellectual disabilities to become confused when experiencing serious emotional stress. Unrelated to a mental disorder, these individuals are predisposed by organic impairments and concrete coping skills to become confused when under severe stress. At times, they may regress in their behavioral presentation because they cannot express their needs (Ghaziuddin, 1988; Matson, 1983; Menolascino & McCann, 1983).

Cognitive disintegration may foster a misdiagnosis of a mental disorder, because individuals may present chaotic thinking, aggressive behavior, and an inability to be in the presence of others, resulting in complete withdrawal. Individuals with intellectual disabilities are often misdiagnosed as suffering from atypical psychosis or schizophrenia because they cannot cope with stress in more acceptable ways. As mentioned previously, when antipsychotic drugs are prescribed under these circumstances, they may aggravate behaviors, resulting in the further misdiagnosis of mental health symptoms.

Baseline exaggeration refers to an increase in severity of preexisting maladaptive behavior due to periods of stress. In a person with intellectual disabilities, a diagnostician may overlook symptoms of a mental disorder because the symptoms exist to a lesser degree at the person's baseline level of functioning. The increase in severity, however, may very well be an indication of a mental disorder.

As Sovner (1986) indicated, the diagnosis of a mental disorder cannot be based solely on the presence of aberrant or maladaptive behaviors. Although symptoms of mental illness are often manifested in maladaptive behaviors, a distinction exists between mental illness and behavioral problems. As described previously, problem behaviors can occur as a result of limitations in an individual's skill development without underlying symptoms of mental illness. As Sovner pointed out, physical discomfort in a nonverbal individual can result in aberrant behavior. The behavior may be eliminated once the cause of the discomfort is resolved. The cause of aberrant behavior is therefore unrelated to mental illness.

Although problem behavior may not indicate the existence of a mental disorder, symptoms of mental illness are often expressed through problem behaviors. For example, Dosen (1988) found psychopathology expressed through maladaptive behaviors (aggression and/or self-injury) in 100% of the cases he studied that were diagnosed with depression. In these cases, the behaviors were presumed by the author to be an expression of symptoms of mental illness.

The process of differentiating between a behavior disorder (the use of inappropriate behaviors to express needs or emotions) and a mental disorder (the use of inappropriate behavior as a symptom of a mental illness as defined in the *Diagnostic and Statistical Manual of Mental Disorders, Fouth Edition*; American Psychiatric Association, 1994) is often complex (Jacobson, 1990; Reiss, 1994). As a result, the accurate interpretation of aberrant behaviors and other symptoms of mental illness in individuals with intellectual disabilities requires the integration of both psychiatric and behavioral observation methods (Evangelista, 1988; Sovner, 1986) along with extensive knowledge of the individual and his or her history. In addition, eliciting information from a variety of sources is helpful to better dissect the behavior and the symptomatolagy and to make a more accurate diagnosis. Translating symptoms into behavioral equivalents of mental health symptoms is also useful (Nezu, Nezu, & Gill-Weiss, 1992; Phillips & Williams, 1975; Sovner & Hurley, 1990). The use of diagnostic equivalents compensates for limits in verbal ability and in self-expression (Sovner & Hurley, 1983).

EFFECTIVE SERVICE DELIVERY SYSTEM

In order to evaluate and treat individuals with intellectual disabilities and problem behaviors, an effective service delivery system must be in place. Three key principles to the provision of effective services are access, appropriateness, and accountability (Beasley, 1997).

Access

For most service planners and advocates, access to care is seen as one of the primary obstacles to overcome in order to promote effective treatment for people with intellectual disabilities. It is defined by the ability of an individual to receive care when and where he or she wants it. Access is also measured by the time it takes to get help when needed. Services must be user friendly, with adequate attention to literacy support strategies, and culturally sensitive.

Appropriateness

Along with access, services must be appropriate. Appropriateness of care is reflected in the ability of service providers to meet the specific needs of an individual. Access to service providers who are inexperienced and untrained can lead to meaningless or even harmful care (Beasley, 1997, 2000). Therefore, rigorous standards and specialized training in diagnosis and treatment of people with intellectual disabilities are essential to improving service performance in order to ensure that appropriate services are delivered.

In evaluating appropriateness of care, the service system must use the proper treatment approaches. An individual can have excellent access to care without receiving appropriate care. Thus, even if the individual has ready access to an inpatient facility during a psychiatric crisis, the services received will not be effective if the treating mental health team does not have an accurate diagnostic and treatment strategy (Beasley & duPree, 2003).

Accountability

The third essential element for effective service provision is accountability. Assessment of services through data collection is crucial to the process. Service systems must be accountable to everyone involved in the provision of care, including funding sources. Outcome measures must be clearly defined, and review of data must be frequent and ongoing (Beasley & duPree, 2003). Outcomes should be realistic and measurable, demonstrate social validity, and be individual centered. Systems must readily adapt to changes in the demands placed on them. Services must also be cost effective. Analysis of data must be used as a barometer of where a service delivery system has succeeded and must guide further development of the system. In addition, data should be multidimensional and should include both qualitative as well as quantitative measures.

SPECIALIZED COORDINATED CARE MODELS

Studies show that people with a dual diagnosis of mental illness (and/or problem behavior) and intellectual disabilities are at greater risk for institutionalization than people diagnosed with an intellectual disability alone (Kearney & Smull, 1992). In addition, empirical evidence shows that people with co-occurring mental illness and intellectual disabilities are more likely to use emergency mental health services and psychiatric inpatient services than other forms of community mental health care (Dorn & Prout, 1993). Experts have attributed these outcomes to a lack of coordination across professional disciplines and a lack of expertise among community mental health practitioners (Fletcher, 1993).

In some cases, the development of model programs with specialized services have occurred with promising results. Most service models emphasize the use of:

- Multimodal approach
- Interdisciplinary team
- Trained personnel
- Family support and education
- Service linkages and cross systems accountability
- Crisis supports
- Ongoing assessment of service outcomes

The results to a 4-year study of 89 individuals at the Sovner Center in Massachusetts found a significant reduction in the use of emergency services over time (Beasley, 2002). Similar findings were found in the literature for other service models. A list of some of the model programs found in the United States is provided in Table 23.6-1.

At the core of coordinated care programs is some form of assessment by specially trained professionals using a multimodal approach. Typically, a dedicated team trained in intellectual disabilities provides assessment, treatment, consultation, and follow-up. Specialist interdisciplinary teams provide services and consultation to other community mental health professionals and primary care physicians. These teams may include a number of professionals such as primary care physicians; neurologists; psychiatrists; psychologists; psychiatric and primary care nurses; social workers, including family support specialists; therapists; and behavioral communications specialists.

Table 23.6-1. Sample programs designed to coordinate mental health care for individuals with intellectual disabilities in the United States

Alaska Cross Systems Approach (Rambow & Arnold, 1996)
Austin-Travis County MHMR Center, Texas (Casner, 1996)
Cambridge Minnesota Regional Support Team (Collond & Weisler, 1995)
Encor, Nebraska (Menolascino, 1989)
Interface, Ohio (Woodward, 1993)
Minnesota Special Services Program (Rudolph, Lakin, Oslund & Larson, 1998)
Rochester Crisis Intervention Program, New York (Davidson et al., 1995)
START/Sovner Center, Massachussetts (Beasley & Kroll, 2002)
Vermont Crisis Intervention Services (Resources for Community Living, 1993)
Woodbridge Project, Connecticut (Beasley & duPree, 2003)

One important mission of many of the specialized coordinated care programs is to promote service linkages in order to facilitate coordination and improvement in existing services (Beasley & Kroll, 2002). Therefore, many services utilized in the context of a service linkage system are independent of one another both administratively and fiscally. Unlike traditional case management, the models using the service linkage approach often have affiliation agreements that are negotiated administratively between systems rather than based on individual service needs alone. This approach is the predominant one used by program models found in North America and Europe to improve the mental health care of individuals with developmental disabilities (Bouras, Holt, Murphy, Brooks, & Xenitidis, 2001).

Another primary goal of coordinated service linkage teams is to prevent the use of emergency mental health and psychiatric inpatient services whenever possible (Beasley & Kroll, 2002). Individuals in crisis may need temporary housing in order to ride out a difficult episode. In many model programs, resources are made available through the service linkage team to fill in service gaps. As a result, most service linkage teams provide emergency consultation and direct support services to enhance the system when needed (e.g., 24-hour crisis support, psychiatry and emergency respite as an alternative to inpatient settings or institutionalization during periods of crisis) (Beasley, Kroll, & Sovner, 1992; Woodward, 1993).

The use of crisis prevention and intervention plans is emphasized to ensure cross systems and interdisciplinary collaboration (Beasley & Kroll, 2002; Colond & Wieseler, 1995; Patterson, Higgins, & Dyck, 1995). The primary function of crisis prevention planning is to diagnose and define problems and to map out a strategy for individuals, their families, and service providers to follow during periods of difficulty (Beasley & Kroll, 2001). An additional function of the planning process is to clarify roles and responsibilities within the service system to ensure ready access to needed services. A primary goal is to ensure the overall system's accountability, and, as a result, crisis prevention planning is an important tool used to improve the community safety net while helping to reduce the strain on an already depleted service system (Beasley, 2002).

Jimmy's story, presented next, demonstrates how a coordinated service system such as those found in model programs throughout the United States works with people with developmental disabilities and problem behaviors and their families. Almost 45% of all people served through model programs live at home with their families.

Jimmy is a 22-year-old man with moderate cognitive disabilities and autism. He has lived with his family all of his life. His parents are in good health and would like to continue to have Jimmy live with them at home. They receive in-home staffing funded through the state Department of Developmental Disabilities but also require other out-of-home support.

Jimmy and his family have tried to obtain family support for many years; however, Jimmy was not able to use traditional out-of-home respite services available to other service recipients because of his ongoing difficulties. In addition to Jimmy's cognitive limitations, he has a history of behavioral problems that include severe self-injury and major property destruction. Over the years, Jimmy received a number of medications to help reduce his behavioral problems, but his family did not think the medications were effective.

Jimmy's family was in a constant state of crisis. His self-abusive behavior and property destruction were so severe and out of control that he was hospitalized in psychiatric facilities on numerous occasions. After each admission, Jimmy seemed worse to his parents. Jimmy's hospital medications would be tapered down to allow Jimmy to "stay awake," but his severe behaviors would return—beginning the cycle of crisis again.

Jimmy and his family were referred to the coordinated services system and the outpatient neuropsychiatric clinic for individuals with developmental disabilities. Upon arrival, the family appeared to be in severe distress. Jimmy's parents expressed doubts that they could continue to manage the situation. Soon after, Jimmy and his family received a number of services through the coordinated service system and the clinic, including diagnostic and treatment planning, crisis prevention and crisis assistance planning, planned respite, parent education, psychiatry, and emergency respite when Jimmy needed out-of-home crisis services.

Since working with the coordinated services team, Jimmy has been diagnosed and successfully treated for obsessive-compulsive disorder and bipolar disorder, and his behavior has improved dramatically. Physical discomfort and medical problems such as constipation and ear infections were also identified as contributing to his distress. Jimmy is monitored and treated by a primary care physician and a developmental specialist who collaborates closely with the team.

Jimmy continues to receive support staffing through a state-funded provider agency in the family home. Members of the coordinated services team provide on-going training and support to his direct service staff members, and they help to monitor signs of Jimmy's mental health service needs. In addition, Jimmy receives out-of-home planned respite at the coordinated service's facility (a four-bedroom home in the community) for one weekend a month. Last summer, his parents were able to take a trip away from home without worrying about Jimmy for the first time in 10 years.

A coordinated services clinician, Edna, attends psychiatric and medical appointments regularly with Jimmy, his direct support person, and his parents to assist in communicating with medical professionals. She also talks with Jimmy's day program provider consistently to ensure that everyone on Jimmy's team communicates about him and his mental health care needs. In addition, Edna makes home visits to assess Jimmy's needs in his natural environment.

Programs like the one just described assist people like Jimmy and his family to live successfully in the community, free from many of the worries that have often been present for people with intellectual disabilities and behavioral health care needs. Jimmy continues to have ongoing challenges; however, he and his family are no longer in constant distress. The system is linked, communication is active, expertise is available, and everyone—especially Jimmy—continues to benefit from the fruits of their efforts.

CONCLUSION

This chapter provides an overview of some of the diagnostic and service issues to consider in addressing the needs of individuals with intellectual disabilities and problem behavior. Clinicians should expect the presenting problems to have multiple and complex etiological and contributing factors (Gardner, 2002). The system as a whole needs to do a better job of training in order to effectively assess and serve individuals with intellectual disabilities, mental illness, and problem behaviors. The training needs of community practitioners have long been identified as an issue affecting the quality of care people with intellectual disabilities may receive (Szymanski & Grossman, 1984).

Despite advances in diagnostic procedures, a tendency remains to overlook a diagnosis of a mental illness in people with intellectual disabilities. Many observers attribute this failure to inadequate training (Hurley, 1996; Reiss, 1982; Sovner, 1986; Szymanski & Tanquay, 1980). In addition, few psychiatric residency programs offer specialty training in intellectual disabilities (Szymanski, Madow, Mallory, Menolascino, & Eidelman, 1991).

In developing and improving services for individuals with intellectual disabilities and problem behavior, planners and policymakers must also assess their capacity and resources as a system of care in order to allow collaboration between clinical and service disciplines to take place. The evidence from program models shows that the ability to actively collaborate, along with expertise to properly assess, treat, and implement strategies to assist individuals, enhances service effectiveness and reduces the reliance on emergency services and inpatient hospitalizations.

REFERENCES

American Psychiatric Association. (1994). *Diagnostic and statistical manual of mental disorders* (4th ed.). Washington, DC: Author.

Barnhill, J., & Hurley, A.D. (2003). Mood disorders and epilepsy. *Mental Health Aspects of Developmental Disabilities, 6,* 36–39.

Beange, H., McElduff, A., & Baker, W. (1995). Medical disorders of adults with mental retardation: A population study. *American Journal on Mental Retardation, 99,* 595–604.

Beasley, J.B. (1997). The three A's in policy development to promote effective mental health care for people with developmental disabilities. *Habilitative Mental Healthcare Newsletter, 16,* 31–33.

Beasley, J.B. (2000). Family caregiving part III: Family assessments of mental health service experiences of individuals with mental retardation in the Northeast Region of Massachusetts from 1994 to 1998. *Mental Health Aspects of Developmental Disabilities, 3,* 105–113.

Beasley, J.B. (2002). Trends in coordinated and planned mental health service use by people with dual diagnosis. In J. Jacobson & R. Fletcher (Eds.), *Contemporary dual diagnosis: MH/MR service models: Vol. II. Partial and supportive services* (pp. 35–51). Kingston, NY: NADD.

Beasley, J.B., & duPree, K. (2003). A systematic strategy to improve services to individuals with coexisting developmental disabilities and mental illness: National trends and the "Connecticut blueprint." *Mental Health Aspects of Developmental Disabilities,* 50–59.

Beasley, J.B., & Kroll, J. (1999). Family caregiving part II: Family caregiver–professional collaboration in crisis prevention and intervention. *Mental Health Aspects of Developmental Disabilities, 2*(1), 22–26.

Beasley, J., & Kroll, J. (2002). The START/Sovner Center Program in Massachusetts. In R.H. Hanson, N.A. Wiesler, & K.C. Lakin (Eds.), *Crisis prevention and response in the community* (pp. 97–125). Washington DC: American Association on Mental Retardation.

Beasley, J.B., Kroll, J., & Sovner, R. (1992). Community-based crisis mental health services for persons with developmental disabilities: The START model. *Habilitative Mental Health Care Newsletter, 11*(9), 55–57.

Benjamin, S. (2000). A neuropsychiatric approach to behavioral issues in epilepsy. *Clinical Nursing Practice in Epilepsy, 1,* 7–12, 97.

Borthwick, S. (1988). Maladaptive behavior among the mentally retarded: The need for reliable data. In J. Stark, F. Menolascino, M. Albarelli, & V. Gray (Eds.), *Mental retardation and mental health: Classification, diagnosis, treatment services* (pp. 3–40). New York: Springer-Verlag.

Bouras, N., Holt, G., Murphy, D., Brooks, B., & Xenitidis, K. (2001). Mental health services for people with learning disabilities. *Psychiatric Bulletin of the Royal College of Psychiatrists, 25,* 323.

Bouras, N., Kon, Y., & Drummond, C. (1993). Medical and psychiatric needs of adults with a mental handicap. *Journal of Intellectual Disability Research, 37,* 177–182.

Bradley, E. (2002). *Guidelines for managing the client with intellectual disabilities in the emergency room.* Toronto: University of Toronto, Surrey Place Centre, Centre for Addiction and Mental Health.

Branford, D. (1997). A follow-up study of prescribing for people with learning disabilities previously in National Health Service care in Leicestershire, England. *Journal of Intellectual Disability Research, 41,* 339–345.

Bregman, J.D. (1991). Current developments in the understanding of mental retardation part II: Psychopathology. *Journal of the American Academy of Child and Adolescent Psychiatry, 30,* 861–872.

Burd, L., Williams, M., Klug, M.G., Fjelstad, K., Schimke, A., & Kerbeshian, J. (1997). Prevalence of psychotropic and anticonvulsant drug use among North Dakota group home residents. *Journal of Intellectual Disability Research, 41,* 488–494.

Campbell, M., & Malone, R. (1991). Mental retardation and psychiatric disorders. *Hospital and Community Psychiatry, 42,* 374–379.

Carlson, G. (1981). Mental disorders and cognitive immaturity. In R.H. Belmaker & H.M. VanPraag (Eds.), *Mania: An evolving concept* (pp. 281–289). New York: Spectrum.

Casner, J.A. (1996). The Austin community support project: A collaborative treatment program provided by Austin state school and Austin-Travis county MHMR center. *National Association of Dual Diagnosis (NADD) Newsletter, 13*(1), 1–4.

Chapman, R.S., & Hesketh, L.M. (2000). Behavioral phenotype of individuals with Down's syndrome. *Mental Retardation and Developmental Disabilities Research, 43,* 340–350.

Charlot, L.R., Doucette, A.C., & Mezzacappa, E. (1993). Affective symptoms of institutionalized adults with mental retardation. *American Journal on Mental Retardation, 98,* 408–416.

Collond, J.S., & Weisler, N.A. (1995). Preventing restrictive placements through community support services. *American Journal of Mental Retardation, 100,* 201–206.

Crisione, T., Kastner, T., Walsh, K., & Nathanson, R. (1993). Managed health care systems for people with mental retardation: Impact on patient utilization. *Mental Retardation, 31*(5), 297–306.

Davidson, P., Cain, N., Sloane-Reeves, J., Giesow, V., Quijano, L., Heyningen, J.V., et al. (1995). Crisis intervention for community based individuals with developmental disabilities and behavioral and psychiatric disorders. *Mental Retardation, 33,* 21–30.

Davidson, P., Cain, N., Sloane-Reeves, J., VanSpeybroeck, A., Segel, J., Gutkin, J., et al. (1994). Characteristics of community-based individuals with mental retardation and aggressive behavior disorders. *American Journal of Mental Retardation, 98,* 704–716.

Davidson, P.W., Morris, D., & Cain, N.N. (1999). Community services for people with developmental disabilities and psychiatric or severe behavior disorders. In N. Bouras (Ed.), *Psychiatric and behavioral disorders in developmental dis-*

abilities and mental retardation (pp. 359–372). New York: Cambridge University Press.

Deb, S., Thomas, M., & Bright, C. (2001). Mental disorder in adults with intellectual disability. 1: Prevalence of functional psychiatric illness among a community-based population between 16–64 years. *Journal of Intellectual Disability Research, 45*, 495–505.

Dorn, T.A., & Prout, H.T. (1993). Service delivery patterns for adults with mild mental retardation at community mental health centers. *Mental Retardation, 31*, 292–296.

Dosen, A. (1988). Community care for people with mental retardation in the Netherlands. *Australia and New Zealand Journal of Developmental Disabilities, 14*, 15–18.

Edelstein, T.M., & Glenwick, D.S. (1997). Referral reasons for psychological services for adults with mental retardation. *Research in Developmental Disabilities, 18*, 45–49.

Emerson, E. (2003). Prevalence of psychiatric disorders in children and adolescents with and without disability. *Journal of Intellectual Disability Research, 47*, 51–58.

Evangelista, L.A. (1988). Comprehensive management of the mentally retarded/mentally ill. In J. Stark, F. Menolascino, M. Albarelli, & V. Gray (Eds.), *Mental retardation and mental health: Classification, diagnosis, treatment services* (pp. 140–146). New York: Springer-Verlag.

Fletcher, R. (1993). Mental illness-mental retardation in the United States: Policy and treatment challenges. *Journal of Intellectual Disability Research, 37*, (Supp. 1) 2–33.

Freeman, R.D., Fast, D.K., & Burd, L. (2000). An international perspective on Tourette syndrome: Selected findings from 3500 individuals in 22 countries. *Developmental Medicine and Child Neurology, 42*, 436–477.

Friedlander, R. (2004). *The association of Tourette syndrome with aggression.* Paper presented at the biannual meetings of the European Association on Mental Illness in Mental Retardation, September, 2004, Rome.

Friedlander, R., Lazar, S., & Klancnik, J. (2001). Atypical antipsychotic use in treating adolescents and young adults with developmental disabilities. *Canadian Journal of Psychiatry, 46*, 741–745.

Gardner, W.I. (2002). *Aggression and other disruptive behavior challenges: Biomedical and psychosocial assessment and treatment.* Kingston, NY: NADD Press.

Gath, A., & Grumley, D. (1986). Behavior problems in retarded children with special reference to Down's syndrome. *British Journal of Psychiatry, 149*, 156–161.

Ghaziuddin, M. (1988). Behavioral disorders in the mentally handicapped: The role of life events. *British Journal of Psychiatry, 152*, 683–686.

Gillberg, C., Persso, E., Grufman, M., & Themner, U. (1986). Psychiatric disorders in mildly and severely mentally retarded urban children and adolescents: Epidemiologic aspects. *British Journal of Psychiatry, 149*, 68–74.

Hastings, R.P, Hatton, C., Taylor, J.L., & Maddison, C. (2004). Life events and psychiatric symptoms in adults with intellectual disabilities. *Journal of Intellectual Disabilities Research, 48*, 42–46.

Hurley, A.D. (1996). Identifying psychiatric disorders in persons with mental retardation: A model illustrated by depression in Down syndrome. *Journal of Rehabilitation, 15*, 6–31.

Hurley, A.D., Folstein, M.F., & Lam, N. (2003). Patients with and without intellectual disability seeking outpatient psychiatric services: diagnoses and prescribing pattern. *Journal of Intellectual Disability Research, 47*, 39–50.

Jacobson, J.W. (1990). Assessing the prevalence of psychiatric disorders in the developmentally disabled population. In E. Dibble & D. Gray (Eds.), *Assessment of persons with mental retardation living in the community* (pp. 19–70). Rockville, MD: National Institute of Mental Health.

Kastner, T., Walsh, K.K., & Fraser, M. (2001). Undiagnosed medical conditions and medication side effects presenting as behavioral/psychiatric problems in people with mental retardation. *Mental Health Aspects of Developmental Disabilities, 4*, 101–107.

Kearney, F.J., & Smull, M.W. (1992). People with mental retardation leaving mental health institutions. In J.W. Jacobson, S.N. Burchard, & P.J. Carling (Eds.), *Community living for people with developmental disabilities* (pp. 183–196). Baltimore: Johns Hopkins University Press.

King, B.H., DeAntoni, C., McCracken, M.T., Forness, S.R., & Ackerland, V. (1994). Psychiatric consultation in severe and profound mental retardation. *American Journal of Psychiatry, 151*, 1803–1808.

Levitas, A., & Gilson, S.F. (2001). Predictable crises in the lives of persons with mental retardation. *Mental Health Aspects of Developmental Disabilities, 4*, 89–100.

Levitas, A.S., Hurley, A.D., & Pary, R.J. (2001). The mental status examination in patients with mental retardation and developmental disabilities. *Mental Health Aspects of Developmental Disabilities, 4*, 2–16.

Lunsky, Y., & Benson, B.A. (2001). The association between perceived social support and strain, and positive and negative for adults with mild intellectual disability. *Journal of Intellectual Disability Research, 45*, 106–114.

Lunsky, Y., Emery, S.F., & Benson, B.A. (2002). Staff and self-reports of health behaviours, somatic complaints, and medication in adults with mild intellectual disability. *Journal of Intellectual & Developmental Disability, 27*, 125–137.

Lunsky, Y., & Havercamp, S.M. (1999). Distinguishing low levels of social support and social strain: Implications for dual diagnosis. *American Journal on Mental Retardation, 104*, 200–204.

Matikka, L.M., & Vesala, H.T. (1997). Acquiescence in quality-of-life interviews with adults who have mental retardation. *Mental Retardation, 35*, 75–82.

Matson, J.L. (1983). Depression in the mentally retarded: Toward a conceptual analysis of diagnosis. *Progress in Behavior Modification, 15*, 57–79.

McCracken, J., & Diamond, R. (1988). Bipolar disorder in mentally retarded adolescents. *Journal of the Academy of Child and Adolescent Psychiatry, 27*, 494–499.

Menolascino, F.J. (1989). Model services for the treatment/management of the mentally retarded-mentally ill. *Community Mental Health Journal, 25*(2), 36–41.

Menolascino, F.J., Gilson, S.F., & Levitas, A. (1986). The nature and types of mental illness in the mentally retarded. *Psychopharmacology Bulletin, 22*, 1060–1071.

Menolascino, F.J., & McCann, B.M. (Eds.). (1983). *Mental health & mental retardation: Bridging the gap* (pp. 3–64). Baltimore: University Park Press.

Nezu, C.M., Nezu, A.M., & Gil-Weiss, M.J. (1992). *Psychopathology in persons with mental retardation: Clinical guidelines for assessment and treatment.* Champaign, IL: Research Press.

O'Neill, R.E., Horner, R.H., Albin, R.W., Sprague, J.R., Storey, K., & Newton, J.S. (1997). *Functional assessment and program development for problem behavior: A practical handbook* (2nd ed.). Pacific Grove, CA: Brookes/Cole.

Patterson, T., Higgins, M., & Dyck, D.G. (1995). A collaborative approach to reduce hospitalization of developmentally disabled clients with mental illness. *Psychiatric Services, 46,* 243–247.

Phillips, I., & Williams, N. (1975). Psychopathology and mental retardation: A study of 100 mentally retarded children. *American Journal of Psychiatry, 132,* 139–145.

Rambow, T.R., & Arnold, M. (1996). Individualized/homogenized/cost effective service model. *National Association of Dually Diagnosed (NADD) Newsletter, 13*(6), 1–4.

Reiss, S. (1982). Psychopathology and mental retardation: Survey of a developmental disabilities day program. *Mental Retardation, 20,* 128–132.

Reiss, S. (1990). Prevalence of dual diagnosis in community-based day programs in the Chicago metropolitan area. *American Journal on Mental Retardation, 94*(6) 578–585.

Reiss, S. (1994). *Handbook of challenging behavior: Mental health aspects of mental retardation.* Worthington, OH: International Diagnostic.

Resources for Community Living. (1993). *Moretown: Vermont Crisis Network.* Unpublished program description.

Riatasuo, S., Taiminen, T., & Solokangas, R.K.R. (1999). Characteristics of people with intellectual disability admitted for psychiatric inpatient treatment. *Journal of Intellectual Disability Research, 43,* 119–127.

Robertson, J., Emerson, E., Gregory, N., Hatton, C., Kessissoglou, S., & Hallam, A. (2000). Receipt of psychotropic medication by people with intellectual disability in residential settings. *Journal of Intellectual Disability Research, 44,* 666–676.

Rudolph, C., Lakin, C., Oslund, J.M., & Larson, W. (1998). Evaluation of outcomes and cost-effectiveness of a community behavioral support and crisis response demonstration project. *Mental Retardation, 36*(3), 187–197.

Rutter, M., Tizard, J., Yule, W., Graham, P., & Whitmore, K. (1976). Research report: Isle of Wight studies, 1984–1974. *Psychological Medicine, 6,* 313, 332.

Singh, N.N., Ellis, C.R., & Wechsler, H. (1997). Psychopharmocoepidemiology of mental retardation: 1966 to 1995. *Journal of Child and Adolescent Psychopharmacology, 7,* 255–266.

Sobsey, D., Sharmaine, G., Wells, D., Pyper, D., & Reimer-Heck, B. (1992). *Disability, sexuality, and abuse: An annotated bibliography.* Baltimore: Paul H. Brookes Publishing Co.

Sovner, R. (1986). Limiting factors in the use of DSM–III criteria with mentally ill/mentally retarded persons. *Psychopharmacology Bulletin, 22,* 1055–1059.

Sovner, R., & Hurley, A.D. (1983). Do the mentally retarded suffer from affective illness? *Archives in General Psychiatry, 40,* 61–67.

Sovner, R., & Hurley, A.D. (1990). Assessment tools which facilitate psychiatric evaluation and treatment. *Habilitative Mental Health Care Newsletter, 9,* 91–98.

Szymanski, L., & Grossman, H. (1984). Dual implications of "dual diagnosis." *Mental Retardation, 22,* 155–156.

Szymanski, L., Madow, L., Mallory, G., Menolascino, F., & Eidelman, S. (1991). *Report of the Task Force on Psychiatric Services to Adult Mentally Retarded and Mentally Disabled Persons* (Task Force Report No. 30). Washington, DC: American Psychiatric Association.

Szymanski, L., & Tanquey, P. (1980). Training of mental health professionals in mental retardation. In L. Szymanski & P. Tanquey (Eds.), *Emotional disorders of mentally retarded persons* (pp. 19–28). Baltimore: University Park Press.

Tardiff, K., & Koenigsberg, H.W. (1985). Assaultive behavior among psychiatric outpatients. *American Journal of Psychiatry, 142,* 960–963.

Van Allen, M.I., Fund, J., & Jurenka, S.B. (1999). Health care concerns and guidelines for adults with Down syndrome. *American Journal of Medical Genetics, 89,* 100–110.

Woodward, H.L. (1993). One community's response to the multi-system service needs of individuals with mental illness and developmental disabilities. *Community Mental Health Journal, 29,* 347–359.

CHAPTER 24

DEVELOPMENTAL THERAPIES AND FUNCTIONAL ASSISTANCE

24.1 OCCUPATIONAL THERAPY

Sharon A. Cermak and Priscilla S. Osborne

Developmental disabilities typically affect multiple areas of an individual's development and several functional areas. In infancy, developmental delays are most apparent in sensory-motor performance skills. Delays in achievement of developmental motor milestones and atypical sensory processing are often the first performance deficits to be noted in the first 2 years of life for children with developmental delays. Acquisition of motor skills is considered essential for the development of mobility, oral-motor, fine motor, and perceptual motor skills. Children with cardiopulmonary or musculoskeleletal problems, children with intellectual disabilities, and children born prematurely typically show developmental delays in the achievement of motor landmarks. Early symptoms of sensory processing disorders may include oversensitivity to and/or lack of awareness of sensory stimuli.

During the toddler years and early childhood years, additional delays may become evident in language and cognitive development. Such delays may have an influence on all performance areas, including activities of daily living (ADL), play, and participation in educational and community-based activities. Cognitive and psychosocial areas are generally the major issues for the adolescents and adults with developmental disabilities. These impairments manifest in difficulty in the major performance areas: ADL, school, work and productive activities, and play and leisure activities.

Professionals from many disciplines work with individuals with developmental disabilities and their families. A child with developmental disabilities benefits most from the collaborative efforts of a team of professionals from multiple disciplines. The specific members of the team are determined by the type and severity of the child's disability, as well as the child's age, support systems, and environments (Case-Smith, 2001). Two disciplines that are most often part of the evaluation and treatment team for children are occupational therapy and physical therapy.

Each of these disciplines is concerned with optimizing the child's function within his or her environment. To that common goal, each of these professions incorporates a family-centered, community-based, and culturally competent approach to practice. Common therapeutic principles include reducing impairments, utilizing the strengths of the child and his or her family, and modifying the environment to optimize the child's function. Each discipline also makes a unique contribution to the care of the individual and to interdisciplinary practice.

Occupational therapy and physical therapy services for children have been influenced by organized advocacy efforts and resulting federal legislation. Access to these services is mandated for children from birth to age 22 through the Individuals with Disabilities Education Act (IDEA) Amendments of 1997 (PL 105-17), Parts B and C. For children younger than 3 years of age, services are outlined in a family-centered service plan, called the *individualized family service plan* (IFSP). Occupational therapy and physical therapy are included as direct services. The administration of birth-to-3 services varies from state to state; however, it is typically the responsibility of the Department of Public Health or the Department of Education.

For children ages 3–22, the *individualized education program* (IEP) delineates the plan to facilitate and support the education of the child. Occupational therapy and physical therapy services are included to the extent that they support the child's education. Services for children from age 3 through the age when the child graduates from high school (or up to age 22) are administered through the Department of Education. Both the IFSP and the IEP may include multidisciplinary services and emphasize service delivery in the child's natural environment and in the least restrictive setting.

In addition to receiving early intervention and/or school-based services, some children with developmental disabilities will also receive occupational therapy and physical therapy services through their health care coverage including Children's Health Insurance Program (CHIP) or Medicaid (Giardino, Kohrt, Ayre, & Welts,

2002). After age 22, services are often provided in community-based programs that are supported by the Department of Mental Retardation and/or the Department of Mental Health.

Although legislation for adults does not specifically address therapy services, it does provide for inclusion of individuals with disabilities within the community, and therapy services may be needed toward that end. The Americans with Disabilities Act (ADA) of 1990 (PL 101-336) prohibits discrimination and ensures equal opportunity for individuals with disabilities. *Olmstead v. L.C.* in 1999 expanded community-based services for individuals with intellectual disabilities. In February 2001, President Bush announced the New Freedom Initiative (U.S. Department of Health and Human Services, 2003), which is a nationwide initiative designed to remove barriers to community living for individuals with disabilities.

In summary, in the United States, federal legislation has greatly influenced the provision of health care, education, and social services for infants, toddlers, children, adolescents, and adults with disabilities. PL 105-17 provides a concept of service continuum for infants, children, and youth with disabilities, with Part B providing guidelines for educational services for children age 3–22, and Part C providing guidelines for early intervention for infants and toddlers. PL 105-17 further specifies that all special education students 14 years of age and older must have individualized transition plans that include specific goals to facilitate their success as adults. PL 101-336, *Olmstead v. L.C.*, and the New Freedom Initiative support equal access and inclusion in community-based programs.

Amanda was adopted from an Eastern European orphanage at 10 months and showed significant developmental delays. She had only been fed from a bottle and was resistant to any foods. She did not accept solid foods until she was 19 months. Amanda received numerous interventions, including occupational therapy, physical therapy, and speech-language therapy. Developmentally, she made excellent progress, and the school felt there was not a need for continued services after early intervention.

At 4-years-old, Amanda started preschool. Her teacher expressed concern because Amanda became very agitated when the class did activities such as fingerpainting, gluing, or playing in the sandbox outside. The teacher also reported that Amanda had difficulty sitting in circle time and became aggressive when other children bumped her. When the noise in the classroom increased, Amanda often hid under the table and covered her ears.

Administration of the Sensory Profile (Dunn, 1999) and an interview with Amanda's mother indicated that Amanda had been an irritable baby who was not cuddly and did not like to be held. Amanda's mother noted frequent gagging problems when she introduced textured foods into Amanda's diet. She reported that Amanda eats only a very limited variety of foods such as custards and plain yogurt, cheese doodles, and macaroni and cheese. Amanda will not eat any food with lumps or grainy textures. Mealtimes are prolonged, often taking 1–1½ hours. Evaluation through parent and teacher interview and observation of Amanda in her preschool classroom indicated that Amanda perceived sensory input such as light touch or loud sounds as noxious, and she evidenced multiple indicators of sensory defensiveness.

Amanda's teacher and parents needed insight into her sensory processing styles and needed to recognize that, rather than exhibiting "behavior problems," Amanda was reacting to the manner in which her nervous system processed sensory information. By understanding Amanda's sensory processing, her teacher and parents could predict situations that may be challenging and make changes in the environment, such as modifying seating placement, offering different activities, and/or preparing Amanda by first providing sensory input that was organizing.

The occupational therapist worked with Amanda's mother to help develop a program to reduce oral hypersensitivity and to expand Amanda's food repertoire. Oral play with rubber toys was suggested to provide oral-motor input to desensitize the oral area and promote tongue and jaw movements (Case-Smith, 2000b). Application of deep pressure around the cheeks and mouth in a game-like fashion was recommended before mealtimes. Amanda's older sister was included in the games. Amanda had been resistant to toothbrushing, and the occupational therapist suggested that these activities might also precede toothbrushing.

Amanda's hypersensitivity to touch was not limited to the oral motor area and feeding but was also evident during classroom activities, which helped to explain why Amanda was resistant to activities such as gluing or fingerpainting. Consultation was provided to Amanda's teacher regarding types of sensory input that were calming and organizing such as deep pressure and proprioception that would precede this type of light touch classroom activities. A "sensory diet" was developed for use in the classroom (Wilbarger & Wilbarger, 2002a, 2002b). Alternate materials such as using a glue stick instead of liquid paste were recommended. In order to help Amanda develop self-regulatory strategies so she was able to participate in home and classroom activities in a more goal-directed way, the Alert Program (Williams & Schellenberger, 1994), a program designed to enhance self-regulation, was incorporated into Amanda's daily routine.

FOCUS AND SCOPE

Occupational therapy helps individuals with developmental disabilities and their families carry out valued daily life activities (Baloueff & Cohn, 2002). Occupational therapy practice is based on an understanding of the interactions among individuals, their activities, and their physical and social environments in order to enable individuals to participate as fully as possible (Case-Smith, 2001). The term *occupation* does not relate specifically to employment. Rather, the term has a broader meaning and "relates to the individual's goal-directed use of time, energy, interest and attention" (Hohlstein & Sprague, 1995, p. 118). This varies as a function of the developmental age and stage of the individual.

The relationship between the individual, the family, the environment, and the tasks that are appropriate for a person's developmental age is dynamic and ongoing with different needs and challenges at different points in time. For example, with a young child, occupational therapy focuses on sensory-motor, cognitive, and communication/interaction skills and the child's ability to engage in play, self-care, social interaction, and school. With an older child, the role of occupational therapy focuses on school; social interaction; supporting community participation, including the development of vocational and life skills; and building support networks. Occupational therapy assists with transition planning for adolescents taking on adult roles and responsibilities (Baloueff & Cohn, 2002).

For adults with developmental disabilities, occupational therapy provides supports and interventions that help individuals "participate in activities of daily living, engage in work activities, enjoy leisure pursuits, and interact socially with other members of the community" (Herge, 2003, p. CE-1). Activities may include increasing access to assistive and universal design technologies, consultation to supported employment programs to enable integration into the workforce, and consultation to community programs to enable individuals with developmental disabilities to participate in health promotion activities.

PROFESSIONAL PRACTICE GUIDELINES

The American Occupational Therapy Association (AOTA), the professional organization of occupational therapy, has published a series of practice guidelines designed to outline the domains and philosophical base of occupational therapy practice as it relates to specific disabilities (Moyers, 1999). In addition to these specific guidelines, AOTA published *The Guide to Occupational Therapy Practice*, which describes "the scope of occupational therapy practice for all individuals experiencing problems or for those at risk for problems in performing the daily activities necessary for functional independence, health, and well-being" (1999, p. 248). This guide includes definitions of the scope of occupational therapy; a model of the occupational therapy process; assessment, evaluation, and intervention approaches; outcome measurement; related terminology; and standards of practice. AOTA (2002) published the *Occupational Therapy Practice Framework: Domain and Process* to describe the domain of occupational therapy, emphasizing its unique perspective on occupation and activities of daily living and the dynamic evaluation and intervention processes that support engagement in occupation.

GOALS

Occupational therapists who work with individuals with developmental disabilities are concerned with enabling the child or adult to participate as fully as possible in society and to meet his or her individual and family goals (Case-Smith, 2000b; Herge, 2003). In early intervention, an important goal of occupational therapy is to support, encourage, and enhance the competence of parents in their role as caregivers. With children, the primary goals are to improve performance of everyday activities and to enhance participation in physical, educational, and social environments (Case-Smith, 2001). Therapeutic intervention focuses on what is meaningful to the child and his caregivers.

Therapists working with adolescents and adults value self-determination and emphasize helping individuals identify their interests and needs and providing skills and supports to meet these needs (Herge, 2003; Herge & Wertz, 2002). The culminating goal of occupational therapy is to facilitate overall well-being and quality of life by supporting an individual's ability to engage in important and meaningful occupations (AOTA, 2002). The goal of intervention is to maximize skill development and active participation, which can be achieved through reducing impairments, promoting wellness and preventing secondary issues, adapting context, and utilizing strengths and resources of the individual and his or her family and/or caregivers.

Cody has cerebral palsy with mild-moderate involvement of upper extremity function. His teacher reported that his poor handwriting was interfering with his performance in school. He was unable to write legibly and could not complete his work in the allotted time. Cody fatigued easily; he failed to stabilize his paper because he used his nonwriting hand to hold his head up.

Cody also demonstrated difficulty with motor planning. He did not have a good awareness of his body in space and had difficulty figuring out how to make his body do what he wanted it to do. Evaluation indicated that Cody had increased tone and decreased strength, both contributing to poor balance and poor stability of his shoulders and arms and to his poor writing skill.

The occupational therapy practitioner focused on improving function by providing strengthening and stability activities. She also incorporated compensatory strategies by adapting Cody's environment (e.g., better positioning of Cody in his chair, adjustment of armrests, frequent movement breaks). The occupational therapist also provided direct intervention for Cody's motor planning difficulty by incorporating sensory integration principles to enhance body awareness and improve motor planning skills (Anzalone & Murray, 2002; Reeves & Cermak, 2002). In addition, the Goal-Plan-Do-Check (Missiuna, 2001) cognitive approach helped Cody learn strategies for handwriting as well as motor skills. If Cody were an older child with the same problems, the occupational therapist might recommend appropriate school accommodations, such as the use of a tape recorder or notetaker and using a computer for writing, perhaps with voice recognition software.

PHILOSOPHY

Occupational therapy is client-centered with a focus on the goals and outcomes that are valued by and meaningful to the client. When working with young children, intervention is family-focused because families provide the central influence in the lives of their children and are the primary social units in which young children live and receive care and nurturing. Parent–professional partnerships are key to the quality of interventions for children. Occupational therapists collaborate with the child and his or her family in developing treatment goals that are important to the family. Parent–professional relationships are greatly enhanced when professionals respect family diversity and cultural backgrounds, communicate clearly, listen to and support families, and believe and trust parents.

When working with adolescents and adults with developmental disabilities, the therapist "functions as a facilitator, respecting the person's choices and providing the support he or she requires to work toward personal goals" (Babola, 2000, p. 125). The treatment planning process is collaborative and individualized toward goals that are meaningful to the individual. When an individual is not able to identify needs and assistance and establish treatment priorities, input is sought from the family and others involved in the individual's daily life.

SETTINGS

Occupational therapists practice in wide variety of settings, including hospitals, rehabilitation centers, mental health clinics, home health care, school systems, early intervention programs, residential centers, extended care facilitates, and community agencies. More than one third of occupational therapists in the United States work in pediatrics, and of those individuals, more than half practice in schools (AOTA, 2000; Rainville, Cermak, & Murray, 1996).

Occupational therapists provide individual intervention, as well as consultative services that foster community participation, prevention, and wellness of individuals and groups (Wilcock, 2003). Occupational therapy intervention may incorporate education, support, direct services, and self-help approaches. Consultation may be provided to individuals with disabilities and their families, care providers, teachers, health professionals, doctors, organizations, communities, or government policy makers (Moyers, 1999).

Within the different settings in which occupational therapists work, services may include direct intervention focused on influencing the biological, physiological, psychological, or neurological processes of the infant, child, adolescent, or adult. Intervention may also include teaching new skills, habits, or behaviors to enable the individual's participation in different contexts. The occupational therapist may suggest adapting the task requirements, using adaptive equipment or assistive technology, or modifying the environment. Disability prevention, education, and health promotion is designed to help individuals avoid the onset of unhealthy conditions, diseases, or injuries (AOTA, 2002). For example, AOTA (2003) developed a brochure and web site on healthy ways to load and wear a backpack to prevent back injuries.

Bethany is an individual with Down syndrome who was in an inclusive vocational program in her high school. During transition planning, Bethany identified that her goal post–high school was "to work" and "to live with friends in my own house." An occupational therapist worked with the team to identify Bethany's strengths and the supports needed for her to obtain and maintain employment and to live independently or in supported living. Although Bethany required only minimal supervision in basic daily living skills (e.g., reminders to shower), she had never used public transportation independently, had not prepared meals or snacks, and had not gone shopping.

Discussion with Bethany's mother indicated that Bethany had never been expected to participate in household chores.

A system of assigned chores was set up at home so that Bethany could begin to learn to wash her clothes and cook simple meals, preparing her for assuming an adult role. At school, Bethany began to work in the school store. Bethany also decided that she would like to learn to use the bus. She and her team decided to begin with using public transportation, instead of the school bus, to go to school. The occupational therapist adapted the Mobility Skills Training Program (McInerney & McInerney, 1992). Training took place in three phases progressing from simulated practice to riding the bus, initially with supervision and eventually independently.

EARLY INTERVENTION AND SCHOOL-BASED SERVICES

Under Part C of PL 105-17, which covers children birth to 3 years, occupational therapy is considered a direct service. Currently, all 50 states have early intervention programs run by a state agency such as the Department of Public Health, the Department of Social Services, or the Department of Education. In early intervention, strong emphasis is placed on family involvement and prevention of problems, not just remediation. Minimizing the potential for developmental delay is the first goal of Part C.

Under federal legislation, all children, regardless of their disability, have the right to a free appropriate public education. According to Part B of PL 105-17, which covers children from age 3 through high school, occupational therapy is a related service provided to a student if it enables the child to participate in and benefit from special education. This requirement means that occupational therapy provided in the schools must be designed to relate to the child's ability to participate in the educational process.

REHABILITATION SERVICES

Many children receive occupational therapy in hospital-based inpatient or outpatient rehabilitation programs, such as services for children who have sustained acute injuries (e.g., traumatic brain injury, burns), as well as for children with more chronic disabilities (e.g., cerebral palsy). Typically, services for adults with developmental delays are provided in community-based programs; however, adults with developmental disabilities may sustain an injury and need rehabilitation services provided in an inpatient facility, on an outpatient basis, or in the home.

COMMUNITY-BASED HEALTH PROMOTION SERVICES

Most individuals with developmental disabilities now reside in communities, and services are provided in the community, in the home, in schools, in employment sites, and in supported living or group homes. Occupational therapists collaborate with an individual with developmental disabilities and others involved in his or her care, including family, caregivers, social supports, case coordinators, and staff, to identify the changing needs of the individual. The therapist may consult on the design and implementation of individual and community-based programs, including provision and training in assistive technology; environmental assessment and adaptation to insure that equipment, services, and sites are accessible; health and wellness programs; and information resources. Occupational therapists also consult with policy and funding agencies and others "to allocate the resources to create environments, technologies and programs that are accessible, inclusive, meaningful, age appropriate, and encourage activity and accommodate people's functional and social needs" (Hammel, 2000. p. 40).

With diabetes and obesity on the rise, fitness and health promotion has become increasingly important for all individuals; however, research indicates that compared with people without developmental disabilities, individuals with such conditions are more likely to lead sedentary lives that can lead to obesity, low cardiac fitness, and increased risk for osteoporosis (Nochajski, 2000, as cited in Herge, 2003). Occupational therapists can develop wellness programs for individuals and provide consultation to industry and community-based programs to optimize health and promote fitness of individuals with developmental disabilities.

REFERRAL TO OCCUPATIONAL THERAPY

Referral for occupational therapy is indicated whenever there is a reason to suspect delay or qualitative impairment in the performance of daily tasks and routines including self-care, play, leisure, work, social interaction, or performance of tasks (Committee on Children with Disabilities, 1996). Referral to occupational therapy is made in a variety of ways. Many states regulate occupational therapy through licensure and regulation laws. Some states determine who may make a referral to occupational therapy and may mandate a referral from a medical doctor. In other states, referrals can be made by a parent, teacher, or other individual involved with the care of a child.

For the infant and young child, referral is typically made for early intervention by the child's pediatrician or parent (Committee on Children with Disabilities, 1999a, 1999b). For example, a parent, caregiver, or pediatrician may be alerted to a possible sensory processing problem when a child has difficulty sleeping, is a poor feeder, is irritable, and startles easily. Referrals may be made directly to the occupational therapist or to an early intervention program. The early intervention team, which includes the occupational therapist as well as the family, decides on the appropriateness of occupational therapy. Some teams incorporate a transdisciplinary model in which one professional assumes the roles of multiple professionals.

In a recent survey, pediatricians identified writing, feeding, and dressing as the most appropriate reasons for referral to occupational therapy (Elwell, 2001). Overall, pediatricians reported observing improvement in 93% of individuals referred for occupational therapy. Observations of improvement were most commonly reported for treatment of sensory sensitivity, sleeping problems, self-injurious behavior, writing, feeding, and dressing problems. In school systems, parents, teachers, another member of the team, or the child's pediatrician may request referral to occupational therapy. Figure 24.1-1 presents a checklist for referral to occupational therapy.

Referral for occupational therapy services for adults can be made in a number of ways. Many adults live in group homes that include occupational therapists as consultants. Several states use individualized budgeting systems that reflect the principles of self-determination whereby individuals select their own services and supports and may choose to include occupational therapy (Herge, 2003). Occupational therapy services for adults with developmental disabilities are typically provided in the form of consultation to programs in which individuals reside and/or work. In most instances, direct occupational therapy is not provided for adults with developmental disabilities unless a specific medical need exists (e.g., injury, stroke) or a change in status occurs (e.g., transition to work, change in living situation) that requires the provision of direct services.

Julio, an individual with intellectual disabilities, recently moved into a group home because his parents were no longer able to care for him. As a resident of the group home, Julio was required to help with household chores, such as setting the table for dinner and taking out the trash. Julio was cooperative and pleasant during chore time but required step-by-step prompting from a staff member or a volunteer to complete his chores. The staff wanted to see Julio do his chores more independently, so they contacted their consulting occupational therapist for suggestions.

The occupational therapist performed an activity analysis for the task of taking out the trash. She noted that the steps for the activity could be performed in a specific, nonvarying order; that is, taking out the trash involved first getting a large garbage bag from the closet, then emptying all the small wastebaskets into the bag, tying the bag closed, and placing the bag into the bin outside. She determined that direct supervision was not required as a safety precaution for the task; however, due to Julio's level of cognitive functioning, he would continue to need some form of cuing or prompting to complete each discrete step of the task in timely manner and to ensure adequate task performance.

The occupational therapist suggested that Julio use an auditory prompting system consisting of a cassette player with headphones and an audiotape for each of his household tasks. She decided to implement the system using the task of taking out the trash. She taped verbal prompts for each step of the task, leaving time for the completion of one step before introducing the next. She incorporated silence, words of encouragement, music, and cues to check the quality of work as filler between instructions for each step. In essence, the occupational therapist "talked" Julio through the task on the audiotape as if she were there with him.

Once the tape was recorded, the occupational therapist walked through the system with Julio. She also trained the staff how to use the audio prompting system with Julio, including how to record instructions appropriately for new tasks and how to determine when ongoing use of the system may no longer be necessary. With practice, Julio became able to take out the trash without staff supervision after being given the tape to insert into his cassette player. Julio's success in using the auditory prompting system for this task led staff members to record additional audiotapes for other household tasks so that Julio could function more independently in the group home.

ASSESSMENT

The goal of evaluation of a child with developmental disabilities is to understand the strengths of the child and his family and areas of concern within the context of the environment in which the child participates. Family members and other team members, such as teachers, are integral to the process. The occupational therapist begins assessment of the child by gaining an understanding of the child's level of participation in daily activities with his or her family and in school with peers and other adults. The therapist, in consultation with the child, the parent, and relevant professionals, identifies what the child needs and wants to do.

Childhood occupations may encompass self-care, play and leisure, education and learning, and socializa-

Referral to occupational therapy

Name of child: ______________________ Date of birth: ______________________

Date of referral: ______________________ Referred by: ______________________

In what capacity do you know this child:

Diagnosis: ______________________

____

Precautions: ______________________

____

Reason for referral: ______________________

____

Areas of concern for which referral is being made (check all that apply)

_____ Activities of daily living _____ Hand skills _____ Parent–child relationships
_____ Play _____ Sports _____ Peer relationships
_____ Leisure _____ Vocational _____ Transitions

Checklist for occupational therapy (preschool through elementary)

Please check the statements that are pertinent.

Gross motor

_____ Seems weaker than other children his or her age; strength not adequate for needed activities
_____ Doesn't have endurance needed for activities
_____ Difficulty with hopping, jumping, skipping, running
_____ Stiff and awkward movements
_____ Clumsy—bumps into others; accident prone
_____ Doesn't understand concepts such as right/left, front/back
_____ Avoids variety of playground activities; may only play on one item
_____ Poor posture; leans against things
_____ Avoids gross motor activities

Fine motor

_____ Difficulty with coloring, drawing, tracing
_____ Performs these activities too quickly and with poor quality
_____ Performs these activities too slowly and cannot finish in allotted time
_____ Work is sloppy or of poor quality
_____ Avoids fine motor activities
_____ Difficulty holding pencil or writing implement
_____ Printing of poor quality
_____ Difficulty with scissor use or other manipulatives
_____ Does not have a preferred hand (check only for children older than 4 years old)

Activities of daily living

_____ Difficulty dressing self or manipulating fasteners
_____ Difficulty with personal grooming

Behavioral

_____ Distractible
_____ Restless
_____ Slow worker
_____ Disorganized
_____ Short attention span
_____ Hyperactive
_____ Difficulty with transitions
_____ Behavior deteriorates when schedule changes

Sensory processing

_____ Overly sensitive to or avoids touch or movement input
_____ Tends to wear only certain types of clothing
_____ Avoids playground activities that involve feet off floor or head tipped back, such as swinging and spinning
_____ Seeks excessive sensory input
_____ Resists being held or cuddled
_____ Very limited food choices; will not eat food with mixed texture

Parent–child relationships

_____ Poor eye-contact with parent or caregiver
_____ Overly anxious; not willing to separate from parent
_____ Overly demanding

Peer relationships

_____ Difficulty making and/or maintaining friendships
_____ Aggressive or bullying
_____ Withdrawn

Figure 24.1-1. Referral to occupational therapy. (*Source:* Dunn, 2000b.)

tion. For older children and young adults, vocational activities and work would be included in the areas addressed by occupational therapy. For adults, emphasis is on activities of daily living, work and leisure. Fitness and health promotion are important to consider at all ages. Understanding the individual's previous history and experiences, patterns of daily living, interests, values, and needs is important in order to determine appropriate intervention (Herge, 2003).

As part of the assessment process, occupational therapists examine whether limitations in participation relate to the child's or adult's abilities, the demands of the tasks or activities, or external factors in the individual's physical or social environment. *Activity analysis* is a process used by occupational therapists to understand activities. In addition to documenting whether the individual is able to perform activities, the occupational therapist examines whether the individual is able to perform at a higher level when given assistance, such as through adapted equipment, assistive technology, modifications of the environment, or the guidance of a skilled adult. Activity limitations are measured by duration, quality of performance, degree of assistance required, safety, and developmental level.

Once activity limitations are identified, the therapist may examine the impairments that are associated with or contribute to limitations in activity and participation. Performance components that are of interest to the occupational therapist are cognitive, sensory, perceptual, motor, and psychosocial. Cognitive components affect the individual's learning as well as his or her perception and attention to the environment. Sensorimotor components include sensory processing, fine and gross motor skills, and neuromuscular abilities such as strength. Psychosocial skills refer to the individual's ability to interact and cope with his or her parents, peers, teachers, and work supervisors as well as in new situations while appropriately managing or regulating his or her behavior.

Assessments generally include interviews, checklists, and observations of the individual's interactions with people and objects in context. Standardized assessments may be either criterion referenced, in which skills are identified, or norm referenced (most often used with children), in which the individual's performance is compared with others in the same age group. An assessment tool such as the Canadian Occupational Performance Measure (COPM) (Law et al., 1998) enables the individual and/or family to identify and prioritize specific individualized goals. Examples of standardized assessments used by occupational therapists are listed in Tables 24.1-1 and 24.1-2, with assessments of activities of daily living listed in Table 24.1-3. Reviews of self-care and independent living assessments and strategies can be found in Babola (2000), Backman and Christiansen (2000), Case-Smith (2000b), and Smith, Benge, and Hall (2000).

INTERVENTION

Occupational therapy focuses on enhancing a child's or adult's ability to perform everyday activities and to participate in multiple environments (Case-Smith, 2001). According to the Committee on Children with Disabilities, "Therapists working with the family, child, and

Table 24.1-1. Examples of developmental assessments frequently used by occupational therapists

Test	Age range	Description
Denver Developmental Screening Test II (Frankenburg et al., 1992)	0–6 years	Test to determine if child's development is within normal range
Miller Assessment for Preschoolers (Miller, 1988)	2 years, 9 months, to 5 years, 8 months	Test of motor, cognitive, language, and behavior skills
First STEP (Miller, 1993)	2 years, 9 months, to 6 years, 2 months	Screening tool for identifying preschool children at risk for developmental delays in cognition, communication, and motor skills
Mullen Scales (Mullen, 1995)	0–69 months	Assessment of language, motor, and perceptual abilities
Hawaii Early Learning Profile (HELP) (Furuno et al., 1994)	0–36 months	Assessment of early infant and child development
Bayley Scales of Infant Development II (Bayley, 1994)	1–42 months	Test of mental, motor, and behavior skills

Table 24.1-2. Examples of tests frequently used by occupational therapists to assess specific areas of development

Test	Age range	Gross motor	Fine motor	Visual-perception	Visual-motor	Sensory integration
Peabody Developmental Motor Scales–Revised (2) (Folio & Fewell, 2000)	0–6 years	X	X			
Beery Visual-Motor Integration, Fifth Edition (Beery, Buktenica, & Berry, 2003)	3–18 years				X	
Test of Visual-Motor Skills–R (Gardner, 1995)	3–13 years				X	
Bruininks Oseretsky Test of Motor Proficiency (Bruininks, 1978)	$4\frac{1}{2}$–$14\frac{1}{2}$ years	X	X		X	
Movement Assessment Battery for Children (Henderson & Sugden, 1992)	6–9+ years	X	X			
Motor Free Visual Perception Test, Third Edition (Colarusso & Hammill, 1996)	4–70+ years			X		
Developmental Test of Visual Perception–Second Edition (Hammill, Pearson, & Voress, 1993)	4–10 years		X	X	X	
Test of Visual Perceptual Skills–Revised (Gardner, 1997)	4–13 years; 12–17 years			X		
Sensory Integration and Praxis Tests (Ayres, (Ayres, 1989)	4;0–8;11 years	X	X	X	X	X
The Sensory Profile (Dunn, 1999)	3–10 years					X
Infant/Toddler Sensory Profile (Dunn, 2002b)	0–36 months					X
Adolescent/Adult Sensory Profile (Dunn & Brown, 2002)	11–65+ years					X

teacher promote a positive functional adaptation to the disability in the context of the child's developmental progress" (1996, p. 308). An occupational therapist may use several frames of reference or theories, often simultaneously, in promoting the individual's development. Developmental, sensorimotor, and sensory integration approaches are used commonly with children.

Play is both a means and an end in occupational therapy. As a means, the occupational therapist incorporates playful qualities into the intervention process because play is an occupation of high relevance and importance to a child. The child who is playing is active, goal directed, and intrinsically motivated. The therapist guides the activity to a point where it becomes a challenge and adapts and modifies the activity to promote the child's success. Activities are incorporated that have meaning and purpose for the child and his or her family. They are graded to present the "just right challenge" to enable the child to successfully respond at the next higher level (Case-Smith, 2001). Play can also be a goal of occupational therapy intervention in that it reflects developmental competencies in cognitive and social areas.

Behavioral approaches including principles of learning are used to teach functional skills. Therapists use compensation/adaptation approaches, such as cues and environmental modifications. Environmental adaptations using both low and high technology are often crucial to the individual's performance and full participation in the community. Assistive technology may be as simple as enlarging a spoon handle to compensate for a weak grasp or teaching a young child to use a switch to activate a toy to learn cause and effect.

Programs for adolescents and young adults with disabilities include the development of vocational interests and skills, focusing on employment preparation (Babola, 2000). Adaptive skills training in areas such as social skills, community mobility, and leisure are essential for enhancing independence in the community. The occupational therapist has an important role in ensuring that the functional needs of the individual are met as he or she makes the transition from the educational environment to a community-based work setting. Adaptive equipment, compensatory techniques, and environmental accommodations are integral parts of practice.

Occupational therapists assist adults with developmental disabilities to live "self-determined lives" (Herge, 2003, p. CE-6) by helping them identify meaningful occupational choices. By working with the individual and his or her caregivers, service providers, and/or health care or employment team, occupational therapists play an integral role in helping adults with developmental

Table 24.1-3. Examples of tools for assessing activities of daily living and instrumental activities of daily living used by occupational therapists

Test	Description
Client's priorities	
Canadian Occupational Performance Measure, Third Edition (Law, Baptiste, Carswell, McColl, Polatojko, Pollock, 1998)	Detects change in individual's self-perception of occupational performance over time; individualized outcomes.
Perceived Efficacy and Goal Setting (PEGS) System (Missiuna, Pollock, & Law, 2004)	Age range of 6–9; assesses child's perception of ability to complete age-appropriate tasks and involves child in goal-setting process.
Children and adolescents	
Pediatric Evaluation of Disability Inventory (PEDI; Haley, Coster, Ludlow, Haltiwanger, & Andrellos, 1992)	Age range of 6 months to 7.5 years; measures capability and performance of functional self-care, mobility, and social function activities.
School Function Assessment (SFA; Coster, Deeney, Haltiwanger, & Haley, 1998)	Examines students' ability to perform important functional activities that support and enable participation in academic environments.
Assessment of Motor and Process Skills (AMPS; Fisher, 1994)	Enables evaluation of person's overall ability to perform activities of daily living and person's motor and process skills.
Vineland II Adaptive Behavior Scales (Sparrow, Cicchetti, & Balla, 2005)	Age range infant to 18 years, 11 months; assesses personal and social functioning.
Functional Independence Measure for Children (WeeFIM; State University of New York at Buffalo [SUNY–Buffalo], 1994)	Age range 6 months to 7 years; assesses independent and dependent behavior and reflects the burden of care for the disability.
Adults	
Assessment of Motor and Process Skills (AMPS; Fisher, 1994)	Enables evaluation of person's overall ability to perform activities of daily living and person's motor and process skills.
Arnodottir OT-ADL Neurobehavioral Evaluation (A-ONE; Arnadottir, 1990)	Identifies neurobehavioral impairments and their relationship to performance in activities of daily living and cortical lesions.
Klein-Bell ADL Scale (Klein & Bell, 1982; Law & Usher, 1988)	Age range 6 to adult; measures independence in activities of daily living.
Barthel Index (Mahoney & Barthel, 1965)	Assesses degree of disability through looking at independence in function.
Functional Independence Measure (FIM; Center for Functional Assessment Research at SUNY–Buffalo, 1993)	For adults; assesses independent and dependent behavior and reflects the burden of care for the disability.
Home Occupation–Environment Assessment (HOEA; Baum, Edwards, Bradford, & Lane, 1995)	Assesses ability to live safely in given environment by addressing behavioral and environmental items.
Milwaukee Evaluation of Daily Living Skills (Leonardelli, 1988)	Assesses functional living skills in people with severe mental illness.
Safety Assessment of Function and the Environment for Rehabilitation (SAFER; Letts, Burtney, Marshall, & McKean, 1998)	Assessment of home safety and function for individuals living in their own homes.

disabilities successfully integrate into their communities, including participation in leisure activities. Therapists develop or recommend appropriate programs and supports to promote community involvement, assess and modify the environments in which the individual lives and interacts, and make recommendations regarding adaptations to activities and/or appropriate assistive technology to support performance (Campbell & Herge, 2000). By serving as advocates for adults with developmental disabilities, occupational therapists aim to provide clients with "more choice, control, and responsibility" (Herge, 2003, p. CE-6), allowing clients to live "self-determined lives" (Herge, 2003, p. CE-6).

Table 24.1-4 lists domains of occupational therapy practice. Further description of the role of occupational therapy with individuals with developmental disabilities are available (Babola, 2000; Bailey, 1994; Campbell & Herge, 2000; Hammel, 2000; Hammel & Nochajski, 2000; Herge, 2003; Herge & Campbell, 1998; Herge & Wertz, 2002; Hotaling, 1998; Kurtz, 2002; Maruyama, Chandler, Clark, Dick, Lawlor, & Jackson, 1999; Reisman, 1993).

Kendra was living in a group home and sustained a fall, resulting in a broken hip. Kendra wanted to return to the group home, but she had limited mobility and was unable to bend. Kendra and her team, which included an occupational therapist, met to discuss modifications needed to enable Kendra to return home.

The occupational therapist suggested some practical techniques to prevent injury to Kendra and other residents, including removing scatter rugs and replacing low-wattage bulbs with high-wattage bulbs to improve lighting. The occupational therapist pointed out that the chair in which Kendra sat was too low and suggested adding a firmer, higher cushion. Kendra's shoes were on the floor in her closet, so a

Table 24.1-4. Domains of occupational therapy practice to support function and participation with individuals with developmental disabilities

Fine motor and hand skills
Sensory processing, sensory integration, and motor planning
Play and leisure activities
Activities of daily living (dressing, feeding, grooming)
Instrumental activities of daily living (community mobility, home management)
Social skills
Behavior management
Fitness and health promotion
Adaptive equipment
Assistive technology
Splinting
Positioning for optimal function
Task and environmental adaptations
Energy conservation
Ergonomics
Training and education
Consultation
Advocacy

hanging shoe bag was recommended so that Kendra would not have to bend down to get her shoes.

Kendra's dresser was rearranged so that the bottom drawers contained infrequently used and out-of-season clothes, and she only needed to use the top two drawers. To make it easier for Kendra to remember the changes, pictures were placed on the dresser drawers indicating the clothing items inside. Kendra was shown how to use a sock aid to help her put her socks on (see Figure 24.1-2).

The occupational therapist ordered a combination raised toilet seat and folding bathtub bench that could be stored and not interfere with the routines of the other residents. The occupational therapist also made several visits to the residence following Kendra's return home to review ADLs to be sure they were performed safely.

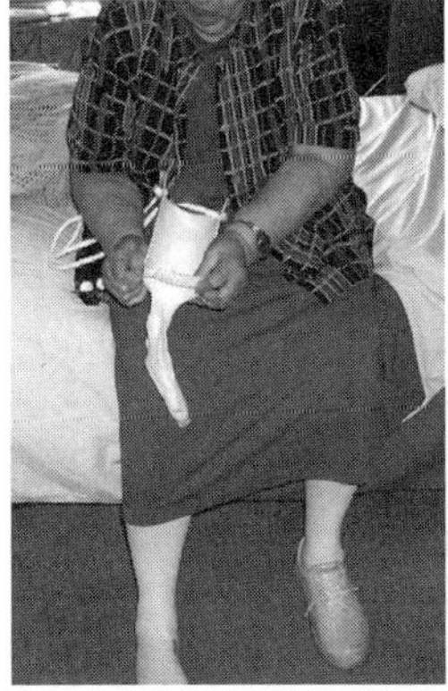

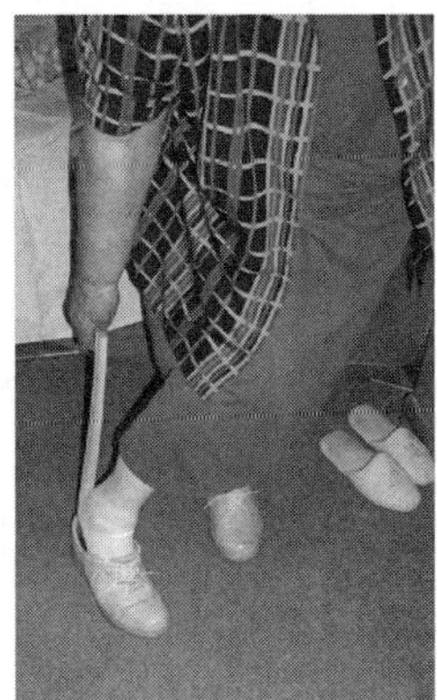

Figure 24.1-2. Kendra using a sock aid to put on her socks (left photo) and a long-handled shoe horn to put on her shoes (right photo).

Providing services in Kendra's home was important to assure carryover of learning (Hotaling, 1998). The occupational therapist also met with the staff of the group home to review precautions and be sure that equipment utilization was presented consistently by all staff.

CONCLUSION

Occupational therapists embrace a client-centered, evidence-based practice model and utilize the best evidence available coupled with clinical reasoning for practice decisions. Numerous outcome studies of early intervention and Head Start programs that include occupational therapy support the effectiveness of these programs (Administration for Child, Youth, and Families, 1983; Guralnick, 1997; Ottenbacher, 1992; Shonkoff & Hauser-Cram, 1987; Shonkoff & Meisels, 2000). Programs with a high level of parental involvement, including guidance and support and suggestions for specific skill development activities to implement at home, were especially effective. Specific occupational therapy parent training programs have also been found effective in enhancing parents' knowledge and practices about child development (Parush & Hahn-Markowitz, 1997) and enhancing children's play skills (Okimoto, Bundy, & Hanzlik, 2000). A home-based weekly occupational therapy program for extremely preterm infants from 6–12 months was found to improve social development at 2 years but did not have a long-term effect on school readiness at 4 years (Salokorpi, Rautio, Kajantie, & Von Wendt, 2002).

The effectiveness of occupational therapy in a school context has been found to enhance performance in a variety of areas including fine-motor skills, upper-extremity use, and handwriting (Bumin & Kayihan, 2001; Case-Smith, 1996; 2000a, 2002; Crocker, MacKay-Lyons, & McDonnell, 1997; Peterson & Nelson, 2003); functional skills (King et al., 1998); attention to task (Fertel-Daly, Badell, & Hinojosa, 2001; Linderman & Stewart, 1999); and powered mobility (Deitz, Swinth, & White, 2002). A systematic review of research to improve upper extremity use that included, but was not limited to, occupational therapy reported positive results (Boyd, Morris, & Graham, 2001). In occupational therapy, both consultation models and direct service models have produced positive effects (Davies & Gavin, 1994; Dunn, 1990, 2000b; Kemmis & Dunn, 1996).

Studies examining the effectiveness of occupational therapy interventions with adolescents and adults with developmental disabilities have found improvements in mobility (McInerney & McInerney, 1992) and in self-identified goals related to transitions to adult roles (Healy & Rigby, 1999). A systematic review of occupational therapy services for older adults (not limited to developmental disabilities) reported positive findings (Carlson, Fanchiang, Zemke, & Clark, 1996). Overall, evidence supports the effectiveness of occupational therapy in enhancing function in individuals with developmental disabilities; however, additional research using controlled trials is warranted.

REFERENCES

Administration for Child, Youth, and Families. (ACYF). (1983). *The effects of Head Start Programs on children's cognitive development.* (ERIC Document No. ED248989).

American Occupational Therapy Association. (AOTA). (1999). The guide to occupational therapy practice. *American Journal of Occupational Therapy, 53*(3).

American Occupational Therapy Association. (AOTA). (2000). *AOTA 2000 Member Compensation Survey.* Bethesda, MD: Author.

American Occupational Therapy Association. (AOTA). (2002). *Occupational therapy practice framework: Domain and process.* Bethesda, MD: Author.

American Occupational Therapy Association. (AOTA). (2003, August 28). *Occupational therapists urge parents to be aware of heavy school backpacks.* Retrieved on November 29, 2003, from http://www.aota.org/backpack/docs/backpack03.pdf

Americans with Disabilities Act of 1990, PL 101-336, 42 U.S.C. §§ 12101 *et seq.*

Anzalone, M.E., & Murray, E.A. (2002). Integrating sensory integration with other approaches to intervention. In A.C. Bundy, S.J. Lane, & E.A. Murray (Eds.), *Sensory integration: Theory and practice.* (2nd ed., pp. 371–394). Philadephia: F.A. Davis.

Arnadottir, G. (1990). *The brain and behavior: Assessing cortical dysfunction through activities of daily living.* St. Louis: Mosby.

Ayres, A.J. (1989). *Sensory Integration and Praxis Tests.* Los Angeles: Western Psychological Services.

Babola, K.T. (2000). Independent living strategies for persons adults with developmental disabilities. In C. Christiansen (Ed.), *Ways of living: Self-care strategies for special needs* (2nd ed., pp. 123–140). Bethesda, MD: American Occupational Therapy Association.

Backman, C., & Christiansen, C.C. (2000). Assessment of self-care performance. In C. Christiansen (Ed.), *Ways of living: Self-care strategies for special needs* (2nd ed., pp. 29–44). Bethesda, MD: American Occupational Therapy Association.

Bailey, D.M. (1994). Technology for adults with multiple impairments: A trilogy of case-reports. *American Journal of Occupational Therapy, 48*(4), 341–345.

Baloueff, O., & Cohn, E. (2002). Introduction to the infant, child, and adolescent population. In E.B. Crepeau, E.S. Cohn, & B.A.B. Schell (Eds.), *Willard & Spackman's occupational therapy* (10th ed., pp. 691–698). Philadelphia: Lippincott, Williams & Wilkins.

Baum, C.M., Edwards, D.F., Bradford, T., & Lane, R. (1995). *Home Occupation-Environment Assessment.* St. Louis: Washington University, Occupational Therapy Program.

Bayley, N. (1994). *Bayley Scales of Infant Development* (2nd ed.). San Antonio, TX: Psych Corp.

Beery, K.E., Buktenica, N.A., & Beery, N.A. (2003). *Developmental test of visual-motor integration* (5th ed.). Los Angeles: Western Psychological Services.

Boyd, R.N., Morris, M.E., & Graham, H.K. (2001). Management of upper limb dysfunction in children with cerebral palsy: A systematic review. *European Journal of Neurology, 8*(Suppl. 5), 150–166.

Bruininks, R.H. (1978). *Bruininks-Oseretsky Test of Motor Proficiency examiner's manual.* Circle Pines, MN: American Guidance Service.

Bumin, G., & Kayihan, H. (2001, June 15). Effectiveness of two different sensory-integration programmes for children with spastic diplegic cerebral palsy. *Disability & Rehabilitation, 23*(9), 394–399.

Campbell, J., & Herge, E.A. (2000). Challenges to aging in place: The elder adult with MR/DD. *Physical and Occupational Therapy in Geriatrics, 18*(1), 75–90.

Carlson, M., Fanchiang, S.-P., Zemke, R., & Clark, F. (1996). A meta-analysis of the effectiveness of occupational therapy for older persons. *American Journal of Occupational Therapy, 50*(2), 89–98.

Case-Smith, J. (1996). Fine motor outcomes in preschool children who receive occupational therapy services. *American Journal of Occupational Therapy, 50*(1), 52–61.

Case-Smith, J. (2000a). Effects of occupational therapy services on fine motor and functional performance in preschool children. *American Journal of Occupational Therapy, 54*(4), 372–380.

Case-Smith, J. (2000b). Self-care strategies for children with developmental disabilities. In C. Christiansen (Ed.), *Ways of living: Self-care strategies for special needs* (2nd ed., pp. 83–122). Bethesda, MD: The American Occupational Therapy Association.

Case-Smith, J. (2001). An overview of occupational therapy for children. In J. Case-Smith (Ed.), *Occupational therapy for children* (4th ed., pp. 2–20). St. Louis: Mosby.

Case-Smith, J. (2002). Effectiveness of school-based occupational therapy intervention on handwriting. *American Journal of Occupational Therapy, 56*, 17–25.

Center for Functional Assessment Research at SUNY Buffalo. (1993). *Functional Independence Measure (FIM).* Amherst, NY: Uniform Data System for Medical Rehabilitation.

Colarusso, R.P., & Hammill, D.D. (1996). *Motor-Free Visual Perception Test (MVPT)* (3rd ed.). Novato, CA: Academic Therapy Publications.

Committee on Children with Disabilities. (1996). The role of the pediatrician in prescribing therapy services for children with motor disabilities. *Pediatrics, 98*, 308–310.

Committee on Children with Disabilities. (1999a). Care coordination: Integrating health and related systems of care for children with special health care needs (RE9902). *Pediatrics, 104*, 978–981.

Committee on Children with Disabilities. (1999b). The pediatrician's role in development and implementation of an individual education plan (IEP) and/or and individual family service plan (IFSP) (RE9823). *Pediatrics, 104*, 124–127.

Coster, W.J., Deeney, T., Haltiwanger, J.T., & Haley, S.M. (1998). *School Function Assessment (SFA).* San Antonio, TX: Psych Corp.

Crocker, M.D., MacKay-Lyons, M., & McDonnell, E. (1997). Forced use of the upper extremity in cerebral palsy: A single-case design. *American Journal of Occupational Therapy, 51*(10), 824–833.

Davies, P.L., & Gavin, W.J. (1994). Comparison of individual and group/consultation treatment methods for preschool children with developmental delays. *American Journal of Occupational Therapy, 48*(20), 155–161.

Deitz, J., Swinth, Y., & White, O. (2002). Powered mobility and preschoolers with complex developmental delays. *American Journal of Occupational Therapy, 56*(1), 86–96.

Dunn, W. (1990). A comparison of service provision models in school-based occupational therapy services: A pilot study. *Occupational Therapy Journal of Research, 10*, 300–320.

Dunn, W. (1999). *Sensory Profile.* San Antonio, TX: Therapy Skill Builders.

Dunn, W. (Ed.). (2000a). *Best practice occupational therapy: In community service with children and families.* Thorofare, NJ: Slack.

Dunn, W. (2002b). *Infant/Toddler Sensory Profile.* San Antonio, TX: Therapy Skill Builders.

Dunn, W., & Brown, C. (2002). *Adolescent/Adult Sensory Profile.* San Antonio, TX: Therapy Skill Builders.

Elwell, E.R. (2001). *Assessing pediatrician knowledge of occupational therapy.* Unpublished master's thesis, Boston University.

Fertel-Daly, D., Bedell, G., & Hinojosa, J. (2001). Effects of a weighted vest on attention to task and self-stimulatory behaviors in preschoolers with pervasive developmental disorders. *American Journal of Occupational Therapy, 55*(6), 629–640.

Fisher, A.G. (1994). *Assessment of Motor and Process Skills. (AMPS).* Fort Collins, CO: AMPS Project.

Folio, M.R., & Fewell, R.R. (2000). *Peabody Developmental Motor Scales–Revised (PDMS–2).* Austin, TX: PRO-ED.

Frankenburg, W., Dodds, J., Archer, P., Bresnick, B., Maschka, P., Edelman, N., et al. (1992). *Denver Developmental Screening Test II.* Denver, CO: Denver Developmental Materials.

Furuno, S., O'Reilley, K.A., Hosaka, C.M., Inasuka, T.T., Allman, T.A., & Zeisloft, B. (1994). *Hawaii Early Learning Profile (HELP).* Palo Alto, CA: Vort Corp.

Gardner, M.R. (1995). *Test of Visual Motor Skills–Revised.* Hydesville, CA: Psychological and Educational Publications.

Gardner, M.R. (1997). *Test of Visual-Perceptual Skills–Revised (TVPS).* Burlingame, CA: Psychological and Educational Publications.

Giardino, A.P., Kohrt, A.E., Ayre, L., & Wells, N. (2002). Health care delivery systems and financing issues. In M.L. Batshaw (Ed.), *Children with disabilities* (5th ed., pp. 707–724). Baltimore: Paul H. Brookes Publishing Co.

Guralnick, M.J. (Ed.). (1997). *The effectiveness of early intervention: Directions for second generation research.* Baltimore: Paul H. Brookes Publishing Co.

Haley, S.M., Coster, W.J., Ludlow, L.H., Haltiwanger, J.T., & Andrellos, P.J. (1992). *Pediatric Evaluation of Disability Inventory (PEDI).* San Antonio, TX: Psych Corp.

Hammel, J. (2000). Assistive technology and environmental intervention (AT-EI) impact on the activity and life roles of aging adults with developmental disabilities: Findings and implications. *Physical and Occupational Therapy in Geriatrics, 18*(1), 37–58.

Hammel, J., & Nochajski, S. (2000). Aging and developmental disability: Current research, programming, and practice implications. *Physical and Occupational Therapy in Geriatrics, 18*(1), 1–4.

Hammill, D.D., Pearson, N.A., & Voress, J.K. (1993). *Developmental Test of Visual Perception–Second Edition (DVTP–2).* Austin, TX: PRO-ED.

Healy, H., & Rigby, P. (1999). Promoting independence for teens and young adults with physical disabilities. *Canadian Journal of Occupational Therapy, 66*(5), 240–249.

Henderson, S.E., & Sugden, D.A. (1992). *Movement Assessment Battery for Children manual.* San Antonio, TX: Psych Corp.

Herge, E.A. (2003, November 17). Beyond the basics to participation: Occupational therapy for adults with developmental disabilities. AOTA Continuing Education Article. *OT Practice*, CE1–CE8.

Herge, E.A., & Campbell, J.E. (1998). The role of the occupational and physical therapist in the rehabilitation of the older adult with mental retardation. *Topics in Geriatric Rehabilitation, 13*(4), 12–21.

Herge, E.A., & Wertz, B. (2002). The role of occupational therapy in health promotion of adults with developmental disabilities. *Developmental Disabilities Special Interest Section Quarterly, 25*(4), 1–3.

Hohlstein, R.R., & Sprague, R.E. (1995). Occupational therapy. In B.A Thyer & N.P. Kropf (Eds.), *Developmental disabilities: A handbook for interdisciplinary practice* (pp. 118–132). Cambridge, MA: Brookline Books.

Hotaling, G. (1998). Rehabilitation of adults with developmental disabilities: An occupational therapy perspective. *Topics in Geriatric Rehabilitation, 13*(3), 73–83.

Individuals with Disabilities Education Act (IDEA) Amendments of 1997, PL 105-17, 20 U.S.C. §§ 1400 *et seq.*

Kemmis, B.L., & Dunn, W. (1996). Collaborative consultation: The efficacy of remedial and compensatory interventions in school contexts. *American Journal of Occupational Therapy, 50*(9), 709–717.

King, G., Tucker, M.A., Alambets, P., Gritzan, J., McDougall, J., Ogilvie, A., et al. (1998). The evaluation of functional, school-based therapy services for children with special needs: A feasibility study. *Physical and Occupational Therapy in Pediatrics, 18*(2), 1–27.

Klein, R.M., & Bell, B. (1982). *Klein-Bell Activities of Daily Living Scale.* Seattle: Educational Resources.

Kurtz, L.A. (2002). Rehabilitation: Physical therapy and occupational therapy. In M.L. Batshaw (Ed.), *Children with disabilities* (5th ed., pp. 647–657). Baltimore: Paul H. Brookes Publishing Co.

Law, M., Baptiste, S., Carswell, A., McColl, M.A., Polatojko, H., & Pollock, N. (1998). *Canadian Occupational Performance Measure (COPM)* (3rd ed.). Toronto: Canadian Association of Occupational Therapists.

Law, M., & Usher, P. (1988). Validation of the Klein-Bell Activities of Daily Living Scale for Children. *Canadian Journal of Occupational Therapy, 55*, 63–68.

Leonardelli, C. (1988). *Milwaukee Evaluation of Daily Living Skills (MEDLS).* Thorofare, NJ: Slack.

Letts, L., Scott, S., Burtney, J., Marshall, L., & McKean, M. (1998). The reliability and validity of the Safety Assessment of Function and the Environment for Rehabilitation (SAFER Tool). *British Journal of Occupational Therapy, 61*(3), 127–132.

Linderman, T.M., & Stewart, K.B. (1999). Sensory integrative-based occupational therapy and functional outcomes in young children with pervasive developmental disorders: A single-subject study. *American Journal of Occupational Therapy, 53*(2), 207–213.

Mahoney, F.I., & Barthel, D.W. (1965). Functional evaluation: The Barthel Index. *Maryland State Medical Journal, 14,* 61–65.

Maruyama, E., Chandler, B.E., Clark, G.F., Dick, R.W., Lawlor, M.C., & Jackson, L. (1999). *Occupational therapy services for children and youth under the Individuals with Disabilities Education Act* (2nd ed.). Bethesda, MD: American Occupational Therapy Association.

McInerney, C.A., & McInerney, M. (1992). A mobility skills training program for adults with developmental disabilities. *American Journal of Occupational Therapy, 46,* 233–239.

Miller, L.J. (1988). *The Miller Assessment for Preschoolers.* San Antonio, TX: Psych Corp.

Miller, L.J. (1993). *First Step.* San Antonio, TX: Psych Corp.

Missiuna, C. (2001). *Children with developmental coordination disorder: Cognitive strategies for success.* Binghamton, NY: Haworth Press.

Missiuna, C., Pollock, N., & Law, M. (2004). *The Perceived Efficacy and Goal Setting (PEGS) system.* San Antonio, TX: Psych Corp.

Moyers, P. (1999). Guide to occupational therapy practice. *American Journal of Occupational Therapy, 53,* 247–322.

Mullen, E.M. (1995). *Mullen Scales of Early Learning.* Circle Pines, MN: American Guidance Service.

Nochajski, S. (2000). The impact of age-related changes on the functioning of older adults with developmental disabilities. *Physical and Occupational Therapy in Geriatrics, 18*(1), 5–21.

Okimoto, A.M., Bundy, A., & Hanzlik, J. (2000). Playfulness in children with and without disability: Measurement and intervention. *American Journal of Occupational Therapy, 54*(1), 73–82.

Ottenbacher, K.J. (1992, Spring). Practical significance in early intervention research: From affect to empirical effect. *Journal of Early Intervention, 16*(2), 181–193.

Parush, S., & Hahn-Markowitz, J. (1997). The efficacy of an early prevention program facilitated by occupational therapists: A follow-up study. *American Journal of Occupational Therapy, 52*(4), 247–251.

Peterson, C.Q., & Nelson, D.L. (2003). Effect of an occupational intervention on printing in children with economic disadvantages. *American Journal of Occupational Therapy, 57*(2), 152–156.

Rainville, E.B., Cermak, S.A., & Murray, E.A. (1996). Supervision and consultation services for pediatric occupational therapists. *American Journal of Occupational Therapy, 50,* 725–731.

Reisman, J. (1993). Using a sensory integrative approach to treat self-injurious-behavior in an adult with profound mental-retardation. *American Journal of Occupational Therapy, 47*(5), 403–411.

Reeves, G.D., & Cermak, S.A. (2002). Disorders of praxis. In A.C. Bundy, S.J. Lane, & E.A. Murray (Eds.), *Sensory integration: Theory and practice* (pp. 71–100). Philadelphia: F.A. Davis.

Salokorpi, T., Rautio, T., Kajantie, E., & Von Wendt, L. (2002). Is early occupational therapy in extremely preterm infants of benefit in the long run? *Pediatric Rehabilitation, 5*(2), 91–98.

Shonkoff, J.P., & Hauser-Cram, P. (1987). Early intervention for disabled infants and their families: A quantitative analysis. *Pediatrics, 80,* 650–658.

Shonkoff, J.P., & Meisels, S.J. (Eds.). (2000). *Handbook of early childhood intervention* (2nd ed.). Cambridge, England: Cambridge University Press.

Smith, R.O., Benge, M., & Hall, M. (2000). Using assistive technologies to enable self-care and daily living. In C. Christiansen (Ed.), *Ways of living: Self-care strategies for special needs* (2nd ed., pp. 333–360). Bethesda, MD: American Occupational Therapy Association.

Sparrow, S.S., Cicchetti, D.V., & Balla, D.A. (2005). *Vineland II Adaptive Behavior Scales.* Circle Pines, MN: American Guidance Service.

State University of New York at Buffalo. (1994). *Functional Independence Measure for Children (WeeFim).* Buffalo: State University of New York at Buffalo.

U.S. Department of Health and Human Services. (2003, October, 16). *The New Freedom Initiative.* Retrieved on November 26, 2003, from http://www.hhs.gov/newfreedom.init.html

Wilbarger, J., & Wilbarger, P. (2002a). Clinical application of the sensory diet. In A.C. Bundy, S.J. Lane, & E.A. Murray (Eds.), *Sensory integration: Theory and practice* (pp. 339–341). Philadelphia: F.A. Davis.

Wilbarger, J., & Wilbarger, P. (2002b). The Wilbarger approach to treating sensory defensiveness. In A.C. Bundy, S.J. Lane, & E.A. Murray (Eds.), *Sensory integration: Theory and practice* (pp. 335–338). Philadelphia: F.A. Davis.

Wilcock, A.A. (2003). Population interventions focused on health for all. In E.B. Crepeau, E.S. Cohn, & B.A.B. Schell (Eds.), *Willard & Spackman's occupational therapy* (10th ed., pp. 30–45). Philadelphia: Lippincott, Williams & Wilkins.

Williams, M.S., & Shellenberger, S. (1994). *"How does your engine run?" A leader's guide to the alert program for self-regulation.* Albuquerque, NM: Therapy Works.

24.2 PHYSICAL THERAPY

Priscilla S. Osborne and Sharon A. Cermak

In the field of developmental disabilities, the focus of the physical therapist is to promote the development of the child's or adult's physical function within his or her family and community. These functional expectations change over time with age and developmental progress. Typically, in infancy, as children gain motor control, they gain stability in varying postures, sitting, quadruped, and standing in the progression to an upright position to interact with others. In addition, mobility is gained as children first move through rolling to crawling and/or creeping, to cruising and walking. With progression through these steps, children gain more independent abilities to sit alone, use their hands for play, move about, and explore their environment.

In preschool age children, motor function advances with the addition of speed, balance, refinement of motor control, and integration of other systems. Once developed, these new additions to skill allow children to use their mobility in a functional manner so that they can run, stop, turn, and manage stairs as well as socially interact through active play with peers. In adolescence and adulthood, muscle strength increases along with the development of skill in sports of interest, allowing for the development of fitness, peer interaction, and enjoyment.

These motor functions are important to all children as they move toward independence in adulthood. For children with disabilities that affect their movement and posture, the development of functional positioning for learning, mobility, social play, and fitness can be difficult. Lack of development in these areas can have an impact on peer interactions and self-esteem and can impinge on the ability to perform autonomously.

In addition to activities that facilitate motor function, all individuals need opportunities that encourage a healthy lifestyle through enjoyment of exercise as a routine of daily life. Sedentary lifestyle and obesity are two issues influencing the health of both children and adults. Establishing the importance of fitness and activity in childhood is a route to a healthier life.

To accomplish these goals, physical therapists work in collaboration with children and adults with developmental disabilities, their families, and community and health providers. The format of the interactions changes with the individual's age and developmental progression as well as the family and community context.

PHILOSOPHY

Family-centered practice is essential in pediatric physical therapy (Kolobe, 1992). Goals are established within the context of both the family's and the child's wishes. Physical therapists work in a collaborative model with the family and child throughout childhood to provide anticipatory guidance, support, and encouragement. In addition, therapists share their professional expertise with the family to optimize the therapeutic intervention and guidance provided to the child through exercise, positioning, and directed play activities incorporated into a home program.

Although the child is always an active participant in physical therapy treatment, he or she becomes more able to actively enter into the therapeutic programming as he or she matures. The interests and desires of the child are an integral part of the intervention process as the child needs to be actively engaged in an activity for learning and change to occur (Campbell, 1997). Treatment is functionally based, and play is an integral part to a child's learning. Care always needs to be taken to provide the adaptive strategies necessary to reduce frustration. For example, if a child is very interested in sitting and playing but not yet able to sit alone, a supportive seat should be provided to adapt for the lack of current function. Sitting alone can continue to be a goal of treatment; however, an adapted strategy can also be employed so that the child's cognitive needs can be met.

PROFESSIONAL PRACTICE GUIDELINES

The Guide to Physical Therapy Practice, Second Edition (2001), was published by the American Physical Therapy Association, the professional organization of physical therapists, to provide guidelines for physical therapy practice. The first edition was published in 1995. The revised version consists of three parts: Part One delineates the scope of physical therapy and describes patient/client management. Part Two delineates preferred physical therapy practice patterns, and Part Three catalogs the tests and measures that are used by physical therapists. In addition to these parts, *The Guide* also provides a definition of *physical therapy* as "a dynamic profession with an established theoretical and scientific base and widespread clinical applications in the restoration, maintenance and promotion of optimal physical function" (2001, P. S13). It addresses physical therapy in both pediatrics and adult care, thus providing physical therapists working in pediatrics with professional guidelines for care.

Sara Beth is a 7-year-old girl who had a stroke at the age of 2 years and had motor coordination difficulties that included dystonia on the right side of her body. When she is nervous, her right arm moves up into overhead flexion at the shoulder and extension at the elbow and flexion at the wrist. Sara Beth did not have physical therapy intervention until the age of 7 years. At first, she was not very interested in participating in these services.

When asked what physical therapy services might help her the most, Sara Beth explained that she needed help at school. Evidently, in the classroom, Sara Beth's hand would move up if she was nervous about a question the teacher was asking. The teacher would assume that Sara Beth was signaling that she knew the answer and would call on her, creating a difficult situation for Sara Beth. The physical therapist set up a procedure with Sara Beth and her teacher that when Sara Beth wanted to answer a question, she would raise her left hand and the teacher would ignore the right hand when it was raised. This solution pleased Sara Beth, and she agreed to work with physical therapy to help get more control over her right arm.

SETTINGS

Providing treatment for children within their usual environment promotes the functional use of their skills. Part C of the Individuals with Disabilities Education Act (IDEA) Amendments of 1997 (PL 105-17) put this concept into legislation. Parts C and B of this law address the issues of children from ages birth to 3 and from 3 to 5, respectively.

For infants and children who are receiving physical therapy treatment as part of an early intervention program, PL 105-17 mandates that services be provided in a natural environment, such as the home, community playgroups, and the playground. Services in the natural environment provide opportunities for integration of children into their community. In addition, treatments become more easily integrated into natural routines. As children enter preschool or elementary school, the school becomes another natural environment. Part B of PL 105-17 provides for physical therapy services as part of school "related services" that will support children with disabilities in the educational environment (McEwen, 2000).

Adolescence should be preparing for independence in the community as well as the workplace. If preparation for these activities is part of the academic plan, the physical therapist may be able to assist the student with physical, motor, and mobility issues in these environments as well. With adults, services may be less of an integral part of their home and work setting and more difficult to obtain. Often, home health or rehabilitation services are used.

Although educationally related physical therapy services are mandated for all children through PL 105-17, at times conflict arises over what part of the service is educationally related. For example, because the need for service must be related to the child's ability to participate in educational services, a child with muscle contractures related to cerebral palsy may have trouble receiving physical therapy treatment through the school. The child's school system may not want to pay for the service because it is not directly related to educational goals, and the child's health insurance company may insist that all services be provided through the school.

MODELS OF SERVICE DELIVERY

Physical therapy services cannot effectively be delivered in isolation, regardless of the individual's age. Direct treatment is always accompanied by consultation services provided to the individual's community. Carry-over of physical therapy goals into the child's usual environment is critical for learning. Functional goals lend themselves well to be carried through by family and providers. For adults with developmental disabilities who depend on their living and work environments, an integrated approach to physical therapy services may become a challenge because these services are less an integral part of the environment.

EVALUATION

The purpose of an evaluation is to gather information concerning the individual's motor function, including areas of strengths, areas of difficulty, and possible impairments to the development of the desired functional motor outcome. If the evaluation is performed outside of the individual's usual environment, information about the individual's typical functioning within his or her usual environment can be gained through interview of the individual and his or her family, teachers, caregivers, and significant others. This information is invaluable in framing both the evaluation results and in proposing intervention strategies. A holistic approach is essential when assessing motor behaviors of a child or adult with developmental disabilities. By working together in an interdisciplinary format, a broad scope of the child's or adult's functioning can be obtained (Shea, 1992).

REFERRAL

Children are most appropriately referred for a physical therapy assessment when motor control issues are known or suspected. For adolescents or adults, a referral may be initiated for a specific problem such as a change in motor function status due to physical or environmental changes, or for reevaluation of adaptive equipment needs. Although many states have Independent Practice Acts for physical therapists, most often a referral to physical therapy is accompanied by a referral from the child's pediatrician or the adult's internist. This situation facilitates communication with the pediatrician and may be necessary for financial coverage of the visits. The referral should clearly state the concern of the referring provider. Of major importance is to obtain from the child or adults and his or her family their primary concern and how the physical therapist can best help them.

EXAMINATION

As with other areas of function, the development of motor skills is complex and requires the integration of multiple biological and developmental systems in a supportive environment. When assessing motor development, all of these factors need consideration. In order to assess a child's ability to function physically within his or her environment, physical therapists must obtain information concerning previous health and developmental progress. Illness, particularly chronic illness, may affect the child's available energy for large motor activities. Developmental history will frame the findings from this evaluation within the context of the child's previous performance and will provide information about other areas of development. As possible, information should be obtained from the family, child, teachers, and community providers (Aylward, 1997).

Tests and measures provide the examiner with data about the physical functioning of the child. In choosing an appropriate measure, the purpose of the testing, the outcome information desired, cultural and ecological factors, and the psychometric properties of the instrument need to be considered (Shea, 1992). Standardized tests can be divided by the purpose of the testing: developmental or functional. Overlapping information is provided by either type of focus.

Developmental Motor Testing

Developmental tests have an underlying foundation in the developmental progression of skills. These testing tools include basic functional skills such as walking, rising from the floor, and stair climbing as well as the development of recreational gross motor play skills such as hopping, jumping, and ball skills. These tests are appropriate for the evaluation of children without major neuromotor coordination difficulties in which movement and posture development are not the focus. For example, for a child with developmental delays, these tests give the examiner a guideline as to where the child is functioning in relationship to peers (see Table 24.2-1).

Cecelia is a 2-year-old girl whose family is concerned that her motor skills are delayed for her age. Cecilia rolled over from her stomach to her back at 6 months of age, sat alone when placed at 12 months of age, and began creeping in quadruped at 18 months of age. She is currently just attempting to pull to stand.

Review of information about Cecelia's health and development are notable for no major illnesses or hospitalizations. Language development has been noted to be delayed as well as Cecelia's development of play skills. The Peabody Developmental Motor Scales–2 (Folio & Fewell, 2000) was used by the physical therapist for assessment of Cecilia's gross and fine motor skills. An age equivalent score was obtained for both the fine motor and the gross motor scales. These scores were compared with the scores in other developmental domains, and motor function was seen to be an area of strength. No movement or postural abnormalities were observed during the testing session or reported by the pediatrician or parents. The physical therapist gave Cecelia's parents suggestions of activities that would help Cecilia move on to the next level of motor function and made plans to monitor her future development.

Functional Motor Testing

Functionally based motor evaluation tools focus on the individual's ability to perform primary functional mobility skills such as walking, running, stair climbing, and transferring skills (see Table 24.2-2). These types of tests are used for children, adolescents, and adults for whom the basic mobility skills are a challenge. Recreational motor activities are important, and some functional tests include gross motor activities as the scale progresses; however, play skills are not the focus of

Table 24.2-1. Examples of tests of motor development

Test	Age range	Description
Bayley Scale of Infant Development: Second Edition: Motor Scale (Bayley, 1994)	1–42 months	Fine and gross motor items combined
Peabody Developmental Motor Scales–2 (Folio & Fewell, 2000)	1–72 months	Separate fine and gross motor scales
Bruininks-Oseretsky Test of Motor Proficiency (Bruininks, 1978)	4.5–14.5 years	Separate fine and gross motor scales; focus on milder coordination disorders
Movement Assessment Battery for Children (ABC; Henderson & Sugden, 1992)	4–12 years	Separate fine and gross motor scales

Table 24.2-2. Examples of tests of motor function

Test	Age range	Description
Gross Motor Function Measure (Russell et al., 1990)	No specific age range	Observational measure
Pediatric Evaluation Disability Inventory (Haley, Coster, Ludlow, Haltiwanger, & Andrellos, 1992)	6 months to 7 years, 6 months	Caregiver report
School Function Assessment (Coster, Deeney, Haltiwanger, & Haley, 1998)	Kindergarten through sixth grade for children with disabilities	Participation within the school setting

these scales. Some functionally based tools are also specific to an environment. For example, the School Function Assessment (Coster, Deeney, Haltiwanger, & Haley, 1998) evaluates the school-age child's ability to manage the school environment and determines the need for services within that specific setting.

Charlie is a 3-year-old boy with the diagnosis of spastic diplegia. He is changing his services from the community early intervention program to the public school system because of his age. The preschool program is interested in Charlie's ability to move about the classroom, sit in circle time, and utilize the other classroom and playground activities. The Gross Motor Function Measure (Russell et al., 1990) was used to provide the teachers and therapists in the new setting information concerning Charlie's gross motor mobility and sitting abilities. In addition, the Pediatric Evaluation of Disability Inventory (Haley, Coster, Ludlow, Haltiwanger, & Andrellos, 1992) was used to provide information not only on Charlie's functional mobility and self-care skills but also on the degree of adaptation necessary to support Charlie's optimal functioning in the classroom.

With the information gained from these measures, the teacher and physical therapist could plan Charlie's seating and mobility needs so that he could fully participate with his classmates. For example, because Charlie cannot sit alone on the floor without support for his back, the mat for circle time was moved from the middle of the room to next to a wall. Charlie and other children could sit with their backs against the wall to listen and participate.

Evaluation of Movement and Postural Patterns

Another emerging motor evaluation tool describes motor development in terms of the changing movement and postural patterns of infants and young children. The purpose of these tests is to evaluate the quality of movement and posture as it changes over the baby's maturation. Often, pictures are provided of typical patterns for comparison (see Table 24.2-3).

The use of these standardized assessment tools provides both a format for comparing the child's performance with a set standard, usually motor abilities of age peers, and the opportunity to observe the child's movement, posture, and coordination as he or she performs a wide constellation of functional and recreational gross motor tasks. Physical therapists use their knowledge about the development and integrity of the biological systems underlying the development of movement to analyze the child's performance at a qualitative level of assessment. Components include muscle tone, muscle strength, joint flexibility, postural reactions, primitive reflex patterns, sensory perception and processing, motor planning, and body coordination skills. Standardized tools exist for the evaluation of most of these components. All of these factors have a developmental component and vary with age.

These systems are thought to provide the building blocks for the development of typical movement and postural abilities. Abnormalities are most significant if framed with the effect they may have on the development of movement and posture and their influence on the development of function. Evaluation components of movement should be framed in function as well as through standardized assessment. For example, passively, muscle tone may be increased; however, functionally, this increase in tone may not be influencing movement at this point in the child's development of motor skill. All of these tools as well as trained observation of the child will help provide information as to the child's development of movement, mobility, and motor skills.

Naturalistic Observation

Each evaluation should include a time of unstructured movement in which the child or adult's movement abilities and posture can be observed in a typical setting. Once allowed the freedom of choice of activity, space, and time parameters, the individual's movement and

Table 24.2-3. Examples of tools that assess movement and postural patterns

Test	Age range	Description
Test of Infant Motor Performance (TIMP; Campbell & Girolami, 1993)	32 weeks postconceptual age to 4 months postterm	Assessment of gross motor movement and postural patterns of the neonate
Alberta Infant Motor Assessment (AIMs; Piper & Darrah, 1994)	Birth to 18 months	Assessment of gross motor movement and postural patterns

posture may be different from that observed under the highly structured activities of standardized testing.

INTERPRETATION

The results of the physical therapy assessment should be considered within the context of the person's other areas of development, health, and environment. The concerns of the parent and child need to be used as the framework for both discussion of results and planning for intervention. Priorities should to be discussed, and the physical therapy finding and recommendations should be framed within those priorities.

INTERVENTIONS

Intervention is based on the outcomes of the assessment and should be oriented to the development of motor function, knowing that motor function includes the development of play, recreational, and fitness skills. When formulating an intervention plan, the physical therapist needs to listen to input from the family, child, school, and other community providers so that goals can be prioritized and framed appropriately within the context of the child's overall development and needs. For this discussion, intervention strategies will be divided into four categories: therapeutic activities, adaptive strategies and equipment, consultation, and education.

Therapeutic Activities

Many theories on which a physical therapist bases treatment take into consideration the motor control issues of the child, the goals of treatment, and how the child best responds. Techniques are based on theories of therapeutic exercise, motor control, motor learning, sensory processing, and developmental progression. Often, modulation of sensory information is used to change motor output. All interventions are formulated with the developmental framework for the child. The goal of the intervention is to promote the development of the best patterns of movement for the child that will optimize movement and minimize the development of secondary impairments.

In many neuromotor disabilities that affect the development of motor function in children and adults, abnormal muscle pull on joints can be a deforming force that causes secondary impairments. New medical treatments provided by physicians, such as the use of Botulinum toxin A injections and the use of intrathecal Baclofen, have been emerging to address this issue for individuals with cerebral palsy. Exercise modalities and positioning have been shown to be effective partners with these new medical therapies in maintaining newly gained range of motion, preventing secondary impairment, and promoting motor function (O'Neil, Fragala, & Dumas, 2003). Range of motion exercises that include passive stretching to the tightened muscles continue to play a role in physical therapy for children and adults with abnormal movement and posture. To optimize effectiveness, passive stretch is combined with positioning, orthotics, splinting, and promotion of active movement.

Modalities may be used to facilitate movement as well. For example, electrical stimulation techniques are being used in conjunction with motor learning and therapeutic exercise to facilitate movement (Maenpaa, Jaakkala, Sandstrom, & von Wendt, 2004). Positioning is another important modality in the treatment of children with motor dysfunction. Positioning is used adaptively to improve function, improve range of motion, strengthen muscle groups, inhibit maladaptive movement, prevent secondary impairments, and promote peer interaction.

Adaptive Strategies and Equipment

Adaptive strategies and equipment are provided to support the individual's function while he or she is working on underlying skills. Often, these types of strategies reduce frustration for the individual, and they always support function. Adaptive strategies may involve wheelchairs, walkers, adaptive seating, orthotics, or alternate ways of performing a task.

The choice of the type of adaptive stroller, seat, or wheelchair that will help the child or adult function best within his or her environment is often a difficult one and requires the entire team's input. Often, the physical therapist leads the team with this process. The field of adaptive equipment and technology is growing very quickly, and it is important that the physical therapist assisting the team with these decisions has specialized knowledge and recent experience in this area to keep up with all of the new options.

Once a decision is made and funding is obtained, changes in the decision process are often not possible. Also, revising of equipment or ordering replacement equipment usually has time limitations set by the insurer. Therefore, with a growing child who has changing needs, therapists must anticipate the child's needs for the future as well as current issues.

Consultation

All treatment with children involves consultation. The physical therapist works with the child's parents, teachers, and other professionals to help provide information for problem solving and carry over of the physical therapy goals into other settings.

Education

Sharing information with the family about their child's movement and postural issues so that the family members become informed consumers and active participants in their child's treatment is an important role for the physical therapist. Anticipatory guidance and teaching of therapeutic or adaptive techniques will optimize the treatment effect for the child and will help the family in understanding what the goals are and how best to help their child accomplish these goals (Shea, 1991). Although physical therapists encourage the family's involvement, the stresses, strains, and time commitments of the family need to be considered and acknowledged. A home program needs to be tailored to the family's needs.

CONCLUSION

Effectiveness studies of treatment techniques to promote movement control in children with developmental disabilities are a focus for the pediatric physical therapy profession at this time. Multiple studies assess the effectiveness of individual techniques for children with specific disabilities. For example, the use of strength training for individuals with cerebral palsy as a method of improving function has been the subject of many studies (Darrah & Fan, 1997). Often, to control variability, these studies are small and discrete. The need for a large, comprehensive study to assess the effectiveness of various techniques for children and adults with cerebral palsy has been identified but is not yet in place.

For both children and adults, fitness is becoming an issue. Obesity is on the rise (U.S. Department of Health and Human Services, 1996). An increasingly sedentary lifestyle is a major cause (Racette, Deusinger, & Deusinger, 2003). Because the cause of obesity is varied, the suggested treatment is as well. Exercise is thought to be an important component to that treatment. Not only is health improved by participation in fitness and recreational physical activities, but also friendships and a more positive attitude toward an inclusive setting are developed (Dykens, Posner, & Butterbaugh, 1998).

Brad is an 8-year-old boy who enjoys being outdoors but prefers sedentary activities such as playing with his handheld videogame system or watching videotapes. Brad has autism, low muscle tone, and strength and sensory processing issues. Since he was 4 years of age, his family has encouraged him to participate in physical activities with his peers in the community. The role of the physical therapist was to help Brad's family consider his strengths in the gross motor area and pair them with his interests to choose a sport. The community soccer team appeared to be a good fit for Brad's skills and interests.

When Brad was 4, his father became one of the coaches for the soccer team to support Brad's participation, and his mother, brother, and two sisters went to every game. He and his father practiced at home. Brad has continued on the soccer team as the children have matured and the game has become more competitive.

The family has been very creative in helping Brad learn the rules, maintaining Brad's safety, and ensuring Brad's participation. The team makes sure Brad has an opportunity to kick at least one goal per game. Brad smiles as he talks about his team and the kicks he has made.

In the past, children and adults with developmental disabilities have had limited opportunities for participation in physical fitness activities (Thomas & Rosenber, 2003). With Healthy People 2010, however, health promotion for everyone is an emphasis. Special Olympics has long been the champion of offering both fitness and recreational opportunities to children with developmental disabilities. Inclusive environments (e.g., community sports leagues) are providing more varied and local community activities for children. Many health clubs are accessible for individuals with developmental disabilities. For children with developmental disabilities, the physical therapist's role can include consulting coaches or families about adaptations that may facilitate the individual's participation and working with the child or adult to help them develop the skills necessary for the desired activity.

REFERENCES

American Physical Therapy Association. (2001). *Guide to physical therapy practice* (2nd ed.). Alexandria, VA: Author.

Aylward, G.P. (1997). Conceptual issues in developmental screening and assessment. *Journal of Developmental and Behavioral Pediatrics, 18,* 340–349.

Bayley, N. (1994). *Bayley Scales of Infant Development* (2nd ed.). San Antonio, TX: Psych Corp.

Bruininks, R.H. (1978). *Bruininks-Oseretsky Test of Motor Proficiency examiner's manual.* Circle Pines, MN: American Guidance Service.

Campbell, S. (1997). Therapy programs for children that last a lifetime. *Physical and Occupational Therapy in Pediatrics, 7,* 1–15.

Campbell, S., & Girolami, G. (1993). *The Test of Infant Motor Performance* (Research ed.). Available from the author.

Coster, W.J., Deeney, T., Haltiwanger, J.T., & Haley, S.M. (1998). *School Function Assessment (SFA).* San Antonio, TX: Psych Corp.

Darrah, J., & Fan, F. (1997). Review of the effects of progressive resisted muscle strengthening in children with cerebral palsy: A clinical consensus on exercise. *Pediatric Physical Therapy, 9,* 12–17.

Dykens, E.M., Rosner, B.A., & Butterbaugh, G. (1998). Exercise and sports in children and adolescents with developmental disabilities: Positive physical and psychosocial effects. *Child and Adolescent Psychiatric Clinics of North America, 7,* 757–771.

Folio, M.R., & Fewell, R.R. (2000). *Peabody Developmental Motor Scales–Revised (PDMS–2).* Austin, TX: PRO-ED.

Haley, S.M., Coster, W.J., Ludlow, L.H., Haltiwanger, J.T., & Andrellos, P.J. (1992). *Pediatric Evaluation of Disability Inventory (PEDI).* San Antonio, TX: Psych Corp.

Henderson, S.E., & Sugden, D.A. (1992). *Movement Assessment Battery for Children manual.* San Antonio, TX: Psych Corp.

Individuals with Disabilities Education Act (IDEA) Amendments of 1997, PL 105-17, 20 U.S.C. §§ 1400 *et seq.*

Kolobe, T. (1992). Working with families of children with disabilities. *Pediatric Physical Therapy, 4,* 57–63.

Maenpaa, H., Jaakkala, R., Sandstrom, M., & von Wendt, L. (2004). Effects of sensory-level electrical stimulation on the tibialis anterior muscle during physical therapy on active dorsiflexion of the ankle of children with cerebral palsy. *Pediatric Physical Therapy, 16,* 39–44.

McEwen, I. (2000). *Providing physical therapy services under Parts B and C of the Individuals with Disabilities Education Act (IDEA) section on pediatrics.* Alexandria, VA: American Physical Therapy Association.

O'Neil, M.E., Fragala, M.A., & Dumas, H.E. (2003). Physical therapy intervention for children with cerebral palsy who receive botulinum toxin A injections. *Pediatric Physical Therapy, 15,* 204–215.

Piper, M.C., & Darrah, J. (1994). *Motor Assessment of the Developing Infant.* Philadelphia: W.B. Saunders.

Racette, S.B., Deusinger, S.S., & Deusinger, R.H. (2003). Obesity: Overview of prevalence, etiology, and treatment. *Physical Therapy, 83,* 276–287.

Russell, D., Rosenbaum, P., Gowland, C., Hardy, S., Lane, M., Plews, N., et al. (1990). *Gross Motor Function Measure.* Ontario, CA: Chedoke-McMasters Hospital.

Shea, A. (1991). Motor attainments in Down syndrome. In Foundation for Physical Therapy, *Contemporary management of motor control problems: Proceedings of the II Step Conference.* Alexandria, VA: Foundation for Physical Therapy.

Shea, A. (1992). Physical therapy. In M.D. Levine, W.B. Carey, & A.C Crocker (Eds.), *Developmental-behavioral pediatrics.* Philadelphia: W.B. Saunders.

Thomas, A.D., & Rosenber, A. (2003). Promoting community recreation and leisure. *Pediatric Physical Therapy, 15,* 232–246.

U.S. Department of Health and Human Services, Centers for Disease Control and Prevention, & National Center for Chronic Disease Prevention and Health Promotion. (1996). *Physical activity and health.* Atlanta, GA: Authors.

24.3 SPEECH, LANGUAGE, AND COMMUNICATION

John M. Costello

"As long as people considered my brain useless and my facial expressions meaningless, I was doomed to remain voiceless," Ruth Sienkiewicz-Mercer wrote (1989). As a nonspeaking woman with cerebral palsy, she spent 16 years in a state institution with the diagnosis of "imbecile" because nobody recognized her attempts to communicate. According to the National Joint Committee for the Communication Needs of Persons with Severe Disabilities,

> Communication is any act by which one person gives to or receives information about that person's needs, desires, perceptions, knowledge or effective state. Communication may be intentional or unintentional, may involve conventional or unconventional signals, may take linguistic or nonlinguistic form, and may occur through spoken or other modes. (2003)

This definition makes it clear that all individuals, *no matter how significant their developmental disabilities,* attempt to communicate. Despite this fact, many medical, clinical, and educational professionals deem individuals with significant developmental disabilities inappropriate for intervention secondary to the extent of their disabilities. Indeed, varied benchmarks of performance or cognitive skill have been highlighted as prerequisites to determine candidacy for communication intervention.

Prior to a communication assessment with Anna, a 27-month-old girl who was born at 25 weeks gestation with a complicated neonatal course, the author reviewed documents from her early intervention team. Under the heading of speech and language, one document stated:

Anna currently does not produce any meaningful speech. Her vocalizations are limited to open vowel sounds and are not produced with communicative intent. Anna does not follow commands or consistently respond to her name. She does not demonstrate cause–effect or consistent intentional social behavior. . . based upon these findings, Anna is a pre-intentional communicator and does not yet have the prerequisites for speech and language. She is currently not eligible for communication services but will be reevaluated before her third birthday.

To address this situation, the American Speech-Language-Hearing Association's (ASHA) position statement regarding the application of restrictive eligibility policies reports that eligibility criteria for communication services and supports "based on a priori criteria violate recommended practice principles by precluding consideration of individual needs" (National Joint Committee, 2003). As detailed in this position statement, criteria historically used to wrongfully preclude candidacy for communication assessment and intervention have included:

(a) discrepancies between cognitive and communication function; (b) chronological age; (c) specific diagnosis or lack of diagnosis; (d) not meeting presumed cognitive or other skills presumed to be prerequisite; (e) failure to benefit from previous communication services and supports; (f) restrictive interpretations of educational, vocational and/or medical necessity; (g) lack of appropriately trained personnel; and (h) lack of adequate funds or other resources.

During the author's assessment of Anna, Anna demonstrated the ability to choose objects of interest from a field of options; consistently selected a switch to activate music; produced intentional vocal behavior to request reoccurrence of a tickling game, and demonstrated numerous natural gestures used to gain attention, socially engage, and reject. If Anna had been denied services until she fit a predetermined mold for readiness, she might well have been considered not eligible for communication services for much of her life. In fact, the assumption that prerequisites must be established prior to initiating services presumes the advent of a *spontaneous combustion of skill.*

ROLE OF SPEECH-LANGUAGE PATHOLOGISTS

The speech-language pathologist may be part of the team for a person with developmental disabilities across the age span. Although the specific goals and focus will change based on individual needs, abilities, and skills, the objective of bridging the gap between what an individual understands (receptive language) and can express (expressive language and speech production) is pervasive. Delays or disorders in development of speech and language may be symptomatic of a variety of developmental disabilities. Early consultation with a pediatrician, audiologist, psychologist, and speech-language pathologist is critical to address diagnosis and treatment of communication disorders.

Aidan is a 6-year-old boy with developmental disabilities of unknown etiology. He is described as social and inquisitive but is characterized by his parents as lazy and obstinate when it comes to speech.

"Aidan can say words if he wants to," Aidan's father explained. "But if he says something, he refuses to say it again. We have heard him say words many times, but then he refuses to say them again."

Indeed, during a motor speech assessment, Aidan was able to produce words and simple phrases and did not demonstrate difficulty with muscle strength or muscle control. Yet, when focus was placed on Aidan's ability to speak and he was asked to repeat the previously produced utterances, Aidan's production was poorly planned and inarticulate.

"See!" exclaimed his father. "He could say it, and now he won't."

On further examination of Aidan's motor speech production, Aidan demonstrated significant difficulty with volitional programming of oral motor movements characteristic of apraxia of speech.

ASSESSMENT CONSIDERATIONS

A child must be able to perceive speech sounds and decode sounds for meaning (auditory processing) in order to develop typical speech and language. The individual must be referred for an audiological assessment when typical speech and language development is in question. Chapters 17.1 and 17.2 provide a detailed examination of hearing screening and hearing disorders.

Speech is the motor activity or the actual production and articulation of sounds, syllables, and words. It can be broken down into specific components, including respiration, phonation, resonation, and articulation. Examining speech production as a sum of these components can be valuable, as it then makes understanding and treating errors or disorders of speech production easier.

Respiration is the flow of air from the lungs, through the larynx, and into the oral and nasal cavity. Phonation is created at the level of the larynx through the process of setting the air traveling through the larynx in motion with the opening, closing, and vibration of the vocal folds. Resonance is the flow of air through the throat, nose, and mouth. Individual differences in the throat, oral, and nasal cavities, including structural anomalies, will affect the quality of resonance and, thus, the quality of an individual's voice. Articulation is the shaping of voice sounds into specific speech sound patterns by the rapid movement of the articulators, including the tongue and lips.

Disorders of speech may be isolated or part of a more complex developmental disorder. Speech disorders include articulation disorders such as substitutions of sounds ("dwink" for *drink*); omissions ("ea" for *eat*), additions ("ba-uh-by" for *baby*), and distortions of sounds; errors of resonance resulting in hypernasal or hyponasal production, errors of rate and rhythm (flat or monotone production); and disorders of phonation affecting pitch, loudness, or smoothness of voice production.

Motor speech disorders or problems in oral-motor movement are more common in individuals with developmental disabilities and may include dysarthria or apraxia of speech. Dysarthria is a neuromotor disorder resulting in poor muscle control as seen in many individuals with cerebral palsy. Apraxia does not involve muscle damage or weakness but is characterized by impaired volitional production of normal articulation and prosody. An individual with apraxia may have difficulty intentionally positioning the articulators for voluntary speech sound production.

Referral for speech therapy is essential for all types of speech and motor speech disorders. Depending on the age of the individual, the specific speech disorder, and the history of treatment/response to treatment, speech therapy may be provided in a variety of manners ranging from intensive one-to-one sessions, to a consultative model of intervention.

Language

Language is a rule-based system that people use to represent their ideas, thoughts, and beliefs. It is the most complex skill acquired, demonstrated, and refined in early life. Very young infants are able to distinguish between sounds in their native language and those of a foreign language, and, in fact, infants as young as 2 days old show a preference for listening to their native language (Werker & Tees, 1999).

The miracle of language development becomes even more evident when considering the complex components of language: form, content, and use (Bloom & Lahey, 1978). The form refers to the structure or the grammar of language. Grammar focuses on combining the *phonemes*, which are the smallest units of sound, with *morphemes*, the smallest units of meaning (e.g., as *-s* at the end of the word to demonstrate plural or *-ing* to denote present progressive), and *syntax*, which is the order in which words are combined to create phrases and sentences. Content refers to the meaning or the *semantics* of the language produced. An individual may use one word or a complete sentence to communicate a thought or idea. Someone with echolalic speech, who repeats spoken words or phrases without communicative intent, may demonstrate good form but little content. Finally, *use* refers to the situations in which one uses language and the pragmatics of use (knowing what to say, how to say it, to whom to say it, and in what situations).

Developmental language disorders may be related to numerous causes, including hearing impairment, prematurity, neurological insult, brain injury, intellectual disabilities, and chromosomal and genetic disorders. Language disorders include the inability to understand spoken language (receptive language disorder), use language appropriately when speaking (expressive language disorder), or a combination of both (communication disorder). According to ASHA (1993), a *language disorder* is an impairment in comprehension and/or use of a spoken, written, and/or other symbol system, that may involve the form, content, and/or function in any combination.

REFERRAL TO A SPEECH-LANGUAGE PATHOLOGIST

A referral should be made for a speech and/or language assessment if an individual does not demonstrate skills commensurate with age peers, is unable to participate functionally, or is frustrated with the inability to successfully communicate (see Table 24.3-1). No minimal age exists for referral to a speech-language pathologist. Infants can benefit from communication intervention if they are at high risk due to a traumatic birth history, demonstrate signs of developmental delays, have a hearing impairment, or demonstrate difficulty with feeding or swallowing.

By the same token, no "lost window of opportunity" exists for language intervention. Young adults and adults of all ages can benefit from intervention that focuses on enhancing expressive and receptive skills and increasing opportunities to successfully interact with unfamiliar communication partners and participate in social opportunities throughout the day. Several commonly used speech and language assessment tools are listed in Table 24.3-2.

Table 24.3-1. General indicators for speech and language evaluation

Age for referral	Indications
Birth to 6 months	Does not respond to voices or environmental sounds
	Does not cry or produce loud/clear voice
3–4 months	Cries only—does not produce comfort sounds (cooing)
	Does not make sounds to let parent know he or she wants or is needed
	Does not visually interact with anyone
1 year	Does not babble or has stopped babbling
	Does not respond to simple phrases/commands (*Come here. Pet the doggie. Get your bottle.*)
	Does not respond to his or her name
	Does not use some words such as *mama, bottle, oh-oh,* or *bye-bye* to communicate by age 15 months and does not use at least 15 words spontaneously by the end of the first year
2 years	Does not use at least 50 different words
	Does not produce simple sentences (*What's that? Mommy go outside.*)
2.5 years	Does not have intelligible speech
	Does not answer simple questions
3 years	Does not use short sentences
	Does not have intelligible speech
	Does not demonstrate understanding of simple concepts (size, color)
	Does not ask *wh-* questions (what, when, or where)
4 years	Has difficulty explaining events
	Has difficulty learning new concepts
	Does not follow two-step directions
	Has difficulty learning new concepts and words
	Does not speak clearly

In addition to formal testing, numerous informal strategies are used to better understand communication skills and strategies. Many people with developmental disabilities across the age span have unique methods of communicating that are only recognized and respected by familiar communication partners. Some of these communication strategies may be inventive gestures, signs, or responses that were created in specific context and continue to be recognized and responded to appropriately by familiar communication partners. Examples of unique communication strategies are shown in Table 24.3-3.

Although these strategies may not be traditional and intervention goals may target establishing more standard strategies of communication, they are nonetheless meaningful communication for the individual. Furthermore, individuals who use such meaningful strategies may become frustrated or angry when communication is not successful or recognized as meaningful. To document nontraditional and inventive communication strategies, a Communication Profile is often recommended (Shane, 1979). This document details communication behaviors (intentional or unintentional) and their referent as reported by the most familiar communication partners. The document is then shared with all educators and service providers so that they can readily recognize and appropriately respond to the nontraditional communication strategy.

COMMUNICATION DISORDERS AND MALADAPTIVE BEHAVIOR

For some people, nontraditional behaviors are not recognized as communicative or are ignored by communication partners. The inability to communicate effectively and have one's needs acknowledged or met may lead to the demonstration of a myriad of maladaptive behaviors ranging from severe withdrawal to serious self-abusive behaviors (see Chapter 23.5). Few physicians, educators, or even family members recognize the possibility that maladaptive behavior may be a communication strategy rather than an organic manifestation.

One tool that investigates this causal link is the Motivation Assessment Scale (Durand, 1988). This tool helps team members recognize what may motivate the maladaptive behavior. It further helps delineate general communication intent including a desire for escape, tan-

Table 24.3-2. Frequently used measures of speech and language skill

Test	Age range (years)	Description
Test of Auditory Comprehension of Language–Third Edition (TACL–3; Carrow-Woolfolk, 1999)	3.0–9.11	Three subtests focusing on understanding structure of spoken language including vocabulary, grammatical morphemes, and elaborated phrases and sentences
Clinical Evaluation of Language Fundamentals–Fourth Edition (CELF–4; Semel, Wiig & Secord, 2003)	5.0–21.0	Multiple subsets focusing on expressive and receptive language
Clinical Evaluation of Language Fundamentals–Preschool (CELF–Preschool; Wiig, Secord, & Semel, 1992)	3–6	Assessment of semantics, morphology, syntax, and auditory memory
Peabody Picture Vocabulary Test–Third Edition (PPVT–III; Dunn & Dunn, 1997)	2.6–22	Test of receptive vocabulary
Expressive One Word Picture Vocabulary Test–Revised (Gardner, 1990)	2.0–15	Test of expressive vocabulary
Goldman-Fristoe Test of Articulation–Second Edition (Goldman & Fristoe, 2000)	2.0–21.0	Test of speech production skills
Receptive–Expressive Emergent Language Test–Third Edition (REEL–3; Bzoch, League, & Brown, 2003)	Birth to 3	Two subtests focusing on receptive responses to sounds and language as reported by parents and expressive assessment of child's current oral language development as reported by parents

gibles, attention, or sensory feedback. Once the motivations have been identified, modifications to demands placed on an individual or appropriate alternative strategies to communication may be introduced. Significant clinical evidence supports the introduction of supplemental or augmentative communication strategies, including the use of sign language, two-dimensional and three-dimensional representations, and simple speech-output technology to replace maladaptive behavior with functional and appropriate communication strategies.

Olivia was referred by a neonatal neurologist at the age of 16 months with a diagnosis of developmental delays secondary to perinatal hypoxic ischemic brain damage and spastic quadriparesis. The focus was to assess Olivia's current communication skills and to introduce strategies to support expressive and receptive language skills. At the time of the initial assessment, Olivia produced minimal vocalizations (mostly "ah" and "ga"), would reach for objects of interest but could not grasp, and had no supported seating with hand and trunk orthotics on order. She ate baby food and required all liquids to be thickened due to insufficient ability to cough and clear.

During the initial assessment, Olivia demonstrated the ability to recognize and discriminate photographs; reach for photographs representing favorite toys while ignoring photographs of less preferred items; hit a switch with simple speech output to "call" her mother; and use simple switch tools to turn on music and other battery and electrical operated devices. At the end of this first meeting during which Olivia's skills and possible goals were detailed, Olivia's mother cried. When asked why, she indicated that Olivia had seen the family pediatrician the day before who exclaimed, "She is severely impaired, and her brain is damaged. This is all you're going to get. Just give her all the love you can."

Olivia was seen by an intervention team, including a speech-language pathologist, two to three times per week until the age of 3. Once in preschool, she continued to work with a speech-language pathologist and clinical/educational team four days per week.

At age 6, Olivia speaks in four-word sentences. She demonstrates mild dysarthria and language learning disabilities, for which she receives speech-language therapy. She loves telling jokes and making her communication partners laugh. She also uses a walker to ambulate and continues to be driven to achieve.

AUGMENTATIVE AND ALTERNATIVE COMMUNICATION

Some people with developmental disabilities are nonspeaking or their speech production is not adequate for functional communication. For these individuals, augmentative and alternative communication (AAC) may be appropriate to support communication. ASHA wrote,

Table 24.3-3. Examples of unique communication strategies

Behavior	Referent
Kicking off shoes	"I want to go home" *Rationale:* A 34-year-old man with significant intellectual disabilities had to remove his shoes before entering his parents home.
Placing hands on cheeks and pushing face back and forth	"No" *Rationale:* Parents and instructors for a 9-year-old boy with Angelman syndrome attempted to teach him to shake his head "no" by physically assisting him to shake his head from left to right. Although he did not learn to shake his head independently, he did learn to put his hands on his cheeks and physically shake his own head from left to right whenever he wanted to refuse or say "no."
Saying, "The night before Christmas."	"I want to go to bed" *Rationale:* A 7-year-old girl with an intractable seizure disorder enjoyed having the book 'Twas the Night Before Christmas read to her before she went to bed when she was 5 years old. After her parents repeatedly read the book to her during the Christmas season, she associated 'Twas The Night Before Christmas with going to bed. Now, she repeats the phrase when she wants to go to bed and is beginning to generalize it as a request to go into her bedroom.
Curling toes of her feet	"I have to go to the bathroom" *Rationale:* A 19-year-old woman with profound intellectual impairments was observed by her mother to curl up her toes prior to soiling her pants. Her mother began to watch for this behavior and take her to the bathroom immediately after observing it. Although the behavior did not appear to be intentional, it was recognized and responded to as communication, resulting in successful use of the bathroom.

"Augmentative communication attempts to compensate (either temporarily or permanently) for the impairment and disability patterns of persons with severe expressive communication disorder" (1989).

AAC can be classified into two distinct categories, unaided communication strategies and aided communication strategies, which may be used singularly or in combination with each other. Unaided strategies require only the use of the body and may include vocalizations, gestures, sign language, and facial expressions. For some individuals, unaided strategies remain the most effective means to support expressive communication, especially if they communicate primarily with familiar partners or with individuals who know the communication strategy (e.g., sign language). Such strategies can be powerful as they do not require the use of a tool and can be readily produced by an individual.

Aided communication strategies incorporate the use of a tool and may necessitate the use of an electronic tool, a nonelectronic tool, or a combination of both electronic and nonelectronic tools. The type and sophistication of an aided system may vary greatly based on the communication skills and needs of the individual with developmental disabilities as well as the scope and diversity of communication partners. For some, an effective nonelectronic aided communication system may incorporate objects or object representations. Other individuals may use picture communication boards or books. Electronic aided communication strategies could be a simple switch that speaks a message when pushed, allowing an individual to call attention or socially engage; a battery-operated device that supports communication of up to 100 messages and more; or a sophisticated microprocessor-based system that supports access to full and generative speech output, full access to writing, and all of the electronic communication conveniences used by people without disabilities, including Internet access and e-mail.

Rick is a 42-year-old man with spastic and athetoid cerebral palsy. He is nonspeaking and nonambulatory and relies on personal care assistance to perform all personal care needs. Through occupational and physical therapy assessment, Rick's most consistent and reliable motor movement was determined to be a right lateral turn of the head; thus, Rick's sole independent control is through a switch mounted on his wheelchair to the side of his head.

Despite significant disability, Rick is able to communicate independently through the use of a sophisticated computer-based system that he controls using a single switch (set Figure 24.3-1). Rick is a college graduate with a degree in special education and is a national and international lecturer on the topic of disability and integration. Furthermore, Rick and his father travel internationally to participate in marathons

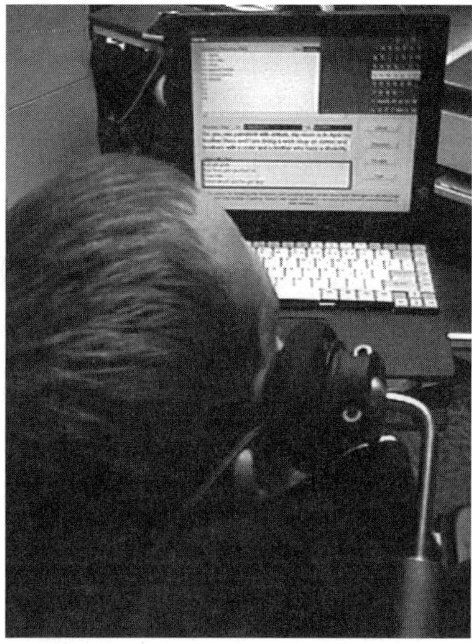

Figure 24.3-1. Rick's most consistent and reliable motor movement was determined to be a right lateral turn of the head.

and triathlons. They enjoy international celebrity as Rick is pushed in his wheelchair in marathons; sits on the front of a custom-made bicycle for bike races, and is pulled in a raft for swim portions of triathlons.

Through Rick's writing and speaking engagements, he delivers the message "I can" to educate people worldwide on issues of disability. Despite his efforts, Rick reported that while recently traveling to participate in an international sports competition, he needed to visit a hospital emergency room secondary to an abrasion he received during a fall. No doctors in the emergency room attempted to communicate with him, even when they were informed that he could understand everything and had a means to communicate—by answering yes/no questions or use of his computer. Medical personnel appeared afraid of interacting with him and, because of his severe physical disability, he was unable to initiate communication. He was treated as if he was a thing being worked on rather than a person who should be consulted on his own medical condition.

"Because I have severe disabilities and could not talk," he said, "they assumed I could not understand or interact."

CONCLUSION

A person's ability to participate in life is intimately connected to his or her success with communication. Without effective communication, cognitive, social, and emotional development are at risk. For a person with a communication impairment, the ability to be recognized as a sentient human being is at risk. Referral for communication intervention, regardless of age, presumed competence, or medical diagnosis is crucial for individuals with communication impairments.

REFERENCES

American Speech-Language-Hearing Association. (ASHA). (1989). Competencies for speech-language pathologists providing services in augmentative communication. *Asha, 31*, 107–110.

American Speech-Language-Hearing Association Ad Hoc Committee on Service Delivery in Schools. (1993). Definition of communication disorders and variations. *Asha, 35* (Supp. 10), 40–41.

Bloom, L., & Lahey, M. (1978). *Language development and language disorders.* New York: John Wiley and Sons.

Bzoch, K.R., League, R., & Brown, V.L. (2003). *Receptive–Expressive Emergent Language Test–Third Edition.* Austin, TX: PRO-ED.

Carrow-Woolfolk, E. (1999). *Test for Auditory Comprehension of Language–Third Edition. (TACL–3).* Circle Pine, MN: AGS Publishing.

Dunn, L.M., & Dunn, L.M. (1997). *Peabody Picture Vocabulary Test–Third Edition. (PPVT–III).* Circle Pines, MN: AGS Publishing.

Durand, V.M. (1988). The Motivation Assessment Scale. In M. Hersen & A.S. Bellack (Eds.), *Dictionary of behavioral assessment techniques* (pp. 309–310). New York: Pergamon Press.

Gardner, M.F. (1990). *Expressive One-Word Picture Vocabulary Test–Revised.* Novato, CA: Academic Therapy Publications.

Goldman, R., & Fristoe, M. (2000). *Goldman-Fristoe Test of Articulation–Second Edition.* Circle Pines, MN: AGS Publishing.

National Joint Committee for the Communicative Needs of Persons with Severe Disabilities. (2003). Position statement on access to communication services and supports: Concerns regarding the application of restrictive "eligibility" policies. *ASHA Supplement, 23*, 19–20.

Semel, E., Wiig, E.H., & Secord, W.A. (2003). *Clinical Evaluation of Language Fundamentals–Fourth Edition. (CELF–4).* San Antonio, TX: Harcourt Assessment.

Shane, H.C. (1979). Approaching communication training with the severely handicapped. In R. York & C. Edgard (Eds.), *Training the severely handicapped* (Vol. IV, pp. 155–179). Columbis, OH: Special Press.

Sienkiewicz-Mercer, R. (1989). *I raise my eyes to say yes.* Wilmington, MA: Houghton Mifflin.

Werker, J., & Tees, R. (1999). Influences on infant speech processing: Toward a new synthesis. *Annual Reviews of Psychology, 50*, 514.

Wiig, E.H., Secord, W.A., & Semel, W.A. (1992). *Clinical Evaluation of Language Fundamentals–Preschool. (CELF–Preschool).* San Antonio, TX: Harcourt Assessment.

24.4 ASSISTIVE TECHNOLOGY

Susan R. Cusack

Medical practitioners must wear many hats in their work with individuals with disabilities. They serve as vital team members, gatekeepers to core funding streams, and conduits of information and resources for families. Most funding sources for assistive technology have a prerequisite for prescriptions, documentation of disabling conditions, and letters of medical necessity. Therefore, medical practitioners are inextricably linked to the process of facilitating access to assistive technology (Mendelson, 1995). The process of identifying, securing, maintaining, and reevaluating the assistive technology needs of individuals is complicated and requires sensitivity and understanding. This chapter explores the relationships among disabilities, technology, federal protections and entitlements, and the increasingly complex role of the medical provider within this context.

From name stamps to laptops, technology helps people with disabilities lead more independent and productive lives. Velcro, large-button calculators, and computers are all part of a continuum of no-tech, low-tech, and high-tech devices that reflect a broad range of *assistive technologies*, a term legally defined as "any item, piece of equipment or product system, whether acquired commercially, off-the-shelf, modified or customized, that is used to increase, maintain, or improve functional capabilities of individuals with disabilities" (PL 100-407).

Assistive technology sounds complicated, scientific, and expensive, but in most cases, it is not. Many assistive technologies are commonly available in office supply and hardware stores. The following are a few examples that can be applied in academic, work, or home settings:

- Remote doorbells found in hardware stores can be used to get someone's attention in another part of a classroom, office building, or home if assistance is needed.
- Inexpensive electronic organizers from an office supply store can help individuals to independently keep track of their daily responsibilities.
- A trackball from computer or office supply stores can be used by someone who is having difficulty managing a traditional mouse for a computer.

While these kind of solutions are simple and easily incorporated into day-to-day activities, there are instances where more complicated solutions are needed. As an individual's needs become more sophisticated, the level of technology increases. The cost and complexity of the supports required to ensure the right technology match also increase. In these instances, the provision of assistive technology devices and services is often tied to a legal mandate or the availability of private insurance or Medicaid.

LAWS SUPPORTING ASSISTIVE TECHNOLOGY

An examination of how federal legislation supports the use of assistive technology at different points in a person's life conveys a fuller understanding of the dynamic between disability and access to technology. Several laws share a common definition for assistive technology and provide varying levels of entitlement to assistive technology. First, Sections 504 and 508 of the Rehabilitation Act of 1973 (PL 93-112) ensure that organizations and employers provide an equal opportunity for individuals with disabilities to participate in and receive program benefits and services (U.S. Department of Health and Human Services, 2003). These laws apply to any programs that receive federal funding, including public schools, municipal programs (arts and recreation), and public hospitals. Section 508 provides individuals with disabilities access to information technology. Although the accountability measures of Section 508 only apply to information technologies that are purchased, developed, and used by federal agencies, the policies and standards that have been developed in support of this legislation have significantly influenced current understanding and best practices about accessible information technology (e.g., web sites, telecommunication products, computers).

The Individuals with Disabilities Education Act (IDEA) of 1990 (PL 101-476) protects the right of children with disabilities, ages 3–21, to receive a free appropriate public education (FAPE). PL 101-476 requires that schools provide students with disabilities the supports and services that they need to gain access to and make progress in the general curriculum in the least restrictive environment possible. These supports and services can include specialized services and assistive technology.

The Technology-Related Assistance for Individuals with Disabilities Act of 1988 (PL 100-407) and the Assistive Technology Act of 2004 (PL 108-364) promote awareness and access to assistive technology at the state level. These laws assert the federal government's belief that technology is a critical tool in promoting independence and productivity for individuals with disabilities. The funding made available through this legislation is allocated to state programs that support consumer awareness and consumer access to assistive technology. A list of state technical assistance projects is available through the Rehabilitation Engineering and Assistive Technology Society of North America (RESNA) at http://www.resna.org/taproject/at/statecontacts.html.

The Americans with Disabilities Act (ADA) of 1990 (PL 101-336) is complementary to, yet broader than, Section 504 of PL 93-112. PL 101-336 inhibits discrimination on the basis of disability in public and private employment sectors, public accommodations, transportation, state and local government services, and telecommunications. It asserts the standard of providing reasonable accommodations to maintain compliance with this law.

ASSISTIVE TECHNOLOGY FOR INFANTS AND TODDLERS

For infants and toddlers, the provision of assistive technology devices and services through PL 101-476 is offered within the context of *natural environments*, or home and community settings that a peer without disabilities would use. "The goal is to enable the child with disabilities to be maximally engaged in and benefit from the same naturally-occurring learning opportunities as would children without disabilities" (Mistrett, 2001, pp. 1–6). Low-tech interventions (e.g., nonskid surfaces to help stabilize a bottle or cup), mid-tech interventions (e.g., single-switch adapted toys), and high-tech interventions (e.g., talking books on the computer) are appropriate for supporting children in their natural environment.

ASSISTIVE TECHNOLOGY FOR SCHOOL-AGE CHILDREN

The U.S. Department of Education reported in 2001 that there were 6.3 million students with disabilities age 3–21 in the public school system. When children enter public school, the legislative emphasis shifts from supporting access to natural environments to promoting access to FAPE in the least restrictive environment possible. PL 105-17 mandates that schools "consider" assistive technology supports and services when developing a child's individualized education program (IEP). Someone on the IEP team should have sufficient knowledge of assistive technology to make an informed decision about its suitability for the student. If assistive technology is considered appropriate but the IEP team is unable to make a final decision about the device, then the team should request an assistive technology assessment for the student (Wyoming Assistive Technology Initiative, 1998).

Assistive technology follows a continuum from simplistic devices, such as a pencil grip that facilitates writing, to more complex strategies, such as voice recognition. That is, devices range from low to high technology, from low to high cost, and from generic to specialized equipment. The National Assistive Technology Research Institute (NATRI) provided the following example of the different types of technology that are available and the ways that they interact with each other to promote learning and independence:

> A high school student who is paralyzed may require a respirator to assist in breathing (medical technology). In a course designed to teach about telecommunications, that individual may use a voice-operated computer (assistive technology) to pursue a tutorial about how to design databases from a software program (instructional technology) that was designed according to principles of near-errorless learning (technology of teaching). As a result of the tutorial, the student will be able to set up a database, enter and retrieve information necessary to function effectively in class (technology productivity tool) and use the Internet (information technology) to locate information that could be stored in the database. (NATRI, 2001)

This student will also use other technologies (low-tech and high-tech) throughout his or her day 1) to manage activities of daily living related to feeding and toileting (e.g., drinking straws, catheters); 2) to support exercise programs, and 3) to control the environment (e.g., environmental control units to turn on lights). Funding to support these additional technologies may be limited. Public schools support the acquisition of technologies used to gain access to the general curriculum, and private insurance or Medicaid subsidize the purchase of medical technologies (respirator, catheters), but the student and his or her family have to find creative ways to acquire the remaining technologies.

ASSISTIVE TECHNOLOGY FOR ADOLESCENTS AND ADULTS

As young people make the transition to adulthood, their need for technology is still vital. Students younger than 21 who still receive supports and services from the public school system are entitled to use assistive technology in the development of skills that support their IEP goals and personal vision. These goals tend to be broader and include objectives related to career development and postsecondary experiences as well as skills related to daily living activities.

New technologies may be suggested during transition that might not have been appropriate at other times during the student's education. For example, a student who has trouble sitting through a full day at school may typically use a modified schedule with summer supports. As the student begins the transition process, other strategies should be explored that are more relevant to adult experiences. In this instance, he or she may begin to use distance education opportunities that provide more flexibility and prepare the student for a typical and more productive postsecondary experience (Canfield & Reed, 2001). Another example is a student who has difficulty writing. Transition should be a new opportunity to shift from the strategy of using a scribe to that of a laptop with voice recognition software in order to gain greater independence and flexibility in postsecondary experiences and in employment.

A final consideration to ensure continuity of support and access to technology is the issue of portability. Each state handles the ownership of technology differently, but in the absence a formal agreement, possession of the technology will revert back to the agency as the student transitions out of the program. The issue of technology portability is a potential problem at all transition points: for children in early intervention making the transition to public school, for young adults making the transition from public school to adult life or postsecondary education, and for postsecondary students making the transition to employment.

Megan is a young woman building a career as a disability rights advocate (see Figure 24.4-1). She has spoken at youth leadership forums and several conferences on the benefits of using technology. Megan uses technology to help her with her speeches and presentations. She currently uses a freeware application called KidBook, a single switch application that simulates a talking book environment. Megan leverages the software's text-to-speech feature to convey her ideas to her audience. The following is a poem that she wrote that reflects her feelings on her life's journey and her path to independence.

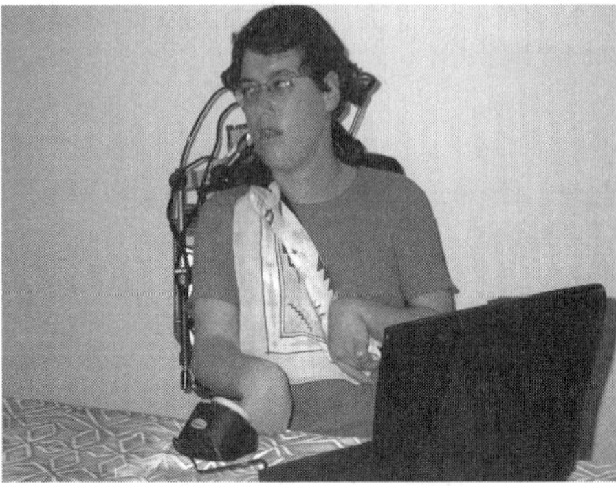

Figure 24.4-1. Megan is a young woman building a career as a disability rights advocate.

Independence
I wander hopefully,
Now anxious for an amazing adventure,
Deciding for myself.
Everything is so good.
Promise that I will be happy.
Everybody that is important, friends and family.
Not being lonely, but
Daring to do things alone.
Empowered to be a self-advocate,
Natural leader,
Confident in choosing.
Ecstatic that my wheelchair gives me independence.

Megan wrote this poem in 1995 when she was a student at Newton North High School in Massachusetts.

EMPLOYMENT

Employers are subject to the criteria of reasonable accommodations under PL 101-336 and PL 93-112, such as modified work schedules, quiet work environments, designated parking spaces, and assistive technologies that enable the qualified employee to perform his or her job. Many employers are very anxious about the cost of accommodating people with disabilities, but interestingly, job accommodations are usually not expensive. According to the Job Accommodation Network (2002), 71% of the job accommodations that they suggested cost less than $500. Examples of job accommodations include alphabet strips and color-coded systems to encourage productivity for a filing clerk with cognitive or visual processing challenges; the use of AlphaSmart (electronic notebook with a liquid-crystal display panel) or a computer-based Instant Messenger system to promote communication for an employee with a hearing loss; or a larger-screen monitor for an employee with a vision impairment.

COMMUNITY INTEGRATION

Although PL 101-336 and other Fair Housing initiatives have been written to protect the civil rights of individuals with disabilities, a recent Supreme Court decision may signal a new opportunity for enforcement of these protections for individuals with severe disabilities. In *Olmstead v. L.C.*, the Supreme Court determined that under certain circumstances PL 101-336 requires states to provide community-based services for individuals with disabilities and holds that "unjustified institutionalization of people with disabilities is prohibited discrimination under the Americans with Disabilities Act" (U.S. Department of Health and Human Services, 2003). This court decision was reinforced by President Bush's New Freedom Initiative, which addresses federal policy barriers that inhibit the full participation of individuals with disabilities in community life.

Both of these actions encourage cross-agency collaboration and coordination with the expectation that working together will lead to more effective utilization of federal resources in support of community integration. Although it is too early to know their full impact, these actions could signal a new trend in the use of technologies that facilitate independence in a community-based environment, particularly if the technologies inhibit institutionalization. Examples of technologies that promote independence in daily living activities and reduce dependency on outside support include personal pagers, adapted bathing and toileting equipment, adapted kitchen utensils and dishes, and environmental controls.

CONSIDERING ASSISTIVE TECHNOLOGY ACROSS THE AGES

Given the estimated 49 million people with disabilities, approximately 13 million people are using some form of assistive technology (Olson & DeRuyter, 2002, as cited in AT/AAC enABLES). These technologies support a variety of sensory, cognitive, and mobility impairments. To help navigate the vast array of technologies available, on-line resources have been developed to make this exploration a little more manageable. One of the most comprehensive resources is ABLEDATA, http://www.abledata.org, a database that contains information on more than 30,000 assistive technology products. The database includes a detailed description of each product, its price, and contact information for the vendor. In searching the ABLEDATA site, or a similar resource, it helps to understand some of the organizational conventions adopted by the industry. Information is usually organized by product type or function. Table 24.4-1 shows assistive technology product categories established by the National Institute of Disability and Rehabilitation Research (NIDRR as cited in U.S. Department of Commerce, 2003).

Table 24.4-1. Assistive technology product categories

Product category	Description
Architectural elements	Door opening/closing devices, door levers, lifts and elevators, ramps, safety equipment
Communication devices	Augmentative and alternative communication (AAC) devices, speech synthesizers, communication boards, board overlays, talking books
Telecommunications	Wireless and corded telephones, text telephones (TTY), amplified telephones, talking pagers
Sensory aids	Noncomputer based devices, such as hearing aids, assistive listening devices, tactile aids for the deaf/blind, alerting devices, and Braille notetakers
Computers	Hardware, software, accessories, including screen readers, large print products, optical character recognition tools, and Braille displays
Environmental controls	Remote-controlled door openers, telephones, lights, and televisions
Aids to daily living	Aids for hygiene, dressing and undressing, toileting, washing, bathing, showering, manicure and pedicure, hair care, dental care, facial and skin care, housekeeping, handling and manipulating products, and orientation
Mobility	Transportation safety, vehicle lifts and ramps, walking/standing aids, wheelchairs, seating systems, other types of wheeled mobility
Orthotics and prosthetics	Spinal orthotic systems, upper/lower limb orthotic systems, hybrid orthotics, upper limb prostheses, upper/lower limb prosthetic systems, nonlimb prostheses, functional electrical stimulators
Recreation, leisure, and sports	Accessible toys, indoor games, arts and crafts, photography, physical fitness, gardening, camping, hiking, fishing, hunting, shooting, sports equipment, musical instruments
Modified furniture and furnishings	Tables, light fixtures, sitting furniture, beds and bedding, adjustable height furniture, work furniture

Source: U.S. Department of Education (2000).

Universal Design

Another dimension of technology that is rapidly working its way into public policy is the notion of *universal design*. Architect Ron Mace introduced the concept as the "design of products and environments to be usable by all people, to the greatest extent possible, without the need for adaptation or specialized design" (Mace as cited in Center for Universal Design, 1997). Universal design has since evolved as a design construct that extends beyond architecture into multiple domains, including learning environments, curriculum, instructional materials, programmatic structures, consumer products, and technologies. It presumes that individuals of varying abilities are the norm and encourages design considerations that are inclusive. Within the context of education, Skip Stahl from Center for Applied Special Technology (CAST) framed the discussion about universal design and curriculum by noting that "assistive technology provides solutions that extend the capabilities of the user. Universal Design provides solutions that extend the capabilities of the curriculum" (Stahl & Cusack, 2002).

The practical ramifications of universal design are played out in the increasing number of generically available technologies that are able to be used by individuals with disabilities without the addition of assistive technology. A confirmation of this trend was reported in a survey of American users of assistive technology, which noted that access to universally designed products and environmental access features reduced the need for assistive technology devices and services for 52% of the survey respondents (Carlson, Ehrlich, Berland, & Bailey, 2001).

Trends in legislation that support the implementation of universal design include the Telecommunications Act of 1996 (PL 104-104), which mandates that telecommunications products and services be accessible to and useable by individuals with disabilities or at least compatible with assistive technology. Although this legislation does not directly provide access to assistive technology, it has gone a long way to facilitate access to education, employment, and community integration through the use of accessible technologies.

One strategic example is the requirement that all televisions be built with closed caption decoding technology. Prior to this legislation, individuals who needed this technology had to buy expensive equipment to access this feature in television broadcasts. Now, this technology not only benefits individuals with hearing impairments, but it also benefits patrons at noisy sports bars and exercise clubs. It is used by parents to foster emerging literacy skills, and it provides a bridge to content for non-English speaking viewers.

Section 508 of PL 104-104 requires federal agencies to make their electronic and information technology accessible to people with disabilities. This law applies to all federal agencies when they develop, procure, maintain, or use electronic and information technology. In addition, federal agencies must give employees with disabilities and members of the public access to information that is comparable to the access available to others. The standards adopted in support of this legislation serve as models of best practice that can be adopted by all information technology designers.

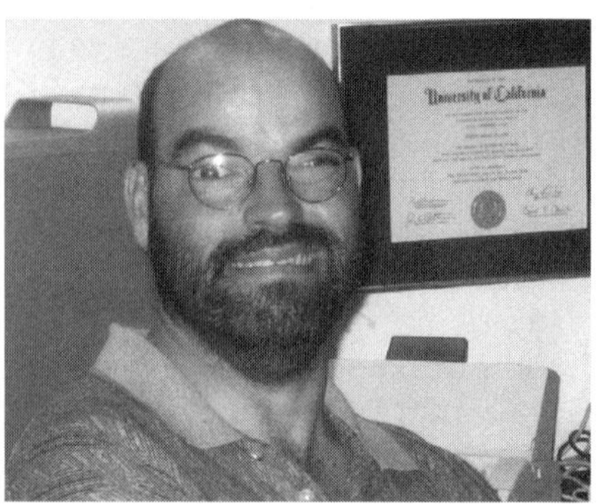

Figure 24.4-2. Dave Clarke is a freelance web development consultant in Boston.

Dave Clarke, a freelance web development consultant in Boston, is aggressively oriented to leveraging universal design in technology (see Figure 24.4-2). Anticipating the need for a rugged and resilient computer, he purchased a Panasonic Toughbook laptop that was originally designed to support contractors in the difficult environment of heavy construction. Dave is also using other features that are native to the computer's operating system to facilitate more efficient keyboarding. He gains access to control panel features like sticky keys, which eliminates the need for simultaneous keystrokes and makes them sequential. He has remapped the keyboard configuration to the Dvorak layout, an ergonomic layout that is more sensitive to keyboarding efficiency than the typical QWERTY layout. Dave also uses the autocorrect feature in Word and Outlook to emulate a type expansion program.

Moving beyond trends, a new policy has emerged with the reauthorization of IDEA in 2004 as the Individuals with Disabilities Education Improvement Act (PL 108-446). The National Instructional Materials Accessibility Standard (NIMAS) requires that publishers adopt a specific digital file format for all textbooks and related print materials. Through NIMAS, all students (age 3–21) with print-based disabilities will have ready access to academic content that can be quickly and easily converted to a format that works best for them, such as Braille or text-to-speech. Inititatives such as NIMAS, accessible information technology, and universal design all work in concert to promote barrier-free and inclusive access to home, school, work, and community environments.

Consumer-Driven Assessment Models

Assistive technology assessments are conducted in a variety of settings; typical providers include hospitals and rehabilitation centers. Each state's Tech Act Agency should have a complete listing of the agencies that provide this kind of service. The process for evaluating an individual's needs is multifaceted and cannot be simplified by aligning a disability type with a specific technology. Preferred models of assistive technology assessment reflect a holistic and person-centered orientation that seeks to actively engage the individual in the process. These models are sensitive to assessing individual needs within the context of the tasks and environment that the technology will be used.

This model is a departure from some of the traditional clinical or hospital-based assessment models in which an individual was evaluated outside the context of his or her natural environment (home, school, work, community settings). The assessment process is enhanced if a multidisciplinary and collaborative team approach is used (Bromley, 2001). Although many clinical settings are adopting the best practice of a multidisciplinary approach, Dr. Howard Shane, Director of the Communication Enhancement Clinic at Children's Hospital Boston, is taking this process one step further by piloting an innovative strategy of using real-time video conferencing to direct and support the assessment, implementation, and adoption of technology in natural setting (Shane & Cordeiro, 2003).

Reimer-Reiss and Wacker suggested the following recommendations should be integrated into all assistive technology assessment and acquisition models:

> A recommended model acknowledges both consumers and professionals as team members. Initially, the consumer is educated about assistive technology choices, financing options, training and resources for maintenance. The consumer then contributes knowledge of his/her personal needs, goals, values and preferences. Solutions are generated through an open exchange of information with all the team members. Finally, the consumer selects the assistive technology that best fits his/her needs. Overall, the findings of this study support two key elements related to successful use of assistive technology. The consumer must be involved in the entire process and the technology must meet an important functional need. (2000, p. 49)

An additional criterion is the establishment of a goal that is linked to measurable outcomes. In articulating a goal, the selection of technology becomes more specific. In establishing outcome measures, the appropriateness of the technology intervention can be assessed and reevaluated.

Michael uses a variety of assistive technologies. His favorite is his bike (see Figure 24.4-3). He experimented with a lot of different bikes and finally settled on one that he saw at the Massachusetts Department of Environmental Management–Universal Access sponsored annual event at the Norratuck bike trail in Northampton, Massachusetts. Michael found a bike that he could use and that he liked from one of the vendors, Bill Darby for Special Purpose Vehicles. The bike he selected was a modified recumbent bike with two-wheels in the front and one in the back.

"It is yellow and cool. I can go to Cumbie's and to get a Dew," he said. "I leave my Mom in my dust."

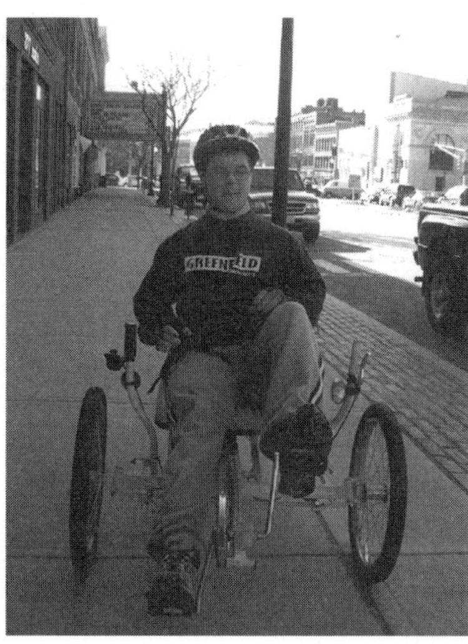

Figure 24.4-3. Michael experimented with a lot of different bikes before he settled on his favorite. (Photo courtesy of Martin A. McGuane, Greenfield, MA, Cable TV.)

The underlying emphasis in all assessment models is to ensure the best match for the individual to the technology. Given that the rate of technology abandonment exceeds 29.3% (Phillips & Zhao, 1993, as cited in Riemer-Reiss & Wacker, 2000), it is important that all participants are sensitive to the many factors involved in the process of technology selection, including those that go beyond alignment of technology and functional needs. These more subtle factors include awareness of the predisposition to using technology, culture, training, and affordability.

Cultural Awareness

According to Jezewski and Sotnik (2002), "Culture sensitivity does not have to do solely with ethnicity. It has to do with the similarities and differences in the values, beliefs and behaviors between the cultural systems of the consumers and the service providers." Most models related to the acquisition of assistive technology are heavily oriented to the consumer and seek to promote outcomes related to independence and self-determination. This orientation, however, may be problematic for some families, particularly linguistically and culturally diverse families. The benefits of meaningful consumer and family involvement in the technology selection and adoption process can be significantly undermined if issues related to family values, cultural influences, and other effects that assistive technology may have on the family are not taken into consideration (Parette & VanBiervliet, 2000).

For example, for some African Americans, a strong sense of community integration may lead to higher preference for blending in. The introduction of assistive technology within this context may be difficult if issues of social inclusion are not addressed with the family (Parette, Huer, & Wyatt, 2002). Within Asian and Hispanic families, where patterns of family interdependence are prevalent, introduction of technologies that foster greater independence and less reliance on the family network may be negatively perceived (Parette & McMahan, 2002). These examples should not be construed as absolutes but as indicators of the necessity of cultural sensitivity in service delivery models.

Funding Options

In spite of legislative action that supports better communication between federal and state agencies, there continue to be substantial gaps in access to technology when looking at the comprehensive needs of an individual with a disability. Access to technology is achievable from birth to 21 via the school system. After age 21, a person can look to employment as a vehicle for gaining access to much-needed technology, but technology is restricted to devices that relate to the individual's job responsibilities. No coordinated service or entity looks *holistically* at the needs of the individual to ensure well-being.

Support for funding assistive technology continues to be dependent on several variables. As the variables shift across a life span, so does the availability of funding. The age of the individual, the person's income, the nature of the disability, the environment that the device will be used in (e.g., home, school, work, community), and the desired outcome of the device (e.g., to inhibit a medical condition, to receive FAPE, to gain independence at home or work, to provide recreation) all affect funding availability. Although the variables may shift, consistent criteria must be followed to secure whatever funding may be available.

The Wyoming New Options in Technology (WYNO) initiative identified the following framework as critical for organizing information and mapping out an individual's access to assistive technology funding. Although this model was developed for Wyoming, the framework is transferable to other states.

1. Define the need.
2. Document the need.
3. Identify the equipment and/or services needed, and secure necessary prescriptions and other justification.
4. Determine if alternative equipment will meet the need.
5. Determine funding sources.
6. Collect and submit the required paper work.
7. Receive authorization.
8. Search for co-payment options.
9. Complete the appeals process.

Funding sources can also be difficult to identify. Although some technologies can be secured through school or places of employment, funding for other technologies may not be that obvious. Table 24.4-2 was generated by the Institute for Community Inclusion at the University of Massachusetts–Boston for the National Center on Workforce and Disability to assist consumers and businesses in addressing alternative funding strategies.

CONCLUSION

According to Hehir, "As the disability movement has demonstrated over and over, there is more than one way to walk, talk, point, read, and write. Assuming otherwise is the root of fundamental inequities" (2002, p. 17). In addition to supporting access to funding and other resources, medical practitioners can broker their networks and facilitate access to traditional (rehabilitation agencies, veterans assistance services, Medicaid) and nontraditional (church and community-based organizations, nonprofit agencies, support groups) resources. In doing so, practitioners are helping consumers and their families gain the knowledge they need to be informed decision makers and become more comfortable with the task before them.

Medical practitioners can also model access considerations and cultural sensitivity within their practices. The following questions may help to contextualize some of these considerations:

- Are pathways in the office of adequate width?
- Are signs in the office appropriate?

Table 24.4-2. Funding sources for assistive technology, equipment, and accommodations

Funding source	Comments	For more information/contact
Employer	Required to fund only if meets criteria for "reasonable accommodation" under the Americans with Disabilities Act (ADA) of 1990 (PL 101-336)	Employer costs can be offset by: ADA Small Business Tax Credit—up to $5,000/year Contact Internal Revenue Service via government pages of telephone book or http://www.irs.ustreas.gov Work Opportunity Tax Credit (WOTC) and Welfare to Work (WtW) Tax Credit—Any employer can receive up to $2,400/employee from WOTC and $8,500/employee from WtW. Contact U.S. Department of Labor via government pages of telephone book or at http://www.doleta.gov/employer/wotc.htm; forms available by calling (877) 828-2050.
Vocational Rehabilitation (VR)	One-Stop partner; must qualify for VR services	VR contact via One-Stop should be able to help.
Medicare	For people who have Medicare health insurance	Contact local Medicare office (government pages of telephone book) or Centers for Medicare & Medicaid Services (CMS) at http://www.cms.hhs.gov
Medicaid	For people who have Medicare health insurance. State may have additional guidelines.	Contact local Medicare office (government pages of telephone book) or CMS at http://www.cms.hhs.gov.
Private insurance	Varies	Check policy and/or contact carrier.
Social Security Work Incentives	IRWE—for people on Supplemental Security Income (SSI) and Social Security Disability Insurance (SSDI) PASS—for people on SSI	Contact local Social Security Administration (SSA) office or call (800) 772-1213; web site: http://www.ssa.gov/work.
Veteran's Affairs (VA)	For people who are veterans or dependents of veterans.	Contact the VA via the government pages of the telephone book or at (800) 827-1000; web site: http://www.va.gov.
Local service, charitable, religious, and civic organizations	Check to see if individual with disability has connection with such an organization.	Local community guides and telephone books often have listings of such organizations.
Private foundations	Application procedures and response times vary significantly.	The Foundation Center; 79 Fifth Avenue, New York, NY 10003; (212) 620-4230; fax: (212) 691-1828; e-mail: library@fdncenter.org; web site: http://fdncenter.org Each state also has a Foundation Center "cooperating collection."

From Institute for Community Inclusion. (2002). *Funding assistive technology and accommodations.* National Center on Workforce and Disability/Adult. Retrieved August 15, 2003, from http://www.onestops.info/article.php?article_id=22; adapted by permission.

- Is medical information available in alternate formats and provided in a way that is culturally sensitive and cognitively accessible?
- Are resources about assistive technology available for patients to review?
- Are there ways to normalize the use of different technologies through modeling (e.g., a communication board with picture symbols to communicate ideas, a flashlight pen to track a sentence in a pamphlet, a poster on the wall that includes users of technology in real-life situations)?

Finally, medical practitioners can be vital participants in the effort to build awareness within the medical community, the public, and the legislature about the complexity of access to assistive technology. In modeling, strategies that encourage access to assistive technology, the integration of universal design considerations, and the commitment to culturally sensitive practices, medical practitioners make a very real contribution to the day-to-day well-being of individuals with disabilities.

REFERENCES

Americans with Disabilities Act (ADA) of 1990, PL 101-336, 42 U.S.C. §§ 12101 *et seq.*

Assistive Technology Act of 2004, PL 108-364, 118 Stat. 1707.

AT/AAC enABLES. (n.d.). *About assistive technology (AT): Who benefits from AT?* Retrieved September 10, 2003, from http://depts.washington.edu/enables/education/about_at.htm

Bromley, B. (2001, March). *Assistive technology assessment: A comparative analysis of five models.* Paper presented at the California State University, Northridge Center on Disability Sixteenth Annual International Conference on Technology and Persons with Disabilities Conference, Los Angeles. Retrieved September 5, 2003, from http://rose.iinf.polsl.gliwice.pl/~kwadrat/www.csun.edu/cod/conf2001/proceedings/0193bromley.html

Canfield, T., & Reed, P. (2001). *Assistive technology and transition.* Wisconsin Assistive Technology Initiative. Retrieved August 15, 2003, from http://www.wati.org/pdf/attransitionpacket.pdf

Carlson, D., Ehrlich, N., Berland, B.J., & Bailey, N. (2001, September 27). *Assistive technology survey results: Continued benefits and needs reported by Americans with disabilities.* Retrieved September 15, 2003, from http://www.ncddr.org/du/researchexchange/v07n01/atpaper/ATpaper.pdf

Center for Universal Design. (1997). *What is universal design? Definition.* North Carolina State University. Retrieved September 5, 2003, from http://www.design.ncsu.edu/cud/univ_design/ud.htm

Hehir, T. (2002, Spring). Eliminating ableism in education. *Harvard Educational Review, 72*(1), 1–29.

Individuals with Disabilities Education Act (IDEA) of 1990, PL 101-476, 20 U.S.C. §§ 1400 *et seq.*

Individuals with Disabilities Education Improvement Act of 2004, PL 108-446, 20 U.S.C. §§ 1400 *et seq.*

Institute for Community Inclusion. (2002). *Funding assistive technology and accommodations.* National Center on Workforce and Disability/Adult. Retrieved August 15, 2003, from http://www.onestops.info/article.php?article_id=22

Jezewski, M., & Sotnik, P. (2002). *Culture brokering: Providing culturally competent rehabilitation services to foreign-born persons. Appendix 1, Table 5.* Retrieved August 20, 2003, from http://cirrie.buffalo.edu/cbrokering.html

Job Accommodation Network. (2002). *Facts about job accommodations.* Retrieved September 10, 2003, from http://www.jan.wvu.edu/media/JANFacts.html

Mendelson, S. (1995, September). New approaches to physician involvement in assistive technology. *Tapping Technology.* Retrieved October 1, 2003, from http://www.mdtap.org/tt/1995.09/art_1.html

Mistrett, S. (2001). *Synthesis on the use of assistive technology with infants and toddlers (birth through age two).* Retrieved August 15, 2003, from http://www.air.org/techideas/reports.html

National Assistive Technology Research Institute. (2001). *Assistive technology resources: Technology types: A complex example.* Retrieved August 24, 2003, from http://natri.uky.edu/resources/fundamentals/types.html

Olmstead v. L.C., 138 F.3d 893 (1999).

Parette, P., Huer, M., & Wyatt, T. (2002, Spring). Young African American children with disabilities and augmentative and alternative communication issues. [Electronic version]. *Early Childhood Education Journal, 29*(3), 201–207.

Parette, P., & McMahan, G. (2002, October). What should we expect of assistive technology? [Electronic version]. *Teaching Exceptional Children, 35*(1), 56–61.

Parette, P., & VanBiervliet, A. (2000, Winter). Family-centered decision making in assistive technology. *Journal of Special Education Technology, 15*(1). Retrieved September 17, 2003, http://jset.unlv.edu/15.1/parette/parette.pdf

Rehabilitation Act of 1973, PL 93-112, 29 U.S.C. §§ 701 *et seq.*

Riemer-Reiss, M.L., & Wacker, R.R. (2000, July–September). Factors associated with assistive technology discontinuance among individuals with disabilities. [Electronic version] *Journal of Rehabilitation, 66*(3), 44–50.

Shane, H.C., & Cordeiro, R.F. (2003, November). *The internet as a service delivery medium for assistive technology: A demonstration project.* Paper presented at the Annual meeting of the American Speech-Language-Hearing Association, Chicago.

Stahl, S., & Cusack, S. (2002, July). *Access, participation & progress: Leveraging universal design and assistive technologies to support all learners.* Presented at the Project MEET Summer Teacher Institute, Springfield, MA.

Technology-Related Assistance for Individuals with Disabilities Act of 1988, PL 100-407, 29 U.S.C. §§ 2201 *et seq.*

Telecommunications Act of 1996, PL 104-104, 110 Stat. 56.

U.S. Department of Commerce. (February, 2003). *Technology assessment of the U.S. assistive technology industry: Market demands for the future.* Retrieved August 20, 2003, from http://www.icdr.us/atreportweb/sec1/market.htm

U.S. Department of Education, National Institute on Disability and Rehabilitation Research. (2000, August). *National classification system for assistive technology devices and services.* Washington, DC: Author.

U.S. Department of Health and Human Services. (2001) *Executive order 13217.* Retrieved September 7, 2003, from http://www.hhs.gov/newfreedom/eo13217.html

U.S. Department of Health and Human Services. (2003) *Your rights under section 504 of the rehabilitation act: What is section 504?* Retrieved September 10, 2003, from http://www.hhs.gov/ocr/504.html

Wisconsin Assistive Technology Initiative. (1998). *Assistive technology consideration.* Retrieved August 15, 2003, from http://www.wati.org/atconsideration.htm

CHAPTER 25

WOMEN'S HEALTH

*Sheryl White-Scott, Deborah Spitalnik,
Yona Lunsky, and Susan Havercamp*

Health care for women with developmental disabilities rests on their status as adults with disabilities, as women, and as women with disabilities. Traditionally, medical and health knowledge about intellectual and developmental disabilities was concentrated in pediatrics. Although intellectual disabilities were originally perceived to be a condition of childhood, people with a full range of developmental disabilities are living longer and need age-appropriate health care delivered by practitioners trained in adult specialties, increasingly including geriatrics. Inaccessible health care and trained professionals may contribute to a lack of identification and treatment of preventable diseases (Spitalnik & White-Scott, 2001).

The routine health care needs of women with developmental disabilities are often overlooked and, in many areas, are unknown. Women face multiple barriers when trying to obtain medical services, often due to a lack of information. The lack of established and validated protocols of care for conditions associated with developmental disabilities may hamper care as well as health care quality improvement efforts.

Women's health has developed into a new area of coordinated health care with attention to specific guidelines and standards of care. Some of the impetus for the development of women's health was self-advocacy by the women's movement in the late 1960s and early 1970s (Boston Women's Health Collective, 1973). This advocacy did not include women with developmental disabilities, whose routine and specialized health care needs are often overlooked by both specialized disability service systems and women's health care providers. Women with disabilities are beginning to organize themselves around health care issues in self-help groups analogous to the early mainstream women's movement and also to hold conferences and other educational events.

The knowledge base about women's health is somewhat limited compared with research on health, including drug efficacy, typically conducted on men. The National Institutes of Health have been working to eliminate these gender disparities in research. Limited research and assessment of the health care needs and clinical management of women with developmental disabilities is available compared with women (or men) without interferences in their development. The Centers for Disease Control and Prevention state projects are expected to increase the knowledge base on the health of women with developmental disabilities.

An additional strand in the consideration of health and health care for women with developmental disabilities is the dual disadvantages of both having a disability and being female. The historical conceptualization, prevalent during the eugenics movement of the late 19th and early 20th centuries, portrayed the "feebleminded female" with her degenerate sexuality as contributing to the moral decay of society (Bragar, 1977). Although long discredited, the taint of this viewpoint has probably contributed to long-held negative views or denial of the sexuality and the sexual and reproductive health of women with developmental disabilities.

This chapter focuses on health care for women with developmental disabilities and reviews current practices and approaches. Addressing the health needs of girls and women with developmental disabilities provides an important opportunity for practitioners to influence health and well-being in their fullest dimensions.

INTRODUCTION

Comprehensive women's health care requires more than just gynecological procedures and should promote self-awareness of one's body, sexuality, health, and well-being (Welner, 1997). A basic understanding of psychosocial issues for women with intellectual and developmental disabilities is an important part of providing optimal health care. Historically, women with intellectual and developmental disabilities were treated as if they were either asexual or sexually irresponsible (Scior,

2000). Women were sterilized without their consent, segregated from men as a means of preventing sexual interactions, and denied any formal sex education. The American Association on Mental Retardation (2004) and The Arc of the United States issued a policy statement on sexuality illustrating a significant philosophical shift. The policy states that "people with MR/DD [intellectual and developmental disabilities], like all people, have inherent sexual rights and basic human needs. These rights and needs must be affirmed, defended, promoted, and respected."

Today, girls and women with intellectual and developmental disabilities are more likely to be provided with sex education; however, they are not necessarily taught how to feel good about their bodies, how to negotiate sexual relationships, or how to express their sexual feelings. They often have a negative self-image and feel that they lack control over their lives and their bodies (McCarthy, 1999). Assumptions about sexual interest or activity cannot be made on the basis of severity of intellectual disabilities. One health clinic survey showed that 50% of adolescent girls with mild intellectual disabilities and 30% of girls with moderate intellectual disabilities were sexually active (Chamberlain, Rauth, Passer, McGrath, & Burket, 1984). Regardless of whether they are involved with a sexual partner, women with intellectual and developmental disabilities have sexual needs and may need support and direction in expressing these needs.

HEALTH EDUCATION

Women with intellectual and developmental disabilities are at increased risk for many health problems, such as osteoporosis, cardiovascular disease, diabetes, and thyroid problems (Rimmer, Braddock, & Fujiura, 1994; Walsh, Heller, Schupf, & van Schrojensein Lantman-de Valk, 2000) and often lack general knowledge about standard medical procedures and activities to promote health (Lunsky, Straiko, & Armstrong, 2003). They may experience pain or discomfort but not know what to do about it. One woman with Williams Syndrome described,

> Ever since puberty I have had a dreadful time with my periods. I have had days of so much pain that all I can do is go to my bed and take a painkiller. All I want is for my periods to stop and disappear all together. (Schwartz, 2000, p. 5)

Physicians should be sensitive to women's comfort level during routine examinations as well as to their health concerns. Anxiety and "noncompliance" in the doctor's office may be due to past sexual abuse (see the section on abuse later in this chapter) or a negative experience during a prior medical examination. The trauma of either can turn a checkup into a horrible, frightening ordeal (Elkins, 1997). For this reason, women must be educated about their health and be informed prior to and following routine examinations. Health education should include instruction on women's anatomy and function, healthy lifestyle choices, health risks and disease, and standard examination procedures. It should also provide women with coping strategies to deal with invasive procedures such as pelvic examinations.

To help prepare for medical examinations, women can be introduced to the health care setting in a nonthreatening manner. Visiting the doctor's office and learning about procedures, speaking with medical staff, and familiarizing oneself with medical instruments can help any woman feel better prepared for her medical care (Elkins, 1997). Finally, women with intellectual and developmental disabilities who have been rewarded for passive and compliant behavior need to be taught how to be more assertive when it comes to their health care. They should be encouraged to ask the doctor questions, they should practice describing health problems and expressing their concerns, and they should take responsibility for their health (Lunsky, Straiko, & Armstrong, 2002).

EXPLOITATION

Women with intellectual and developmental disabilities are vulnerable to exploitation across the life span by professionals, community members, family, and other people with disabilities. Rates of sexual abuse, for example, are higher for these women than for any other disability group. Their heightened vulnerability comes into play whenever they are treated by medical professionals. Clinicians must be sensitive to potential abuse in a woman's past, and hypervigilant about potential abuse that may be ongoing. A supportive and accepting attitude is essential for women to feel comfortable disclosing potential abuse and feel safe if they choose to or are able to discuss their situation.

All women with intellectual and developmental disabilities need to learn about safe sex practices at a level that is meaningful to them. This instruction should include finding the appropriate time and place for sexual activity and knowing how to protect oneself from disease or unwanted pregnancy. Women must understand the importance of and their right to give consent to sexual activity, including the knowledge that one can change her mind about engaging in sex at any time. Even women who appear educated may be misinformed. One young woman with mild intellectual disabilities reported to her doctor that she did not use condoms with her boyfriend because he told her that birth control pills would protect her from any diseases. Only when she learned about symptoms of sexually transmitted diseases (STDs) in a women's health class did she discover that she had contracted an STD from this man.

An important aspect of sex education is the practical side of negotiating sexual relations. One woman with intellectual and developmental disabilities explained,

> I do not like all of the confusing feelings that I have about sex. For me, knowing the basics is not enough because sometimes I just do not feel what other people feel. Occasionally what is supposed to be pleasurable has turned out instead to be painful. (Schwartz, 2000, p. 5)

Women should be taught to be assertive about their comfort level and sexual needs. They should feel ownership over their bodies, understanding that they have the right to refuse sex at any time, even if the partner is someone they have been intimate with before. One of the most important concepts for a woman with intellectual and developmental disabilities to learn is that her body is private and should only be touched with permission. This message can be reinforced during checkups by asking permission and informing the woman what is going to happen prior to invading her personal space.

Women (and men) should learn that if someone touches them in a way that they do not like, they should seek help by telling someone whom they trust. Outside of the doctor's office, women can learn that their bodies are private by being given privacy when changing clothes or bathing. If a woman requires assistance taking a bath, for example, she could bathe with bubbles so that she feels more protected.

Finally, women need to learn that discussing sexuality is part of a comprehensive medical assessment. Physicians should never assume that a woman is not sexually active and, when asking about sexual activity, physicians should realize that the woman might prefer to discuss such issues in private and not with agency staff or family who may have accompanied her to the doctor's visit. Physicians may need to learn about relevant sexuality policies endorsed by the woman's service agency and about the caregivers' attitudes toward sexuality, particularly when such attitudes do not correspond with the views of the woman. How caregivers respond to the sexual expression of a woman they support has important consequences for the woman's health and self-esteem (Valenti-Hein & Dura, 1996).

ABUSE

As noted in the prior section, women with developmental disabilities are more likely than women without disabilities and men with developmental disabilities to experience sexual abuse (Stromsness, 1993). Wilson and Brewer (1992) reported that women with intellectual and developmental disabilities were 10.7 times more likely to be sexually assaulted than other women. According to the University of Alberta Violence and Disability Project (Sobsey, 2000), of 100 sexually abused women and adolescent girls with intellectual and developmental disabilities, nearly half reported repeated sexual assaults (more than 10 incidents). Only 8.3% of the offenders were strangers, with the most common perpetrators being family friends, service providers, other people with disabilities, and family members. Ninety-five percent of the women suffered social, emotional, and physical harm from the assault but only 20% received appropriate counseling or therapy (Mansell, Sobsey, & Calder, 1992). Thus, sexual abuse was reported to be frighteningly common for women with developmental disabilities, and inadequate treatment was the norm.

Women with intellectual and developmental disabilities have a greater risk than the general population of being victims of physical violence (Wilson & Brewer, 1992). Little is known about intimate partner violence, but it may be quite common among the minority of women with intellectual and developmental disabilities who have intimate partners. Carlson (1998) interviewed women with intellectual and developmental disabilities and found that many of women were physically abused, threatened, controlled, insulted, blamed, and isolated from others by their partner. A lack of social support, low self-esteem, and weak assertiveness skills made it difficult for these women to leave the abusive relationship or seek help.

Caregiver abuse and abuse from peers have also been documented for women with intellectual and developmental disabilities (Sobsey, 2000). On occasion, such violence is severe enough to lead to death, but more often subtle forms of violence or coercion take place. Women with intellectual and developmental disabilities may not think that they have a right to more humane treatment or may fear losing services if they report the abuse. As a consequence of their intellectual disabilities, they may also be more compliant and anxious to please those they perceive as authorities (Spitalnik & White-Scott, 2001).

Amy is a 24-year-old woman with moderate intellectual disabilities. She came to the attention of social services when she was referred to a work program after graduation from high school. Work supervisors immediately noticed that Amy was very shy and suspicious of new people; displayed an exaggerated startle response to loud noises or sudden movements; and sometimes had visible bruises on her arms, face, and neck.

Initially, she insisted that the bruises were self-inflicted or she explained them away as evidence of her clumsiness. After several months, however, Amy admitted that she suffered ongoing emotional, physical, and sexual abuse at the hands of her grandfather. With the support of her supervisors at work, Amy was able to contact the authorities and moved from her grandfather's home into a group home.

Four years later, Amy still worked and had moved from the group home into a supervised apartment. She loved her apartment and valued her privacy, but she complained of frequent nightmares in which her grandfather forced her to live with him. She would wake from these nightmares in a panic and would be unable to fall back to sleep. Occasionally, she caught a glimpse of a man at a store and thought that it was her grandfather. When this happened, she ran out of the store very upset, shaking, crying, and hyperventilating.

With appropriate supports and mental health services, Amy was able to overcome her abusive past. She was diagnosed with posttraumatic stress disorder and treated with anxiolytic medication and individual psychotherapy. She was also taught specific strategies to cope with her fear. Emotion recognition, relaxation training, and problem-solving skills helped her to feel more aware and in control of her feelings. She now reports that her nightmares have decreased and she rarely feels frightened or thinks about her past abuse.

Physicians should be aware of this potential for abuse at the hands of staff, peers, or family and be prepared to intervene as required. For example, Amy's bruising was only brought to the attention of medical professionals after it was noted by her care staff.

Helping women avoid or escape abusive situations can occur at both at the individual and societal level (see Carlson, 1997, for further detail). At the individual level, predisposing personal characteristics can be targeted, such as dependency, overcompliance, and low self-esteem. Skill deficits can be addressed by teaching the woman to solve problems, behave assertively, and seek help. Women who are victims of abuse would likely benefit from individual therapy to help them cope with feelings of guilt, vulnerability, and anxiety. These services were of great benefit to Amy.

At the societal level, appropriate services for abuse victims with intellectual and developmental disabilities must be developed. This process may involve training personnel at existing facilities (e.g., rape crisis centers) to work with women with intellectual disabilities. Once appropriate services are in place, advocacy will be needed to ensure that victims have access to services (e.g., social services, criminal justice services, health and medical agencies, housing/employment services) in a timely manner.

Efforts to prevent abuse and exploitation should be directed at all levels of the service delivery system. First, health care providers should teach and reinforce assertiveness in individuals with developmental disabilities. They should ask permission before touching a woman during an exam and respect her level of comfort. They should also reassure the woman that she can always talk to the doctor in private, if desired. In addition, health care providers must be vigilant to signs of abuse, including changes in behavior (e.g., anxiety, fearfulness, secretiveness, sleep disturbances) as well as physical signs such as bruising. Second, parents and service providers need to be educated about the vulnerability of women with developmental disabilities to exploitation so they are alert to risky situations and early warning signs of abuse. Third, health care providers should monitor the stress level of parents and caregivers. They may recommend respite services to help caregivers avoid burnout, thereby lowering the abuse potential of the environment.

MENTAL HEALTH

Prevalence estimates place the rate of "dual diagnosis" or co-occurrence of intellectual disabilities and mental health problems at 39%, generally higher than that of the general population (Maxmen & Ward, 1995; Reiss, 1982). This apparent vulnerability has been attributed to biological risk factors including seizure and genetic disorders as well as social risk factors, such as social strain and low levels of social support. In the general population, women are recognized to be more vulnerable to certain psychiatric disorders than men (Culbertson, 1997). Epidemiological studies report no differences in the overall rate of psychiatric disturbance in men versus women; however, differences were found in the prevalence of specific disorders across gender (Kessler, McGonagle, & Zhao, 1994; Robins & Regier, 1991).

Women are twice as likely to have mood and anxiety disorders, whereas men tend to have more difficulties with substance abuse and antisocial behaviors (Kessler et al., 1994; Robins & Regier, 1991). Women are also more likely to report physical symptoms of distress, such as headaches and fatigue, than men. When gender differences were examined in adults with developmental disabilities, similar trends were reported (e.g., Benson, 1985; Heiman & Margalit, 1998; Koller, Richardson, Katz, & McLaren, 1983; Lunsky & Benson, 2001; Meins, 1993; Reiss, 1982; Reiss, 1988; Reiss & Trenn, 1984; Reynolds & Miller, 1985). Schizophrenia and bipolar disorder are reported to occur with equal frequency in men and women in the general population (American Psychological Association, 1994; Castle, 2000; Walsh, 1998) and in individuals with intellectual and developmental disabilities (Glue, 1989; Benson, 1985; Reiss, 1982).

Identifying Mental Health Problems

Physicians should be aware that there is a strong bias against reporting mental health problems in women with intellectual and developmental disabilities (Borthwick-Duffy, 1994). They should guard against this bias when conducting their evaluation. Referrals to mental health service are biased in favor of certain types of mental health or behavioral problems, partially due to the fact that very few individuals with developmental disabilities initiate the referral process themselves (Fletcher, 1993; Nezu & Nezu, 1994). As many individuals with developmental disabilities have a limited ability to provide an accurate self-report, their referral for mental health services largely depends on the ability of family members and program/service staff to recognize the presence of behavioral and emotional disturbance.

Aggression and other acting-out behaviors attract attention and evoke a referral more often than do symptoms of sadness or withdrawal (Charlot, Doucette, & Mezzacappa, 1993; Edelstein & Glenwick, 1997; Ghaziuddin, 1988; Stack, Haldipur, & Thompson, 1987). This referral bias has implications for women's mental health because men are more likely to display acting-out behaviors, whereas women are more likely to have depressive or anxious symptoms (Benson, 1985; Day, 1985; Reiss, 1982). Therefore, women's mental health problems tend to go unrecognized and untreated.

Mental health screening should be part of routine care for individuals with developmental disabilities. Brief screening instruments are available to detect mental health problems based on informant ratings (The Reiss Screen for Maladaptive Behavior, Reiss, 1988; PAS-ADD Checklist, Moss et al., 1998). Mental health problems may present differently in women with intellectual and developmental disabilities. Women may be more likely to express their emotional distress through somatic complaints (Lunsky, 2003). A stomachache may be that woman's way of communicating that she is too anxious to go to work, for example.

It may be necessary to take extra time to build rapport with the woman with intellectual and developmental disabilities so that she feels comfortable expressing her feelings. She may think that it is wrong to say that she is feeling sad, not realizing that all people can experience negative emotions. Particularly if some of her emotional difficulties relate to women's issues, she may prefer to discuss her concerns with another woman present, such as a social worker or nurse practitioner, which was the case for Amy, who needed to feel very safe before she could disclose the sexual abuse that was happening to her.

Physicians should be alert to the following changes as possible indicators of emotional strain: changes in interests or activity level; decrease in adaptive skills; decrease in self-esteem; changes in health, hygiene, or appearance; exacerbation of problems with communication, attention, memory, or learning; changes in sleep or appetite; unusual mood or emotional expression; or changes in relationships or sexual expression. Such information may not be available without the cooperation of caregivers, particularly when the person with the disability has communication impairments. Therefore, health care professionals need to work closely with caregivers to obtain observations, documentation, and objective measures of behavioral changes.

Physicians should be sensitive to the fact that women with developmental disabilities may react strongly to stressors that appear minor, such as a change in staffing or routine. In fact, stress reactions frequently explain the onset or exacerbation of emotional or behavior problems for women in the general population and for women with intellectual and developmental disabilities (Walsh et al., 2000). When suffering a loss, women with intellectual and developmental disabilities experience grief and bereavement like anyone else. Unfortunately, service providers tend to minimize the impact of such loss. Physicians should ask about any life or relationship changes that might precede or coincide with the behavior change.

Treatment Issues

Mental health and behavior problems in individuals with intellectual and developmental disabilities respond to the same interventions that have proven effective in the general population (i.e., psychotherapy, especially behavior therapy and cognitive-behavior therapy, and psychotropic medication). Prior to prescribing medication, other possibilities should be considered, such as increasing the woman's social network, providing suggestions to her and her caregivers, and helping to reduce the stress in her immediate environment. It was helpful for Amy, for example, to escape the abusive environment of her grandfather's home and to receive the emotional support of her supervisors at work.

Communication problems may limit not only the reporting of symptoms but also the use of certain therapeutic techniques. Psychotherapy outcome data for women (and men) with intellectual and developmental disabilities is lacking (Prout, Chard, Nowak-Drabik, & Johnson, 2000). In the general population, women report differences in therapeutic gain and side effect profiles from psychotropic medications (Fitzgerald & Seeman, 2000). Unfortunately, very little attention has been paid to gender issues in response to medication for people with intellectual and developmental disabilities (e.g., Reiss & Aman, 1998; Rinck, 1998).

Obtaining some information from women with communication impairments is difficult unless it is explicitly monitored and documented by caregivers, including ratings of activity, appetite, lactation, weight gain, and sleep patterns. Because women with intellectual and developmental disabilities are unlikely to self-report symptoms of emotional distress, physicians should consider their emotional state as part of their routine health checkup. Also, physicians should review current medications, possible interactions, and side effects on a regular basis, including how medications interact with menstrual cycles.

Mental Health Promotion

The area of women's mental health is not just about women's struggles with mental illness but also about how women can lead healthy emotional lives. Mental health promotion is an important part of general health promotion for women with intellectual and developmental disabilities. An important role of the physician may involve education of caregivers, both family members and direct support workers. Services and resources need to be offered to caregivers who may be misinformed about women with intellectual and developmental disabilities and their mental health. Caregivers could be taught, for example, how to recognize mental health problems as well as how to encourage the woman to express emotions and mental health concerns.

Service providers should also be educated about the major risk factors for mental health problems in women and about the tendency to underestimate mood and anxiety disorders. They should learn how to ask women with developmental disabilities about their feelings and how to encourage them to get help without feeling stigmatized.

GYNECOLOGICAL ISSUES ACROSS THE LIFE SPAN

Women with developmental disabilities have a similar average age of menarche as women in the general population, and most women with developmental disabilities appear to have regular menstrual cycles (Walsh et al., 2000). Clinicians need to know the features of pubertal development in girls and young women and to document them as accurately as possible as there are a variety of clinical conditions that have associated irregularities in onset. Chapter 19 reviews precocious puberty and delayed puberty in detail. These conditions include chromosomal and nonchromosomal syndromes; individuals with severe central nervous system involvement (either congenital or acquired); and those on medications, especially psychotropic and antiepileptic drugs.

Management of the menstrual and contraceptive needs of young women with intellectual disabilities is similar in most cases to the management of women without disabilities. Grover reviewed 107 women with intellectual disabilities, and only 2 women required surgical intervention. Surgical management, endometrial ablation, or hysterectomy was required after all medical interventions had failed and heavy irregular bleeding affected quality of life (Grover, 2002).

Menstruation

Menstrual irregularities are a very common reason for referral to the primary care provider. A menstrual chart is a vital record for all women to keep and especially those dependent on others for their care. The chart in Figure 25.1 is an example drawn from the Personal Health Record developed by The Centre for Developmental Disability in Victoria, British Columbia (Burbidge, 2003). Filling in this chart on a monthly basis, including to indicate missed periods, will help establish a menstrual history and a pattern of irregular versus regular menses. In all cases, an individual assessment with history, physical exam, and appropriate lab tests should be completed.

Year	Jan.	Feb.	Mar.	April	May	June	July	Aug.	Sept.	Oct.	Nov.	Dec.
1												
2												
3												
4												
5												
6												
7												
8												
9												
10												
11												
12												
13												
14												
15												
16												
17												
18												
19												
20												
21												
22												
23												
24												
25												
26												
27												
28												
29												
30												
31												

Figure 25.1. Menstrual chart to be used when a woman experiences problems with periods or problems that may be linked to menstrual cycles. Insert any relevant letters from the key into the square for that day. Make new codes if required. Common codes include *N* = normal flow, *L* = light flow, *H* = heavy flow, *C* = clots or flooding, *P* = pain, *D* = distressed, *S* = seizure, *A* = aggressive, *I* = Irritable, and *B* = bloating.

Amenorrhea

Distinguishing between primary and secondary amenorrhea is important. *Primary amenorrhea* is defined as

No periods by age 14 in the absence of growth or development of secondary sexual characteristics.

No period by age 16 regardless of the presence of normal growth and development with the appearance of secondary sexual characteristics (Pletcher & Slap, 1999).

Secondary amenorrhea is defined as

In a woman who has been menstruating, the absence of periods for a length of time equivalent to a total of at least three of the previous cycle intervals or 6 months of amenorrhea.

The woman's history is a crucial element in making the distinction between types of amenorrhea. The usual onset of menarche in the United States is 12 years with a range of 10.5–15 years. If the girl is in this age range, the physician can reasonably adopt a wait-and-see approach. If a girl is 16 years of age or older and has never had a period, a workup should be instituted as soon as possible. Primary amenorrhea can result from a range of causes. Initial workup should include history, physical with assessment of pubertal development, and possibly chromosomal studies. Tables 25.1 and 25.2 present an overview of causes and characteristics. A more detailed discussion and workup can be found in a standard gynecology textbook.

If a girl or woman has had a period in the past and is no longer menstruating, then a workup for secondary amenorrhea should begin. Secondary amenorrhea is common and often due to emotional, behavioral, and medication effects. The history, including medications, is a key element in determining the cause for secondary amenorrhea in women with disabilities. Table 25.3 provides a quick overview of testing and common diagnosis for secondary amenorrhea for clinicians. A more extensive review and management can be found in current gynecological textbooks or in consultation with a gynecologist.

The absence of a known history of sexual activity in women with developmental disabilities should not preclude a pregnancy test because of the possibility of sexual abuse. Clinical assessment requires a comprehensive history with information obtained from the woman. When appropriate, the history should be obtained from family members or support personnel for women with more severe intellectual disabilities.

The continuity of providers is essential for all individuals, but especially with women with more severe disabilities who are nonverbal. The provider can become familiar with alternative methods of communication. Challenging behaviors or changes in behavior can be documented along with the menstrual chart to try to correlate cycles with behavior changes. Premenstrual symptoms may present as behavior changes in women with developmental disabilities. Charting should be done for at least 2–3 months to see if there is a correla-

Table 25.1. Primary amenorrhea and delayed puberty

Diagnosis	Breast	Pubic	Uterus	Genotype
Ovarian dysgenesis	–	–	+	XO
Pseudohermaphrodite	–	–	+/–	XY
Constitutional delay	–	–	+	XX
Androgen insensitivity	+	–	–	XY
Ovarian failure	–	–	+	XX
Chronic illness	–	–	+	XX

Key: – = absent; + = present.

Adapted from *Pediatric Clinics of North America, 46,* Pletcher, J.R., & Slap, G.B., Adolescent gynecology, Part I—Common disorders, 505–518, Copyright 1999, with permission from Elsevier.

Table 25.2. Primary amenorrhea and normal puberty

Diagnosis	Breast	Pubic	Uterus	Genotype
Ovarian failure	+	+	+	XX
Chronic illness	+	+	+	XX
Pregnancy	+	+	+	XX
Outflow obstruction	+	+	+	XX
Müllerian agenesis	+	+	–	XX

Key: – = absent; + = present.

Adapted from *Pediatric Clinics of North America, 46,* Pletcher, J.R., & Slap, G.B., Adolescent gynecology, Part I—Common disorders, 505–518, Copyright 1999, with permission from Elsevier.

Table 25.3. Approach to secondary amenorrhea

Laboratory tests	Diagnosis
Increased human chorionic-gonadotropin	Pregnancy
Increased luteinizing hormone/ follicle stimulating hormone, decreased estrogen	Ovarian failure
Normal luteinizing hormone/ follicle-stimulating hormone, normal estrogen	No endometrium
Decreased luteinizing hormone/ follicle-stimulating hormone, decreased estrogen	Extensive differential diagnosis
Increased androgens	Polycystic ovarian syndrome, congenital adrenal hyperplasia, tumor

Adapted from *Pediatric Clinics of North America, 46,* Pletcher, J.R., & Slap, G.B., Adolescent gynecology, Part I—Common disorders, 505–518, Copyright 1999, with permission from Elsevier.

tion. Interventions should be individualized; medications or natural supplements may be beneficial.

Effects of Medication on Menstrual Cycle

The side effects of medications are common reasons for amenorrhea. Antipsychotic and antiepileptic drugs are widely taken by individuals with developmental disabilities. Prolactin levels are often elevated due to treatment with the older antipsychotic medications. Some of the new antipsychotic medications have mild or no effect on prolactin.

Chronic elevation of prolactin can result in decreased follicular and luteinizing hormone release, leading to declines in ovarian function. This decline may result in amenorrhea or infertility, which may increase age-related disorders associated with reduced estrogen levels (Walsh et al., 2000). Hyperprolactinemia can result in galactorrhea, amenorrhea or oligomenorrhea, infertility, hirsutism, acne, vaginal dryness, and atrophy. Osteoporosis may also result most probably due to gonadal dysfunction rather than excessive prolactin.

Women with developmental disabilities on antipsychotic medications should have their prolactin level checked as part of their ongoing clinical monitoring. A normal prolactin level at baseline can be monitored along with ongoing labs. Mildly elevated prolactin levels should be rechecked in the morning with the individual at rest. Elevated levels, in the absence of an obvious explanation, require evaluation of the pituitary with neuroimaging of the sellar region. Gadolinium enhanced magnetic resonance imaging (MRI) is the procedure of choice, computerized axial tomography (CAT) scan is a reasonable alternative if MRI is unavailable (see Table 25.4).

If no mass lesion is found, monitoring prolactin level with no treatment is a reasonable approach. Decreasing dosage of antipsychotics or switching to a newer prolactin-sparing atypical antipsychotic may be helpful clinical interventions. If galactorrhea and/or abnormal periods are present with an elevated prolactin and a normal MRI, a dopaminergic agonist (e.g., bromocriptine) can be used for symptomatic relief. Dopamine agonist have been used to reverse hyperprolactinemia but may exacerbate psychiatric symptoms (Goroll & Mulley, 2002). If pregnancy is not desired, oral contraceptives are an alternate option. Consultation with an endocrinologist can be done at any stage of the workup or during management if additional assistance is required. Coordinated management and communication among the primary medical provider, subspecialist, and psychiatrist provides the best clinical care. Additional research is required to assess present practice, test for the least invasive medication, and determine the long-term implication of the use of antipsychotic medications (Wieck & Haddad, 2002)

Table 25.4. Management of hyperprolactinemia

Level (ng/mL)	Cause	Action
20–100	Normal pulse	Monitor clinically and repeat as needed
	Hypothyroidism	Recheck as needed
	Psychotropics	Recheck as needed
100–200	Microadenoma	Magnetic resonance imaging
< 200	Mass	Magnetic resonance imaging

Adapted from *Pediatric Clinics of North America, 46,* Pletcher, J.R., & Slap, G.B., Adolescent gynecology, Part I—Common disorders, 505–518, Copyright 1999, with permission from Elsevier.

Ginny is a 55-year-old woman with severe intellectual disabilities, challenging behaviors, and arthritis. Her behavior has recently become more aggressive and self-abusive. Her periods were previously regular but have been irregular for the past 6 months. She has not been able to have a gynecological exam completed due to her behaviors. Ginny has no menses chart or other past medical/gynecological history.

An initial review of Ginny's history revealed no additional information. She was new to the agency with limited information but was taking multiple psychiatric medications, including Lithium, Klonopin, Tegretol, Depakote, and Risperdal. Her exam was limited but revealed no grossly abnormal findings. Ginny's labs were significant for a white blood cell count of 2,600 with normal differential, decreased platelet count of 100,000, Tegretol level of 11 (nl 4–12), and Depakote level of 128 (nl 50–100). A pelvic sonogram noted that her uterus was present and intact, and her ovaries were both visualized and normal. No abnormalities were noted, although the exam was limited. A mammogram was attempted but was unsuccessful.

The recommendation was made to monitor Ginny's menses with a menses chart and to have Ginny's psychiatrist reevaluate her present medications and intervention due to her abnormal labs. A follow-up clinical visit for reevaluation of Ginny's gynecological status was scheduled in 3 months. During those 3 months, Ginny's psychiatric medications were changed. At the following clinic visit, Ginny's lab values had returned to normal, and her menstrual cycles for the last 2 months had been regular. Regular visits with her primary care doctor would continue for monitoring.

Fertility and Reproduction

Fertility rates are not significantly different for women with intellectual disabilities alone. Certain genetic syndromes may have an impact on fertility. Fertility will be affected if genital organs or hormonal levels are altered by genetic syndromes. For example, only a few births have been documented in women with Down syndrome (Walsh et al., 2000).

Physical disabilities or the impact of chronic disabilities may affect the ability to conceive and carry to term. Physiologic changes during pregnancy include decreased mobility, fluid retention, bladder function, and increased urinary tract infections. These issues can be compounded in women with physical disabilities during pregnancy. Management with a knowledgeable obstetrician/gynecologist can help a women with physical disabilities have a successful pregnancy. Dr. Welner's (1999) review, *A Provider's Guide for the Care of Women with Physical Disabilities and Chronic Medical Conditions*, gives an overview of potential complications and management strategies to assist practitioners in the care of women with physical disabilities.

The prevalence of contraception and use of different methods remains generally unknown in women with intellectual and developmental disabilities (Servais et al., 2002). Studies assessing the hormonal status during menstrual cycles in women with cognitive disabilities have methodological problems including small sample size, sampling of only a few cycles, and lack of control for the stage of menstrual cycle in which the blood sample was drawn (Walsh et al., 2000). More research is required to evaluate the menstrual cycle in women with disabilities. Evidence does suggest that the majority of women with cognitive disabilities fall within the range of normal hormonal functioning.

The need and use of contraceptives varies depending on the individual. Women with severe disabilities who are not likely to be sexually active have less of a need for contraception. Women with milder disabilities will need contraception depending on their level of sexual activity. Multiple birth control methods are available to women with developmental disabilities. Historically, sterilization and therapeutic amenorrhea were methods of birth control used for women with developmental disabilities (Huovinen 1993; Smith & Polloway, 1993). Clinical and legal practices now protect the rights of women with disabilities, ensure women's right to choose, and monitor interventions used for women who are unable to choose for themselves.

The evaluation and method selected should be done with the individual and his or her provider. Health providers need assistance with training and patient information for all levels of disabilities. A clinician cannot make an assumption about the need for contraception based solely on the level of impairment. Pictures or samples of methods of contraception are helpful in discussing options with women with intellectual disabilities.

Menopause and Aging

Menopause, a natural part of the life cycle for women, is defined as the absence of a menstrual period for 12 consecutive months. Menopause can occur as early as age 35 and as late as 59. The average age for menopause in the United States is between 50 and 52. Menopause before the age of 40 is considered early.

A family history with the ages of menopause for first-degree relatives may be helpful in predicting the approximate age of menopause for women with developmental disabilities. Research in the area of menopause and women with a range of developmental disabilities is still needed. Studies suggest that women with Down syndrome and epilepsy may reach menopause at an earlier age than women in the general population (Schupf et al., 1997).

The symptoms experienced at menopause vary from woman to woman. Symptoms commonly experienced with menopause include hot flashes, sweating, insomnia, heart palpitations, itchy skin, backaches, joint pain, headaches, bloating, weight gain, thinning hair, and the growth of facial hair. The physiologic changes that occur with menopause may not be understood by women with developmental disabilities. Behavior changes can occur because of the physiologic changes.

Clinicians need to use history, physical examination, and lab tests to assist with diagnosing menopause. History should review, in particular, menstrual history, menses chart, medications, psychosocial history, and detailed review of systems. Physical examination should include weight, general appearance, hirsutism, nipple discharge, signs of hypothyroidism, and adrenal disease. Lab tests to evaluate hormonal status should initially consist of follicle-stimulating hormone and luteinizing hormone. If elevated, confirmation with a low estradiol level can confirm ovarian failure (see Table 25.3) A full evaluation to eliminate other medical or psychiatric etiologies is also required before menopause is accepted as the cause of behavior changes.

Physiological Changes and Medical Conditions Associated with Menopause Menopause with estrogen deficiency can increase the risk of estrogen-related health conditions including heart disease, depression, breast cancer, and dementia. Little or no research has been done with women with intellectual disabilities. Preventive screening for older women with developmental disabilities should continue especially if they are on hormonal replacement. Osteoporosis is an example of a disease that requires ongoing screening and intervention with aging.

Osteoporosis is a disease in which bones become fragile and more likely to break. Risk factors for osteoporosis include advanced age, family history of osteoporosis, Caucasian or Asian ethnicity, very thin or small stature, physical inactivity, early menopause, limited dietary intake of calcium or vitamin D, high alcohol and/or coffee intake, excessive dieting, excessive weight loss, and smoking. Women with developmental disabilities may be at increased risk of osteoporosis because of inactivity due to mobility impairments and/or sedentary lifestyles, long-term use of medications including anticonvulsants, excessive thyroid hormones and steroids, amenorrhea, and early menopause. Screening should be done based on risk factors, and treatment should be determined from the results.

Prevention of osteoporosis is the best intervention. Dietary intake of calcium should be recommended throughout life. Supplements can be a source of calcium. Close attention should be paid to the other medications taken when calcium is added to the regimen. Calcium can bind medications taken at the same time and limit their bioavailability. Exercise, weight loss, smoking cessation, hormonal replacement therapy, decreased caffeine intake, and decreased alcohol intake are all modalities that can be used to prevent osteoporosis.

Management of Menopause Treatment of menopause is specific to the individual and the symptoms. Symptomatic relief can include diet, exercise, natural supplements, and hormonal replacement. Management should be based on guidelines developed for women in the general population until research supports alternate management.

The risks and benefits of hormonal replacement should be evaluated for each woman as clinically indicated. Interactions with other medications should also be reviewed. Additional research will help to clarify recommendations and interventions that work best for women with developmental disabilities.

Complementary and alternative medicine (CAM) is growing in popularity within the United States. Limited research exists on the efficacy of CAM in the general population, and little or no research exists on CAM in individuals with developmental disabilities. Individuals or family members may be interested in using CAM for common conditions, including premenstrual syndrome, menopause, breast cancer, depression, arthritis, pregnancy, and lactation. A full review of herbal treatments is beyond the scope of this chapter; however, Table 25.5 lists common herbs used for premenstrual syndrome and menopause.

CAM is not without risk. For example, evening primose oil should be used in caution in individuals with seizures or on antipsychotic medications. Health professionals need to ask individuals and family members about the use of CAM. It is often overlooked or not disclosed because it is thought to be nonmedical or not acceptable to health professionals. The National Institutes of Health, National Center for Complementary & Alternative Medicine (NCCAM) will provide research trials to evaluate utilization and efficacy. Individuals with developmental disabilities need to be included in trials to assess interventions. Providers need to become informed about the risk and benefits of CAM to assist in comprehensive management for all women.

Table 25.5. Complementary treatments for premenstrual syndrome and menopause

Premenstrual syndrome
Evening primose oil
Chaste tree berry
St. John's wort, B vitamins, calcium, diuretic herbs
Valerian, Black haw
Don Quai (less information available and less studied for premenstrual syndrome)
Diet, exercise, meditation, relaxation
Menopause
Don Quai
Black cohosh
Soy
Wild yam
Sage
Nettles
Ginseng
Calcium
Vitamin E
B vitamins
Red clover

Source: National Center for Complimentary and Alternate Medicine (2005)

CLINICAL ASSESSMENT

Stella is a 32-year-old woman with mild intellectual disabilities, seizure disorder, scoliosis, and speech impediment due to cleft lip repair. She recently moved out of a group home setting and now lives with her boyfriend. She is managing her own medications, appointments, and medical care. Stella continues to have occasional seizures but states that she is compliant with her medications.

Stella is due for her gynecological exam but now lives 20 miles away from her primary care doctor, who used to perform her gynecological exam in his office and explain the different parts of the exam with words she could understand. The exam room was comfortable and familiar. The new primary care doctor does not do gynecological exams and has referred Stella to the gynecologic clinic for an exam.

Stella was upset. She yelled at her primary care doctor, "You are my doctor! You know me and my problems. Another doctor won't understand me and know how to do my exam!"

The recommendation was made to provide training with the new primary care doctor about specific needs for Stella's gynecological exam. Stella and the primary care doctor agreed to do this.

Routine health care for women with developmental disabilities involves evaluation of gynecological issues. Huovinen (1993) evaluated gynecological problems for women with intellectual disabilities in Finland. Reasons for gynecological consultation were therapeutic amenorrhea, gynecological status monitoring, vaginal discharge, and abnormal bleeding patterns. Grover (2002) reviewed 107 women with intellectual disabilities referred for gynecological services during a 9-year period. Consultation was requested for complaints including menorrhagia, irregular menses, dysmenorrhea, amenorrhea, need for advice or information, and the need for contraception. Medical management was successful in the majority of referrals, only 2 of the 107 women required surgical intervention after failure of several medical approaches. Ongoing review or specialist gynecological care was not indicated in 68% of the young women.

Primary care practitioners can provide an initial assessment of common presenting gynecological complaints. Referral to a gynecologist by practitioners should occur when the clinical issue requires additional evaluation and interventions beyond the scope of the practitioner. Resources and additional training for primary health care professionals about management of gynecological issues will allow for improved care. Identification of knowledgeable gynecological practitioners can provide the next level of care when needed. Additional research can evaluate the effectiveness of primary care management and gynecological interventions.

Gynecological History

Women with developmental disabilities present unique challenges for medical providers. They may not have information about the dates of menarche, family history, dates of gynecological surgery, or previous gynecological evaluations. This situation may be particularly true for women in community residences or congregate living situations apart from their family. Information about previous gynecological history and exams should be obtained prior to the visit or during the scheduled visit from the individual, responsible family member, or support staff.

If the woman is unable to give the history, a family member of support person who is familiar with the individual's history should be present. In many situations, the history remains inadequate and incomplete because of a lack of information. The medical record should reflect the history available, so if there is no past information, this situation should be documented at the baseline visit. A copy of the pertinent medical information should be given to the individual or surrogate for future providers. Any surgical interventions, adverse medication events, or successful treatments for common disorders are helpful to document and retain for the future.

A notebook or binder is a simple solution to keeping medical records. If a computer is accessible a computerized log of visits, pertinent exams, and tests should be kept for future reference. The clinician can educate parents or caregivers of younger women with developmental disabilities and young women themselves about the importance of documentation of significant events like puberty, menarche, menstrual cycle, and impact of medications for use by future health care providers. This activity is especially important for women with severe disabilities who are unable to communicate verbally and for women with intellectual disabilities, including memory impairments.

The use of pictures, diagrams, models, and peer support groups are a few of the interventions available to assist in educating women about pelvic exams. A friend, family member, or support person may be helpful for the individual's comfort. The woman should always be asked first if she would like assistance or if she would prefer to be alone during the exam. For women with more severe cognitive disabilities, the clinician along with caregivers can determine what would be most appropriate. Physicians should not assume that staff or family members automatically stay during the exam. If necessary, there should be sufficient health personnel to complete the exam with the woman independently. Again, this situation requires planning prior to the initial visit for the best outcome.

Music and adjustment of lighting are additional sources of comfort for individuals who may be anxious about the exam. Mirrors for the individual's use are helpful tools to educate and inform the individual about the gynecological exam. Presedation with mild oral antianxiety agents (e.g., Ativan, Valium) can be considered on an individual basis. A review of previous reactions including paradoxical reactions to medications must be completed, and a recent medical examination with allergies, vital signs, physical, labs, and complete medication list should be obtained prior to using sedation.

Appropriate training for personnel in BCLS and ACLS certification as well as resuscitation equipment should be on hand in case of an adverse effect. If an individual is sedated, proper monitoring of vital signs, including pulse oximetry by medical staff, should be available. The individual should not be left alone or fed until fully alert and responsive. If sedation is utilized, then prior planning should be done with other practitioners to coordinate other needed exams during the same administration of sedation.

Marjory is a 24-year-old woman with cerebral palsy, severe spasticity, severe intellectual disabilities, urinary incontinence, constipation, and recurrent vaginal infections. Her spasticity makes it difficult to position her on a standard exam table to complete the speculum exam. Her recurrent vaginal infections are most likely secondary to urinary pooling and urinary incontinence.

Marjory's parents are concerned about sexual abuse due to her limited ability to communicate and protect herself. Over the years, they and medical staff have established a comfortable routine and have been successful in completing the exam. A special hydraulic table to make transferring and positioning easier for women with physical disabilities makes the exam table more accessible.

Marjory recently moved into a group home setting after living at home with her parents for her entire life. Her mother states that she appears happy and that it is a lovely setting. The staff members are wonderful, and the group home is run by the same agency that Marjory attends for day program. Marjory's mother is concerned about an increase in vaginal infections with multiple caregivers now responsible for Marjory and about the possibility of sexual abuse. She has requested ongoing gynecological exams with the same provider even though it is different from the agency provider due to the sensitivity of the providers and the accessibility.

The recommendation was made to collaborate and continue regularly scheduled gynecological exams until training could be done for the new physicians and staff. These exams included ongoing assessment for sexual abuse. Everyone was willing to participate in the training. The long-range plan will be to coordinate the care with the new provider once training is completed.

Sexually Transmitted Diseases

Assessment of the risk, screening, treatment, and prevention of sexually transmitted diseases is an integral part of gynecological care. The rate for STDs in adults with developmental disabilities has not been well documented. Information on the rates of human immunodeficiency virus (HIV) in adults with developmental disabilities in the United States is also limited (Walkup, Sambamoorthi, & Crystal, 1999). Educational programs geared to women with developmental disabilities must be adapted to account for alternate learning styles and the impact of intellectual disabilities (Walsh et al., 2002). Research is needed to develop and evaluate the effectiveness of HIV prevention strategies and interventions for people with developmental disabilities (Brown & Jemmott, 2002).

Physical Examination

Comprehensive medical management of women with developmental disabilities includes a full assessment of mind and body. A natural sequence is to have the physical exam and gynecological exam done by the same provider, if possible. This practice is especially helpful when a woman has severe physical disabilities and is difficult to transfer to an exam table. The physical exam should include a full assessment of the entire body at least once a year. The clinical setting should be fully accessible with additional assistance available as needed. Ideally, the schedule should allow for the additional time it may take to assist the woman with behavioral, emotional, or physical needs that may arise during a gynecology exam.

The woman's age and history should be used to determine what exams are indicated. The standard gynecological exam includes a breast exam, abdominal exam, pelvic exam, and rectal exam. If the woman is younger than 18 and not sexually active, the menstrual history along with assessment of pubertal changes should be sufficient. If the woman is older than 18 and not sexually active, the history, breast exam, and pelvic exam are indicated. An internal exam with speculum should be done if no baseline pap exists or if there are vaginal complaints, menstrual irregularities, or questions of sexual abuse.

Women with developmental disabilities may be fearful of pelvic exams or any medical interventions because of a lack of understanding, fear, previous medical interventions, or past abuse. Women with intellectual disabilities who have been taught that "no one touches your private parts" may have difficulty understanding the changed circumstances when a health provider is examining her in the health setting. Common emotions range from fear, anger, hostility, and aggression. Patience, education, and natural supports are necessary to assist women with developmental disabilities and complete a pelvic exam (Elkins, 1997). Women who are very uncomfortable with medical interventions may benefit from behavioral therapy to help them understand the procedures and to cope with their emotional reactions. A curriculum, *Women Be Healthy*, is available to help women understand, prepare for, and manage anxiety surrounding breast and cervical cancer screening (Lunsky et al., 2002).

All women should be assessed for sexual abuse regardless of level of functioning and testing should be completed as indicated (e.g., gonorrhea, chlamydia, HPV testing). Screening for STDs, including syphilis, gonorrhea, chlamydia, and HIV, is dependent on the individual. The clinician should assess the individual's needs based on her history and physical exam.

Specific equipment in office settings like the hydraulic exam table, full range of metal speculums (pediatric, adolescent, and adult), and halogen lights improves the level of comfort. The accessibility during pelvic exams is also enhanced. If a pelvic exam cannot be successfully completed, a pelvic sonogram may provide an alternate assessment. Transvaginal sonogram provides the best assessment but may present similar difficulties to complete as a pelvic exam. Sedation, including oral, intravenous, or general anesthesia must be individualized with an assessment of the risks and benefits. A referral to a gynecological specialist, preferably a practitioner with previous experience with women with developmental disabilities, should be considered at any time there is a clinical issue or concern beyond the scope of the primary provider. A baseline exam with a gynecological specialist can also be considered if indicated. A team approach with a primary care provider and a gynecological specialist can provide comprehensive management for a woman with more complicated gynecological issues.

Preventive Health Care Screening

Jackie is a 38-year-old woman with moderate intellectual disabilities, Prader-Willi syndrome, and depression who went to her physician for a routine mammogram screening. Her mammogram showed a suspicious area of microcalcifications. She was referred to a breast surgeon for further intervention. Jackie's mother reported no history of breast cancer in the immediate family, but the biopsy was positive. Jackie had a mastectomy and received chemotherapy.

Jackie's mother was concerned about Jackie's understanding of her illness and about her picking at the site of the mastectomy due to her habit of skin picking and self-abusive behaviors. Jackie and group home staff attended informational sessions about breast cancer and spoke with breast cancer survivors to help educate everyone about the disease. Jackie's psychiatrist, internist, and oncologist have worked with her to develop a coordinated holistic approach to her current health care needs. The psychiatrist added medications to assist with the obsessive-compulsive aspects of the skin picking, and the internist worked with staff to identify early signs of infection and preventive interventions. The oncologist worked with the family and staff to provide the chemotherapy in a comfortable setting, and training about Jackie's particular needs was provided to medical staff administering the chemotherapy.

Jackie successfully completed chemotherapy and experienced no reoccurrence of the breast cancer. She still has occasionally episodes of skin picking. The staff and family monitor her closely, and serious infections have been avoided. Ongoing counseling and psychiatric management are part of her treatment plan.

Referrals for mammography should be made to a facility that uses low-dose equipment and adheres to high standards of quality control. Standards have been established by the Mammography Quality Standards Act of 1992 (PL 102-539), a federal law mandating that all mammography sites in the United States be accredited through a process approved by the U.S. Department of Health and Human Services (2002). Table 25.6 summarizes the current screening recommendations. Routine screening for breast cancer every 1–2 years with mammography alone or mammography and clinical breast examination is recommended for women age 50–69.

The evidence is conflicting for mammography at ages 40–49, and there is no evidence regarding benefit for women older than age 75, with mammography to be utilized at the discretion of the physician. Women with disabilities are living longer, and many women with disabilities have not been pregnant. Nulliparity is one of the associated risk factors for breast cancer (Davies & Duff, 2001). A medical provider must use his or her clinical judgment along with an individual's assessment to determine testing in these age ranges in women with developmental disabilities.

In the 1994 Disability Survey and the Health Promotion/Disease Prevention, supplement mammography testing in the previous 2 years in women 40 years or older with three or more functional limitations was 49.8%. In women 50–64, the rate was 61%. This population is not an exact match with women with developmental disabilities, but there are similar barriers to their access to preventive health screening. Barriers to obtaining mammograms for women with intellectual dis-

Table 25.6. Recommended breast cancer screening

Screening method	Age group	Frequency
Breast self exam	20 and older	Each month after menstrual period
Physical exam by health provider	20–40	Every 3 years
	40 and older	Yearly
Mammogram	40–49	Every 1–2 years
	50 and older	Yearly

Adapted from *Pediatric Clinics of North America, 46,* Pletcher, J.R., & Slap, G.B., Adolescent gynecology, Part I—Common disorders, 505–518, Copyright 1999, with permission from Elsevier.

abilities include lack of awareness by health providers, difficulty with anxiety, challenging behaviors, difficulty with patient instructions, and accessibility of equipment. Lack of patient education about preventive health care screening recommendations is an additional barrier.

Solutions often come from women with disabilities. Information sharing about prevention screening, education of health care providers to the needs of women with disabilities, user-friendly instructions about mammograms, and self-help groups are possible responses to certain barriers. Clinical research and data collection will assist in specific guidelines or adjustments required from preventive clinical guidelines.

Cervical Cancer Screening

Regular pap tests are recommended for all women who are or have been sexually active and who have a cervix. Pap tests should be performed at least every 2 or 3 years after two negative pap smears. Initial pap smears should begin once an individual is sexually active or at or about 18 years of age. The frequency of pap smears should be based on individual risk factors for cervical cancer.

Women who have never engaged in sexual intercourse are at low risk for cervical cancer and therefore may not require screening. The issue of screening women with developmental disabilities for cervical cancer if they are not sexually active would be based on the clinician's discretion. Women should still be evaluated for risks of other abnormalities or cancer including fibroids, ovarian cysts, ovarian cancer, and uterine cancer. The documentation of no sexual activity would be critical. When in doubt, until further evidence is presented, screening should occur consistent with stated recommendations.

Elderly women do not appear to benefit from pap testing if repeated cervical smears have been consistently normal; however, insufficient evidence is available to recommend for or against an upper age limit. This decision should be made after discussion between the individual or surrogate and the health care provider. Women who have undergone a hysterectomy with removal of the cervix do not benefit from pap testing unless it was done because of cervical cancer. If the cervix remains, continued testing is necessary.

Pap smears that cannot be completed for women with developmental disabilities due to challenging behaviors require individual assessment. Assistance from friends or family may be helpful, desensitization, patient education, music, or pictures may be helpful. As previously mentioned, the *Women Be Healthy* curriculum is available to prepare women to participate actively in breast and cervical cancer screening (Lunsky et al., 2002). The use of oral sedation to assist with anxiety or challenging behaviors can be considered depending on the clinical setting and assessment of woman's risk. Baseline testing under anesthesia would require an evaluation of the risks and benefits of the possible results obtained versus the risk of anesthesia.

In the national studies evaluating women older than 18, 67% had pap smears within the last 3 years. In a study of women with functional limitations related to physical activities from the 1994 Disability Survey and the Health Promotion/Disease Prevention supplement, 61% of women with three or more functional limitations had pap smears within the last 3 years. The barriers to pap testing in women with developmental disabilities are similar to barriers to mammograms. Lack of trained health professionals, lack of awareness of preventive health screening by patients, lack of accessible exam tables, and challenging behaviors. Improvements in the screening rates for women with developmental disabilities will be assessed by tracking rates of pap smears, increased education of health professionals, patient education, accessible equipment, and behavioral interventions.

CONCLUSION

The need for improved health care delivery systems for women with developmental disabilities is a reality throughout the country. The health care management of women with developmental disabilities is an evolving field. The team approach of coordinated care involving the woman, regardless of her level of disability; caregivers; family members; health professionals; and support staff is the best way to deliver health care services. The increased awareness and education about the needs of women with developmental disabilities should lead to an improvement in their health care and quality of life.

Women with intellectual disabilities are living longer, and little research is available on the perceptions of health and aging. A preliminary report of perceptions of older women with intellectual disabilities reported that women held mostly negative perceptions of aging, had misconceptions and limited knowledge regarding age-related physical and psychosocial changes, expressed a desire for more information about their bodies, wanted explanations of health service procedures, tended not to identify as having a disability, lacked information on health understanding of potential consequences, and lacked information and autonomy regarding personal rights and empowerment in managing their own health (Brown & Gill, 2002). Women with intellectual disabilities require more information and better-quality health care to improve their health. Healthy living is more then just biomedical interventions. Attention to the psychosocial well-being of women with intellectual disabilities is a major part of healthy living.

REFERENCES

American Association on Mental Retardation. (2004, Dec. 3). *AAMR/Arc position statements: Sexuality.* Retrieved from http://www.aamr.org/Policies/pos_sexuality.shtml

American Psychiatric Association. (2004). *Diagnostic and statistical manual of mental disorders* (4th ed.). Washington, DC: Author.

Benson, B.A. (1985). Behavior disorders and mental retardation: Associations with age, sex, and level of functioning in an outpatient clinic sample. *Applied Research in Mental Retardation 6,* 79–95.

Borthwick-Duffy, S. (1994). Epidemiology and prevalence of psychopathology in people with mental retardation. *Journal of Consulting and Clinical Psychology, 62,* 17–27.

Boston Women's Health Collective. (1973). *Our bodies, our selves.* Boston: Author.

Bragar, M.C. (1977). *The feebleminded female: An historical analysis of mental retardation as a social definition, 1890–1920.* Unpublished doctoral dissertation, Syracuse University.

Brown, A., & Gill, C. (2002). Women with developmental disabilities health and aging. *Current Women's Health Reports, 2,* 219–225.

Brown, E., & Jemmott, L. (2002). HIV prevention among people with developmental disabilities. *Journal of Psychosocial Nursing, 40,* 15–21.

Burbidge, M. (2003). *Personal health records for people with developmental disability.* Retrieved from http://www.cddh.monash.org/clinical/phr/phr.html

Carlson, B.E. (1997). Mental retardation and domestic violence: An ecological approach to intervention. *Social Work, 42,* 79–89.

Carlson, B. (1998). Domestic violence in adults with mental retardation: Reports from victims and key informants. *Mental Health Aspects of Developmental Disabilities, 1,* 102–112.

Castle, D.J. (2000). Women and schizophrenia: An epidemiological perspective. In D.J. Castle, J. McGrath, & J. Kulkarni (Eds.), *Women and schizophrenia* (pp. 19–34). Cambridge, England: University of Cambridge Press.

Chamberlain, A., Rauth, J., Passer, A., McGrath, M., & Burket, R. (1984). Issues in fertility control for mentally retarded female adolescents: I. Sexual activity, sexual abuse and contraception. *Pediatrics, 73,* 445–450.

Charlot, L.R., Doucette, A.C., & Mezzacappa, E. (1993). Affective symptoms of institutionalized adults with mental retardation. *American Journal on Mental Retardation, 98,* 408–416.

Culbertson, F.M. (1997). Depression and gender: An international review. *American Psychologist, 52,* 35–31.

Davies, N., & Duff, M. (2001). Breast cancer screening for older women with intellectual disabilities living in community group homes. *Journal of Intellectual Disability Research, 45*(3), 253–257.

Day, K. (1985). Psychiatric disorder in the middle-aged and elderly mentally handicapped. *British Journal of Psychiatry, 147,* 660–667.

Edelstein, T.M., & Glenwick, D.S. (1997). Referral reasons for psychological services for adults with mental retardation. *Research in Developmental Disabilities, 18,* 45–59.

Elkins, T.E. (1997). Reproductive health care for women with mental handicaps. *The Contraception Report, 8*(4), 4–11.

Fitzgerald, P., & Seeman, M.V. (2000). Women and schizophrenia: Treatment implications. In D.J. Castle, J. McGrath, & J. Kulkarni (Eds.), *Women and schizophrenia* (pp. 95–110). Cambridge, England: University of Cambridge Press.

Fletcher, R.J. (1993). Mental illness and mental retardation in the United States: Policy and treatment challenges. *Journal of Intellectual Disability Research, 37,* 25–33.

Ghaziuddin, M. (1988). Referral of mentally handicapped patients to the psychiatrist: A community study. *Journal of Mental Deficiency Research, 32,* 491–495.

Glue, P. (1989). Rapid cycling affective disorders in the mentally retarded. *Biological Psychiatry, 26,* 250–256.

Goroll, A.H., & Mulley, A.G. (2002). *Primary care medicine recommendations.* Philadelphia: Lippincott, Williams & Wilkins.

Grover, S. (2002). Menstrual and contraceptive management in women with an intellectual disability. *Medical Journal of Australia, 176*(3), 108–110.

Heiman, T., & Margalit, M. (1998). Loneliness, depression, and social skills among students with mild mental retardation in different educational settings. *Journal of Special Education, 32,* 154–163.

Huovinen, K. (1993). Gynecological problems of mentally retarded women. *Acta Obstetricia et Gynecologica Scandinavica, 72,* 475–480.

Kessler, R.C., McGonagle, K.A., & Zhao, S. (1994). Lifetime and 12-month prevalence of DSM–III–R psychiatric disorders in the United States: Results from the National Comorbidity Study. *Archives of General Psychiatry, 51,* 8–19.

Koller, H., Richardson, S., Katz, M., & McLaren, J. (1983). Behavior disturbance since childhood among a 5-year birth cohort of all mentally retarded young adults in a city. *American Journal of Mental Deficiency, 87,* 386–395.

Lunsky, Y. (2003). Depressive symptoms in intellectual disability: Does gender play a role? *Journal of Intellectual Disability Research, 47,* 386–395.

Lunsky, Y., & Benson, B.A. (2001). Association between perceived social support and strain, and positive and negative outcome for adults with mild intellectual disability. *Journal of Intellectual Disability Research, 45,* 106–114.

Lunsky, Y., Straiko, A., & Armstrong, S. (2002). *Women be healthy.* [Revised by S. Havercamp, K. Kluttz-Hile, & P. Dickens]. Chapel Hill: North Carolina Office of Disability and Health.

Lunsky, Y., Straiko, A., & Armstrong, S. (2003).Women behealthy: Evaluation of a health intervention by women with intellectual disabilities. *Journal of Applied Research in Intellectual Disabilities, 16,* 247–254.

Mammography Quality Standards Act of 1992, PL 102-539, 106 Stat. 3547.

Mansell, S., Sobsey, D., & Calder, P. (1992). Sexual abuse treatment for persons with developmental disabilities. *Professional Psychology: Research and Practice, 23,* 404–409.

Maxmen, J.S., & Ward, N.G. (1995). *Essential psychopathology and its treatment* (2nd ed.). New York: Norton & Co.

McCarthy, M. (1999). *Sexuality and women with learning disabilities.* London: Jessica Kingsley.

Meins, W. (1993). Prevalence and risk factors for depressive disorders in adults with intellectual disability. *Australia and New Zealand Journal of Developmental Disabilities, 18,* 147–156.

Moss, S., Prosser, H., Costello, H., Simpson, N., Patel Rowe, S., Turner, S., & Hatton, C. (1998). Reliability and validity of the PAS-ADD Checklist for detecting psychiatric disorders in adults with intellectual disability. *Journal of Intellectual Disability Research, 42,* 173–183.

National Center for Complimentary and Alternate Medicine. (2005). *Health information.* Retieved from http://nccam.nih.gov/health/

Nezu, C.M., & Nezu, A.M. (1994). Outpatient psychotherapy for adults with mental retardation and concomitant psychopathology: Research and clinical imperatives. *Journal of Consulting and Clinical Psychology, 62,* 34–42.

Office of the Surgeon General. (2002). *Closing the gap: A national blueprint to improve the health of persons with mental retardation.* Rockville, MD: U.S. Department of Health and Human Services.

Pletcher, J.R., & Slap, G.B. (1999). Adolescent gynecology, Part I—Common disorders. *Pediatric Clinics of North America, 46,* 505–518.

Prout, H.T., Chard, K.M., Nowak-Drabik, K.M., & Johnson, D.M. (2000). Determining the effectiveness of psychotherapy with persons with mental retardation: The need to move toward empirically based research. *NADD Bulletin, 3,* 83–86.

Reiss, S. (1982). Psychopathology and mental retardation: Survey of a developmental disabilities mental health problem. *Mental Retardation, 20,* 128–132.

Reiss, S. (1988). *The Reiss Screen for Maladaptive Behavior–test manual.* Worthington, OH: IDS Publishing.

Reiss, S., & Aman, M. (1998). *Psychotropic medication and developmental disabilities: The international consensus handbook.* Columbus: The Ohio State University Nisonger Center.

Reiss, S., & Trenn, E. (1984). Consumer demand for outpatient mental health services for mentally retarded people. *Mental Retardation, 22,* 112–115.

Reynolds, W.M., & Miller, K.L. (1985). Depression and learned helplessness in mentally retarded and non-mentally retarded adolescents: An initial investigation. *Applied Research in Mental Retardation, 6,* 295–306.

Rimmer, J.H., Braddock, D., & Fujiura, G. (1994). Cardiovascular risk factor levels in adults with mental retardation. *American Journal on Mental Retardation, 98,* 510–518.

Rinck, C. (1998). Epidemiology and psychoactive medication. In S. Reiss & M. Aman (Eds.), *Psychotropic medication and developmental disabilities: The international consensus handbook.* Columbus: The Ohio State University Nisonger Center.

Robins, L.N., & Regier, D.A. (1991). *Psychiatric disorders in America: The epidemiological catchment area study.* New York: Free Press.

Schupf et al. (1997). Early menopause in women with Down syndrome. *Journal of Intellectual Disability Research, 41,* 264–267.

Schwartz, P. (2000). Living with a disability: A service user's account. *Clinical Psychology Forum, 137,* 5.

Scior, K. (2000). Women with disabilities: Gendered subjects after all? *Clinical Psychology Forum, 137,* 6–10.

Servais, L., Jacques, D., Leach, R., Conod, L., Hoyois, P., Dan, B., et al. (2002). Contraception of women with intellectual disability: Prevalence and determinants. *Journal of Intellectual Disability Research, 46*(2), 108–119.

Smith, J.D., & Polloway, E. (1993). Institutionalization, involuntary sterilization, and mental retardation: Profiles from the history of the practice. *Mental Retardation, 31,* 208–214.

Sobsey, D. (2000). Faces of violence against women with developmental disabilities. In W. Abramson, E. Emanuel, V. Gaylor, & M. Hayden (Eds.) *Impact: Feature issue on violence against women with developmental or other disabilities.* Minneapolis: University of Minnesota, Institute on Community Integration.

Spitalnik, D.M., & White-Scott, S. (2001). Health care needs of adults with mild cognitive impairments. In A.J. Tymchuk, K.C. Larkin, & R. Luckasson (Eds.), *The forgotten generation.* Baltimore: Paul H. Brookes Publishing Co.

Stack, L.S., Haldipur, C.V., & Thompson, M. (1987). Stressful life events and psychiatric hospitalization in mentally retarded patients. *American Journal of Psychiatry, 144,* 661–663.

Stromsness, M. (1993). Sexually abused women with mental retardation: Hidden victims, absent resources. *Women and Therapy, 14,* 139–152.

Valenti-Hein, D., & Dura, J.R. (1996). Sexuality and sexual development. In J. Jacobson & J. Mulick (Eds.), *Manual of diagnosis and professional practice in mental retardation* (pp. 301–310). Washington, DC: American Psychological Association.

Walkup, J., Sambamoorthi, U., & Crystal, S. (1999). Characteristics of persons with mental retardation and HIV/AIDs infection in a statewide Medicaid population. *American Journal on Mental Retardation, 104,* 356–363.

Walsh, A., (1998). Women and mood: Biological considerations. In S.E. Romans (Ed.), *Folding back the shadows: A perspective on women's health* (pp. 165–176). Otago, New Zealand: University of Otago Press.

Walsh, P.N., Heller, T., Schupf, N., & van Schrojenstein Lantman-de Valk, H. (2000). *Healthy aging—adults with intellectual disabilities: Women's health issues.* Geneva: World Health Organization.

Welner, S.L. (1997). Gynecologic care and sexuality issues for women with disabilities. *Sexuality and Disability, 15,* 33–40.

Welner, S.L. (1999). *A provider's guide for the care of women with physical disabilities and chronic medical conditions.* Chapel Hill: North Carolina Office on Disability and Health.

Wieck, A., & Haddad, P. (2002). Hyperprolactinaemia caused by antipsychotic drugs. [Editorial]. *British Medical Journal, 324,* 250–252.

Wilson, C., & Brewer, N. (1992). The incidence of criminal victimization of individuals with an intellectual disability. *Australian Psychologist, 27,* 114–117.

CHAPTER 26

GERIATRICS

Kathryn Pekala Service,
Carl V. Tyler, Jr., and Matthew P. Janicki

Improvements in health, hygiene, and nutrition have led to a growth in the number and proportion of older individuals and a remarkable increase in life expectancy. In the United States, the current life expectancy is 79.4 for women and 73.9 for men (Anderson & DeTurk, 2002). Policies and practice have been designed for most of the 20th century with a youthful society in mind (United Nations, 2003), particularly in the field of intellectual and developmental disabilities, where programs have often focused on such issues as prevention, early intervention, and school inclusion. Furthermore, as stated by Ansello and Janicki, "the demographic evolutions in the developed nations have produced millions of older people without necessarily producing aging-related expertise to go along with them" (2000, p. 5). The aim of this chapter is to describe the nature of older people with intellectual and developmental disabilities, their physical aging health issues and needs, and select social aging issues facing them and their caregivers. Stories illustrate the difficulties of medical diagnosis and treatment; the complexities involved with gaining access to community resources; and the efforts necessary to maximize function while preserving autonomy as individuals with intellectual and developmental disabilities age.

DEMOGRAPHICS

The absolute number of aging adults with intellectual and developmental disabilities has increased, and a significant increase has also occurred in their life expectancy. Earlier estimates were that 4 or 5 out of every 1,000 people older than the age of 60 had an intellectual or developmental disability (Ansello & Janicki, 2000). In 2000, an estimated 641,000 adults with developmental disabilities were older than 60 (Heller, Janicki, Hammel, & Factor, 2002). In 2002, about 75% of all older adults with intellectual disabilities were in the 40- to 60-year-old age group; expectations are that the 60 years and older group will increase threefold by 2020 (Janicki, 2002).

With the same advances in health, education, and technology, people with intellectual disabilities are also surviving into old age and living longer, even into their eighth and ninth decades (see Figure 26.1) (Hogg, Lucchino, Wang, & Janicki, 2001). Similarly, those individuals who, in the past, had been documented as having a lower life expectancy (e.g., individuals with Down syndrome) are also living longer. The average age of death for adults with Down syndrome is in the mid 50s, with 25% of individuals still alive at age 65 years (Baird & Sadnovnick, 1989; Janicki, Dalton, Henderson, & Davidson, 1999; Yang, Rasmussen, & Friedman, 2002).

PRINCIPLES OF GERIATRIC MEDICINE

Homeostasis refers to the ability of biological systems to maintain a stable internal environment. Aging involves homeostenosis, a decline in the ability of each organ system and the body as a whole, to maintain homeostasis. An increased vulnerability to stress and illness occurs because of a corresponding reduction of physiologic reserve. Homeostenosis occurs very gradually, generally beginning in the third decade of life. The rate of decline varies in each individual and in each organ system within an individual and is influenced by genetics, diet, environment, and lifestyle.

From this basic understanding of aging follows a number of core principles in geriatric medicine:

1. *As individuals age, they become more dissimilar from each other.* Talking about the "average 70-year-old," or saying, "What do you expect at that age?" becomes less and less meaningful.

2. *An abrupt decline in function should always be assumed to be due to disease or illness, not aging.* Decline due to aging alone tends to occur gradually and imperceptibly.

3. *The rate of decline with aging can be modified by lifestyle modifications and treatment of known illness.* Individuals

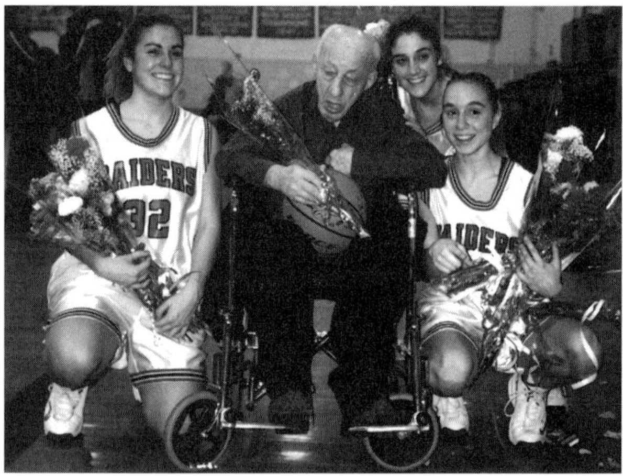

Figure 26.1. Intergenerational activities are valued in the field of aging. This girls' basketball team honored one of their favorite fans, Simon, on his 91st birthday, by presenting him with a basketball, team shirt, and team picture. (Used by permission from Shane Covey, *Athol Daily News*.)

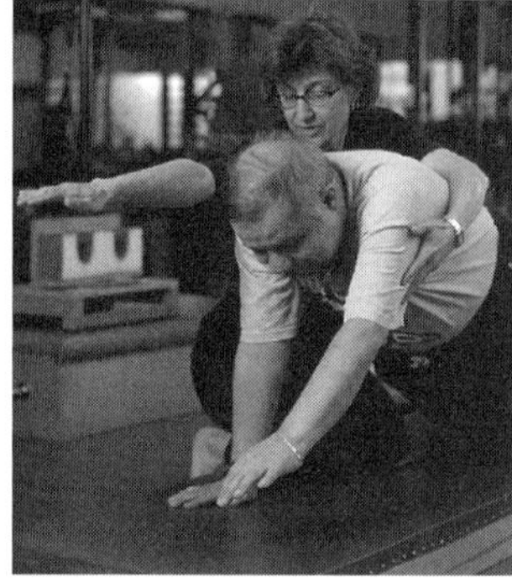

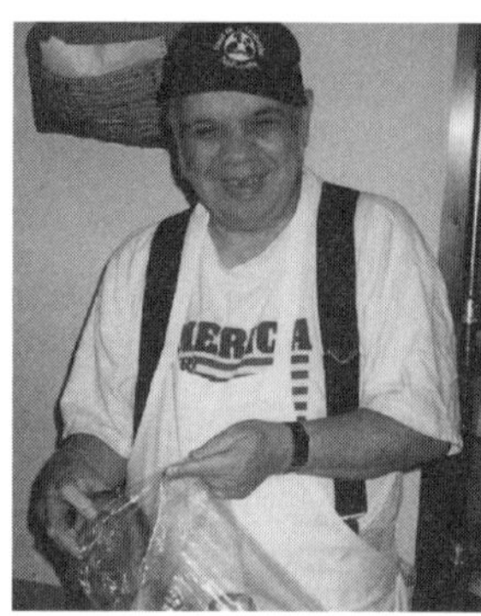

Figure 26.2. Reflecting improved health and changes in society, the younger cohorts, or young-old, such as Bruce (age 62), are exercising more, volunteering more, and continuing to work for a salary. (Left photo courtesy of Lynne Squadrille.)

can still accrue health benefits by stopping smoking, becoming more physically active, or controlling blood pressure.

4. *Disease and illness often present in atypical ways.* Older adults may have pneumonia without a cough or fever, myocardial infarction without chest pain, or depression without tearfulness.
5. *Multiple organ system dysfunctions, chronic diseases, acute illness, nutritional deficiencies, and psychosocial stressors operate together to cause impairments.* Functional improvement may not occur unless all relevant factors are identified and addressed.
6. *Successful aging is not just about physical health.* It includes maintaining engagement with life through relationships and productive activities.

INFLUENCES ON THE AGING PROCESS

With certain exceptions, people with intellectual and developmental disabilities experience the same physical process of aging (influenced by genetics) as individuals without lifelong disabilities (Davidson, Heller, Janicki, & Hyer, 2003; see Figure 26.2). Similar to the general population, the health status of aging people with intellectual disabilities can also be affected by disease, disuse, and suboptimal health promotion and disease prevention practices. Many losses in function have been erroneously attributed to the inevitable consequence of aging, when in fact they occur because of physical inactivity and resultant deconditioning; malnutrition; obesity; and substandard diagnosis and treatment of acute and chronic medical conditions. A number of factors have an impact on a person's health in older years: lifelong health and lifestyle patterns of poor nutrition or dental care, lack of physical activity, obesity, smoking, limited access to health care, poor hygiene practices, poverty, abuse, violence, neglect, and inadequate social networks and education (Davidson, Heller, et al., 2003; Janicki, 2002; Walsh & Murphy, 2002).

GERIATRIC SYNDROMES

Older adults are also prone to the development of one or more health problems termed "geriatric syndromes." Each of these syndromes has its own differential diagnosis and clinical methodology for assessment and management. Table 26.1 lists conditions commonly defined as geriatric syndromes. Individuals involved in the health care of older adults with intellectual and developmental disabilities should be familiar with these syndromes and ensure that these conditions are fully evaluated and properly treated. Although some individuals with intellectual and developmental disabilities may have experienced some of these conditions at an earlier age, the etiologies and management strategies for these problems can change with age.

LIFE EXPECTANCIES

A number of risk factors have been associated with a reduced life expectancy in individuals with intellectual and developmental disabilities, including cerebral palsy with severe motor and functional impairments (Davidson, Heller, et al., 2003; Evenhuis, Henderson, Beange, Lennox, & Chicoine, 2001; Strauss, Cable, & Shavell, 1999); epilepsy with refractory seizures; chronic upper respiratory infections; heart conditions; infections; choking; reduced mobility; dependency in eating and toileting; and severe to profound intellectual disabilities (Hayden, 1998). Although premature death is not caused directly by a lower functional level, many concomitant health problems are common in people with severe disabilities (Eyman & Borthwick-Duffy, 1994). Studies have also demonstrated similarities between the leading causes of death (cardiovascular, respiratory, and neoplastic diseases) for both the general population and individuals with intellectual disabilities (Janicki, Davidson, et al., 2002; Patja, Molson, & Iivanainen, 2001).

AGING AND SPECIFIC SYNDROMES

Specific genetic syndromes may be associated with characteristic aging trajectories. For example, Down syndrome is associated with a shorter life expectancy and a higher risk for dementia compared with individuals with intellectual disabilities from other causes. This fact reinforces the potential value, throughout the life span, of diagnosing the precise etiology for an individual's developmental disability. Periodic review of the clinical literature is necessary to maintain an up-to-date knowledge of the health problems associated with specific syndromes in later life (Tyler & Edman, 2004). Individuals diagnosed with known syndromes should be encouraged to enlist in disease-specific registries, to enable clinicians and researchers to better understand and document syndrome-specific health care needs throughout the life span.

Table 26.1. Common geriatric syndromes

Dementia
Delirium
Urinary incontinence
Falls
Dizziness
Syncope
Hearing impairment
Visual impairment
Osteoporosis/osteomalacia
Malnutrition
Feeding problems
Pressure ulcers
Sleep problems

COMMON AGE-ASSOCIATED CONDITIONS

Older individuals with intellectual disabilities may have similar (Kapell et al., 1998) or even higher rates of age-related conditions than older adults without lifelong disabilities (Evenhuis et al., 2001). Common age-associated conditions may have different etiologies and, therefore, a different focus of intervention in individuals with intellectual and developmental disabilities. For example, in adults with intellectual and developmental disabilities, osteoporosis appears to occur at an earlier age and is probably more often related to antiepileptic drug use, hypogonadism, and suboptimal calcium and vitamin D intake (Tyler, Snyder, & Zyzanski, 2000). Management of osteoporosis, then, should include consideration of antiepileptic medications with lesser impact on bone mineral density, identification and treatment of hypogonadism, and assurance of optimum vitamin D and calcium intake.

DEMENTIA

Dementia refers to a group of neurodegenerative disorders causing impairments in multiple cognitive functions, including memory, speech and language, praxis, and executive functioning. The most common age-associated dementias are Alzheimer disease, followed by vascular dementia, dementia of the Lewy body type, and dementia associated with Parkinson disease. Individuals with Down syndrome carry an unusually high risk for developing Alzheimer-type dementia. Although the prevalence of dementia in the general population is about 6% at age 60, it estimated to be as high as 50% for individuals with Down syndrome at the same age (Janicki, Heller, Seltzer, & Hogg, 1995).

Recognition of dementia in individuals with intellectual and developmental disabilities requires a knowledge of their baseline cognitive and adaptive functioning. In individuals with a higher premorbid level of functioning, initial symptoms of dementia may be memory impairment, reduced verbal output, and temporal disorientation; whereas for those with a lower premorbid level of functioning, typical early symptoms of dementia may be apathy, inattention, diminished alertness, slowing of movement, and decreased social interaction (Janicki et al., 1995; Lai & Williams, 1989).

Individuals with intellectual and developmental disabilities carry a risk of both underdiagnosis and overdiagnosis of dementia. As the association between Down syndrome and dementia becomes more widely appreciated, individuals with Down syndrome who manifest changes in cognitive and adaptive functioning may not receive an adequate evaluation for other disorders that can mimic dementia or exacerbate the functional impact of it. Figure 26.3 outlines a typical evaluation for functional decline. Most commonly, an interplay of several medical, psychiatric, and social-environmental factors, not dementia, is responsible for decline. Even if dementia is eventually diagnosed, comorbid medical and psychiatric conditions deserve recognition and treatment to avoid premature deterioration. Ellie's story exemplifies how easily behavior change is "misdiagnosed" as dementia.

Staff had learned that Down syndrome is a risk factor for Alzheimer disease and readily attributed 52-year-old Ellie's resistance to getting in and out of the van that brought her to work as behavior problems secondary to dementia. After an evaluation to rule out other correctable conditions, they later learned that osteoarthritis in Ellie's knees made the transfer action painful. With appropriate treatment, Ellie's resistance disappeared.

PREVENTIVE HEALTH CARE

Guidelines for preventive health care in individuals age 65 and older have been established by the American Geriatric Society, the United States Preventive Services Task Force, the American College of Physicians, and the American Academy of Family Physicians. These groups concur in some, but not all, of their recommendations. Individuals and their families, health care professionals, and service providers are faced with deciding whose guidelines to follow.

As is the case with health care decisions in other contexts, more health care is not necessarily better health care. Certain screening decisions (e.g., the use of digital rectal exam and serum prostate specific antigen testing for prostate cancer screening) are based on the ability to clearly communicate with the individual the specific risks, benefits, and uncertainties of a specific screening methodology. Many individuals with intellectual and developmental disabilities will need assistance with making these more complicated screening decisions.

Known comorbidities also influence preventive health care recommendations. Individuals with certain primary health problems may, over time, develop additional health problems as a consequence of the primary disorder. These complications are termed *secondary conditions* (see Chapter 4). Thoughtful preventive care practices established in early life can prevent the emergence of these secondary conditions in later life, or at least minimize their severity and functional impact (Janicki et al., 1999). For instance, as mentioned previously, seizure disorders requiring chronic antiepileptic drug use increase the risk of osteoporosis and osteomalacia. Thus, bone mineral density testing should be conducted earlier than would otherwise be recommended on the basis of age alone.

Along with generic preventive services based on age and gender, additional preventive care may be necessary because of syndrome-specific health risks. The Down Syndrome Preventive Medical Checklist is one example of additional screening recommendations based on health risks associated with an etiologic diagnosis (Cohen, 1999). Further individuation of preventive health care must account for estimated life expectancy, individual and family values, previous screening history, family and personal medical history, and general health status. Table 26.2 is a list of recommendations for preventive health screening in older adults with intellectual and developmental disabilities.

CHRONIC DISEASE

Chronic diseases that are prevalent among older adults include arthritis, hypertension, heart disease, chronic obstructive pulmonary disease, diabetes, cerebrovascular disease, atherosclerosis, and cancer (Schretzman & Strumpf, 2002). Many significant chronic diseases go unrecognized in adults with intellectual and developmental disabilities (Beange, McElduff, & Baker, 1995; Kapell et al., 1998). Complexities of diagnosis include difficulties with health care provider–patient–ancillary informant communication, fear and inability to perform medical tests (e.g., mammography, pulmonary function testing), and difficulty with accessing primary and specialty medical care. More frequent health care contacts are often necessary to uncover disease. Table 26.3 lists common diagnoses in older adults that are frequently overlooked. Changes in residence or in primary care physician often represent opportunities for complete review of health status, accrual of complete health information database, institution of previously neglected preventive health services, and a fresh perspective on the functional impact of chronic diseases (Tyler & Bourguet, 1997). Many hospitals and health insurance carriers offer chronic disease management programs that benefit older adults with congestive heart failure, asthma/chronic obstructive pulmonary disease, diabetes, or coronary heart disease.

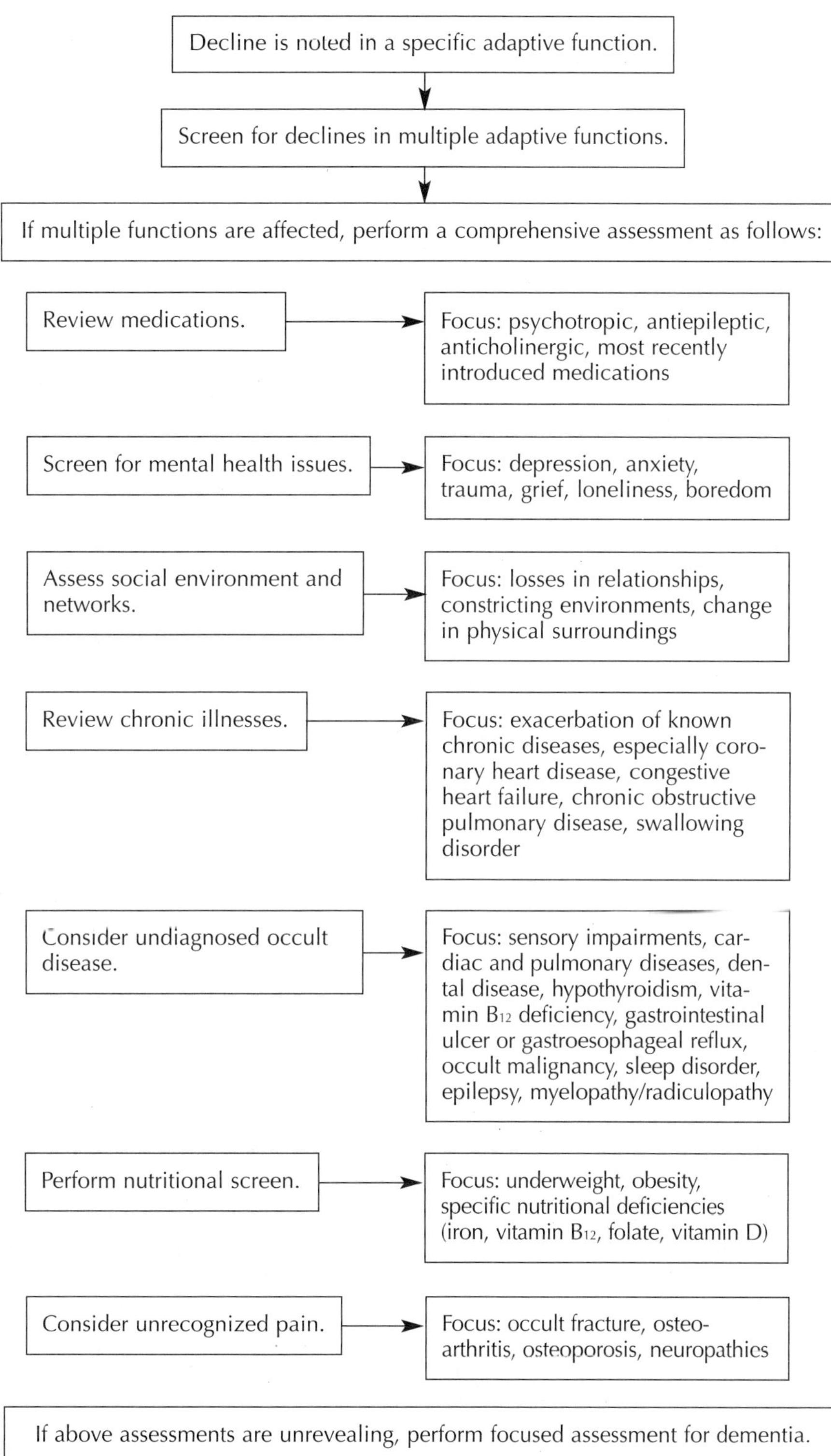

Figure 26.3. Algorithm for evaluation of function decline. (From Tyler, C.V. [1999]. *Medical issues for adults with mental retardation/developmental disabilities.* Homewood, IL: High Tide Press; reprinted by permission.)

PHARMACOTHERAPY

Appropriate prescribing is one of the most important, and difficult, areas of geriatric medicine. With aging, the emergence of chronic diseases, and the ever-expanding number of new pharmacotherapies, more medications are prescribed, and there is a greater risk for prescriber errors. Any symptom in an older adult, particularly an adult with an intellectual and/or communicative impairment, should be considered an adverse drug effect until proven otherwise. Failure to recognize adverse drug effects may result in the inappropriate prescription of even more medication, a dangerous process termed the *prescribing cascade.*

Medications with greater likelihood for side effects include cardiovascular drugs, all psychotropic medications (especially sedative/hypnotics, antipsychotics, and anxiolytics), antiepileptic drugs, and drugs with anticholinergic properties (e.g., gastrointestinal and urinary antispasmodics; muscle relaxants; many psychoactive and cardiovascular medications). Dangerous drug interactions frequently involve warfarin, digoxin, angiotensin converting enzyme inhibitors, and theophylline. Handheld computers equipped with pharmacotherapy programs that detail drug side effects, dosages, and drug interactions can be immensely helpful in averting errors in clinical practice. Experts in the fields of geriatrics and pharmacotherapy periodically publish a list of medications, termed the *Beers Criteria,* that are potentially inappropriate for use in older adults (Fick, Cooper, Wade, Waller, Maclean, & Beers, 2003). Individuals who are prescribed these higher risk medications should be carefully assessed to assure that they are achieving therapeutic goals without adverse effects. According to Henderson,

> Long-term adverse effects of chronic pharmacotherapies may lead to devastating functional impairments by late life. For example, the antiepileptic drugs phenytoin and phenobarbital are associated with two metabolic bone diseases, osteoporosis and osteomalacia, that increase risk for fragility fractures. Some anti-psychotic medications are associated with osteoporosis, through their effect on prolactin levels and gonadal function. (2002)

Bernard is a 68-year-old man who had a lifelong history of poorly controlled seizures. After living in group homes, he was able to move into a home with a family. Over time, he lost a number of activities of daily living (ADL) skills and the ability to ambulate independently. Initially, this loss of skills was believed to be due to some "dementing process," and his brother, who was his guardian, felt that Bernard was not safe in this home setting. He arranged to have Bernard moved to a nursing home. Bernard started to attend a day habilitation program while living in the nursing home and regained some of his ADL skills and engaging personality; however, he never regained his former mobility skills and even needed a mechanical lift to transfer. His dementia diagnosis was later discarded and replaced by a diagnosis of phenytoin encephalopathy.

As Bernard's story illustrates, drug-induced movement disorders are particularly important to recognize as early as possible. Phenytoin encephalopathy, characterized by progressive cognitive impairment and cerebellar atrophy, is attributed to excessive plasma levels of unbound phenytoin (Iivanainen, 1998). More commonly, the chronic use of antipsychotics is associated with several types of movement disorders, including parkinsonism, tardive dyskinesias, and tardive dystonias. These complications of therapy may not manifest until the offending drug is withdrawn or dosage decreased. Older adults prescribed psychotropics or antiepileptics should undergo routine systematic clinical observation for abnormal movements.

COMPREHENSIVE GERIATRIC ASSESSMENT

Some adults may benefit from the expertise of specialists in geriatric medicine and/or from a multidisciplinary comprehensive evaluation process termed *comprehensive geriatric assessment,* or CGA (Gallo, Fulmer, Paveza, & Reichel, 2000; Henderson & Davidson, 2000). Individuals typically referred for these services include older adults with multidomain functional declines, recurrent hospitalizations, multiple chronic diseases with frequent decompensations, multiple geriatric syndromes, or the threat of institutionalization. CGA is conducted by a team of geriatric specialists, including a geriatrician, geriatric nurse practitioner, social worker, occupational therapist, and physical therapist and may include a geropsychiatrist, podiatrist, or other health professionals.

Some geriatric assessment clinics may not have much specific experience or training in the care of older adults with developmental disabilities. They may be prone to familiar clinical errors such as "diagnostic overshadowing," misclassification of self-talk as a psychotic symptom, or overdiagnosis of dementia in individuals with Down syndrome. CGA has not been extensively studied specifically in older adults with intellectual and developmental disabilities, but in the general geriatric population, these assessments have been demonstrated to improve function and to reduce hospitalizations and nursing home placements.

Table 26.2. Periodic health evaluation guidelines for older adults with intellectual and developmental disabilities

Target conditions and risks	Assessment (yearly unless otherwise specified)
Sensory impairments	
Visual impairment	Conduct visual acuity test, glaucoma screen, and ophthalmoscopy every 1–2 years.
Hearing impairment	Perform otoscopy and audiometry every 1–2 years.
Cardiovascular diseases	
Hypertension	Check blood pressure.
Atrial fibrillation	Assess heart rhythm.
Inadequate physical activity	Review physical activity habits, and provide exercise counseling.
Hyperlipidemia	Perform a fasting lipid profile baseline, and repeat as the occasion arises.
Cancer screening	
Colon cancer	Conduct fecal occult blood testing yearly along with flexible sigmoidoscopy every 5 years or colonoscopy every 10 years.
Breast cancer	Perform mammography every 1–2 years and a clinical breast exam yearly.
Cervical cancer	No screening is necessary if the woman has no history of sexual intercourse. No further screening is necessary if the woman has had a hysterectomy for noncancer indications. May cease Pap smears after age 65 if the woman has no history of human papilloma virus (HPV)/abnormal Pap smears and has three documented normal Pap smears. Continue annual Pap smears if HPV is positive.
Skin cancer	Perform a clinical skin examination.
Prostate cancer	Screening by prostate-specific antigen (PSA) remains controversial. Discuss potential risks, benefits, and limitations.
Ovarian cancer	No adequate screening methodologies are yet available, including bimanual pelvic examinations and CA-125 monitoring.
Lung cancer	Offer smoking cessation counseling. No adequate screening methodologies are yet available.
Nutritional issues	
Obesity	Perform a body mass index (BMI).
Malnutrition	Perform a BMI and nutrition screening.
Osteoporosis	Assure that the individual has 1,500 mg. daily calcium intake and 800 IU daily vitamin D intake. Conduct baseline bone mineral density testing, and repeat as the occasion arises.
Oral cavity diseases	Have a dentist perform an examination.
Mental health issues	
Depression	Screen for depression.
Sleep	Assess sleep for interval changes.
Social isolation	Assess changes in social network.
Abuse	Screen for physical, sexual, and psychological abuse or neglect.
Substance abuse	Screen for alcohol, drug, and tobacco use.
Functional changes	
Cognitive impairments	Screen for interval changes in cognitive function.
Mobility impairments	Screen for interval changes in mobility.
Adaptive functioning impairments	Screen for interval changes in adaptive functioning.
Falls	Screen for interval events.
Incontinence—fecal and urinary	Screen for interval changes in continence.
Immunizations	
Tetanus/diphtheria	Give a primary series, then once every 10 years.
Pneumococcal	Give at age 65, then review indications for a booster.
Influenza	Give annually.
Hepatitis B	Give a primary series if unvaccinated, and review indications for a booster.
Advance planning	
Advance directives	Review and update advance directives. Specify a person to assist with decision making.

Table 26.3. Underrecognized common health problems in older adults with intellectual and developmental disabilities

Coronary artery disease
Congestive heart failure
Peripheral arterial disease
Chronic obstructive pulmonary disease
Osteoporosis
Osteoarthritis
Spinal stenosis
Podiatric problems
Dental caries
Periodontal disease
Malnutrition
Dehydration
Anxiety disorders
Depression
Gastroesophageal reflux disorder

Source: Tyler (1999).

FUNCTIONAL DECLINE

Careful medical assessment is required whenever an aging adult with intellectual and developmental disabilities manifests a decline in adaptive functioning. This decline can be either in self-care or ADL skills (e.g., dressing, bathing) and/or other skill areas based on physical or cognitive performance. Functional decline may be described by those who provide the care as changes in social skill quality or types rather than as losses of specific ADL skills (Henderson & Davidson, 2000). Ava's story reveals the complex dynamics among the presentations of the problem(s) and care management issues.

A consultation was requested for Ava, a 77-year-old woman who lived with minimal external support in her own apartment after moving out of a state school 30 years ago. She reportedly had a long history of poor hygiene, and, a few years ago, personal care homemaker services were secured through the local elder service agency. In addition to receiving help at home, Ava attends an adult day health program. She uses local public transportation and walks with a cane within town with no difficulties. Ava is quite verbal and speaks simply but accurately about current world events. Her known diagnoses were hypertension and non–insulin-dependent diabetes, both of which had been controlled with medications.

Two years ago, a consultant psychiatrist prescribed antipsychotic medication for what he interpreted as command hallucinations related to a probable dementia. As more time was spent with Ava, it was determined she may have a hearing impairment based on the loudness of the television, her lack of consistent responses, and her vague responses. Former providers succinctly noted that, "She probably can't hear real well, but she gets along okay. . . that's just Ava." Subsequent tests revealed a severe bilateral hearing loss. Hearing aides were obtained, and Ava used them consistently. Her antipsychotic medication was slowly discontinued with success.

Concealed medical morbidities often manifest as behavioral symptoms (Davidson, Janicki, Ladrigan, Houser, Henderson, & Cain, 2003). Diverse medical conditions, adverse drug effects, untreated pain, and psychosocial issues all can result in functional decline (see Table 26.4). Concurrent and even interrelated conditions have the potential to cause disability (Henderson & Davidson, 2000; Service & Hahn, 2003). Common clinical errors include inappropriately attributing functional decline to age or to the intellectual disability itself, a form of diagnostic overshadowing.

STAFF TRAINING AND EDUCATION

Individuals who never required environmental modifications or adaptive equipment in younger years may benefit from these supports in later life. Staff may need education about the types of modifications and assistive devices available in order to identify opportunities for their use. They may appreciate general information about aging and more specific information about age-associated diseases, their management, and their prognosis. (See Table 26.5 for list of training resources.) As health-related issues emerge, staff may require specific cognitive and skill training in monitoring health conditions, such as blood pressure measurement, finger-stick glucose testing, or recognition of signs and symptoms of congestive heart failure. Younger staff may learn best about the experience of aging through simulation experiences.

"Until you showed us in that sensitivity training what is happening to Jane's eyes as she was getting older, by having us wear those glasses and such, I really couldn't understand when she had problems doing things and really thought her behaviors were just attention seeking" one staff member said after participation in Aging-Sensitivity Training taught by nurses, physical, speech, and occupational therapists that simulated changes of aging for the participants. "I think that now, with your suggestions, we can better support her."

HEALTH PROMOTION

Adults with intellectual disabilities, like adults in the general population, have high rates of obesity and sedentary lifestyle (Janicki et al., 2002). Being overweight

Table 26.4. Common contributors to declines in adaptive functioning in older adults with intellectual and developmental disabilities

Visual impairment
Hearing impairment
Adverse medication effect
Depression
Adjustment disorders
Grief
Suboptimal epilepsy management
Unrecognized pain
Malnutrition
Unrecognized cardiac disease
Unrecognized pulmonary disease

Source: Tyler (1999).

and having little physical activity can lead to insulin resistance, which predisposes individuals to diabetes, coronary heart disease, stroke, and peripheral vascular disease. In addition, obesity can greatly compound the functional impairments related to arthritis, spasticity, and cardiopulmonary diseases. Any meaningful health promotion program must assist at-risk individuals in losing weight and increasing physical activity.

Many factors affect an older person's participation in health promotion activities, including socioeconomic factors; beliefs and attitudes of the person; informal and formal networks; the meaning of the activity; encouragement by family, direct care staff, and health care providers; and motivation and access to resources (Service & Hahn, 2003). Health promotion, therefore, is more than clinical recommendations and programmatic services and involves such fundamental issues as social involvement and inclusion.

Table 26.5. Internet resources about age-associated diseases

American Academy of Family Physicians—http://www.aafp.org
American Association on Mental Retardation—www.aamr.org.
American Geriatrics Society—http://www.americangeriatrics.org
American Medical Directors Association—http://www.amda.com
American Society on Aging—http://www.asaging.org
Administration on Aging—http://www.aoa.gov
Gerontological Association of America—http://www.geron.org/
International Association on Scientific Study of Intellectual Disabilities, Special Interest Group (SIRG) on Aging—http://www.iassid.org
John A. Hartford Foundation—http://www.jhartfound.org
John A. Hartford Foundation Institute for Geriatric Nursing—http://www.hartfordign.org/links/
National Council on the Aging—http://www.ncoa.org
National Institute on Aging—http://www.nia.nih.gov
Nutrition Screening Initiative—http://www.aafp.org/nsi.xml
Rehabilitation Research and Training Center on Aging with Developmental Disabilities (RRTCADD)—http://www.uic.edu/orgs/rrtcamr/
United States Preventative Services Task Force—http://www.ahcpr.gov/clinic/uspstfix.htm

PSYCHOSOCIAL CONSIDERATIONS

Older adults with intellectual disabilities are influenced by others in their social network; by their gender; by the social-cultural context; and by their own physical, emotional, and intellectual disabilities (Edgerton, 1994). According to Thorpe, Davidson, and Janicki (2001), scant empirical data is available about the normal psychological developmental process throughout the life span of individuals with intellectual disabilities. People with intellectual disabilities have restricted social roles and fewer networks and opportunities to learn tasks associated with aging. Thus, life changes such as bereavement may have a greater impact with more adverse outcomes.

GRIEF AND LOSSES

Aging is truly a two-edged sword. As people with intellectual disabilities live longer, they also experience the joys and sorrows of aging (Ludlow, 1999). They may experience decline or loss in functional abilities (or hard-earned skills) from aging or chronic illness; loss of family, friends, and staff members; residential transitions; changes in opportunities; or lack of choice-making. Secondary losses may result from major primary losses. Small changes (or losses) in the ability of the older person to perform daily activities or in the ability of the caregiver to provide support can have an impact on major life decisions (Gallo et al., 2000). Thus, the actual and potential dilemmas are the same with people who have intellectual disabilities as they are with the general population (Service & Hahn, 2003), as is demonstrated in Celeste's story.

For the past 12 years, Celeste, age 80, has been living with Clara in Clara's home. This situation was set up through an adult family (foster) care program managed by the area agency on aging. Celeste attends an adult day health program 5 days a week. Recently, she has been experiencing problems with gait and balance and frequently needs to void during the night. Even with a bedside commode, she often sustains bruises from injuries while attempting to transfer to the commode chair at night. When a baby monitor was utilized, Clara's sleep was so disrupted that she could not function the following day. Regulations and costs prohibited employment of a separate nighttime caregiver. It appeared a residential move would be necessary.

DEMENTIA CARE

Losses associated with dementia are particularly challenging in that philosophically those who work in the field of intellectual disabilities are used to helping people grow, learn and develop new skills (Janicki & Dalton, 1999; Janicki et al., 1995; Service, Lavoie, & Herlihy, 1999; Wilkinson & Janicki, 2002). With dementia, even maintenance becomes impossible. One model of care that considers factors related to care practices is ENCEPS (Janicki, McCallion, & Dalton, 2002). *E* stands for *early screening and diagnosis.* An accurate diagnosis is necessary for management and planning. A referral to a neurologist, geriatrician, geropsychiatrist, or memory clinic may assist with diagnosis, classification, and staging of the dementia. Comorbid conditions must be identified and treated.

C stands for *clinical supports.* Local Alzheimer Association chapters and hospital-based or outpatient geropsychiatric services may assist staff and families with difficult behavior management issues. The pharmacotherapies provided to individuals with dementias are increasingly complex. Multiple cognitive-enhancing drugs are now available and used in combination. Antipsychotic, antidepressant, and anxiolytic medications are useful to treat specific psychiatric symptoms as they emerge during certain stages of the disease. Some individuals may benefit from consultation with a geropsychiatrist or psychopharmacologist (Prasher, Adams, Holder, & the Down Syndrome Ageing Study Group, 2003). Some anticonvulsants used for seizures may compound cognitive decline (see Tsiouris, Patti, Tipu, & Raguthu, 2002).

E stands for *environment modifications.* Changes to the environment can enhance safety and preserve existing skills (see Hutchings, Olsen, & Ehrenkrantz, 2000). *P* stands for *program adaptations.* The focus of care from fostering skill development to maintaining function and supportive care may be difficult for many staff (and families) to understand and requires ongoing training and support. The process of dementia is inexorably progressive but affects each individual uniquely, at different rates, and with variable constellations of psychiatric symptoms and problematic behaviors. Particular behaviors represent very meaningful feelings, but standard functional behavioral analysis may not yield useful strategies for behavioral management, particularly the "usual" behavioral modification therapies. Programmatic planning requires a systems-oriented approach that explicitly identifies and analyzes the complex relationships (and impact on routines, meanings, and behaviors) of individuals with dementia and everyone around them.

S stands for *specialized care.* As dementia progresses, caregivers change their focus to physical care and comfort for the individual. Discussion regarding end-of-life issues should begin soon after the initial diagnosis, not in the later stages of dementia. People must learn how to let go while finding ways to remain connected. The philosophy of this type of care is often quite different for staff of intellectual and developmental disabilities agencies (Service et al., 1999). Hospice care can be very helpful to those in the support network (Janicki, McCallion, et al., 2002; Service, 2002).

END-OF-LIFE ISSUES

Issues with death and dying are increasingly being discussed and planned for (see Botsford & Force, 2000; Luchterhand & Murphy, 1998). There is a growing recognition and acknowledgement that people with intellectual disabilities experience grief and recognize and understand loss (Dowling & Hollins, 2003; Ludlow, 1999) and that, for many, grief may be expressed through behaviors. End-of-life care needs to be proactive. Planning and discussions should occur earlier in the life span and be reinforced throughout one's life. Preparation includes information, inclusion, and detail regarding the end of life. Likewise, the understanding of bereavement is increasingly being addressed for people with intellectual disabilities.

Interventions for bereavement can be provided either individually or in groups but need to be designed according to the individual's understanding, presenting symptoms, physiological functioning, and support systems (Stoddart, Burke, & Temple, 2002). The use of rituals (e.g., attending funerals and memorial services) with support and such tools as memory books are particularly meaningful and tangible. Eloise's story illustrates the dynamics within the social networks and the historical context that converge at these emotional times.

Eloise was 55-years-old when she died suddenly of a stomach volvulus. Although she was ambulatory, she was nonverbal and used hand-over-hand assistance for almost all of her ADLs, except eating. She had been admitted to a state school at age 10. No one could remember any family involvement after her admission. After the funeral, staff, who had been resentful of the family's recent reinvolvement, went to Eloise's 80-year-old mother's home.

Eloise's mother reminisced with staff about Eloise's early years and admitted, "It was hard times for us. We were poor, and there was no help, and I had other children to raise. We did the best we could. The doctors told us to put her away and to forget about her. But I never, never did. I thought about her, my daughter, every single day in my life, every single day."

As people age, there are increasing situations for decisions to be made regarding their health care treatment (see Midwest Bioethics Center et al., 1996). Although it is beyond the scope of this chapter to fully discuss this issue, early questions such as "Who is this person, and what really matters to him or her?" will help to guide surrogates in the determination of some personal, emotional, and very complicated decisions.

Excellence in end-of-life care necessitates careful recognition and treatment of pain. Individuals with intellectual and developmental disabilities are at risk for suboptimal pain management. Rare instances of congenital insensitivity to pain have been generalized into a myth that people with intellectual and developmental disabilities do not feel pain. Frequently, individuals experience a delay in diagnosis of painful conditions, such as cancer, fractures, and arthritis. Direct care staff and health care providers may have difficulty developing means to assess pain in individuals with communicative impairments. Cognitive, psychological, and behavioral factors may interfere with an individual's willingness to honestly report his or her pain experience.

Sophie was 62 years old and living with her mother and several siblings when she was diagnosed with stage IV squamous cell carcinoma of the head and neck. She underwent gastrostomy tube placement to assist with feeding while undergoing radiotherapy, which she ceased after several treatments. Home hospice services were initiated. When Sophie's family physician made a house call, Sophie was alert and restless and had not slept for 2 days. When questioned about Sophie's pain medications, Sophie's sister explained that the hospice nurse had only authorized them to give Tylenol because Sophie would shake her head "No" whenever the hospice nurse asked her if she wanted something stronger. The family physician began morphine, and Sophie became less restless and was able to sleep. The hospice nurse and family were counseled to observe Sophie's behavior and sleeplessness as indicators of pain, rather than her response to questions.

The ideas of choice and self-determination, which are based on the principle of autonomy, are integral in the field of intellectual disabilities. Even today, the autonomy of older adults is often compromised by unproven assumptions about the older person's capacity for decision making. Because this situation is historically similar for people with developmental disabilities, individuals with intellectual and developmental disabilities who reach old age are in "double jeopardy" of disfranchisement from the decision-making process.

The term *assisted autonomy*, proposed by Ansello and Janicki (2000), describes a process in which individuals make their choices through negotiation with and assistance of others. This process does not contradict an aging person's fundamental need for respect, care, meaning, and social connectedness. It also recognizes individuals within a social and historical context and the importance of values, beliefs, and health care practices of different cultures (Service & Hahn, 2003), as illustrated by Ladislav's story.

Ladislav was an 88-year-old man who had moved into a group home 15 years ago after living in a state institution, where he had been since the age of 13. He had been diagnosed as status post encephalitis and had undergone surgical repairs of fractures in both hips. Ladislav had suffered from mild hearing loss, constipation, a history of gastrointestinal bleeding, and Parkinson disease for the last 25 years. He used a wheelchair and used thumbs up or down to indicate choices.

Ladislav had chronic aspiration causing recurrent pneumonias. His staff worked with him to complete an advance directive. The legal means in his state was the use of a health care proxy, and Ladislav named his brother, Josef, as his agent. He had the capacity to make informed decisions and decided that he did not want to have a feeding tube. Following a hospitalization for pneumothorax, he decided to go home to die. He returned to his group home with hospice services and died peacefully surrounded by his caregivers, some of whom had worked directly with him for 30 years.

EXTERNAL ENVIRONMENT/COMMUNITY

Residential settings for older people with intellectual disabilities are considerably diverse and include the family home, nursing homes, adult family or foster care, supported and independent living arrangements, licensed intermediate care facilities and group homes, and other congregate living facilities managed within the elder network. The range of day program models include senior centers, social day care and adult day health, individual retirement programs, and continuance of work either full or part time. Residential and day programs will evolve and change as the characteristics and needs of each age cohort evolve and change. The importance of social support for health, and the fragility of support that is characteristic of many older persons, is well documented and has implications for the service delivery system and management of health needs.

Although many of the similarities between the two specialties of aging and developmental disabilities have been noted, there still exist many differences, particularly within the service delivery system. Each agency has its own operational policies, terminology, funding qualifications, criteria for eligibility for different types of service, and philosophy and priorities of care (Hacker, McCallion, & Janicki, 2000). There have been increasing cross-agency collaborations such as training and coordination of efforts, as is summarized in Margaret's story.

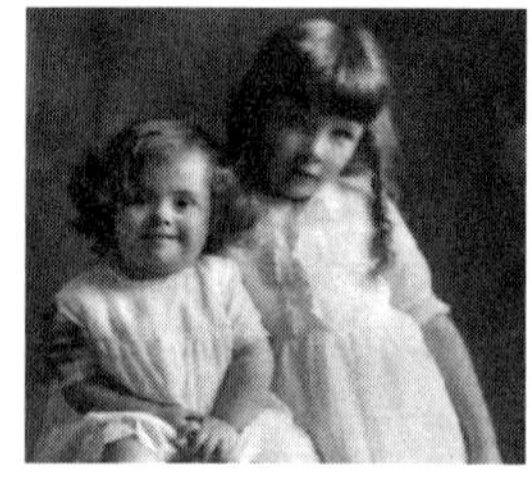

a

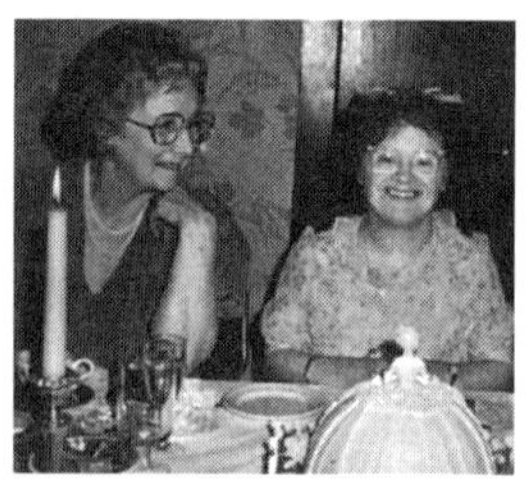

b

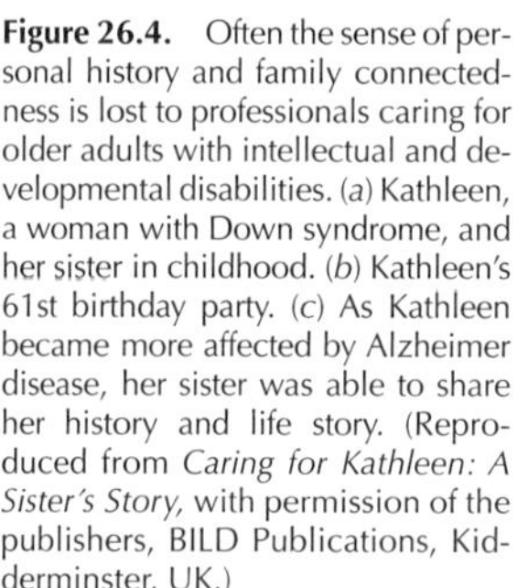

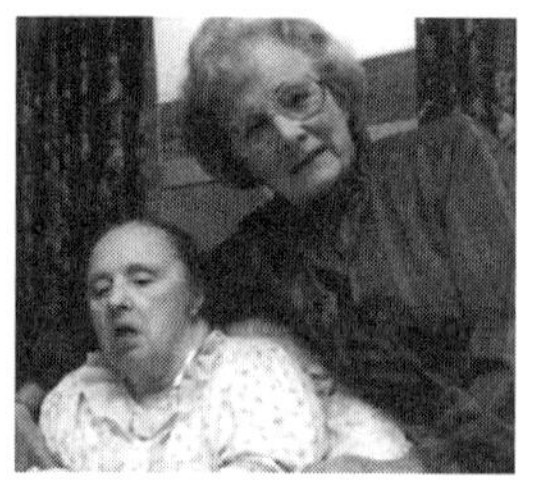

c

Figure 26.4. Often the sense of personal history and family connectedness is lost to professionals caring for older adults with intellectual and developmental disabilities. (*a*) Kathleen, a woman with Down syndrome, and her sister in childhood. (*b*) Kathleen's 61st birthday party. (*c*) As Kathleen became more affected by Alzheimer disease, her sister was able to share her history and life story. (Reproduced from *Caring for Kathleen: A Sister's Story,* with permission of the publishers, BILD Publications, Kidderminster, UK.)

Margaret is a 68-year-old widow with numerous physical and psychological health problems who lives in a subsidized apartment. She receives some individual support services through the local intellectual and developmental disabilities agency. After her hospitalization for an embolectomy, she required daily anticoagulation therapy with intensive medication monitoring. Margaret only wanted to "go home" and refused to return anywhere other than her apartment. Regulations prevented the intellectual and developmental disabilities agency from direct medication administration. Margaret did not meet the criteria for skilled nursing care through the local Visiting Nurses Association. Finally, a nearby adult day health program was located whose program registered nurse would assume medication management, frequent health assessments and monitoring, and help with a much-needed weekly shower.

THE AGING FAMILY

The social environment is an important factor in healing and the promotion of optimum health and function. As people with intellectual disabilities age, their support may come from either formal networks, which are usually government-sponsored professional services, or informal networks, which are the nuclear family, extended kin, friends, and neighbors. These informal support networks are usually small, dense, and predominantly family members (Bigby, 2000).

Families are the major providers of supports for adults with intellectual disabilities (Heller et al., 2002; see Figure 26.4). Research indicates in the United States that 76% of adults with intellectual and developmental disabilities of all ages live at home (Fujiura, 2001) and that more than 25% of their family caregivers are older than 60. This growing phenomenon of aging families has generated its own special concerns and issues for health care providers. Both positive and negative aspects exist regarding caregiving and interdependence of adults with intellectual disabilities and their family members (see Heller et al., 2002), as witnessed by Zeke's situation.

Zeke, age 50, resides with his 71-year-old mother (who is his guardian) and an unmarried sister, Carol, who is age 52. Zeke's sister, Carol, works in a fast food restaurant and assists her mother in the management of the household. They all live in a low-income housing project. Zeke spent 15 years in a residential school and moved back to living with his family about 25 years ago.

Zeke is ambulatory and is fairly healthy, but he has a controlled seizure disorder and at times experiences constipation. Zeke needs verbal and some physical assistance with his ADLs. He communicates with a few words, using mostly vocalizations and gestures. In addition, Zeke may have autism.

About 3 years ago, when Zeke's mother began to have heart problems, social workers felt that it might ease her caregiver burden if Zeke was enrolled in a day habilitation program. Zeke began attending the program, where he was assisted with various skill developments. The day program, however, frequently reported that Zeke's hygiene was poor.

Six months ago, a vacancy occurred in a four-person group home in town, and Zeke was suggested to fill the vacancy. The other three men who already lived there attended the same day program and appeared to be compatible with Zeke. Because of Zeke's mother's apparent growing frailty and Carol's chronic exhausted demeanor, the case manager believed that she was being proactive in planning for Zeke;

however, the family procrastinated on the decision to permit him to move, even after a number of positive visits. The case manager finally realized that the basis for their reluctance was that they were very dependent on Zeke's government benefits to make their ends meet.

Zeke's mother stated, "I'm his mother, and Zeke really does okay with us now. When I'm gone, Carol will just take over if there aren't any other places open."

Zeke's mother's statement illustrates the dilemma faced by many low-income families whose dependence on the benefits of their relative with a disability is at odds with pursuing the best interests of their relative. In Zeke's case, no clear-cut solution existed—the continued intactness of family (and potential sacrifice of Zeke's immediate well-being) weighed against the potential disintegration of the family (and Zeke's entry to a life on his own). Yet, these types of dilemmas are common, as depicted by the comments of a 79-year-old mother of a 45-year-old daughter with Down syndrome, "I don't know what I'd do without my Annie. She helps me out with errands and such, is good company, keeps me young, and gives me a reason to get up in the morning!"

Many parents will avoid succession planning (i.e., who will care their child after they are gone) and permanency planning in areas of legal (e.g., guardianship), financial, or residential concerns. The lifelong perception of parental responsibility often blocks the initiation of planning for the future and the extent and nature of any planning (formal and informal) is varied along a continuum (see Bigby, 2000; Janicki, 2002). Sibling relationships have been shown to be complex and multifaceted, to vary across the life span, and to be influenced by the family dynamics and milieu (see Seltzer, Greenberg, Krauss, Gordon, & Judge, 1997). As with all families, the family history, the nature of the characteristics, particular family dynamics, and negotiated commitments all have an impact on the individual and his or her networks in a multitude of ways.

Illustrative of this concept are the comments of a 68-year-old sister (and guardian) of Isabelle, a 64-year-old woman with Down syndrome who was diagnosed 5 years ago with Alzheimer disease. Isabelle's older sister personally paid for expensive adaptations to her home to accommodate her sister's changing needs. She continues to advocate for everything possible to be done for her sister, who is now in the end stage of the disease and has a feeding tube and tracheostomy, which the sister manages.

The sister has noted, "I promised Mama that I would always care for Isabelle. She is a child of God, and they always told us that she wouldn't live long, but look what we have done. She may be my cross to bear, but she is my sister, and I have and will do what I need to do for her to live."

Parental illness, incapacity, death, or even retirement can contribute to a major life transition for the adult child and for the other family members or informal networks. It can be both a period of broad opportunities and vulnerabilities due to a lesser quality of supports and the loss of familiar informal supports (Bigby, 2000). This situation has many implications both for the informal and formal networks (particularly with service provision) with many challenges and opportunities for health care providers in assessment, interventions, and treatments (Service & Hahn, 2003). Celeste's situation illustrates this dynamic.

Celeste needed to move from Clara's home. She was offered a single room in a group home with 24-hour staffing and regular nursing consultation. Although it was 20 miles from her previous residence, Celeste could still attend the adult day health program as she had done for 16 years. Her niece, Lisa, whose family Celeste visited on some holidays, became more involved, and she wanted her aunt to stay closer to her.

There were many discussions with Celeste and Lisa about the benefits of that group home. Celeste frequently changed her mind about her choice, but she finally decided to go into a nursing home, which was in the same town as her niece. Because of regulations and massive costs, she would not be able to attend the day health program. Celeste shared a tiny room with two other women and had minor disagreements about the television that they shared. She also expressed fear because a confused resident frequently came into her room. As opportunities arose, Celeste was asked about moving, and she still vacillated.

When Lisa was approached, she tersely said, "I don't know why you keep pestering us. All the other family members have written her off but me. Either me, my husband, or my kids visit Aunt Celeste every day. Staff can come and go, but we are her family. It beats a private room in a fancy home and is more important than the day program. How come you can't understand that?"

CONCLUSION

Successful aging requires adaptation to many life changes. Components of successful aging have been defined as: 1) avoiding disease and disability; 2) maintaining optimum physical and cognitive functioning; and 3) maintaining engagement with life (Rowe & Kahn, 1998). The first generation of individuals with intellectual and developmental disabilities are surviving to old age, many of whom may meet the criteria for successful aging.

Many of the impairments previously attributed to old age are now understood to be treatable diseases and preventable secondary conditions. Many of the health burdens currently carried by older adults are the consequence of undiagnosed disease, institutionalization, and neglect. Optimizing health and function in later years requires considerable time, effort, and commitment on the part of individuals, families, and service and health care providers; creative utilization of aging service networks; and thoughtful future planning.

Every advancement in general knowledge about health and aging begs the question "Does this apply to older adults with intellectual and developmental disabilities, too?" Each generation of older adults will carry its own unique history and experience. So, too, must individuals who work with each generation shift and adapt to the unique needs and circumstances of the older adults they serve.

REFERENCES

Anderson, R.N., & DeTurk, P.B. (2002). *United States life tables, 1999: National vital statistics reports.* Hyattsville, MD: National Center for Health Statistics. Retrieved August 24, 2004, from http://www.cdc.gov/nchs/

Ansello, E.F., & Janicki, M.P. (2000). The aging of nations: Impact on the community, the family, and the individual. In M.P. Janicki & E.F. Ansello (Eds.), *Community supports for aging adults with lifelong disabilities* (pp. 3–18). Baltimore: Paul H. Brookes Publishing Co.

Baird, P.A., & Sadovnick, A.D. (1989). Life tables for Down syndrome. *Human Genetics, 82*(3), 291–292.

Beange, H., McElduff, A., & Baker, W. (1995). Medical disorders of adults with mental retardation. *American Journal of Mental Retardation, 99*, 595–604.

Bigby, C. (2000). Informal support networks of older adults. In M.P. Janicki & E.F. Ansello (Eds.), *Community supports for aging adults with lifelong disabilities* (pp. 55–70). Baltimore: Paul H. Brookes Publishing Co.

Botsford, A.L., & Force, L.T. (2000). *End of life care: A guide for supporting older people with intellectual disabilities and their families.* Albany, NY: NYSARC.

Cohen, W.I. (Ed.). (1999). Health care guidelines for individuals with Down syndrome: 1999 revision. *Down Syndrome Quarterly, 4*(3).

Davidson, P.W., Heller, T., Janicki, M.P., & Hyer, K. (2003). *The Tampa Scientific Conference on Intellectual Disability, Aging, and Health.* Chicago: University of Illinois at Chicago, Rehabilitation and Research Training Center on Aging with Developmental Disabilities.

Davidson, P.W., Janicki, M.P., Landrigan, P., Houser, K., Henderson, C.M., & Cain, N.N. (2003). Associations between behavior disorders and health status among older adults with intellectual disability. *Aging & Mental Health,* 7(6), 424–430.

Dowling, S., & Hollins, S. (2003). Coping with bereavement: The dynamics of intervention. In P.W. Davidson, V.P. Prasher, & M.P. Janicki (Eds.), *Mental health of adults with intellectual disabilities* (pp. 166–178). Oxford, England: Blackwell Publishing.

Edgerton, R.B. (1994). Quality of life issues: Some people know how to be old. In M.M. Seltzer, M.W. Krauss, & M.P. Janicki (Eds.), *Life course perspectives on adulthood and old age* (pp. 53–66). Washington, DC: American Association on Mental Retardation.

Evenhuis, H., Henderson, C.M., Beange, H., Lennox, N., & Chicoine, B. (2001). Healthy ageing—Adults with intellectual disabilities: Physical health issues. *Journal of Applied Research in Intellectual Disabilities, 14*(3), 175–194.

Eyman, R.K., & Borthwick-Duffy, S.A. (1994). Trends in mortality rates and predictors of mortality. In M.M. Seltzer, M.W. Krauss, & M.P. Janicki (Eds.), *Life course perspectives on adulthood and old age* (pp. 93–105). Washington, DC: American Association on Mental Retardation.

Fick, D.M., Cooper, J.W., Wade, W.E., Waller, J.L., Maclean, J.R., & Beers, M.H. (2003). Updating the Beers Criteria for potentially inappropriate medication use in older adults: Results of a U.S. Consensus Panel of Experts. *Achieves of Internal Medicine, 163*, 2716–2724.

Fray, M.T. (2000). *Caring for Kathleen: A sister's story about Down's syndrome and dementia.* Kidderminster, United Kingdom: British Institute of Learning Disabilities.

Fujiura, G. (2001). *Family demography: Emerging policy challenges.* Paper presented at the Invitational Research Symposium on Aging with Developmental Disabilities: Promoting Healthy Aging, Family Supports, and Age-Friendly Communities, Chicago.

Gallo, J.J., Fulmer, T., Paveza, G.J., & Reichel, W. (2000). *Handbook of geriatric assessment* (3rd ed.). Gaithersburg, MD: Aspen Publishers.

Hacker, K.S., McCallion, P., & Janicki, M.P. (2000). Outreach and assistance using Area Agencies on Aging. In M.P. Janicki & E.F. Ansello (Eds.), *Community supports for aging adults with lifelong disabilities* (pp. 439–455). Baltimore: Paul H. Brookes Publishing Co.

Hayden, M.F. (1998). Mortality among people with mental retardation living in the United States: Research, review, and policy applications. *Mental Retardation, 36*(5), 345–359.

Heller, T., Janicki, M.P., Hammel, J., & Factor, A. (2002). *Promoting healthy aging, family support, and age-friendly communities for persons aging with developmental disabilities: Report of the 2001 Invitational Research Symposium on Aging with Developmental Disabilities.* Chicago: University of Illinois at Chicago, Rehabilitation Research and Training Center on Aging with Developmental Disabilities. Available at http://www.uic.edu/orgs/rrtcamr/

Henderson, C.M. (2002, December). *Function, aging, and selected (common) older-age related conditions in adults with developmental disabilities.* Paper presented at the First International Conference on Aging Persons with Developmental Disabilities, Tampa, Florida.

Henderson, C.M., & Davidson, P.W. (2000). Comprehensive adult and geriatric assessment. In M.P. Janicki & E.F. Ansello (Eds.), *Community supports for aging adults with lifelong disabilities* (pp. 373–386). Baltimore: Paul H. Brookes Publishing Co.

Hogg, J., Lucchino, R., Wang, K.Y., & Janicki, M.P. (2001). Healthy aging—Adults with intellectual disabilities: Aging and social policy. *Journal of Applied Research in Intellectual Disabilities, 14*(3), 229–255.

Hutchings, B.L., Olsen, R.V., & Ehrenkrantz, E.D. (2000). Modifying home environments. In M.P. Janicki & E.F. Ansello (Eds.), *Community supports for aging adults with lifelong disabilities* (pp. 243–256). Baltimore: Paul H. Brookes Publishing Co.

Iivanainen, M. (1998). Phenytoin: Effective but insidious therapy for epilepsy in people with intellectual disability. *Journal of Intellectual Disability Research, 42*(Suppl. 1), 24–31.

Janicki, M.P. (2002, March). *Current tendency and future directions of community care for people with aged intellectual disabilities.* Paper presented at the International Seminar on Welfare of Persons with Disabilities: Aged persons with disability—Community Care and Quality of Life, Tokyo.

Janicki, M.P., & Dalton, A.J. (Eds.). (1999). *Dementia, aging, and intellectual disabilities: A handbook.* Philadelphia: Taylor & Francis.

Janicki, M.P., Dalton, A.J., Henderson, C.M., & Davidson, P.W. (1999). Mortality and morbidity among older adults with intellectual disability: Health services considerations. *Disability and Rehabilitation, 21*(5/6), 284–294.

Janicki, M.P., Davidson, P.W., Henderson, C.M., McCallion, P., Taets, J.D., Force, L.T., Sulkes, S.B., Frangenberg, E., & Ladrigan, P.M. (2002). Health characteristics and health services utilization in older adults with intellectual disability living in community residences. *Journal of Intellectual Disability Research, 46*(4), 287–298.

Janicki, M.P., Heller, T., Seltzer, G., & Hogg, J. (1995). *Practice guidelines for the clinical assessment and care management of Alzheimer and other dementia among adults with mental retardation.* Washington, DC: American Association on Mental Retardation.

Janicki, M.P., McCallion, P., & Dalton, A.J. (2002). Dementia-related care decision-making in group homes for persons with intellectual disabilities. *Journal of Gerontological Social Work, 38*(1/2), 179–195.

Kapell, D., Nightingale, B., Rodriguez, A., Lee, J.H., Zigman, W.B., & Schupf, N. (1998). Prevalence of chronic medical conditions in adult with mental retardation: Comparison with the general population. *Mental Retardation, 36*(4), 269–279.

Lai, F., & Williams, R. S. (1989). A prospective study of Alzheimer's disease in Down syndrome. *Archives of Neurology, 47,* 849–853.

Luchterhand, C., & Murphy, N. (1998). *Helping adults with mental retardation grieve a death loss.* Philadelphia: Taylor & Francis.

Ludlow, B.L. (1999). Life after loss: Legal, ethical and practical issues. In S.S. Herr & G. Weber (Eds.), *Aging, rights and quality of life: Prospects for older people with developmental disabilities* (pp. 189–221). Baltimore: Paul H. Brookes Publishing Co.

Midwest Bioethics Center & University of Missouri–Kansas City, Institute for Human Development Task Force. (1996). Health care treatment decision-making guidelines for adults with developmental disabilities. *Bioethics Forum,* 1–8.

Patja, K., Molson, P., & Iivanainen, M. (2001). Cause-specific mortality of people with intellectual disability in a population-based, 35-year follow-up study. *Journal of Intellectual Disability Research, 45*(1), 30–40.

Prasher, V.P., Adams, C., Holder, R., & the Down Syndrome Research Group. (2003). Long term safety and efficacy of donepezil in the treatment of dementia in Alzheimer's disease in adults with Down syndrome: Open label study. *International Journal of Geriatric Psychiatry, 18,* 549–551.

Rowe, J.W., & Kahn, R.L. (1998). *Successful aging.* New York: Pantheon.

Schretzman, D., & Strumpf, N.E. (2002). Principles guiding care of older adults. In V.T Cotter, & N.E. Strumpf (Eds.), *Advanced practice nursing with older adults* (pp. 5–25). New York: McGraw-Hill.

Seltzer, M.M., Greenberg, J.S., Krauss, M.W., Gordon, R.M., & Judge, K. (1997). Siblings of adults with mental retardation or mental illness: Effects on lifestyle and psychological well-being. *Family Relations, 46,* 395–405.

Service, K.P. (2002). Considerations in care for individuals with intellectual disability with advanced dementia. *Journal of Gerontological Social Work, 38*(1/2), 213–224.

Service, K.P., & Hahn, J.E. (2003). Issues of aging: The role of the nurse in the care of older people with intellectual and developmental disabilities. *Nursing Clinics of North America, 38,* 291–312.

Service, K.P., Lavoie, D., & Herlihy, J.E. (1999). Coping with losses, death, and grieving. In M.P. Janicki & A.J. Dalton (Eds.), *Dementia, aging and intellectual disabilities: A handbook* (pp. 330–357). Philadelphia: Taylor & Francis.

Stoddart, K.P., Burke, L., & Temple, V. (2002). Outcome evaluation of bereavement groups for adults with intellectual disabilities. *Journal of Applied Research in Intellectual Disabilities, 15,* 28–35.

Strauss, D., Cable, W., & Shavelle, R. (1999). Causes of excess mortality in cerebral palsy. *Developmental Medicine and Child Neurology, 41,* 580–585.

Thorpe, L., Davidson, P., & Janicki, M. (2001). Healthy aging—Adults with intellectual disabilities: Biobehavioural issues. *Journal of Applied Research in Intellectual Disabilities, 14*(3), 218–228.

Tsiouris, J.A., Patti, P.J., Tipu, O., & Raguthu, S. (2002). Adverse effects of phenytoin given for late-onset seizures in adults with Down syndrome. *Neurology, 59,* 779–780.

Tyler, C.V., & Edman, J. (2004). Down syndrome, Turner syndrome, and Klinefelter syndrome: Primary care throughout the lifespan. *Primary Care: Clinics in Office Practice, 31*(3), x–xi, 627–628.

Tyler, C.V., Snyder, C.W., & Zyzanski, S. (2000). Screening for osteoporosis in community-dwelling adults with mental retardation. *Mental Retardation, 38*(4), 316–321.

Tyler, C.V., & Bourguet, C. (1997). Primary care of adults with mental retardation. *Journal of Family Practice, 44*(5), 487–494.

United Nations, Department of Economic and Social Affairs, United Nations Secretariat. (2003, January 15). *Implications for an ageing society.* Retrieved September 29, 2003, from http://www.un.org/esa/socdev/ageing/ageimpl.htm

Walsh, P.N., & Murphy, G.H. (2002). Risk and vulnerabilities: Dilemmas for women. In P.N. Walsh & T. Heller (Eds.), *Health of women with intellectual disabilities* (pp. 154–169). Oxford, England: Blackwell Publishing.

Wilkinson, H., & Janicki, M.P. (2002, March). The Edinburgh Principles with accompanying guidelines and recommendations. *Journal of Intellectual Disability Research, 46*(3), 279–284.

Yang, Q., Rasmussen, S.A., & Friedman, J. M. (2002). Mortality associated with Down's syndrome from 1983 to 1997: A population-based study. *Lancet, 359*(9311), 1019–1025.

Chapter 27

Severe and Profound Disabilities

27.1 Complex Medical Problems

I. Leslie Rubin

A review of the last half century of care for individuals with severe and profound disabilities reveals that our society has raised the standard for care for this vulnerable population. Individuals with severe and profound disabilities represent a relatively small group but have significantly greater needs and thus place a greater demand on the knowledge, time, finances, and organizational processes of the health care delivery system. For purposes of discussion, looking at disability terms that are in current and familiar use is helpful. Exploration of the terms *mental retardation/intellectual disability* and *cerebral palsy* lead to different bodies of literature from different clinical and service delivery universes, but they nevertheless reveal similar information. The term *children with special health care needs*, as used in pediatrics, helps to illustrate the increased needs of such individuals from their families, providers of heath care and other services, and society as a whole.

In an examination of the health care needs of adolescents using the 1984 National Health Interview Survey, Newachek (1989) found that more than 6% of adolescents, or nearly 2 million nationwide, suffered some degree of disability or limitation in their usual activities that year. This group of adolescents was shown to have three times as many physician contacts annually and to spend nine times as many days hospitalized as their counterparts without disabilities. In addition, one in every seven adolescents with disabilities was found to be uninsured, thus exposing their families to significant financial risks. In the 1999–2000 national Medical Expenditure Panel Survey, Newacheck et al. (2004) found that 7% of U.S. children with disabilities used many more services than their counterparts without disabilities. They spent eight times as many days in the hospital, had six times as many nonphysician professional visits, and had almost 10 times as many home health provider days that translated into four times as many health care expenditures and twice as many out-of-pocket expenses. If this generic perspective of "children with special health care needs" demonstrates the increase in need for and utilization of services, then how much more will the need for services be when the underlying clinical condition is more severe and more complex.

Although there clearly are common functional, neurological, medical, educational, and social conditions that are associated with having severe and profound disabilities, each individual must be examined and understood as an individual. Health care providers must be familiar not only with the underlying etiological factors and the neurological and medical features of the person but also with his or her personality. Subtle physiological, emotional, and behavioral manifestations may express changes in the person's physiology and clinical conditions. These factors are important both for their respect due to the individual (as Crocker points out in Chapter 27.2) but also from the perspective of providing optimal health care. This latter is particularly significant in appreciating nuances in underlying physiological stability as well as underlying health status that alert a clinician to look for a clinical condition that is responsible for the change, identifying and treating it early, and thus preventing unnecessary and potentially serious complications.

Individuals with severe and profound disabilities include children and adults with severe and profound intellectual disabilities and/or severe cerebral palsy. These conditions are consequences of severe central nervous system (CNS) dysfunction. Figure 27.1.1 illustrates how etiology and functional outcome can be viewed in relation to the CNS. At the simplest level, the functional manifestations of the CNS are in the motor, cognitive, and behavioral domains. Additional functional impairments are seen in other neurological domains that include

- Sensory—especially vision and hearing
- Smooth muscle—especially gastrointestinal tract
- Complex integrative functions—eating and swallowing and the oral expression of speech

Individuals with developmental disabilities can be characterized by functional ability in five areas, and each functional area requires a thorough analysis for its clinical implications:

1. Ability to communicate
2. Ability to eat (feed self, chew, and swallow)
3. Ability to control bowel and bladder function
4. Ability to change position
5. Ability to use an arm or hand

Individuals with severe and profound disabilities are

- Less likely to be able to communicate effectively
- Less likely to be able to eat independently
- More likely to need assistance in feeding
- More likely to have difficulty in chewing and swallowing
- More likely to be fed by a gastrostomy feeding tube
- Less likely to have bowel and bladder control
- Less likely to be able to change position (e.g., roll over)
- Less likely to be able to use an arm or hand

These individuals not only have significant functional impairments, but they also are more likely to have associated neurological and sensory conditions. In a study by the Centers for Disease Control and Prevention (Mervis et al., 1995), children with more severe intellectual disabilities were one and a half times more likely to have an additional disability, more than two times more likely to have a seizure disorder, almost three times more likely to have cerebral palsy, and four times more likely to have a visual impairment (see Table 27.1-1).

The more severe the CNS insult or compromise, the more severe and complex the functional implications will be for the individual and the more likely the individual is to have a larger number of complicating factors. These factors confer on the individual not only functional limitations in mobility, learning, speech and communication, and sensory input and interpretation, but also greater implications on health and well-being. Individuals with severe and profound disabilities are more likely to have multiple medical problems that require multiple specialty providers, medications, hospitalizations, and surgeries and result in an increase in cost and reduction in life expectancy.

In a study in Washington State, Medicaid claims data for 310,977 children from birth to age 18 years who were enrolled at any time in fiscal year 1993 were examined. Ireys, Anderson, Shaffer, and Neff (1997) looked at the entire population of children and then at a set of children with eight chronic medical conditions including cerebral palsy, spina bifida, and muscular dystrophy. They found that children with one of the eight selected conditions incurred mean expenditures four times that of *all* Medicaid-enrolled children, and mean payments associated with the selected conditions ranged from 2.5 times to 20 times more than payments to *all* children. This figure translated into the statistic that approximately 10% of children accounted for approximately 70% of the payments in general *and* in each diagnostic grouping. For most conditions, inpatient stays accounted for the greatest proportion of expenditures; for some conditions—particularly cerebral palsy—transportation, durable equipment, home nursing, inpatient and outpatient services, primary and specialty medical care, surgeries, and medication-related services accounted for substantial proportions of total expenditures, reflecting the needs of this group of children.

Table 27.1-1. Number of children with other developmental disabilities, by severity of intellectual disability

	Mild ID	Severe ID
Other developmental disabilities	n = 331	n = 110
Any other developmental disability	37	59
Epilepsy	22	48
Cerebral palsy	14	35
Vision impairment	3	12
Hearing impairment	2	1

Key: ID = intellectual disabilities.

From Mervis, C.A., Decoulf, J.P., Murphy, C.C., & Yeargin-Allsopp, M. (1995). Low birthweight and the risk for mental retardation later in childhood. *Paediatric and Perinatal Epidemiology, 9,* 455–468; adapted by permission.

ETIOLOGICAL FACTORS

In a review of the etiological diagnoses of children with severe neurologic disabilities, Plioplys (2003) found approximately 50% of causes were prenatal, 30% were perinatal, and 20% were postnatal. The major etiological factors of severe and profound disabilities include

1. Neurodegenerative disorders that have progressive and increasingly complex medical problems. Neurodegenerative conditions represent the cause of only about 3%–4% of severe and profound disabilities and typically result in early death for the individual (see Chapter 7 and Lindsey's story later in this chapter).
2. Syndromes of multiple congenital anomalies with severe CNS compromise and other organ system

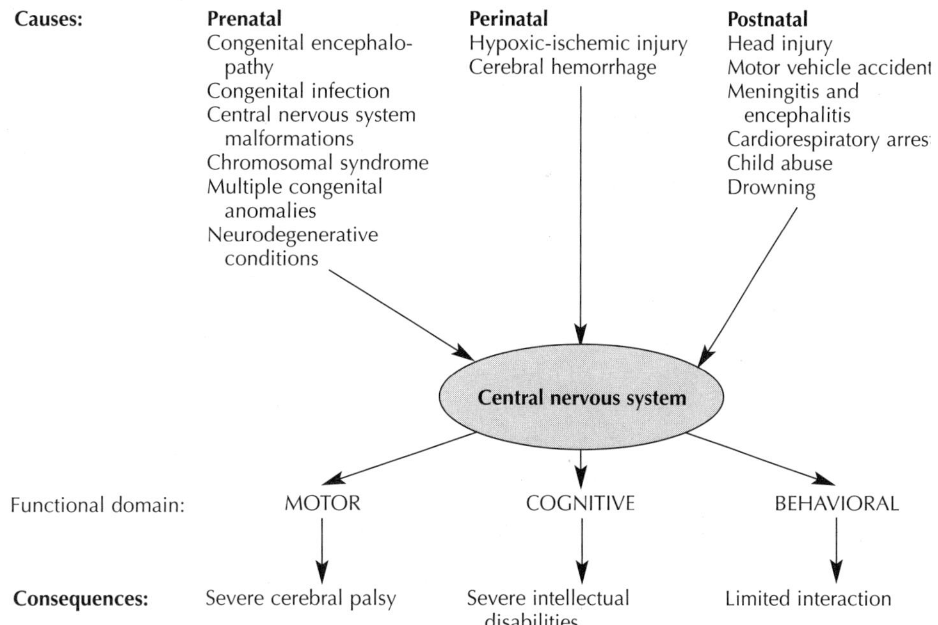

Figure 27.1-1 Etiological perspective of severe and complex disabilities (From Rubin, I.L., [1992]. Diagnosis and disabilities. *Journal of Intellectual Disability Research, 36,* 1–8; adapted by permission.)

involvement (see Chapter 8.2). Prenatal conditions cause the highest percentage of severe and profound disabilities. Where mortality and morbidity exist along a continuum, it is interesting to note that in the Annual Summary of Vital Statistics (Martin, Kochanek, Strobino, Guyer, & MacDorman, 2005) the leading cause of infant mortality for 2002 was congenital malformations (20%), with conditions related to short gestation and low birth weight coming a close second (17%).

3. Conditions that are associated with more severe insults to the CNS, most significantly of hypoxic ischemic insults or intraventricular hemorrhage in the perinatal period secondary to extreme prematurity (see Chapter 10).

INCREASE IN PREVALENCE OF SEVERE DISABILITIES

Advances in science and technology and the application of this knowledge to the management of challenging medical problems have resulted in an increased survival for infants and children with the more severe and complex conditions described previously. This has been most dramatically seen in the situation of infants of extremely low birth weight (see Chapter 10). As more of these infants are surviving, the number of infants and children with the more severe disabilities has also increased. Wilson-Costello, Friedman, Minich, Fanaroff, and Hack (2005) demonstrated an increase in the survival of infants born with extremely low birth weight and gestational age between 1982–1989 and 1990–1998 from 49% to 67% and a corresponding significant increase in overall rates of neurologic abnormalities mainly in the finding of cerebral palsy and sensory impairments, particularly hearing. More to the point, the mean Psychomotor Development Index also decreased significantly.

In addition, there is an emerging appreciation that children with severe and profound disabilities are living longer because of greater understanding of the associated medical conditions, improved management strategies, and enhanced knowledge of treating professionals, all resulting in better medical care. This finding bears out the importance of what has been learned from experience in dealing with the medical conditions of children and adults with severe and profound developmental disabilities and demonstrates the enhanced knowledge and commitment of treating professionals to provide optimal health care to this vulnerable group of people.

LIFE EXPECTANCY

Reports of life expectancy for individuals with developmental disabilities (Blair, Watson, Badawi, & Stanley, 2001; Hutton, Colver, & Mackie, 2000; Williams & Alberman, 1998) clearly demonstrate that the more severe the individual's neurological impairment, the shorter his or her life expectancy; however, this complex situation requires a very thoughtful approach. The first challenge is to define the population in order to standardize the data (e.g., those individuals who were able to eat by themselves or move about relatively well have a higher life expectancy than those who require tube feeding and have seriously limited independent movement). Next, it is important to define the circumstances, that is, where and when was the data collected, what was the time period being investigated, where did the individuals live, and what services did they receive.

Data by Eyman, Grossman, Chaney, and Call (1993) presented a rather limited life expectancy for children with the severe and profound disabilities relating to their relative abilities in communicating, eating, and moving, but the data were gathered from a cross-section of the population in California from 1980–1991 and reflected earlier clinical practices that were relatively unenlightened. The unspecified quality of medical care across a wide range of settings reflects a wide range of quality of services. A later analysis by Plioplys (2003) looked at the a similar population but from a later time period, 1985–1996, and with a more stable set of environments and health care delivery systems. Plioplys found a more positive outlook with a greater survival and longer life expectancy for comparable populations. This increase in life expectancy was attributed to improved medical care for people with developmental disabilities and an increased awareness of these individuals' health care needs by their families, caregivers, and providers as well as medical and nursing professions, all of which resulted in improved access to medical care and prompt medical response. Thus it is important to look at health and life expectancy not only in terms of underlying clinical conditions but also in terms of the quality of care being provided to the individual as well as to groups of individuals.

When reports began to appear that certain groups of individuals with disabilities had a higher mortality in the community than in institutional settings (Strauss, Eyman, & Grossman, 1996), suggesting that institutional care was better than community care, concern was raised that the data, taken at face value, would result in a return to institutional care (see Chapter 6.9). This interpretation was an oversimplification and led to emotional reactions rather than thoughtful analysis. The probable basis for the finding was that placements in the community did not take into consideration the complex set of infrastructural elements that had evolved in institutional settings during the period of institutional reform. Although plans and preparations were made for safe transitions from institution to the community for most individuals, there were unforeseen elements that compromised the care that the individuals received and that resulted in an unexpected risk for morbidity and mortality.

The real concern is that individuals with severe and profound disabilities and complex medical problems should be regarded as being "medically fragile" in that their stable health status is critically dependent on constant attention to many details and factors that depend on a stable health care infrastructure and a set of knowledgeable and sensitive caregivers and health care providers. Transition from one setting to another for a medically fragile individual should take into consideration many factors, and a careful and thoughtful transition is more likely to succeed if more time and thought and communication is spent on the process.

Jamie (whose story is presented later in the chapter) was a teenager who had been living at home all of his life. When he was transferred to a skilled nursing facility, his mother lamented that he suffered medical problems that he had not suffered at home. After a period of time, the staff at the facility became more familiar with Jamie and his nuances. As a result, his condition stabilized.

Having learned lessons from these experiences and the findings of emerging reports, as a society, we are able to reduce the morbidity and mortality for all individuals who are either at risk for developmental disabilities or who have existing disabilities and are able to diminish the likelihood of complications and secondary conditions that compromise quality of life and life expectancy.

CAUSES OF MORTALITY

Reports of deaths can be limiting in their singular and familiar language (Williams & Alberman, 1998). Death certificates, which form the documentary basis for recording causes of death, are generally written by physicians who are present at the death or who are called on to validate the death. Their final diagnostic determinations can be relatively arbitrary and may reflect the immediate cause of death (e.g., pneumonia, peritonitis) or the underlying condition (e.g., Down syndrome, cere-

Table 27.1-2. Causes of death

Respiratory	59%
Unknown/inadequate explanation	11%
Status epilepticus	9%
Infections	5%
Accidents	3%

From Blair, E., Watson, L., Badawi, N., & Stanley, F.J. (2001, August). Life expectancy among people with cerebral palsy in Western Australia. *Developmental Medicine and Child Neurology, 43*(8), 508–515; adapted by permission.

bral palsy). If one considers the specific medical conditions that cause death rather than the underlying condition, then the most common cause of death is due to respiratory causes, which occur three to four times more often in individuals with severe and profound disabilities than in individuals with mild or moderate disabilities (see Table 27.1-2).

In contrast, deaths as a result of accidents are reported to occur three to four times more in individuals with the milder degrees of developmental disabilities than in individuals with severe and profound disabilities, primarily because individuals with severe and profound disabilities are less mobile and, therefore, are at less risk for accidents. Congenital anomalies account for the second most common cause of death in all children age 1–4 years behind accidents, the third most common cause in the age group 5–9 years, and the fourth most common in the age group 10–14 years (Martin et al., 2005). These findings suggest that infants with severe and profound disabilities are more likely to die at a younger age than those with less severe disabilities. Seizures are sometimes said to be a cause of death, but some clinicians feel that the underlying condition is more significant.

Be that as it may, a single diagnostic label does not provide the full understanding of the disease process that ultimately ends in death. A survey of 17 deaths that occurred in a community setting (Rubin, 1997) found that not all deaths could be easily determined (see Table 27.1-3). Consider the following stories to get a sense of some of the complicating factors involved.

Table 27.1-3. A survey of 17 deaths that occurred in a community setting

Deaths that occurred as a result of unpredictable events and not apparently related specifically to medical management = 3
Deaths that occurred unexpectedly without any clear antecedents = 3
Deaths associated with premorbid signs and symptoms = 4
Deaths associated with symptoms that could potentially have been seen as significant in retrospect = 4
Deaths that are not clear because there was limited information = 3

Source: Rubin (1997).

Forty-one-year-old Ned had profound intellectual disabilities, obsessive-compulsive disorder, incontinence, recurrent weight loss, and recurrent respiratory problems with aspiration pneumonias and an episode of respiratory failure a year ago. He also had a recent history of dramatic weight loss and acute pulmonary distress. Ned was described as being asymptomatic until 4 days before he died. His appetite was poor with coughing spells, difficulty breathing, and sleep disturbance. He was coughing with much expectoration, and wheezing was noted the next morning.

Ned was treated with cough medication. He was described as having a stable day and night, with regular appetite during the next day. He then began to have a persistent and increasing cough, with deep shallow respirations and a low-grade fever. His pulse oxygen saturation was 83%.

Ned was taken to the local hospital emergency room where he was treated with intravenous antibiotics. He suddenly became agitated, and, while trying to stand up, he suddenly collapsed and died. Autopsy revealed diffuse acute bilateral pulmonary hemorrhage with bilateral pulmonary and pericardial adhesions.

Chronic lung disease and recurrent pneumonias, commonly associated with aspiration, are the most common cause of death in individuals with severe developmental disabilities and complex medical problems. Ned clearly had a history of recurrent respiratory problems, including an episode of respiratory failure and a recent history of weight loss. The underlying process to explain these symptoms is unclear, but Ned did develop respiratory symptoms that required aggressive management. His autopsy revealed both the acute fatal finding of pulmonary hemorrhages as well as the chronic evidence in the pulmonary and pericardial adhesions.

Leroy was 34 years, 9 months old. He had severe intellectual disabilities and a complex seizure disorder that was very difficult to manage on four anticonvulsant medications (e.g., 67 seizures were recorded during a 1-week inpatient hospital stay). He also had a history of gastroesophageal reflux with Barrett's metaplasia, status post gastrostomy feeding tube and fundoplication, and was on H2 Blockers. He also had frequent urinary tract infections requiring antibiotics. Nursing notes did not indicate anything unusual before Leroy's death. There was an hourly note of his sleeping status, then a note of absent breathing and heart rate. No autopsy was performed.

Leroy's underlying medical complexity, including his complex seizure disorder, which was very difficult to manage, was associated with a sudden and unexpected death. This is a not uncommon situation and is not possible to anticipate or prevent. The fact that there was no autopsy makes it difficult to determine if there was another condition that could potentially have been identified and treated.

Twenty-four-year-old Vince had severe intellectual disabilities, autism, seizures, attention-deficit/hyperactivity disorder, and self-injurious behavior. Vince seemed to be in his usual state of health until around 5.30 P.M., when he started crying and running around with his fingers in his mouth. He also was hitting his head and cheek until they were red and picking at his neck until it bled, so he was taken to the hospital. He was examined and discharged (there were no notes of details of the findings or a treatment plan).

When he returned to his residence, Vince was checked regularly through the night at 20–30 minute intervals. At 6.40 A.M., he was found to have blue lips, no pulse, and no breathing movements. Cardiopulmonary resuscitation was instituted, and 911 was called.

Vince was intubated by paramedics and resuscitated. He was then transferred to the hospital, where he died despite aggressive treatment. No autopsy was performed.

Vince's situation is particularly challenging as it chronicles unusual and dramatic behavior in an individual with a history of self-injurious behavior that indicates distress. His pattern of behavior possibly gave a clue to the source of distress. He was appropriately taken to the emergency room for evaluation and management, but the medical staff there did not find a good enough medical reason to admit him or do a workup. Without the autopsy to determine the cause of his distress and death, it is very difficult to know what could or should have been done to prevent his death. It does speak, however, to the need to aggressively evaluate the situation when an individual who has limited communication presents with a dramatic nonverbal expression of distress and challenges clinicians to use the resources available to try to determine the cause (see Tables 23.1-3 and 23.1-4). It also speaks to the need to train physicians in the medical management of individuals with developmental disabilities who are nonverbal and who may present in unusual ways.

These stories are presented to provide important lessons and are particularly instructive if analyzed and discussed with clinical providers. Where possible, it is advisable to obtain an autopsy to assist in the understanding of pathological processes that will help in the management of future patients and improve overall care, or at least hold a morbidity and mortality discussion on each case.

MEDICAL NEEDS

There are several ways of looking at the health care needs of individuals with severe and profound disabilities. Medical needs will be manifest in three ways:

1. Needs that are associated with a specific genetic or nongenetic syndrome, such as Down syndrome or Prader-Willi syndrome (These are discussed in greater detail in each of the sections of Chapter 8 and 9).

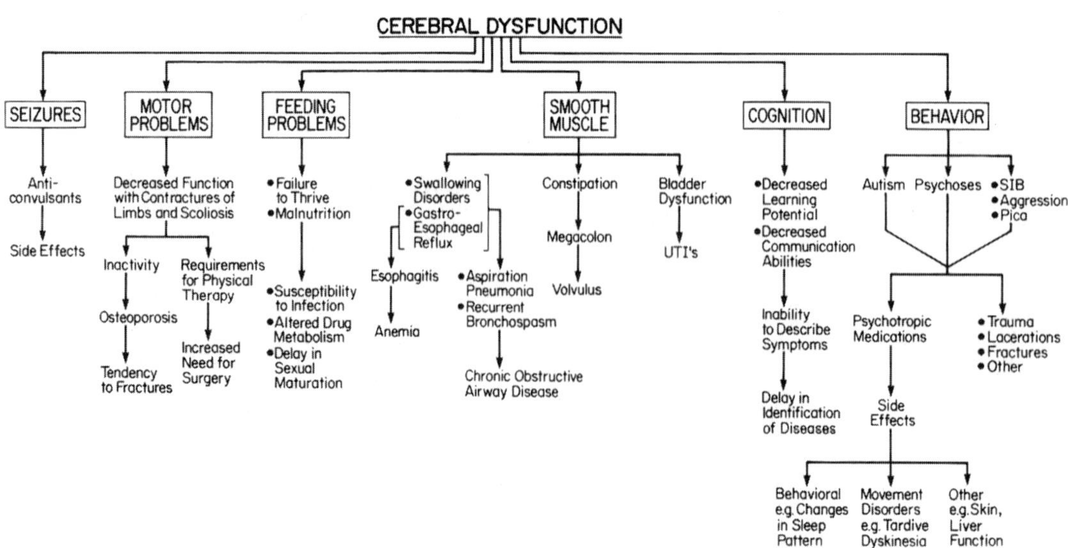

Figure 27.1-2. Underlying pathophysiologic processes of cerebral dysfunction. (*Key:* SIB = self-injurious behavior; UTI = urinary tract infection.)

2. Needs associated with specific organ system dysfunction, including aging, and treatment modalities such as medications (These are dealt with in the organ system–specific chapters, and conditions associated with aging are explored in Chapter 26).
3. Needs associated with the consequences of brain dysfunction (see Figure 27.1-2).

This chapter deals exclusively with the consequences of CNS dysfunction and their natural history.

The clinical characteristics of children and adults with severe and profound disabilities can be seen in Table 27.1-4. Percentage data for some conditions for which the author had previous surveys are shown and represent a composite. The importance is not in the details but in the perspectives: *The more severe the disabilities, the more likely the medical complications.*

Table 27.1-4. Clinical characteristics of children and adults with severe and profound disabilities

Neurology	
Seizures	85%
Spastic cerebral palsy	62%
Hypothermia	11%
Sensory impairment	
Vision	26%
Hearing	37%
Orthopedic	
Scoliosis	77%
Hip dysplasia	38%
Frequent fractures	17%
Osteoporosis	—
Gastrointestinal	
Feeding disorders	65%
Gastroesophageal reflux	51%
Gastrostomy feeding tubes	59%
Chronic severe constipation	65%
Hemorrhoids	4%
Respiratory	
Aspiration pneumonia	28%
Asthma	20%
Tracheostomies	1%
Skin	
Decubitus ulcers	< 1%
Behavioral and psychiatric conditions	
Self-injurious behaviors	11%
Pica	12%
Hospitalizations	65%
Surgeries	
Gastrointestinal	60%
Orthopedic	34%
Eye	12%
Ear, nose, and throat	10%
Ventriculoperitoneal shunt	8%
Hernia	5%
Other	12%

Note: These data reperesent a compilation of data from Rubin (1989) and Rubin, Rubin, Carter, and Westerman (2002).

Monitoring and Maintaining Health

Individuals with severe and profound disabilities require constant attention from all care providers, including parents, other direct care providers, therapists, teachers, and nurses. The multiplicity and complexity of these individuals' health care needs means that care must be provided in an organized and structured manner with clear guidelines. At a day-to-day level, health is maintained through continual attention to hygiene, feeding, bowel and bladder function, skin care, and position. Caregivers administer medication and assist the individual in moving about the environment using adaptive equipment, including wheelchairs.

Care providers should be well-trained and experienced, knowledgeable, and able to attend to any changes in health status. In addition, prevention strategies are necessary to not only assure maintenance of health but also to prevent untoward threats to well-being. Because of the individual's limited ability to move, communicate, or indicate need, pain, distress, or desire, care providers must be attuned to subtle nuances and changes in the individual's physiology and behavior in order to identify changes early and to respond appropriately in order to prevent delays and complications. Charts recording bowel movements, seizures, menstrual cycles, and sleep patterns can indicate when there is a change in health status. Because it is very likely that an individual will experience changes in care providers, charts make sure that all providers are aware of what is happening and provide continuity of care. A form that reflects an individual's basic physiological parameters as well as patterns of movement behavior, communication, and socialization is extremely helpful (see Figure 27.1-3).

Health Care Infrastructure

A stable and predictable set of quality health care services must be in place to assure that any threat to the individual's health and well-being will be appropriately managed. The elements of this infrastructure include trained nurses; primary health care providers; specialty health care providers; accessible and available emergency services with appropriately trained personnel; and a hospital with the necessary specialized personnel to manage hospital stays for acute illnesses, surgical pro-

1. **List of medical problems:**
 ____
 ____
2. **List of medications:**
 ____
 ____
3. **List of familiar providers:**
 ____
 ____
4. **Basic health parameters:**
 Vital signs ______________
  Pulse ______________
  Blood pressure ______________
  Basal temp ______________
  General color ______________
  Pattern of sweating ______________
 General level of activity ______________
 Pattern of eating/feeding ______________
  Tube or oral ______________
  Behavior before ______________
  Response after ______________
 Pattern of bowel movements ______________
5. **General reaction to stress:**
 Pain ______________
 Discomfort ______________
 Malaise ______________
 Noise ______________
6. **General likes and dislikes:**
 Activities ______________
 People ______________
 Events ______________
 Quiet time ______________
7. **Patterns of communication:**
 Sound ______________
 Facial expressions ______________
 Limb movement ______________

Figure 27.1-3. Early clinical identification profile.

cedures as needed, and intensive care if needed. Ideally, appropriately trained and competent nurses, and expert primary and specialty care providers are based at a tertiary care hospital, and a medical home would be part of the infrastructure.

The provision of health care is not merely the domain of nurses and physicians, but encompasses and incorporates many elements at many levels, the most critical being the development of systems that assure, monitor, and maintain health and an information system to track all of the elements (see Figure 27.1-4). Other important elements in the delivery of health care include personal lifestyles, environmental adaptations, skilled and caring personnel (e.g., nurses), and availability and accessibility of an array of services.

Social opportunities include communication (speech therapy, augmentative communication strategies), adaptive behavior (life experiences, behavior management strategies), and community integration (recreation, transportation).

The delivery of health care cannot be seen in isolation and requires not only the assembly of practical strategies, personnel, and equipment, but also a set of principles and values that drive the quality of the health care being delivered.

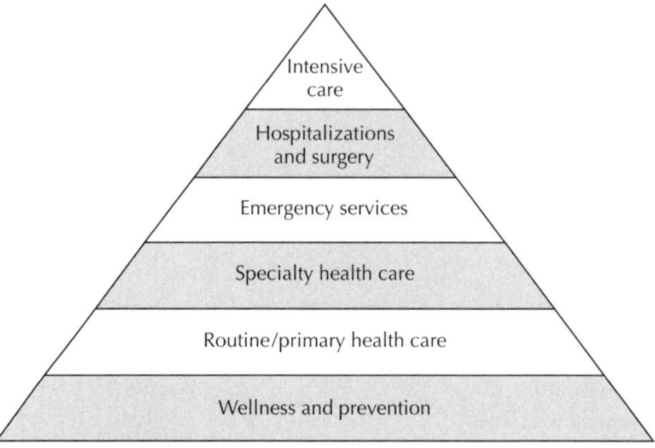

Figure 27.1-4. Health care infrastructure.

Considering the multiplicity and complexity of the clinical conditions listed previously, it might be helpful to examine one individual, Jamie, and explore the elements that evolved in his care.

Jamie was born at 36 weeks gestation weighing 2.87 kg. His mother had premature rupture of membranes. Jamie was delivered by cesarean section secondary to fetal distress as a result of cephalopelvic disproportion. In the immediate neonatal period, he acquired Group B *Streptococcus* meningitis, and was on a ventilator for 11 days with 100% oxygen.

At age 15 years, Jamie had a list of diagnoses that included

- Severe cerebral palsy with quadriplegia
- Scoliosis
- Severe intellectual disability
- Seizure disorder
- Reactive airway disease
- Gastrostomy feeding
- Temperature instability

The following represents a comprehensive review of his medical records, which reflect organ system disorders and medical management.

- *Pulmonary*—Jamie requires regular visits to his pulmonologist and has had recurrent respiratory problems. The visits have been annual and intermittent on an outpatient basis as well as consultation during hospitalization. He has had numerous chest x-rays to diagnose and follow the pneumonias. Pulmonary medications have included bronchodilators, steroids, inhalation therapies for the reactive airway disease, and antibiotics for the intermittent infections.
- *Neurology*—Jamie is seen by his neurologist every 6 months on a scheduled basis but more frequently when his seizures are out of control. He has also had electroencephalograms as the situation has required. He has been on a number of antiepileptic medications including phenobarbital, valproic acid, carbamazepine, phenytoin, and diazepam, which is used on an as needed basis.
- *Gastroenterology*—Jamie is followed frequently by his gastroenterologist for his gastroesophageal reflux and frequent episodes of upper gastrointestinal bleeding. He had an endoscopy for diagnostic purposes and subsequently required a gastrostomy feeding tube and a fundoplication. He has also had a chronic problem with constipation, which has required frequent abdominal x-rays to assess the degree of his constipation and the effects of the treatments. His medications for gastrointestinal problems have included proton pump inhibitors, promoters of gastric motility, and laxatives.
- *Orthopedics*—Although he was followed by his orthopedist every 6 months when he was younger, Jamie is now followed annually. He requires orthoses on an ongoing basis to maintain position. He also requires a wheelchair that needs to be modified to suit his growth and changing posture and position. Jamie has had numerous x-rays of his hips, spine, and other joints and has had soft tissue surgeries.
- *Hospitalizations*—Jamie has had numerous hospitalizations for hypothermia, respiratory and gastrointestinal disorders, seizure management, and surgeries.

COMPUTERIZED MEDICAL RECORDS

Given the inherent medical complexity and the need for multiple providers of care in multiple settings, this would be an ideal situation for the development of a computerized medical record to benefit the individuals being served as well as the providers and coordinators of the services. There are a number of proprietary systems available but none that has become universally applied. We will not go into any discussion of the different systems but will suggest that each service delivery system needs to determine which programs best suit the particular practice and its participants and then make it work.

STRESSES ON FAMILIES

There is no question that there are significant stresses on families who have children (of any age) with developmental disabilities or other chronic medical conditions (see Chapter 5), but those children who have the most severe and complex conditions are obviously more demanding of time, energy and finite resources, which range from the emotional to the financial to the simple notion of time. In addition to the usual challenges of costs of care (Rasell, Bernstein, & Tang, 1994), dealing with insurance, schools, and social life, there are the medical appointments, emergency room visits at all hours, hospitalizations, and surgeries, along with often life-threatening situations requiring intensive care (see Chapter 29). There are also very difficult decisions that need to be made by families that revolve around medical care, surgical procedures, how to budget time and money, how to include the whole family in activities, placement in residential settings, and end-of-life decisions (see Chapter 30). Family constellations and cultures are also critically important in framing diagnostic and therapeutic approaches. Having knowledge is not enough; at times, situations require much experience, sensitivity, and delicacy (see Chapter 27.2).

Presented next are a set of four vignettes, each of which was chosen to reflect a different aspect of care relating to clinical challenges, difficult decisions families have to make, and how families have coped and adapted to the challenges. After all, no child or adult can be seen in isolation. There are families, friends, and communities, and, as was said by the mother of a child with cerebral palsy, "If it takes a village to raise a child, it takes a metropolitan area to raise a child with developmental disabilities."

Jamie was living at home with his parents and siblings. His mother was his care coordinator and ardent advocate. She had secured appropriate medical attention and established for her son a set of specialty care providers and educational and recreational opportunities. His father was in the construction business and built a suite for him at home. The family had to purchase appropriate adaptive equipment and transportation for him, including a wheelchair and vehicle.

His mother had secured the necessary home nursing coverage to help care for him and monitor him at night. The family went on vacations together. At age 16, Jamie developed Type I diabetes, which complicated his management at home, and he needed to move to a skilled nursing facility. Below is a letter his mother wrote explaining the situation.

Hi,

I hope all is well with you and your family. This letter is to bring you up to date with Jamie's progress. We placed him at Skilled Nursing Facility (SNF) when he was 17 years old. When he turned 16, he was diagnosed with Type I diabetes, which significantly complicated his care. His increasing growth, increased medical care, and the financial complications convinced us that it was the best choice for him.

I remember you telling me that keeping him at home as long as possible would most likely be the best thing for him. In the 17 years that he lived at home, he was only hospitalized five times. Unfortunately, once we placed him, he didn't do very well at all. In fact, he was hospitalized for 4 months, and we almost lost him numerous times. He also had two more hospitalizations after that. I think that SNF is a good place, but Jamie's complicated care makes it tough for him to live at a facility. At home, he had me being able to oversee all his care and provide consistency in his care. His primary care pediatrician and the other doctors have worked hard to make sure that Jamie's care plan works for him. We are hoping next year will be a better year.

He is now 18. We are so thankful we had him with us for 17 years. His brothers and sisters love him. We would have never made it all those years if I did not get on track when I was younger and connected with all the specialists. I still count on the support of his orthopedic surgeon, gastroenterologist, neurologist, and pulmonologist.

Thanks for your support over the years.

Happy Holidays!
Mrs. N and family

In the next story, Sarah's father discusses the decision to place his daughter in a skilled nursing facility, the economics of making sure services are provided, the challenging decision around whether to do surgery or not, frustrations around dealing with tertiary care centers, and the value of direct care service providers.

In 1991, our then 3-year-old daughter contracted viral encephalitis and spent 4 months at The Children's Hospital. Her clinical course was complicated by a cardiorespiratory arrest requiring tracheostomy and gastrostomy feeding, and $1.2 million later, she was transferred to a secondary level hospital for rehabilitation. Despite 4 months of rehabilitation, she regretfully made little clinical progress. Over the months, it became apparent that she would need intense nursing services for the rest of her life.

After wrestling with whether or not we should attempt to raise her at home, it soon became clear that extensive modifications of our basement would be necessary for the placement of suctioning apparatus and oxygen, together with 24-hour-a-day nursing services. After painful deliberation, we decided that Sarah would live in a skilled nursing facility that is affiliated with a local teaching hospital not far from our home so that we could visit frequently.

Sarah has remained relatively well, requiring about three or four emergency admissions to The Children's Hospital over the last 15 years for pain control, pneumonia, and fractures. Her day-to-day stay at the skilled nursing facility is relatively smooth. After 15 years, she is well known to all the staff, and we are very comfortable calling day and night to get little updates on her progress and "how she is doing."

Her medical insurance is covered by a private payer for the first 100 days every year, and, in mid April, this switches to Medicaid. The additional monies from the private insurer serve to cover some of her costs at the skilled nursing facility. In addition, the town in which we reside pays money for her education at the facility.

One of the more harrowing decisions needed in regard to Sarah's health care was the decision whether to have spinal surgery for scoliosis. In preparation for soliciting appropriate opinion on these issues, we sent, ahead of time, detailed medical records and x-rays to the orthopedic offices. After 2 visits and lengthy discussions, we were relieved to decide that the surgery was not absolutely necessary for her.

Although we have been very satisfied with the level of medical care, this large, busy facility often shows symptoms of inadequate communication between staff, which at times becomes distressing. On one visit, we discussed Do Not Resuscitate Orders on one admission with five different people. There are delays in service, particularly in the emergency room (where we once spent 18 hours looking into a change in her mental status). The service can be impersonal, and one expects this because of the changing nature of large urban hospitals; however, for the most we are very happy with the technical aspects of the care and advice given at The Children's Hospital, but we are always relieved to return to home—the skilled nursing facility—where the majority of the nursing aides are recent immigrants from third-world countries, taking their first steps in these United States and only too delighted to be given the opportunity to enter the work market and prove themselves as worthy employees.

Without their dedication and service, I often wonder who would change Sarah's diapers and bathe her and wash her hair each day. Both her parents and her siblings are grateful for the fact that there is somewhere that Sarah can call home.

The following story is about a 14-year-old boy, Drake, who has a history of poor weight gain, recurrent episodes of pneumonia, and severe scoliosis. The challenge of making a decision about placing a gastrostomy tube (G tube) is complicated by his complex clinical condition and by his family constellation.

Drake is a 14-year-old boy with a history of developmental delay of unknown etiology and cerebral palsy. Drake's family consists of his mother, who has mild intellectual disabilities and his grandmother, who is blind. Drake was first seen at the Cerebral Palsy Clinic with spastic quadriplegia, severe scoliosis, a seizure disorder, limited social interaction, and failure to thrive. His whole family regularly accompanies him to the clinic. Drake was admitted to the hospital for a workup and nutritional rehabilitation. During his hospitalization, Drake's family was with him the entire time.

After discharge, Drake was followed regularly in the clinic and seemed to be making progress. Over the past 3 months, he had two episodes of pneumonia necessitating admission and has lost weight. On close questioning of his family, he is not eating as much as he was before; he is coughing more and is more sleepy. He has also lost weight.

Consideration is given to placing a G tube. To Drake's family, the placement of the G tube is a dramatic and invasive procedure and will prevent the pleasurable and nurturing opportunity for the family to feed him. Although it is expected that his nutritional status will improve and will promote the adolescent growth spurt, there is real concern that this growth spurt may result in a dramatic increase in his scoliosis, which will then raise the question of spinal surgery.

Drake's situation is not an unusual complex dilemma that families face, and it requires very thoughtful discussion and may require repeated visits for clarification and planning. The decision to place a G tube is complicated enough, but Drake's family and cultural background require extraordinary and thoughtful consideration.

The final story deals with terminal complications associated with a progressive neurodegenerative disorder. There is an unfortunate reality of limitations in medical treatment for some situations, but a network of support systems, such as 24-hour nursing services at home and hospice, provide an invaluable benefit to individuals and their families.

Lindsey was a 10-year-old girl who had been diagnosed as having cerebral palsy but whose clinical course gradually and clearly became more complicated, suggesting a neurodegenerative disorder. Her mother had concerns about pain, tachycardia, gastrointestinal motility, and Lindsey's future outcome. The following is a response to her drafted by her Medical Home pediatrician.

1. From the time when Lindsey was admitted to The Children's Hospital late January with the Duodenal Hematoma, her baseline condition has changed. She is now less resilient and more fragile. As you are aware, she endured a rocky course for 3 months as an inpatient with multiple changes and clinical crises. Her condition did improve to the extent that she could go home, but unfortunately, not to the state of health and strength that she had enjoyed before the acute event and hospitalization in late January. In addition, since returning home, her condition has necessitated two brief hospitalizations, one for a fever and the second for episodes of hypoxemia. She is now home again, and not only does she not appear to be better, but she actually appears to be more fragile.
2. From her long and complicated history and clinical course, we have reason to believe that she has a condition that is progressive, and in the process, she is physically and physiologically becoming less able and less resilient and more medically complicated. The magnetic resonance imaging she had at the last visit shows significant loss of brain tissue, which is consistent with a "neurodegenerative" disorder. As you recall, we did have her seen by a geneticist a few years ago and had an extensive metabolic workup, including a muscle biopsy to look for mitochondrial disorders, with no positive findings. As yet, we do not have a characterization of the underlying pathophysiological process that is causing her to lose function.
3. Unfortunately, we do not have any good answers on how best to manage some of her unusual clinical presentations without incurring further complications from the treatments. We will obviously continue to try to do all we can to help by trying to find out why she has the symptoms she has and what to do about them, but as you have been frustrated to discover, our knowledge and abilities are limited, despite the extensive testing, multiple hospitalizations and multiple specialty physicians and other resources.
4. As she is becoming more medically complicated and fragile, and our professional and academic resources are limited in what can be offered, and also considering the progressive nature of her conditions, it may be appropriate at this point to contact Hospice and explore what they can offer. This may be a difficult step to contemplate because of its implications, but as we have discussed over the past week, the likelihood of dramatic improvement is small, and, as her condition appears to be progressive, there are limits as to what can be done. You have thoughtfully and ably articulated the responses to a dramatic change in her status—the "DNR" order—which spells out clearly what should and should not be done in the event of a medical emergency. We need to continue to try to help her in any way we can with the knowledge and technology we have available, at the

same time we need to be sure she is free of pain and suffering and that you have the support you need to take care of her at home and adjust to the changed reality.

The outcome of Lindsey's story is that she went home with 24-hour around-the-clock nursing care and required two emergency room visits and one hospitalization for temperature instability and tachycardia. Approximately 2 months after this letter was drafted, Lindsey died at home. An autopsy was performed, and the final neuropathological report read: "Progressive neurodegenerative disorder, most likely mitochondrial encephalopathy (specific disorder undetermined) with necrotizing lesions with vascular prominence, vacuolation, and basal ganglia, cerebellum, and brainstem nuclear degeneration."

CONCLUSION

The management of individuals with severe and profound disabilities and their families requires a thorough knowledge of the medical conditions that can arise and an understanding of the inherent complexity and interaction between the different conditions. Providers must also know the treatment and intervention strategies necessary to improve health and well-being and the potential adverse outcomes of the interventions. An appreciation of the infrastructure of services necessary is critical to optimal delivery of care; this group of individuals requires a committed primary care provider or medical home (American Academy of Pediatrics, 2002), a set of expert specialty care providers and specialty care settings, which must have a working knowledge of the health care needs and treatment options. Providers must also know how to communicate the knowledge and understanding to families, caregivers, and other care providers and how to deal with a complex system of health care delivery. Most important, providers need a sensitive understanding of not only the health care needs of each individual but also the subtleties of the emotional life of the individual and his or her family and community.

REFERENCES

American Academy of Pediatrics. (2002). AAP policy statement: The medical home. *Pediatrics, 110*(1), 184–186.

Blair, E., Watson, L., Badawi, N., & Stanley, F.J. (2001). Life expectancy among people with cerebral palsy in Western Australia. *Developmental Medicine and Child Neurology, 43*(8), 508–515.

Eyman, R.K., Grossman, H.J., Chaney, R.H., & Call, T.L. (1993). Survival of profoundly disabled people with severe mental retardation. *American Journal of Disease in Childhood, 147,* 329–336.

Hutton, J.L., Colver, A.F., & Mackie, P.C. (2000). Effect of severity of disability on survival in north east England cerebral palsy cohort. *Archives of Disease in Childhood, 83*(6), 468–474.

Ireys, H.T., Anderson, G.F., Shaffer, T.J., & Neff, J.M. (1997). Expenditures for care of children with chronic illnesses enrolled in the Washington State Medicaid Program, fiscal year 1993. *Pediatrics, 2,* 197–204.

Martin, J.A., Kochanek, K.D., Strobino, D.M., Guyer, B., & MacDorman, M.F. (2005). Annual summary of vital statistics—2003. *Pediatrics, 115,* 619–634.

Mervis, C.A., Decoulf, J.P., Murphy, C.C., & Yeargin-Allsopp, M. (1995). Low birthweight and the risk for mental retardation later in childhood. *Paediatric and Perinatal Epidemiology, 9,* 455–468.

Newacheck, P.W. (1989). Adolescents with special health needs: Prevalence, severity, and access to health services. *Pediatrics, 84*(5), 872–881.

Newacheck, P.W., Inkelas, M., & Kim, S.E. (2004). Health services use and health care expenditures for children with disabilities. *Pediatrics, 114*(1), 79–85.

Plioplys, A.V. (2003). Survival rates of children with severe neurologic disabilities. *Seminars in Pediatric Neurology, 10,* 120–129.

Rasell, E., Bernstein, J., & Tang, K. (1994). The impact of health care financing on family budgets. *International Journal of Health Services: Planning, Administration, Evaluation, 24*(4), 691–714.

Rubin, I.L. (1989). Management of children and adults with severe and profound central nervous system dysfunction. In Rubin, I.L., & Crocker, A.C. (Eds.), *Developmental disabilities: Delivery of medical care for children and adults.* Philadelphia: Lea & Febiger.

Rubin, I.L. (1992). Diagnosis and disabilities. *Journal of Intellectual Disability Research, 36,* 1–8.

Rubin, I.L. (1997). *Review of deaths in Hissom Consent Decree, Oklahoma.* Unpublished manuscript.

Rubin, A., Rubin, I.L., Carter, K., & Westerman, S. (2002). *Survey of children with CP from an inner city clinic.* Poster presentation at the American Association on Mental Retardation Annual Meeting.

Strauss, D., Eyman, R.K., & Grossman, H.J. (1996). American predictors of mortality in children with severe mental retardation: The effect of placement. *Journal of Public Health, 86*(10), 1422–1429.

Williams, K., & Alberman, E. (1998). Survival in cerebral palsy: The role of severity and diagnostic labels. *Developmental Medicine and Child Neurology, 40,* 376–379.

Wilson-Costello, D., Friedman, H., Minich, N., Fanaroff, A.A., & Hack, M. (2005). Improved survival rates with increased neurodevelopmental disability for extremely low birth weight infants in the 1990s. *Pediatrics, 115,* 997–1003.

27.2 EXCEPTIONALITY

Allen C. Crocker

In friendships and care assignments for some individuals with developmental disabilities, workers are at times struck with the notable degree of personal exceptionality that is present. The perception of differentness need not be a defining feature, but it is culturally pertinent, brings richness, and calls for understanding and sharing. Workers are drawn close by special needs, including medical ones, and find themselves in a vigorous learning environment. The setting also has an element of wonder in it, and some special individuals emerge as unforgettable. Such an individual was Bobby, who was 26 years old at the time his course was previously presented (Crocker, 1998), and with whom this author has had a relationship since Bobby was 2 years old.

Bobby has serious expression of spastic quadriplegia with very limited and arduous assisted walking after numerous orthopedic operations. He is nonverbal; he can work a yes–no switch but not more complicated assignments. His mental age in adulthood has adaptive skills at the level of somewhere around 1 year of age.

With family agreement, I interviewed his child care workers, teachers, therapists, and social workers, who had known him well for different periods of his life. Noting the extraordinary modification of his activities that was present, these supporters were asked how they viewed Bobby's life. Reponses included such affirmations as

- "It's a good life."
- "His life has quality. To society maybe not, but it does to family and friends."
- "It's incredible, so much love, everyone has gained."
- "He's successful in his own reference frame. Bobby loves Bobby's life."
- "His life is uplifting. Many have come to care about him."
- "He has a strong sense of life. He's aware of his impact."

Some of the same colleagues were further asked about what Bobby has taught them. Their answers again showed substantial effects.

- "He's taught me about love and struggle and devotion."
- "He made me realize that I had something that I could contribute."
- "One must look at a person's strengths. Don't assume he doesn't understand."
- "The responses may be less, but you get it, and it makes you feel good."
- "He taught me there is more to other people than you first see."
- "People of all skill levels can be happy. He makes me feel better about my life."

A young lady named Danielle has Rett syndrome. She was 11 years old at the time of an earlier report (Crocker, 1998). Her developmental limitations are profound. She underwent the decline in function commonly seen for children with this disorder in toddlerhood; her course has been thoughtfully supported by a resourceful and loving family. Communication is based on a small repertoire of physical signs and gestures (she throws a cup on the floor to express thirst; she sits on the couch if she is tired). Danielle can do a little walking. Exchange is rich within her family circle.

Bogdan and Taylor (1989) have observed and warmly reflected on the notable personal features of many individuals with severe or profound cognitive disabilities, and they provide assistance in identification of the most basic elements of humanness. In conversation with Danielle's parents, I considered some of these central capacities. Four are delineated by Bogdan and Taylor. The first is *attribution of thinking*, which can refer to elements separate from language and also to nonstandard or idiosyncratic cognition. Recognition of "smartness" may use its own idioms (and other intelligences). In this regard, Danielle's father noted that she understands about 50 words, recognizes 10–20 people, and laughs when yelled at.

The second element of special interest is *expression of individuality*. This refers to the persistence of likes and dislikes, feelings and motives, and a unique personality. Included here for Danielle would be her love of music tapes, her enjoyment at watching other kids in action, and her pleasure in acting up when taken to stores.

The third item in Bogdan and Taylor's tabulation of the social construction of humanness is *reciprocation*. This speaks to giving back or contributing something to a relationship. Is there companionship? Does the caregiver get to feel rewarded from having made a contribution? For her part, Danielle brings a smile to everyone and responds to people.

The last item asks whether the person has a *social place*. Is he or she part of a social unit and taking part in processes and rituals? Does the person have special roles? Will the person be missed? Danielle's parents affirmed that Danielle is indeed in the middle of things and is definitely happy. Hence, in many ways, she rates highly in this thoughtful inventory of life attributes.

This author made another visit to see Bobby and Danielle and their families 7 years later. Bobby was now 33, challenged, but happy and mostly well. He had PCA (personal care attendant) help in the morning, arrived at his day program, and remained a "people person." He had no real walking, but he did use his stander. His comprehension was appreciable, but he had no words. His family commented that his "goals are less elevated now." His parents' health problems had been serious (including malignancy). Danielle was now 19 years old and loved football games (and villains on television). She had had some surgical intervention to assist walking. She had a PCA, school, swimming, and therapeutic riding. She was also making more vocalizations. Her laughter is an important part of the household.

LOOKING WITH NEW EYES

People who are building relationships with exceptional individuals may see lifestyles and singularities that at first are bewildering and even uncomfortable. Such items later become blended into the persona. They are territories that may be part of disability or may be simply personal variation. To some extent, irrespective of age group, there are half dozen areas of special concern:

1. *Lack of self-care*—Individuals can have diffuse disability and may not be able to dress, feed, or toilet themselves. They may have a compelling dependency on others throughout their lives.

2. *Communication challenge*—The integrated function of language expression (and even reception) is predictably limited when development is seriously compromised. Obviously, a broad universe of alternatives exists to verbal language, some of which may be called on for understanding.

3. *Aberrant behavior*—Unusual behavior can be an element of communication, a response to confusing signals, simple self-stimulation, the drive of sensory urges, or regrettable blockade. Bizarre repetitive or stereotypic behavior including rocking, twirling, and posturing may be seen; self-injury is the most distressing.

4. *Complicating health problems*—If developmental gains are much reduced, the probability of there being coexisting bodily abnormalities are appreciable (especially in hereditary or malformation syndromes). Relevant conditions would be seizures, bowel function troubles, chronic infection, visual impairment, reduced hearing, cutaneous problems, and secondary phenomena.

5. *Limitation of ambulation or other gross motor function*—Personal care and opportunities for learning may be specifically restricted by movement problems. Some individuals with major disabilities in cognitive function, however, may have wonderful motor skills (including "bolting").

6. *Greater commitment for teaching*—Some individuals with multiple challenges or reduced incidental learning may elicit caregivers to bring forward special communication and support. Important stories are heard of superior companionship and teaching. Unique values are transmitted, in each direction. (Crocker & Nelson, 1992).

This section explored the world of individuals for whom needs are very great. This consideration assuredly has crucial messages for everyone, for it speaks of an aspect of human interaction in which much growth and understanding is required. This tale is well captured in the famous quotation of Marcel Proust, "The real voyage of discovery consists not in seeking new landscape, but in having new eyes."

Gunnar Dybwad (1999) reflected on the utilization of a "profound" characterization of special needs, or "profound mental retardation" as was employed a generation ago. He agreed that *profound* was an apt description for individuals with very involved disabilities and spoke of significant gains from creative training programs and environmental change. He noted that severe concurrent physical impairments are common (as mentioned previously) and relevant to function. These elements may respond to remediation. He urged that the specific term *profound mental retardation* be abandoned and the broader representation of *profoundly disabled* be substituted.

EFFECTS OF EXCEPTIONALITY

For our comrades with significant differentness, there are life activity implications that derive therefrom. It is appropriate to pause and reflect on the mechanisms and circumstances for these impacts and to regard the possible systems for relevant support. Four regions are prominent in these considerations (Crocker, 1998):

Modification of Achievement or Performance

Modification of achievement or performance is a basic component of development that can be measured and viewed in relation to thoughtful standards. It should be remembered that the final effects of constraints in intelligence are modulated by concurrent attainments in adaptation. If expectations remain low, elements of self-fulfilling prophesy will intrude on performance.

Requirement for Services

Assistance is needed for the affected person and his or her family to realize best progress, and pursuit of these services can be a major determinant in planning location and enrollment. Everyone utilizes services (and guidance); for people with disabilities, however, these services are more urgent.

Participation in Life Events and Sequences

Participation in life events and sequences refers to involvement in the usual experiences of growth and daily living. In recent times, administrators and advocates have strived to assure as conventional an environment as possible—with attention to normalization, communitization, least restrictive environment, access, inclusion, and other integrating modes, with varying success. Many declarations of rights speak to such experiences and contracts.

Connectedness

A most significant and elemental component of a person's existence is meaningful alliances with a variety of other people, which can get sacrificed in specialized programs. Historically, clinicians did not give priority to membership in the larger fellowship. The evolution of this movement, and the leadership of self-advocates, have been important here. Perske has spoken for many years about the crucial value of the "Circle of Friends"; friendship is an elusive though precious happening.

RADICAL HOSPITALITY

Jason is a 20-year-old man who has Down syndrome, in an astonishing fashion with autism and Tourette syndrome. He fulfills his voluntary job by recycling trash at the First Parish Church of Sudbury, MA. On one Sunday, he went up to the worship service and sat in his invariable seat by the window. Rev. Katie Lee Crane, the pastor, was gladdened. Her words that morning included references to gates, welcoming, and hospitality. She thought of the concepts of Radical Hospitality, and her conversations about that idea with Fr. Daniel Homan, a Benedictine monk. Rev. Crane believed that:

- Hospitality is about accepting responsibility for the care of strangers, the ones at our gate, and those who are a world away.
- Hospitality is a call to revere what is sacred in every person.
- Hospitality is the way we come out of ourselves. It is the first step toward dismantling the barriers of the world.
- Hospitality is the act of a recklessly generous heart.

Similarly, Fr. Homan (Homan & Pratt, 2002) advocated that:

- Hospitality tops the list of what is valued in a monastery because people are valued, and an equal dignity for all is assumed.
- Hospitality requires not grand gestures, but open hearts.
- In the monastic image of the world, we are all guests, we are all travelers, we are all a little lost, and we are all looking for a place to rest a while.
- Hospitality makes room even for the one who is frighteningly different. Hospitality treats people respectfully.

ADOPTION

A heartening model of voluntary engagement in the care and support of children with serious developmental challenges is that of special needs adoption. This component of child welfare activity has become notably successful and well established (McKenzie, 1993). I am familiar with a local program carried out by Project Impact in Boston. Barbara Pine visited 52 families who had adopted 114 children with Project Impact. The children had a variety of significant developmental disabilities. Most of the families had had biological children at an earlier time; of the adopted children, 41% came from foster care (Lightburn & Pine, 1996).

It was striking that there were no disruptions of adoptions. Most families were highly satisfied with the experience; two thirds of them adopted more than one child. Interviews with the parents showed them to have a strong sense of coherence and to be motivated to achieve in difficult situations. The children's extensive needs for care did not have a negative impact on family life. Quite the contrary, most of the families spoke of the joy and meaning their children had brought to their lives.

ACCEPTANCE

Robert Bogdan and Steven Taylor of the Center on Human Policy (Special Education) at Syracuse University, in a series of presentations, have contributed some gentle insights on the "sociology of acceptance." In these, they have looked at the bonding elements that facilitate sustained positive relations between individuals with intellectual disabilities and typically developing people (Bogdan & Taylor, 1987; Taylor & Bogdan, 1989). These elements are in contrast to the analysis of negativity by Goffman (stigma) and Becker (outsiders). Bogdan and Taylor employ *acceptance* as a generic term that captures the human outreach and encompasses affection and respect.

In the view of Bogdan and Taylor, there are four primary routes to a state of acceptance. *Family* is obviously a prominent facilitator, in which family values supercede differences. Family is the most pervasive link in society. It may be incorporated in part in service programs and other collaborations. *Religious* motivations can be a result of a religious social movement or commitment to beliefs about service. The individual's deviance may be an incentive, expressed in compassionate terms. Certain residential programs are founded on particular religious philosophies.

Humanitarian forces are evident in a concern for needs as viewed by humanism, civil rights, or the helping professions. In some settings of human services, meaningful ties with individuals with disabilities may on occasion replace "affective neutrality." More extensive involvement by individuals who are advocates can occur, starting with efforts to improve the quality of life. *Friendship* may be built by individuals liking one another. The differences can become unimportant, with positive attributes more central, or the difference may make a person more special or interesting.

CONCLUSION

Notable degrees of individual difference can in fact foster the development of rich personal alliances. Interactions that at first feel less familiar become warm and gratifying. By embracing a spirit of hospitality, one can appreciate exceptionality and foster an environment of acceptance in which individuals with disabilities are valued for their humanness and the qualities they have to offer.

REFERENCES

Bodgan, R., & Taylor, S. (1987). Toward a sociology of acceptance: The other side of the study of deviance. *Social Policy, 18*, 34–39.

Bogdan, R., & Taylor, S.J. (1989). Relationships with severely disabled people: The social construction of humanness. *Social Problems, 36*, 135–148.

Crocker, A.C. (1998). Exceptionality. *Developmental & Behavioral Pediatrics, 19*, 300–306.

Crocker, A.C., & Nelson, R.P. (1992). Mental retardation. In M.D. Levine, W.B. Carey, & A.C. Crocker (Eds.), *Developmental-behavioral pediatrics* (2nd ed., pp. 500–509). Philadelphia: W.B. Saunders.

Dybwad, G. (1999). Whom do we call mentally retarded? In M.A. Allard, A.M. Howard, L.E. Vorderer, & A.I. Wells (Eds.), *Ahead of his time: Selected speeches of Gunnar Dybwad* (p. 19). Washington, DC: American Association on Mental Retardation.

Homan, D., & Pratt, L.C. (2002). *Radical hospitality: Benedict's way of love.* Brewster, MA: Paraclete Press.

Lightburn, A., & Pine, B.A. (1996). Supporting and enhancing the adoption of children with developmental disabilities. *Children & Youth Services Review, 18*, 139–162.

McKenzie, J.K. (1993, Spring). Adoption of children with special needs. *The Future of Children*, 63–76.

Taylor, S.J., & Bogdan, R. (1989). On accepting relationships between people with mental retardation and non-disabled people: Toward understanding of acceptance. *Disability, Handicap & Society, 4*, 21–36.

CHAPTER 28

INFECTIOUS DISEASES

Harry L. Keyserling

Throughout history, infectious diseases have been the leading cause of death, particularly in infants and children. Tuberculosis, pertussis, typhoid, pneumonia, cholera, malaria, rheumatic fever, measles, and acute gastroenteritis were common at the beginning of the 20th century. Major advances in sanitation that provided clean water and food sources, decreased household crowding, universal vaccination programs, and the discovery of antimicrobial agents have resulted in significant improvements in life expectancy. Public health activities such as disease surveillance, epidemic investigation, quarantine, and isolation policies have contributed to decreases in the infectious disease burden.

Nevertheless, normal social activities facilitate the spread of infectious agents from person to person. For many infections, the highest risk of transmission occurs shortly before the onset of symptoms, preventing the opportunity to isolate infected individuals for disease control. Viral respiratory infections occur 6–8 times per year in children younger than 2 years of age. In addition, annual influenza epidemics cause symptomatic disease in 30%–60% of school-age children and are a substantial cause of mortality in the elderly. Acute gastroenteritis occurs in one fourth of the U.S. population each year.

As children develop, their risk of serious infection decreases as a result of improved hygiene, better motor control, and the maturation of their immune responses. The elderly are also at increased risk of serious infections related to the senescence of the immune system, multiorgan deterioration, poor hygiene, and neuromuscular deficiencies.

MECHANISMS THAT PREDISPOSE TO INFECTIONS

Central nervous system dysfunction associated with developmental disabilities can result in a variety of anatomic and physiological disturbances that may predispose directly and indirectly to an increased risk for infections and may complicate diagnosis and treatment. Physiologic dysfunctions include impaired innate or adaptive immune responses, abnormal respiratory ciliary kinetics, and disorders in gastrointestinal motility and urinary tract function. Anatomic abnormalities of the eustachian tube, respiratory tract, urinary tract, and spleen also predispose to increased or more severe infections.

Motor impairments lead to poor control of pharyngeal musculature. Normal protective respiratory responses are compromised, resulting in increased risk of otitis media, sinusitis, bronchitis, and pneumonia. Recurrent aspiration pneumonia is likely with severe motor impairment. In addition, immobility results in muscle contractures, decubitus ulcers, and cutaneous infections such as cellulitis and skin abscesses. Lower spinal cord dysfunction causes neurogenic bladders, resulting in stasis of urine, bladder colonization, and urinary tract infections.

Some etiological conditions may have additional predisposing factors. Chromosome abnormalities and inborn errors of metabolism may suppress granulocyte function and cellular and humoral immunity. Traumatic brain injury may lead to direct inoculation of bacteria, causing a wound infection, subdural hematoma, meningitis, or brain abscess. In addition, severe central nervous system dysfunction may result in ineffective central temperature control that makes infections more difficult to diagnose. Poor communication skills and sensory impairments may delay a definitive diagnosis of focal infections.

PERINATAL INFECTIONS

Tory was a term infant born to a mother with an uneventful pregnancy. Immediately after delivery, she was noted to have microcephaly and a petechial skin rash. Additional findings included hepatosplenomegaly and choreoretinitis on physical examination. Laboratory evaluation was negative for syphilis, rubella, and toxoplasmosis; however, cytomegalovirus (CMV) was isolated from a urine culture. Magnetic resonance imaging of Tory's brain demonstrated periventricular calcifications. Tory was treated for 6 weeks with intravenous ganciclovir. She will be followed closely for hearing and visual impairments and general neurologic development.

Congenital infections may be acquired by the transplacental route or during labor and delivery. In addition, breast milk is a common route of infection for human immunodeficiency virus (HIV). Unfortunately, women may not exhibit evidence of infection during pregnancy, and early gestational infections are more likely to cause brain insults than third-trimester infections. Most congenital infections are manifested by multiorgan involvement.

Prior to the introduction of a rubella vaccine, congenital rubella syndrome caused significant morbidity and mortality. In 1964, there were 10,000–20,000 cases of congenital rubella in the United States. Manifestations of congenital rubella include cataracts, retinopathy, glaucoma, patent ductus arteriosus, peripheral pulmonic artery stenosis, sensorineural hearing loss, behavior disorders, meningoencephalitis, and intellectual disabilities. Infants with congenital rubella may shed the virus in their urine for as long as 1 year; these infants are contagious and should be isolated to prevent transmission to susceptible family members and other contacts. Universal childhood immunization recommendations in the United States have virtually eliminated congenital rubella (Cooper & Alford, 2001), and several countries are initiating national immunization programs to eradicate rubella.

Congenital CMV occurs in 1%–2% of deliveries. Most of the infections are asymptomatic. As many as 20% of infected infants will develop symptoms. The most common cause of nongenetic sensorineural hearing loss in the United States is congenital CMV. Neurologic problems include microcephaly, intracranial calcifications, chorioretinitis, intellectual disabilities, seizures, and motor impairments (Stagno, 2001).

Congenital toxoplasmosis occurs in the neonates of about one third of women who acquire infections during pregnancy. Estimated annual cases in the United States are 1,000–3,500. As many as one half of cases will have evidence of neurologic disease—intracranial calcifications, microcephaly, hydrocephalus, seizures, and intellectual disabilities. Three quarters will have chorioretinitis (Remington, McLeod, Thulliez, & Desmonts, 2001).

Neonatal herpes infections usually are caused by exposure of the infant to maternal genital infections during delivery. Other sources of infection are maternal oral secretions or exposure to areas of the body of infected individuals that are shedding the herpes virus. Annual disease estimates for the United States are 300–1,000 cases. As many as one half of infected infants will have central nervous involvement including chorioretinitis, encephalitis, seizures, and paralysis. Even with early therapy, neurologic sequelae are common (Kohl, 1997).

HIV became identified as a cause of perinatal infections in the 1980s. Disease burden in some parts of the world such as sub-Saharan Africa is reported as high as 40% of pregnant women. In the United States, the majority of HIV infections in children occur by mother-to-infant transmission either in utero, at delivery, or via breast feeding. With no intervention, transmission rates are 15%–35% percent. When women are diagnosed prenatally and appropriate antiviral therapy is administered to the mother and infant, transmission rates can be decreased to 2% percent.

Central nervous system involvement is frequent in untreated children. As many as 60% of children with advanced HIV disease will have neurologic dysfunction. Problems include impaired brain growth, generalized weakness, ataxia, seizures, and myoclonus. Most of these children will develop progressive encephalopathy, causing loss of developmental milestones and dementia. Therapy with antiretroviral regimens consisting of multiple drugs can prevent or reverse neurologic impairment (Borkowsky, 2004). Additional pathogens that are rare causes of developmental disabilities include syphilis, tuberculosis, and varicella.

COMMON INFECTIONS

Viral upper respiratory infections are not necessarily more frequent in individuals with developmental disabilities but may be more likely to result in secondary bacterial sinusitis, otitis media, bronchitis, and pneumonia. For example, children with Down syndrome have an increased risk of otitis media because of shortened and horizontal eustachian tubes. Cleft palate also predisposes to otitis media secondary to palatal insufficiency. Children with oral motor disorders are unable to handle oral secretions, leading to increased episodes of otitis media.

Upper Respiratory and Middle Ear Infections

Bacterial pathogens isolated from middle ear infections include *Streptococcus pneumoniae*, *Haemophilus influenzae*, *Moraxella catarrhalis*, and group A *Streptococcus*. First-line therapy should be amoxicillin (90 mg/kg per day, in two divided doses). If the individual does not respond to amoxicillin, then second line therapy would include amoxicillin-clavulanate (90 mg/kg per day of amoxicillin component in two divided doses), cefdinir (14 mg/kg per day in one dose or two divided doses), cefpodoxime (10 mg/kg per day, once daily), cefuroxime (30 mg/kg per day in two divided doses), or ceftriaxone (50 mg/kg per day for 3 days) (Subcommittee on Management of Acute Otitis Media, 2004).

Pneumonia

Rasheed was a 5-year-old boy diagnosed with Duchenne muscular dystrophy at 6 months of age. He had a 2-day history of cough, fever, and chest pain in October. There was no evidence of rhinorrhea or pharyngitis, but Rasheed had had numerous prior admissions for respiratory infections. A chest x-ray showed a right middle lobe opacity. Blood cultures from admission were negative. Intravenous ceftriaxone and clindamycin were administered. After 2 days, Rasheed became afebrile and was discharged to complete a 7-day course of oral amoxicillin/clavulanate. An annual influenza vaccine was administered to him and all family members.

Aspiration pneumonia is increased in children with motor disorders and those with gastroesophageal reflux (see Chapters 14.1, 14.2, and 15). Common etiologies of pneumonia in children include respiratory viruses such as influenza, respiratory syncytial virus (RSV), metapneumovirus, parainfluenza, and adenoviruses. Bacterial pathogens include *Streptococcus pneumoniae*, *Mycoplasma pneumoniae*, *Haemophilus influenzae*, and group A *Streptococcus*. *Staphylococcus aureus* is causing an increasing number of severe community-acquired pneumonias that often are methicillin resistant. Mild pneumonia could be treated with a combination of a macrolide and amoxicillin. More severe pneumonia should be treated with vancomycin and a third-generation cephalosporin. For aspiration pneumonia, anaerobic coverage should be added as well. Clindamycin or other antibiotics effective against anaerobes are also typically administered.

Gastrointestinal Infection

Gastrointestinal infections may be more common because of poor hygiene. The risk of dehydration is increased in children with neurologic or muscular impairments.

Urinary Tract Infection

Diagnosis of pyelonephritis or cystitis may be more difficult in children with neurogenic bladders because symptoms of dysuria, frequency, and urgency may be difficult to illicit. Therefore, complaints of fever and/or abdominal pain must be evaluated for urinary tract infections.

Central Nervous System Infections

Ventriculitis or meningitis may follow shunting procedures for hyrocephalus. Empiric therapy for shunt infections should cover gram positive organisms such as *S. aureus* or other staphylococcal species and gram negative enterics. Vancomycin and third-generation cephalosporin are the preferred regimen.

Skin

Immobility causes decubitus ulcers and skin necrosis predisposing to cutaneous infections such as cellulitis, impetigo, and skin abscesses. Common organisms are *S. aureus* and group A *streptococcus*. Empiric therapy must be effective against methicillin-resistant *staphylococcus*.

EVALUATION OF FEBRILE INDIVIDUALS

For individuals who are febrile, an appropriate history should be obtained including travel, food and water exposure, contact with ill family or friends, and review of systems for evidence of a focus of infection. Careful examination of the ears, nasopharynx, and skin should be conducted. Blood cultures should always be obtained in children with congenital heart disease. If the individual is tachypneic, a chest x-ray is recommended. In individuals with ventricular shunts, a shunt tap should be considered if there is erythema or tenderness along the shunt tract, peritonitis, irritability, lethargy, seizure activity, or meningismus.

Table 28.1. Hand hygiene recommendations

Clean hands:
Before, during, and after food preparation
Before and after meals
After use of the bathroom
After handling animals or animal waste
When your hands are visibly soiled
After diaper changes or contact with oral secretions
Before and after patient contact
Hand hygiene technique:
Alcohol-based formulations are preferred over soap and water.
Rub hands vigorously together and scrub all surfaces.
Continue the process for 10–15 seconds.
Allow hands to air dry or dry with a towel.

Recommended Childhood and Adolescent Immunization Schedule UNITED STATES • 2005

Vaccine ▼ / Age ▶	Birth	1 month	2 months	4 months	6 months	12 months	15 months	18 months	24 months	4–6 years	11–12 years	13–18 years
Hepatitis B[1]	HepB #1	HepB #2			HepB #3				HepB Series			
Diphtheria, Tetanus, Pertussis[2]			DTaP	DTaP	DTaP		DTaP			DTaP	Td	Td
Haemophilus influenzae type b[3]			Hib	Hib	Hib	Hib						
Inactivated Poliovirus			IPV	IPV	IPV					IPV		
Measles, Mumps, Rubella[4]						MMR #1				MMR #2	MMR #2	
Varicella[5]						Varicella			Varicella			
Pneumococcal[6]			PCV	PCV	PCV	PCV			PCV / PPV			
Influenza[7]					Influenza (Yearly)				Influenza (Yearly)			
Vaccines below red line are for selected populations												
Hepatitis A[8]									Hepatitis A Series			

This schedule indicates the recommended ages for routine administration of currently licensed childhood vaccines, as of December 1, 2004, for children through age 18 years. Any dose not administered at the recommended age should be administered at any subsequent visit when indicated and feasible.

■ Indicates age groups that warrant special effort to administer those vaccines not previously administered. Additional vaccines may be licensed and recommended during the year. Licensed combination vaccines may be used whenever any components of the combination are indicated and other components of the vaccine are not contraindicated. Providers should consult the manufacturers' package inserts for detailed recommendations. Clinically significant adverse events that follow immunization should be reported to the Vaccine Adverse Event Reporting System (VAERS). Guidance about how to obtain and complete a VAERS form are available at **www.vaers.org** or by telephone, **800-822-7967**.

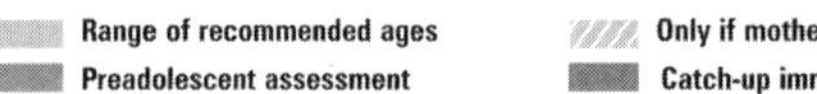

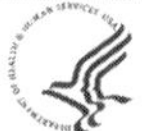

DEPARTMENT OF HEALTH AND HUMAN SERVICES
CENTERS FOR DISEASE CONTROL AND PREVENTION

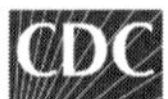

The Childhood and Adolescent Immunization Schedule is approved by:
Advisory Committee on Immunization Practices www.cdc.gov/nip/acip
American Academy of Pediatrics www.aap.org
American Academy of Family Physicians www.aafp.org

Footnotes
Recommended Childhood and Adolescent Immunization Schedule
UNITED STATES • 2005

1. **Hepatitis B (HepB) vaccine.** All infants should receive the first dose of HepB vaccine soon after birth and before hospital discharge; the first dose may also be administered by age 2 months if the mother is hepatitis B surface antigen (HBsAg) negative. Only monovalent HepB may be used for the birth dose. Monovalent or combination vaccine containing HepB may be used to complete the series. Four doses of vaccine may be administered when a birth dose is given. The second dose should be administered at least 4 weeks after the first dose, except for combination vaccines which cannot be administered before age 6 weeks. The third dose should be given at least 16 weeks after the first dose and at least 8 weeks after the second dose. The last dose in the vaccination series (third or fourth dose) should not be administered before age 24 weeks.

   Infants born to HBsAg-positive mothers should receive HepB and 0.5 mL of hepatitis B immune globulin (HBIG) at separate sites within 12 hours of birth. The second dose is recommended at age 1–2 months. The final dose in the immunization series should not be administered before age 24 weeks. These infants should be tested for HBsAg and antibody to HBsAg (anti-HBs) at age 9–15 months.

   Infants born to mothers whose HBsAg status is unknown should receive the first dose of the HepB series within 12 hours of birth. Maternal blood should be drawn as soon as possible to determine the mother's HBsAg status; if the HBsAg test is positive, the infant should receive HBIG as soon as possible (no later than age 1 week). The second dose is recommended at age 1–2 months. The last dose in the immunization series should not be administered before age 24 weeks.

2. **Diphtheria and tetanus toxoids and acellular pertussis (DTaP) vaccine.** The fourth dose of DTaP may be administered as early as age 12 months, provided 6 months have elapsed since the third dose and the child is unlikely to return at age 15–18 months. The final dose in the series should be given at age ≥4 years. **Tetanus and diphtheria toxoids (Td)** is recommended at age 11–12 years if at least 5 years have elapsed since the last dose of tetanus and diphtheria toxoid-containing vaccine. Subsequent routine Td boosters are recommended every 10 years.

3. ***Haemophilus influenzae* type b (Hib) conjugate vaccine.** Three Hib conjugate vaccines are licensed for infant use. If PRP-OMP (PedvaxHIB® or ComVax® [Merck]) is administered at ages 2 and 4 months, a dose at age 6 months is not required. DTaP/Hib combination products should not be used for primary immunization in infants at ages 2, 4 or 6 months but can be used as boosters after any Hib vaccine. The final dose in the series should be administered at age ≥12 months.

4. **Measles, mumps, and rubella vaccine (MMR).** The second dose of MMR is recommended routinely at age 4–6 years but may be administered during any visit, provided at least 4 weeks have elapsed since the first dose and both doses are administered beginning at or after age 12 months. Those who have not previously received the second dose should complete the schedule by age 11–12 years.

5. **Varicella vaccine.** Varicella vaccine is recommended at any visit at or after age 12 months for susceptible children (i.e., those who lack a reliable history of chickenpox). Susceptible persons aged ≥13 years should receive 2 doses administered at least 4 weeks apart.

6. **Pneumococcal vaccine.** The heptavalent **pneumococcal conjugate vaccine (PCV)** is recommended for all children aged 2–23 months and for certain children aged 24–59 months. The final dose in the series should be given at age ≥12 months. **Pneumococcal polysaccharide vaccine (PPV)** is recommended in addition to PCV for certain high-risk groups. See *MMWR* 2000;49(RR-9):1-35.

7. **Influenza vaccine.** Influenza vaccine is recommended annually for children aged ≥6 months with certain risk factors (including, but not limited to, asthma, cardiac disease, sickle cell disease, human immunodeficiency virus [HIV], and diabetes), healthcare workers, and other persons (including household members) in close contact with persons in groups at high risk (see *MMWR* 2004;53[RR-6]:1-40). In addition, healthy children aged 6–23 months and close contacts of healthy children aged 0–23 months are recommended to receive influenza vaccine because children in this age group are at substantially increased risk for influenza-related hospitalizations. For healthy persons aged 5–49 years, the intranasally administered, live, attenuated influenza vaccine (LAIV) is an acceptable alternative to the intramuscular trivalent inactivated influenza vaccine (TIV). See *MMWR* 2004;53(RR-6):1-40. Children receiving TIV should be administered a dosage appropriate for their age (0.25 mL if aged 6–35 months or 0.5 mL if aged ≥3 years). Children aged ≤8 years who are receiving influenza vaccine for the first time should receive 2 doses (separated by at least 4 weeks for TIV and at least 6 weeks for LAIV).

8. **Hepatitis A vaccine.** Hepatitis A vaccine is recommended for children and adolescents in selected states and regions and for certain high-risk groups; consult your local public health authority. Children and adolescents in these states, regions, and high-risk groups who have not been immunized against hepatitis A can begin the hepatitis A immunization series during any visit. The 2 doses in the series should be administered at least 6 months apart. See *MMWR* 1999;48(RR-12):1-37.

Figure 28.1. Recommended childhood and adolescent immunization schedule. Available from http://www.cdc.gov/nip/recs/child-schedule.htm#printable

Stool cultures may be useful if diarrhea is present. In individuals with urinary abnormalities, a urine culture should be obtained by bladder catherization if no other infection is identified. An unspun gram stain of freshly collected urine may provide a rapid diagnosis of pyelonephritis or cystitis.

INFECTION CONTROL ISSUES

Individuals with developmental disabilities may be cared for in institutional settings and are likely to have frequent hospitalizations. Colonization with resistant organisms results from repeated courses of antibiotics and exposure to crowded outpatient facilities and hospital environments. Rigorous hand hygiene is the first line of defense to prevent acquisition of pathogenic organisms (see Table 28.1).

Children with most respiratory, enteric, cutaneous, and systemic infections should not attend outpatient group activities until after the contagious period has passed or until antimicrobial medications have been administered. Specific recommendations for isolation precautions and time periods are available (Garner, 1996). Although children with congential CMV may be shedding the virus from urine, CMV infections are common in young children, and no specific precautions need to be instituted except for good hand hygiene.

Children with herpes simplex infections may have recurrent oral or skin lesions. They do not need to be excluded from group settings. The skin lesions should be covered with an impervious dressing until the lesions crust. Children with abnormal behaviors, such as frequent biting, may require restrictions in their activities.

Children with disabilities should receive the recommended childhood immunizations unless there are medical contraindications (see Figure 28.1). Annual influenza vaccine should be administered to both the children and all other family members. Prophylactic antibiotics should be administered for recurrent urinary infections or urologic abnormalities. Prophylaxis for recurrent otitis media is generally not recommended.

Antibiotic Resistance and Appropriate Use of Antimicrobial Agent

Because antibiotics have been widely prescribed since the 1940s, bacteria have become more resistant to multiple antibiotics. Some pneumococci are resistant to most oral agents including amoxicillin, cephalosporins, macrolides, trimethoprim-sulfamethoxazole, and quinolones. Seven studies have demonstrated that recent antibiotic use is a risk factor for invasive pneumococcal disease (Dowell & Schwartz, 1997).

Since 2000, community-acquired methicillin resistant *staphylococcus* (CA-MRSA) has increased to more than 50% in many areas of the country. Cellulitis, adenitis, bone and joint infections, endocarditis, pericarditis, abscesses, and pneumonia may be caused by CA-MRSA. Alternative regimens, including trimethoprim-sulfamethoxazole, clindamycin, linazolide, and vancomycin, should be used when staphylococcal infections are suspected.

The Centers for Disease Control and Prevention and the American Academy of Pediatrics have published many clinical guidelines promoting the judicious use of antibiotics. These programs have been successful, but continued education and modification of practice patterns will decrease development of more antibiotic-resistant organisms (American Academy of Pediatrics, 2003). Although decreased use of antibiotics in children with developmental disabilities may be impossible due to their high risk of serious bacterial infections, decreased community use will reduce the national burden of antibiotic resistant organisms.

CONCLUSION

Evaluating and treating infections in children with developmental disabilities is challenging. Physiologic and anatomic abnormalities predispose to increased infections. Pulmonary and urinary infections may be life threatening. Poor hygiene compounds the problem. Evaluation of febrile illnesses is difficult because of limitations in communication and sensory impairments. Primary prophylaxis with vaccines, vigilant infection control practices, and prompt institution of antibiotics when appropriate will improve outcomes.

REFERENCES

American Academy of Pediatrics. (2003). Antimicrobial agents and related therapy. In L.K. Pickering (Ed.), *Red book: 2003 report of the committee on infectious diseases* (26th ed., pp. 693–787). Elk Grove Village, IL: American Academy of Pediatrics.

Borkowsky, W. (2004). Acquired immunodeficiency syndrome and human immunodeficiency virus. In A.A. Gershon, P.J. Hotez, & S.L. Katz (Eds.), *Infectious diseases of children* (pp. 1–30). St. Louis: Mosby.

Cooper, L.Z., & Alford, C.A. (2001). Rubella. In J.S. Remington & J.O. Klein (Eds.), *Infectious diseases of the fetus and newborn infant* (pp. 347–388). Philadelphia: W.B. Saunders.

Dowell, S.F., & Schwartz, B. (1997). Resistant pneumococci: Protecting patients through judicious antibiotic use. *American Family Physician, 55*, 1647–1654.

Garner, J.S. (1996). Hospital infection control advisory committee: Guidelines for isolation precautions in hospitals. *Infect Control and Hospital Epidemiology, 17*, 53–80.

Kohl, S. (1997). Neonatal herpes simplex virus infections. *Clinics in Perinatology, 24*, 129–150.

Remington, J.S., McLeod, R., Thulliez, P., & Desmonts, G. (2001). Toxoplasmosis. In J.S. Remington & J.O. Klein (Eds.), *Infectious diseases of the fetus and newborn infant* (pp. 205–346). Philadelphia: W.B. Saunders.

Stagno S. (2001). Cytomegalovirus. In J.S. Remington & J.O. Klein (Eds.), *Infectious diseases of the fetus and newborn infant* (pp. 389–424). Philadelphia: W.B. Saunders.

Subcommittee on Management of Acute Otitis Media. (2004). Diagnosis and management of acute otitis media. *Pediatrics, 113*, 1451–1465.

CHAPTER 29

INTENSIVE CARE: A NARRATIVE

Robert J. Graham

Children and adults with developmental disabilities are a growing segment of the general population throughout the United States (Federal Interagency Forum on Child and Family Statistics, 2000; Pope & Tarlov, 1991). Technological advancements, both in the hospital and homecare settings, and expanding knowledge about disease physiology have allowed individuals with developmental disabilities to thrive. Broader care options and better appreciation of the rewards of raising and working with individuals with disabilities have fostered their integration and, ultimately, contributions to their respective families and communities.

As the population of individuals with developmental disabilities increases in number and complexity, medical care providers are challenged with meeting their special health care needs. Routine health maintenance has a different meaning when, for example, it encompasses management of antiepileptic medications, ventilator strategies, and special nutritional needs and restrictions, not to mention a lifetime of unique experiences for both the individual and his or her primary caregivers. The spectrum of medical need is obviously quite broad. Certain developmental disabilities also lead to specific medical vulnerabilities and, unfortunately, increased hospitalizations for some of these individuals. A smaller group of those with developmental disabilities may also require more frequent admission to an intensive care unit (ICU) because of the complex nature of their health care needs and their sometimes tenuous constitutions (Dosa, Boeing, Ms, & Kanter, 2001; Graham, Dumas, O'Brien, & Burns, 2004).

In general terms, intensive care providers are charged with the task of understanding multiple system pathophysiology, determining the best means of delivering oxygen to vital tissues, and meeting metabolic needs while identifying and treating the inciting insult. When an individual has antecedent medical issues, additional obstacles must be addressed. Thus, individuals with developmental disabilities represent some of the greatest challenges and potential rewards of comprehensive critical care.

In the author's recent year-long study, children with congenital neurodevelopmental disabilities constituted one quarter of all admissions to one pediatric critical care unit (Graham et al., 2004). Representation likely varies depending on the size of the care center and referral base. Acknowledgement and understanding of these individuals, however, is important for all care providers. As medical resources allow for greater mobility, individuals with developmental disabilities and complex histories will increasingly be seeking care beyond urban centers, whether on vacations or living in a rural setting.

This chapter focuses on the challenges of caring for individuals with developmental disabilities and their families in the critical care setting. The format strays from a traditional text, following the hospitalization of a single person, Willie. Utilizing a narrative outline illustrates a number of the unique issues surrounding critical care in the context of developmental disabilities. The intent is not to review all aspects of intensive care management but rather to prompt readers to consider how developmental disabilities may lead to variation in disease manifestations and response to therapies and, perhaps, influence the intensive care experience as a whole.

It is not unusual in the ICU to observe the evolution of a disease or physical insult. Helping the individual and his or her family cope with the disease experience can be difficult. This process may be even more challenging with individuals with developmental disabilities and concurrent, chronic health care needs, as they often enter the ICU with an extensive history of positive and negative medical experiences. Their conditions also may not follow a typical course. Health-related quality of life and individual, or family, autonomy must be recognized and respected.

When progressing through the narrative, the reader will recognize some obvious transition points in Willie's health status and consequently his care. Such shifts in

Special thanks goes to Willie's mother for her consent to document his history as well as for her dedication. In addition, Willie's primary nurse team in the ICU must be recognized for their comprehensive and compassionate care

care paradigms are usually not so clear, and the personality of an individual ICU has an impact on the course of events. I hope, however, that readers will reflect on this chapter when caring for individuals with developmental disabilities at all stages of their lives.

Like many young adults with chronic health care needs, Willie continued to seek care at a pediatric facility despite his chronologically advanced age of 25 years. Pediatric care providers perpetuate such relationships due to personal attachments, continuity of care, and "expertise" in what were often exclusively childhood conditions. Nevertheless, adult care providers and facilities are increasingly assuming care responsibilities for individuals with developmental disabilities. By anticipating such transitions, sharing knowledge, and embracing the spirit of topics discussed in this chapter, clinicians can provide optimal care for this special group of individuals, whether in the intensive care or outpatient setting.

INTENSIVE CARE UNIT AS A RESOURCE FOR INDIVIDUALS WITH SPECIAL HEALTH CARE NEEDS

Willie was a 25-year-old man with Hurler-Scheie Syndrome, or mucopolysaccharidosis I H/S (Jones, 1997; see also Chapter 7.2). Early in the summer, he transferred from his chronic care facility to a tertiary pediatric care hospital for evaluation and treatment of skin breakdown over his exceptionally large ventral hernia. The purulent wounds, his copious tracheal secretions, and his general dysmorphic appearance were striking and initially off-putting for some of my fellow staff members. However, as we grew to know Willie, his sense of humor, his love for his mother, his ability to compensate for severe physical limitations, and his desire to live touched us tremendously and left a more lasting and positive impression. He taught us about his life with a developmental disability.

Due to the natural progression of his underlying disorder, Willie had developed a combination of upper airway obstruction and restrictive lung disease. These conditions required his use of continuous positive airway pressure (CPAP) via a tracheostomy at night. Thus, despite the fact that he was near his baseline state of health, Willie was admitted to the critical care unit. In many hospitals, intensive or intermediate care settings are the best means of optimizing safety and centralizing resources and staffing. Like Willie, many of our patients with developmental disabilities depend on medical technology and require admission to the ICU even for routine care. Unfortunately, this situation can cause a Catch-22 because individuals with chronic and complex medical needs often contend for the same time, equipment, and space as acutely ill, "critical" patients.

Willie's history was remarkable for his diagnosis with mucopolysaccharidosis at age 15 months in the context of evaluation of an abdominal wall hernia. He became progressively more affected throughout his childhood, accumulating effects in almost every organ system. A tracheostomy was placed when he was 8 years old secondary to airway obstruction. He subsequently had multiple bronchoscopies and laser excision of tracheal mucopolysaccharide deposits (last at age 19 years). Willie underwent ventriculoperitoneal (VP) shunt placement and cervical laminectomy at age 18 years for communicating hydrocephalus and was resuscitated from a significant respiratory arrest during one hospitalization.

In following with the evolution of Hurler-Scheie Syndrome, Willie had visual impairment secondary to corneal clouding, hearing loss, and developmental delay. In addition, he lived with a marked kyphoscoliosis, restrictive lung disease, and a history of congestive heart failure with mitral and aortic valve stenosis and mitral regurgitation. He had a prominent and persistent abdominal wall hernia even after multiple surgeries, neurogenic bladder, and a remote history of seizure activity corresponding with acute hydrocephalus. Despite all of these impairments and disabilities, Willie was a contributing member of his family and community. He had completed school and participated in the Special Olympics (see Figure 29.1).

Such a history is not unusual in the ICU, where multiorgan system interaction is the forte of ICU care providers. Individuals with developmental disabilities, however, demand special attention. The intricacies and natural history of Willie's underlying disease coupled with a lifetime of medical intervention made his care regimen unique. Parents and primary care physicians often can anticipate potential questions and minimize areas of confusion by providing a medical "passport" or

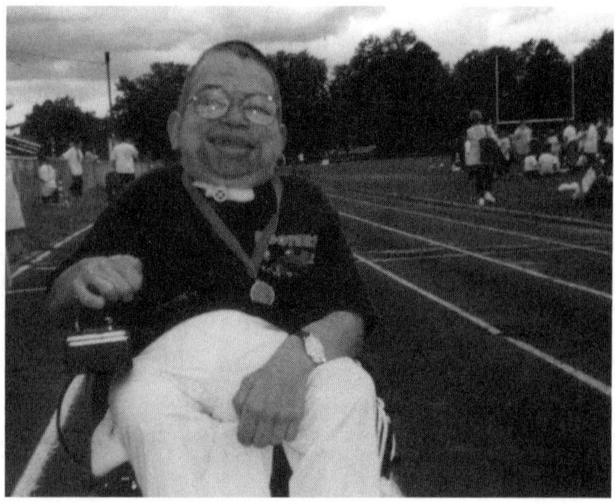

Figure 29.1. Willie participated in the Special Olympics.

brief summary (see Table 29.1). This document can be very helpful to the medical care team but also can supplement the often repeated inquiries during the admission process.

Review and management of such cases as Willie's present great learning opportunities for critical care providers and trainees even when not confronted with acutely "critical" illness. For example, Willie challenged the pediatric residents with a variety of questions. "How does restrictive and obstructive pulmonary disease affect long-term cardiac function?" "What are signs of VP shunt malfunction?" "Does intermittent bladder catheterization prevent infection and subsequent upper tract damage?" "How do the kidneys compensate for chronic respiratory insufficiency?"

In all disciplines, delivering optimal care is dynamic. Maximizing the individual's and parents' satisfaction depends on communication during the initial evaluation and throughout the course of treatment. Because the majority of individuals in the ICU have a limited ability to provide their own history, clinicians depend on a variety of other sources. Parents, written and electronic medical records, radiography, care providers from chronic care or rehabilitation facilities, primary physicians, and specialists may need to be contacted during the ICU course as direct patient interaction is impaired by sedation, pain, acute processes, intubation, or chronic impairment.

Table 29.1. Medical passport and historical information

Primary diagnoses
Secondary diagnoses
Updated medication list with dosing, milligram concentrations, timing, and indications for as needed medications
Oxygen needs, ventilator, continuous positive airway pressure, or bilevel positive airway pressure settings if applicable
Allergies and adverse responses to medications and foods (with descriptions)
Immunization history (including flu vaccine, pneumococchal vaccine, and respiratory syncytial virus prophylaxis)
Diet regimen and fluid supplements or restrictions
Approximate developmental level versus chronologic age and specific behavioral and communication issues
Basic therapy regimen and goals from physical, occupational, and speech therapies as well as adaptive equipment needs (e.g., orthoses, communication boards, helmets)
Past surgical interventions and recovery issues
Resuscitation status
Primary contact information of family and physician care providers

Note: This table is not a comprehensive or prioritized list and could be adapted for the individual.

Communication with Willie certainly posed a challenge: his hearing loss led nurses and staff to yell at the bedside; respiratory insufficiency dampened his vocalization around the tracheostomy; and his developmental delay, although mild, was also an obstacle depending on one's level of comfort with individuals with physical and mental limitations. Willie's mother served as his primary voice and was an invaluable resource for managing day-to-day issues as well as his overall course.

In many ways, Willie's initial ICU admission was not atypical. Hospitalization allowed for care of the primary concern, ventral hernia care, as well as reevaluation by his subspecialty care providers. The ICU care team consulted general surgery, the wound care nurse specialist, nutrition, and otolaryngology while updating pulmonary, urology, and neurosurgery. Cardiology had recently performed an echocardiogram as an outpatient, revealing mild mitral valve regurgitation and stenosis, mild aortic valve stenosis, but good biventricular function. Bacterial endocarditis prophylaxis was recommended, and cardiology cleared Willie for the operating room. The ICU staff served as care coordinators. Although this role is often time consuming and tedious, a critical care approach is uniquely suited to weigh the utility and impact of diagnostic procedures, interventions, and anticipatory measures for individuals with developmental disabilities and potentially fragile constitutions.

TRANSITION TO A GENERAL HOSPITAL WARD

After a week in the ICU, Willie was transferred to a general inpatient ward in anticipation of surgical repair of his ventral hernia. Preparing for this move, however, was no small task. Staff considered safety and monitoring as well as Willie's generally high maintenance care needs. Willie, however, demonstrated competency in sounding his own call alarm if distressed, and he tolerated long intervals without positive pressure airway support or suctioning. His ventral wall ulceration also appeared to be slowly responding to local therapies. A clear management plan had been outlined by the wound care specialist in conjunction with his primary surgeon. Thus, he appeared sufficiently stable for the transfer.

Willie and his mother both were pleased with the decision to transfer to the floor. The move was not only a sign of progress, but they welcomed the change of environment. Critical care units are designed to optimize monitoring and to facilitate any necessary interventions. Unfortunately, due to noise, confined space, lack of privacy, and minimal personal amenities, these units are not always comfortable for individuals or their visitors. Willie's sleep cycles, diet, and activities were obviously affected by these conditions. In addition, being in the intensive care has a psychological impact. Although some people may feel reassured and comforted by the smaller nursing-to-patient ratios and support, others may feel a loss of autonomy as well as fear—justified or not—that they may never leave the ICU.

Willie's progress on the wards continued slowly. An operative date was tentatively set for hospital day 18. There was some uncertainty as his abdominal wall wounds might still be "too purulent for mesh repair." Social work followed up with Willie's mother. The duration of hospitalization was placing a strain on her. She voiced growing frustration that hospital staff seemed no closer to fixing Willie's abdomen. A single parent, she was balancing work and the need to be with Willie. The hospital patient care coordinator also noted that Willie's skilled nursing facility would only reserve his bed until the first of the month, 3 days after the proposed surgery date. Whether Willie's mother was aware of this predicament, care providers recognized that this situation could certainly have an impact on Willie's projected length of stay.

Preoperative evaluation pressed ahead. The Neurosurgery Service requested a head computerized axial tomography and routine shunt series for operative clearance. The Pulmonary Service provided recommendations for CPAP management and optimal medication regimen. Willie's primary otolaryngologist followed along with the pulmonologist in anticipation of diagnostic bronchoscopy while in the operating room. Anesthesia reviewed his extensive history and previous operative experiences thoroughly.

In more emergent circumstances, such a luxury is not often afforded the anesthesiologist, emergency room physician, or intensivist. Special considerations, however, must be made when preparing to induce anesthesia (see Table 29.2) and manage a potentially difficult airway (see Table 29.3). In addition, if the individual has a tracheostomy, the physician should determine the age of the stoma and obtain a replacement tracheostomy tube of the appropriate size, cuff, and design. Some artificial airways are custom made or metal reinforced, limiting options and factoring into safety of exchange. Physicians should always consult an airway specialist if they are concerned that a fiberoptic scope, Parson's blades, bougies, light-wands, tube exchangers, or other devices should be used or available. Issues may also arise when coordinating transports between care facilities for individuals with developmental disabilities or chronic medical issues, affecting the composition of the transport team and necessary equipment and medication.

Willie was going to receive general anesthesia, with induction through his tracheostomy. Invasive venous and arterial monitoring lines would be placed once he was sedated. The possibility of an epidural for intra and postoperative pain management was also discussed, although it was unclear if this would be feasible given Willie's degree of scoliosis. Orders were written to hold enteral feeds, and plans were made for recovery in the ICU.

Table 29.2. Considerations for anesthetic induction in individuals with developmental disabilities

Review acute history and medical passport as thoroughly as possible (see Table 29.1).
Review past anesthetic and surgical history and recovery issues.
Recognize that the hospital setting, separation from care providers, and paradoxical reaction to preoperative medications may produce significant dysphoria.
Be aware that a history of gastroesophageal reflux or delayed gastric emptying, primary or secondary, may necessitate a rapid sequence induction.
Identify individuals with higher risk of malignant hyperthermia (e.g., diagnoses of Duchenne muscular dystrophy, osteogenesis imperfecta, myelomeningocoele, myotonia congenita, neuroleptic malignant syndrome), and utilize appropriate paralyzing agent and "clean technique."
Assess cardiac function and cardiopulmonary interaction given the myocardial depressant effect of most volatile (inhaled) and some parenteral anesthetics. Remain vigilant to syndrome-related congenital heart lesions, repaired or unrepaired.
Be aware of possible reactive airway disease if there is a history suggestive of recurrent aspiration.
Employ intracranial pressure precautions in individuals with hydrocephalus, craniosynostosis, or other high-risk conditions.
Determine baseline hepatic and renal function in anticipation of potential medication clearance issues.

Note: This table is a partial review of an anesthetic evaluation. Consult an anesthesiologist or review a comprehensive anesthesia text for specific issues.

Sources: Jones, 1997; Stoelting, Dierdorf, and McCamman, 1988.

ACUTE-ON-CHRONIC CARE

CODE BLUE! CODE BLUE! 4:05 A.M. on Willie's operating room date, the ICU team responded to the overhead emergency page. Willie was seizing and apneic. Ventilation and oxygenation were managed via Willie's tracheostomy, but obtaining intravenous (IV) access was difficult.

In controlled circumstances, as opposed to a resuscitation scenario, airway and vascular access in individuals with developmental disabilities can prove challenging. As noted previously, craniofacial and laryngo-tracheal anomalies may make bag–mask ventilation difficult and intubation prohibitive outside of the operative setting. Past history of IV or arterial access attempts, distorted anatomy, baseline vasomotor tone, and habitus, small or large, often factor into success or failure of securing vascular access (see Table 29.4).

Table 29.3. Anatomic variations contributing to airway management decisions

Head size and development (e.g., assess for midface hypoplasia as in Crouzon syndrome and maxillary hypoplasia in Rubinstein-Taybi syndrome)
Neck mobility (e.g., atlanto-axial instability associated with Down syndrome or mucopolysaccharidoses, foramen of magnum abnormalities associated with achondroplastic dwarfism or Chiari malformation, limited extension individuals with Klippel-Feil syndrome or following cervical spinal fusion)
Nare patency (e.g., CHARGE association)
Mandibular size and mobility (e.g., micrognathia in Treacher Collins syndrome, Pierre Robin sequence, trisomy conditions, and Turner syndrome; retrognathia as in velo-cardio-facial syndrome; prognathia as seen in Sotos and Crouzon syndromes)
Dentition
Tongue (e.g., relative or true macroglossia in Down and Beckwith-Wiedemann syndromes or mucopolysaccharidoses)
Cleft lip and palate (consider spontaneous ventilation and equipment to aid in visualization of the larynx)
Pharyngeal tone, tonsil and adenoid hypertrophy
Tracheal stenosis or malacia in individuals with a history of intubation

Note: This table is a partial review of congenital anomalies affecting airway management. Consult an anesthesiologist or review more comprehensive texts for specific issues

Source: Jones, 1997.

Table 29.4. Special vascular access considerations

Fear or aversive conditioning may be heightened for individuals with developmental disabilities because of limited understanding, pain, and past experiences, thus adding to the difficulty of obtaining vascular access. Sedation may facilitate efforts, but one must be wary of airway protection. Use topical analgesics when possible.
Tracheostomies or other past surgical intervention in the neck may alter the relative position of the jugular veins, carotid arteries, and airway.
Contractures limit sites for attempting lines and maintenance of lines once they are obtained.
Scoliosis may dramatically alter the position of the subclavian veins, leading to a greater likelihood of pneumothorax.
Past vascular access, thromboses, cardiac catheterizations, or surgical cut-downs may limit sites.
Actual habitus must be considered rather than age-appropriate or ideal size when choosing catheters (e.g., too long of a central venous catheter inserted into the subclavian may result in a proximal port that is intrathoracic but not intravascular).
Some syndromes are commonly associated with vascular anomalies (e.g., Klippel-Feil and Klippel-Trenaunay-Weber syndromes).

Willie received two doses of lorazepam of 3 mg each before his IV line infiltrated. He was given rectal diazepam followed by 3 mg more of lorazepam once a new IV was placed. Willie's seizures continued. A loading dose of fosphenytoin was given. Complete blood count, electrolytes, and blood cultures were sent, and serum glucose was 98. Neurosurgery accessed Willie's VP shunt reservoir to check for elevated intracranial pressure and to sample cerebrospinal fluid. A forth dose of lorazepam was given as well as antibiotic coverage with 2 g of ceftriaxone. Willie stopped seizing after approximately 45 minutes. His return to the ICU was not going to be as planned.

Acute events in the context of a complex history often support extensive diagnostic evaluation. Depending on the underlying disease states, a person with disabilities may not be able to compensate for even a mild metabolic or infectious stressor (Kanter, 1998). Physical impairments or chronic conditions can cloud a clinician's interpretation of obvious signs and symptoms (e.g., temperature or hemodynamic instability with hypothalamic dysfunction, chronic lung disease with persistent auscultatory and radiographic abnormalities) and potentially distract them from a significant problem. Limitations in communication, again, can be an obstacle.

Following Willie's resuscitation and initial cerebrospinal fluid and blood sampling, further evaluation included emergent brain computerized tomography, blood and urine cultures, and repeated serochemistries. No clear events had occurred during his hospitalization that could account for the seizure. Willie received broad-spectrum antibiotics, pending culture results, and continued on antiepileptic medications.

The only remarkable aspects of his workup were shunt cerebrospinal fluid counts with 15 white blood cells, 940 red blood cells, elevated protein at 109 mg/dL, glucose of 93 mg/dL, and a Gram stain showing no organisms. Willie remained hemodynamically stable but was notably obtunded and required full ventilator support. This seizure was his first in many years. He had, in fact, not been on any antiepileptic medications for more than 5 years.

Electroencephalogram revealed paroxysmal lateral epileptiform discharges (PLEDs) suggesting possible herpetic encephalitis. Acyclovir was added. Magnetic resonance imaging showed mild changes in bilateral hippocampal regions with restricted diffusion.

Where did the ventral hernia and wound fall in terms of prioritization now? The ICU team was tending to new issues with possible viral versus bacterial encephalitis, fluid shifts of unclear etiology, diminishing renal function, hyponatremia, changes in antiepileptic medications, and respiratory support needs with a persistent right lower lobe process. Otolaryngology evaluation showed significant upper airway obstruction and pulmonary edema. Prominent mucopolysaccharide deposits were found distal to the tracheostomy as well as a large accumulation near the carina, creating a "ball-valve" effect of one of the mainstem bronchi. Repeat laser excision was too risky.

Airway options were discussed with Willie's mother, but the otolaryngology staff expressed concern that Willie may "succumb to his illness." Although Willie was slightly more responsive, his mental status remained markedly depressed nearly 1 week after the seizure episode. Serial electroencephalograms showed waxing and waning right-sided

PLEDS, but leukopenia and nephrotoxicity prompted the team to discontinue Acyclovir after 7 days of therapy.

The ICU staff grappled with daily management issues, responding to acute changes and integrating consultation recommendations. Willie's primary nursing team, however, always provided poignant perspectives on Willie's overall status and maintained the focus on the family's goals.

Many ICUs have adopted the primary nurse and mutual care model, recognizing its contribution to comprehensive care. A primary nurse, although obviously attuned to the basic care issues, also becomes more invested and aware of the individual's needs and eccentricities. The nurse often forms a tight relationship with family members and, consequently, may provide a good barometer to gauge stressors on the individual and family.

As the most consistent presence at the bedside, Willie's primary nurse was an invaluable resource. She recognized even the smallest changes in the ventral wounds and knew when Willie was uncomfortable. Her role as intermediary with Willie's mom, however, was most significant as multiple care and consulting services visited Willie.

For individuals who have recurrent hospital admissions, primary nursing assignments may even be included on the medical "passport." As staffing allows, such continuity will likely facilitate care and enhance satisfaction. It was evident throughout Willie's hospitalization that his mood waxed and waned in accordance with the schedule of his primary team.

On hospital day 25, Willie was further from having his hernia repair than he had been on admission. The ICU attending remarked in a progress note that it was "important to determine what level of care he and his family wish."

Discussions about resuscitation status or advanced directives are often clarified in the ICU. For individuals with chronic conditions, such issues can be anticipated. It is often better if dialogue between the individual, family, and primary care provider is initiated in a less-urgent setting.

Willie and his mother had clearly thought about this decision previously. His mother stated that Willie was still to receive full resuscitation efforts if there was an acute decompensation. She understood the gravity of the situation but wished to continue as she and Willie had discussed before the admission.

Over the next several days, Willie became more lucid and interactive. No additional seizures were noted, and Willie did not have any adverse response to the anticonvulsant regimen. The etiology of his acute decline remained elusive. Ventilator support weaned to CPAP at night and mist collar when awake. A trial with a Poissy-Muir valve was attempted to allow Willie to talk, but his pulmonary mechanics were still too borderline. A second operative date was set. The ICU roller coaster appeared to have leveled out.

OPPORTUNITY FOR REASSESSMENT

Anesthesia's preoperative evaluation was updated. Otolaryngology had decided to perform a rigid bronchoscopy with potential removal of obstructive soft tissue near Willie's carina. Willie's mother was pleased to proceed, but nursing, social work, and pastoral care notes reflected the strain she was enduring, balancing issues at home, work, and the hospital. Willie's wheelchair was being repaired in anticipation of his postoperative resumption of normal activities. General surgery and the ICU team had some final discussions about testing Willie's readiness for wound revision and hernia reduction. An abdominal binder was tried the evening before Willie's operation.

An individual with combined chronic obstructive and restrictive pulmonary disease, recurrent aspiration pneumonia, and moderate cardiac dysfunction might not tolerate a decrease in functional residual capacity and tidal volumes. The abdominal binder forced the contents of the hernia up against the diaphragm. Not surprising, Willie's oxygen requirement and CPAP settings both increased dramatically with the binder in place. He was not comfortable and complained of a sensation in his airway as though he needed to be suctioned. The trial was viewed as a failure but was informative. Operative plans were put on hold, and a multidisciplinary family meeting was scheduled instead. With great reluctance, nursing, fellows, and attending surgeons, broke the news to Willie's mother.

Although difficult to arrange and often time consuming, team meetings can be very productive, especially for individuals with developmental disabilities. They allow input from all providers, family members, and the individual, when possible.

Willie's meeting began with discussion about concrete issues, airway concerns, and the difficult interaction between hernia reduction and respiratory status. Although fixing Willie's wounds would address infectious risks, comfort, mobility, and body-image, Willie would require an increase in chronic ventilator support. Willie's perceived quality of life needed to factor into the decision-making process. His mother held Durable Power of Attorney through an advance directive, but Willie was his own agent for health care decisions, as long as his competency could be acknowledged.

Decisional capacity, informed consent, and patient assent are essential concepts when providing appropriate and legal health care (American Academy of Pediatrics, 1995). Determining comprehension and eliciting expression of understanding and preferences for adults and children with developmental disabilities poses substantial challenges. For many, parental or proxy consent suffices, but health care providers must respect the decision-making abilities or shared responsibilities that an individual with disabilities may hold.

In light of Willie's seizure episode and protracted recovery, formal evaluation was necessary. Consequently, discussions about any surgical options, resuscitation status, and end-of-life care were deferred. Minor changes in management were made over the next several days. It was clear that the abdominal binder compromised Willie's comfort. Screaming into Willie's hearing aid and standing inches from his face, psychiatry and the ICU fellow discussed circumstances with Willie. He understood everything. The hernia could not be fixed at this time, but a bronchoscopy was recommended.

The risk versus benefits of potential interventions were reviewed. Willy expressed that he was depressed; however, he was not anxious about an operation despite the possibility of ventilator dependence and even death. If there was the possibility of improved respiratory function, then he wanted to pursue all options. With competency established, Willie's mother updated the health care proxy, and the consulting services weighed the options. Stabilization of Willie's airway obviously took priority.

Forty-three days after admission, Willie went to the operating room for bronchoscopy. Pulmonary and Otolaryngology coordinated simultaneous evaluations. Findings included both significant fixed and dynamic airway obstruction. Measurements were taken for a custom tracheostomy. Willie, again, was weaned slowly from ventilator support, but his primary nurses noted more complaints of "air hunger."

At a follow-up family meeting, team members decided that the sequence of events should be to obtain the custom tracheostomy, retry the abdominal binder, and then proceed with wound revision and hernia repair. The extent of Willie's skin breakdown varied. There were increasing regions of devitalized tissue, but these regions were not compromising him. Willie expressed interest in eating by mouth, and psychiatry adjusted Willie's antidepressant regimen.

As with many long-term patients, many of the ICU staff became very connected with Willie and his mother. They were invested in his care beyond the routine assignments. One of Willie's primary nurses outlined *Willie's Daily Agenda,* including activities of daily living, telephone calls, and therapies, to give Willie some semblance of control. Residents, respiratory therapists, nurses, fellows, and other staff joined Willie in his struggle. He and his mom were realistic and agreed that they would likely transition to a comfort care paradigm if they had any more difficulties.

The new tracheostomy tube seemed to take forever to arrive. In the interim, the ICU team grappled with recurring fluid shifts as well as an evolving abdominal wound infection. Antibiotics were started, and the hernia appeared to be expanding. Two weeks after going to the operating room, Willie received his new tracheostomy tube. It fit and bypassed his tracheal lesions, terminating only a half centimeter above the carina. This tube, however, was as much of a curse as it was a blessing. Although Willie could literally breathe easier, he hated the new tracheostomy. It was not fenestrated. It also offered more resistance, and he could not talk. His quality of life was deteriorating quickly because he was also experiencing more abdominal pain and discomfort.

REDIRECTION

Prediction models for ICU mortality, such as APACHE (Knaus et al., 1991) and PRISM (Pollack, Patel, & Rüttiman, 1996; Pollack, Ruttimann, & Getson, 1988), have not been validated for individuals with severe developmental disabilities. Due to chronic medical conditions, subpopulations with developmental disabilities are likely to be at higher risk of morbidity and mortality. Few care providers, however, would have predicted that the ICU would be transitioning to end-of-life care 2 months after Willie's admission.

Hollistic Care Service and the Pain Treatment Team were consulted. An assisted communication device was obtained to help Willie express his needs. Transferring to a different facility to focus on comfort was discussed, but Willie's status declined rapidly. He escalated to full controlled ventilation. The abdominal hernia continued to expand further, causing more pain and secondary problems. Systemic venous drainage appeared to be compromised with increasing ascites and diminishing renal function. The hernia was actually interfering with VP shunt function through obstruction of distal drainage. Patient- and nurse-controlled analgesia with morphine was implemented.

One evening, Willie pulled himself off the ventilator. It was unclear whether this event was intentional or just a product of Willie's growing disorientation and agitation. Everyone realized that cumulative insults had taken their toll on Willie.

Willie's mother was clearly struggling. The team learned that she had a previous child, Willie's older brother, who had succumbed to complications of the same Hurler-Scheie syndrome at age 5 years old. Cumulative insults had obviously taken their toll on his mom as well. She, like other families caring for individuals with disabilities, had encountered and survived life-threatening episodes in the past. Thus, differentiating and believing that her son had truly reached the end was difficult, if not impossible.

Willie's mother discussed her feelings openly. Willie was suffering too much. The ICU team engaged the hospital's Advance Care Team to discuss potential options to optimize Willie's end-of-life care and support his mother with these decisions.

On hospital day 65, Willie expressed desire to have his ventilator support withdrawn. His wishes were discussed extensively with all of his family. The ventilator was removed, and Willie died comfortably with his mother sitting next to him.

OUTCOMES

Fortunately, Willie's story is not representative of the majority of critical care outcomes for individuals with developmental disabilities. Disposition in this setting, however, is often complicated. Recovery from surgery and acute medical illness can be quite protracted in individuals with chronic medical conditions.

Assessing readiness for extubation, for example, can be difficult. An individual with even moderate delay, with or without sedation in place, may not be able to follow commands and perform volitional pulmonary function testing. Alternative approaches may be helpful in children and adults when communication is not optimal.

In 2002, Randolph and colleagues published results of a multicentered trial that attempted to standardize extubation criteria for all individuals based on oxygen saturations and requirements, mode of ventilation, tidal volumes, and respiratory rate. Investigators accounted for age and size variability and eliminated effort-dependent variables (Randolph et al., 2002). Because this type of evaluation is independent of cooperation, it may be particularly useful when caring for individuals with developmental disabilities.

If an individual is felt to have reached a plateau in recovery, he or she is sometimes deemed to be at *new baseline.* Care providers must be cautious in using this term prematurely, as such branding may alienate the individual and his or her family and may not be accurate (Steele, 2000). Depending on the nature and chronicity of the individual's disabilities, it may take a long time for a child with a disability to resume his or her developmental path or for an adult to realize his or her own premorbid status. Engaging a family early in the hospital course is usually the best course to determine their perspective on quality of life and care issues.

Hospitals have tried various models of coping with the challenges surrounding disposition. Some facilities have adapted transitional, or step-down units, to provide subacute care, permitting technologic support outside of the ICU. Other ICUs have close relations with rehabilitation centers that allow for continued medical care with the addition of comprehensive occupational, physical, speech-language, and psychiatric therapies as well as the advantage of time.

Some families elect to continue the recovery process at home. The availability of home care nursing is highly variable; however, the burgeoning advancements in portable ventilators, monitors, and home care services allow for individuals to make the transition to more familiar environments. As with Willie, consideration can also be made for transfer to an alternative care setting, or hospice, for end-of-life care, where the objective is comfort and family support versus recovery.

Ironically, difficulties with placement and prolonged hospitalization, although troublesome, could actually be viewed as being a product of the ICU's success. Willie and his mother, for example, were familiar with the ICU. In my study of children with congenital neurodevelopmental diagnoses in the ICU, 309 children accounted for 427 annual admissions (Graham et al., 2004). The "frequent flier" cohort evokes many questions about the relationship of pediatric critical care practice and children's chronic health issues (Nicholson, 2004).

Overall mortality rates for critical care units across the United States are relatively low. Pediatric units range from 2% to 10%, whereas adult units experience 5% to 40% death rates (Knaus, 1993; Tilford, Roberson, Lensing, & Fiser, 1998). Individual units vary dramatically depending on volume, patient mix, and level of acuity (Gemke, 1995; Glance, 2000). Children with comorbidities have higher mortality risk (Seferian et al., 2001; Tomaske, Bosk, Eyrich, Bader, & Niethammer, 2003), but the contribution of developmental diagnoses may be overestimated (Graham et al., 2004).

As part of research trials, quality assurance and improvement efforts, resource utilization evaluations, and other endeavors, intensive care providers have looked to other outcomes indices beyond survival to gauge the success of interventions and care systems. Standard outcome tools include length of stay, ventilator or ventilator-free days, medication requirements, and serial severity of illness scores. Depending on the nature of the insult, investigators may focus on specific physiologic measures, such as pulmonary function testing, neurologic batteries, or developmental assessments for children, including the Vineland Adaptive Behavioral Scale (Sparrow, Balla, & Cicchetti, 1984). More holistic measures include health-related quality-of-life scores, such as the Short Form-36 (Ware, 2003) and the Child Health Questionnaire (Landgraf et al., 1998), functional independence measures, and global function scores, like the Pediatric Overall Performance Category (Fiser, 1992; see Table 29.5). All of these measures, however, have limitations, and the applicability for individuals with developmental disabilities is even more problematic.

Had Willie survived his ICU course, how would one assess his outcome? Most outcomes scores, whether based on daily function, basic physiology, or complex neuropsychiatric performance, assume a "normal" baseline. Comparison with preadmission status is usually not available. As previously noted, recovery times are often prolonged; thus, determining the best time for assessment may be difficult. Lack of sensitivity to detect change as well as potential ceiling or floor effects may also be troublesome depending on the tool. Pediatric patients with developmental disabilities pose an even greater challenge, as they are moving targets. Even when delayed, development is dynamic; therefore, an outcome tool would ideally compare an individual to him- or herself and to population norms and would track the individual according to developmental patterns.

Ultimately, efforts to follow individuals with developmental disabilities are needed to optimize their comprehensive care. Although formal follow-up and outcomes evaluation are difficult, this process would be potentially informative and rewarding. ICU staff are often amazed to see how well individuals do following hospitalization. Anecdotes, however, do not necessarily—and should not—alter practice of medicine, but they do enhance morale and alter perspectives.

Table 29.5. Outcome measures in the intensive care

Single concept or disease-specific measures—mortality, length of stay, ventilator-free days, readmission rates, pulmonary function tests, biologic indices (e.g., interluekin levels), and extent of extremity amputation

Predictive models as outcome surrogates—Acute Physiology, Age, Chronic Health Evaluation (Knaus, et al., 1991); Pediatric Risk of Mortality score (Pollack, Patel, & Ruttiman, 1996; Pollack, Ruttimann, & Getson, 1988); and Score for Neonatal Acute Physiology (Richardson, Gray, McCormick, Workman, & Goldmann, 1993)

Severity of illness scores as outcome surrogates—Multiple Organ Dysfunction Score (Marshall et al., 1995); Sequential Organ Dysfuntion Assessment (Vincent et al., 1996); and Therapeutic Intervention Scoring System–28 (Miranda, de Rijk, & Schaufeli, 1996)

Quality of life scales—Short Form 36 (Ware, 2003); Child Health Questionnaire (Landgraf et al., 1998); Sickness Impact Profile (Lipsett et al., 2000); and Health Utilities Index–Mark I, II, & III (Feeney, Furlong, & Torrance, 2003)

Rehabilitation and physical function scales—New York Heart Association Functional Class (Criteria Committee of the New York Heart Association, 1994); Glascow Outcome Score (Jennett & Bond, 1975); Rancho Los Amigos Brain Injury Scale (Hagen, Malkmus, & Durham, 1972); and Disabilities Rating Scale (Choi et al., 1998)

Developmental/health status measurements—return to work or school; Functional Status IIR (Stein & Jessop, 1990); Functional Independence Measure (Keith, Granger, Hamilton, & Sherwin, 1987; Msall et al., 1994); and Vineland Adaptive Behavioral Scales (Sparrow, Balla, & Cicchetti, 1984)

Neuropsychological assessments—Wisconsin Card Sorting Test (Berg, 1984) and Wechsler Memory Scale (Weschler, 1997)

Specific measures designed for the critical care setting—Pediatric Overall Perfomance Category (POPC; Fisher, 1992) and Pediatric Cerebral Performance Category (PCPC; Fisher, 1992)

Note: This table is a sample of adult and pediatric outcome measures utilized by critical care investigators. Each measure could be critiqued, especially with respect to the applicability to individuals with developmental disabilities.

CONCLUSION

From the moment of first encounter to final disposition, whether end-of-life care or discharge to home, individuals with developmental disabilities present significant challenges to the intensive care team. Willie's story illustrates many of these complexities. His acute-on-chronic medical issues contributed to pathophysiologic dilemmas. Willie's cumulative medical experiences and exposures combined with his mother's journey influenced therapeutic options and decision making. Limitations in communication posed barriers in many aspects of his care. Hospitalization can be quite prolonged, and coordination of care is time consuming. Because of such complexities, however, the comprehensive care perspective of most intensive care settings is uniquely tailored for the care of the special and growing population of individuals with developmental disabilities.

REFERENCES

American Academy of Pediatrics, Committee on Bioethics. (1995). Policy statement: Informed consent, parenteral permission, and assent in pediatric practice. *Pediatrics, 95*(2), 314–317.

Berg, E.A. (1984). A simple, objective technique for measuring flexibility in thinking. *Journal of General Psychology, 39,* 15–22.

Choi, S.C., Marmarou, A., Bullock, R., Nichols, J.S., Wei, X., & Pitts, L.H. (1998). Primary end points in phase III clinical trials of severe head trauma: DRS versus GOS. *Journal of Neurotrauma, 15,* 771–776.

Criteria Committee of the New York Heart Association. (1994). *Nomenclature and criteria for diagnosis* (9th ed.). Boston: Little, Brown, & Co.

Dosa, N.P., Boeing, N.M., Ms, N., & Kanter, R.K. (2001). Excess risk of severe acute illness in children with chronic health conditions. *Pediatrics, 107*(3), 499–504.

Federal Interagency Forum on Child and Family Statistics. (2000). *America's children: Key national indicators of well-being 2000.* Washington, DC: Author.

Feeney, D.H., Furlong, W., & Torrance, G.W. (2003). *Health Utilities Index I, II, and III.* Retrieved from http://www.health utilities.com

Fiser, D.H. (1992). Assessing the outcome of pediatric intensive care. *Journal of Pediatrics, 121*(1), 68–74.

Gemke, R.J. (1995). Comparative assessment of pediatric intensive care: A national multicenter study. Pediatric Intensive Care Assessment of Outcome (PICASSO) Study Group. *Critical Care Medicine, 23*(2), 238–245.

Glance, L.G. (2000). Effect of mortality rate on the performance of the Acute Physiology and Chronic Health Evaluation II: A simulation study. *Critical Care Medicine, 28*(10), 3424–3428.

Graham, R.J., Dumas, H.M., O'Brien, J.E., & Burns, J.P. (2004). Congenital neurodevelopmental diagnoses and an intensive care unit: Defining a population. *Pediatric Critical Care Medicine, 5*(4), 321–328.

Hagen, C., Malkmus, M.A., & Durham, M.A. (1972). *The Rancho Los Amigos Scale.* Retrieved from http://www.neuro skills.com/index.html?main+tbi/rancho.html

Jennett, B., & Bond, M. (1975). Assessment of outcome after severe brain damage. *The Lancet, 7905*(1), 480–484.

Jones, K.L. (1997). *Smith's recognizable patterns of human malformation.* Philadelphia: W.B. Saunders.

Kanter, R.K. (1998). Control of breathing and acute respiratory failure. In B. Fuhrman & J.J. Zimmerman (Eds.), *Pediatric critical care* (pp. 529–537). St. Louis: Mosby.

Keith, R.A., Granger, C.V., Hamilton, B.B., & Sherwin, F.S. (1987). The Functional Independence Measure: A new tool for rehabilitation. *Advances in Clinical Rehabilitation, 1,* 6–18.

Knaus, W.A. (1993). Variations in mortality and length of stay in intensive care units. *Annals of Internal Medicine, 118*(10), 753–761.

Knaus, W.A., Wagner, D.P., Zimmerman, J.E., Bergner, M., Bastos, P.G., Sirio, C.A., et al. (1991). The APACHE III Prognostic System: Risk prediction of hospital mortality for critically ill hospitalized adults. *Chest, 100*(6), 1619–1636.

Landgraf, J.M., Maunsell, E., Speechley, K.N., Bullinger, M., Campbell, S., Abetz, L., et al. (1998). Canadian-French, German, and UK versions of the Child Health Questionnaire: Methodology and preliminary item scaling results. *Quality of Life Research, 7,* 433–445.

Lipsett, P.A., Swoboda, S.M., Campbell, K.A., Cornwell, E., III, Dorman, T., & Pronovost, P.J. (2000). Sickness impact profile score versus a modified short-form survey for functional outcome assessment: Acceptability, reliability, and validity in critically ill patients with prolonged intensive care unit stays. *Journal of Trauma, Injury, Infection, and Critical Care, 49*(4), 737–743.

Marshall, J.C., Cook, D.L., Christou, N.V., Bernard, G.R., Sprung, C.L., & Sibbald, W.J. (1995). Multiple organ dysfunction score: A reliable descriptor of a complex clinical outcome. *Critical Care Medicine, 23,* 1638–1652.

Miranda, D.R., de Rijk, A., & Schaufeli, W. (1996). Simplified therapeutic intervention scoring system: The TISS-28 items—results from a multicenter study. *Critical Care Medicine, 24*(1), 64–73.

Msall, M.E., DiGaudio, K., Rogers, B.T., LaForest, S., Catanzaro, N.L., Campbell, J., et al. (1994). The Functional Independence Measure for Children (WeeFIM): Conceptual basis and pilot use in children with developmental disabilities. *Clinical Pediatrics, 33,* 421–430.

Nicholson, C.E. (2004). Pediatric critical care for children with congenital neurodevelopmental diagnoses. [Editorial]. *Pediatric Critical Care Medicine, 5*(40), 407–408.

Pollack, M.M., Patel, K.M., & Ruttimann, U.E. (1996). PRISM III: An updated pediatric risk of mortality score. *Critical Care Medicine, 25*(5), 743–752.

Pollack, M.M., Ruttimann, U.E., & Getson, P.R. (1988). Pediatric risk of mortality (PRISM) score. *Critical Care Medicine, 16*(11), 1110–1116.

Pope, A.M., & Tarlov, A.R. (1991). *Disability in America: Towards a national agenda for prevention.* Washington, DC: Institute of Medicine.

Randolph, A.G., Wypij, D., Venkataraman, S.T., Gedeit, R.G., Meert, K.L., Lucket, P.M., et al. (2002). Effect of mechanical ventilator weaning protocols on respiratory outcomes in infants and children: A randomized controlled trial. *Journal of the American Medical Association, 288*(20), 2561–2568.

Richardson, D.K., Gray, J.E., McCormick, M.C., Workman, K., & Goldmann, D.A. (1993). Score for neonatal acute physiology (SNAP): A physiologic severity index for neonatal intensive care. *Pediatrics, 91,* 617–623.

Serefian, E.G., Carson, S.S., Pohlman, A., et al. (2001). Comparison of resource utilization and outcome between pediatric and adult intensive care unit with patients. *Pediatric Critical Care Medicine, 2*(1), 2–8.

Sparrow, S.S., Balla, D.A., & Cicchetti, D.V. (1984). *Vineland Adaptive Behavior Scales.* Circle Pines, MN: American Guidance Service.

Steele, R.G. (2000). Trajectory of certain death at an unknown time: Children with neurodegenerative life-threatening illnesses. *Canadian Journal of Nursing Research, 32*(3), 49–67.

Stein, R.E., & Jessop, D.J. (1990). Functional Status II(R): A measure of child health status. *Medical Care, 28*(11), 1041–1054.

Stoelting, R.K., Dierdorf, S.F., & McCamman, R.L. (1988). *Anesthesia and co-existing disease.* New York: Churchill Livingstone.

Tilford, J.M., Roberson, P.K., Lensing, S., & Fiser, D.H. (1998). Differences in pediatric ICU mortality risk over time. *Critical Care Medicine, 26*(10), 1737–1743.

Tomaske, M., Bosk, A., Eyrich, M., Bader, P., & Niethammer, D. (2003). Risk of mortality in children admitted to the paediatric intensive care unit after haematopoirtic stem cell transplantation. *British Journal of Haematology, 121*(6), 886–891.

Vincent, J.L., Moreno, R., Takala, J., Willatts, S., DeMendonca, A., Bruining, H., et al. (1996). The SOFA (Sepsis-related Organ Failure Assessment) score to describe organ dysfunction/failure. *Intensive Care Medicine, 22,* 707–710.

Ware, J.E. (2003). *The SF-36 health survey.* Retrieved from http://www.sf-36.com/tools/sf36.shtml

Wechsler, D. (1997). *Wechsler Memory Scale–Third Edition.* San Antonio, TX: Harcourt Brace.

CHAPTER 30

END-OF-LIFE CARE

Sandra L. Friedman

This chapter addresses end-of-life issues for individuals with severe developmental disabilities and complex medical problems. Families often have many questions regarding end-of-life care: When are issues regarding resuscitation decisions addressed? Who should be involved in the decision-making process? What are the distinctions between medical treatment and resuscitation? Is there a difference between palliative care and hospice care? Should nutrition and hydration be altered or discontinued? What happens if there is a difference of opinion regarding how the care plan should be implemented? Can decisions regarding the care plan be changed, and if so, by whom? Newman's story presents a number of relevant issues to consider regarding end-of-life care.

Newman was an 8-year-old boy diagnosed with Hunter Syndrome (mucopolysaccharidoses II, see Chapter 7.2). He lived with his parents, grandmother, and older brother. His devoted family experienced difficulty acknowledging the progressive nature of his metabolic disorder, despite explanations regarding the anticipated course of his medical problems.

Over the years, Newman's medical and cognitive functioning deteriorated. His family initially provided most of his care; however, they later needed to obtain some in-home nursing coverage for additional assistance. Newman's last cognitive assessment approximately 1 year prior revealed that he was functioning in the range of severe intellectual disabilities. Despite his worsening status, he displayed pleasure in the presence of other people, particularly his family members.

Newman experienced significant upper and lower respiratory tract symptoms, abdominal distention due to organomegaly, and a history of cardiomyopathy with multiple cardiac valvular abnormalities. He had required tracheostomy tube placement, due to worsening airway obstruction from accumulating mucopolysaccarides and tissue in his trachea. He also had undergone ventriculoperitoneal shunt for obstructive hydrocephalus. Newman received all of his nutrition via gastrostomy tube. At this point, he was nonambulatory, nonverbal, and incontinent.

Multiple specialists provided his medical care, and Newman required many medications for his cardiac, pulmonary, and gastrointestinal problems. He had been hospitalized frequently to treat his progressive condition, particularly the worsening of his upper airway obstruction and reactive airway disease. His parents had always wanted aggressive medical management provided for him, to which he had usually responded favorably. They also had desired full resuscitation for him, in the event of cardiopulmonary arrest.

Ultimately, little more could be done to ameliorate Newman's worsening airway obstruction. He frequently appeared uncomfortable and was less interactive with others. After long and difficult discussions with Newman's primary care provider regarding the expectation that death was imminent, Newman's family decided to change his resuscitation status to Do Not Resuscitate (DNR). They continued to want him to be treated for acute, reversible illnesses. They also continued to want him to be fed and hydrated.

One of his medical providers had suggested that hospice care be provided so that Newman would be comfortable during his final days, to which the family agreed. They decided to transfer him out of the acute hospital setting; however, it had become more difficult for the family to manage his care at home. Newman was therefore admitted to a pediatric skilled nursing facility, where he would receive ongoing care.

The staff at the pediatric skilled nursing facility was familiar with providing palliative care at the end of life, although they had not previously worked directly with a hospice agency. Upon Newman's admission, a hospice worker from the local agency met with the physicians, nursing staff, and the family. Pain management issues were reviewed. She suggested that his feeds and hydration be discontinued.

The family was not ready to discontinue hydration and feeds, and the providers at the skilled nursing facility were also not comfortable with those recommendations. As they did not yet know Newman or his family, they wanted some time to develop relationships with them. Newman, therefore, continued to receive his usual therapies, medications, and feeds, as well as narcotic medication for provision of comfort.

Even though Newman's parents were intellectually aware that their son would soon die, emotionally they did not seem to accept the fact, as they continued to hold onto the hope that somehow he would improve. The family met frequently with the social work staff, as well as other providers. Over the course of several weeks, Newman's need for narcotic medication to provide comfort increased. He also became less tolerant to any type of fluids provided via his gastrostomy tube. His fluids and medications, with the exception of morphine, were ultimately discontinued, due to markedly reduced gut motility and abdominal distension. Newman expired 2 days later, which was approximately 4 weeks after his time of admission.

HISTORICAL PERSPECTIVE

Issues regarding end-of-life care for individuals with disabilities are fraught with high emotional tension when presented with the backdrop of the previous abuses directed toward individuals with intellectual and other disabilities. Many are familiar with "medical" experiments performed during the Nazi regime, whereby people were forced to endure potentially life-threatening conditions, with the anticipated results of death. Eugenics was also used by the Nazis and actually was legalized for people with intellectual and developmental disabilities in the United States in the early 20th century. Although these procedures decreased significantly after World War II, the laws were not repealed in the United States until the 1960s (Diekema, 2003; Wehmeyer, 2003). The Belmont report was prepared as a response to some of the abuses seen in this country to lay foundations for the ethical treatment of all people, with particular emphasis on the most vulnerable individuals (National Commission for Protection of Human Subjects, 1979).

Just as social advances toward safeguarding the dignity of human life have been made, so have medical advances been developed in the ability to extend human life. Concepts such as quality of life and medical futility have been discussed when considering treatment options, particularly when there is a high likelihood of death as a potential outcome (Burn & Truog, 1997; Gordon, 2003). Although individuals have the right to refuse treatment, there also is concern that these rights may be abused toward those citizens who are not able to defend themselves well or articulate their wishes (Commonwealth of Massachusetts, 1999).

Debates have occurred regarding the extent of entitlement to medical care that citizens in general should be provided. The United States does not at this time have universal medical coverage or a single payer system, as do a number of other countries. Therefore, people have their medical costs covered by private insurance, managed care programs, government programs, or they pay out of pocket. Many individuals with significant developmental disabilities require government subsidy for medical care. As such, medical coverage is generally provided for acute situations and hospitalizations. Although certain medications may require prior approval and certain treatments may not be allowed, most medical conditions are covered (Kaiser Commission on Medicaid Facts, 2001a, 2001b).

Individuals with developmental disabilities who are living in the community, however, may lack access to medical services (Office of the Surgeon General, 2002). Some providers do not accept or limit the number of individuals who are funded by Medicaid. Some individuals may not have the means to travel to a medical provider's office, and some offices are not adequately able to accommodate the needs of people with disabilities. There continues to be a need for accessible, quality health care in the community that is both preventive and treatment oriented (Shavelle & Strauss, 1999; Strauss, Ashwal, Shavelle, & Eyman, 1997). The medical home for children with special health care needs, as supported by the American Academy of Pediatrics (AAP), underscores the need to provide assistance for the child and family in all phases of medical care. Although challenges exist to deliver such care to all children, efforts are being made to develop programs of medical care that are accessible, family centered, continuous, comprehensive, coordinated, compassionate, and culturally sensitive (AAP Policy Statement, 2004; Moore & Tonniges, 2004).

In addition, significant advances in medical care have resulted in longer life spans for the population in general and for individuals with disabilities in particular (American Association on Mental Retardation [AAMR], 2003; Lawhorne, 1999). Despite the advances in medical management, including factors such as use of enteral feeds, advances in antibiotic coverage, and more aggressive treatment to improve pulmonary function, individuals with severe intellectual disabilities and special health care needs are still expected to have a lower life expectancy compared with the general population (Chaney & Eyman, 2000; Strauss, Shavelle, & Anderson, 1998; Strauss, Shavelle, Anderson, & Baumeister, 1998). The lower their cognitive level, the more likely they will have chronic medical conditions.

Functional abilities, such as those related to voluntary motor skills and ability to feed oneself, have been found to be strong predictors of life span (Smith, Camfield, & Camfield, 1999). As such, individuals with lower functional status are more likely to die at a relatively early age (Shavelle & Strauss, 1999; Strauss, Kastner, Ashwald, & White, 1997). Ideally, families should be prepared to address end-of-life decisions prior to acute, life-threatening events.

DEFINITIONS, GENERAL ISSUES, AND PREFERENCES

End-of-life care addresses issues regarding the type of medical and related care that is provided to an individual when death is a probable outcome. Decisions are made regarding the degree or intensity of medical treatments and interventions. Sometimes, individuals indicate choices even before life-threatening events take place, just as choices and changes in plan are often made during an acute event itself. At some point in the medical management, particularly when death is imminent, individuals may also elect to forego potential treatment and only wish that comfort measures be provided (Ethics Advisory Committee, 1999; Fordyce, 2001; Heffner, Barbieri, & Casey, 1996; Miller & Miller, 2003; Wolfe, Freiber, & Hilden, 2002).

Certainly, personal preferences need to be taken into account when addressing end-of-life issues, as each person presents with a unique combination of social, religious, and experiential factors that may affect decisions, in addition to the medical condition per se (Contro, Larson, Scofield, Sourkes, & Cohen, 2002; Gillick, 2000; Wolfe et al., 2002). Individuals who are not capable of providing informed consent generally rely on a surrogate decision maker, who may have been designated to make such decisions via a formal legal document (AAP Committee on Bioethics, 1998; Ackerman & Kemle, 1999; Cantor & Pearlman, 2003; Cogen, Patterson, Chavin, Landsberg, & Posner, 1992). In that respect, an individual's level of cognitive functioning must be considered. Ethical dilemmas may also arise regarding what is in the best interest of the individual and who should be the one making those decisions if a person is not able to speak for him- or herself.

As the demographics of society have changed, much has been written regarding end-of-life issues for elderly adults, particularly with reference to health care proxies and living wills (see Table 30.1; Cantor & Pearlman, 2003; Friedman, Helm, & Marrone, 2003; Gordon, 2001; Gordon & Soklowski, 2002; Heffner et al., 1996). In the pediatric population, medical, ethical, and legal factors have been taken into account in the management of children with severe, irreversible problems, such as in the management of end-stage cancer, brain injury, congenital anomalies, and complications of the very premature infant (Cantor & Pearlman, 2003; Chaney & Eyman, 2000; Heffner, Barbieri, Fracica, & Brown, 1998; Wolfe et al., 2002).

End-of-life issues for individuals with developmental disabilities have many similarities to these other

Table 30.1. Basic definitions for terms associated with end-of-life care

Advanced directives—health care proxies, durable power of attorney for health care, or living wills, indicating an individual's preferences in the event of a future life-threatening illness or condition.

Cardiopulmonary resuscitation (CPR)—medical intervention in the event of cardiac or pulmonary arrest, including chest compressions, artificial means of ventilation, ventilator use, cardiopressor and other medications, defibrillation, and other extraordinary life-sustaining measures.

Competence—ability of an adult, 18 years or older, to make sound legal, medical, financial, and personal decisions for him- or herself. The court makes the determination of competence based on medical, cognitive, and functional assessments of a person's ability to independently care for his or her needs.

Do Not Resuscitate (DNR) orders—document written by a physician, in conjunction with the designated legal decision maker, to withhold CPR in the event of cardiopulmonary arrest. DNR does not refer to cessation of treatment of acute, reversible medical conditions. An individual may have a DNR order and yet continue to be treated for illness such an upper and lower respiratory tract infections, urinary tract infections, orthopedic problems, and so forth.

Health care proxies—document written by a competent adult in anticipation of a circumstance whereby he or she no longer has the ability to make health-related decisions. Another competent adult is appointed to make such medical decisions. Health care proxies may not be written by or for an individual with a guardian. They may also be referred to as power of attorney for health care.

Hospice care—provision of palliative care as well as personal and family support, with the focus on the dying process; the individual is anticipated to die within a certain time period. Comfort measures are an integral component in hospice care, as is bereavement support for the surviving family.

Living will—document written by a competent adult to indicate his or her preferences for medical intervention, or lack thereof, in the event that he or she is not able to directly communicate to physicians or family members.

Palliative care—multidisciplinary support focused on the particular serious medical condition and attending to the medical, emotional, spiritual, and cultural needs of the individual. Comfort measures are provided, which may or may not temporarily prolong life, although they will not cure the condition.

Redirection of care—in instances when providing aggressive medical management may not be in a person's best interest, the goals of care are changed from curative to provision of comfort measures.

Surrogate decision maker—person or persons with the responsibility to make treatment decisions for individuals who are not competent to do so themselves. For individuals younger than 18 years of age, the parents or court-appointed guardian have that responsibility. The courts may appoint guardians—often parents—when an individual reaches adulthood and is not considered competent. In some states, it is permissible for family members without formal legal authority to make decisions for an adult who is not able to do so. A specific order of priority (e.g., spouse, adult child, parent) is followed.

Withholding and withdrawal of care—legally equivalent terms whereby withholding certain life-sustaining measures are not initiated (withholding) or stopped after they have been started (withdrawal).

Sources: Commonwealth of Massachusetts, 1999; Ethics Advisory Committee, 1999; Fogg, 1995; Moses and Mousoufi, 2003; Pituro, 2003; Partnership for Caring, 2003.

groups and also pose a unique combination of factors. In some respects, similarities can also be drawn between those individuals with severe developmental disabilities and complex medical problems, and with adults with acquired, advanced dementia. In both groups, individuals may be nonverbal, nonambulatory, incontinent, unable to eat orally, and dependent on others for all of their daily living needs (Friedman, Helm, & Marrone, 1999; Lawhorne, 1999; Nusbaum, 2001). Due to their debilitated condition, they are at increased risk of acquiring, and succumbing to, infections. They also are not capable of providing informed consent for decisions related to their own medical care.

Just as similarities exist in these groups, so do very distinct differences. Unlike an adult counterpart with acquired dementia, a child with severe to profound intellectual disabilities and multiple medical problems has likely not yet lived a full life. He or she has not been able to express personal wishes regarding intervention in the event of a life-threatening illness. Usually, a parent or guardian has been responsible for management decisions. Even children and adolescents with end-stage cancer, whose parents are the legal decision makers, are frequently part of the decision-making processes, with information provided to them appropriate to their developmental level (Heffner et al., 1996; Wolfe et al., 2002). In these and other potentially life-threatening conditions, physicians seek to obtain assent from children and adolescents, that is, their willingness to accept treatment (AAP Committee on Bioethics, 1998; Burn & Truog, 1997; Kunin, 1997).

A backdrop of changing political, social, economic, and legal conceptualizations and policies exists regarding individuals with disabilities (AAMR, 2003; Friedman et al., 1999). Certainly, individuals with developmental disabilities should be presented with information that is understandable to them and should be part of the decision-making process, if possible. In instances in which another party has been deemed the legal guardian, efforts need to still be made to include the individual in the discussion of medical management decisions at a level that is understandable (Commonwealth of Massachussetts, 1999). At times, however, an individual with developmental disabilities will not be capable of being part of the decision-making process.

DECISION MAKER

In this context, questions have also arisen regarding who is the best decision maker for end-of-life care (AAP Committee of Bioethics, 1998; Burn & Truog, 1997; Gordon, 2001, 2003; Gordon & Sokolowski, 2002). Certainly, past abuses directed toward individuals with disabilities have underscored the need to value all human life and respect everyone's civil rights. Who is to speak for those who cannot speak for themselves? Should that responsibility be given to the parent, guardian, other caregivers, doctors, the court system, the insurance company, or government agencies? Who decides when treatment is futile? Should futility even be considered in the decision-making process? Who determines when the anticipated outcome does not warrant aggressive management? What are the desired outcomes?

Generally speaking, parents are provided with the legal responsibility of decision maker until their children become 18-years of age (Ethics Advisory Committee, 1999; Gillick, 2000). They usually seek guardianship when their child with intellectual disabilities turns 18 years of age and, as a result of an evaluation process, the court determines that the child is not capable of caring for his or her basic needs and making informed decisions (Commonwealth of Massachusetts, 1999). If parents are not able to assume that responsibility, then another family member or designated individual may be able to seek guardianship. It is assumed that the parent or guardian is acting in the individual's best interest and is actively involved in the process of making decisions for him or her.

If health care providers do not agree with parental decisions and an impasse develops regarding what is in the best interest of the person with intellectual disabilities with regards to medical management, the issue may be presented to the Ethics Committee at a hospital or other medical facility. The Ethics Committee reviews pertinent information and meets with all parties involved to better understand the context of the issues and to provide recommendations. Sometimes, however, options within the health care system have been exhausted, and all parties involved cannot reach a mutually agreeable decision. In those rare instances, the right of a parent or guardian to make such decisions may be legally challenged (Ethics Advisory Committee, 1999).

The decision maker is assumed to not only act in the best interest of the person for whom he or she assumes responsibility, but also to make decisions reflecting the presumed wishes of that person. Elderly adults with acquired cognitive disabilities may have communicated their wishes to family members, determined who should have power of attorney, designated health care proxies, and/or written living wills. Interestingly, some have found that surrogates' choices in those types of situations may not necessarily reflect those of the individual who is ill (Cogen et al., 1992).

When an individual has never been able to express those wishes, the situation becomes more complicated. A person's medical condition, its acuity, and the understanding of this information may have an impact on decisions (Ackermann & Kemle, 1999; Contro et al., 2002; Gordon, 2003; Gordon & Sokolowski, 2002; Kunin, 1997). Similarly, the personal frames of reference of the decision makers, as well as age, etiology for disability, and impression of quality of life of the person with the disability, may also potentially influence such decisions (Commonwealth of Massachusetts, 1999; Friedman, 2000; Wolfe et al., 2002).

Health care proxies per se need to be written by a competent adult who designates another competent adult to serve as his or her agent in the event that he or she can no longer make such decisions. Health care proxies do not apply to individuals with guardians. When a legal guardian has not been appointed for an individual with intellectual disabilities, the court may then provide a substituted judgment, making decisions on behalf of the individual. For adults, health care decisions may be also made by a health care agent, if so deemed by the court with a proxy document (Commonwealth of Massachusetts, 1999).

PHYSICIAN'S ROLE

The physician generally has the responsibility of speaking to a family regarding end-of-life issues (Gordon, 2001). He or she also designates a patient's resuscitation status in the medical orders of the hospital or nursing home, based on the desires of the person responsible for making the medical decisions (Burn & Truog, 1997, Heffner et al., 1998). These orders need to be renewed at the time of each hospital admission and ideally should be reviewed on a regular basis for those individuals residing in long-term care facilities. DNR orders apply to individuals who are hospitalized or residing in other facilities, such as nursing homes, where physicians write medical orders as a means to implement the care of patients. The DNR order, per se, therefore, does not apply to those individuals residing in the community setting.

Some individuals or family members previously carried letters signed by physicians with the hope that the paramedics and other first responders would honor the DNR preference in the event that an emergency situation occurred within the community. Due to the practical and medical-legal issues that arose with this practice, most states have implemented programs whereby individuals have official documents or bracelets to indicate DNR preference outside of the hospital setting. In Massachusetts, the Department of Public Health is responsible for such a program, designated as the Comfort Care Program/DNR Verification Program (Massachusetts Department of Public Health, 2002). If a person experiences cardiopulmonary arrest while out in the community for activities such as recreation, shopping, or in transit to a medical appointment, the paramedics would honor the designated preference not to undergo resuscitation efforts, such as cardiopulmonary resuscitation (CPR), defibrillation, mechanical means to breathe, or use of medications to affect cardiac function. To participate in this program, specific forms need to be completed and signed by the legal decision maker (e.g., competent adult, parent, or guardian) as well as the treating physician. These programs vary from state to state.

Ordinarily, end-of-life issues are not part of general pediatric practice and may also not be regularly addressed in the routine care of adults. Hospitals that accept Medicare and Medicaid funds are required by federal law to provide information to patients regarding advanced directives and the right to refuse treatment upon admission. Each state has its own laws regarding the application of advanced directives as they pertain to adults (Ethics Advisory Committee, 1999; Moses & Mousoufi, 2003; Partnership for Caring, n.d.). Certainly, when adults are acutely ill with a serious medical condition, it is not unusual for desires for medical intervention to be addressed (Byock, 1999; Heffner et al., 1996; Heffner et al., 1998).

Consideration of various treatment and intervention options are often addressed when caring for children with special health care needs in all settings. Ideally, consideration of end-of-life issues should also be broached prior to a time of crisis. For individuals who reside at home, physicians may not initiate these discussions until the time of a major, acute illness. End-of-life discussions, however, may be part of the care plan for individuals of all age groups who reside in long-term nursing facilities (Kelly, 2003). Federal regulations for long-term care facilities mandates that facilities have policies and practices in place consistent with their state laws regarding end-of-life issues, as they apply to residents of the facility (Fogg, 1995).

When a person is hospitalized or resides in a long-term care facility, the physician has the responsibility to communicate the care plan to other members of the care team (Heffner et al., 1996; Heffner et al., 1998). Differences of opinion among caregivers and family members may occur, however, regarding the recommended management. Different parties may believe that their opinion addresses the best interest of the patient. A physician or other caregiver, such as a nurse, may refuse to provide treatment if he or she is uncomfortable with the care plan or requests for certain interventions. Ongoing communication is imperative between all of those involved, and alternatives should be provided to the family with the hope of being able to find a resolution to the differences.

Frida was a 17-year old adolescent with severe intellectual disabilities and cerebral palsy secondary to congenital brain malformations. She had resided in a pediatric skilled nursing home since soon after birth. Her parents had been told that she would not live more than a few years at best. Frida's father had always been the primary decision maker. He visited Frida and was in contact with the staff of the facility on a regular basis.

Frida was nonverbal, nonambulatory, and incontinent. She was able to show pleasure and displeasure, was socially interactive, and demonstrated the ability to steer her wheelchair by herself for short distances. Although she ate all of her foods by mouth, her feeding skills were notably impaired. These difficulties were most apparent when she was ill, as it was difficult for her to ingest adequate fluids and food intake.

Frida also experienced gastroesophageal reflux (GER) with frequent regurgitation. She was thin and anemic and experienced associated lower respiratory tract symptoms. Her father did not want her to undergo surgical procedures (e.g., fundoplication with gastrostomy tube placement) that might have the effect of prolonging her life, although he did want her to be comfortable. Her father also wished that Frida be treated for potentially reversible conditions. Frida's father and the treating physician discussed treatment and end-of-life options. Her father felt strongly that in the event of cardiopulmonary arrest, he did not want resuscitation measures to be provided, as he felt that Frida would suffer unduly.

Frida began to demonstrate worsening GER with episodic blood-streaked emesis, despite aggressive medical management. She was treated intermittently for aspiration pneumonia and required episodic hospitalization for dehydration and intravenous antibiotic administration during periods of illness. After several hospitalizations, Frida's father decided that he did not want her transferred to an acute care facility in the event of acute esophageal bleeding or deterioration. He wished that medical care would be provided at the skilled nursing facility only, which could potentially include oral antibiotics, hydration, and feeds. Other medical treatments, such as oxygen by mask and pulmonary toilet, could also be provided.

The staff caring for Frida had grown very fond of her through the years and wanted more aggressive management of her medical problems. The treating physician, nurse, and other direct staff were not comfortable with her father's preferences. They believed that, without surgery, she would be at greater risk for a variety of medical complications. If she experienced a significant bleed, they also had concerns about treating her in a palliative manner. They felt that surgery would improve Frida's quality of life, with decreased discomfort and other symptoms, and would potentially prolong her life. Risks, however, were associated with general anesthesia and surgery, and there was some uncertainly regarding surgical outcome.

A multidisciplinary team met, and the social worker and physician also spoke to the father. A resolution could not be reached to which all parties were comfortable. The dilemma was then brought before the Ethics Committee who had the responsibility for reviewing such issues and rendering an opinion. The Ethics Committee directed their attention to the following issues:

- Is the parent's decision reasonable (risk vs. benefit of intervention)?
- How do the principles of nonmaleficience (do no harm) and beneficence (do good) apply?
- What is the implication of the parent's wish not to prolong the life of his or her son or daughter?
- When is nutrition considered to be extraordinary versus supportive care?
- Under what circumstances is challenging the parent's prerogative to make decisions regarding his or her child appropriate?

After meeting with Frida, her father, and the staff, as well as reviewing the medical history and issues at hand, the Ethics Committee did feel that the father had indeed demonstrated true commitment to Frida's best interest through the years. He did not want his daughter to suffer, although he did not want to prolong her life. If Frida were to die, her father wanted her to be surrounded by those who loved her rather than with unfamiliar personnel in an Emergency Room or Intensive Care Unit. Frida had experienced difficulty adjusting to new situations in the past and was notably more content in her familiar settings. She also was felt to be at considerable surgical risk if she were to undergo a surgical procedure for acute bleeding, or even for fundoplication with gastrostomy tube placement. The father's stance was, therefore, felt to be reasonable, albeit different than those caring from Frida on a daily basis. The staff accepted the findings of the Ethics Committee and continued to work closely with Frida's father (Friedman et al., 1999).

Sometimes, medical and nursing teams do not feel that they could in good conscience carry out a family's wishes. In those instances, care may be sought in another medical facility. In this situation, however, the staff was quite attached to Frida and did not want her to be cared for elsewhere. If they had not felt comfortable caring for her in the manner so deemed by her father, they could have also used legal means to assist in resolving these issues (Ethics Advisory Committee, 1999).

TREATMENT, RESUSCITATION DECISIONS, AND REDIRECTION OF CARE

Individuals with disabilities need to be provided with the same choices as others regarding request for, or refusal of, treatment (Nelson, 2003). The medical provider is responsible for explaining treatment options in a manner that is understandable to the individual or to the surrogate decision maker. An individual must understand the risks and benefits of these types of decisions so that an informed decision can be made. The three essential parts to informed consent delineated in the Belmont Report for research that also apply to informed consent in the clinical setting are 1) information, 2) comprehension, and 3) voluntariness (National Commission for the Protection of Human Subjects, 1979). The physician needs to be able to provide information regarding the medical treatment or lack thereof, risks and benefits, alternative interventions, and opportunities to ask questions. He or she also needs to be able to provide such information in a manner that is understandable to the individual(s) making the decisions. Consent needs to be voluntarily given by the individual and not coerced in any manner. Questions should be answered, and additional resources or other opinions offered, as indicated by the situation. As families have diverse frames of reference, there is more than one way to approach many medical issues, particularly those dealing with the end-of-life care (Friedman et al., 2003; Wolfe et al., 2002).

A distinction that is often misunderstood is the difference between resuscitation decisions and treatment. *Resuscitation* refers specifically to medical intervention intended to restart or augment the heartbeat and breathing in the event of cardiopulmonary arrest. In those situations, CPR is initiated (e.g., chest compressions, bag and mask, intubation with mechanical ventilation). If an individual has a DNR order, CPR is not provided; however, an individual with a DNR order can continue to receive oxygen by mask, as opposed to actual assistance with the breathing process. Treatment for acute illnesses and infections can also occur. Comfort measures should always be provided to all individuals, regardless of their resuscitation status.

In some instances when death is imminent or soon anticipated, goals of care may be redirected from curative to comfort only (Ethics Advisory Committee, 1999). Palliative care continues to focus on the disease process and may continue to provide some treatment, although not with the intent of curing the illness (Fordyce, 2001). Hospice care incorporates palliative care, with the emphasis on the dying process (Moses & Mousoufi, 2003). Tube feeding, hydration, and medication administration may be discontinued and considered treatments (Fordyce, 2000; Nusbaum, 2001). Some believe that a dying person does not actually experience hunger or thirst, and feeding at the end of life actually provides more potential discomfort than benefit (Gillick, 2000; McCann, Hall, & Groth-Junker, 1994). The issue of hydration and nutrition remains one that many providers are uncomfortable discontinuing, even in situations in which it may be considered legally and medically appropriate (Lin, 2003; Taylor, 2001).

The law needs to protect the individual rights of all people, particularly those who are least apt to be able to protect themselves. The Massachusetts Department of Mental Retardation's policy on end-of-life issues, "Life-Sustaining Treatment for Adults with Mental Retardation," states that individuals with intellectual disabilities should have the right to treatments and informed choices with family support. Decisions such as redirection of care need to be made with respect for an individual's autonomy, dignity, and comfort. Their policy considers DNR orders to be appropriate if one has a terminal illness, the diagnosis of persistent vegetative state, or if CPR is felt to cause more harm than good (Commonwealth of Massachusetts, 1999). Many individuals with severe medical problems do not survive resuscitation efforts, and some believe that the resuscitation process may actually be more harmful than beneficial (Gordon, 2003; Nelson, 2003).

Physicians need to know the definition of DNR and be comfortable speaking to families regarding therapy and resuscitation options. The risks versus the benefits of CPR need to be considered. Individual providers need to become familiar with variation among state laws concerning end-of-life issues. Although some families feel that physician-assisted suicide or euthanasia may be reasonable in certain situations, it is not legal or practiced in the United States, with the exception of Oregon (Daskal, Houghan, & Sachs, 1999; Moses & Mousoufi, 2003). Certainly, those who are least able to advocate for themselves need to be carefully protected in all situations.

Discussing the specifics of pain management for dying patients is beyond the scope of this chapter. Suffice it to note that treatment of pain and discomfort needs to be provided aggressively and urgently. Some care providers have been uncomfortable with providing narcotic medication for comfort, concerned about the possibility of drug addiction, which bears no relevance when someone is dying. Concerns may also be voiced that potential respiratory depression may result, hastening death, and thus a form of euthanasia. The ethical principle of double effect, however, has been cited to clarify the rationale for providing needed comfort and reduction of suffering. Providers generally abide by the overriding principle of doing no harm (nonmaleficience) and the principle of doing good (beneficence).

Sometimes when acting in the patient's best interest to relieve suffering, there may be a secondary effect of doing some harm (Beauchamp & Childress, 2001). In those instances, the intention should not be that of harm, and the good should clearly outweigh potential harm. Giving medication to alleviate pain may be provided to make a dying person comfortable, with the secondary effect of potential respiratory depression. The goal is to make a person more comfortable and not to harm the individual, which is very different from euthanasia, which has as its goal to hasten death (Lawhorne, 1999).

CONCLUSION

Families, particularly those of individuals who are not capable of providing informed consent, need to feel that their wishes are heard and understood. Care providers have an obligation to know the options of care, social policy, and potential legal avenues that may be needed by the family to support that care. They also need to be comfortable counseling families, providing compassionate and effective end-of-life care, and diminishing pain and suffering (Contro et al., 2002). Physicians who care for dying individuals need to be knowledgeable and capable of providing effective and swift pain management. The experiences and history of each family should be understood so that the priorities and needs of all involved can be met with dignity.

The trend of increasing life expectancy will hopefully lead to increased social, nursing, and medical support in the community, as more people are cared for at home (Ackermann & Kemle, 1999; Shavelle & Strauss, 1999). Community physicians and other care providers will need to be able to better individualize care around end-of-life issues and to counsel individuals and families in a timely manner. Families should anticipate issues and discuss options with all those involved. End-of-life care for children should be further developed within the context of the medical home, and adequate reimbursement needs to be in place to support these crucial services. Social policy needs to continue to protect those who are more apt to be subject to abuses, yet also allow choices to be made that are comparable to the general population.

Each individual comes with his or her own experiences, concerns, beliefs, and opinions. It is important that there be ongoing respect and communication so that all individuals and their families receive the needed support and caring at the end of life.

REFERENCES

Ackermann, R.J., & Kemle, K.A. (1999). Death in a nursing home with active medical management. *Annals of Long Term Care, 7*(8), 313–319.

American Academy of Pediatrics Committee on Bioethics. (1998). Informed consent, parental permission, and assent in pediatric practice. *Pediatrics, 98*(20), 314–317.

American Academy of Pediatrics Policy Statement. (2004). The medical home. *Pediatrics, 113*(5), 1545–1547.

American Association on Mental Retardation. (2003). *National goals, state of knowledge and research agenda for persons with intellectual and developmental disabilities: Keeping the promises. Findings and recommendations.* Washington, DC: Author.

Beauchamp, T.L., & Childress, J.F. (2001). *Principles of bioethics* (5th ed.). New York: Oxford University Press.

Burn, J.P., & Truog, R.D. (1997). Ethical controversies in pediatric critical care. *New Horizons, 5*(11), 72–84.

Byock, I.R. (1999). End of life care: A public health crisis and opportunity for managed care. *American Journal of Managed Care, 7*(12), 1123–1232.

Cantor, M.D., & Pearlman, R.A. (2003). Advance care planning and long-term care facilities. *Journal of the American Medical Directors Association, 4*(2), 101–107.

Chaney, R.H., & Eyman, R.K. (2000). Patterns of mortality over 60 years among persons with mental retardation in a residential facility. *Mental Retardation, 38*(3), 289–293.

Cogen, R., Patterson, B., Chavin, S., Landsberg, L., & Posner, J. (1992). Surrogate decision-maker preferences for medical care of severely demented nursing home patients. *Archives of Internal Medicine, 152*, 1885–1888.

Commonwealth of Massachusetts, Department of Mental Retardation. (1999). *Life sustaining treatment for adults with mental retardation* (DMR Policy No. 99). Boston: Author.

Contro, N., Larson, J., Scofield, S., Sourkes, B., & Cohen, H. (2002). Family perspectives on the quality of pediatric palliative care. *Archives of Pediatric and Adolescent Medicine, 156*(1), 14–19.

Daskal, F.C., Houghan, G.W., & Sachs, G.A. (1999). Physician-assisted suicide: Interventions with patients with dementia and their families. *Annals of Long Term Care, 7*(8), 293–298.

Diekema, D.S. (2003). Involuntary sterilization of person with mental retardation: An ethical analysis. *Mental Retardation and Developmental Disabilities Research Reviews, 9*(1), 21–26.

Ethics Advisory Committee. (1999). *Membership handbook.* Boston: Children's Hospital.

Fogg, R. (1995). *Nursing home regulations. Survey, certification, enforcement manual.* Washington, DC: Thompson.

Fordyce, M. (2001). At the end of life. *Annals of Long Term Care, 9*(3), 80–84.

Fordyce, M. (2000). Dehydration near end of life. *Annals of Long Term Care, 8*(5), 29–33.

Friedman, S.L., Helm, D.T., & Marrone, J. (1999). Caring, control, and clinician's influence: Ethical dilemmas in developmental disabilities. *Ethics & Behavior, 9*(4), 349–364.

Friedman, S.L., Helm, D.T., & Marrone, J. (2003). Ethical dilemmas in developmental disabilities. *Directions in Rehabilitation Counseling, 4*(6), 57–69.

Friedman, S.L. (2000, May). *Factors that impact resuscitation decisions for children with severe developmental disabilities and complex medical problems.* Paper presentation at the annual meeting of the American Association on Mental Retardation, Washington, DC.

Gillick, M.R. (2000). Rethinking the role of tube feedings in patients with advanced dementia. *New England Journal of Medicine, 342*(3), 206–210.

Gordon, M. (2001). Whose life is it and who decides? A dilemma in long-term care. *Annals of Long Term Care, 9*(11), 32–41.

Gordon, M. (2003). CPR in long-term care: Mythical benefits or necessary ritual? *Annals of Long Term Care, 11*(4), 41–49.

Gordon, M., & Sokolowski, M. (2002). When is refusal of lifesaving therapy a refusal? *Annals of Long Term Care, 10*(10), 21–24.

Heffner, J.E., Barbieri, C., & Casey, K. (1996). Procedure specific do-not-resuscitate orders. Effect of communication on treatment limitations. *Archives of Internal Medicine, 156*, 793–797.

Heffner, J.E., Barbieri, C., Fracica, P., & Brown, L.K. (1998). Communicating do-not-resuscitate orders with computer-based system. *Archives of Internal Medicine, 158*, 1090–1095.

Kaiser Commission on Medicaid Facts. (2001a). *Medicaid's role for the disabled population under age 65.* Washington, DC: The Henry J. Kaiser Family Foundation.

Kaiser Commission on Medicaid Facts. (2001b). *Medicaid's role in long term care.* Washington, DC: The Henry J. Kaiser Foundation.

Kelly, E. (2003, April). The challenges of improving palliative care in the nursing home. *Long Term Care Interface*, 27–31.

Kunin, H. (1997). Ethical issues in pediatric life-threatening illness: Dilemmas of consent, assent, and communication. *Ethics & Behavior,* 7, 43–57.

Lawhorne, L.W. (1999). Avoidable and unavoidable decline—naturalness of dying: The nursing home dilemma. *Annals of Long Term Care,* 7(8), 309–312.

Lin, R.J. (2003). Withdrawing life-sustaining medical treatment—a physician's personal reflection. *Mental Retardation and Developmental Disabilities Research Reviews, 9*(1), 10–15.

Massachusetts Department of Public Health. (2002). *Comfort Care, Emergency Medical Service. Do Not Resuscitate (DNR) Order Verification Program.* Boston: Author.

McCann, F.M., Hall, W.J., & Groth-Junker, A. (1994). Comfort care for terminally ill patients: The appropriate use of nutrition and hydration. *Journal of the American Medical Association, 272*(16), 1263–1266.

Miller, K.E., & Miller, M. (2003). Challenges in end of life pain management. *Annals of Long Term Care, 11*(4), 26–32.

Moore, B., & Tonniges, T.F. (2004). The "every child deserves a medical home" training program: More than a traditional continuing medical education course. *Pediatrics, 113*, 1479–1484.

Moses, J., & Mousoufi, M. (2003, May). *Advanced directives and palliative care.* Interactive Poster Presentation at American Association on Mental Retardation Annual Meeting, Chicago.

National Commission for the Protection of Human Subjects of Biomedical and Behavioral Research. (1979). *The Belmont report: Ethical principles and guidelines for the protection of human subjects of research.* Washington, DC: Department of Health, Education, and Welfare.

Nelson, L.J. (2003). Respect for the developmentally disabled and forgoing life-sustaining treatment. *Mental Retardation and Developmental Disabilities Research Reviews, 9* (1), 3–9.

Nusbaum, N.J. (2001). Feeding tubes: Ethical decision making in theory and practice. *Annals of Long Term Care, 9*(11), 20.

Office of the Surgeon General. (2002). *Closing the gap: A national blueprint to improve the health of persons with mental retardation.* Rockville, MD: U.S. Department of Health and Human Services.

Partnership for Caring. (n.d.). *Partnership for Caring glossary of terms.* Retrieved August 31, 2003, from http://www.partnershipforcaring.org

Pitturo, M. (2003, April). Bordeaux long-term care's supportive palliative care program. *Caring for the Ages*, 26–29.

Shavelle, R., & Strauss, D. (1999). Mortality of persons with developmental disabilities after transfer to community care: A 1996 update. *American Journal on Mental Retardation, 104*(2), 143–147.

Smith, S.W., Camfield, C., & Camfield, P. (1999). Living with cerebral palsy and tube feeding: A population-based follow-up study. *Journal of Pediatrics, 135*, 307–310.

Strauss, D., Ashwal, S., Shavelle, K., & Eyman, R.K. (1997). Prognosis for survival and improvement in function in children with severe developmental disabilities. *Journal of Pediatrics, 131*, 712–717.

Strauss, D., Kastner, T., Ashwald, S., & White, J. (1997). Tube feeding and mortality in children with severe disabilities and mental retardation. *Pediatrics, 99*, 358–362.

Strauss, D.J., Shavelle, R.M., & Anderson, T.W. (1998). Life expectancy of children with cerebral palsy. *Pediatric Neurology, 18*, 143–149.

Strauss, D., Shavelle, R., Anderson, T.A., & Baumeister, A. (1998). External causes of death among persons with disability: The effect of residential placement. *American Journal of Epidemiology, 147*, 855–862.

Taylor, P.R. (2001). Decision making in long-term care: Feeding tubes. *Annals of Long Term Care, 9*(11), 21–26.

Wehmeyer, M.L. (2003). Eugenics and sterilization in the heartland. *Mental Retardation, 41*(1), 57–60.

Wolfe, J., Frieber, S., & Hilden, J. (2002). Caring for children with advanced cancer. *Pediatric Clinics of North America, 49*, 1043–1062.

Section III

Values and Quality of Care

CHAPTER 31

PREVENTIVE HEALTH CARE

Allen C. Crocker

Since the 1970s, there has been a growing resolve to affect the occurrence of disability or developmental impairment in young children, to the degree that it has become a cultural movement (Alexander, 1998; Crocker, 1982, 1992). This outreach was supported in part by the real growth in the knowledge base but equally or more by deeply felt social concerns. Efforts in this area have been significantly fruitful. Much of the achievement in prevention has had a biomedical foundation, with striking effects. Phenylketonuria and galactosemia are countermanded early; congenital hypothyroidism is overcome. Measles encephalitis and Hib meningitis are vastly reduced. The care of infants in the newborn intensive care unit is assisted (including babies who might have had erythoblastosis). Car seats are lifesaving; genetic counseling may give valuable insight.

Other preventive activity may be environmental or institutional, with strategic effects. Reduction in teen pregnancy (and supports for the young women when needed) is important, as is developmental screening and the whole world of early intervention. Family supports help when disability is present, including those planned via a medical home. Reduction in exposure to lead has made important gains.

The field has gone on to become more searching and resourceful, as exemplified by vastly expanded territories of newborn screening (inborn errors of metabolism; see Chapter 7.1), new work with fetal surgery (congenital anomalies; see Chapter 8.2), and experiments in gene transfer (single gene disorders). There is real excitement in the successes being achieved currently in universal newborn hearing screening (congenital deafness; see Chapter 17.1) and the addition of folic acid to enriched grain products for baked goods (neural tube defects; Centers for Disease Control and Prevention, 2004). Our society has a philosophy of benevolent intervention and human assistance, which reaches out to areas such as infection control, injury prevention, best diet, favorable lifestyle, problem solving, and training.

CONSERVING THE HEALTH OF ADULTS

Since about 1990, significant emphasis has been placed on the concept of *secondary conditions* as a means of identifying extended or complicating components of disability syndromes (see Chapter 4). These considerations were analyzed in depth in the pioneer volume by Pope and Tarlov (1991). Secondary conditions represent a particular challenge for the care provider—some of them are capable of prevention by earnest planning; many of them eventually become part of the total health care needs for individuals with developmental disabilities. Secondary conditions are a marker of the basic vulnerability of many people in the field. They are also an area of important research needs.

The most recent in a series of national guides (published in 10-year intervals) for health care and prevention planning is that of *Healthy People 2010* (National Center on Birth Defects and Developmental Disabilities, 2001). This substantial production, generated with the collaboration of multiple individuals and agencies, provides a thoughtful listing of goals and objectives with particular consideration of public need and incomplete prior attention. Items included in *Healthy People 2010* are likely to be involved in federal projects and public discussion. Of the 28 chapters or topic areas in *Healthy People 2010*, Chapter 6 is most directly related to disability and secondary conditions. Discussion and data are on surveillance, mental health, social programs, wellness, assistive technology, barriers, and life satisfaction. Other chapters pick up the expected health issues of arthritis, osteoporosis, diabetes, nutrition, heart disease, and family planning.

Personal fitness is a broadly respected but incompletely realized achievement in the health pursuit territory (see Chapters 4, 14.1, and 25). Rimmer captured it well in his wonderful book:

> This is perhaps one of the greatest times in American history to take advantage of the tremendous publicity that physical

activity has received in terms of impacting the health of children, adults, and seniors with mental retardation. For years we have been listening to health professionals advocate for higher quality physical activity programs. Unfortunately, sedentary activity continues to dominate the lives of most Americans, including people with retardation. Professionals, staff, and caregivers must lead the charge in educating people with mental retardation about the value of a physically active lifestyle. (2000)

A report from the Surgeon General has noted that physical inactivity is a major contributor to disease. The level of health risk resulting from inactivity is similar to the risk from smoking. The recommendation was that everyone should be moderately active for 30 minutes per day, preferably every day of the week. Rimmer (2000) noted that less than 10% of adults with intellectual disabilities engage in physical activity a minimum of 3 days per week. Most activities chosen for leisure time activity were sedentary in nature, such as watching television or listening to the radio.

Another area of contemporary concern in prevention of disabilities is one preeminently of public, rather than personal, action. For enhancement of our larger planning interest, some brief notes are included in this review. This relates to possible *environmental toxicities* that may have been or are currently in the world of individuals with developmental disabilities. Thoughtful scholars in the field urge that greater cultural and scientific reflection be given to "pollution, toxic chemicals, and mental retardation" for their possible contribution to present dilemmas. An important conference on this topic took place in Wisconsin in July 2003. Excerpts from the summary give an indication of the speculations in consideration:

We know that more toxic chemicals are being put into our environment every year.

We know that our chemical body burden for some chemicals is increasing.

We know that some neurotoxicants can affect brain and nervous system development in children.

We know that a large percentage of occurrences of mental retardation are likely to have more than a single cause and that several causes can interact including genetics, infections, chemical toxicants, birth and other trauma, and hormonal factors.

We know that exposure levels that were formerly considered to be safe for lead, mercury, and PCBs, have since been proven to disrupt normal brain development; safe exposure levels have been revised downward.

We know that timing is important, that exposure to neurotoxicants during key vulnerable periods of brain development at levels that do not impact adults can cause permanent neurodevelopmental limitations later in life.

And we know that the fetal brain may be susceptible to some neurotoxic exposures that do not have comparable effects postnatally at similar dosages. (American Association on Mental Retardation, 2004)

It is instructive to review *mortality reports* as these reflect encroaching disease and the ambient need for preventive health care. Current statistics from the Massachusetts Department of Mental Retardation (2002) show the agency population to be having longer survival than might be expected. Seventy-five percent of the enrollees are now between 25 and 64 years, but 9% are older than 75 (the so-called "old old"). Inevitably, the mortality rate climbs steadily, with a sharper rise after about 60 years. Female survival is such that women become a substantial majority after age 70. Residence in a nursing home has the highest mortality, as is conditioned by several factors.

Charting of causes of death indicates that heart disease is by far the leading vulnerability (about 21% of the total). Aspiration pneumonia is second (12%); this is sometimes a difficult determination. A complex situation with septicemia is third, and following this are cancer, Alzheimer disease, and influenza and pneumonia. Accidents are low, as is stroke. In the general population mortality statistics for the state and country, heart disease is also first. Cancer and stroke are second and third. Accidents and diabetes are prominent.

A records review is made within the Massachusetts Department of Mental Retardation regarding clinical events and possible lessons on particular deaths. From the Mortality Committee, Sharon Oxx, the departmental Director of Health Services, commented that certain circumstances are regularly the most common for difficult final courses in individuals with developmental disabilities—namely, we see again and again the presence of aspiration, severe constipation, dehydration, and/or seizures.

DEVELOPING A PREVENTIVE HEALTH CARE SYSTEM

There is a lively challenge to utilize the growing knowledge base in health care for individuals with developmental disabilities and to construct guidelines for gentle, continuing intervention that will have preventive outcomes. This chapter describes some valuable resources that can assist in this mission. Having elements

Procedure	19–24 years	30–39 years	40–49 years	50–64 years	65+ years
Health maintenance visit (height and weight measurement)	Annually	Annually	Annually	Annually	Annually
LABS AND SCREENINGS					
Cancer screening					
Breast cancer (mammography)	Clinical breast exam and self-exam instruction as appropriate. Mammography not routine except for patients at high risk. Accurate and detailed history and family history will identify risk factors.		Clinical breast exam and self-exam instruction as appropriate. Mammography every 1–2 years, at discretion of physician.	Clinical breast exam and self-exam instruction as appropriate. Annual mammography.	Mammography annually through age 69 years. Age 70 years and older, annually at discretion of physician.
Cervical cancer (Pap smear)	Every 1–3 years, at physician's discretion.				May be omitted after age 65 if previous screenings were consistently normal.
Colorectal cancer	Not routine except for patients at high risk.			Fecal occult blood testing annually and sigmoidoscopy every 5 years OR colonoscopy every 10 years.	
Prostate cancer	Not routine.		Not routine except for patients at high risk. Risk factors include: family history and African-American ancestry.	At physician's discretion after discussion of risks and benefits of available screening strategies (prostate-specific antigen, digital rectal examination).	
Skin cancer	Periodic total cutaneous examinations targeting populations at high risk for malignant melanomas. Periodicity at physician's discretion.				
Other recommended screenings					
Hypertension	At least annually	Annually	Annually	Annually	Annually
Cholesterol	Every 5 years or at physician's discretion.				At physician's discretion.
Diabetes (Type II)	At least every 5 years until age 45. Every 3 years after age 45. Fasting glucose screen for individuals at high risk. Risk factors include: family history of premature congenital heart defect, hypertension, diabetes mellitus, peripheral atherosclerosis or carotid artery disease, current cigarette smoking, or high density lipoprotein > 35 mg/dl.				
Liver function	Annually for Hepatitis B carriers. At physician's discretion after consideration of risk factors, including long-term prescription medication.				
Osteoporosis	Bone density screening when risk factors are present: long-term polypharmacy, mobility impairments, hypothyroid, postmenopausal women. Periodicity of screening at physician's discretion. Annually counsel about preventative measures including dietary calcium and vitamin D intake, weight-bearing exercise, and smoking cessation.				Counsel elderly patients about specific measures to prevent falls.
Infectious disease screening					
Chlamydia and sexually transmitted diseases	For all sexually active men and women, screen annually < 25 years; > 25 years, screen annually if at risk.	Annually if at risk. Risk factors include inconsistent use of barrier contraceptives, new or multiple sex partners in last 3 months, new partner since last test, history of sexually transmitted disease, and partner who has had other sexual partner(s).			

(continued)

Figure 31.1. Massachusetts Department of Mental Retardation Health Screening Recommendations.

Figure 31.1. *(continued)*

Human immunodeficiency virus	Periodic testing if at risk and testing of pregnant women at increased risk.				
Hepatitis B and C	Periodic testing if risk factors present.				
Tuberculosis	Tuberculin skin testing every 1–2 years when risk factors present. Risk factors include residents or employees of congregate setting, close contact with people known or suspected to have tuberculosis.				
Sensory screening					
Hearing assessment	Screen annually. Reevaluate if hearing problem is reported or change in behavior is noted.				
Vision assessment	Screen annually. Reevaluate if vision problems are reported or change in behavior is noted.				
Eye exam for glaucoma	Every 3–5 years in high-risk patients. At least once in patients with no risk factors.		Every 2–4 years	Every 2–4 years	Every 1–2 years
MENTAL AND BEHAVIORAL HEALTH					
Depression	Screen annually for sleep, appetite disturbance, weight loss, general agitation.				
Dementia	Monitor for problems performing daily activities.		In individuals with Down syndrome, annual screen after age 40.		
Immunizations					
Influenza vaccine	Annually	Annually	Annually	Annually	Annually
Pneumococcal vaccine	Once				
Hepatitis B vaccine	Once. Reevaluate antibody status every 5 years.				
For individuals with Down syndrome (in addition to above recommendations)					
Thyroid function test	Every 3 years (sensitive thyroid-stimulating hormone)				
Cervical spine x-ray to rule out atlanto-axial instability	Obtain baseline as adult. Recommend repeat if symptomatic, or 30 years from baseline.				
Echocardiogram	Obtain baseline if no records of cardiac function are available.				
General counseling and guidance					
Prevention counseling	Annually counsel regarding prevention of accidents related to falls, fire/burns, choking.				
Abuse or neglect	Annually monitor for behavioral signs of abuse and neglect.				
Preconception counseling	As appropriate, including genetic counseling, folic acid supplementation, discussion of parenting capacity.				
Healthy lifestyle	Annually counsel regarding diet/nutrition, incorporating regular physical activity into daily routines, substance abuse.				

of a preventive health care system can be expected to bring some equity to care for individuals with disabilities. This will assure use of modern techniques and a degree of quality control. Preventive thinking can also be a unifying force that gives guidance equally to service-providing agencies, planning groups, families, and advocates. The specifications of preventive care can help to fill in where there are some restrictions in technical aspects (e.g., incomplete histories, language limitations, changes in service providers).

An energetic and well-considered project in this regard has been undertaken by Gail Grossman, Assistant Commissioner for Quality Management of the Massachusetts Department of Mental Retardation. In a dedicated training manual on health promotion, a series of resources has been provided for use in the community and facilities, and key examples are presented next (Grossman, 2003). The screening guidelines draw particularly on materials of the planning group, Massachusetts Health Quality Partners (2003). The material

HEALTH RECORD

Massachusetts Department of Mental Retardation

DATE: __/__/__

(To be completed or updated at the ISP and brought to all new medical contacts)

Name ____________ **Likes to be called** ____________

D.O.B. ________ **Soc. Sec #** ________ **Religion:** ____________

Address ____________

____

Tel. # ____________

Health Insurance (type & numbers)
Primary: ____________
Secondary: ____________

Consent Status: ☐ Can give own consent ☐ Consent from guardian ☐ **Unable to give own consent and no guardian**
Name ____________ Tel. # ____________

Resuscitation Status: ☐ DNR ☐ Full Resuscitation
If DNR, is comfort care form available ☐ Yes ☐ No ☐ Unknown

Health Care proxy ☐ No ☐ Yes Name ____________ Tel. # ____________

Agency Responsible for Providing Care? ☐ **No** ☐ **Yes** ____________ **Tel #** ____________
(Name of Agency/Primary contact person)

Emergency Contacts
#1 Name ____________
Tel. ____________
#2 Name ____________
Tel. ____________

Medications: ☐ Medication sheet/record attached
Or ☐ List attached

Pharmacy: Name: ____________ Tel: ________
Address: ____________

Allergies: Medications: ____________
Food/Environmental: ____________

Current Medical Problems & Diagnosis: ____________

____
____
____
____
____

Communication:
☐ Able to Communicate
☐ Communication Difficulties/Uses Verbalizations
☐ Communication Difficulties/Uses Gestures
☐ Not Able to Communicate Needs
☐ Unable to Use Call Bell

Vision:
☐ Normal
☐ Low Vision
☐ Blind
☐ Wears Glasses

Hearing:
☐ Normal
☐ Hard of Hearing
☐ Deaf
☐ Hearing Aid

Supportive Devices:
☐ Padded side rails
☐ Splints
☐ Braces
☐ Helmet
☐ Other ________

Toileting Ability:
☐ Continent
☐ Needs Assistance
☐ Incontinent
☐ Catheterized
☐ Other________

Medical Administration:
☐ Independent/Self Medicates
☐ Medication Administered by Staff

Dining/Eating:
☐ Independent
☐ Needs Assistance
☐ Totally Dependent
☐ Fed Through a Tube
☐ Other ________

Diet Texture:
☐ Regular
☐ Chopped
☐ Ground
☐ Puree
☐ Thicken Liquid

Diet type: ________
____

Ambulation:
☐ Independent __Steady __Unsteady
☐ Needs Assistance __1 person __2 people
☐ Ambualtion Aids __Walker __Cane __Crutches
☐ Wheelchair
☐ Non-Ambulatory

Personal Hygiene:
☐ Independent
☐ Special Needs ________

Oral Hygiene:
☐ Independent
☐ Special Needs

Head of Bed Elevated:
☐ Yes
☐ No

SPECIAL NEEDS

Usual Response to Medical Exams: ☐ Cooperates ☐ Partially Cooperates ☐ Resistant ☐ Fearful

☐ Sedation for clinical visits (Explain): ____________

☐ Special positioning required for examination (Explain): ____________

☐ Double staffing required for assistance with exams (Explain): ____________

☐ Requires limited waiting periods for exams

☐ Prefers early day appointments ☐ Prefers end of day appointments

☐ Special communication device/method (Explain): ____________

Pain Response: ☐ Normal ☐ Unique (Explain): ____________

(continued)

Figure 31.2. Massachusetts Department of Mental Retardation Health Record.

Figure 31.2. *(continued)*

MEDICAL PROVIDERS

Primary Care	Subspecialist/Type:
Name ______ Tel. # ( ) ______	Name ______ Tel. # ( ) ______
Address ______	Address ______
Dental Care	**Subspecialist/Type:**
Name ______ Tel. # ( ) ______	Name ______ Tel. # ( ) ______
Address ______	Address ______
Eye Care	**Subspecialist/Type:**
Name ______ Tel. # ( ) ______	Name ______ Tel. # ( ) ______
Address ______	Address ______

Living Status: ☐ Group Home ☐ Own Family ☐ Independent ☐ Home Sharing/Shared Home ☐ Other ______

Marital Status: ☐ Single ☐ Married ☐ Other ______

Work/Day Program Status: ☐ Community Day Support ☐ Day Habilitation ☐ Regular job ☐ Sheltered workshop

Nursing Supports available: ☐ In home ☐ In home 24 hr ☐ Nursing Coordination ☐ Access to VNA

IMMUNIZATIONS

Date of last TETANUS ______ ☐ Unknown ☐ Allergic ☐ Never

Date of last FLU SHOT ______ ☐ Unknown ☐ Allergic ☐ Never

Date of last PNEUMOVAX ______ ☐ Unknown ☐ Allergic ☐ Never

Date of last HEPATITIS B VACCINE

Primary Series (3 shots) ______ ☐ Unknown ☐ Allergic ☐ Never

Booster ______ ☐ Unknown ☐ Never

Date of last MEASLES/MUMPS/RUBELLA (MMR) ______ ☐ Unknown ☐ Allergic ☐ Never

List any other vaccinations and date (e.g., Lyme, Hepatitis A, Varicella, etc.)

______

______

TUBERCULOSIS SKIN TEST (PPD):

Have you ever had a positive skin test for tuberculosis? ☐ Yes ☐ No ☐ Unsure

If yes, was any treatment given? ☐ Yes (describe) ______ ☐ No

Date of last PPD ______

PAST MEDICAL HISTORY

☐ **Medical history not released by parent/guardian**
For information, contact: Name ______________ Relation ______________
Tel # ______________ Address ______________

SURGICAL:

List all previous surgeries and dates (most recent first):
____
____
____

List any serious trauma or broken bones:
____
____
____

Any previous problems with anesthesia? ☐ No ☐ Yes (describe) ______________

GYNECOLOGIC (women only):

Age menstruation started ______________ Age menstruation stopped ______________ ☐ Still menstruating
Date of last PAP smear ______________ ☐ Unknown ☐ Never
Any history of abnormal PAP smear? ☐ No ☐ Yes (describe below) ______________
Date of last mammogram ______________ ☐ Unknown ☐ Never

MEDICAL: List all serious medical illnesses (e.g. pneumonia, heart attack) and ongoing medical problems (e.g., diabetes, high blood pressure, epilepsy)
____
____
____
____

PSYCHIATRIC: List all major behavioral & psychiatric diagnoses (e.g., depression, schizophrenia, self-injurious behavior)
____
____
____
____

PRIOR EVALUATIONS:

Date of last EYE EXAM ______________ ☐ Unknown ☐ Never
Date of last DENTAL EXAM ______________ ☐ Unknown ☐ Never
Date of last BONE DENSITOMETRY (checks bone thickness) ______________ ☐ Unknown ☐ Never
Date of last SIGMOIDOSCOPY or COLONOSCOPY ______________ ☐ Unknown ☐ Never
(scope examination of large intestine)

FAMILY HISTORY

Father: Deceased? ☐ Yes Age at and cause of death:
☐ No Current age: ______________

Mother: Deceased? ☐ Yes Age at and cause of death:
☐ No Current age: ______________

List all brothers and sisters with information about their age and health:
____
____
____

Is there any familiy history of:

DIABETES	☐ Unknown	☐ No	☐ Yes
HIGH BLOOD PRESSURE	☐ Unknown	☐ No	☐ Yes
HIGH CHOLESTEROL	☐ Unknown	☐ No	☐ Yes
HEART DISEASE	☐ Unknown	☐ No	☐ Yes
OSTEOPOROSIS	☐ Unknown	☐ No	☐ Yes
COLON POLYPS	☐ Unknown	☐ No	☐ Yes
CANCER	☐ Unknown	☐ No	☐ Yes

What Type? ______________
____

Are there any other diseases that "run in the family"?
☐ Unknown ☐ No ☐ Yes (give details below)
____
____
____

Has there been any genetic counseling in the family?
☐ Unknown ☐ No ☐ Yes (give details below)

Result: ______________
____
____

(continued)

Figure 31.2. *(continued)*

Massachusetts Department of Mental Retardation

Chronological List of Medical Events & Contacts:

Please list all surgeries, hospitalizations, procedures, vaccinations, etc. and attach to the back of the *Health Record* (Example: injuries, x-rays, tests)

Date	**Information** [include name of hospital or M.D.]

derives from leading texts (Massachusetts Department of Public Health, Massachusetts Hospital Association, Massachusetts Medical Society, Massachusetts League of Community Health Centers), 11 major health plans, and several medical schools and professional groups. The "Health Screening Recommendations" from the manual are available as two condensed pages for ready display and reference (see Figure 31.1). In clinical use, the priority for pursuit of individual items can be based on the person's age, gender, risk status, general health, and availability of support systems. Inevitably, the areas of special sensitivity will be malignancy, cardiovascular signs, diabetes, osteoporosis, sensory function, thyroid activity, and immunity.

The manual urges that physicians request that a Health Review Checklist be prepared before either the annual physical examination or episodic visits to the health care provider. This form can be completed by the family, agency nurse, or knowledgeable staff and should include notes on current symptoms or signs (filed as observations, not judgments) and information on sleeping, eating, respiratory concerns, seizures, headaches, mobility, and behavior. Use of the checklist is strategic for carrying out the office or clinic systems review. Also given is an outline of personal preparations for the medical visit (including a medication list).

There is much at stake in the techniques for recordkeeping. Figure 31.2 is a specialized Health Record. Its front sheet can serve as the "portable record," with other pages added as needed. Discipline is required to keep these notes up-to-date. It may be advisable to maintain this file in several locations. One hopes that the elusive elements of past experience and efforts can be thoughtfully preserved; the Health Record is a gold mine of ongoing information. Material from the Health Record, the Health Review Checklists, and the Health Care Encounter Forms can also be used at times of personal planning, such as when service providers and support staff put together documents like the individualized service plan (ISP).

Attention should be given to certain signs of significance, such as choking, aspiration, decline in skills, behavior change, activity of chronic health conditions, or the development of new ones. Utilizing health record information in ISP formulation can be instructive to agency personnel regarding the relationship of health care goals to general program goals. It also verifies that the periodic medical review did occur on schedule.

NOTES ON PREVENTIVE SERVICES

The considerable energy that is currently devoted to preventive care is exemplified by the supporting literature. Without question, the most valuable resources are those from the U.S. Preventive Services Task Force (*Guide to Clinical Preventive Services, Third Edition*, 2002), where detailed information is given on several hundred screening procedures, counselings, and immunizations. It is apparent that quality improvement efforts are very strong in prevention work now. Outreach being done in the field of developmental disabilities obviously gains directly from work in the generic field of prevention.

Important conceptual understanding of disability, its significance, and its prevention was provided in the work of the Institute of Medicine in a 2-year study project published in 1991 (Pope & Tarlov, 1991). This valuable work provided modern statistics and underlined the need for a dynamic disability model (pathology, impairment, functional limitation, disability). It was shown that preventive efforts, including prevention of secondary conditions, must acknowledge the sequence and interdependency of the components of the disabling process.

Table 31.1. Everyday lives principles

Choice—in the decisions of life: choice of jobs, friends, recreation, where and with whom to live

Control—of relationships, money, transportation, services, medicine and staff

Permanency—with a life in the community among family and friends; no fear of returning to the institution

Security—protection for those who have difficulty in communicating; competent services; and safety in the community

Freedom—of movement and from stigma

Prosperity—freedom from poverty and a chance to be successful

Individuality—by having a name and a personal history and by making a difference; having dignity and status

Relationships—with friends, family, and partners

Recognition—of abilities, capacities, and gifts

Privacy—of records, files and histories; protection from being labeled and the option of living alone

Citizenship—as part of the community, having a feeling of belonging, partnership in dreams and beliefs; playing a part in decisions which affect you

Passion—in advocates and self-advocates to fight and dream together

Reprinted from Philadelphia Coordinated Health Care. (1998). *Health promotion for people with developmental disabilities: A guide to optimizing health.* Philadelphia: Department of Public Health.

CONCLUSION

Finally, it is of significance to reflect on an ultimate supportive environment that can enrich the personal circumstances of individuals with special needs. Philadelphia Coordinated Health Care (1998) has gathered the "Everyday Lives Principles" that can implement good life progress and serve the preventive hopes (see Table 31.1). The values are extraordinary.

REFERENCES

Alexander, D. (1998). Prevention of mental retardation: Four decades of research. *Mental Retardation and Development Disabilities Research Reviews, 4*, 50–58.

American Association on Mental Retardation. (2004). *Pollution, toxic chemicals, and mental retardation: Framing a national blueprint for health promotion and disability prevention.* Washington, DC: Author.

Centers for Disease Control and Prevention. (2004). *Spina bifida and anecephaly before and after folic acid mandate.* Retrieved July 29, 2005, from http://www.cdc.gov/mmwr/PDF/wk/mm5317.pdf.

Crocker, A.C. (1982). Current strategies in prevention of mental retardation. *Pediatric Annals, 11*, 450–457.

Crocker, A.C. (1992). Data collection for the evaluation of mental retardation prevention activities: The fateful forty-three. *Mental Retardation, 30*, 302–317.

Grossman, G. (Ed.). (2003). *Health promotion and coordination initiative: Training and resource manual.* Boston: Department of Mental Retardation.

Massachusetts Department of Mental Retardation. (2002). *Mortality report.* Boston: University of Massachusetts Medical School.

Massachusetts Health Quality Partners. (2003). *Guidelines: Adult preventive care recommendations.* Boston: Author.

National Center on Birth Defects and Developmental Disabilities. (2001). Vision for the decade. In *Healthy People 2010.* Atlanta, GA: Centers for Disease Control and Prevention.

Philadelphia Coordinated Health Care. (1998). *Health promotion for people with developmental disabilities: A guide to optimizing health.* Philadelphia: Department of Public Health.

Pope, A.M., & Tarlov, A.R. (Eds.). (1991). *Disability in America.* Washington, DC: National Academies Press.

Rimmer, J.H. (2000). *Achieving a beneficial fitness: A program and a philosophy in mental retardation.* Washington, DC: American Association on Mental Retardation.

U.S. Preventive Services Task Force. (2002). *Guide to clinical preventive services* (3rd ed.). Alexandria, VA: International Medical Publishing.

CHAPTER 32

CONCEPTS OF HOLISTIC CARE

Linda L. Barnes and David L. Coulter

The term *holistic* was coined by Jan (Christiaan) Smuts (1870–1950) to refer to care that attended to all aspects of a person. It lingered in the vernacular, coming into its own in the 1970s, as patients, health reformers, alternative medicine practitioners, and some physicians wrestled with how to define a more encompassing vision of care. Frequently, holism has been articulated as attention to "body, mind, and spirit," and contrasted with biomedicine's historical focus on physiology. Each of these parts is represented as intrinsically interconnected and understandable only in relation to the whole.

Yet, this tripartite formulation of the person—although it corrects for prior exclusions—still omits critical dimensions of human experience. This chapter reviews a meaning-centered holistic model with which to gain a deeper understanding of how individuals, their families, and their clinicians locate the experience of a chronic condition. It also discusses two systemic approaches to assessment, concluding with an integrative model of intervention. Holistic care, as this chapter uses the term, refers to care provided in ways that account for the different aspects of each of these frameworks.

MEANING-CENTERED MODEL

A chronic condition, such as a disability, does not simply *happen* in the life of a person, family, community, or culture as a neutral event; it is also assigned meanings. To understand what a particular condition signifies in the life of a given individual and his or her family members, it is useful to consider seven factors: 1) paradigms of Healing, understood as forms of ultimate human possibility; 2) interpretations of Suffering and Affliction; 3) concepts of a person and all of the parts that comprise him or her; 4) understandings of illness, sickness, and disease; 5) the range of interventions considered appropriate or necessary; 6) the kinds of practitioners available in a given context; and 7) the different aspects of efficacy (see Barnes, 2003; Barnes, Plotnikoff, Fox, & Pendleton, 2000).

Paradigms of Healing

Paradigms of Healing—with a capital *H*—refer to an understanding of ultimate human possibility that may either occur during a person's life or following one's death. Many of these paradigms originate in the world's religious traditions. Healing, in such contexts, represents the tradition's deepest hope and promise. It may be a way of talking about a person's relation to a highest reality, whether that be known as God, Yahweh, Allah, Atman, Nirvana, Obatala, kamis, Tian, or another name. It may take the form of salvation, a place in Heaven, life in a World to Come, Paradise, Nirvana, freedom from cycles of rebirth, immortality, sagehood, revered ancestral status, remaining alive in human memory, or something else that is not related to any particular tradition.

Healing, understood in this way, makes everything else about human life relative. It functions as the frame of reference within which someone may interpret the rest of his or her experience, including the meaning of health in this lifetime. The influence of such visions of ultimate possibility are often read back into how people conduct their lives, leading them to try to live in ways that will bring about this Healing.

Different members of a family may share a paradigm of Healing, but each member will still make individual sense of what it means personally to him or her. It is also possible that members of a family may hold different paradigms. Moreover, health providers bring their own understandings of Healing. Rarely, however, are these frames of reference ever discussed in relation to a chronic condition, even though they may lie at the heart of how people engage in the daily experience of chronicity as patients, family members, or clinicians.

Although not universally the case, most of the world's religious and spiritual traditions and related systems of healing represent some aspects of Healing as occurring after death. Death, therefore, becomes not only an end, but also a transition—a threshold, marking a change of state. In contrast, biomedicine is a healing tradition that has no way of talking about what follows death because the demise of the body represents the closing off of the sphere of biomedicine intervention. As a result, death can only represent failure and is often experienced as such by biomedical clinicians. Some clinicians, of course, engage their own spiritual worldviews in tandem with their biomedical training, in ways that provide them with multiple perspectives on the situation.

I cared for an infant boy who was fine until, at 2 months, he had an acute apneac episode that left him with severe brain damage. After a month in the intensive care unit (ICU), his family faced difficult choices. It had become clear he would not recover and that the damage to his brain was irreversible. The family and I talked at considerable length about the different possibilities. I told them that one option was to perform a tracheostomy and a gastrostomy and to transfer him to a pediatric rehabilitation hospital for further care.

"Are there other options?" said his mother.

"We can withdraw life support," I said.

I suppose some neurologists would have presented these choices in reverse order, but for me—given my own life and faith orientation and the fact that I knew the family was Roman Catholic—it was important to present the choices in a way that respected these values. Their parish priest had been a frequent visitor to the ICU and had helped them through the difficult weeks their son had spent there. When it came time for the family to consider whether they wanted to withdraw their son's life supports and let him die, the priest reassured them that their decision was reasonable and acceptable within their faith.

The ICU doctors gave the parents the time they needed to have their entire extended family visit and say goodbye. Everyone agreed that it was time to let the baby go, to be somewhere else. On the day he died, his sister wrote a letter saying, "He will go up to God where he will suffer no longer. He will be in God's loving and caring hands for the rest of his life and forever. And even though his presence is not with us, he is still a part of our family. We will be together forever." Her letter demonstrated how the religious context of the family's decision provided a frame of reference in which they could release their son in a way that they interpreted as being for his benefit.

Paradigms of Suffering and Affliction

Paradigms of Suffering and Affliction represent explanations for why suffering and affliction happen[1]. Again, these paradigms are often rooted in religious traditions, and nuanced by particular cultural settings. Many traditions, for example, explain Suffering as the fruits of earlier actions or as a sign of judgment, punishment, and/or testing. The explanation may reiterate core narratives of a tradition: Some early individuals behaved in a forbidden way, for example, as a result of which all subsequent humans suffer. According to a tradition such as Buddhism, the very nature of reality is characterized by impermanence. Nothing lasts. The human desire to hold on to things is therefore always frustrated, causing Suffering. Consequently, Suffering constitutes a fundamental human experience, until one learns how to disengage from its causes. Generally, paradigms of Suffering and Affliction are offset by paradigms of Healing. The former attempt to explain why we suffer, the latter offer possible responses and ultimate alternatives.

Such paradigms may frame how each party interprets specific experiences like disability or other forms of chronicity. A paradigm surfaces when a parent asks why a particular condition has affected *their* child. "Am I being punished, Doctor? Am I being tested?" Actual experience, however, may lead individuals to reject a paradigm as inadequate to account for a particular reality and to struggle to find some other reason for why that reality is happening. "No God could be that cruel to an innocent child. There has to be another explanation!" In such cases, the person is still searching for a paradigm adequate to the experience.

Some of these paradigms may be experienced as punitive. If a family is told, for example, that God doesn't give them more to bear than they can handle, it is hard for them not to think, "If we were stronger, would our beloved family member not have had to live with this disability? Would he still be alive now?" God may be represented as indifferent or punishing—and families have a hard time believing in a God like that. Yet the paradox of many traditions is that the sacred is represented as both merciful and loving and as a force of judgment that is sometimes terrifying (Carman, 1994). The challenge for individuals and their families may involve navigating their way through such paradoxes.

Parts of Personhood

Virtually no tradition defines a person only in relation to bodily dimensions. Even biomedicine includes "mind," although often in relation to neurological structures. American popular culture, through the influence of New Age thought, has oriented many people to conceptualize "the whole person" as a combination of body, mind, and spirit. Illnesses are then classified accordingly, as *physical*, *mental*, and less clearly specified *spiritual* conditions. Because these categories have taken such deep root

[1]It is important to note that we recognize that words like *suffering* and, often, *burden* have been used in ways that have been harmful and damaging to people with disabilities and their families. Here, however, we use *Suffering* as a term commonly employed in the study of world religions in relation to existential questions.

in the culture, they can seem self-evident. But not every culture or tradition understands body, mind, and spirit to be the only parts or aspects constituting a person.

In Western cultures, biomedicine, with its anatomical foundations, has always emphasized the materiality of the body. The power of this anatomical perspective has been so strong that Western traditions more interested in life forces, subtle energies, or other aspects of "vitalism" have frequently been marginalized. Relatively few people know that many modern complementary and alternative medicine practices have a longstanding history in the broad field of American medicine. From the perspective of vitalism, the body is not simply a bounded system of physical structures.

Likewise, in some other medicine traditions, the key element may be a vital force rather than material structures. In traditional Chinese medicine, for example, *qi* (pronounced "ch'ee") is a subtle force that has both energetic and material dimensions. All reality consists of *qi*. Rocks are *qi*, winds and clouds are *qi*, blood is *qi*, and so is everything else about the body and all its subtle aspects. Indeed, rather than structures, the system emphasizes patterns of process, change, and transformation. A clear division between "body" and "mind," therefore, does not pertain. Even though there are words for both things, their meanings are not the same.

For that matter, some traditions would add in one or more souls (which may be differentiated from the spirit). Here, the religious tradition involved makes a difference. "Soul" in the Christian tradition is not the same thing as "soul" in the Confucian tradition. If the culture or tradition views reincarnation as a process intrinsic to human life, then a person is conceptualized not only in terms of this life, but of previous lives that may underlie who he or she is. In some West African traditions, when elders die, they reincarnate back into the family line. Grandchildren may then be recognized not only as themselves, but also as a returned grandparent.

Each aspect of personhood is inflected by cultural norms of human development. These norms impose expectations as to how each aspect is imagined to unfold over time. It is against such norms—or images of "normalcy"—that variations are assessed. In light of these norms, certain valued qualities are fostered, certain qualities may be overlooked, and other qualities or characteristics may be rejected or condemned. Early developmental milestones such as sitting up may be encouraged differently in different cultures. Cultures that say "You can't spoil a baby" have notions about what *spoiling* means. Ideas of how children should develop govern approaches to breast feeding, toilet training, expected interactive behaviors, and the like. If the aspects of personhood are formulated as body, mind, and spirit, then physical, mental, and spiritual differences are vulnerable to being positioned along related value scales.

One particularly powerful and normative model of personhood privileges the stand-alone individual, the person who has successfully "individuated." The ideal is expressed through expectations that one of the tasks of young adulthood is the ability to separate from one's family and strike out on one's own. Neo-Piagetians such as Robert Kegan (1982) nuanced the argument, suggesting that only by differentiating oneself from something can one enter into relationship with it. Still, the emphasis is on becoming an autonomous individual—*not* an ideal in all cultures, some of which value the capacity to sustain interconnectedness over the model of individual autonomy.

In India, for example, Valentin Daniel (1984) posited the metaphor of the "fluid self"—a self immersed in its relationships with others, without the felt need for clear-cut boundaries. In Confucian thought, the *self* is understood as the center of a network of relationships. One cultivates oneself to become a profound person but can only do so in the context of each of those relationships (Tu, 1985). For systems that view family, clan, tribe, or analogous networks as the ground from which a person emerges and finds meaning, the relational and communal is yet another intrinsic part of the person. In some African systems, this interconnecting thread is voiced in saying, "*I* am, because *we* are."

Candace Cole-McCrea, describing her experience as someone with disabilities in a Native American community, recalled that "my value and potential as a human being were never questioned or doubted. By definition, as a human being, I was seen as gifted, regardless of my physical condition. The question was only: How was I gifted?" (Cole-McCrea, 2001, p. 91). Her culture simply assumed that she would make a contribution to humanity.

The aspects of personhood, the expectations of how each aspect should express itself over time, the notion of the individual as autonomous or profoundly communal—each variable is a circle within other circles. The person who lives with disabilities or a chronic condition sits at the center of all them. Surrounding the person, and impinging on all of these other factors, may be the paradigm of suffering and affliction, with its calls and responses of "Why?" The outermost and most encompassing circle, however, may be the paradigm of Healing, of ultimate human possibility, which takes on deepened meanings in light of disability and chronicity.

A Haitian family brought their 20-year-old son with intellectual disabilities to see me. I explained to his mother that she would have to go before a judge to be awarded guardianship.

Given that her son became legally recognized as an adult at the age of 18, I said that the guardianship would authorize her to take care of him. She looked at me as though I were an idiot—how could I imagine that she and her family would not continue to care for him?

I found myself laughing, and saying, "Yes, it's a stupid American law," realizing that from the perspective of many other cultures, it would be self-evident that the family would remain involved. They would not require the relationship to be legally defined. This instance was one of different understandings of personhood—the one viewing the young man as an autonomous choice-making individual whose rights had to be protected and the other seeing him as part of a network of relationships in which all parties had roles and responsibilities.

A final point in relation to the developmental significance of disabilities: Growing up with disabilities is quite different from acquiring one in adulthood. Many people, for example, are prone to see someone in a wheelchair and think, "I would never want to be like that. My life would not be worth living if that happened to me." If, however, one has grown up using a wheelchair, one has never known a different way of living. One of the authors (Dr. Coulter) has first-hand experience with regard to hearing loss:

I have had a hearing loss most of my life. It was first discovered during routine screening when I entered kindergarten. Fifty years later, I can still remember being taken out of the classroom and walking up the hall to have my hearing tested. I learned years later that I had a significant hearing loss, so I assume this is why they kept testing me. Indeed, I have a moderate to severe loss in my left ear, covering all the speech frequencies, and a mild high-frequency loss in my right ear.

I was able to compensate well enough to be successful in life. I learned to hold a telephone to my right ear instead of my left, because otherwise I could not hear what people were saying. I learned to sit with people on my right side, so I could hear them. Without doing so consciously, I learned to read people's lips as they were talking, so I could understand them better. At the same time, I learned to focus and tune out distracting stimuli. So, during my training in pediatrics, I found that I could concentrate on the tasks at hand.

Dr. Coulter found that some of his life activities were made more difficult, yet he was never diagnosed as having a disability, nor was he particularly aware of missing anything. In recent years, he got a hearing aid and realized that he was now hearing sounds that others around him were taking for granted. Indeed, he now realizes that he did have a disability but was not really aware of it. Because he did not grow up thinking of himself as someone with a disability, it was not part of his self-concept. As he later came to see, people must not project their own fears about what their lives would be like if they lost some cherished ability (e.g., mobility, hearing, vision, intelligence) onto people who have fashioned full and satisfying lives in the absence of such abilities.

The point is not always readily apparent to even the most well-intentioned caregiver. It speaks to the significance of the disability over time in the person's concept of who he or she is—something that caregivers must learn to see through the eyes of the person with disabilities. Dr. Coulter was able to succeed on his own terms without thinking of himself as being disabled and without being considered disabled by society. What if other people considered as having disabilities were able to succeed on their own terms in the same way?

Illness, Disease, and Chronic Conditions

Why does it matter to know how the parts of personhood are conceptualized? The answer is that if clinicians do not know the parts of a person, they do not know all the ways a person can get sick or be afflicted. Generally, each aspect of a person is conceptualized as susceptible to particular kinds of illness or affliction. Etiologies and causal factors point, on the one hand, to broader paradigms of suffering. Indeed, the individual version of a disability or chronic condition may be experienced as the personalized enactment of paradigms of suffering and affliction. On the other hand, they also point to the specifics of the aspect that is afflicted. For example, a woman may view her cerebral palsy as a test, even as she conceptualizes its causes in neurological terms.

The situation is particularly challenging when the nature and cause of a given problem are unclear within the systems with which the individual, family, or clinician is familiar. Not knowing how to define a condition makes it difficult to understand its implications or to know how to respond to it. The anxiety related to that form of limbo is different from the anxieties related to defining a condition and determining what can be done in response.

Things also get complicated when the parties involved conceive of the person in different and even conflicting terms. A now classic example is Ann Fadiman's (1997) narrative about a Hmong child, Lia Lee, in *A Spirit Catches You and You Fall Down.* From infancy, Lia suffered from epilepsy. According to her pediatricians, for whom her physiology and neurology were the key aspects involved, the initial problem arose in these domains and needed to be addressed in these domains. For Lia's parents, however, a radically different key aspect involved Lia's souls, which could be stolen or lost. For them, the seizures represented evidence that this worst of outcomes had occurred. Similarly, in traditional Chinese thought, each person had 11 souls, all of them various forms of *qi*. After death, certain souls entered the ground with the corpse. If not properly attended to, they could become hungry ghosts and afflict the descendant who was neglecting them.

Another way to explain the point is that, just as notions of personhood are socially, culturally, and religiously constructed, so are ideas about disability and chronicity. How 18th- or 19th-century European and American clinicians constructed understandings of disability was directly related to how they thought about a person as a physiological entity, a moral agent, and even as a child of God. The notion, for example, of "moral imbecility" would seem unconscionable today. None of these understandings could be separated from normative ideas about personhood.

As Turmusani explains of disability in the Middle East, in some contexts it:

> Is often perceived as divine intervention or work of evil spirit (Jinn)... implying impurity and indifference on the part of people who have impairments. In the long run those with impairments are made to feel less than others. The birth of [a] disabled child brings shame and blame to family members especially mothers. These perceptions lead to negative attitudes towards disabled people and result in isolation and invisibility of the person who has impairment. (2001, p. 74)

A parallel argument can be made about one's own particular locations in time and space. As Turmusani's example illustrates and as Gaventa suggested, "Different cultures and settings place different values and interpretations on what might appear to be the 'same' human ability, disability, or behavior" (2001, p. 31). For example, a young woman experienced the new onset of seizures. Her mother said, "She can't be having seizures—they come from the Devil, and I'm a religious woman. There cannot be seizures in my family."

That disabilities can be construed differently is evident in the differences between the several versions of the Federal definition included in the Developmental Disabilities Services and Facilities Construction Amendments of 1970 (PL 91-517) related to eligibility criteria. In all of these versions, the person is conceptualized as a citizen with a potential claim on benefits. According to social contract theory, citizens with disabilities have a particular claim on societal resources because of their disability. The original version of the Act defined developmental disabilities in categorical terms, which means that one had a disability if one could be diagnosed with a particular category or disorder such as mental retardation, cerebral palsy, epilepsy, or another neurological disorder (e.g., blindness, deafness, autism or learning disability) that is "closely related" to mental retardation in terms of treatment needs. This categorical approach was rejected in 1978, and a new functional approach was promulgated. In the Rehabilitation, Comprehensive Services, and Developmental Disabilities Amendments of 1978 (PL 95-517), a *developmental disability* is defined as a severe, chronic disability that is attributable to a mental or physical impairment, that is manifested before age 22 years and is likely to continue indefinitely, that results in substantial functional limitations in three or more areas of major life activity (self-care, language, learning, mobility, self-direction, capacity for independent learning, and/or economic self-sufficiency), and that reflects the individual's need for supports and services for an extended duration.

The distinction between categorical and functional approaches to defining disability reflects a fundamental change in how individuals with disabilities are conceptualized. Categorical approaches locate the disability within the person who has a specific neurological disease or disorder. Functional approaches locate the disability within the interaction between the individual's needs and the demands of the social environment (Luckasson et al., 1992). Disability is now thought of as a problem in functioning because of this interaction.

The World Health Organization (WHO) classifies diseases and disorders according to the International Classification of Diseases (1993) and classifies problems in functioning according to the International Classification of Functioning (2001). Diseases and disorders may increase the risk of problems in functioning but are conceptually distinct from them. Note that in the original categorical list of developmental disabilities, some are now classified as diseases or disorders (epilepsy, cerebral palsy, blindness, deafness) and some are now classified as problems in functioning (mental retardation, autism, learning disabilities).

This distinction was further clarified in the American Association on Mental Retardation's latest definition and classification of *mental retardation* (Luckasson et al., 2002). Etiology was conceptualized as the presence of one or more of a variety of interacting biomedical, social, behavioral, and educational risk factors, whereas disability was conceptualized as the expression of limitations in individual functioning within a social context that represents a substantial disadvantage to the individual. Classification of individuals with mental retardation involves five dimensions, including intellectual abilities, adaptive behavior, functioning (participation, interactions and social roles), health, and context (environments and culture). No one dimension alone is sufficient to describe the person, and all are necessary. According to this view, a person with mental retardation is a person first (a valued member of society) who happens to have certain specific problems in functioning within society for a variety of reasons (classified in the five dimensions), and who needs supports and services in order to function optimally as a member of society.

Each set of definitions envisions a person from a different angle—that is, each is based on a different *anthropology*, or theory of the person. Correspondingly, each constructs the issue differently. Likewise, each understands "development" differently over the life span of a person.

Related Interventions

Just as people classify health conditions in different ways, they also identify specific interventions as appropriate and/or necessary for each one. The identification of necessary or desirable interventions is culturally shaped. It may seem self-evident, for example, that if a person breaks a bone, he or she goes to a hospital emergency room or orthopedist to have it set, with related follow-up. For members of the majority culture, however, it might seem less self-evident that one might go, instead, to a traditional bone setter, get acupuncture to promote healing, and go for a divination reading to understand why that particular accident happened to that particular person at that particular time and to learn what needs to be done to correct a deeper problem. Without attention to all three aspects, this hypothetical individual might argue that real healing cannot be expected.

As Donald Schön and Martin Rein (1994) and have suggested, *how* a problem is framed is also directly related to what people think can and should be done for it. What should be done for it is, in turn, related to each of the aspects discussed so far. Each therapy touches on these multiple levels, with different layers of hope, expectation, and things at stake. The hopes and expectations are tied in both with normative ideas of personhood and, in the case of individuals with disabilities, with how the disability is construed.

Care providers must learn how individuals and their families have conceptualized the individual's situation and how all involved have defined what needs to be done in order to attain a better understanding of where one's care fits in the larger scenario. To recognize these different dimensions allows the provider to grasp a patient- and family-centered view of holistic care, which will vary from individual to individual and from family to family. It increases the likelihood of developing an integrative approach to care in which different kinds of interventions can complement one another.

A good model for such an integrative approach has been developed by pediatrician Kathi Kemper, who observed:

> Different kinds of practitioners have different theories, rely on different treatments, and often compete rather than cooperate with one another. It doesn't have to be this way. Rather than being therapy-centered, polarized, and competitive, healing can be child-centered, integrated, cooperative, and holistic. (2003, pp. 1–2)

Kemper (1996) posited four broad categories of therapies that allow one to integrate biomedical interventions with complementary and alternative therapies of different kinds: 1) biochemical, 2) biomechanical, 3) lifestyle, and 4) bioenergetic (see Table 32.1). Biochemical interventions include pharmaceutical medications, over-the-counter medicines, herbs, and nutritional supplements. Biomechanical therapies involve external manipulations or interventions such as massage, physical therapy, chiropractic, osteopathy, and surgery. Lifestyle-related therapies include nutrition, exercise, modifica-

Table 32.1. Integrative therapies

Biochemical	Lifestyle	Biomechanical	Bioenergetic
Medications	Nutrition	Massage	Acupuncture
Herbs	Exercise	Physical therapy	Therapeutic touch
Nutritional supplements	Environment	Spinal manipulation (chiropractic, osteopathy)	Healing touch
			Laying on of hands
	Mind–body	Surgery	Reiki
			Qigong
			Prayer and ritual
			Homeopathy

Source: Kemper, 2003.

tions to the individual's environment, and mind–body therapies such as biofeedback. Bioenergetic therapies are predicated on theories of subtle energies and include homeopathy, traditional Chinese medicine (e.g., acupuncture), Therapeutic Touch and Healing Touch, laying on of hands, Reiki, and *qigong*. They also include prayer and ritual.

When asking a family about the kinds of interventions they may have been trying, or would like to include in the care of a patient, these four categories prove particularly useful. Like everything else, each one has specific cultural variations and expressions. Herbs as used by a middle-class European American family, purchased at a health-food store, are likely to be quite different from those used by a family that has recently emigrated from the Caribbean. Similarly, ideas of health-related food and diet will probably differ, as will understandings of spirituality and religion, insofar as these may be understood to contribute to the individual's and family's well-being. The different kinds of therapies are each related to a particular kind of change they are hoped to bring. Each represents a domain of potential transformation.

Clinicians know that people go to other practitioners—the literature says that some 40% of Americans seek complementary therapies in general. Why would it not be the case for families with a member who lives with disabilities? I had a patient from Jamaica—a nice man with a wonderful family. He developed neurofibromatosis, a disease that produces tumors. A large tumor grew on his upper arm, so he went to see specialists who told him that it was so bad that they would need to amputate his arm.

He and his family came to see me. I told them that an amputation was not medically necessary. They said, "The tumor is ugly, but we can live with it." I offered a number of possible medications to help with the discomfort.

The family decided, instead, to go to an herbalist, who gave them an herbal tea. They said that it smelled and tasted nasty but were certain that it helped. They chose this option over medications. I appreciated their telling me about it.

The *Physicians' Desk Reference* now actually recognizes possible interactions between herbs and pharmaceuticals. Drug inserts sometimes now include such possibilities.

Related Caregivers

The different kinds of intervention are related to different kinds of practitioners, clinicians, and caregivers (some of them religious and/or traditional). Just as it is important to know the kinds of therapies an individual and family feel are important, it is useful to know the different kinds of practitioners they may choose to involve in the individual's care. In the best of all worlds, the biomedical provider is aware of these other practitioners and may even establish some connection with them in the interest of the individual.

The role of the community as a caregiver may also be important to ask about. For some families, the combined effects of modernity and sometimes of cultural dislocation have compromised the availability of communities that once helped with taking care of the person with disabilities. The challenges of the disability may be experienced even more deeply in the awareness of this absence.

Moreover, the roles played by the clinician may be varied in ways that can be challenging, albeit potentially rewarding. For example, enculturation into the profession of medicine varies, even in an apparently uniform field. Physicians generally practice medicine the way they were taught in medical school and residency, with different treatment approaches tightly related to different diagnoses. If their program emphasized Problem-Based Learning, or narrower understandings of evidence-based medicine, it may have shaped their attitudes toward issues such as complementary/alternative medicine or spirituality. It may present a challenge to be open to the range of meanings an individual and family assign to such practices.

Biomedical training also often privileges *doing* over *being there*, and *curing* over *caring*, making it more difficult for the provider to recognize the value of his or her simple presence. One's technical skills may be crucial at various points in the care of the particular person, but one's capacity to function as a Healer is also tested and, hopefully, deepened. To think of oneself as a Healer can mean situating one's own work differently, allowing one to engage in Healing at different levels of meaning—leading to the question of efficacy.

Meanings of Efficacy

People commonly ask whether a therapeutic intervention has "worked"; however, this apparently simple question can hold many meanings. For example, which aspect of personhood was suffering and to what was the suffering attributed? What intervention or interventions were deemed necessary, and what was expected of each one? In the case of a disability or a degenerative disease, the meanings become even complex and nuanced. If the larger framework of Healing is factored into the picture, then the most meaningful kinds of change—of "working"—may be understood to happen after the person's death. The expectation of some life after death modifies the time frame of Healing. Other frameworks of hope operate similarly.

Efficacy is another way of talking about change that is recognized and valued. We suggest that, to grasp the different meanings of efficacy involved in a situation, one must know how both Healing and Suffering are understood; must understand the concept of the person at work, along with *which* aspect of the person is viewed as having been affected; and must know how the person and his or her family envisions all the necessary healers and interventions, in order for both healing and *Healing* to happen.

One must also recognize the ways in which one's own understandings of efficacy grow out of frameworks that may or may not be the same as those of individuals and their families. Indeed, when one does not discern the differences between one's own frameworks and those of individuals and their families, one ends up at cross-purposes. When all parties can bring together their respective visions of Healing and emerge with a shared vision that draws on the best of each set of hopes and possibilities, then that process, itself, is part of Healing.

In the lives of people with disabilities, transformation and Healing all take on their meanings within the framework of the disability and of the particular person. The range of possibilities is a particularized one, related directly to who *this* person is and what abilities and potential he or she has. In the context of poor outcomes and even impending death, as in the case of a person with a degenerative disease, efficacy may involve changes in how people locate meaning in the situation. It may simply mean everyone's being present—including clinicians who are interested and available. Sometimes, simple presence is healing within the larger frame of all lives being valuable, even though nothing else in the outcome changes. Indeed, one way to understand Healing lies in how one values the person being healed—the value, that is, that is assigned to that life within a moral economy.

SYSTEMIC CONTEXTS

Each of the seven dimensions discussed previously is located within larger systems and circles of involvement. A person with disabilities lives at the center of many spheres of influence, each of which informs the particulars of the seven categories. These spheres, together, can be conceptualized as the specific cultural frame. Three different models, developed by Maria P. P. Root, Robert Saper, and William Gaventa, help to discern such frames.

Root (1999), for example, provides an ecological model that encourages clinicians to ask about how such variables as gender, race, social class, personal traits, family economies, support structures, and the challenges of acculturation (for families who have relocated) constitute the systemic contexts in which the person with disabilities lives. Although Root's particular interest is in the influences on racial identity development—and in addition to the importance of this aspect of the person's experience—such factors also figure in a person's cultural formation. Likewise, the caregiver is also personally shaped by such variables, influencing how he or she views and engages with these systemic dimensions in the individual's life. Root's model (see Figure 32.1) allows one to view more explicitly the added challenges to an individual and family members who occupy one or more socially targeted positions, including being a woman, being someone with a minority sexual orientation, being part of a racial/ethnic minority, having a low socioeconomic class status, being a recent immigrant, and belonging to a religious tradition that may suffer stigmatizing in the media or in popular perception.

Such forms of targeting constitute what medical anthropologists have characterized as *structural violence*. The term refers to social structures and systems that have perpetrated and perpetuated unequal access to resources and justice for different groups in the United States (Kleinman, Das, & Lock, 1997). Such inequities have been buttressed throughout American history by economic, political, legal, and religious influences, taking their toll on individual bodies. When therapeutic interventions focus solely on individual bodies, however, they overlook the structural and ideological underpinnings of the individual's poor health—what are really individual expressions of social conditions. No disability occurs in a vacuum, making it crucial to situate each one in its complex cultural frame. As the following narrative illustrates, the convergence of many factors play out in a person's health, just as a constellation of systemic and social supports is essential in response.

Doug's mother Mary Beth was 25 when she became pregnant. Mary Beth had had a difficult history that included physical and sexual abuse when she was a teenager. She became addicted to heroin and entered a drug treatment program when she was 20 but relapsed a year later. During the years before she became pregnant with Doug, she lived with a number of different men and had children with them, all of whom were removed by the Department of Social Services.

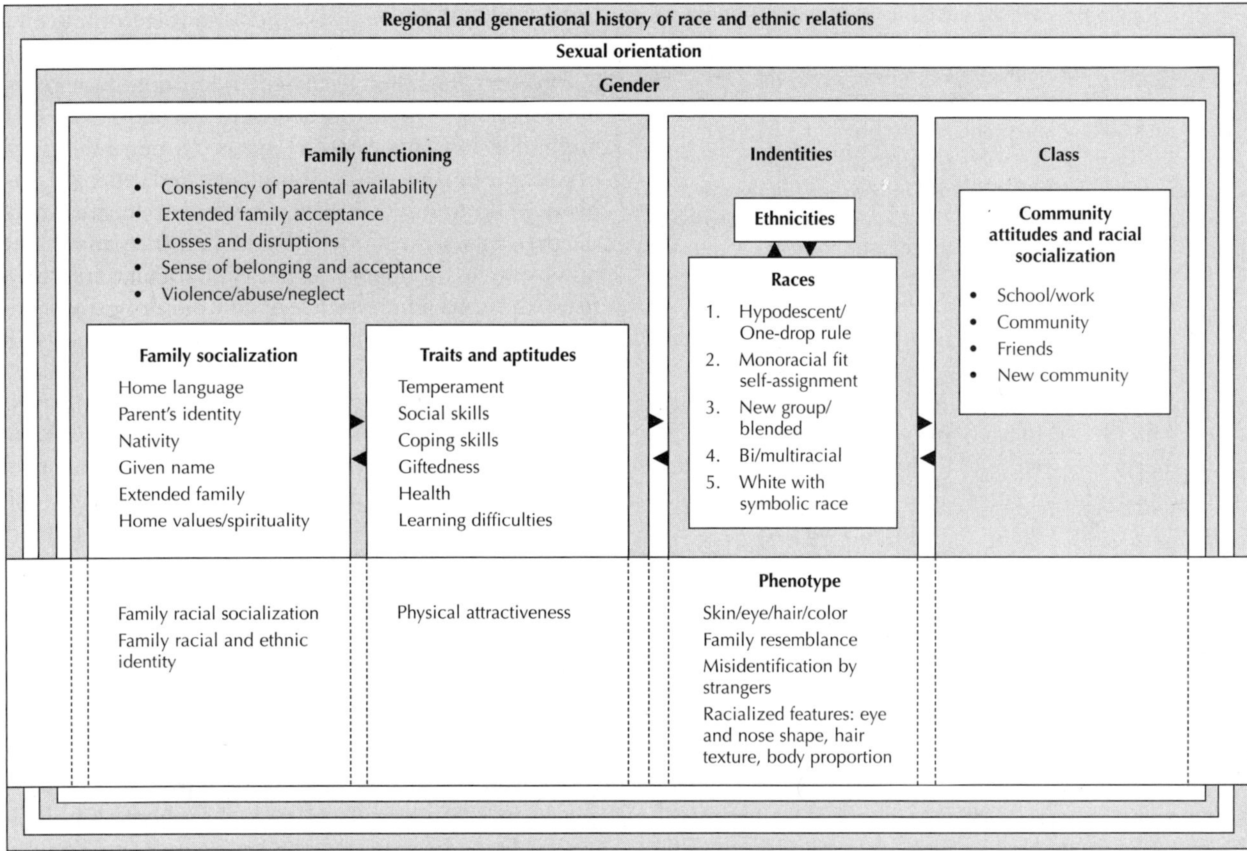

Figure 32.1. Root's ecological framework for understanding multiracial identity development. (From Root, M. [2004]. Multiracial families and children: Implications for educational research on multicultural education [2nd ed., p. 116]. San Francisco: Jossey-Bass. © Maria P.P. Root, Ph.D., 2002.)

She finally stopped taking drugs but could not stop drinking or smoking cigarettes. When she learned that she was 2 months pregnant with Doug, she sought treatment for her alcoholism.

Doug was born at full term but weighed only 5 lb, 2 oz at birth. The delivering obstetrician immediately noticed the baby had problems and transferred him to the neonatal intensive care unit, where the pediatricians recognized the facial features of fetal alcohol syndrome. When Doug showed signs of cardiac problems, the pediatricians obtained cardiologic evaluation that showed the presence of serious congenital heart disease. Doug underwent cardiac surgery at 2 weeks of age that partially corrected the abnormality, but further surgery was anticipated when he got older.

Mary Beth made daily visits to the hospital and stayed in contact with her social worker. She had found an apartment and was receiving financial support from several social service agencies. After considerable discussion, the decision was made to discharge Doug to his mother. Plans were made for frequent visits from the social worker and a visiting nurse, and Doug was referred to the local early intervention program.

Doug and Mary Beth did well for about 6 months, and the visiting nurse felt she could cut back to monthly monitoring visits. A new social worker's caseload was too great to allow frequent visits. Mary Beth took Doug to all of his doctor visits and made sure he got all of his immunizations.

When Doug was 15 months old, Mary Beth moved in with her new boyfriend, Bill. Unfortunately Bill soon became abusive and would beat Mary Beth when he was drunk. After a while, Mary Beth started drinking again. She did not enroll Doug in the early intervention program and missed several of Doug's doctors' appointments.

Finally, when Doug was 28 months old, Mary Beth left Bill and went to live in a shelter with Doug. During the next 6 months, she completed treatment for alcoholism, took parenting classes, and went through a job training program. Doug received medical care from the shelter's free clinic but did not receive early intervention services because the local service provider did not consider him to have a stable address.

When Doug was 3, Mary Beth graduated from the job-training program and landed a job as a secretarial assistant at the local women's clinic, where she felt she had a lot of support from the staff. She helped start a women's support group there. With her income, she was able to get an apartment nearby. She realized Doug needed help and talked to the clinic's doctors, who referred her to an excellent pediatrician in the community who accepted Medicaid.

The pediatrician referred Doug to the Developmental Assessment Clinic at the hospital, where he was determined to have significant delays in cognitive, language, and gross and fine motor development. He was referred to the cardiologist for further management of his congenital heart disease and to the local public school system for enrollment in special education. Mary Beth and Doug were finally safe, secure, stable, and surrounded by caring friends and professionals who could give them the support they needed.

Robert Saper has suggested another integrative ecological model that conceptualizes a person as intersecting spheres of body, mind, spirit, and social world (see Figure 32.2). In assessing how Affliction and Suffering become specific in a person's life, each of these spheres provides an entrée into inquiry. Together, they allow for a comprehensive history taking that addresses the many facets of an individual's life. Moreover, by envisioning each sphere as intersecting, one is better able to *see* how the various factors affect each other. For example, if a family has entered the United States as a consequence of economic or political violence, every member will be affected not only by the trauma of the relocation, but also by the change in support structures along with the challenges of navigating new cultural challenges. These social dimensions will spill over into how the family is able to address the physical and other challenges of the one member's disability.

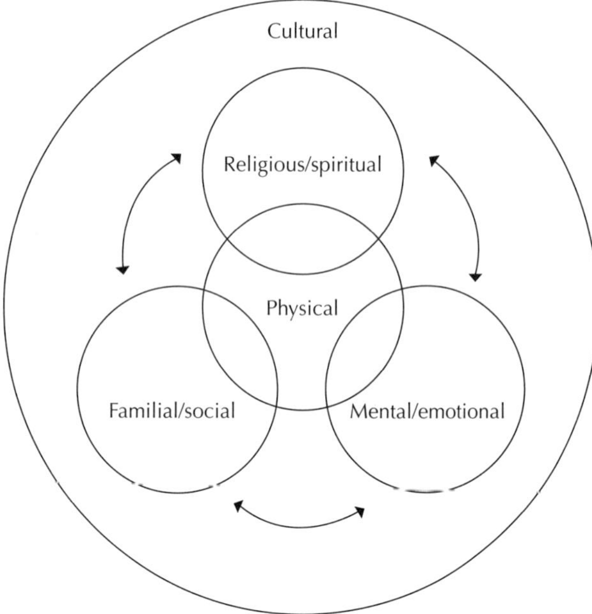

Figure 32.2. Robert Saper's ecological model that conceptualizes a person as intersecting spheres of body, mind, spirit, and social world. Courtesy of Robert Saper, M.D., M.P.H. All rights reserved.

Finally, the model has the advantage of allowing one to arrive at a more integrative approach to care. It is, of course, based on a particular concept of the parts, or aspects of a person. Yet, it also suggests how one might develop similar models to account for other ways of conceptualizing the person and related approaches to history taking and therapeutic responses. Regardless of the particulars, the model includes family members and other sources of support—what William Gaventa refers to as "the crucial importance of community embeddedness," better allowing the clinician to explore the available resources that will do the most good (2001, p. 43). Within each of these frames, one asks, "What *are* the abilities of the person with the disability?"

Gaventa's model (see Table 32.2) includes many of these variables, overlapping with Saper in its attention to the spiritual dimensions of an individual's and family's experience and worldview. Gaventa, himself building on the work of others, argued that "spirituality is a major way of finding meaning, coping, understanding, changing, and motivating. Whether or not one believes that spirituality is 'substantive' or 'real' part of human experience, we cannot ignore its functional role" and pervasive presence in each of the other variables (2001, p. 35).

Likewise, spirituality—however it is understood—is present in all individuals, including those with intellectual disabilities or those who are, neurologically speaking, in a persistent vegetative state. Coulter posited that one must learn to look at each individual as "a person with the 'breath of life' of human consciousness," rather than succumbing to more superficial characteristics (2001, p. 4). A second step involves learning to look at the other person as a human being like oneself, recognizing that just as one experiences spirituality, so does that other person, regardless of whether it looks familiar. "The purpose of this second look is to try to enter into the other person's point of view, to try to experience the other person's subjectivity, to try to appreciate

Table 32.2. Gaventa's model of holistic and spiritual assessment

Holistic assessment	Spiritual assessment
Biological (medical) decisions	Belief and meaning
Psychological dimension	Vocation and obligations
Family systems dimension	Experience and emotion
Psycho-social dimension	Courage and growth
Ethnic/racial/cultural dimension	Ritual and patience
Social issues dimension	Community
Spiritual dimension	Authority and guidance

From Gaventa, W. (2001). Defining and assessing spirituality and spiritual supports: A rationale for inclusion in theory and practice. In W.C. Gaventa & D.L. Coulter (Eds.), *Spiritual and intellectual disability: International perspectives on the effect of culture and religion on healing body, mind, and soul* (p. 34). New York: Haworth Pastoral Press; reprinted by permission.

what it means to the other person to be alive" (Coulter, 2001, p. 6). The third way of looking locates the ground of all existence in that other person—that same transcendence that is at the heart's core of our own spirituality. To engage in all three ways of looking at another person is to go beyond any and all of the boundaries that appear to divide us.

CONCLUSION

The challenge is to engage with an individual, a family, and a person's network of care in ways that take into account these different dimensions and that understand that holistic care is going to mean different things in each case. The function of models is to tease out the particulars in a given life in order to understand both which kinds of care and intervention best fit and in what ways. The vision suggested is a complex one—not always a welcome thought to overworked care providers—because the realities of the whole person are complex. When one practices seeing all of them, however, one finds that each of the pieces comes more and more naturally into focus, even as all of them together move and shift, as in a kaleidoscope.

The image of pieces in motion is an especially important one insofar as talking about processes over time. Part of the job of a caregiver in his or her role as healer is to help a person, a family, and a network develop a lifetime perspective with an understanding of all that is possible. Naturally, what is possible—including the full potential and possibility of the person with disabilities—undergoes change and transformation over time as well.

REFERENCES

Barnes, L. (2003). Spirituality and religion in health care. In J.A. Bigby (Ed.), *Cross-cultural medicine* (pp. 237–268). Philadelphia: American College of Physicians.

Barnes, L., Plotnikoff, G., Fox, K., & Pendleton, S. (2000). Religious traditions, spirituality and pediatrics: Intersecting worlds of healing: A review. *Journal of the Ambulatory Pediatric Association, 106*(4), 899–908.

Carman, J. (1994). *Majesty and meekness: A comparative study of contrast and harmony in the concept of God.* Grand Rapids, MI: W.B. Eerdmans.

Cole-McCrea, C. (2001). Cultural/spiritual attributions as independent variables in the development of identity and potential for personals of exceptionality: A case study of North American Christianity and Native American religious influence. In W.C. Gaventa & D.L. Coulter (Eds.), *Spiritual and intellectual disability: International perspectives on the effect of culture and religion on healing body, mind, and soul* (pp. 87–98). New York: Haworth Pastoral Press.

Coulter, D. (2001). Recognition of spirituality in health care: Personal and universal implications In W.C. Gaventa & D.L. Coulter (Eds.), *Spiritual and intellectual disability: International perspectives on the effect of culture and religion on healing body, mind, and soul* (pp. 1–11). New York: Haworth Pastoral Press.

Daniel, E. (1984). *Fluid signs: Being a person the Tamil way.* Berkeley: University of California Press.

Developmental Disabilities Services and Facilities Construction Amendments of 1970, PL 91-517, 84 Stat. 1316.

Fadiman A. (1997). *The spirit catches you and you fall down.* New York: Noonday Press.

Gaventa, W. (2001). Defining and assessing spirituality and spiritual supports: A rationale for inclusion in theory and practice. In W.C. Gaventa & D.L. Coulter (Eds.), *Spiritual and intellectual disability: International perspectives on the effect of culture and religion on healing body, mind, and soul* (pp. 29–48). New York: Haworth Pastoral Press.

Gaventa, W., & Coulter, D. (Eds.). (2001). *Spirituality and intellectual disability: International perspectives on the effect of culture and religion on healing body, mind, and soul.* New York: Haworth Pastoral Press.

Kegan, R. (1982). *The evolving self: Problem and process in human development.* Cambridge, MA: Harvard University Press.

Kemper, K. (1996). Separation or synthesis: A holistic approach to therapeutics. *Pediatrics Review, 17*(8), 279–283.

Kemper, K. (2003). *The holistic pediatrician* (2nd ed.). New York: Quill.

Kleinman, A., Das, V., & Lock, M. (Eds.). (1997). *Social suffering.* Berkeley: University of California Press.

Luckasson, R., Borthwick-Duffy, S., Buntinx, W., Coulter, D., Craig, E., Reeve, A., et al. (2002). *Mental retardation: Definition, classification and systems of supports* (10th ed.). Washington, DC: American Association on Mental Retardation.

Luckasson, R., Coulter, D., Polloway, E., Reiss, S., Schalock, R., Snell, M., et al. (1992). *Mental retardation: Definition, classification and systems of supports* (9th ed.). Washington, DC: American Association on Mental Retardation.

Rehabilitation, Comprehensive Services, and Developmental Disabilities Amendments of 1978, PL 95-602, 92 Stat. 2955.

Root, M. (1998). Experiences and processes affecting racial identity development: Preliminary results from the biracial siblings project. *Cultural diversity and mental health, 4*(3), 237–247.

Root, M. (1999). The biracial baby boom: Understanding ecological constructions of racial identity in the 21st century. In R. Sheets & E. Hollins (Eds.), *Racial and ethnic identity in school practices: Aspects of human development* (pp. 67–89). Mahwah, NJ: Lawrence Erlbaum Associates.

Schön, D., & Rein, M. (1994). *Frame reflection: Toward the resolution of intractable policy controversies.* New York: Basic Books.

Tu, W. (1985). *Confucian thought: Selfhood as creative transformation.* Albany: State University of New York Press.

Turmusani, M. (2001). Disabled women in Islam: Middle Eastern perspective. In W.C. Gaventa & D.L. Coulter (Eds.), *Spiritual and intellectual disability: International perspectives on the effect of culture and religion on healing body, mind, and soul* (pp. 73–85). New York: Haworth Pastoral Press.

World Health Organization. (1993). *International classification of diseases and related health problems* (10th ed.). Geneva: Author.

World Health Organization. (2001). *International classification of functioning, disability and health (ICF).* Geneva: Author.

CHAPTER 33

ETHICAL CARE

Peter J. Smith and David L. Coulter

This chapter presents a short overview of the history of medical ethics, outlines two of the most important systems of ethical thought, offers an ethical system *from within* the field of developmental disabilities, and discusses an ethical dilemma in light of the prior sections. We recognize that, because of its nature as a review, this chapter will not fully develop these important topics or pursue fully the questions raised. It should, however, provide a good starting point for individuals in the field of developmental disabilities, and the reference list should allow for further development of this topic by interested readers.

ANCIENT TRADITION

Within the Western tradition, medical care often is traced back to the Greek physician Hippocrates and the community gathered around him. Who precisely created the code of conduct that is represented in the Hippocratic oath is unclear, but this oath and other ancient oaths (and the ethical systems that they imply) are as old as the medical profession. In addition, as medical care and the societies surrounding it have developed, so have the ethical systems that inform it.

One of the dominant influences on medical ethics for the last 2,000 years in the Western world has been the Christian Church. Within this tradition grew the field of Moral Theology, which allowed for lengthy debates by its scholars that fostered the development of complex ethical systems. From earlier Roman seeds, the Church's ethicists developed a complex paradigm now know as *natural law* (see Table 33.1), which was a system of thinking that did not rely on overt religious belief but rather drew its inspiration from the idea that the "natural" world had a predetermined order. Usually, the order was supposed to have been arranged by God, but this determination has been dropped by some who otherwise endorse the system.

All people, including healers, were required to refrain from "unnatural" acts and to direct their energies toward upholding and preserving natural relationships. This ancient system is still very influential today (explicitly and implicitly) for many thinkers, especially within Christian groups (particularly Roman Catholicism); however, it would not be considered by most commentators as the dominant one today. The current state of medical ethics is briefly discussed in the next section.

CURRENT STATE OF MEDICAL ETHICS

The first step in understanding the current state of medical ethics is to examine the underlying assumptions and predispositions of the larger society. Simply stated, the current consensus in Western countries is that culture and society ought to be structured, as articulated by Thomas Jefferson in 1776, on the foundations of life, liberty, and the pursuit of happiness. Because of this orientation, the conception of *liberty* implies freedom *from* oppressive restrictions.

This framework is based on the definition that *personhood is determined by an ability to choose.* Over time, liberal society has responded to criticisms regarding membership and has greatly expanded its definition of a citizen; however, it has not been able to expand the definition beyond the strict limits that are inherent in its conception of citizens as competent choice makers. Therefore, the framework sees any individuals who do not fit into this rubric as defective and needing to be fixed. In addition, the modern American bioethics movement, starting with the Nuremberg Trials at the end of World War II, was born within a worldview that not only mistrusted previous systems but also saw the need to safeguard individuals from the domination of larger entities.

Principle-Based Ethics

Within the contemporary discussions of bioethical issues in Western liberal society, the dominating system of thought is based on two foundational assumptions that are drawn from the larger culture. First, ethics is

Table 33.1. Description of natural law

Natural law has taken many forms during the 23 centuries of its development and has had a diverse multitude of proponents (religious and secular). Its enduring resilience has stemmed from three factors:

1. Its appeal to universal reason allows it to transcend time and geography while retaining an ability to analyze contemporary questions.
2. Its core formulations reflect a basic humanism that is genuinely egalitarian.
3. Its potential for use by both the powerful and the weak adds an authentic check against trends toward domination and subjectivity.

The Encyclopedia of Bioethics (D'Arcy, 1987, p. 1133) suggested "six theses, one or more of which each version of natural has affirmed and argued":

1. Some things are right or wrong, or good or evil, by their very nature. Good and right things are obligatory while wrong and evil things are forbidden.
2. Things that are right and wrong are known to be so by every adult.
3. Special arguments (e.g., the action is against a person's rights) can prove some actions to be right or wrong.
4. Man-made laws must conform to natural law to be viable.
5. Every viable social organization must develop rules of conduct based on the experience of being human and the nature of world.
6. An intrinsic relationship may exist between law and morality. Many theories (e.g., those of Aquinas and Locke) propose that a single theory can provide a framework for both laws and morals.

An even more basic distillation of the natural law philosophy suggests that two simple questions are the basis of formulating all natural law arguments: What does it mean to be a person? and What does it mean to be a person in society? This philosophy presupposes that

1. These questions can be answered
2. Reasonable people (regardless of their culture, time period, or personal experiences) will be able to come to a consensus on their answers.
3. The answers will be formulated in a continuing body of (usually unwritten) collective knowledge that informs the ongoing discussion of contemporary ethical problems.

brought to focus at points of tension or conflict, usually represented though use of real or theoretic problematic situations. It relies on only minimal conceptions of what constitutes health, society, and common interest:

> Standard bioethics, by which I mean the family of secular approaches that are dominant in the English-speaking world, is a product of modernity, and the moral task of modernity is to resolve conflicts between competing interests in order to secure social cooperation without appeal to robust views of the good. The agenda of standard bioethics, at the risk of oversimplification, follows accordingly: for every new issue that arises in biomedical research and care its task is to safeguard individual autonomy, calculate potential risks and harms, and determine whether or not a just distribution will follow. (McKenny, 1997, p. 8)

Second, moral dilemmas are best resolved by objective application of universal principles by thoughtful (and preferably disinterested) actors. Although there is much debate and discussion about exactly what constitutes a moral dilemma, what are the universal principles that ought to be applied to a dilemma, and how these general principles become relevant for the particularities of each situation, consensus has been reached about the methodology and overall approach of principle-driven bioethics (the most often quoted example of this position is *Principles of Biomedical Ethics* by Beauchamp & Childress, 2001).

Virtue Ethics

Another contemporary ethical system, *virtue ethics*, also has both ancient roots and strong claims of universality:

> Probably every society has identified certain human characteristics as being especially praiseworthy and worth cultivating, while also identifying others as vices, which are morally corrupt, contemptible or otherwise undesirable. These traditions of virtues, in turn, have frequently given rise to systematic reflection on what it means to be virtuous. (Porter, 2001, p. 96)

Traces of this type of thinking started at least in Greek antiquity. Later, Roman culture included a vision of the virtues, especially as developed by the philosophical tradition of the Stoics and promoted by the great orator and public official, Cicero (106–43 B.C.), which focused on acting according to right reason. During the Christian era, the most influential promoters of virtues have been Augustine of Hippo (A.D. 354–430) and Thomas Aquinas (c. 1225–74 B.C.). Augustine built on the Roman premise that there is one foundation for virtue; however, instead of using wisdom or reason, he placed love of God at the foundation. In contrast, Aquinas (n.d.) introduced virtues as falling under the classification of habits: "Therefore human virtues are habits" (I.II.55.1c)

Contemporary virtue ethicists (e.g., see Pellegrino's [1985] *The Virtuous Physician*) often specifically define themselves as *not* attempting to create systems that promote virtuous *actions* but rather creating environments and expectations that help foster virtuous *individuals:*

> Renewed interest in virtue ethics arises from a dissatisfaction with the way we do ethics today. Most discussions about ethics today consider major controversial actions. . . .Virtue ethicists are different. We are not primarily interested in particular actions. We do not ask, 'Is this action right?' 'What are the circumstances around an action?' Or, 'What are the consequences of an action?' We are simply interested in persons. We believe that the real discussion of ethics is not the question 'What should I do' but 'Who should I become?' In fact, virtue ethicists expand that question into three key, related ones: 'Who am I?' 'Who ought I to become?' 'How am I to get there? (Keenan, 1997, p. 84)

PROPOSAL OF "EXCEPTIONAL ETHICS"

The underlying goal of this chapter is to begin the process of seeing the work of ethics not as impeded by the difficulties of accounting for differences but rather as enhanced by the adoption of a perspective centered on otherness. The concept of *exceptionality* is familiar to most English speakers and generally carries positive overtones (see Chapter 27.2). It was introduced into the field of disability studies in the lectureship address to the Society of Developmental and Behavioral Pediatrics on September 28, 1997:

> Most of us handle variation, or exceptionality, on what might be called a 'dose-related' basis. In some measured element, whether it be something like IQ [score], or height, or visual acuity, or whatever number you wish to use, if the individual under discussion deflects by one standard deviation, we commonly refer to this as a 'borderline' state. We react to it good-naturedly, and very often take the person to lunch. If, on the other hand, the individual varies by two standard deviations, we now acknowledge by convention, in most of our fields, that this is abnormality. Our response there, very often, is that our service mode kicks in and we begin to think of how we are going to affect or ally ourselves with that person in a more lasting way. If the individual we are discussing varies by four or five standard deviations, in this arbitrary item that we are referring to, this is what might be called 'assertive abnormality.' Here is where we very commonly become personally uncertain. This is true low incidence, and it will be with that area that a great deal of the matter in discussion will be concerned. (Crocker, 1998, p. 300)

Several significant points are contained within this proposal. First, all attempts to differentiate between individuals, *by the very nature of the task*, ignore shared humanity. Therefore, every measurement ought to be considered as arbitrary and incomplete. Of course, the reification of abstract classification systems is so common that it can be imperceptible for those who operate within the conceit. The use of the conjoined term *defective child* instantly causes the hearer to focus on the "defect" that implies differentness rather than *child*, which points to the overwhelming majority of facets of the individual that are shared with the hearer.

Second, through the process of dividing people through these arbitrary distinctions, the entrenched classifications diminish the likelihood of sharing across boundaries. In essence, some current paradigms sharply restrict ideas of personhood and emphasize competition, whereas the new model hopes to encourage both the rediscovery of broad diversity within the conception of "people" and stimulate renewed forms of basic human cooperation.

Third, by choosing the term *exceptional*, an emphasis is placed on those individuals who are "assertively abnormal." The simple fact is that they are rare and therefore *necessarily require* a recalibration of expectations and assumptions. This shift will be required whenever they are encountered within statistical comparisons, whenever they resist definition by law or public policy, and whenever they bump up against personal attitudes that had been formed in their absence. By definition, a system of ethics that is centered on exceptionality will need to be flexible and dynamic and will find unusual confrontations to be enriching rather than detracting: "We and the parents, faced with difference in a young person, are obliged to reset our priorities, our reference frame, and to use new vision" (Crocker, 1998, p. 300).

Health care is increasingly faced with conflicts that have "never been seen before" and, therefore, needs an ethical framework with just this type of adaptability. Simply stated, individuals with disabilities prophetically remind all observers that *in times of vulnerability and being served, strong bonds between people are formed.* For example, who can doubt the love of a parent, spouse, or friend who has served during times of illness, suffering, old age, or infancy? Ironically, exceptional people are blessed with the paradoxical talents of both asserting their uniqueness and insisting on their connectedness within their very nature.

Having begun the work of defining the term *exceptional*, the next step is to trace an outline of the overarching canons for this new ethic. Preliminary work in this area has already begun to take shape. Drawing on a psychological perspective, one of the most influential (and enduring) figures in the field of disability studies, Wolf Wolfensberger, suggested that any new construction whose goal is to protect and value people already devalued or at risk of being devalued ought to start with a perspective that ennoblement of the individual must be understood within a context. He labeled this endeavor as *Social Role Valorization* and defined it by suggesting that it "implies, as much as possible, the use of culturally valued means in order to enable, establish, and/or maintain valued social roles for people"(1985, p. 61). Later, he defined success in the following endeavor:

> One can say that the goal of Social Role Valorization has been achieved if a person is accorded valued roles, life conditions, experiences, valued participations, autonomy, and choices that are available to at least the majority of other people of the same age and sex, *and* if these things have been accorded because the person is seen as valuable. Because these things are not attainable in full for every person, it is important to keep in mind the qualifying phrase "as much as possible" in the social role valorization definition. (1985, pp. 71–72)

Valuing a person for his or her social role may not be enough, however. How can one learn to value all individuals, even those whose social roles are quite limited, just because they exist? Coulter (2001) introduced the concept of *spiritual valorization* to explain how one can value the spirituality that is present in all individuals, including individuals with profound disabilities (e.g., Miguel, described next). Spiritual valorization can be learned by applying the "three ways of looking," in which one seeks to know the other person as a spiritual being like oneself and value in him or her what one values in oneself. In this sense, spiritual valorization is a foundation for an exceptional ethic, in that it values the spiritual existence of exceptional individuals to the same extent as other members of the human community (Coulter, 2004).

Ethical Dilemma

Miguel was a baby born with an anterior encephalocele, which meant that a large portion of his brain was wrapped in a sac that grew outside his forehead and had to be surgically removed in the first days of life to prevent an infection and death. After surgery, his medical difficulties were many, and he required both a gastrostomy tube for eating and a tracheostomy to protect his airway. His brain was not only smaller than average, but it showed signs of significant abnormalities, causing him to have profound intellectual disabilities and making even the basic function of maintaining a stable body temperature difficult for him at times.

Most of the nurses and doctors taking care of Miguel thought that he should be allowed to die peacefully. They recommended that a *Do Not Resuscitate* order be placed in Miguel's chart, but his parents disagreed. His parents were a young, unmarried couple; they were also both immigrants to the United States. They loved Miguel and wanted him to live.

Every available medical and technological option was used to keep Miguel alive and as comfortable as possible. This process was not easy, though. Many people involved in Miguel's care voiced strong opposition to working with him. Not only was he medically fragile and technologically dependent, but his body, especially his face, had been physically transformed by his congenital malformation and subsequent surgeries.

In addition, relationships with Miguel's family were difficult. His parents had very different lives and perspectives from his medical care team: they did not speak English as their first language, they were devoutly religious, and Miguel's father was often disruptive and unpleasant to the hospital staff. Some suspected him of using drugs. Finally, some staff found out that Miguel's mother had been told that her son's problems were God's punishment for her out-of-wedlock pregnancy, that his suffering was her "cross to bear," and to try to fight "God's will" would further compound her sin.

Many questions are raised by Miguel's story, but they boil down to two basic questions (which are actually the two basic questions in most ethical dilemmas): "What ought to be done?" and "Who decides?" The assumptions that are brought into the struggle to answer these questions will usually shape the inquiry in such a way that any "facts" or "truths" that are offered will not symmetrically counter the arguments of another commentator (in effect, they will be "talking past each other"). For example, some within the natural law tradition may suggest that the crucial issue to be decided is whether the care offered to Miguel beyond feeding him is "extraordinary" and, therefore, not obligatory. Others, working within the concept of deductive principles, might suggest that what is important is a determination of Miguel's "best interests" (a second-best substitute for his autonomous choice, which will never be known). Because of the difficulty of the task, virtue ethicists might see the need for caregivers to learn to serve this individual and family as part of the formation of virtuous clinicians. The answer to "what ought to be done" hinges on who is designated (actively, by default, or by accident) as the person or group who "gets to decide." Therefore, all ethical conflicts eventually devolve into a power struggle over decision making.

An ethics perspective that starts with exceptionality would reject the premise shared by all of these approaches that Miguel's story represents a failure that needs "fixing." Rather, an exceptional ethic would recognize in this family and situation an opportunity for everyone to grow more human. Growth does not imply simplicity, clarity, or comfort (ask the parent of any adolescent!); however, it implies that Miguel should be seen as a teacher instead of as a burden. Exceptional ethics would encourage those involved to stop seeing Miguel's medical care as a waste of time, money, and effort and to begin to see his care as an opportunity to learn. In addition, by restructuring the terms and attitudes of the care team, the clinicians not only change themselves, but they also change Miguel from a monster to a mentor and his parents from enemies to fellow humans who are caught in this difficult situation. "What ought to be done?" and "Who decides?" are still practical, and ultimately unavoidable, questions; however, the rancor over the decision is lessened or eliminated because people involved all can recognizably gain from the experience.

In addition, an exceptional ethic would *not* endorse or suggest answers to the questions *a priori*. Either limiting treatment *or* pushing forward aggressively may be acceptable answers (and who decides could be answered variously). What an exceptional ethic would insist on is that 1) Miguel has intrinsic value, and 2) he must be respected as a fellow human. Furthermore, an exceptional ethic would mandate awareness in the medical team that Miguel can potentially teach them about themselves on a level and to a degree at least as profound as they help him. The ethic does not mandate what should be done, but it does color the course of action that is pursued.

CONCLUSION

Ethical inquiry is frequently misunderstood as the pursuit of the "right" answers to tough questions. In addition, medical ethics is often erroneously thought to have started in the 20th century. Instead, ethics represents an area of thought and debate as old as civilization itself that attempts to help people live together more happily and draw deeper meaning from their lives. Contemporary medical ethics in the Western world is frequently dominated by paradigms that emphasize a very limited understanding of personhood that is centered on individual liberties. People with disabilities (especially children and individuals with intellectual disabilities) are poorly served by these systems. An exceptional ethic would change this situation for the better by emphasizing the universality of dependence and the need for vulnerability for growth and full self-actualization. It would mandate respect for all humans and would not seek limits on personhood. This respect, however, would not imply general answers to questions that necessarily depend on contextual details. It should be hopeful and encouraging.

REFERENCES

Aquinas, T. (n.d.). *Summa theological.* I.II.55.1c.

Beauchamp, T.L., & Childress, J.F. (2001). *Principles of biomedical ethics* (5th ed.). New York: Oxford University Press.

Coulter, D.L. (2001). Recognition of spirituality in health care: Personal and universal implications. *Journal of Religion, Disability, and Health, 5,* 1–11.

Coulter, D.L. (2004, June). *Peace-making is the answer to death-making.* Paper presented at the Annual Meeting of the American Association on Mental Retardation, Philadelphia.

Crocker A.C. (1998). Exceptionality. *Developmental and Behavioral Pediatrics, 19*(4), 300–305.

D'Arcy, E. (1987). Natural law. In W. Reich (Ed.), *The encyclopedia of bioethics* (Vol. III, p. 1133). New York: Macmillan.

Keenan, J.F. (1997). Virtue ethics. In B. Hoose (Ed.), *Christian ethics: An introduction* (p. 84). London: Chapman.

McKenny, G.P. (1997). *To relieve the human condition: Bioethics, technology, and the body* (p. 8). Albany: State University of New York Press.

Pellegrino, E.D. (1985). The virtuous physician, and the ethics of medicine. In E.E. Shelp (Ed.), *Virtue and medicine* (pp. 237–255). The Hague, Netherlands: D. Reidel Publishing.

Porter, J. (2001). Virtue ethics. In *The Cambridge companion to Christian ethics* (p. 96). Cambridge, England: Cambridge University Press.

Wolfensberger, W. (1985). An overview of social role valorization and some reflections on elderly mentally retarded persons. In M.P. Janicki & H.M. Wisniewski (Eds.), *Aging and developmental disabilities: Issues and approaches* (pp. 60–72). Baltimore: Paul H. Brookes Publishing Co.

CHAPTER 34

ABUSE AND NEGLECT

Randell Alexander

Abuse may impair an individual's future health and well-being. Individuals who have been abused benefit most from multidisciplinary assessment. In this respect, abuse has a strong resemblance to many other issues involved with working with people with developmental disabilities. In addition to a resemblance of form, there is a strong overlap between the actual abuse of people and developmental disabilities.

This chapter focuses primarily on child abuse as a form of maltreatment that intersects with developmental disabilities. Much more is known about the abuse of children than individuals in other age groups, and much is known about the relationship between developmental disabilities and the abuse of children. Adults, however, may have both developmental disabilities and a history of child abuse—sometimes one being the cause of the other. Both may have lifelong consequences and are too often misunderstood or even missed by some clinicians.

CHILD ABUSE

Child abuse is a widespread public health problem that has been described as a national epidemic (U.S. Advisory Board, 1995). It is a major cause of acquired developmental disabilities, has an extensive impact on pediatric and adult quality of life, and is strongly associated with many of the leading causes of adult disability and death (e.g., smoking, alcoholism, chronic depression, greater than 50 sexual partners, history of sexually transmitted disease, adult rape, intravenous drug use, attempted suicide, severe obesity, physical inactivity, cancer, diabetes, hepatitis), including early death (Felliti et al., 1998). Child abuse occurs probably 2–4 times more frequently than developmental disabilities, has a spectrum of severity, and, as mentioned previously, often benefits from the efforts of a multidisciplinary management team. The effects may last a lifetime.

Definition

Child abuse has a variety of definitions for different professions. Thus, *child abuse* may be defined in one field but not upheld in another. For example, even though a court finds that child abuse has not occurred, the child's medical record may still list the diagnosis of child abuse. Thus, child abuse may be dependent on the different viewpoints of various professions as well as their determination of the situation.

Within the legal arena, child abuse has different definitions in juvenile versus criminal court, and definitions may vary between states. Iowa, for example, is one of the only states to consider exposure to illegal substances to be a form of child abuse (Iowa Code 232.68f). Child abuse statutes historically have been some of the most changeable laws, with frequent changes in reporting procedures, definitions, and agency functioning. Against this backdrop, professionals find it impossible to keep track of each legal particular. In addition, legal definitions of abuse are not the same as a diagnosis by another profession. For example, the medical field may consider a child to have been neglected in contexts where legal sanctions may not apply (e.g., child not wearing a seatbelt; parents smoking around a child with asthma). Thus, a definition of child abuse that is more broadly and universally applicable would be: Any action or lack of action between a child and a caregiver which results in nonaccidental harm to the child's physical, emotional, and/or developmental state. Note that for most child abuse, the emotional and/or developmental consequences are the ones that cause long-term harm.

Types

Child abuse is divided into three main categories: neglect, physical abuse, and sexual abuse. Emotional abuse and emotional neglect are subsumed under neglect unless specifically designated. Cultural considerations influence how child abuse is viewed. For example, in the

1970s, a child suffering injuries because he or she was not restrained in a seatbelt was considered an accident. Now, this situation might be considered neglect. Various cultural medical practices (e.g., coining) may cause an intentional injury and be considered by some to be of no medical value, but they may not be seen as the equivalent of physical abuse.

Statistics

Child abuse is one of the more pervasive conditions of childhood. According to the U.S. Department of Health and Human Services (2003), in 2001 approximately 903,000 children were substantiated as having been abused in the United States. These numbers consist of children reported to child protective services (CPS) and for whom sufficient evidence was found to confirm that abuse occurred. No expert in the field, however, believes that these numbers represent the true occurrence of abuse. For every child reported and substantiated as having been abused, probably 3–5 times as many victims exist about whom nothing is ever heard. For the nearly 1 million children substantiated as having been abused in 2001, however, the primary form of abuse was neglect (57%), followed by physical abuse (19%) and sexual abuse (10%). The rest of the abuse situations fell into minor categories. Of course, some of the victims had multiple forms of abuse. Overall, the rate of child abuse was about 12.4 per 1,000 children per year in the United States.

Besides being the most frequent form of abuse, neglect fatalities are also about equal to physical abuse fatalities. Although "official" estimates of child abuse fatalities typically range around 1,200–1,300 children per year (U.S. Department of Health and Human Services, 2003), the actual rate is estimated to be at least 2,000 per year (U.S. Advisory Board, 1995). The lower numbers are derived from data from the 50 states' CPS systems; however, some children die without CPS involvement, and child death review teams routinely find that CPS numbers are considerable underestimates. Thus, child abuse is among the largest causes of death during early and middle childhood.

Child abuse is also estimated to be responsible for about 18,000 serious disabilities per year (Baladerian, 1991). The emotional and developmental toll is considerable and often not well examined. The cost of child abuse in the United States has been estimated by Prevent Child Abuse America (2001) to be approximately $94 billion annually—probably a conservative estimate.

Child Abuse Leading to Developmental Disabilities

Child abuse affects the brain emotionally and developmentally but may also have a direct physical effect on it. Early experiences with violence can lead to selection of certain hormonal and neurobiological adaptations useful perhaps to the adverse environment but dysfunctional in the normal world (Frank, Klass, Earls, & Eisenberg, 1996; Perry, 1994; Developmental Disabilities Assistance and Bill of Rights Act of 1975 [PL 94-103]). Neglect can lead to deletion of neuronal responses (and likely neurons themselves) for stimuli that are infrequent or not experienced (Alexander, Levitt, & Smith, 2001; National Center on Child Abuse and Neglect, 1993; Westcott, 1991).

Of course, the most direct physical effect is overt brain damage. Abusive head trauma is responsible for about 80% of child abuse deaths; however, many survivors suffer significant brain damage. In an urban cerebral palsy clinic, Diamond and Jaudes (1983) found that 9% of the children had cerebral palsy because of physical abuse, 9% had cerebral palsy before being abused, and in 2% of the cases, it was not possible to say which came first.

At 1½ months of age, Tracy was admitted for focal seizures. Computed tomography (CT) and magnetic resonance imaging (MRI) were normal. Fundoscopic examination was also normal, and she was discharged after 5 days.

Three weeks later, she was admitted to the hospital in cardiorespiratory arrest. The history was that she fed well and seemed "fine" for several days before admission. According to her mother, that morning she suddenly turned blue and quit breathing. No history of trauma was elicited. Tracy was intubated, and her pulse was restored.

Tracy's pupils were fixed and dilated. Numerous bilateral retinal hemorrhages were seen. A lumbar puncture showed bloody fluid that did not clear (subarachnoid bleeding). CT showed acute large subdural hemorrhages in the right fronto-parietal-temporal area. Parietal encephalomalacia apparently reflected a prior event (probably related to the events 3 weeks prior). An MRI the next day showed large bilateral hemorrhages surrounding both cerebral hemispheres and extending into the interhemispheric fissure bilaterally (see Figure 34.1). A head CT conducted 9 days later revealed continued large subdural hemorrhages and considerable cerebral volume loss (see Figure 34.2). The skeletal survey was normal.

Tracy subsequently had placement of a gastrostomy tube and a tracheostomy tube. One year later, she had little purposeful activities, had severe spastic quadriplegia, and continued to have both tubes. Her mother pled guilty to child endangerment.

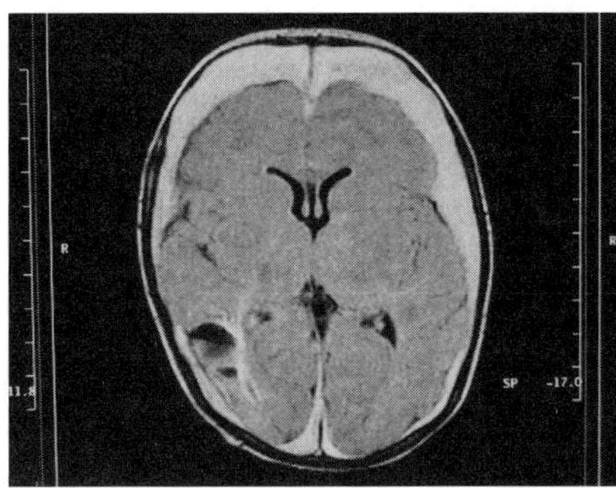

Figure 34.1. Magnetic resonance imaging taken the day after the second admission. Note the large acute subdural hemorrhages in the frontal areas extending around the hemispheres and into the interhemispheric fissure bilaterally. An area of encephalomalacia is seen in the right parieto-occipital area.

Shaken baby syndrome has a death rate of approximately 25% (Alexander et al., 2001). All survivors seem to have at least minimal developmental problems, but most survivors have moderate to severe disabilities (Ewing-Cobbs et al., 1998; Ewing-Cobbs, Prasad, Kramer, & Landry, 1999). For what might appear to be a similar amount of brain damage, shaken baby syndrome typically has a worse developmental outcome. In Tracy's situation, she apparently had been shaken enough to present with seizures 3 weeks prior but not enough to cause sufficient findings to indicate abusive trauma. The shaking episode on the day of her admission was more severe, resulting in medically evident findings and her severe outcomes. With the severity of the brain damage, a child in this condition almost invariably dies of pneumonia within several years (secondary to secretions, lack of a good cough reflex, and general immobility). Such cases are often prosecuted at a later date as murder.

Child death review teams often struggle with deaths secondary to neglect. Not only are such deaths relatively common, but they often elicit different reactions from various professionals on such teams. Some may see a given case as an "accident" while others view it as serious neglect worthy of prosecution. The number of deaths ascribed as neglect therefore is an underestimate of what probably transpires. Child death review teams therefore frequently categorize the degree to which a death is preventable: definitely, possibly, and not realistically preventable.

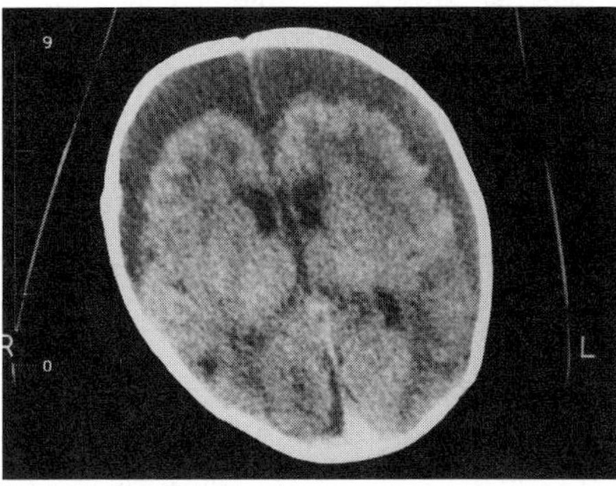

Figure 34.2. Computed tomography taken 9 days later revealed continued large subdural hemorrhages and considerable cerebral volume loss.

Trudy left her 6-month-old boy, Niko, in the bathtub for "just a minute" to go to another room to answer the phone. Upon return, she found Niko face down in the water. He was unresponsive and not breathing. Emergency medical services quickly responded, determined that Niko had a very slow heart rate, and intubated him on the scene.

Upon arrival in the emergency room, Niko had a Glasgow Coma Scale score of 6 (range of 3–15). After a week in the pediatric intensive care unit, he was able to be extubated and transferred to a rehabilitative unit. CT of his head showed large areas of infarcts involving both frontal and parietal lobes. Developmental evaluation 2 years later showed Niko to have moderate spastic quadriplegia and moderate intellectual disabilities.

Although some of the physicians initially thought of this incident as an accident and Trudy as a victim of this tragedy, the case was ultimately reported to CPS. Trudy later pled guilty to misdemeanor child endangerment and received 3 years probation.

Neglect is often more difficult to label as abuse than more overt, deliberate actions. Nevertheless, the consequences are as lethal and devastating as any other form of abuse. In many cultures, the reason for abuse (or a crime) is perceived as important, rather than the abuse considered by itself. Because physical abuse is purposeful (i.e., has an explicit motive), it is often thought to be worse than neglect, which often is not purposeful. Seen from the point of an injured or dead child, such distinctions may not be meaningful.

Other than a physician, a child might not see any professional prior to school enrollment. Therefore, the physician must be alert for signs of developmental problems so that intervention might occur in time to maximize the child's potential. Likewise the physician should be alert for signs of possible physical abuse or neglect so that, if present, interventions can minimize subsequent damage. Unfortunately, the physician may not see the child or be in a position to notice the abuse when it occurs.

A neighbor was concerned about seeing Miles and Randi playing outdoors on a cold November day. The young children wore only tee shirts, had no shoes, and were outside for several hours. CPS was called.

On visiting, CPS determined that Miles and Randi were 2 and 3 years of age and that their mother was the only adult in the home. On questioning, their mother admitted that she had become frustrated with the children's behavior and locked them outside so that she could get some relief.

An inspection of the home revealed 9-month-old Andy in a crib in a darkened room. The house was not only cluttered but filthy. The kitchen sink and counters had numerous dirty dishes with caked-on food that appeared to have been there for days or weeks. Some roaches were observed. The refrigerator contained only a stick of butter, ½ bottle of catsup, and a bottle with some milk that smelled sour. Several cans of food were found in a cupboard, but no formula was in the house.

CPS staff had difficulty walking from one room to another because of piles of clothes, boxes, and debris on the floor. A very strong odor came from the bathroom, where there was a filthy toilet that did not flush. All three children were noted to have black dirt under their fingernails and a strong odor.

The children were examined in the medical clinic. Andy had dry, somewhat brittle hair. He was below the 5th percentile for weight for height (i.e., failure to thrive), was hypotonic, and had poor eye contact. He could not yet roll over from back to front or sit. Review of birth records showed that he was 7 lb at birth and had a normal examination. This examination was the last medical encounter he had. Miles reported that his mother left Andy alone in the crib all day and did not take him out.

Records showed that both parents were high school graduates in regular classes. Developmental testing shortly after foster care placement showed Andy to be functioning at the 2-month-old level on all domains. Testing 6 months later showed some catch-up, but Andy's standard scores on cognitive and motoric testing remained around 60. Speech and language was the greatest delay with later testing at 4 years of age.

Miles and Randi had lesser delays initially and had only a few smaller delays at long-term follow-up. Their mother apparently had an exacerbation of her bipolar disorder after the birth of Andy, and her care for her children seriously deteriorated thereafter. Medical and developmental specialists concluded that Andy had suffered such severe lack of stimulation that brain development was compromised as a result. Some of the damage was permanent.

Animal studies and human experience (e.g., Romanian orphanages) have repeatedly shown that lack of calories and sensory and motor stimulation can have permanent consequences (Alexander et al., 2001; Kerr, Black, & Krishnakumar, 2000; National Center on Child Abuse and Neglect, 1993). Although children with failure to thrive can sometimes make a good recovery (Kessel, Tal, Jaffe, & Even, 1996), in Andy's case, the plasticity of his brain to compensate for lesser deprivations was exceeded. All children removed to foster care should receive a thorough developmental evaluation as the incidence of developmental disabilities is relatively high. In situations such as Andy's, developmental testing shortly after foster care and then repeated several months later may show "catch-up growth" in development further documenting the impact of the neglect on the child.

Child Abuse in Children with Disabilities

Children with developmental disabilities are at higher risk of child abuse and neglect (Sullivan, Brookhouser, Knutson, Scanlan, & Schulte, 1991; Westcott, 1991). The National Center on Child Abuse and Neglect (1993) found an approximate two-fold increase in the risk of child maltreatment in children with disabilities compared with those without disabilities. The degree of extra risk, however, is not certain because the definitions of child abuse and developmental disabilities in various studies may vary. Thus, the exact percentages may not be as important as the general trend and the mechanisms that underlie it.

For example, children with physical disabilities may spend more time with a caregiver. This situation alone increases the probability of abuse. In addition, some disabilities require extra attention or work that may be beyond the willingness of the caregiver. Some children with swallowing dysfunctions (e.g., with some degree of cerebral palsy) require extra time for oral feedings. For a child who needs 30 minutes to consume sufficient calories, a caregiver with a 10-minute attention span for feeding may be a serious mismatch.

Some cases of failure to thrive in this context are not so much due to deliberate neglect, but rather due to a parent who is not up to the task. Yet the effect on the child is the same. Having to change a diaper past the age when most children are toilet trained, having a child with irritable personalities secondary to a particular condition or syndrome, caring for a child with significant cognitive impairments, and the presence of other differences in a child might prove stressful in a susceptible parent who then physically abuses or neglects a child in one form or another. Perpetrators may have the perception that children with communication problems are less likely to tell that they have been abused or are less likely to be believed if they do tell.

An aide who had tended regularly to a 12-year-old girl, Stephanie, with spastic quadriplegic cerebral palsy, profound intellectual disabilities, and few verbalizations, was under investigation of possible sexual abuse in an institutional setting. No meaningful interview of Stephanie was possible. Given Stephanie's spasticity, physical unattractiveness, and unpleasing personality, some of the investigators initially believed that it was virtually unlikely that anyone would have sex with her. Forensic genital examination by a child abuse pediatrician, however, revealed sperm in her vagina.

Stereotypes of who might be the perpetrator or victim of any form of abuse are unsupported by data and are dangerous assumptions. Even in children who have good verbal skills, the lack of a history is not evidence that something did not occur. Children with developmental disabilities may prove frustrating to a caregiver, and caregivers may be tempted to give the child too much medication (chemical restraint), engage in ever-increasing punishment, or to learn to ignore a child in need of basic needs.

A 9-year-old girl, Mackenzie, had myelomeningocele and required a wheelchair for ambulation. She had mild intellectual disabilities and considerable behavior problems, including unpredictable aggression. She attended a fourth-grade inclusive classroom. Classroom problems arose periodically when other children walked by Mackenzie and were punched, hit, or bitten without any apparent provocation. Mackenzie's inappropriate yelling and cursing were also problematic.

Subsequently, Mackenzie's wheelchair was anchored in place, and other desks were moved outside of her "range." Her verbalizations continued to be disruptive. The teacher began to use "time-outs"—moving Mackenzie behind a screen in the back of the room when disruptions occurred. About 4 months later, the teacher was reported for abuse.

Review of the extensive logs kept by the teacher showed that initially the time-outs lasted for 5 minutes and occurred about once a day. Over weeks to months, the length of the timeouts gradually progressed from 5 minutes to 15 minutes to 30 minutes and eventually to several hours. Mackenzie was moved from behind the screen to a small, empty room in the back. At the end, she spent essentially the whole day in the back room without supervision, with no catheterization, and sitting in soiled and wet clothes.

Neglect was substantiated. The teacher had been regarded as one of the best in the system but was suspended pending completion of a remedial plan to intensively complete an internship and educational program in developmental disabilities and to understand how a person might progressively slide into such abusive patterns.

Gradual acquiescence and participation in ever-increasing punishments is a very common human experience. Neglect often starts slowly. Because it is often gradual, it may be difficult to recognize. In the same way that pilots must sometimes rely on their instruments and not their senses (which are susceptible to gradual distortions of direction and rotation), people working with individuals with disabilities must use written instruments and peer review to maintain best practice in disciplinary situations. Group homes and residential institutions use protocols and peer review in an attempt to avoid abusive practices, such as overuse of restraint, locked rooms, and medicines in doses that are unduly chemically restraining. Physicians and other professionals must be careful that in their management of children with disabilities, they do not endorse physical abuse or neglect of the children by their parents (Ryan, Salbenblatt, Schiappacasse, & Maly, 2001).

Medical Conditions that May Be Misunderstood

Children with developmental disabilities sometimes have characteristics that confuse caregivers and some professionals not familiar with the conditions. This situation may be especially true for children with syndromes that may cause stereotyped physical or behavioral traits.

Jae-eun was born at normal birth weight. She fed poorly in the nursery but was sent home with her mother. On subsequent well-child checkups, Jae-eun was noted to be a poor feeder and to be steadily dropping percentiles by only gaining weight very slowly. The physician instructed Jae-eun's mother on how to prepare a higher caloric formula. Nevertheless, Jae-eun's weight gain was poor. Her mother was seemingly resistant to medical suggestions, and her compliance was suspected to be poor. At the 6 month visit, Jae-eun weighed only 11 lb—considerably below the 5th percentile.

The case was reported to CPS, and Jae-eun was hospitalized. During the hospitalization, Jae-eun's weight gain continued to be poor. Hypotonia was noticed, and Neurology was consulted. The neurologist clinically diagnosed Prader-Willi syndrome, and Genetics confirmed the diagnosis. Jae-eun was returned home to her parents with specialized feedings and experienced improved weight gain thereafter. Her CPS case was closed.

Children with Prader-Willi syndrome are born with significant hypotonia that is also reflected as poor feeding. Most children with Prader-Willi syndrome require some form of supplemental feeding assistance (e.g., nasogastric tube feedings) in the first few months of life (see Chapter 9.4). This poor feeding can lead to failure to thrive despite the best efforts of the parents. Physicians must monitor a child's weight, make efforts to ensure proper caloric intake, and hospitalize a child who does not gain sufficiently to determine what the problem is. Although some parents of a child with Prader-Willi syndrome may be neglectful, most simply have difficulty with feeding that transcends normal resources and techniques. In Jae-eun's case, her mother's attitude was presumed to be the issue, and the correct diagnosis was perhaps delayed.

Management of a child with a particular syndrome should mean that the professional understands any associated behaviors and conditions that might affect interactions. Lack of knowledge or misunderstanding opens the possibility of occasionally serious mistreatment.

Buck, a 16-year-old boy with Prader-Willi syndrome, had moderate intellectual disabilities and a short attention span. He weighed about 300 lb. Family and physicians found him to be usually happy and easygoing. He only rarely had behavior problems (consisting of moderate tantrums—usually about food or change of routine). Within the last school year, however, two episodes of concern occurred with one of the school's teachers.

The first occurred when the teacher attempted to take some food away from Buck at lunchtime. Buck grabbed the teacher's wrist as he attempted (unsuccessfully) to take his food back away from her. The second episode occurred about a month later when the teacher was angry with Buck for failing to comply with a demand that she made for him to perform a task. She stood inches away from his face and pointed her finger "in his face." He grabbed her arm and pushed it away from him. The teacher did not suffer injuries with either of the episodes. About 3 months later, the teacher brought charges of assault against Buck. The case is currently pending.

Individuals with Prader-Willi syndrome have a seemingly insatiable appetite—presumably based on a hypothalamic dysfunction. Coupled with behavioral characteristics that include stubbornness and irritability when someone intrudes too closely and is bossy, Buck's reaction was completely predictable. His attempt to protect his food and to have the teacher back off was misinterpreted as offensive initiatives. By her actions, the teacher actually caused emotional harm to Buck.

A series of complaints in a school for the deaf resulted in an external investigation. The complaints alleged that children were receiving bruises at the hands of the staff. All of the children were interviewed separately with the help of sign language interpreters not connected with the school. Staff members were interviewed, and records were reviewed.

Some bruises were recorded, consisting primarily of grab marks, but a few involved the face or other parts of the body. Some were caused by the staff, but some were caused by fellow students. No other significant injuries were found. Investigation revealed that staff and students would sometimes engage in animated conversation on nonpunitive topics. Without the ability to hear, someone not looking or walking away would not know that he or she was being summoned without being grabbed. In addition, some instances involved hand gesticulation with sign language that inadvertently resulted in another party being hit. Ultimately, none of the instances were judged to be abusive.

An understanding of the nature of sign language, the need to get a person's attention when he or she is not looking, and the occasional "excitability" of communication may occasionally lead to some inadvertent and minor bumps. Such situations should be evaluated to be sure that abusive intent was not an issue. Some physicians refer to "inflicted injuries" when they mean "abusive injuries"—this case demonstrates the limitations with the term *inflicted*, which may not be an abusive act.

Evaluating physical injuries in the context of child abuse usually means considering the effect of the child's age. Thus, infants younger than 6 months of age rarely have bruises because they are not developmentally capable enough to sustain sufficient self-induced accidental forces. A 3-year-old, however, typically has bruises on surfaces with underlying bone (e.g., shin) from running into objects in the environment. Yet, if the 3-year-old has a developmental disability such that he or she is not ambulatory, bruises might not be expected. Thus, chronological age is a proxy, but developmental age and abilities are the true keys to the nature of how many injuries should be interpreted.

Seventeen-year-old Craig was admitted to a developmental disabilities inpatient unit for further evaluation of seizures, feeding problems, and for a decubitus ulcer. He had severe cerebral palsy (spastic quadriplegia) and profound intellectual disabilities. Craig was transported in a wheelchair but could not operate it himself, even with intensive adaptations. He had a gastrostomy tube for feeding and spent most of his time lying in a bed, requiring essentially total nursing care.

During one shift, a nurse reported that he was lifting Craig to turn him over and both felt and heard his femur snap. Hospital authorities were contacted, including the child abuse pediatrician. X-rays were taken of the leg and other bones (skeletal survey). No other injuries were seen; however, the review with the pediatric radiologist showed the bones to be "washed out"—a degree of osteopenia not seen unless there has been considerable bone loss. A number of laboratory studies (e.g., renal studies) were conducted but were unrevealing as to any issue about the fracture.

The child abuse pediatritian concluded that Craig had an advanced degree of osteopenia secondary to extreme disuse and that his bones were secondarily fragile. No abuse was felt to have occurred. Normal handling represented a risk for further fractures. Additional precautions were subsequently taken with his care, and his nursing home was advised.

Investigating the origin of an unexpected injury is reasonable. In Craig's situation, a careful review of the circumstances and an understanding of the dynamics of bone loss in children who do not ambulate led to the determination that the staff member was not abusive or negligent. Had this situation involved a 3-year-old with a similar condition, residual prenatal contribution to bone formation would have made such a pathologic fracture unlikely.

Other Considerations

Children with intellectual disabilities at times may be more impulsive and socially "dis-inhibited." Although this behavior often is accompanied by friendliness, sometimes children may express sexually inappropriate behaviors, creating a challenge for community service providers. In one survey of 243 community agencies who provided services to individuals with developmental disabilities, the most common types of offensive behaviors were seen in public situations, in situations that inappropriately involved others, and in situations that involved minors (Ward, Trigler, & Pfeiffer, 2001). Such behaviors could also be viewed as sexually abusive or as reflecting a child who is exhibiting such behaviors as a consequence of having been sexually abused. Distinguishing between these possibilities and developing the skills and resources to appropriately manage such issues is a difficult challenge.

Interviewing children with developmental disabilities can at times be difficult. Child Advocacy Centers are specialized sites (in more than 400 communities) in which forensic interviewing by specially trained social workers or psychologists aids police and CPS in the determination as to whether abuse, especially sexual abuse, occurred. These centers are also a starting point for the provision of further counseling for those in need. For those children with serious cognitive or language impairments, such interviewing can be difficult and may be greatly assisted with the help of a developmental specialist.

Out-of-Home Care

When a family is overwhelmed with intensive care of their child, one option in some communities is temporary respite care. A study of respite care for children with developmental disabilities in Iowa revealed a significant decrease in Parenting Stress Index scores after participation (Cowen & Reed, 2002). It was found that the occurrence of child abuse was significantly related to the life stress, social support, and service level during the period of enrollment. Adequate respite care in a community is one option to help prevent child abuse.

Child abuse is a major reason that children enter into foster care. To enter foster care, requires juvenile court (or its equivalent) to find that the child is so significantly abused or at risk that continued placement in the home is unacceptable. Thus, many children have already accumulated significant adverse experiences prior to foster care, and many of these children have developmental disabilities (American Academy of Pediatrics, 2000). Earlier identification of those at developmental risk would be valuable, but the legal system is rarely sophisticated enough to accommodate this.

Children entering foster care are vulnerable to poor health including acute and chronic illnesses, mental health problems, growth and developmental problems, and difficulty obtaining services (Kools & Kennedy 2003). Multiple foster care placements often aggravate these issues. The American Academy of Pediatrics (2000) recommended that foster children receive comprehensive assessment and periodic reassessment by pediatricians and child development specialists, yet this assessment is uncommon. One reason is lack of expertise; another is limited resources.

A study by Giardino, Hudson, and Marsh (2003) illustrated the difficulties faced in service provision. This study was conducted in an Abuse Referral Clinic for Children with Disabilities to determine the outcome of children receiving complete outpatient evaluations. The children's special needs spanned a wide range of behavioral, physical, and developmental/cognitive conditions. After the evaluations, 18% of the children were determined to be abused, 13% were at high risk, 25% were at low risk of abuse, and 44% were not abused. The billing collection rate was 14% for an average reimbursement of $38 per child. Of the 25 cases that were referred for outpatient mental health counseling, only 48% had complied. Thus, medical reimbursement is poor, mental health services were frequently recommended but often not used, and the family compliance was overall poor.

Against this backdrop, it is not surprising that children who have been abused or are entering the foster care system do not receive services that might make a substantial difference in their lives. The result, even more so in the many instances where such a specialized clinic does not exist, is that children with disabilities who have been abused receive substandard management. The system of care seems to perpetuate harm to the children.

ADULT ABUSE

In comparison with child abuse, little is known about the relationship between adult abuse and developmental disabilities. Although extrapolation from childhood may lead to a conclusion that an adult with disabilities is at higher risk of abuse by another person, outside of examples within abusive institutions little has been done to study this possibility. Further extrapolation may suggest that some cases of adult abuse may cause disabilities. Although undoubtedly true for individual cases (e.g., a beating with brain damage), no known systematic study exists to show the extent or characteristics of this relationship.

Some laws deal with the abuse of dependent adults, defined as people older than 18 years who must rely on others to meet some of their basic needs (e.g., physical, financial). An example may include an adult with quadriplegia who depends on others to turn him frequently in his bed to avoid bed sores. Failure to do so exposes the adult to risk of improper healing, sepsis, or death. In addition to neglect of those with disabilities (e.g., as occurs in some nursing homes), physical abuse is likely vastly underreported.

A similar problem presents itself with older adults with disabilities related to medical conditions or with extreme age. Their vulnerability (financial problems, physical inability to resist) may by coupled with a frequent legal need that the person must actually pursue charges. (In contrast, a child with injuries has no legal standing about whether charges are pressed.) An immense opportunity presents itself to future researchers to learn more about the complex interactions between family members in this age range.

Abuse of adults may also be an extension of abuse that began at an earlier time. Not only teenagers, but young adults sometimes continue to be physically and sexually abused by parents. The possible relationship of disabilities to these behaviors has not been carefully studied. In turn, sometimes families are seen in whom older adults suffer from physical abuse by their grown progeny—the same individuals who, when they were children, were beaten by the parents. Sometimes men do not physically fare as well with age as their wives—and some wife abusers are beaten in their old age by the very women they used to abuse. Although these examples of retribution may be understandable, they are fundamentally as wrong as the original abuse and have as their basis the notion that someone stronger or with less disability than another may then act abusively.

CONCLUSION

Child abuse and developmental disabilities are intimately related both as cause and effect for each other. Each is often a complex condition that benefits from specialized, multidisciplinary diagnosis and management. Specialists in developmental disabilities and in child abuse can also help to prevent situations where lack of understanding of the child's condition or the suspected abuse can lead to erroneous conclusions or treatment. More widespread centers of expertise and better reimbursement are vital in achieving progress with these tragic and often preventable conditions.

Although research involving child abuse and developmental disabilities should be accelerated, an even larger gap in knowledge exists with adult abuse and disabilities. Extrapolation of concepts learned about children may be very useful, but it is reasonable that there may be differences with adults who have been abused and have disabilities. Only when the entire spectrum of a person's life is carefully examined will the consequences of abuse and developmental disabilities be clearly understood and the means to mitigate them be most apparent.

REFERENCES

Alexander, R., Levitt, C., & Smith, W. (2001). Abusive head trauma. In R. Reece & S. Ludwig (Eds.), *Child abuse: Medical diagnosis and management* (2nd ed.). Philadelphia: Lippincott, Williams & Wilkins.

American Academy of Pediatrics, Committee on Early Childhood, Adoption and Dependent Care. (2000). Developmental issues for young children in foster care. *Pediatrics, 106*, 1145–1150.

Baladerian, N.J. (1991). *Abuse causes disabilities: Disability and the family.* Culver City, CA: SPECTRUM Institute.

Cowen, P., & Reed, D. (2002). Effects of respite care for children with developmental disabilities: Evaluation of an intervention for at risk families. *Public Health Nursing, 19*, 272–283.

Developmental Disabilities Assistance and Bill of Rights Act of 1975, PL 94-103, 100 Stat. 840, 42 U.S.C. §§ 6000 *et seq.*

Diamond, L.I., & Jaudes, P.K. (1983). Child abuse in a cerebral-palsied population. *Developmental Medicine and Child Neurology, 25*, 169–174.

Ewing-Cobbs, L., Kramer, L., Prasad, M., Canales, D., Louis, P., Fletcher, J., et al. (1998). Neuroimaging, physical, and developmental findings after inflicted and noninflicted traumatic brain injury in young children. *Pediatrics, 102*, 300–307.

Ewing-Cobbs, L., Prasad, M., Kramer, L., & Landry, S. (1999). Inflicted traumatic brain injury: Relationship of developmental outcome to severity of injury. *Pediatric Neurosurgery, 31*, 251–258.

Felitti, V.J., Anda, R.F., Nordenberg, D., Williamson, D.F., Spitz, A.M., Edwards, V., et al. (1998). Relationship of childhood abuse and household dysfunction to many of the leading causes of death in adults. *American Journal of Preventive Medicine, 14*(4), 245–253.

Frank, D., Klass, P., Earls, F., & Eisenberg, L. (1996). Infants and young children in orphanages: One view from pediatrics and child psychiatry. *Pediatrics, 97*, 569–578.

Giardino, A., Hudson, K., & Marsh, J. (2003). Providing medical evaluations for possible child maltreatment to children with special health care needs. *Child Abuse & Neglect, 27*, 1179–1186.

Kerr, M., Black, M., & Krishnakumar, A. (2000). Failure-to-thrive, maltreatment and the behavior and development of 6-year-old children from low-income, urban families: A cumulative risk model. *Child Abuse & Neglect, 24*, 587–598.

Kessel, A., Tal, Y., Jaffe, M., & Even, L. (1996). Reversible brain atrophy and reversible developmental retardation in a malnourished infant. *Israel Journal of Medical Sciences, 32*, 306–308.

Kools, S., & Kennedy, C. (2003). Foster child health and development: Implications for primary care. *Pediatric Nursing, 29*, 39–41, 44–46.

National Center on Child Abuse and Neglect. (NCCAN). (1993). *A report on the maltreatment of children with disabilities.* National Clearinghouse on Child Abuse and Neglect Information, Administration for Children and Families, U.S. Department of Health and Human Services (Westat/James Bell Associates, Contract No. 105-89-1630).

Perry, B. (1994). *Neurobiological sequelae of childhood trauma: Post-traumatic stress disorders in children.* Washington, DC: American Psychiatric Press.

Prevent Child Abuse America. (2001). *Total estimated cost of child abuse and neglect in the United States: Statistical evidence.* Retrieved from http://www.preventchildabuse.org/learn_more/research_docs/cost_analysis.pdf.

Ryan, R., Salbenblatt, J., Schiappacasse, J., & Maly, B. (2001). Physician unwitting participation in abuse and neglect of person with developmental disabilities. *Community Mental Health Journal, 37*, 499–509.

Sullivan, P., Brookhouser, P., Knutson, J., Scanlan, J., & Schulte, L. (1991). Patterns of physical and sexual abuse of communicatively handicapped children. *Annals of Otology, Rhinology & Laryngology, 100*, 188–194.

U.S. Advisory Board on Child Abuse and Neglect. (1995). *A nation's shame: Fatal child abuse and neglect in the United States.* Washington, DC: U.S. Department of Health and Human Services.

U.S. Department of Health and Human Services. (2003). *Child Maltreatment 2001.* Washington, DC: Author.

Ward, K., Trigler, J., & Pfeiffer, K. (2001). Community services, issues, and service gaps for individuals with developmental disabilities who exhibit inappropriate sexual behaviors. *Mental Retardation, 39*, 11–19.

Westcott, H. (1991). The abuse of disabled children: A review of the literature. *Child: Care, Health and Development, 17*, 243–258.

CHAPTER 35

UTILIZATION, COST, AND FINANCING

Arnold Birenbaum and Herbert J. Cohen

This chapter analyzes the utilization, expenditures, and financing of health care for individuals with developmental disabilities throughout their life span. At the onset of life, families of children born at biological risk or with established developmental disabilities are subject to multiple hazards. Financing children's medical care is a significant stress for families and part of an array of major pressures, such as consequent interpersonal and family distress, informational requirements about chronic illness and disability, and threats to parental confidence in their ability to solve current and future child-related problems (Guralnick, 1997).

These family stresses are compounded by a rapidly changing health care system. The promotion of managed care during the 1990s has generated concerns among policy makers and health services researchers, as well as parents, that families of children with special health care needs may not be able to gain access to specialty care. In a national survey, investigators found that more than one third of children with autism, more than one fifth of children with intellectual disabilities, and more than one fifth of children with other disorders had problems obtaining needed care from specialty physicians. Getting referrals from primary care physicians and locating specialists with the appropriate experience were some of the difficulties cited by parents (Krauss, Gulley, Sciegaj, & Wells, 2003).

This chapter explores what is known about the relationship among utilization, expenditures, and financing of health care for individuals with developmental disabilities. The use of reliable and accurate data from national data sets, where possible, helps to determine whether access to health services is available and to make recommendations for adequate and equitable financing of these services. As with the population of the United States in general, access to care for people with developmental disabilities is affected by the availability of insurance coverage. Similarly, individuals who have become eligible for Medicaid or Medicare, by virtue of their disabilities, pay far less out-of-pocket than those who are privately insured or who are among the uninsured. Individuals with multiple secondary conditions are far more expensive to care for than individuals with single developmental disabilities.

The absence of health insurance can have a deep impact on people with disabilities. The struggle to obtain health care at a time when care has become very expensive has been shown to affect these individuals in several ways. According to the 1998 Harris survey of 1,000 adults with disabilities, which was conducted for the National Organization on Disability, one in four adults postponed getting health care that they thought they needed in the past year because they could not afford it; one in three had no insurance benefits that would pay for special equipment, therapies, or medicine; and almost one in five could not get covered by commercial health insurance because they had a disability or preexisting condition. Lack of insurance also can have an impact on institutions that furnish uncompensated care to those with the most severe disabilities. The existing payment system has made no provisions to deal with these most expensive consumers of hospital care. Furthermore, medical and hospital providers alike are rarely able to make up for losses incurred in caring for these individuals by cross-funding from the well insured.

A particular problem in providing care is the financial loss that threatens the continued existence of academic medical centers. Consider the reports in the *Boston Globe* in March and April 2001, by Kowalczyk and Barnard respectively, regarding the extraordinary financial deficits incurred by Boston Children's Hospital for certain admitted individuals for whose care public insurers furnish poor compensation. The 965 out-of-state children sent to this famous tertiary care facility, one that often deals with the most medically complex cases, led to losses of $4 million in 2000. One New Hampshire baby alone, born with severe birth defects that include blindness, deafness, intellectual disabilities, heart deformities, and gastrointestinal abnormalities, cost Children's Hospital $79,450 because the Granite State's Medicaid reimbursement was not sufficient to cover the costs of hospital services (Kowalczyk, 2001). In another high-maintenance situation, while the Commonwealth of Massachusetts sought a residential school placement for a 15-year-old with intellectual disabilities, his 10-month stay at Children's Hospital cost $619,451. Because most of the care for this adolescent was not regarded as medically necessary, Massachusetts Medicaid did not pay for most of the hospital stay.

Physicians in private practice face similar threats to their financial solvency. Insured individuals have always helped to cross-fund the uncompensated care given to individuals without insurance and those who cannot afford to pay the usual and customary fees established by providers. As states face severe deficits, legislatures and governors retain fee schedules for Medicaid patients that were established years ago, uncorrected for inflation; or lawmakers refuse to pay for "optional" services, such as physical therapy, which many people with disabilities depend on to maintain functioning.

Consequently, physicians in fee-for-service practices are pressed not to depend too heavily on Medicaid patients to generate income. Medicare is a better payer than Medicaid because it is closer to the usual and customary fees established by consensus among physicians in a particular locality; however, Medicare participation requires physicians to accept discounted payments for services rendered, although they are never at rates as low as those found in Medicaid. In addition, the managed care plans that enroll most commercially insured Americans have touched more than 90% of private practice physicians. The Center for Studying Health Systems Change found that doctors averaged 13.1 managed care plan contracts in 2001 (Strunk & Reschovsky, 2002). Managed care plans, when seeking cost effectiveness, may trade access to "covered lives" (as enrollees are designated) in exchange for physician acceptance of discounted fees.

Discounting means that private-practice physicians need to see more individuals per day to meet their expenses and support themselves. In managed care arrangements, individuals who take a great deal of time to examine, as is the case with many people with developmental disabilities, may mean that fewer individuals can be seen in any given day. Physicians may limit the number of people with disabilities they include in their patient panel.

The plight of tertiary care institutions and physicians in private practice, such as those affected by the kinds of dilemmas depicted previously, is discouraging for many families with relatives with developmental disabilities. Although most hospital admissions for people with developmental disabilities or office-based procedures do not require costly services, a persistent concern among health care policy experts is the lifelong financing problems of families with members with serious chronic illness or disability. Ongoing policy debates on the cost of care for people with disabilities, the impact of managed care on service delivery to these individuals, and the appropriate roles of private and public insurance in paying for their health care have generated few remedies for financially burdened individuals and their families (Birenbaum & Cohen, 1993).

Despite the lack of progress since the 1990s in arriving at affordable mechanisms for equitable financing for the health care of people with developmental disabilities, there is some promise that these problems will be addressed. The 2001 Surgeon General's Conference on Health Disparities and Mental Retardation renewed interest in improving the organization, delivery, and financing of health services to individuals with developmental disabilities (Office of the Surgeon General, 2002). Accurate data collection and careful estimates of costs are needed. The results of such research will provide health care financing information in support of family-centered, community-based, comprehensive care. With good estimates of utilization of services throughout the life span, state and federal lawmakers can more fully understand the potential benefits from private insurance reforms and public programs.

A lack of baseline data on utilization, expenditures, and financing reflects the general fragmentation found in the world of health care. Too often, the data available come from studies performed at service locales (e.g., clinics, hospitals) rather than from probability sampling for the entire population. Clinicians learn about those who get care more than about those who do not have access to such care. They learn about the problems of those who are easy to reach—the conveniently sampled—rather than from data that includes the full range of problems of a representative sample of people with developmental disabilities. Funded by the federal government, national health utilization and expenditure surveys apply probability sampling to create an opportunity to capture an accurate picture of the entire population. In other words, every household has an equal chance of being randomly selected for participation.

1994–1995 NATIONAL HEALTH INTERVIEW DISABILITY SUPPLEMENT

Population-based information is developed from household surveys where questions can be asked pertaining to service use, costs, and financing. In the 1994–1995 National Health Interview Survey (NHIS) (Larson, Lakin, Anderson, Kwak, & Lee, 2000), a unique 2-year supplement was administered to collect data on individuals with disabilities who were not living in institutionals.

This disability supplement (NHIS-D) collected data that described the demographic characteristics of these individuals, their health status, functional limitations, and supports and services. This monumental endeavor has produced, and continues to produce, reports on utilization of services by individuals with disabilities.

An elaborate screening scheme was part of the disability supplement. What follows is a very abbreviated version of what took place during the household interview. People with intellectual disabilities were found in several ways: 1) by direct identification by a household member that someone with intellectual disabilities resided there; 2) by indirect inference, as when a household member noted that intellectual disabilities was a cause of an age-specific activity limitation for another household member (e.g., placement in special education classes); or 3) when this condition was mentioned in the interview as a cause of limited functioning (e.g., getting along with others).

Medical classification was also utilized to identify people with intellectual disabilities. If an International Classification of Disease (ICD) code for mental retardation was the reason for a doctor's visit or the receipt of related services, such as occupational therapy, then the designation of intellectual disabilities was applied to that individual. In addition, when an individual was reported to have a condition frequently associated with intellectual disabilities—autism, cerebral palsy, Down syndrome, spina bifida, hydrocephalus, or other related conditions—then a follow-up question concerning significant functional limitations in learning was asked.

In the supplement to the NHIS, developmental disabilities were identified through a multistaged process involving the seven areas of functional limitation found in the federal developmental disabilities definition (See PL 95-602, sec. 102[7]). These areas included significant limitations in: 1) self-care, 2) expressive or receptive language, 3) learning, 4) mobility, 5) self-direction, 6) capacity for independent living, and 7) economic self-sufficiency. A detailed discussion of the process of developing these measures of intellectual and developmental disabilities can be found in Larson et al. (2000).

The research team from the University of Minnesota generated a number of important findings. In the 2-year sample period, 3,076 individuals with intellectual or other developmental disabilities were identified out of a total survey of 48,000 households. Larson, Lakin, Anderson, and Kwak (2001) estimated that, based on this sample, 3,887,158 individuals with intellectual and/or developmental disabilities lived in households, or 1.49% of the population of the United States. The true number of individuals with intellectual and developmental disabilities cannot be known without a costly and unaffordable enumeration of every household by survey teams that would administer the disability supplement as a screening tool along with the regular NHIS. Therefore, this estimate has a statistical error rate that is small and acceptable.

Although most philosophies of rehabilitation and habilitation encourage and promote independence, productivity, and inclusion, adults as well as children with intellectual and developmental disabilities live with relatives at a rate two times greater than people without these conditions (Larson et al., 2001). Functional limitations were, by definition, found frequently in the intellectual and developmental disabilities sample for those older than age 18 in economic self-sufficiency and independent living, whereas learning and self-direction were limited for disproportionately large numbers of children as well as adults. Language limitations, mobility, and personal care limitations were also evident in the intellectual and developmental disabilities sample.

Health care needs, based on self-reporting on health status, were an extensive population-based problem for individuals with intellectual and developmental disabilities. Sample members with intellectual and developmental disabilities, or their proxies, reported being in fair or poor health 24.5% of the time, as compared with 9.8% of the respondents without intellectual and developmental disabilities in the NHIS.

> Only 42% of people with MR/DD [mental retardation and/or developmental disabilities] (or their proxies) reported that their health was very good or excellent, while 67% of the sample without mental retardation and/or developmental disabilities reported having very good or excellent health. (Larson et al., 2001, p. 3)

As can be seen in Table 35.1, Medicaid participation by the subsample of individuals with intellectual and developmental disabilities was strong—these individuals were nine times more likely to be receiving Medicaid support than the comparative population.[1] Medicaid eligibility is extended in most states when a child or an adult is deemed eligible for Supplemental Security Income (SSI), an income support program for individuals designated as unable to support themselves temporarily or permanently due to disability (Lakin, Polister, Prouty, & Smith, 2001).

The data from the NHIS Disability Supplement allowed the University of Minnesota research team to de-

[1]Population estimates require that the standard error of estimate be established. Larson, Laken, Anderson, and Kwak (2001) presented the standard error as the relative standard error (RSE). As the authors state, "The RSE was computed by dividing the standard error of estimate by the population estimate and multiplying the result by 100. Since the NHIS-D is a survey administered to a sample of people from the population rather than to every person in the U.S., we can only estimate the true number in the population with a particular characteristic" (2001, p. 2).

Table 35.1. Self-reported health status and services for the U.S. noninstitutionalized population

Characteristic	People with ID/DD			Percent people without ID/DD	Chi square
	Est. pop.	RSE	Percent		
Self-reported health status					
Excellent	810,760	4.6%	21.2%	38.0%	502.52**
Very good	797,143	4.8%	20.8%	29.2%	
Good	1,283,506	3.5%	33.5%	23.1%	
Fair	588,580	5.2%	15.4%	7.1%	
Poor	349,548	7.0%	9.1%	2.7%	
Participation in government health programs					
Medicaid	1,550,987	3.9%	45.6%	8.8%	563.82**
Medicare	479,245	6.7%	14.0%	12.8%	3.17
Both Medicare and Medicaid	223,813	9.8%	6.6%	1.0%	76.94**
Mental health (for adults)					
Uses psychotropic medication	406,231	6.8%	10.5%	2.4%	138.04**

Key: *p < .05; ** p < .01; Chi square = a measure of statistical significance; Est. pop. = estimated population; ID/DD = intellectual and developmental disabilities; RSE = relative standard error.

From Larson, S., Lakin, C., Anderson, L., & Kwak, N. (2001). Characteristics and services used by persons with MR/DD living in their own homes or with family members: NHIS-D analysis. *MR/DD Data Brief, 3*(1), 3; reprinted by permission.

termine whether people with intellectual and/or developmental disabilities were greater users of in-hospital services during the 12-month period of observation and had more doctor visits during a 2-week look-back period than people without these diagnoses. As can be seen in Table 35.2, people with intellectual and/or developmental disabilities in the sample had more short-term hospital episode days per capita than the comparison group. In particular, the percentage of people with these diagnoses who had 3- to 5-day hospital stays was far greater than among those without a diagnosis of intellectual and/or developmental disabilities (Anderson, 2002).

Overall, use of mental health services in a 12-month period for people 18 and older with intellectual and developmental disabilities was also greater than for people without disabilities. Although the difference be-

Table 35.2. Number of short-stay hospital episode days in the last year, excluding delivery, and number of doctor visits in previous 2 weeks reported in the 1994–1995 National Health Interview Survey for people with and without intellectual and developmental disabilities

	People with ID/DD			People without ID/DD			
	Est. pop	Percent	RSE	Est. pop.	Percent	RSE	X^2
Number of days in hospital							82.59**
None	3,433,388	88.33%	2.53%	240,953,658	93.80%	0.96%	
1–2	384,480	9.89%	6.11%	14,790,579	5.76%	1.26%	
3–5	55,721	1.43%	16.13%	1,049,995	0.41%	3.78%	
6–10	7,193	0.19%	##	71,720	0.03%	13.72%	
11+	6,378	0.16%	##	9,906	0.00%	##	
Total	3,887,158			256,875,857			
Number of doctor visits							139.95**
None	2,853,190	73.40%	2.76%	218,254,837	84.97%	0.96%	
1–2	860,678	22.14%	4.70%	34,708,433	13.51%	1.16%	
3–5	123,363	3.17%	12.99%	3,102,408	1.21%	2.48%	
6–10	33,090	0.85%	20.19%	685,660	0.27%	5.22%	
11+	16,838	0.43%	30.34%	124,520	0.05%	11.00%	
Total	3,887,158			256,875,857			

Key: ** p > 0.01; ## = RSE greater than 30%; Est. pop. = estimated population; ID/DD = intellectual and developmental disabilities; RSE = relative standard error.

Source: Anderson, Larson, Lakin, and Kwak (2003).

tween the two samples regarding inpatient admissions was not statistically significant, the following comparisons showed statistically significant differences and found people with intellectual and developmental disabilities using more services than the comparison sample in terms of: 1) number of nights spent in inpatient care; 2) any outpatient mental health care; 3) months of outpatient care; 4) total outpatient visits; and 5) regularity of visits to a psychiatrist (Anderson, 2002; see Table 35.3 for exact differences). An additional mental health finding, found in Table 35.1, shows that adults with intellectual disabilities are 2.5 times more likely to use psychotropic medications than people without intellectual disabilities.

FINANCING HEALTH CARE FOR SEVERE DEVELOPMENTAL DISABILITIES

Prior to the use of NHIS-D, it was very difficult to use census data to identify individuals with intellectual and/or developmental disabilities. Therefore, an analysis of how income might affect access to services for a particular disorder (e.g., cerebral palsy) was not possible. Even the highly regarded NHIS-D might not generate samples of sufficient size for different categories of disability to do appropriate analyses on utilization, cost, and financing. Still, national surveys do have the quality of *representativeness*—a characteristic missing from single site specialty clinic studies with

Table 35.3. Mental health services in the past 12 months of noninstitutionalized people 18 and older with or without intellectual and/or developmental disabilities from the 1994–1995 National Health Interview Survey, Disability Followback Survey

	People with ID/DD		People without ID/DD		
	Est. pop.	Percent	Est. pop	Percent	X^2
Inpatient admissions					NS
1–2	1,539,438	98.7%	40,160,167	99.8%	
3–5	9,730	0.6%	46,924	0.1%	
6–10	1,363	0.1%	4,787	0.0%	
11+	9,121	0.6%	10,312	0.0%	
Total	1,559,652		40,222,189		
Number of nights spent in inpatient care					10.97**
1–2	1,504,768	96.5%	39,798,154	98.9%	
3–5	6,716	0.4%	67,176	0.2%	
6–10	6,334	0.4%	91,408	0.2%	
11+	41,874	2.7%	265,452	0.7%	
Total	1,559,692		40,222,189		
Any outpatient mental health care					24.06**
Yes	246,445	16.3%	2,937,004	7.5%	
No	1,262,111	83.7%	36,147,597	92.5%	
Total	1,508,555		39,084,601		
Months of outpatient care					25.80**
1–2	1,334,241	85.5%	37,857,781	94.1%	
3–5	63,098	4.0%	876,645	2.2%	
6+	162,313	10.4%	1,487,764	3.7%	
Total	1,559,652		40,222,189		
Outpatient visits					25.52**
1–2	1,330,216	85.3%	37,718,619	93.8%	
3–5	42,448	2.7%	582,128	1.4%	
6–10	31,569	2.0%	427,488	1.1%	
11+	155,420	10.0%	1,493,955	3.7%	
Total	1,559,652		40,222,189		
Regularly sees psychiatrist					39.84**
Yes	198,028	32.8%	1,686,034	9.7%	
No	406,202	67.2%	15,614,186	90.3%	
Total	604,230		17,300,219		

** $p < 0.01$; Est. pop. = estimated population; ID/DD = intellectual and developmental disabilities; NS = not statistically significant.
Source: Larson, Lakin, Anderson, and Kwak (2001).

the unrepresentative, albeit highly convenient, samples for study.

To compensate for the weaknesses of these two approaches, the authors, along with Dorothy Guyot (Birenbaum, Guyot, & Cohen, 1990), conducted a national study of health care costs, utilization, and financing of individuals with severe developmental disabilities. With Special Project of Regional and National Significance (SPRANS) funding from the Maternal and Child Health Bureau (MCH-B) more than 17 years ago, and with supplemental funds from the Administration on Developmental Disabilities and the National Institute on Mental Health, this goal was accomplished through data collection at 12 community sites in every region of the United States, for children, adolescents, and young adults with autism or severe intellectual disabilities. This multisite study is still being cited in the literature on costs, utilization, and financing of health services for individuals with severe disabilities and is considered a model for learning directly about this subject.

What follows is a brief report of this 4-year national study on health care for people with developmentally disabilities. The 1985–1986 data collected from 308 children and young adults younger than age 25 with autism and from 326 with severe or profound intellectual disabilities produced some interesting findings and contrasts concerning cost of medical and health care, financing, and utilization of these services. Space limitations do not permit further discussion of the elaborate methodology used to assure a representative sample by virtue of a national data gathering effort. The logic of this procedure is still valid because large, randomly drawn national samples now generate adequate samples of individuals with disabilities, as previously discussed, but may not generate adequate samples of individuals with low-prevalence conditions (e.g., muscular dystrophy).

The selection of sites for data gathering was guided by information on state Medicaid generosity, mean income of families, percentage of families with private insurance, and number of physicians relative to the size of the population. Although this data was not a probability sample, the study avoided the pitfalls found in using convenience samples drawn from individuals at specialized outpatient health care facilities. To find families eligible for the study, a wider net was cast, using the census of children in need of special education in 11 school districts in 9 states. Table 35.4 presents the locations and their characteristics where data collection took place.

The findings regarding annual physician visits and hospital discharges were compared with national data from the 1980 National Medical Care Utilization and Expenditure Study, the 1986 NHIS, and the 1987 National Medical Expenditure Survey. An individual's annual number of physician visits is defined as the sum of all visits to physicians' offices, hospital outpatient departments, and emergency rooms. Children and young adults with autism visited physicians, on average, about 4 times per year, about the same as the national average of 3.6 visits for those from birth through age 24. By contrast, children and young adults with severe intellectual disabilities averaged about 9 visits per year.

Two thirds of the children with severe intellectual disabilities had physical impairments, which accounted for their high visit levels. Note that preschool children went to hospital clinics, where specialists were avail-

Table 35.4. Data collection sites in terms of the four criteria for stratifying the sampling frame

Site	Family income	Generous Medicaid	Private insurance	Number of physicians
Morris County, NJ	High	High	High	High
Wayne County, MI, excluding Detroit	High	High	High	Low
Suffolk County, NY	High	High	Low	—
Jefferson County, AL, excluding Birmingham	High	Low	—	High
Eleven counties in central Iowa	High	Low	—	Low
Detroit, MI	Low	High	High	—
Fresno City, CA	Low	High	Low	High
Fresno County, CA	Low	High	Low	Low
Dallas, TX, and Birmingham, AL	Low	Low	—	High
Jacksonville, FL	Low	Low	Low	Low

From Birenbaum, A., Guyot, D., and Cohen, H.J. (1990). *Health care financing for severe developmental disabilities* (Monograph 14, p. 13). Washington, DC: American Association on Mental Retardation; reprinted by permission.

able, at about five times the average rate, but went to physicians' offices at about twice the rate. The ability to walk half a mile was associated with low use of medical services, and, in contrast, high users did not have this ability.

The annual number of short-term hospital stays is a standard measure of health care utilization. Not only may hospitalization indicate the presence of a serious medical condition in the child, but also it is the major health care expenditure for American children despite its rare occurrence. The children in this study who lived at home were more frequent users of in-hospital care than the average child. Ten percent of the children with autism in the 5–17 age group were hospitalized during the year, compared with 3% of all children. Another measure of hospital use is based on the frequency of hospital discharges per 1,000 people in the population. The discharge rate in 1986 for all American children ages 5–17 was 38 per 1,000 children, but for children with autism, it was about 100 per 1,000 children, and for children with severe intellectual disabilities, it was about 400 per 1,000 children, due to the high incidence of secondary conditions.

Some characteristics that predict health care use in the population at large also hold true for children with disabilities. The mother's educational attainment predicts higher use of preventive and habilitative care and lower use of emergency room services. African American children were less likely to receive medical attention than Caucasian children. Lack of insurance predicted lower health care usage.

Information on utilization and costs were provided by parents in telephone interviews. The information received was checked, where possible, against the records of health care providers and insurers. The following dollar amounts are corrected for inflation and represent 2003 dollars, derived from the Consumer Price Index created by the Department of Labor. Nevertheless, some important findings generated at that time are still relevant to discussions about how payment is made for services for these individuals. The highlights with regard to expenditures are:

- None of the children had expenditures in excess of \$86,000, and very few reached \$48,000.
- The average annual expenditure for children with autism was about \$1,720 and about \$2,941 for young adults, compared with the \$716 average cost at that time for all American children. Children with autism received an average of four physician visits annually, slightly above the average for children in the general population. Hospitalization accounted for one third the health care expenditures among children with autism, but for two thirds among young adults with the disorder.
- For children and young adults with severe intellectual disabilities, the average expenditure on health care was about \$6,880, due to physical impairments in two thirds of the children. Children averaged about 12 physician visits annually, whereas individuals older than 18 averaged 8 visits. Children were hospitalized about eight times the national rate for all children, and for young adults, the rate was about twice that of their age peers.
- For people with autism and people with intellectual disabilities, preventive or habilitative services were of little use, and, consequently, these services were a tiny fraction of health care expenditures. For individuals whose primary physicians judged that they would benefit from physical or speech therapy, less than one quarter were receiving these services. This frequency included services from day programs to promote habilitation or activities of daily living and public school programs.
- Inequities abounded in the financing of health care. Almost 20% of the parents of children with severe or profound intellectual disabilities and 10% of the parents of children with autism had experienced refusals or limitations in the health insurance that they could buy for their child. In both disability groups, about 15% of those with private insurance had policies that specifically excluded coverage for some of the child's health care, usually due to preexisting condition stipulations, a limitation on claims still found today.
- Because the individuals with autism in this study were from families with higher incomes than were those with intellectual disabilities, they were twice as likely to be privately insured.
- Seven percent of the children with autism and 4% of those with severe or profound intellectual disabilities surveyed had no health insurance. The percentage of the uninsured who did not visit a physician in the 12-month study period was three times higher than for insured individuals.
- Only 60% of all children had routine dental examinations within the 12-month study period, a worse record than the average American child.
- Income differences between the two groups of families are dramatically revealed when out-of-pocket

expenses are compared. For children with autism, the average out-of-pocket expenses for health and personal care was almost $1,720, about 3% of family income, but about 2% of families had expenses greater than 15% of their income. Families with a child with severe or profound intellectual disabilities typically spent almost $3,440 out-of-pocket, an average of 7% of their income, but as many as 10% spent more than 15% of their total income. Medical debts more than $3,440 were held by 1% of the families with children with autism and 5% of the families with children with severe or profound intellectual disabilities.

Although these data reflect the health system of 1986–1987, with greater dependency on inpatient and less ambulatory care than exists today, people with disabilities continue to be more likely to use inpatient care than other sectors of the population (see Walsh, Kastner, and Criscione, 1997). Moreover, because they were and still are often enrolled in Medicaid, an insurance program with few restrictions on access to hospital admissions and lengths of stay, they may have been attractive to providers. Despite these dynamics related to different financing, families of members with severe disabilities still complain of difficulties in obtaining care and receiving coverage for complex and expensive procedures. A focus group of parents of adults with severe developmental disabilities conducted in 1995 found that health maintenance organizations were particularly unwilling to pay for specialists outside of the plan and for some kinds of durable medical equipment (Birenbaum, 1999).

DISABILITY AND UTILIZATION OF HEALTH CARE SERVICES

To what extent do the findings on utilization of health care services for people with developmental disabilities mirror the trends found among all people with disabilities? The population of the United States, for analytic purposes, can be divided into those with disabilities and those without. Furthermore, amongst the population with intellectual and developmental disabilities, it is important to determine the prevalence of secondary conditions and their costs by comparing individuals with intellectual and/or developmental disabilities with and without such additional conditions.

The resettling of individuals with developmental disabilities from residential facilities to various forms of community living (e.g., group homes, apartment living) spurred a number of research efforts to determine what the additional onus on the health care system might be if individuals who formerly lived in institutions would be receiving their health care in the community. Ziring and his colleagues (1988) concluded that it would be erroneous to assume that the generic health care system could meet all of the health care needs of individuals transferred from state residential facilities to the community.

Although no prospective studies of the impact of deinstitutionalization on the health care system followed this prediction of an overload of demand for services, a number of studies have assessed the health care needs of people with developmental disabilities and have determined that these individuals have a greater number and variety of health care needs than the average population of the same gender and age. Beange, McElduff, and Baker (1995) reported in a population study in Sydney, Australia, of medical disorders of adults with intellectual disabilities that the rates of utilization of services were higher than for the general population. They found that in comparison to randomly selected adults between the ages of 20 and 50 years, a similar age group of individuals with developmental disabilities had significantly increased cardiovascular risk factors, rates of medical consultation, rates of hospitalization, and mortality. The research sample had a mean of 5.4 medical disorders per person, only half of which had been detected before this medical assessment.

Epilepsy is one of the comorbid conditions found to be disproportionately more frequent among people with developmental disabilities. It also adds to the cost of medical care. Burke and his colleagues (1999) found that among individuals with developmental disabilities living in institutions, epilepsy was a significant contributor to additional medical costs. Retrospective measures of costs, using two separate methods of attribution, on 50 people with epilepsy in a population living in a residential facility and 50 without epilepsy living in the same facility found that costs attributed to epilepsy were between $825 and $918 for a 6-month period. According to Burke et al., "The following categories accounted for cost: personnel (47%), drugs (40%), hospitalizations (9%), and laboratories/procedures (4%)" (1999, p. 148).

The cost and utilization of services has been studied by Walsh and Kastner and their associates, using data derived from New Jersey through a commercial health care data management firm that tracks all hospitalizations in that state. In comparison with people without disabilities, the acute care hospitalizations during alternate years between 1983 and 1991 for people with developmental disabilities showed increases in admissions (56%) and hospital days (42%) (Walsh et al.,

1997). Total hospital charges for people with developmental disabilities increased by 206%—a rate that was twice that for people without disabilities who were hospitalized. They also found that a relatively small number of individuals hospitalized accounted for most of the hospital days used and charges incurred. Care coordination services did reduce hospital admissions and length of stay for individuals with developmental disabilities who were followed prospectively in this study.

Care coordination was also found to offset costs for individuals seen at the Developmental Disabilities Center at Morristown Memorial Hospital in New Jersey. With this service in place at the annual average cost of $668 for care coordination for people with severe intellectual disabilities, the designers of this project were able to demonstrate not only that the health care of individuals in the program was improved, but also that fewer resources (i.e., hospital days) were required to provide optimal care (Criscione, Kastner, O'Brien, & Nathanson, 1994).

The data from the NHIS of 1989 were analyzed by LaPlante, Rice, and Wenger (1995) to determine if people with a limitation in activity due to chronic illness or impairment, a way of defining disability, are more likely to see physicians than those not limited in activity. They also wanted to determine if insurance coverage increased physician contacts. Disability and/or the lack of insurance coverage are powerful predictors of physician use.

Adults who are unable to perform their major activity (paid work or keeping house), contact their physicians more than 20 times a year. By contrast, people who are not limited in their major activity have 3.9 contacts a year. Lack of insurance coverage also affects physician contacts. Uninsured adults unable to perform their major activity have 25% fewer physician contacts than those with insurance—15.6 versus 20.9 contacts. Among adults not limited in activity, physician contacts are 47% fewer for those without insurance than for those with insurance—2.3 versus 3.9 contacts (LaPlante et al., 1995).

Similar results were found when hospital stays were compared among those with and without limits in activities and for those with and without health insurance. Note that these findings were compiled before managed care enrolled many Americans. Although it is likely that *uninsurance*, a term introduced by the Institute of Medicine (2002), will fuel the same lower utilization rates today as they did in 1989, research needs to be done to see whether individuals with limitations in activities who are in managed care plans have as many physician contacts as in the past or as many hospital stays.

Restrictions in activity are often associated with two or more disabling conditions. In a subsequent analysis of 1992 NHIS data, Trupin and Rice found that "People with multiple disabling conditions have poorer health and use more medical services than those with only one condition" (1995, p. 1). Furthermore, the average number of bed-disability days more than doubles for those reporting two or more conditions as compared with those individuals reporting only one condition.

Medicaid and Medicare cover half of all the medical expenditures for people with disabilities. Trupin, Rice, and Max, using data from the 1989 NHIS, found that "Public programs account for 37 percent of medical expenditures for adults aged 18 to 64 with disabilities, as compared to 11 percent for those without" (1995, p. 3). Although out-of-pocket expenditures account for a lower proportion of all medical expenditures for people with disabilities than for those without, people with disabilities spend out-of-pocket more than twice the dollar amounts of those without disabilities. This amount is especially noteworthy because those with limitations in activities are more likely to be at lower income levels than those without limitations in activities (McNeil, 1997, 1998).

The previous discussion noted that people with disabilities are heavy users of medical services and that they often demand access to care when it is denied. Advocacy organizations that are disability related, including The Arc and United Cerebral Palsy, have been at the forefront of efforts to gain coverage for services. Moreover, providers of special educational services, vocational rehabilitation and training, personal assistance, independent living centers, group homes, and health care tailored to people with disabilities also find it important to locate and sustain financial support for their activities. Moreover, corporations that produce durable medical equipment and supplies that assist individuals with disabilities to perform various functions of daily living are enthusiastic about increasing access to services and appliances. Skeptics have suggested that, although independence and productivity might be the goals for each individual, these producers and providers are more interested in stable markets for their products, services, and interventions (Albrecht, 1992).

DIFFERENCES IN UTILIZATION OF SERVICES AMONG CHILDREN

Studies of children with disabilities and/or with chronic conditions that require extra attention are good sources of information about the disproportionate need for health services. An epidemiologic profile of children with special health care needs used a new definition of these individuals to analyze the data available from the 1994 NHIS-D. This definition included children with chronic physical, developmental, behavioral, and emotional conditions, as well as those who also used health or related services beyond those ordinarily used by children (Newacheck et al., 1998).

The researchers analyzed the 1994 NHIS-completed interviews with parents responsible for more than 30,000 children younger than age 18. When compared with all children combined and children without special health needs, children with special health care needs had a higher rate of use of health services, as measured according to the number of physician contacts annually, percent hospitalized, and the average annual hospital days per 1,000 children. This population not only used health services more than the comparison groups but were also more likely to have bed days due to illness and higher rates of school absence also due to illness, as can be seen in Table 35.5.

Not all children with special health care needs had equal access to services or had all their health care needs met. Newacheck and his colleagues (1998) also found that children from low-income families who were uninsured had lower access to services than children with public or private insurance. Compared with their insured counterparts, they were four times as likely not to have a usual source of care (22% vs. 5%); had about half as many physician contacts as all children with insurance per year (5 vs. 11 contacts); and were almost three times more likely to have unmet health needs as insured children with special health care needs.

Data collected for administrative purposes also allows for expenditure analyses. Using 1992 Medicaid claims data from California, Georgia, Michigan, and Tennessee, Kuhlthau and her colleagues (1998) compared expenditures for children who were supported by the SSI program with other Medicaid eligible children. Despite the fact that the SSI sample contained children with relatively severe mental health, physical, or developmental disabilities, the sample had relatively modest Medicaid expenditures. Among those within the study population who were SSI eligible and had high expenditures, some children had several chronic comorbidities (hence, the following percentages are expressed as ranges): 15%–26% were children with intellectual disabilities; 17%–29% were children with epilepsy; 21%–38% were children with cerebral palsy; 5%–13% were children with congenital anomalies of the nervous system; 6%–12% were children with muscular disorders (e.g., muscular dystrophies); and 8%–19% were children with spina bifida. The children with the high expenditures were more likely to use hospital and long-term care, accounting for more than half of the mean expenditures. Among the high users, a small proportion accounted for a very large part of the Medicaid expenditures.

The data collected by states supply researchers with a substantial data set for analysis to determine expenditures. In one study of 310,997 children from the state of Washington that was led by Ireys (Ireys, Anderson, Shafferr, & Neff, 1997), 18,233 had one of eight conditions (e.g., cerebral palsy, muscular dystrophy, spina bifida) that were regarded as potentially expensive. Medicaid claims data from 1993, analyzed by Ireys and his colleagues to calculate expenditures compare children with one of eight selected chronic health conditions. Average expenditures for these children with special health care needs were $3,800 per child compared with $955 for all Medicaid-enrolled children. Mean payments associated with the selected conditions ranged from 2.5 to 20 times more than payments for all children. Approximately 10% of children accounted for approximately 70% of the payments in general and in each diagnostic grouping.

Table 35.5. Utilization of health services and health status for children with special health care needs in the United States in 1994

Health status			
Average annual bed days due to illness	2.8	6.1	2.0
Average annual school Absences due to illness	3.6	7.4	2.0
Use of health services			
Average annual physician contacts	3.3	6.4	2.6
Percent hospitalized in past year	3.1	7.4	2.2
Average annual hospital days per 100 children	225.0	691.0	122.0

OUT-OF-POCKET EXPENSES

Children and adults with developmental disabilities may also be underinsured as well as uninsured. The degree to which families spend out-of-pocket was noted in the summary of the national study of health care financing for children with severe developmental disabilities conducted by Birenbaum, Guyot, and Cohen (1990). More recent national surveys of parents confirmed these results. Private insurance often places annual or lifetime caps on the amounts paid out to beneficiaries for various services, and because of the frequency of usage of services, families of children with special health care needs may also, even when insured, spend more on co-payments, deductibles, and premiums.

Krauss and her colleagues (2000) found that more than 20% of the parents in their national survey of families of children with special health care needs paid more than $3,000 per year out-of-pocket for services that were not insured. More than half of the families reported severe financial impacts resulting from their child's health needs, and families with commercial insurance were more likely to report these burdens than families who were eligible for Medicaid. Among those with a commercial policy, more than 40% of the families had a "wrap around" coverage from secondary insurers, primarily based on Medicaid eligibility because of excessive medical expenses.

FAMILY COSTS BEYOND HEALTH SERVICES

As was seen in the beginning of this chapter through the 1994 NHIS-D data, no matter what their age, the vast majority of children and adults with developmental disabilities live with their families. The broad range of services that they require are more likely to be paid for by Medicaid and Medicare than by private insurance. The shift to public insurance makes rehabilitation services more accessible than in private commercial insurance policies; however, some gaps still exist in coverage that even public insurance will not address because it may involve subsidizing families to furnish direct care to their dependent family members. In the monograph *Health Care Financing for Severe Developmental Disabilities*, Birebaum, Guyot, and Cohen (1990) answered the following questions because they had implications for understanding whether family support would be cost effective:

- How much do parents spend on babysitting, home modification, and other services and adaptations when a child with severe developmental disabilities lives at home?
- How do these total amounts compare with the cost of providing 24-hour-a-day care for children with severe intellectual disabilities or autism living in residential facilities?
- Are total amounts different or are they the same as the costs accrued for individuals with severe intellectual disabilities and autism?
- What do parents give up (opportunity costs) when they provide in-home care?

A tabulation accounted for all out-of-pocket expenses for each family who maintained children with these severe disabilities at home. Included were expenses to modify and repair homes; modify or acquire vehicles that could accommodate a wheelchair; and procure additional child care services, including special summer camp programs.

Parents reported whether their children age 10–24 years could take care of themselves at home alone. According to the respondents, only one third of the 308 members of the study population with autism could take care of themselves, even for a few minutes. Among individuals with severe and profound intellectual disabilities, less than one fifth could take care of themselves. Only one fourth of these 10- to 24-year olds received regular care from someone outside the household—about half from a relative who contributed the service. Among those who had help in child care, the lowest 25% used less than 6 hours per week and the highest 25% used more than 40 hours per week.

Opportunity costs, among other things, are earnings that were not achieved because parents were busy taking care of a child with severe disabilities. These losses were dramatically illustrated with comparisons between the employment status of mothers whose children with severe intellectual disabilities lived in residential placement and mothers whose children lived at home. Almost 80% of the mothers whose children lived in residential care were employed part time (one fourth) or full time (three fourths) whereas only 50% of mothers whose children lived at home held a job.

For mothers of children with developmentally disabilities living in residential care, the proportion working full time was about 40%, not far below the national average. The indirect costs in income of the children's chronic disabilities due to the mothers' foregoing work were substantial. These differences in income were likely to have promoted serious consequences for families. In a study specific to low-income single mothers, Wolfe and Hill (1995) reported that the presence of children with disabilities in the family discouraged working. (See Chapter 5 for a discussion of the psychosocial consequences of disability, particularly the impact of developmental disabilities on family life.)

Since the 1980s, some community alternatives to institutional placement have become available. Family support can come in innovative forms, including care-at-home, fueled by the Medicaid Waiver program, discussed later, that is available throughout the life span of individuals with developmental disabilities. Although long-term care is less health-oriented than residential in character, one of these new programs, funded by Medicaid—Home and Community-Based Services—deserves special discussion as a way of supporting family and community living.

HOME AND COMMUNITY-BASED SERVICES

As a part of the Omnibus Budget Reconciliation Act of 1981 (PL 97-35), the Home and Community-Based Services (HCBS) Waiver Program was conceived, through the provision of less-costly alternatives, as a way of containing the increasing costs of institutional care paid for from federal revenues. The funding authority for this program came from the Social Security Act Amendments of 1981 (PL 95-123) wherein states could receive Medicaid matching funds to provide HCBS Waivers to individuals who otherwise would receive care in a hospital, nursing home, or intermediate care facility. What is truly unique about this program was permission by the Center on Medicare & Medicaid Services (CMS) to state Medicaid programs to allow them to pay for clinically appropriate nonmedical services, including case management; home modification; homemaker/health aide services; personal care services; and adult day health, habilitation, and respite care. Other services, subject to approval by CMS could be requested by states because they are needed by HCBS Waiver participants to avoid being placed in a medical facility (e.g., nonmedical transportation, in-home support services, special communication services, minor home modifications, adult day care).

The original purpose of the HCBS Waiver program was to dampen the demand for intermediate care facilities placements by making other, more affordable community-based services available to low-income individuals with chronic disabilities and illnesses. The creators of the program also recognized that many individuals at risk of being placed in long-term care facilities could be cared for in their homes and communities, preserving their independence and ties to family and friends at a cost no higher than that of institutional care. Indeed, in fiscal year 2000, approximately 35% of the recipients of HCBS Waivers, mostly adults, lived in the homes of their families, and an additional 16% lived in their own homes and received personal assistance, supervision, and support (Lakin et al., 2001).

Under the HCBS Waiver program, the U.S. Department of Health and Human Services allows states to finance community services through Medicaid for people with developmental disabilities who would otherwise typically be in intermediate care facilities (Castellani, 1987). Designed to divert the flow of individuals from the community into expensive intermediate care facility programs, the HCBS Waiver programs were operating in 48 states by 1992 (Smith & Gettings, 1992). By 1991, $1.7 billion was spent on this program, with 65% of the total going for care of individuals with intellectual disabilities (Miller, 1992). By 1995, all 50 states were participating in the HCBS Waiver program, and, as reported by Lakin and colleagues, "between June 30, 1999 and June 30, 2000 HCBS [Waiver] recipients increased by 11.1% (or 29,173) to 291,003 individuals" (2001, p. 100). Accompanying this increase in individuals served by this program was a dramatic decrease in the number of individuals in large intermediate care facilities.

The HCBS Waiver accounts for only a small percentage of total expenditure on community services in the United States, but it grew rapidly during the 1980s, making it the largest source of federal funds for community services by 1994. The program promotes individualized service options and family supports, administered by the state intellectual and developmental disabilities agency through direct payments to service providers. Included among these services are habilitation services, respite care, family counseling, equipment to promote adaptation or safety, architectural adaptation of the home, in-home training, education, behavior management, and recreational services (Braddock & Fujiura, 1991).

The program does not provide complete support for an individual living in the community. Medicaid law does not allow HCBS Waivers to finance the cost of room and board, usually a cost met by HCBS Waiver recipients through SSI. Consequently, because of this prohibition and some other factors, the expenditures on a per capita basis for individuals receiving HCBS Waivers in the states, compared with residents of intermediate care facilities, are very modest.

HCBS do not come cheap, even when they are less expensive than intermediate care facility services. Fiscal year 2000 expenditures for Medicaid waiver services for individuals with developmental disabilities were $9.644 billion. The mean expenditure per recipient of HCBS Waivers was $33,141 in fiscal year 2000. Still, the program may yield substantial benefits and savings. Aside from keeping people with intellectual and developmental disabilities out of institutional care and in more normalizing settings, the program may also offset other costs such as health care in the form of hospital admissions and lengthy stays.

Similar results may be found when at-risk children who receive early intervention services are compared prospectively with those who do not receive them when it comes to health care resource utilization and expenditures. Unfortunately, at this point in time, there is no cost-benefit analysis for early intervention that has verified this possible outcome. Nor is it likely in the foreseeable future because it would be against the law to deny early intervention services to any eligible child. Therefore, no comparison study of early intervention versus no services is possible.

POLICY IMPLICATIONS AND RECOMMENDATIONS

Some important policy implications are derived from this chapter's summary of utilization, expenditures, and financing. First, most studies point to the fact that a small percentage of people with developmental disabilities account for most of the health care expenditures. This fact is particularly true for children. Managed care plans in the commercial sector and Medicaid are reluctant to take the risk for high-maintenance individuals with developmental disabilities because they are unsure of what the costs will be to them. Transportation expenses alone to receive care and therapies could be costly, if these are required as part of a managed care plan. Comprehensive studies on large populations, using sampling techniques that insure that every appropriate individual has an equal chance to be in the study are required to make accurate risk-adjustment calculations so that insurers will include these expensive individuals, or states may have to reinsure these plans or create a financial pool from all existing managed care plans to handle these rare but expensive individuals.

Second, the health care requirements for children, adolescents, and adults with developmental disabilities should be viewed broadly in order to include personal care, family support, and transportation needs. A healthy, typically developing 5-year-old may only require an annual medical checkup. A 15-year-old boy with spina bifida, however, may need corrective surgery, physical therapy, the installation of a home elevator, a special vehicle for transportation, and a sitter who can perform clean intermittent catheterization. We believe that it is appropriate to regard all of these services as health care related because, in the absence of a health condition, none of them would be necessary for the 15-year-old. Coverage for these special circumstances should be part of all comprehensive insurance policies. Case management should also be covered to permit coordination of the whole gamut of necessary care.

Third, financing should promote family-centered care. The family should be regarded as the unit for receiving services. The tendency of Americans in the 21st century to look at individuals without seeing them as members of families results in a distorted view. Specifically, believing that excellent services have been supplied to a child with severe intellectual and physical disabilities because he or she receives appropriate schooling when family members obtain no assistance in bearing the physical, mental, emotional, economic, and social responsibilities for the child's care is unrealistic. When parents are empowered, they should be able to call on services to assist them in keeping their son or daughter with disabilities in their home beyond childhood. The natural desire of parents to nurture their children during their growing years should be especially encouraged for children whose progress is measured in centimeters. Whenever families decide that they can no longer furnish care in the home, the transition to a residential placement should be facilitated. Therefore, comprehensive insurance coverage should provide for more than traditional medical care.

Fourth, financing and organizing of family supports and subsidies should be administratively simple. Long-term care needs should be included in comprehensive thinking about children with severe developmental disabilities. Just as fresh thinking about long-term care for older adults includes new ways to expand home care, so thinking about children with chronic conditions should include many varieties of child care and family services. Medicaid eligibility rules deem that the family income belongs to the child during the first month, but thereafter, only the child's own income and assets, typically nil, share in the payment. The paradox of this situation is that home care is cost effective from a societal perspective but costly to family members because they must either find the free caregivers among relatives or pay the entire bill themselves. If a single source were to pay for both long-term residential care and for its substitutes, then the payer would have monetary incentive to provide a range of child care, home care, day programs, and respite services as alternatives to residential care. This recommendation fits the national trend of toward reducing the number of young adults entering institutions.

Fifth, Medicaid has been expanded to increase the use of HCBS. Medicaid waivers have been a flexible, but complicated, method for states to obtain permission from the CMS to use federal funds for services provided outside of institutions. For people covered by a HCBS Waiver, the state has two freedoms: 1) to provide specific services not included in the mandatory or optional state services, and 2) to decline to provide those services to others served by Medicaid. The CMS has preferred not to issue new HCBS Waivers but to encourage states to use their options flexibly. In many states, HCBS Waivers are difficult to obtain.

Sixth, financial support for families is a necessity because of all of the care that families provide. Support for unpaid caregivers comes in three forms: tax credits or deductions (the federal government child and dependent care tax credit); direct payments to family members (the Michigan program of family support); and direct services to the unpaid provider (ranging from training to respite). Families may also gain eligibility for a child with developmental disabilities through a certification process for SSI.

Tax breaks are always unobtrusive and often inequitable but easy to administer. The long-standing federal tax deduction for individuals who are blind may need to be expanded to those with severe hearing loss, for example. The federal dependent care income tax credit, which applies to all children younger than age 15 and to spouses with disabilities, may need to apply to older children with disabilities and frail elderly relatives.

Family financial support programs have the merit that they give families flexibility to meet their needs as they define them. An impressive example is the Michigan family support program for children younger than 18. Families of children with severe intellectual disabilities, children with intellectual and physical disabilities, or children with autism are eligible for a subsidy of $225 per month as long as the family income is less than $60,000. The program started in 1984 and now supports more than 3,000 families. The initial hope that a substantial number of families would bring their children younger than 18 home from residential placement proved to be false. Only 60 children have returned home (Wayne State University, 2002). Most likely, other forms of community placements were found for those people with developmental disabilities who were once in residential care (e.g., foster family care, apartment living, group homes). Nevertheless, the fundamental reason to mount such programs remains unchallenged—they improve existing family life, even when they fail at promoting reintegration.

CONCLUSION

The current focus on achieving independence for people with disabilities neglects the members of their households. The people who share a household with a person with a serious disability are laden with cares beyond those of most people. If public policy addressed the immediate family as the unit that needs services due to a member's disability, then respite services and other family supports would be common, rather than the rarity we found them to be. Empowerment of people with disabilities cannot ignore those who provide day-to-day care. Therefore, society must find an expanded mechanism to assist families to shoulder their special burden.

REFERENCES

Albrecht, G.A. (1992). *The disability business: Rehabilitation in America* (Vol. 190). Newbury Park, CA: Sage Library of Social Research.

Anderson, L. (2002). *Analyses of the 1994–1995 National Health Interview Survey Disability Supplement.* Unpublished data from the Research and Training Center on Community Living, University of Minnesota.

Anderson, L., Larson, S.L., Lakin, K.C., & Kwak, N. (2003). Health insurance coverage and health care experiences of persons with disabilities in the NHIS-D. *MD/DD Data Brief, 5*(1), 13–14.

Barnard, A. (2001, April 24). A costly wait for special ed. *Boston Globe*, pp. A1, A12.

Beange, H., McElduff, A., & Baker, W. (1995). Medical disorders of adults with mental retardation: A population study. *American Journal on Mental Retardation, 99*, 595–604.

Birenbaum, A. (1999). *Disability and managed care: Problems and opportunities at the end of the century.* Westport, CT: Praeger Publishers.

Birenbaum, A., & Cohen, H.J. (1993, April). On the importance of helping families: Policy implications from a national study. *Mental Retardation, 31*(2), 67–74.

Birenbaum, A., Guyot, D., & Cohen, H.J. (1990). *Health care financing for severe developmental disabilities: Monograph 14.* Washington, DC: American Association on Mental Retardation.

Braddock, D., & Fujiura, G. (1991). Politics, public policy and the development of community mental retardation services in the United States. *American Journal on Mental Retardation, 95*(4), 369–387.

Burke, T.A., McKee, J.R., Pathak, D.S., Donahue, R.M.J., Parsuraman, T.V., & Batenhorst, A.S. (1999). Cost of epilepsy in an intermediate care facility for persons with mental retardation. *American Journal on Mental Retardation, 104*(2), 148–157.

Castellani, P. (1987). *The political economy of developmental disabilities.* Baltimore: Paul H. Brookes Publishing Co.

Congressional Budget Office. (1988). *Estimated costs and provisions of H.R. 3454 and H.R. 5233: Staff working paper.* Washington, DC: Congress of the United States.

Criscione, T., Kastner, T.A., O'Brien, D., & Nathanson, R. (1994, February). Replication of a managed health care initiative for people with mental retardation living in the community. *Mental Retardation, 32*(1), 43–52.

Guralnick, M.J. (1997). *The effectiveness of early intervention.* Baltimore: Paul H. Brookes Publishing Co.

Institute of Medicine, Committee on the Consequences of Uninsurance, Board of Health Care Services. (2002). *Health insurance is a family matter.* Washington, DC: National Academies Press.

Ireys, H.T., Anderson, G.F., Shafferr, T.J., & Neff, J.M. (1997, August). Expenditures for care of children with chronic illnesses enrolled in the Washington State Medicaid Program, fiscal year 1993. *Pediatrics, 100*(2), 197–204.

Kowalczyk, L. (2001, March 4). Cost of a child's care: Children's loses millions on out-of-state patients. *Boston Sunday Globe*, pp. A1, A10.

Krauss, M.W., Gulley, S., Leiter, V., Minihan, P., & Sciegaj, M. (2000). *Report on a national survey of the health care experiences of families with special health care needs.* Waltham, MA: Brandeis University.

Krauss, M.W., Gulley, S., Sciegaj, M., & Wells, N. (2003, October). Access to specialty medical care for children with mental retardation, autism, and other special health care needs. *Mental Retardation, 41*(5), 329–339.

Kuhlthau, K., Perrin, J.M., Ettner, S.L., McLaughlin, T.J., & Gortmaker, S.L. (1998, September). High expenditure children with supplemental security income. *Pediatrics, 102*, 610–615.

Lakin, K.C., Polister, B., Prouty, R.W., & Smith, J. (2001). Utilization of and expenditures for Medicaid Institutional and Home- and Community-Based Services. In R.W. Prouty, G.A. Smith, & K.C. Lakin (Eds.), *Residential services for persons with developmental disabilities: Status and trends through 2000* (pp. 90–119). Minneapolis: University of Minnesota, Research and Training Center on Community Living/Institute on Community Integration.

LaPlante, M.P., Rice, D.P., & Wenger, B.L. (1995, May). Medical care use, health insurance, and disability in the United States. *Disability Statistics Abstract*, 8.

Larson, S., Lakin, K.C., Anderson, L., & Kwak, N. (2001, April). Characteristics of and services used by persons with MR/DD living in their own homes or with family members: NHIS-D analysis. *MR/DD Data Brief, 3*, 1–12.

Larson, S., Lakin, K.C., Anderson, L., Kwak, N., Lee, J.H., & Anderson, D. (2000, April). Prevalence of mental retardation and/or developmental disabilities: Analysis of the 1994/1995NHIS-D. *MR/DD Data Brief, 2*, 1–12.

McNeil, J.M. (1997). *Americans with disabilities: 1994–1995—Table 8.* Washington, DC: U.S. Census Bureau. Available from http://www.census.gov/hh . . . pp/disab9495/ds94t8.html

McNeil, J.M. (1998). *Americans with disabilities.* Washington, DC: U.S. Census Bureau. Available from http://www.census .gov/hh . . . p/disab9495/asc9495html

Miller, N.A. (1992, Winter). Medicaid 2176 Home and Community-Based Waivers: The first ten years. *Health Affairs, 11*, 162–171.

National Organization on Disability. (1998). *Americans with disabilities still face sharp gaps in securing jobs, education, transportation and in many areas of daily life.* Washington, DC: National Organization on Disability.

Newacheck, P.W., Strickland, B., Shonkoff, J.P., Perrin, J.M., McPherson, M., McManus, M., et al. (1998, July). An epidemiologic profile of children with special health care needs. *Pediatrics, 102*, 117–140.

Office of the Surgeon General. (2002). *Closing the gap: A national blueprint for improving the heath of individuals with mental retardation.* Washington, DC: U.S. Department of Health and Human Services.

Omnibus Budget Reconciliation Act (OBRA) of 1981, PL 97-35, 95 Stat. 357.

Smith, G.A., & Gettings, R.N. (1992). *Medicaid funded Home and Community-Based Waiver Services for people with disabilities.* Alexandria, VA: National Association of State Mental Retardation Program Directors.

Social Security Act Amendments of 1981, PL 97-123, 95 Stat. 1659.

Strunk, B.C., & Reschovsky, J.D. (2002, November). *Kinder and gentler: Physicians and managed care, 1997–2001* (Tracking Report No. 5.) Washington, DC: Center for Studying Health Systems Change.

Trupin, L., & Rice, D.P. (1995, June). Health status, medical care, and number of disabling conditions in the United States. *Disability Statistics Abstract*, 9.

Trupin, L. Rice, D.P., & Max, W. (1995, November). Who pays for the medical care of people with disabilities? *Disability Statistics Abstracts*, 13.

Walsh, K.K., Kastner, T., & Criscione, T. (1997). Characteristics of hospitalizations for people with developmental disabilities: Utilization, costs and impact of care coordination. *American Journal on Mental Retardation, 101*(5), 505–520.

Wayne State University, Developmental Disabilities Institute. (2002). *Family Support Subsidy Study update.* Final report submitted to the Michigan Developmental Disabilities Council.

Wolf, B.L., & Hill, S.C. (1995). The effect of health on the work effort of single mothers. *Journal of Human Resources*, 30, 42–62.

Ziring, P.R., Kastner, T., Friedman, D.L., Pond, W.S., Barnett, M.L., Sonnenberg, E.M., et al. (1988, September 9). Provision of health care for persons with developmental disabilities living in the community: The Morristown model. *Journal of the American Medical Association, 260*(10), 1439–1444.

CHAPTER 36

INTERNATIONAL EXPERIENCES IN HEALTH CARE

36.1 INTERNATIONAL CONSULTATION

David T. Helm, Alfred Brann, Jr., and I. Leslie Rubin

From 1980 to 2000, approximately 850,000 people arrived each year to the United States from foreign countries (Jezewski & Sotnik, 2001), and by 2003, 33.5 million foreign-born individuals resided in the United States, representing 11.7% of the total U.S. population (U.S. Census Bureau, 2003). Issues of cultural competence and the perplexities surrounding working with individuals who are not of the same culture can pose dilemmas for clinicians. This chapter presents two case studies that have important implications for working with individuals on a cross-national basis as well as with individuals now living in the United States who may have immigrated or arrived via refugee status.

Individuals, centers, organizations, and countries who have developed knowledge and expertise in the understanding and care of individuals with developmental disabilities have been participating in consultations to countries where there is a concern to improve the situation for their citizens with developmental disabilities. This consultation has been most notable in the countries of the Former Soviet Union because in all Soviet societies a considerable stigma was attached to any form of disability. The prejudice in these societies continues and is directly linked to lack of information, making it difficult to attract attention to the problems of children and adults with disabilities. Consequently, initially there were no services available for people with disabilities, and due to economic hardship, a large number of children have been abandoned and institutionalized in state orphanages. This chapter presents consultation projects in Armenia and Georgia that serve to illustrate the situations in those countries, the questions and concerns of their citizens, the consultation process, and the outcomes of international consultation.

ARMENIA

From 1996 to 1998, David T. Helm and other faculty from the Institute for Community Inclusion at Children's Hospital, Boston participated in a series of consultations on the health care of individuals with disabilities in the Republic of Armenia. The proposal, which was initiated in 1995 by an Armenian nurse practitioner living in the United States, was to provide training for a group of physicians from Armenia who were interested in learning more about children with developmental disabilities. Funding was secured from the United Armenian Fund–Children of Armenia Reaching Peaks. The project supported a training course for four Armenian physicians to come to the United States for a 10-week period to be exposed to the current philosophies and practice in providing services for children and adults with developmental disabilities. The program that was developed combined the goals of the visiting physicians with the expectations of the funding entity.

The Armenian team included a neurologist/director of a hospital, a pediatrician/neurologist, a pediatric neurologist/geneticist, and a child psychiatrist. The team arrived late September 1996 for an 8-week program in Boston and Atlanta, Georgia, and was joined by the Vice Minister of Health of Armenia for a week of meetings focused on administrative planning, culminating with the entire group traveling to Washington, D.C., for additional discussions with nongovernmental organizations (NGOs) and governmental leaders in the field.

The expectations of the Armenian team included

- Receiving training in specific medical techniques
- Finding out new ideas for treatment and prevention
- Learning more about the American system of health care for children with developmental disabilities

The American team had the following goals:

- Training a cadre of physicians on working with children with developmental disabilities and their families

- Developing plans for a "Developmental Center" in Yerevan to provide diagnosis, training, and support
- Helping to develop a survey that would identify individuals with developmental concerns
- Helping to provide assistance to other ministries (education, recreation, welfare) to work to change their perception and support for individuals with developmental disabilities and their families at a national level

The program of study was rigorous and consisted of visiting ongoing clinics, attending preestablished didactic sessions and a series of workshops designed specifically for their training, and visiting community programs. Debriefing by the Project Coordinator allowed for fuller explanation of conceptual practices, clarification of underpinning value-based activities, and a translation of jargon and Americanisms that they may have been exposed to during the day. The training activities included introduction to topics on the system of services, program design, curriculum design, rights to treatment, family violence, employment, and the use of natural supports.

The Armenian team shadowed U.S. clinicians working in clinics dealing with 1) children with a variety of developmental disabilities (e.g., autism, Down syndrome, Williams syndrome), 2) infants who were at risk for disability, 3) children age 3–5 years with developmental delays, and 4) genetics and neuropsychology. They also attended clinics that focused on children with functional difficulties (e.g., feeding, swallowing). These daily clinical experiences allowed them a window from which to view current diagnostic practice as well as family-centered approaches to working with the families.

The team visited programs in the community twice each week that included a pediatric residential center, an early invention program, a community hospital program, and a large community-based human service organization. In addition, they met with community leaders in the disability field including the directors of parent organizations, Special Olympics, and the local Arc. In Atlanta, they were able to visit the Centers for Disease Control and Prevention.

The arrival of the Armenian Vice Minister of Health signaled the Armenian government's stamp of approval. This minister was a solid supporter of individuals with disabilities and was attempting to alter the way the Armenian system responded to various unmet needs. His schedule focused on discussions of system change, needs of families, and needs of children and included meetings with state and local administrators as well as leading Armenian Americans working in the health care fields. The delegation then went to Washington, D.C., to talk to foundation directors, U.S. policy makers, and various NGO executives, among others, about developing funding and information streams to bolster their efforts.

Reflections on the Program

In retrospect, the training activities were somewhat overwhelming for the Armenian team. It was easy to assume that since everyone spoke English—some better than others—that information and communication was flowing. The relatively open and informal style of the American team was not familiar to the Armenians, who were trained under much more formal teacher–pupil relationships. The leap from Neurological Children's Hospital #6 in Yerevan, Armenia, to Children's Hospital Boston was immense. The American team had not yet seen the Armenian facility, so they could not imagine the extent of the differences. The cultural shock from a system where there is a daily struggle to find adequate medicines (even aspirin), clean sheets, and curtains, to one of the most advanced and equipped facilities in the world had to be unsettling for the Armenian team, yet taken for granted by the American team. In addition, although American values toward individuals with disabilities were openly discussed, the Armenian team had a difficult time leaping into American culture.

After the Training

The Armenian team was enthusiastic and felt empowered upon their return to Armenia. They were dedicated to change and to making progress—they had learned a significant amount during their 10-week stay and were eager to implement changes. The first setback came suddenly and had a significant impact on their efforts. The Armenian Vice Minister of Health died unexpectedly of a massive heart attack. His support and leadership vanished. His forward thinking ideas were not widespread. Political will to change was no longer in the mix; the team would have to do it alone.

The realities of everyday life, the poverty, and the lack of resources made change difficult, if not impossible; however, Armenia was a country of postearthquake and postwar reality in which the number of people with disabilities had increased drastically. At the same time, several international organizations arrived in the country with intentions of developing rehabilitation services for people with disabilities, and several NGOs and parents of children with disabilities were beginning to become politically active. Thus, the political landscape had begun to change in various ways. In addition, given their experiences during the training period, the Armenian team began to introduce language, concepts, and practices that tried to push governmental progress as well. Proposals were made, discussions were held, and efforts to change were promulgated continuously from the United Armenian Fund and other supporters to provide more and better services for children with disabilities and their families.

The international scene was also an outside factor working on the side of progressive change—the "global child," rights for people with disabilities, and treatment of youth were all in the spotlight at this time through efforts of the United Nations, UNICEF, the World Health Organization, and other international initiatives. The Armenian team was working at Neurological Children's Hospital #6 and was in communication with the Children of Armenia Reaching Peaks (CARP) project; together they worked to create a follow-up opportunity to advance their cause on a larger scale.

Visit to Armenia Two Years Later

In August 1998, the American team was invited to participate in a conference on children with disabilities to be held at American University in Yerevan (see Figure 36.1-1). After considerable negotiations and efforts of the Project Director, funding was secured, passports and visas were arranged, and a program was developed. The schedule of events included two 2-day conferences along with numerous visits to facilities and meetings with health officials. The initial conference consisted of an Inter-Ministerial Joint Conference for Childhood Disabilities, co-sponsored by the Ministries of Health and Education.

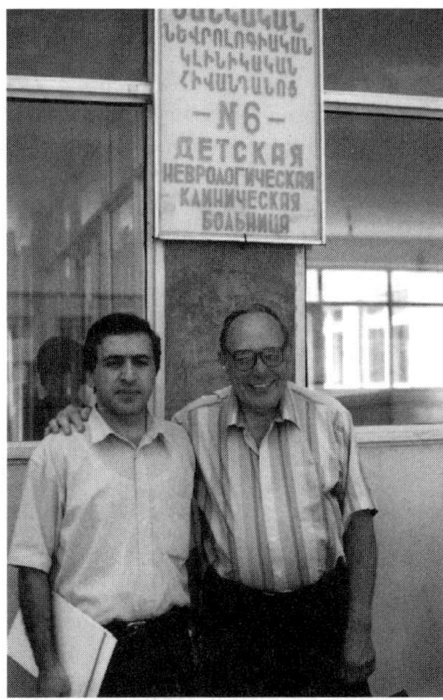

Figure 36.1-1. The American team was able to travel to Armenia to visit the Armenians whom they had trained in the United States.

The keynote address was given by the Special Rapporteur of the United Nations Commission for Social Development on Disability and included representatives from both cosponsoring Armenian ministries as well as UNICEF and the United Nations. The focus was on the *Standard Rules on the Equalization of Opportunities for Persons with Disabilities*, a United Nations document endorsed by more than 50 countries at that time but unsigned by the Republic of Armenia. The goal was to garner universal acceptance by Armenia of a similar, but more Armenia-focused, document created by participants at the conference and to send a signed copy of it to the Armenian Premier for his endorsement. At the end of those 2 days, an escorted caravan drove to meet the Premier for the signing. Much enthusiasm and anticipation was generated from this gesture.

In addition, 2 days of Pediatric Workshops on Developmental Disabilities were organized by the Armenian team and directed toward physicians and community leaders representing the NGOs throughout Armenia with representatives from the Departments of Health and Education and the United Nations. The goal was to challenge those in attendance to develop more family-centered and child-supportive services. The American team began by reviewing causation and health care management for children who had one of the major syndromes. They then outlined a framework on how to develop and work as an interdisciplinary team and raised issues of prevention of secondary conditions, collaborating with education and medical personnel, as well as developing system changes that would support these kinds of ideas. The simultaneous translation from English to Armenian, or vice versa, facilitated the broadcast and exchange of ideas, and a slide presentation in dual languages was appreciated.

The ideas were well received on the surface, but many local obstacles were pointed out. The starting point for many was steeped in suspicion of government and a fundamental lack of understanding of children with disabilities (i.e., the real abilities and potential of the children). There was also a dearth of practical experience (e.g., of 150 physicians in the audience, when asked by a show of hands how many had worked with or seen a child with Down syndrome, less than a handful acknowledged that they had). The shame and stigma of disability, as well as the inheritance and continued influence of Soviet corrective defectology, continued to hamper the effort to address values and practices based on full and valued participation by all.

Part of the American team's consultation efforts also included visiting community programs and meeting with health care officials. They visited two orphanages, a rehabilitation hospital, the Ministry of Health, and the city of Yerevan Public Health Department. They also met with officials from UNICEF, OXFAM, and other NGOs and talked at length with the UN Special Rapporteur on Disabilities about next steps in the process of change and how best to make progress. These visits were particularly helpful for the American team to better and more fully understand the cultural process, the existing Armenian system, and how change was viewed and could be facilitated.

The American team also visited Neurological Children's Hospital #6. The hospital was sparse in all ways. Supplies, facilities, and general resources were thin. The only area of abundance was the Armenian team's enthusiasm to implement new ideas and to try to have an impact on their local scene. The American team's ideas for change and implementation were beginning to be undertaken but in modest confines. The cultural exchange had been translated into local realities in ways that the Americans could not fully anticipate without seeing the facilities and reflecting on the attitudes and social milieu in which those changes needed to occur. The ultimate goal to create the Children's Developmental Evaluation Center (CDEC) was delayed as the Armenian team waited for broader supports from the Ministry. They were, however, engaging in more interdisciplinary teamwork, becoming more family- and child centered, and developing outreach efforts to lay the groundwork for broader system changes that they hoped would occur in the not too distant future. The following year, the Armenain team began creating their own CDEC.

Impact and Lessons Learned

Our trip to Armenia was exciting and thought provoking as well as disturbing and frustrating. We were all in uncharted waters. Our journey into the Armenian health care system evoked a great deal of excitement as well as angst. We didn't fully appreciate at the time that we were entering a realm fraught with potential cultural clashes and subtle misunderstandings. We knew that the people we were to work with spoke English, had medical degrees, and were interested in learning about health care practices for children with disabilities and their families. They were interested in changing a system that had become obsolete from decades of Soviet-style medical "defectology" and a social system of stigma and shame associated with having children with disabilities. The poverty of the post-Soviet Armenia, along with antiquated images of individuals with disabilities were major contributing factors holding back social change; however, the desire of the individuals and the enthusiasm of their U.S. sponsors were positive influence for change.

Both the Armenian and the American teams changed their views of the world and how they practiced medicine as a result of their experience. Those who are consulting with international visitors or who travel abroad to provide technical assistance and consultation can learn from this experience as well. When visitors observe a clinician's work settings, shadow his or her workday, or attend his or her classes and seminars, the clinician should keep in mind that the foundation of information with which the visitors arrive is contextually based and emanates from their experiences and settings and the realities of their clinical and academic experience. These experiences create a filter through which they hear and absorb the information the clinician imparts. The visitors must translate new information to fit into their working context, and the translation process changes the information. This change is an unavoidable artifact of translation, and yet, if the clinician is attuned to it, he or she can minimize what is lost in translation. By checking in with visitors, the clinician can help decipher and articulate new material to fit the visitors' environments and contexts.

When clinicians travel to locations that are foreign to them, they need to again consider the fact that their experience within the context of their work setting (bounded by institutional, cultural, and social differences) will alter the meaning of the information they receive. Even the underlying values of their ideas may be in jeopardy of misinterpretation. For instance, clinicians know how difficult it is to effectively develop and work in interdisciplinary teams in the United States, to collaborate across disciplines, and to share resources. They need to be reticent of the competitive element of professional work and how personal recognition (perhaps egos) and turf building can get in the way of these goals. When resources are scarce, these boundaries may be even more difficult to cross. Clinicians must be cognizant of this process and actively work to circumvent these barriers.

The goal of coalition building and collaboration is made more difficult in the developmental disabilities field where cultural bias and stigma may relegate individuals with disabilities to a lower social status. To overcome social and cultural viewpoints is a difficult assignment that requires sensitivity to cultural nuances. Many of these attitudes continue to be barriers to progress in the United States as well. American clinicians need to provide support to those they work with who are trying to implement changes in their countries. One way to do this is to continually look for and nurture relationships with cultural brokers, that is, to work with those to whom the culture is known and familiar, or, those who are part of the culture and have access and status to help change efforts. For example, the American team worked with individuals who served as the link between the Armenian and American cultures and could act as cultural brokers to assist in the translation process and to clarify new concepts and ideas. This help was a critical component of the successes both teams enjoyed.

TBILISI, GEORGIA

As Director of the World Health Organization Coordinating Council of Atlanta, Alfred Brann had worked in many countries around the world, including the Former Soviet Union and, specifically, in the Caucasus. He had worked with the countries' Ministries of Health, with their hospitals and medical schools, and with a number of NGOs. In 1999, he was asked by an NGO, The First Step (TFS), operating in Former Soviet Georgia to assist in the investigation of a number of deaths of children with disabilities living in a particular orphanage and to develop a set of recommendations for improving the situation for children with disabilities in Georgia.

TFS is a private charitable NGO made up of dedicated Georgians and foreign nationals that was established to address the serious problems of children with developmental disabilities living in horrendous conditions in state institutions in the Republic of Georgia. The TFS Mission Statement says: "Its mission is to improve the level of care and living conditions for disabled children, and to remove the stigma that Georgian society continues to attach to physical and mental imperfections in children." In Georgia, four state institutions exist for children with disabilities, and approximately 250 children still live in intolerable conditions with no opportunity to develop their potential and have a decent life. TFS works with UNICEF and a number of other NGOs to alleviate this situation.

The following is an excerpt of a report from TFS on the situation in the Kaspi Orphanage.

> Kaspi is a tragedy. While most of the 82 children's institutions in Georgia strive to give children the special attention they need, the Kaspi Orphanage stands out for its omissions and negligence. In 1994, 24 children reportedly died because of these horrific conditions. The state of the orphanage is alarming, particularly in terms of the quality of care provided the children. Numerous visits by donors and concerned observers have shown that the children live in a social, psychological, and emotional void. The orphanage is, essentially, a "storage facility."
>
> The children at Kaspi have been labeled as either physically or mentally handicapped, and restrictions are placed on their opportunities to develop and grow toward their potential. The management at Kaspi considers a blind or deaf child, or a mentally impaired one, as incapable of learning. A child with epilepsy is regarded and treated as handicapped. And some of the diagnoses of physical handicaps appear suspect.

To give the children the emotional and medical care they need, TFS planned to establish a care center in Tbilisi to be a home and child care center offering model care for children with intellectual and physical disabilities as well as specialized training for caregivers. Within the next 2 years, TFS planned to design and build the facility and to develop a cadre of professionals who would provide specialized care to these troubled children and who, in turn, would train other caregivers throughout Georgia. The staff would be trained in modern techniques for the treatment and rehabilitation of children with disabilities.

A report extracted and adapted from correspondence from Keti Nemsadze and Lisa Kaestner informed Dr. Brann and his team members that TFS needed a specialist who could assist them in starting to answer the following questions:

1. To what extent is it appropriate/possible to keep all the children at Kaspi together, given their variety of ages and disabilities?
2. What staff composition would be most appropriate to help these children develop to their full potential?
3. In the longer term, as the new center is able to accept new admissions, what sort of medical profile should the center target? (Keeping in mind that our objective is to assist children, who in the Soviet system would have been institutionalized for life, to participate to the fullest extent possible in their communities.)
4. What sort of out-patient services would the center be able to provide with its full-time staff?

Response to The First Step's Request

In November 1999, Dr. Brann's team visited Tbilisi and the Kaspi Orphanage and met with a number of individuals and organizations to help understand the extent of the problem, to appreciate the existing resources and progress, and to offer recommendations for the next steps to be taken in improving the situation for the children and their families. The major part of Kaspi was one old large building where, the team was told, a total of 74 "children" with an age range from 4–17 years lived, but a review of census revealed that the children had an age range of 5–22 years. Fifty-five individuals were present at the time, 12 were at home with their families, and 7 were inpatients at Children's Hospital #3 in Tbilisi. The team was told that there had been six hospitalizations in the past year: three for infections and three for trauma (one fractured arm, one fractured leg, and one laceration). Team members were also told that 12 children with epilepsy were evaluated about a year ago by a neurologist in Tbilisi with special funding and that there has been no reported follow-up.

The facility was old and in poor condition. The dining room was being plastered and painted. Three or four small tables with about four chairs each were in the dining room. In the kitchen, the electricity was not working, so the cooks had to use a small wood stove for a pot of beans and a pot of rice. Team members were shown a can of beef and told it would be added to the rice. They saw many large empty rooms with big windows, some with no glass. The vestibule of the building was dark.

Team members were ushered into a small room approximately 10 m x 3 m. The room was smoky with a small wood stove in the center with an exhaust pipe leading to a window. A low grate approximately 2 ft high was located on two sides of the stove. An estimated 35 children of varying ages, with varying levels of intellectual disabilities and self-stimulatory behavior, occupied the further half of the room, spilling over the middle where the stove was situated. Some staff people were in the room near the stove in states of inactivity and noninvolvement.

In all, this experience was very disturbing for the team and confirmed the descriptions of Kaspi that were reported by TFS. The team could then appreciate the fact that an initiative had been taken to admit a group of children who had been most vulnerable to the Children's Hospital #3 and that their conditions had improved. Indeed, one individual who had previously been admitted from Kaspi had spent time at the hospital, had gained weight, and had been subsequently returned to Kaspi. She then returned to Children's Hospital #3 in a state of severe malnutrition after about a year, having suffered the loss of all the weight she had previously gained.

In addition to the visit to Kaspi, the clinicians were able to tour the hospitals and facilities and meet with a variety of people involved in the care of children:

- Staff and faculty of Children's Hospital #3
- Staff and faculty of Republican Children's Hospital
- Staff and faculty of The Treatment and Educational Center of Child Neurology and Neurorehabilitation
- Co-Founder of TFS and members of the TFS board
- Minister of Maternal and Child Health
- Minister of Social Affairs

Some progress had already been made:

- Evaluation of the seizures of the 12 children with epilepsy at Kaspi by the Neurorehabilitation Center in 1998
- Rehabilitation of children from Kaspi in 1997 and again in 1999 at Children's Hospital #3
- Development of the Neurorehabilitation Center
- Development of a Child Development Training Program within the Department of Pediatrics at the Republican Children's Hospital
- Collaboration between psychologists and physicians who were beginning to evaluate the children at Kaspi
- Involvement at the Ministry level
- Interest of business and NGOs in this project

Recommendations

Considering the present conditions that existed for the children of Kaspi and the upcoming winter months, the team strongly advised TFS to creatively develop plans that would ensure that the children of Kaspi were kept well fed, warm, and safe. This endeavor would require collaboration between all active programs, be they clinical, governmental, private, or nongovernmental organizations. The team's following suggestions would be helpful as a start but should also be seen as part of a longer-term solution for the country.

- Check on the families of the 12 children from Kaspi who were reported to be at home with their families when the team visited, and see what the families would need to keep the children at home permanently.
- Keep the 7 children currently at Children's Hospital #3 at the hospital for the duration of the winter, and DO NOT return them to Kaspi. Instead, look for alternative placements.
- Identify other children who are malnourished and vulnerable, and transfer them to a warmer, safer, and more nurturing place as soon as possible, before the winter becomes fierce.

- Identify those children and young adults who are most intellectually and socially competent, and find more suitable living and working environments for them.
- Document the interventions at Children's Hospital #3 for the groups of children from Kaspi to use as the beginning of a protocol for developing a program of rehabilitation. Document the weight gains of the children who came from Kaspi to Children's Hospital #3 as a record of the benefit of this placement, including the weight of the child who returned to Kaspi and was brought back to Children's Hospital #3. Keep a photographic record of how the children looked and, if possible, a videotape of their behavior when they arrived compared with when they have the benefit of a warm, safe, and nurturing environment.
- Explore and document the needs of the children while they are at Children's Hospital #3 so that an appropriate and child-specific long-term plan can be developed for the placement of each child from the hospital.
- Use the material gathered on the children who were at Children's Hospital #3 to develop a protocol for intervention for the children with developmental disabilities that can be modified and applied to children from other places.

At the time, the team's recommendations built on TFS's existing program development and also introduced two important elements—a Task Force and collaboration of services.

The Task Force, which would be led by TFS, would consist of representatives from the various programs and organizations involved with the children of Kaspi:

- TFS
- Children's Hospital #3
- Republican Children's Hospital
- The Neurorehabilitation Center
- Faculty from the Department of Pediatrics in Developmental Pediatrics
- Ministries of Health, Social Affairs, Education
- Elected officials
- Business sector
- Clergy
- Parents of children with disabilities
- Other providers of care
- Other agencies and organizations

The Task Force would review the team's recommendations and adapt the recommendations to the existing resources and realities. It would also coordinate and integrate the various participants in the process and institute plans to affect change. Finally, the Task Force would ensure a smooth and safe transition of the children from Kaspi into the community.

Considering that children with developmental disabilities are likely to have significant and often multiple and serious associated medical problems, the team strongly advised that all resources be utilized to maximize efficacy and efficiency, which would require collaboration between active groups that are currently involved with aspects of the care:

- At a funding level, the Ministry of Social Affairs should collaborate with the Ministry of Health.
- At the level of provision of care and training, Children's Hospital #3, the Republican Children's Hospital, and the Department of Neurology and Neurorehabilitation should work collaboratively.
- NGOs should be active participants in the process.

Ultimately, all programs and organizations would need to be involved at all levels to work together and develop a coordinated and concerted plan of action to ensure the health and well-being of the children and their families in the society in the most effective and efficient manner.

The team also made the following recommendations toward the long-term improvement of children in orphanages:

- Reduce the census at orphanages (institutions) through planned appropriate discharge.
- Once alternative programs are developed, do not admit any more children into an orphanage after a certain date.
- Reduce the number of orphanages toward a goal of eventual elimination of the institutional system except for children with very rare and complicated medical conditions.
- Establish a center from which the program will operate, including clinical space for evaluation and rehabilitation/therapies, a training space for the optimal management of the children at home in the community, and a capacity for interdisciplinary academic training of professionals for leadership roles in providing care for children with developmental

disabilities and helping to develop systems of care in collaboration with governmental and nongovernmental organizations.

The team recommended transforming orphanages during the phase-out period into more healthy environments for children by actively reducing the number of children in the orphanages through discharge and transfer to more favorable settings that approximate a home environment. Also, the team advised against building other institutions and recommended looking at existing resources and developing a generic health care delivery system. For the children from orphanages, the team thought it may be better to bring them into society through a foster care system. Creating a foster care system would entail identifying potential foster care providers, training foster care providers to provide nurturing care in the home setting, and monitoring the children in the foster homes very closely.

In addition, TFS could focus on the Kaspi Orphanage as a pilot project. It could establish and identify funds for the project, evaluate the current nutritional status and health care needs of all children involved with Kaspi, and use the information obtained by the evaluation of the children to determine the configuration of a health care delivery system required to meet the needs of the diverse group of children according to the current guidelines for health supervision as outlined by the Ministry of Health. TFS could build in a monitoring system to assure the health and safety of the children and create an education system for the children. It could also build into the system the potential for finding permanent homes for the children either with their own families or with foster families.

Outcomes

Since its establishment in 1998, TFS has developed a wide range of services for children with disabilities. Initially, TFS concentrated on the basic needs of children in institutions such as nutrition, health care, and psychosocial rehabilitation. The program is now concentrated on four main areas. This first is TFS Village, which is located in Digomi, a suburb of Tbilisi. It has one operational cottage and two more cottages that will be ready for occupation in February 2005. The first cottage is a residence for 12 children with disabilities evacuated from the Kaspi orphanage. The second cottage will serve as another residential house, accommodating an additional 12 children with disabilities. The third cottage will serve as a child care center and school for 36 children with severe disabilities.

TFS village is based on a family model according to which the children are under the care of a house mother and aunts. The goal of the village is to equip children who have lived most of their lives in institutions with the knowledge and habits necessary for independent living. Based on international best practice, TFS professional staff has developed a Functional Skills Development Program that aims to teach life skills to enable children to live independently or semi-independently and adapt to life in society. The objective is to reintegrate, foster, or provide alternative community-based services to an increasing number of children and to provide developmental services to children still living in institutions.

In addition to medical rehabilitation, the provision of specialized education for children with disabilities is one of the prime objectives of TFS. In February 2005, TFS will open a school/child care center for 36 children with severe disabilities. Ten of these children will be from the TFS residential program, and the remaining 26 openings are for children living with their families. TFS has trained special teachers and psychologists, and two classes have already been initiated in a temporary site, Children's Hospital #2 in Tbilisi. When the third new cottage is available, the school/child care centre will be moved to TFS Village.

TFS also launched the first integrated classes for children with disabilities in two state schools in Tbilisi and Zugdidi. This pilot project will integrate children with disabilities into the standard school system while also offering specialized teaching. The program has been very successful, and, funding permitting, TFS intends to expand it in the coming year.

TFS formed a partnership with Dr. Givi Chikobava and his organization, Aisi, to create a Rehabilitation and Social Adaptation Center for children and young adults requiring special care. This center opened in September 2004 and is serving some 40 children, teenagers, and young adults with mild to moderate disabilities. TFS doctors continue to provide medical assistance to all the children in these locations, monitoring their health condition and providing emergency services where necessary.

In cooperation with the Ministry of Health, Labor, and Social affairs, TFS has surveyed the remaining state orphanages and has created a database of children living in these institutions. TFS is working closely with the various Ministries to create the legal framework for the effective deinstitutionalization of these children and has succeeded in returning 10 children to their biological families. In summary, TFS now has the capacity to provide for 24 children in residential care and more than 120 children in child care centers. With the continued and increasing support of donors, TFS will be able to offer services to a larger number of children with disabilities. The ultimate goal of TFS is to help the Georgian authorities to drastically decrease the number of children in institutions and prevent new children from being institutionalized.

CONCLUSION

As American clinicians open their minds about American practices and work more with people from diverse cultures, they need to remain sensitive to the contextual overlay they bring to interactions as well as those brought by people from different cultures. Lessons learned on the international front can also be put to good use on the local scene. Awareness of cultural values and expectations that are different puts clinicians in a position to understand how their work may be interpreted and thus better arm themselves to work more effectively with people from most cultures.

Change on an individual or family basis begins with an open mind and a willingness to learn from families and the people with whom one works. Change on a broader basis often requires finding entry points where ideas and support for change can occur. By finding mutual goals and aspirations, these cultural exchange opportunities can flourish. Clinicians need to constantly switch the automatic pilot off to effectively explore the new cultures they come in contact with.

REFERENCES

Jezewski, M.A., & Sotnik, P. (2001). *Culture brokering: Providing culturally competent rehabilitation services to foreign-born persons.* Buffalo, NY: State University of New York, University of Buffalo, Center for International Rehabilitation Research Information and Exchange.

Tobis, D. (1999, April). *Moving from residential institutions to community-based services in Eastern Europe and the Former Soviet Union.* Report prepared for the World Bank. Available from the World Bank, 1818 H Street NW, Washington, D.C. 20433.

U.S. Census Bureau. (2003). *Foreign-born population in the U.S. 2003.* Washington, DC: Author.

36.2 INTERNATIONAL ADOPTION

Lisa Albers Prock

Adoption of children into families is recognized as ideal in optimizing the long-term health and development of infants and young children who are permanently separated from their birth parents (Johnson, 2002). An estimated 125,000 or more children are adopted each year in the United States through international, foster care, private agency, independent, and step-parent adoptions, with a trend toward increasing international adoptions. In 2004, 22,884 children were internationally adopted by U.S. parents, representing nearly a 300% increase in children adopted internationally from 1993 (8,333 adoptions) to 2004 (see Figure 36.2-1). The majority of children adopted internationally in 2004 were born in China, Russia, Guatemala, South Korea, Ukraine, and Kazakhstan—with only South Korea and Guatemala having a history of international adoption for more than a decade (U.S. State Department, 2004).

Mona's parents met her for the first time when she was 2½ years of age and living in an orphanage in Russia. According to information provided to her family prior to their trip to adopt her, Mona was the third child born to her parents. Because of her congenital heart disease (transposition of the great vessels) and difficulty with eating and growing, her birth parents had placed her in an orphanage at several weeks of age. Before they met Mona, Mona's parents knew that she was very small and had delayed development. They also knew her heart problems had been repaired and expected that her growth and development would "catch up" after joining their family.

Although international adoption has occurred in the United States for more than half a century, many aspects of the process are dynamic, including parents' reasons for adopting children and adoptive children's countries of origin, age at adoption, and reasons for adoption eligibility. Political, economic, and child welfare conditions in children's countries of origin have a dramatic impact on the reasons for and the trends in age and health of children eligible for adoption. For example, in the early 1990s, the end of the Cold War and the opening of China to the West corresponded with an increase in children such as Mona adopted from institutions in Eastern Europe and the former Soviet Union and China into Western countries.

Mona's brother, Noah, joined the family at 8 months of age when he arrived at the airport in Boston from Korea. They recognized him from his preadoptive referral pictures and had followed his growth for months, but his parents were still amazed at his size and apparent health as he was larger than Mona was at 2½ years.

Children enter the process of international adoption for a variety of reasons and with various types and length of substitute care in institutions or foster homes.

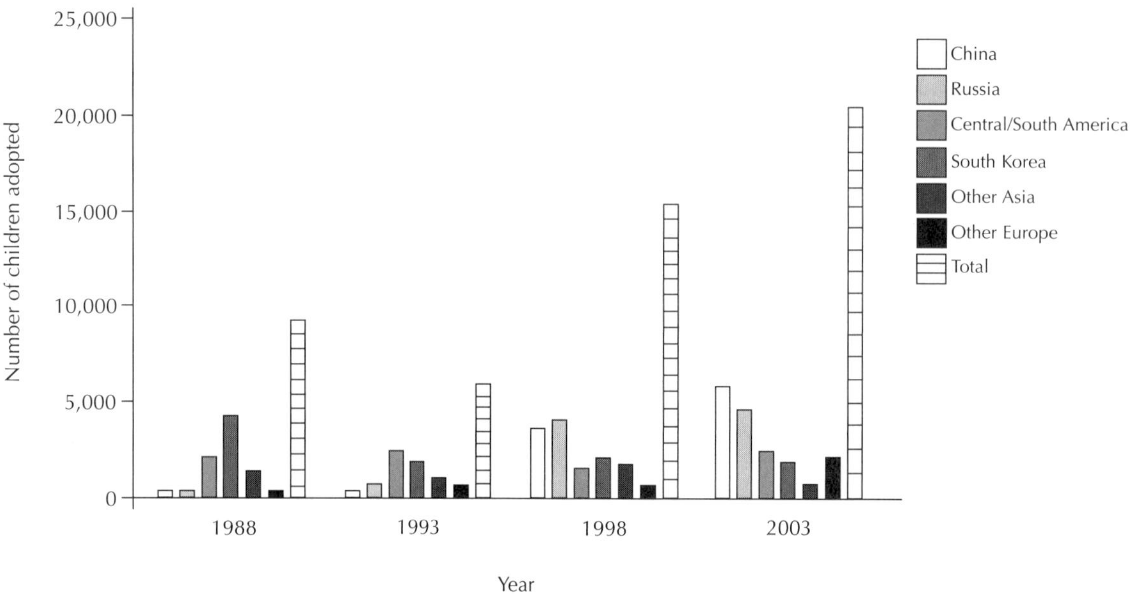

Figure 36.2-1. International adoption statistics 1988–2003. (*Source:* U.S. State Department, n.d.)

Preadoptive care, which is related to both child welfare policies and the economy of the child's home country, affects the child's long-term health and development. Children adopted internationally in 2004 were on average older and more likely to have resided in an institution prior to their adoption than children adopted a decade earlier (Johnson & Dole, 1999). In China, the "one child family policy" and the strong preference for male offspring have led to a preponderance of infant girls being "abandoned" and subsequently internationally adopted. In Korea or Guatemala, single birth mothers, such as Noah's mother, often work with social workers during an untimely pregnancy to plan for their child's adoption. In many countries, families overwhelmed by poverty or alcohol or other substance abuse may leave their infants in hospitals at the time of birth or parental rights may be voluntarily or involuntarily terminated because of substantiated severe abuse or neglect of a child. Currently, foster care is the national norm for children such as Noah who are awaiting adoption in Korea and Guatemala while Eastern Europe, Russia, and China primarily provide care for children such as Mona in orphanages.

CLINICAL CHALLENGES

Preadoptive information

Families who adopt children internationally may be provided with limited or no information about their child's history, current health, and well-being prior to traveling to bring them home or meeting them at the airport in the United States. Written medical records, abstracted information from a child's medical record, lab results, social history information, pictures, and videotapes may be part of the information shared with families preadoptively. Families may be encouraged by their adoption agency to seek consultation with a medical professional or they may elect to do this themselves as part of their decision-making process. Both professionals and families reviewing preadoptive information must realize that what is recorded may not be the complete or accurate picture regarding a child. Knowledge of contemporary political and health concerns in a child's home country is important when considering the possible health of a prospective adoptive child.

Information about a birth mother's health prior to the delivery of her child is typically sparse. Prenatal care may not have occurred. Sometimes children may be described as being born prematurely, although often their mothers have not had any prenatal care. Therefore, gestational age may be estimated solely based on birth size, leading to a report of "premature birth" rather than a more accurate "intrauterine growth retardation." For example, prenatal care in Korea may occur in the context of a mother's deciding to place her child for adoption and residing in a facility for expectant mothers. In China, however, the mothers of a large majority of children being internationally adopted do not seek care during or after their pregnancy.

Given the frequently limited information about maternal health during a pregnancy, considering the typical health risk factors of individuals residing in a country, and particularly what these factors may mean for a prospective adoptive child, is helpful. For example, without prenatal care, both mother and unborn child may have untreated infections such as syphilis or human immunodeficiency virus (HIV). Without mothers' knowledge of hepatitis B infection or access to secondary prevention (i.e., hepatitis B immune globulin), children may be prenatally or perinatally infected.

Prospective parents may ask health care providers if there are specific health risks for children adopted from specific countries. In general, all children adopted internationally have lived in a developing country with concomitant infectious and environmental risk factors. Infectious disease risks may relate to maternal history (e.g., hepatitis C with maternal drug use) or the endemic disease rate in a country (e.g., hepatitis B in most Asian countries). In addition, many children have lived in an institution and are at additional risk for infectious diseases, growth difficulties, and developmental delays.

Several days after Mona arrived home in the United States, she met her cardiologist. An echocardiogram revealed that she needed to have additional surgery to repair her cardiopulmonary vessels. The hope was that after her surgery she would be less fatigued with eating and would gain weight; however, she continued to have little interest in eating or drinking anything other than liquids via her bottle. Several months after Mona's surgery, Mona's mother read information about fetal alcohol syndrome and wondered if Mona may have this disorder, given her heart problems and difficulties gaining weight. In addition, Mona's parents had recently learned that her birth parents drank.

Prenatal Substance Exposure

Prenatal exposure to alcohol or other substances may not be reported or questioned prior to a child's referral for adoption. The absence of information about prenatal alcohol exposure, such as a report that a birth mother was not on the "alcoholic registry" in Russia, does not mean that no prenatal alcohol exposure occurred. Although the prevalence of alcohol-related concerns is not easy to determine in many countries, the combination of ubiquitous alcohol consumption and significant levels of unemployment and poverty contribute to frequent use of alcohol (including during pregnancy) by individuals in many parts of the world.

For example, in the former Soviet Union and much of Eastern Europe, alcohol use is common. Public health awareness of the impact of drinking during pregnancy is limited, and, therefore, a child's risk of presenting with symptoms of prenatal alcohol exposure is an important consideration. The average adult in Russia is estimated to consume 38 liters of 100% proof alcohol per year, and 30% of the adult population may chronically abuse alcohol in the Russian Federation (Johnson, 2002). More ominously, there has been a 48.1% increase in alcoholism among women of child-bearing ages. In girls ages 15 to 17 years, 80%–94% drank "sometimes," and 17% drank "often." As a result, it is reasonable to assume that an increased number of children from these countries would be at risk for prenatal alcohol exposure. In addition, factors correlated with alcohol consumption may also contribute to a child's abandonment and termination of parental rights leading to a child's placement for adoption.

Birth Information

Information about a child's condition during or following his or her birth may not be available prior to or following adoption. Women who are planning for the adoption of their children may seek medical services around the time of delivery, but many women who do not disclose their pregnancy may deliver at home without any assistance. Infants delivered at home and then brought to an orphanage or abandoned with limited information may be at risk for hypoxia or infections such as neonatal tetanus. Children with congenital anomalies such as cardiac problems, limb abnormalities, cleft lip, and/or palate are at increased risk of being placed in an institution and later referred for adoption. In Mona's case, her medical concerns reportedly led her family to place her in an orphanage and ultimately to relinquish their parental rights.

Preadoptive Neglect and Abuse

All internationally adopted children have a birth family who was not able to care for them, either because of significant poverty or parental limitations due to mental health concerns, substance abuse, or abuse/neglect leading to termination of parental rights. Many children also reside in an institution prior to adoption. As a result of the limited caregiving they have experienced, children who have resided in an institution (e.g., hospital, orphanage, baby home) prior to adoption may face extra challenges beyond those of children who have only resided with foster parents prior to adoption. Both historical and contemporary studies confirm a correlation between a child's length of time residing in an institution prior to adoption and later developmental, behavioral, and emotional concerns (American Academy of Pediatrics, 2003; Federici, 1998; LeMare, 2001; O'Connor & Rutter, 2000; O'Connor, Rutter, Beckett,

Keaveney, & Kreppner, 2000; Rutter, 1995; Rutter et al., 1999; Rutter, O'Connor, & Thomas, 2004). Published studies examining child development after institutionalization are not able to differentiate the impact of general lack of stimulation from the specific absence of an attachment figure; however, ascribing all detrimental effects of early institutionalization to maternal deprivation is clearly a gross and inaccurate simplification.

Similar to many children with a history of institutional care, Mona was one of 20–30 children assigned to be fed by a single caregiver. As an infant, she often had her bottle propped on rags in her crib. As a toddler, she learned to run to the table and protect her bowl when an adult brought soup twice per day.

The conditions experienced by any child residing in an institution are extremely complex and vary between institutions, within any given institution over time and with any specific child's institutional experience. In general, orphanages that have been associated with optimum child health and development have been described as providing children with adequate nutrition and health care; having a lower caregiver ratio (3:1 vs. 10:1); having a lower total number of caregivers over the life of the child; and having caregivers who recognize and respond to the distress and vocalizations of children. Gunner, Bruce, and Grotevanat (2000) suggested three levels of privation that may have an impact on a child within an institutional setting: 1) basic nutritional, hygiene, and medical needs; 2) stimulation and opportunity to interact with the environment in a way that supports motor, cognitive, language, and social development; and 3) stable interpersonal relationships allowing children to develop an attachment relationship with a consistent caregiver.

Although these levels of privation may be theoretically described, they are not independent factors in real-life experiences. Nevertheless, an appreciation of the different levels of support required for optimal child development prepares adoptive parents for the challenges of children residing in an institution in early infancy and childhood. The degree of privation suffered by any child who resided in an institution is essentially impossible to determine but may be significant. Provision for a child's basic needs can be observed and reflected in a child's growth parameters, although ensuring adequate interpersonal relationships within busy institutional settings is much harder. A child's relatively good growth trajectory implies improved likelihood of additional caregiver attention beyond feeding.

Typically, even children who have a history of residing in an institution prior to their adoption and who have significant developmental, behavioral, and/or emotional challenges after adoption have not been described to have significant developmental disabilities to their preadoptive parents.

Mona's parents expected that she would have growth and developmental delays after adoption, but they expected that these were "mild' based on preadoptive reports and assurances they had received. Shortly after adoption, Mona began to sit and crawl, and she began babbling. When Mona had her first early intervention visit at 31 months, her parents were shocked to learn that she was still developmentally at the level of a 6- to 9-month-old. They wondered how they could help her catch up and when her rocking, head banging, and hand flapping would diminish.

In addition to the difficulties that are inherent in orphanage living, including malnutrition, emotional neglect, and lack of emotional connection with a caregiver, international adoptees may be exposed to a number of risk factors prior to or following birth. Prenatal history often is unknown or incompletely reported to families. The prevalence of alcoholism in the former Soviet Union contributes to an increased risk of fetal alcohol syndrome. In addition, environmental toxins (e.g., lead, which affects brain development) have been reported for children adopted from China (Centers for Disease Control and Prevention, 2000).

Long-Term/Longitudinal Studies

Health and development outcomes of children internationally adopted by U.S. families began to be reported in the late 1980s (Hostetter, Iverson, Dole, & Johnson, 1989). Initial reports focused on growth patterns and infectious diseases after adoption. Children internationally adopted into the United States are not followed as a single cohort; hence, the majority of information reported in the medical literature describing the health and development of international adoptees involves case series reported from specialty clinic populations. Descriptive data, however, is available from national data sets examining national cohorts of international adoptees in Scandinavia and Sweden.

A review of the literature describing diverse clinical populations of internationally adopted children suggested that children who are internationally adopted have a 2–3 times greater chance of school difficulties, psychiatric problems, and relationship difficulties than their nonadopted peers (Cederblad, 2003). Limited information is available about the current epidemiology of significant developmental disorders in international adoptees; however, the likelihood of significant concerns appears to be proportional to age at adoption. One study in Denmark (Raunskov, Nord, Ellegaard, & Primdahl, 2001) described a cohort of children adopted in 1992–1993 as reported via parent questionnaire 6–7 years after adoption (92% parent response rate). According to parental report, at ages 7–10 years of age, 81% of the children were assessed to be functioning without any problems; 13% had lasting, moderate difficulties (e.g., learning, attention, language problems); and 6% had severe disturbances (e.g., intellectual disabilities, autism, cerebral palsy). A greater proportion of moderate difficulties was found among children who were older at the time of adoption (35% for children adopted after 3 years of age vs. 10% for children under 2 year of age).

Although a number of investigators have focused on aspects of health and development of children adopted internationally, two well-designed longitudinal epidemiological studies conducted in the United Kingdom and Canada provide the clearest picture of the impact of severe deprivation characteristic of Romanian orphanages in the early 1990s on child health and development (see Table 36.2-1). Consistent with earlier studies, length of time in institutional care is associated with the degree of growth failure and the likelihood of ultimate "catch-up growth" for children adopted from institutions. Both the British and Canadian longitudinal studies of children adopted from Romania demonstrate a "dose–response" relationship between the length of institutionalization and both the reduction of cognitive abilities in preschool and early school years and the risk of disturbed attachment behaviors.

Mona entered an inclusive preschool program at 3 years of age. Her parents observed that during the first 2 years she was enrolled, she seemed to make less progress than most of her peers with respect to speaking and understanding language. When Mona's family attended an annual reunion for families of children adopted from Russia, they learned of other children who were still having difficulties with using language and who also still rocked and flapped their hands at times. Some of these children had been diagnosed with an attachment disorder, sensory integration dysfunction, or autism.

Attachment Difficulties and "Quasi-Autistic" Behaviors

The importance of an infant's early relationships with his or her caregivers(s) in providing a solid foundation for future interpersonal relationships and healthy emotional development cannot be underestimated. Adoptive families often hear much from professionals and other parents about the potential for attachment disorders in their adopted children. A review of web sites and written publications aimed at foster and adoptive families reveals numerous checklists that can lead families to attribute a number of their child's developmental or behavioral characteristics to an attachment disorder.

Zeanah and Boris provided an excellent discussion of the history of conceptualizing and assessing the disturbances and disorders of attachment in early childhood (Zeanah, 2000, 2003; Zeanah & Boris, 2000). Certainly, children residing in abusive and/or neglectful homes or orphanages are at risk for not having an attuned caregiver responding to their expressed needs in infancy and early childhood; however, the long-term implications of these early interactions may be modulated by many factors including a child's temperament, a child's innate resilience, or additional environmental factors—all of which are extremely difficult to measure. In addition, prediction of future interpersonal strength or difficulties is rarely as elegantly simple as ascribing all of a child's difficulties to an early attachment difficulty.

Atypical behaviors of children in institutions have been well described, including reduced interpersonal interactions, language delays, and self-stimulatory behavior leading to a "quasi-autistic" behavior pattern (Federici, 1998; O'Connor & Rutter, 2000; O'Connor et al., 2000; Rutter at al., 1999). Many children demonstrate self-stimulatory behaviors (head banging, rocking, hand flapping) shortly after adoption from an institution, but most children's symptoms diminish over time or are restricted to bedtime or times of boredom. Some children, such as Mona, continue to fulfill diagnostic criteria for an autism spectrum disorder well beyond their transitional postadoptive period.

ROLE OF PEDIATRIC PROVIDERS

Mona's parents had not realized that they could seek professional consultation prior to Mona's adoption regarding her health and development, but they did take advantage of this information prior to adopting Noah. Mona's cardiac condition had been described in her preadoption physical, but the neurologic sequelae of long-term hypoxia prior to her surgery were not described or discussed with her parents. In contrast, Mona's parents reviewed Noah's monthly physical examinations, laboratory results, and growth parameters with their pediatrician in the months before his adoption.

Preadoption Preparation

Pediatric providers may work with families before, during, or after the process of adopting a child internationally. Before adopting their child, families may

Table 36.2-1. Developmental and behavioral outcomes—Romanian longitudinal studies

	English and Romanian Adoptees Study*	Canadian Study**
Type of study	Stratified random sample	Cohort follow-up
Study population	**Romanian adoptees** (*n* = 155) Three study groups by months of institutionalization preadoption: • Less than 6 months (*n* = 58) • 6–24 months (*n* = 59) • 24–42 months (*n* = 48) **Control group** (*n* = 52) Domestic adoption, less than 5 months institutionalization preadoption	**Romanian adoptees** (*n* = 75) Study groups based on age at adoption: • Younger than 4 months old (*n* = 29) • Age 8–24 months • Older than 24 months **Control group** (*n* = 46) Canadian born, not adopted
Analysis compares	Each of three groups with controls and with each other: • Domestic U.K. adoption • Romanian adoption < 6 months 6–24 months 24–42 months	Romanian orphans adopted after 8 months of age Early adoptees younger than age 4 months at adoption Late adoptees older than 8 months at adoption Control group who were not adopted
Schedule of follow-up assessments	At 4 years of age if child was adopted when younger than 24 months old At 6 years of age for all children	Time 1—median 11 months in adoptive/birth home Time 2—median 39 months in adoptive/birth home
Cognition	Assessed at adoption using the Denver Developmental Screening Test II (Frankenburg et al., 1992) and McCarthy Scales for Children's Abilities (McCarthy, 1972) • 59% of study population had a developmental quotient (DQ) less than 50 Assessed at age 6 years with the McCarthy Scales for Children's Abilities; percent of study population with McCarthy General Cognitive Index (GCI) less than 80: • Control group—2% • Children with less than 6 months of institutionalization—2.3% • Children with 12–24 months of institutionalization—12.0% • Children with 24–42 months of institutionalization—32.6% Cognitive impairments correlate with head circumference	Assessed with the Stanford-Binet Intelligence Scale, Fourth Edition (Thornndike, Hagan, & Sattler, 1986) for mean IQ score 3 years after adoption: • Younger than 4 months at adoption—no difference from control • 8–24 months at adoption—mean IQ score = 90 (65–127) • Older than 24 months at adoption—mean IQ score = 69 (52–98)
Attachment	Percent of children with disorganized attachment patterns: • Control group—3.8% • Children with less than 6 months of institutionalization—8.95% • Children with 6–24 months of institutionalization—24.5% • Children with 24–42 months of institutionalization—33.3%	Percent of children with insecure attachment: • Nonadopted—42% • Older than 8 months at adoption—63%
"Quasi-autistic" features	6% of children experienced "quasi-autistic symptoms." 6% of children experienced "mild symptoms of autism."	At Time 2, 41% of Romanian orphans continued stereotypical behaviors.
Behavioral concerns	Percent of children with severe inattention/overactivity: • Control group—9.6% • Children with less than 6 months of institutionalization—13.6% • Children with 6–24 months of institutionalization—32.1% • Children with 24–42 months of institutionalization—38.6%	At Time 2, 29% of Romanian orphans had externalizing behavior concerns.

*Sources: Rutter (1995, 1999, 2004); O'Connor (2000); O'Connor (2000).

**Sources: Ames (1997); LeMare (2002).

have specific questions about the meaning or lifelong implications of their child's medical diagnosis. Parents may ask providers to review preadoptive information (medical record abstracts, physical examination data, developmental checklists, pictures, and/or videotapes). Preadoptive information available to families prior to adoption varies widely with respect to quantity and quality of information.

In Eastern Europe and the former Soviet Union, medical terms may not be applied in the way that a Western-trained physician would expect. For example, diagnoses of "perinatal encephalopathy" and "hypoxic ischemic encephalopathy" are commonly used for children with unknown perinatal history or reportedly normal delivery but suggest risk factors for the child that may range from true hypoxia to absence of prenatal care or a cephalohematoma. "Diagnoses" described on a medical document from the former Soviet Union describing a child may be simply an abstraction from a list in the medical record rather than a description of current concerns. Although families may be concerned about a benign physical finding they see on a preadoptive picture, they may not appreciate the significance of relative microcephaly for a child's risk of chronic developmental challenges.

Additional information gathered during the preadoptive process is not always helpful to families in planning for their child's future needs. Reported developmental milestones or laboratory values may later prove to be inaccurate. As in Mona's case, families may not have received accurate information from referral agencies about the serious long-term challenges. Preadoptive consultations with prospective parents also provide an excellent opportunity to discuss the importance of having family members immunized for hepatitis B (regardless of child's reported hepatitis B status) and of having updated immunizations (there have been several measles outbreaks among families of recently adopted children) prior to adopting a child.

The web site for the Centers for Disease Control and Prevention (http://www.cdc.gov/travel/) provides excellent recommendations regarding travel for families as well as recommendations specific for internationally adopted children (http://www.cdc.gov/travel/other/adoption.htm). Providers should also be aware that although an immigration physical performed by a designated physician in the child's birth country is required for all children who are internationally adopted in order to receive a visa for travel, this examination is solely to complete legal requirements and screen for certain communicable diseases or serious physical and intellectual disabilities. The immigration physical should not be considered comprehensive, as a child's clothing may not even be removed for the examination.

Immediate Postadoption Medical Evaluation

Routine medical screening for possible infectious diseases and other health concerns are recommended within 2 weeks of adoption for all internationally adopted children. A complete history and physical examination performed during an initial postadoption visit may reveal concerns not known or reported prior to adoption. Any birthmarks, scars, bruises, or evidence of past physical or sexual abuse should be carefully documented in the child's medical record. Parents may question their child's true birthday as a date of birth may have been assigned based on a best estimate at the time of his or her abandonment. Most physicians with international adoption experience routinely wait at least 1 year prior to reassigning any birth date based on changes in a child's growth, development, bone age, and dental age. Reduced weight, height, and head circumference in comparison to age-expected norms are commonly reported after international adoption.

The American Academy of Pediatrics (2003) provides recommendations for screening children for infectious diseases after international adoption (see Table 36.2-2). In addition to screening for infectious diseases, children should be evaluated for possible congenital anomalies, evidence of trauma/abuse, anemia, growth concerns, lead exposure, hearing or vision impairments, and developmental delays. Shortly after a child arrives home, parents are generally most concerned about their child's possible infections; growth parameters; developmental profile; and understanding their child's eating, sleeping, and behaviors. All families benefit from parental support, empowerment, and healthy attachment of parent to child, but this is particularly important in the setting of adoption.

Common Medical Concerns

Infectious diseases are relatively common for children after international adoption. Screening for infectious diseases continues to evolve, and the *American Academy of Pediatrics Red Book* (2003) provides recommendations for both routine screening for possible infectious concerns (see Table 36.2-2) and treatment if necessary. Intestinal pathogens have been reported in 15%–35% of internationally adopted children. For children who demonstrate growth solidly within the normal range and present with no gastrointestinal symptoms, screen-

Table 36.2-2. Screening recommendations after international adoption

Recommended for all international adoptees	Comments
Complete blood count with indices	Anemia, thalassemia, eosinophilia
Lead level	Lead exposure common in many countries
Hepatitis B profile	HBsAg, anti-HBs, anti-Hbc; consider retest at 6 months
Human immunodeficiency virus (HIV)	Consider retesting in 6 months
Venereal disease research laboratory and/or rapid plasma reagin tests	Regardless of maternal/child treatment history for syphilis
Intestinal pathogens	At least one sample for ova and parasites
Tuberculin skin test	Regardless of known/suspected BCG status
Hearing and vision screen	Age appropriate
Developmental screen	Age appropriate
Consider	
Hepatitis C antibody	Especially for children from Asia and the former Soviet Union
Varicella, immunization titers	See chapter text
Newborn screen/thyroid function tests	Recommended for all children younger than 1 year and those with delays or failure to thrive
Urinalysis	Once before school age
Giardia Lamblia, Cryptosporidium parvum, *Helicobacter pylori*	Consider these based on child's age and clinical presentation

Source: American Academy of Pediatrics (2003).

ing one stool sample for ova and parasites is probably adequate. For children with significant growth failure or persistent gastrointestinal symptoms, three stool samples and checking antigens for *Giardia lamblia* and *Cryptosporidium parvum* are recommended.

Syphilis exposure, infection, and/or treatment is frequently reported in preadoptive records. Screening for possible infection (preferably with both a nontreponemal and a treponemal test) is recommended for all children regardless of their reported exposure and treatment status prior to adoption. Although not common, several children reportedly found to be negative for HIV infection in their birth countries have been found to be positive upon evaluation for HIV infection in the United States.

Evidence of acute or chronic hepatitis B infection (anti-HBs positive) has been reported in 1%–5% of international adoptees. All children who are anti-HBs positive should be evaluated for possible chronic hepatitis B infection and should be assessed for biochemical evidence of chronic liver disease as a guide for possible treatment. Screening for hepatitis C is recommended for children adopted from China, Russia, Eastern Europe, and Southeastern Asia as well as for any child with a history of maternal drug use or receipt of blood products.

Latent tuberculosis infection has been reported in 0.6%–1.9% of international adoptees. Children who are found to have a positive tuberculin skin test (> 10 mm; > 5 mm if known to have been exposed to tuberculosis) should have a chest x-ray. Suspected or known BCG vaccination is not a contraindication for administering a tuberculin skin test (TST). Although BCG vaccine has been documented to decrease a child's risk of systemic infection with tuberculosis, primary infection is not prevented.

Children in many countries receive BCG vaccines because they reside in a country with a high risk of tuberculosis exposure. In addition, orphanage caretakers have been documented as a significant source of tuberculosis infection for international adoptees. One relative contraindication to placing a TST is a weeping BCG scar (BCGitis). Treatment decisions for a child with a TST in duration between 5 mm and 10 mm if BCG has been given or is suspected requires a consideration of the risks and benefits of treatment versus nontreatment.

Significantly elevated blood lead levels from environmental lead exposure have been reported in internationally adopted children (D.E. Johnson, personal communication, 2004). Lead exposure may result from a variety of sources, including leaded gasoline exhaust, ceramic ware, and traditional medicines. All internationally adopted children should be screened for lead exposure, with follow-up and treatment based on standard guidelines (see http://www.cdc.gov/nceh/lead/lead.htm).

Children may have immunizations documented as given in their birth country, but the accuracy of the reporting and the efficacy of the vaccines administered have been questioned. Immune responses to vaccines administered to international adoptees in their birth countries may be incomplete, and a significant percentage of children lack adequate immunity despite satisfactory vaccination records. As a result, international adoptees should either be reimmunized or tested for evidences of vaccine-preventable diseases (e.g., hepatitis B, diphtheria, tetanus, polio, measles, mumps, rubella) to ascertain the children's immune status on arrival in the United States and to guide decisions about revaccination (American Academy of Pediatrics, 2003).

Growth Monitoring

Poor linear growth is one of the most commonly identified concerns for children after international adoption). Psychosocial growth failure (psychosocial dwarfism) while living in institutions and a surge in growth after adoption are typical for children adopted internationally. For children reared in institutions in Russia, China, and Romania, linear growth potential has been described to be lost at a rate of approximately 1 month per 2–3 months of institutionalization (Johnson, 2002; Johnson et al., 1992).

The syndrome of relative height suppression with weight-for-height more preserved, involves a reduced secretion of growth hormone (GH), blunted GH response, and cell resistance to growth factor similar to neuroendocrine markers in childhood or early onset depression or major depression in adulthood. These neuroendocrine markers demonstrate improvement toward a normal response only 3 weeks after being removed from the deprived environment. Neuroendocrine effects of privation have also been postulated to affect the early onset of puberty with decreased final adult stature as described particularly in girls adopted from institutions in India. For children not accelerating their growth velocity toward the typical growth curve within 1–2 months of adoption, further evaluation of a possible organic cause of growth failure is warranted

Child Development, Language, and Behaviors

The medical concerns of children who are internationally adopted and an approach to screening for them after adoption have been well described (Albers, Johnson, Hostetter, Iverson, & Miller, 1997; Hostetter et al., 1989; Johnson, 2000, 2002; Johnson & Dole, 1999; Miller, 1999, 2000; see Table 36.2-2); however, the developmental and behavioral needs of internationally adopted children and their families are less well known in the community of professionals working with families prior to and following adoption (Federici, 1998; Verhulst, Althaus, & Versluis-Den Bieman, 1990, 1992). Monitoring a child's developmental progress and behavior after international adoption is crucial to providing timely intervention and support for families. After adoption from an institution, children frequently demonstrate developmental delays and self-stimulatory behaviors such as rocking, head banging, or wiggling and staring at their hands. In the first few months after adoption, rapid developmental progress along with a decrease in self-stimulatory behaviors should occur.

Developmental concerns are to be expected for children who have been institutionalized, neglected or abused, severely malnourished, or denied developmental stimulation. Developmental expectations may also vary across cultures (i.e., infants may be swaddled, never placed on the floor), which may limit a child's developmental progress at the time of adoption. Nutrition and developmental stimulation do help a great deal but may not completely resolve a child's delays. Parents may be surprised to learn that their child's "developmental delays" will not always resolve with food and a loving family.

Infants with developmentally delays typically make at least 2 months of developmental progress in 1 month after adoption. Early intervention services are strongly recommended for children with severe developmental delays or if parental support seems indicated. Most parents welcome the option of a developmental assessment and ongoing monitoring and therapy if indicated.

Language development in a second language (English) has been described in infants adopted from Eastern Europe as occurring along a trajectory similar to that of native language development in English. Unlike other immigrant children who continue to speak their primary language, international adoptees lose their first language in parallel with gaining a second one. A study by Glennen and Masters (2002) examined the language development of infants and young children adopted from Eastern Europe and concluded that the majority of infants and toddlers adopted from Eastern Europe develop English according to the same language growth trends seen for nonadopted English-speaking peers; however, predictable language delays continued through age 36 months and increased in magnitude with increasing age at adoption.

No comment was made as to the trajectory of language development for children older than 36 months of age or with respect to higher-order language development. These children have not yet entered school, when increased demands for understanding and using complex higher order language is important. As a result of their findings, Glennen and Masters suggested that any child who is not progressing rapidly should be referred immediately for speech and language services (see Table 36.2-3). Professionals working with international adoptees should use caution in generalizing this study's results, as sample reporting bias (Internet ascertainment via parent support group) and significant overrepresentation of children adopted at younger than 12 months of age may not reflect the experience of all international adoptees.

Table 36.2-3. Recommendations for speech and language referral

Age at adoption	Speech and language referral recommended
Younger than 12 months	Refer the child the same as if he or she were a primary English language speaker.
13–18 months	Refer the child if he or she is not producing 50 words or two-word phrases at 24 months.
19–24 months	Refer the child if he or she is not using English by 24 months and 50 words or two-word phrases by 28 months.
25–30 months	Refer the child if he or she is not using English within several weeks at home or is not speaking 50 English words or two-word phrases by 31 months.

Source: Glennen and Masters (2002).

Older children who are adopted internationally after speaking a native language face additional challenges as they lose their primary language while acquiring a new language (Federici, 1998; Gindis, 2000). Particularly for children with previous knowledge of their native language, assessment of a child's language abilities at the time of adoption is helpful in gauging the language support a child requires in educational and social settings. For school-age children, a nonverbal cognitive assessment may be helpful in determining a child's optimal school placement. Functional receptive language is initially acquired, but more robust language in the school-age child may take years to fully develop.

Learning difficulties and attentional concerns are particularly common in children with a history of institutionalization, alcohol exposure, or malnutrition. This situation is particularly true for children older than 3 years of age. Although English as a second language (ESL) services may be helpful, additional language remediation is often necessary for older adoptees who may have a primary language disorder (Federici, 1998; Gindis, 2000). Although many children make significant gains after adoption, some children continue to have severe developmental concerns. Children may present with possible congenital developmental challenges, but regardless of genetic vulnerability to developmental concerns, children's level of functioning may be also be negatively affected by preadoptive neglect, malnutrition, or toxic exposures.

A child's emotional and behavioral profile postadoption is related to a number of factors, including the child's temperament, parental temperament, preadoption environment, abuse, health, and postadoptive adjustment. Some common behaviors of concern to parents include self-stimulatory behaviors (i.e., head banging, rocking) that can be expected to diminish with time. Gorging on food or refusal to eat is relatively common. Sleeping patterns may initially be erratic given time zone changes, novelty of sleeping alone versus in an institutional setting, and having the option to do something other than lying in bed. Parents appreciate an explanation of concrete goals for eating and sleeping behaviors, and they may need additional support to reduce sleeping and eating concerns.

Parents may also raise concerns about a possible attachment disorder, possible physical or sexual abuse, or psychiatric concerns given their child's preadoptive history. Generally, younger adoptees form a strong relationship with and reliance on their new parents within a week of meeting them, although signs of difficulties with attachment are more common in even young adoptees (see Table 36.2-1). Indiscriminate friendliness is common in older international adoptees and can be both disturbing to the family and a safety risk for the child.

Symptoms of depression manifested at an age-appropriate level, perhaps including irritability and somatic complaints, are also common after adoption. Clarification of these concerns requires longitudinal monitoring and often the assistance of other professionals for diagnosis or treatment. Understanding a child's cognitive and emotional profile, as well as any underlying neurologic difficulties, is critical to describing a treatment plan that addresses emotional or interpersonal difficulties. Treatment of significant trauma or severe attachment-related difficulties requires a multidisciplinary approach to assist families and children and should incorporate a variety of treatment modalities, including individual, family, and group therapeutic approaches. Families may ask about "holding therapies," which are widely advertised in public forums to address attachment disorders in adopted children. No peer-reviewed assessment of holding therapies has been reported, and several deaths have resulted from holding therapy–associated interventions. Further considerations regarding the diagnosis of attachment disorders and numerous interventions promoted to address these concerns from infancy through adolescence are discussed in a recent practice parameter (American Academy of Child and Adolescent Psychiatry, 2005).

CONCLUSION

An overwhelming majority of families surveyed after international adoption would recommend international adoption (98%), but a large percentage (42%) report they would do so again with reservations (D.E. Johnson, personal communication, 2004). Increased stressors have been reported in families who have internationally adopted. Predictors of parenting stress after adoption from Romanian institutions related both to aspects of the child's behavior (attachment security and behavioral problems) and to family variables (income, number of Romanian children adopted, and the mother's age) (Ames, 1997). An understanding of parental expectations prior to international adoption as well as the implications of early childhood deprivation and abuse are crucial to assisting families to foster the optimal development of their children well after they have joined loving and supportive homes.

REFERENCES

Albers, L.H., Johnson, D.E., Hostetter, M.K., Iverson, S., & Miller, L.C. (1997). Health of children adopted from the former Soviet Union and Eastern Europe: Comparison with preadoptive medical records. *Journal of the American Medical Association, 278*(11), 922–924.

American Academy of Pediatrics. (2003). *American Academy of Pediatrics Red Book.* Elk Grove Village, IL: Author.

Ames, E. (1997). *The development of Romanian orphanage children adopted to Canada. Final report to the National Welfare Grants Program: Human Resources Development Canada.* Burnaby, British Columbia: Simon Fraser University.

Cederblad, M. (2003). *Adoption—But at what cost?* Stockholm: Government Offices of Sweden.

Centers for Disease Control and Prevention. (2000, February 11). Elevated blood lead levels among internationally adopted children—United States, 1998. *Morbidity & Mortality Weekly Report, 49*(5), 97–100.

Federici, R. (1998). *Help for the hopeless child: A guide for families.* Washington, DC: Federici.

Frankenburg, W.K., Dodds, Archer, P., Bresnick, B., Maschka, P., Edelman, N., & Shapiro, H. (1992). *The Denver Developmental Screening Test II* (2nd ed.). Denver, CO: Denver Developmental Materials.

Gindis, B. (2000). Language-related issues for international adoptees and adoptive families. In T. Tepper, L. Hannon, D. Sandstrom (Eds.), *International adoption: Challenges and opportunities.* Meadowlands, PA: Parents Network for the Post Institutionalized Child.

Glennen, S., & Masters, M.G. (2002). Typical and atypical language development in infants and toddlers adopted from Eastern Europe. *American Journal of Speech-Language Pathology, 11*(4), 417–433.

Gunnar, M.G., Bruce, J., & Grotevanat, H.D. (2000). International adoption of institutionally reared children: Research and policy. *Development and Psychopathology, 12,* 677–693.

Hostetter, M.K., Iverson, S., Dole, K., & Johnson, D. (1989, April). Unsuspected infectious diseases and other medical diagnoses in the evaluation of internationally adopted children. *Pediatrics, 83*(4), 559–564.

Johnson, D.E. (2000). Medial and developmental sequelae of early childhood institutionalization in Eastern European adoptees. In C.A. Nelson (Ed.), *Minnesota Symposia on Child Psychology: Vol. 31. The effects of early adversity on neurobehavioral development* (pp. 113–162). Minneapolis: University of Minnesota Press.

Johnson, D.E. (2002). Adoption and the effect on children's development. *Early Human Development, 68*(1), 39–54.

Johnson, D.E., & Dole, K. (1999, April). International adoptions: Implications for early intervention. *Infants & Young Children, 11*(4), 34–45.

Johnson, D.E., Miller, L.C., Iverson, S., et al. (1992). The health of children adopted from Romania. *Journal of the American Medical Association, 268,* 3446–3451.

LeMare, L. (2001, April 10–13). *Follow-up on the Romanian Adoptee Study.* Presentation given at Joint Council on International Children's Services, Washington, DC.

McCarthy, D.A. (1972). *McCarthy Scales of Children's Abilities.* New York: Psych Corp.

Miller, L. (1999). Caring for internationally adopted children. *New England Journal of Medicine, 341*(20), 1–3.

Miller, L.C. (2000). Initial assessment of growth, development, and the effects of institutionalization in internationally adopted children. *Pediatric Annals, 29*(4), 224–232.

O'Connor, T.G., & Rutter, M. (2000). English and Romanian Adoptees Study Team: Attachment disorder behavior following early severe deprivation: Extension and longitudinal follow-up. *Journal of the American Academy of Child and Adolescent Psychiatry, 39,* 703–712.

O'Connor, T.G., Rutter, M., Beckett, C., Keaveney, L., & Kreppner, J. (2000). The English and Romanian Adoptees Study Team: The effects of global severe privation on cognitive competence: Extension and longitudinal follow-up. *Child Development, 71,* 376–390.

Raunskov, J.-U., Nord, L., Ellegaard, V., & Primdahl, M. (2001). *A survey of the health conditions of all foreign adoptive children placed in Denmark through Adoption Centre in 1992 and 1993.* Paper presented September 29, 2000, at the Nordic Research Conference "35 Years with Intercountry Adoptions," Goteborg, Denmark. Retrieved April 26, 2005, from http://www.nia.se/publi/ovrigt/abst.pdf

Rutter, M. (1995). Maternal deprivation. In M.H. Bornstein (Ed.), *Handbook of parenting: Vol. 4. Applied and practical parenting* (pp. 3–31). Mahwah, NJ: Lawrence Erlbaum Associates.

Rutter, M., Andersen-Wood, L., Beckett, C., et al. (1999). Quasi-autistic patterns following severe early global privation. *Journal of Child Psychology and Psychiatry, and Applied Disciplines, 40*(4), 537–549.

Rutter, M., O'Connor, T., & Thomas, G. (2004). Are there biological programming effects for psychological development? Findings from a study of Romanian adoptees. *Developmental Psychology, 40*(1), 81–94.

Thorndike, R.L., Hagen, E.P., & Sattler, J.M. (1986). *Stanford-Binet Intelligence Scale* (4th ed.). Chicago: Riverside.

U.S. State Department. (2004). *Immigrant visas issued to orphans coming to the U.S.* Retrieved April 26, 2004, from http://travel.state.gov/family/adoption/stats/stats_451.html

U.S. State Department. (n.d.). *International adoption.* Retrieved June 28, 2005, from http://travel.state.gov/family/adoption/stats/stats_458.html

Verhulst, F.C., Althaus, M., & Versluis-Den Bieman, J.H.M. (1990). Problem behavior in international adoptees: II. Age at placement. *Journal of the American Academy of Child and Adolescent Psychiatry, 29*, 104–111.

Verhulst, F.C., Althaus, M., & Versluis-Den Bieman, J.H.M. (1992). Damaging backgrounds: Later adjustment of international adoptees. *Journal of the American Academy of Child and Adolescent Psychiatry, 31*, 518–524.

Zeanah, C. (2003, November). *Attachment disorders in children.* Presentation given for the American Academy of Pediatrics National Conference and Exhibition, New Orleans.

Zeanah, C. (2000). Disturbances of attachment in young children adopted from institutions. *Journal of Developmental and Behavioral Pediatrics, 21*, 230–236.

Zeanah, C., & Boris, N. (2000). *Handbook of infant mental health* (2nd ed.). New York: Guildford Press.

INDEX

Page numbers followed by *f* indicate figures; those followed by *t* indicate tables.